Head and Neck Surgery

System requirement:
- **Windows XP or above**
- **Power DVD player (Software)**
- **Windows media player 10.0 version or above (Software)**

Accompanying DVD ROM is playable only in Computer and not in DVD player.

Kindly wait for few seconds for DVD to autorun. If it does not autorun then please do the following:
- Click on my computer
- Click the **drive labelled JAYPEE** and after opening the drive, kindly double click the file **Jaypee**

DVD CONTENTS

- **Repair of CSF leak from lateral wall of sphenoid sinus**
  Dr MV Kirtane

- **Uses of microdebrider**
  Dr Samir Bhargava

- **Endoscopic DCR**
  Dr Samir Bhargava

- **Cancer of the nasopharynx with biopsy**
  Dr Chris de Souza

- **Epistaxis caused by granuloma from middle turbinate**
  Dr Chris de Souza

- **Endoscopic DCR with follow-up after 1 year**
  Dr Chris de Souza

Head and Neck Surgery

Volume 1

- Rhinology
- Facial Plastics

Editor-in-Chief

Chris de Souza MS DORL DNB FACS (USA)
Visiting Assistant Professor in Otolaryngology
Dept. of Otolaryngology, SUNY Brooklyn, New York, USA
Visiting Assistant Professor in Otolaryngology, LSUHSC Shreveport, Louisiana, USA
ENT and Skull Base Surgeon, Tata Memorial Hospital, Mumbai, India
ENT Surgeon, Lilavati Hospital, Holy Family Hospital, Holy Spirit Hospital, Mumbai, India

Editors

RHINOLOGY

Chris de Souza MS DORL DNB FACS (USA)
Visiting Assistant Professor in Otolaryngology
Department of Otolaryngology, SUNY Brooklyn, NY,
USA
ENT and Skull Base Surgeon
Tata Memorial Hospital, Mumbai, India

Gady Har-El MD FACS
Chairman, Department of Otolaryngology
Head and Neck Surgery, Lenox Hill Hospital
Professor of Otolaryngology and Neurosurgery
SUNY–Downstate, New York, USA

FACIAL PLASTICS

Fred Stucker MD FACS
Jack W Pou Professor and Chairman
Department of Otolaryngology, Louisiana
State University, Shreveport, Louisiana, USA

Cherie-Ann O Nathan MD FACS
Professor and Vice Chairman
Department of Otolaryngology, Louisiana
State University, Shreveport, Louisiana, USA

ONCOLOGY

Anil D'Cruz MS DNB
Professor and Head
Department of Head and Neck Surgery
Tata Memorial Hospital, Mumbai, India

Pankaj Chaturvedi MS FAIS FICS
Associate Professor
Department of Head and Neck Surgery
Tata Memorial Hospital
Mumbai, India

LARYNGOLOGY

Abir K Bhattacharyya
MS DNB FACS FRCS (Eng) FRCS (ORL)
Consultant ENT and Head and Neck Surgeon
Associate Director of Medical Education (Surgery)
Whipps Cross University Hospital, London E11 1NR, UK
Hon. Senior Lecturer, Institute of Laryngology and
Otology, London, UK
Consultant ENT Surgeon
High Commission of India, London

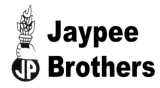

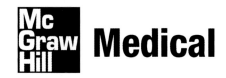

© 2010, Jaypee Brothers Medical Publishers
First published in India in 2009 by

Jaypee Brothers Medical Publishers (P) Ltd.

Corporate Office
4838/24 Ansari Road, Daryaganj, **New Delhi** - 110002, India, +91-11-43574357

Registered Office
B-3 EMCA House, 23/23B Ansari Road, Daryaganj, **New Delhi** 110 002, India
Phones: +91-11-23272143, +91-11-23272703, +91-11-23282021,
+91-11-23245672, Rel: +91-11-32558559 Fax: +91-11-23276490, +91-11-23245683
e-mail: jaypee@jaypeebrothers.com, Website: www.jaypeebrothers.com

First published in USA by The McGraw-Hill Companies, 2 Penn Plaza, New York, NY 10121.
Exclusively worldwide distributor except South Asia (India, Nepal, Sri Lanka, Bhutan, Pakistan,
Bangladesh, Malaysia).

Set ISBN 978-0-07-171981-0 • MHID 0-07-171981-4
Volume 1 P/N: 9780071719773 • 0071719776
Volume 2 P/N: 9780071719797 • 0071719792
DVD P/N: 9780071719780 • 0071719784
Box P/N: 9780071719803 • 0071719806

To

Our Parents, Wives, Children
Our Patients and Teachers

Contributors

Abir K Bhattacharyya
MS DNB FRCS FRCS (ORL)
Consultant ENT and
Head and Neck Surgeon
Whipps Cross University
Hospital, London
Honorary Senior Lecturer, Institute
of Laryngology and Otology, London

Adash Vasanath MD
Resident
Department of Otolaryngology
Tufts University School of Medicine
Tufts-New England Medical Center
Boston, Massachusetts, USA

Adel K El-Naggar MD PhD
Department of Pathology
Head and Neck Section
MD Anderson Cancer Center
University of Texas, Houston, USA

Adorján Ferenc Kovács MD DMD PhD
Associate Professor
Klinik für Kiefer-und Plastische
Gesichtschirugie, Klinikum der
Johann Wolfgang Goethe-
Universität, Frankfurt am Main
Germany

Ahmed Kara MD
Head and Neck Department
Center Oscar Lambret, Lille, France

Ajit Pai MS MCh
Research Fellow
Tata Memorial Hospital
Mumbai, India

Aldo C Stamm MD PhD
Professor
Department of Otolaryngology and
Head and Neck Surgery
Federal University of
São Paulo, Brazil
Director, ENT São Paulo Center
Hospital Professor Edmundo
Vasconcelos, São Paulo, Brazil

Alyssa G Rieber MD
Fellow, Medical Oncology
University of Texas MD Anderson
Cancer Center, Houston, Texas, USA

Amir Minovi MD
Chief Resident, Department of
Otorhinolaryngology—Head, Neck
and Facial Plastic Surgery
Klinikum Fuldag AG, Teaching
Hospital of the Philipps-University
Marburg, Fulda, Germany

Amita A Bagal MD

Anand K Devaiah MD FACS
Assistant Professor, Department of
Otolaryngology – Head and Neck
Surgery and Neurological Surgery
Boston University School of
Medicine, Boston, Massachusetts
USA

Ananda Prasad MD PhD
Distinguished Professor of
Medicine, Wayne State University
Detroit, Michigan, USA

Andrea Bolzoni MD
Department of Otolaryngology
University of Brescia, Italy

Anil D'Cruz MS DNB
Professor and Head
Head and Neck Department
Tata Memorial Hospital
Mumbai, India

Anil Dewan MD
Head and Neck Oncology
Reconstruction
Pennsylvania State University
College of Medicine, Hershey, PA

Anil T Ahuja FRCR
Professor, Chairman
Department of Diagnostic
Radiology and Organ Imaging
The Chinese University of Hong Kong

Ann D King FRCR
Professor, Department of
Diagnostic Radiology and
Organ Imaging
The Chinese University of Hong Kong

Ann M Gillenwater MD
Associate Professor
Department of Head and Neck
Surgery, MD Anderson Cancer
Center, University of Texas
Houston, Texas, USA

Anthony E Magit MD FAAP
Associate Clinical Professor of
Otolaryngology and Pediatrics
University of California at San Diego
School of Medicine, Children's
Hospital and Health Center of
San Diego, San Diego, USA

Ashutosh Kacker MD
Associate Professor, Department of
Otolaryngology—Head and Neck
Surgery, New York Presbyterian
Hospital, Weill-Cornell Medical
College, New York, USA

B Schick
Department of Otolaryngology
Head and Neck Surgery
University Erlangen-Nürnberg
Germany

Bachi T Hathiram MS DORL DNB
Associate Professor, Department of
ENT and Head and Neck Surgery
TN Medical College and BYL Nair
Charity Hospital, Mumbai, India

Bevan Yueh MD MPH
University of Washington
Department of Otolaryngology
Head and Neck Surgery
Seattle, USA

Bhagwati Krishnan PhD
Nursing Superintendent
Tata Memorial Hospital, Mumbai, India

Bhavin G Jankharia DMRD MD
Jankharia Imaging Center
Mumbai, India

Brad Woodworth MD

Brendan C Stack Jr MD FACS
Associate Professor and Director of
Head and Neck Oncology/
Reconstruction
Pennsylvania State University
College of Medicine
Hershey, PA, USA

Brent A Senior MD
Division of Rhinology
Allergy and Sinus Surgery
Department of Otolaryngology/Head
and Neck Surgery
University of North Carolina at
Chapel Hill, North Carolina, USA

Brian E Emery MD FACS
Department of Otolaryngology
Head and Neck Surgery
University of Maryland Medical
System, Baltimore, Maryland, USA

Brian F Perry MD
Department of Otolaryngology
Head and Neck Surgery
University of Virginia Health System
Charlottesville, Virginia, USA

Cecily S Ray MPH
Senior Research Assistant, Healis
Sekhsaria Institute of Public Health
Navi Mumbai, India

Cesare Piazza MD
Department of Otolaryngology
University of Brescia
Spedali Civili of Brescia
Brescia, Italy

Chaitanya Divgi MD
Professor
University of Pennsylvania
Chief, Nuclear Medicine and Clinical
Molecular Imaging
Hospital of the University of
Pennsylvania, USA

Cherie-Ann O Nathan MD FACS
Professor and Vice Chairman
Department of Otolaryngology
Louisiana State University
Shreveport, Louisiana, USA

Chris de Souza
  MS DORL DNB FACS (USA)
ENT Consultant, Lilavati Hospital
Holy Family Hospital
Tata Memorial Hospital
Mumbai, India

Christophe Le Tourneau
Department of Medicine
Institut Gustave-Roussy
Villejuif, France

Christopher GL Hobbs
  BSc MBBS MRCS DLO
Royal College of Surgeons
Research Fellow
Laryngeal Research Group
University of Bristol, Bristol, UK

Christopher J O'Brien
Professor
Head and Neck Cancer Institute
Royal Prince Alfred Hospital
Sydney, Australia

Collin S Karmody FRCSED
Professor of Otolaryngology
Tufts University School of Medicine
Tufts-New England Medical Center
Boston, Massachusetts, USA

Dale A Baur DDS MD
Colonel
US Army Residency Program
Director and Chief, Maxillofacial
Surgery Service
Eisenhower Army Medical Center
Fort Gordon, USA

Dan M Fliss MD
Professor and Chairman
Department of Otolaryngology
Head and Neck Surgery
Tel-Aviv Sourasky Medical Center
Tel-Aviv, Israel

Daniel C Daube Jr MD
Consultant Cosmetic Surgeon
Gulf Coast Facial Plastics
ENT Center, Panama City
Florida, USA

Daniel M Zeitler MD
Resident, Department of
Otolaryngology, New York University
School of Medicine
New Bellevue Hospital
New York, USA

Danielle Elliott
Department of Pathology
Head and Neck Section
MD Anderson Cancer Center
University of Texas, Houston, USA

David J Adelstein MD
Department of Hematology and
Medical Oncology
Cleveland Clinic Foundation
Cleveland, Ohio, USA

Devon H Graham III MD FACS
Clinical Assistant Professor
Department of Otolaryngology
Head and Neck Surgery
Tulane University School of
Medicine, New Orleans
Louisiana, USA

Devyani Lal MBBS MD
Resident
Department of Otolaryngology
Head and Neck Surgery
Loyola University Health System
Illinois, USA

Dimitrios Moraitis MD
Head and Neck Services
Memorial Sloan-Kettering Cancer
Center, York Avenue
New York, USA

DS Grewal MS FACS
Professor and Head, Department of
ENT and Head and Neck Surgery
TN Medical College and BYL Nair
Charity Hospital, Mumbai, India

Edmund HY Yuen FRCR
Radiologist, Apex MRI Center
Limited, Hong Kong

Edward H Farrior MD
Consultant Plastic-Reconstructive
Surgeon, Tampa, Florida, USA

Edward S Kim MD
Assistant Professor
Department of Head and Neck
Thoracic Medical Oncology
University of Texas MD
Anderson Cancer Center
Houston, Texas, USA

Edward W Chang MD
Consultant Facial Reconstruction
Surgeon, Palo Alto, California, USA

Eric M Genden MD FACS
Associate Professor and
Acting Chairman
Department of Otolaryngology and
Associate Professor
Center for Immunobiology, Mount
Sinai School of Medicine, USA

Ernest A Weymuller Jr MD
Department of Otolaryngology
Head and Neck Surgery
University of Washington
Seattle, WA, USA

Etai Funk MD

Eugene N Myers
MD FACS Hon FRCS (ED)
Professor and Eye and Ear
Foundation Chairman
Department of Otolaryngology
University of Pittsburgh School of
Medicine, The Eye and Ear Institute
Pittsburgh, PA, USA

Eva Lunderskov MD

Francis P Ruggiero MD
Head and Neck Oncology
Reconstruction
Pennsylvania State University
College of Medicine, Hershey, PA

François Lüthi
Attending Physician
Multidisciplinary Oncology Center
University of Lausanne Hospitals
Lausanne, Switzerland

Frank D Vrionis MD PhD
Associate Professor of Neurosurgery
Director, Complex Spine Surgery
Skull Base Surgery and Department
of Neurosurgery, University of South
Florida College of Medicine Neuro-
oncology Program, H Lee Moffitt
Cancer Center and Research
Institute, University of South Florida
College of Medicine, Tampa
Florida, USA

Frans JM Hilgers
Chairman
Department of Head and Neck
Oncology and Surgery
The Netherlands Cancer Institute
Plesmanlaan
Amsterdam and Institute of Phonetic
Sciences (ACLC)
University of Amsterdam Herengracht
Amsterdam, The Netherlands

Fred J Stucker MD FACS
Jack W Pou Professor and Chairman
Department of Otolaryngology
Head and Neck Surgery
Louisiana State University
Health Science Center, Shreveport
Louisiana, USA

Gouri Pantvaidya
Assistant Professor
Department of Head and Neck Surgery
Tata Memorial Hospital
Mumbai, India

Gady Har-El MD FACS
Professor of Otolaryngology and
Neurosurgery, State University of
New York, Downstate Medical
Center, Brooklyn, New York, USA

Gary Y Shaw MD FACS
Associate Clinical Professor
University of Health Sciences
Kansas City, Missouri, USA

Giorgio Peretti MD
Assistant Professor
Department of Otolaryngology
University of Brescia
Spedali Civili of Brescia
Piazza Spedali Civili 1
25123 Brescia, Italy

Giulio Cantù MD
Chief, Head and Neck Surgical
Department, Istituto Nazionale
Tumori, Milan, Italy

Gregory A Grillone MD FACS
Department of Otolaryngology
Head and Neck Surgery
Boston University School of Medicine

Gregory S Weinstein MD
Professor and Vice Chairman
Director, Division of
Head and Neck Cancer
Department of Otorhinolaryngology
Head and Neck Surgery
University of Pennsylvania, USA

Guy J Petruzzelli MD PhD MBA FACS
Professor, Otolaryngology
Head and Neck Surgery
Professor, General Surgery
Section of Endocrine Surgery
Chief-Head and Neck Oncology
Service, Cardinal Bernardin Cancer
Center, Loyola University Health
System, Illinois, USA

Guy Kenyon MD FRCS FRCS (Ed)
Whipps Cross University Hospital
London, UK

Hannes Braun MD PhD
Department of Otorhinolaryngology
Head and Neck Surgery, University
Medical School, Graz, Austria

Heinz Stammberger MD PhD
Department of Otorhinolaryngology
Head and Neck Surgery, University
Medical School, Graz, Austria

Henning A Gaissert MD
Assistant Professor
Massachusetts General Hospital
Blake, Fruit Street, Boston, MA, USA

Hermes C Grillo
Professor, Thoracic Surgery
Massachusetts General Hospital
Harvard Medical School
Boston, Massachusetts, USA

Hugo Canhete Lopes MD
Department of Otolaryngology
Hospital Professor Edmundo
Vasconcelos, São Paulo, Brazil

IB Tan
Department of Head and Neck
Oncology and Surgery
The Netherlands Cancer Institute
Plesmanlaan, Amsterdam
The Netherlands

Itzhak Brook MD MSc
Professor of Pediatrics and
Medicine, Georgetown University
School of Medicine
Washington, DC, USA

J David Osguthorpe MD

J Peter Rodrigues MS FICS DORL
Honorary Head
Department of Otolaryngology
St Georges Hospital

Jain George P MS MCh
Clinical Fellow in Neurosurgery
Department of Neuro oncology
H.Lee Moffitt Cancer Center and
Research Institute, University of
South Florida College of Medicine
Tampa, Florida, USA

James Reidy
Professor and Chairman
Department of Head and Neck
Surgery, Roswell Park Cancer
Institute, Buffalo
New York, USA

Jamie A Cesaretti MD
Assistant Professor
Department of Radiation Oncology
Mount Sinai School of Medicine
New York, USA

Jan S Lewin PhD
Associate Professor
Department of Head and
Neck Surgery
The University of Texas
MD Anderson Cancer Center
Houston, Texas, USA

Jason G Newman MD
Assistant Professor
Department of Otorhinolaryngology
Head and Neck Surgery
University of Pennsylvania, USA

Jatin P Shah
Professor and Chief
Head and Neck Memorial Sloan-
Kettering Cancer Center
New York, USA

Jay O Boyle MD
Director, Fellowship Training Program
Head and Neck Surgery Service
Memorial Sloan-Kettering Cancer
Center, York Avenue
New York, USA

Jeanette Boohene MD
Department of Palliative Care and
Rehabilitation Medicine, UT MD
Anderson Cancer Center
Houston, Texas, USA

Jean-Louis Lefebvre
Head and Neck Department
Center Oscar Lambret, Lille, France

Jeeve Kanagalingam

Jeffrey G Neal MD

Jeffrey H Spiegel MD
Chief, Facial Plastic and
Reconstructive Surgery
Associate Professor
Department of Otolaryngology
Head and Neck Surgery, Boston
University School of Medicine, USA

Jern-Lin Leong FRCS (GLASG)
Consultant, Department of
Otolaryngology, Singapore General
Hospital, Singapore

Jesus E Medina MD FACS
Paul and Ruth Jonas
Professor and Chairman
Department of Otorhinolaryngology
The university of Oklahoma Health
Sciences Center, Oklahoma City
Oklahoma, USA

John Pickett PhD
Department of Medical Physics
Barts and the London NHS Trust
London, UK

John R Jacobs MD
Professor, Wayne State University
Department of Otolaryngology and
Head and Neck Surgery, Detroit MI
USA

John S Rubin MD FACS FRCS
Royal National Throat, Nose and Ear
Hospital, London, UK

Johnny Kao MD
Assistant Professor
Department of Radiation Oncology
Mount Sinai School of Medicine, USA

Jolie Ringash MD MSC FRCP (C)
Princess Margaret Hospital
University Health Network
University of Toronto, Toronto
Ontario, Canada

Jonathan AT Sandoe
MBCh Phd FRCPATH
Consultant Microbiologist, Leeds
Teaching Hospitals NHS Trust
Honorary Senior Lecturer
University of Leeds, UK

Jonathan M Owens MD

Joseph I Helman DMD
Clinical Professor and Chairman
Department of Oral and Maxillofacial
Surgery, University of Michigan, USA

Joseph K Salama MD
Chief Resident, Department of
Radiation and Cellular Oncology
University of Chicago, USA

JV Divatia MD
Professor
Department of Anesthesia
Critical Care and Pain
Tata Memorial Hospital
Mumbai, India

Kazim Sahin
Department of Animal Nutrition
Faculty of Veterinary Science
Firat University, Elazig, Turkey

Kevin C McMains MD
Assistant Professor of
Otolaryngology, University of Texas
Health Science Center at San
Antonio, San Antonio, Texas, USA

KT Wong FRCR
Consultant, Department of
Diagnostic Radiology and Organ
Imaging, Prince of Wales Hospital
Hong Kong

L Kapoor
Department of ENT, Head and Neck Surgery, Whipps Cross University Hospital, London, UK

LM Sneddon
Research Associate, University of Newcastle upon Tyne, UK

Laura Locati MD
Head and Neck Cancer Medical Oncology Unit
Cancer Medicine Department
Istituto Nazionale Tumori
Milan, Italy

Lauren L Patton DDS FDS RCS (Ed)
Professor, Department of Dental Ecology, School of Dentistry
University of North Carolina
Chapel Hill, USA

Lena Hijazi FRACS
Whipps Cross University Hospital
London, UK

Lisa Licitra MD
Chief, Head and Neck Cancer Medical Oncology Unit
Cancer Medicine Department
Istituto Nazionale Tumori, Milan, Italy

Letícia Schmidt Rosito
Otorhinolaryngologist, Fellow of the Otorhinolaryngology Service
Hospital de Clínicas de Porto Alegre
Rio Grande do Sul, Brazil

M Greenwood
Consultant and Honorary Senior Lecturer, University of Newcastle Upon Tyne, UK

Marc Bassim MD

Maria J Worsham PhD FACMG
Professor, Director of Research
Department of Otolaryngology
Head and Neck Research, Henry Ford Health System, Detroit, MI, USA

Mariana Magnus Smith
Otorhinolaryngologist, Fellow of the Otorhinolaryngology Service
Hospital de Clínicas de Porto Alegre
Rio Grande do Sul, Brazil

Mark Izzard
Otolaryngology
Head and Neck Surgery
University of Auckland and
Consultant Otolaryngologist
Head and Neck Surgeon
Counties-Manukau DHB, New Zealand

Martin J Citardi MD FACS
Professor-Chairman
Department of Otorhinolaryngology
Head and Neck Surgery
University of Texas Medical School
Houston, Texas, USA

Mathew Karen MD
Consultant, Winchester Facial Cosmetic Surgery
Winchester, Virginia, USA

Matthew S Russell MD
Department of Otolaryngology
Head and Neck Surgery, Boston University School of Medicine, USA

Meher Ursekar DMRD MD

Michael S Benninger MD
Department of Otolaryngology
Head and Neck Surgery
Henry Ford Hospital, Detroit Michigan, USA

Michael T Milano MD PhD
Assistant Professor
Department of Radiation Oncology
University of Rochester

Mike Papesch FRACS

Miriam R Robbins
Department of Oral Medicine
New York University College of Dentistry, NY, USA

Moshe Ephrat MD FACS
Assistant Clinical Professor
Albert Einstein College of Medicine
Bronx, New York, USA
Assistant Clinical Instructor
Mount Sinai School of Medicine
New York, USA

Mukta R Bapat MD DM
Consultant Gastroenterologist
Institute of Advanced Endoscopy
Mumbai, India

Nadim B Bikhazi MD
Department of Otolaryngology
Ogden Clinic, Ogden, Utah, USA

Neil M Vora MD
Department of Otolaryngology
Head and Neck Surgery
Louisiana State University Health Science Center Shreveport
Louisiana, USA

Nicholas Reading MRCP FRCR
Consultant Radiologist, Whipps Cross University Hospital, London

Nilesh R Vasan
University of Oklahoma Health Sciences Center
Department of Otorhinolaryngology
Oklahoma City, Oklahoma, USA

Omer Kucuk
Department of Medicine
Division of Hematology-Oncology
Center for Molecular Medicine and Genetics, Wayne State University School of Medicine
St. Antoine, Detroit, MI, USA

Ozlem E Tulunay MD
Fellow, Wayne State University School of Medicine, Department of Otolaryngology, Head and Neck Surgery, Detroit, MI, USA

Pablo Mojica-Manosa MD
Fellow, Head and Neck Surgery
Roswell Park Cancer Institute
Elm and Carlton Streets
Buffalo, New York, USA

Pankaj Chaturvedi MS FAIS FICS
Associate Professor
Department of Head and Neck Surgery
Tata Memorial Hospital
Mumbai, India

Paolo Bossi MD
Head and Neck Cancer Medical Oncology Unit, Cancer Medicine Department, Istituto Nazionale Tumori, Milan, Italy

Patrick J Bradley MBA FRCS
Professor of Head and Neck Surgical Oncology

Department of Otorhinolaryngology
Head and Neck Surgery
Nottingham University Hospitals
Queens Medical Center Campus
Nottingham, UK

Patrizia Olmi MD
Department of Radiotherapy
Istituto Nazionale Tumori, Milan, Italy

Paul Johnson MD
Resident Physician
Department of Otolaryngology
Head and Neck Surgery, New York
Presbyterian Hospital, Weill-Cornell
Medical College, New York, USA

Pete S Batra MD
Section Head, Nasal and Sinus
Disorders, Head and Neck Institute
Cleveland Clinic Foundation
Cleveland, Ohio, USA

Peter A Adamson MD FRCSC FACS
Consultant Cosmetic Facial
Surgeon, Toronto, Ontario, Canada

Peter Andrew

Peter J Catalano MD FACS
Associate Professor
Otolaryngology, Boston University
Boston Massachusetts, USA
Chairman, Department of
Otolaryngology – Head and Neck
Surgery, Lahey Clinic, Burlington
Massachusetts, USA

Philip Abraham
Consultant Gastroenterology and
Hepatology
P D Hinduja National Hospital and
Medical Research Center
Mahim, Mumbai
Professor, Department of
Gastroenterology, King Edward
Memorial Hospital, Parel
Mumbai, India

Prakash C Gupta DSc FACE
Director, Healis Sekhsaria Institute
of Public Health, Navi Mumbai, India

Priya Ranganathan MD DNBE
Assistant Professor
Department of Anesthesia
Critical Care and Pain
Tata Memorial Hospital, Mumbai, India

Purushothaman Sen MSc MS DNB FRCS
Specialist in ENT, Whipps Cross
University Hospital, London, UK

Pushkar Mehra BDS DMD
Director, Department of Oral and
Maxillofacial Surgery
Boston University Medical Center
and Boston Medical Center
Associate Professor, Vice Chairman
Department of Oral and Maxillofacial
Surgery, Boston University School of
Dental Medicine, Boston, USA

RA Ord MD DDS FRCS FACS MS
Professor and Chairman
Department Oral-Maxillofacial
Surgery, University of Maryland
Greenebaum Cancer Center
Baltimore, Maryland, USA

RJ Lowry
Senior Lecturer, University of
Newcastle upon Tyne, UK

Rajeev T MS DORL
Chief Resident, Department of ENT
and Head and Neck Surgery
TN Medical College and BYL Nair
Charity Hospital, Mumbai, India

Rakesh K Chandra MD
Assistant Professor
Director Division of Nasal and Sinus
Disorders, Department of
Otolaryngology
Head and Neck Surgery
University of Tennessee Health
Science Center Memphis
Tennessee, USA

Ralph P Tufano MD FACS
Associate Professor
Director of Thyroid and
Parathyroid Surgery
Division of Head and Neck
Surgical Oncology
Department of Otolaryngology
Head and Neck Surgery
Johns Hopkins School of Medicine
Baltimore, Maryland, USA

Randall P Morton
Professor of Otolaryngology
Head and Neck Surgery
University of Auckland and
Consultant Otolaryngologist

Head and Neck Surgeon
Counties-Manukau DHB
New Zealand

Ravindhra G Elluru MD PhD
Cincinnati Children's Hospital
Medical Center
Division of Otolaryngology
Head and Neck Surgery and
University of Cincinnati College of
Medicine, Department of
Otolaryngology/Head and Neck
Surgery, Cincinnati, Ohio, USA

Ravindra M Mehta MD FCCP DABSM
Assistant Professor of Medicine,
Division of Pulmonary/Critical Care/
Sleep Disorders Medicine, Brooklyn
VA Medical Center, State University
of New York, Brooklyn, NY, USA

Rebecca E Fraioli MD

Renuka A Bradoo MS DORL
Professor and Head
Department of ENT and
Head and Neck Surgery
LTM Medical College and General
Hospital, Mumbai, India

Ricard Simo
Consultant Otorhinolaryngologist
Head and Neck Surgeon, Guy's and
St Thomas Hospital
London, Honorary Senior Lecturer
and Clinical Advisor, Guy's King's
and St Thomas' Medical and Dental
School, London, UK

Richard R Orlandi MD
Associate Professor
Division of Otolaryngology
Head and Neck Surgery
University of Utah School of
Medicine, Salt Lake City, Utah, USA

Ricardo Persaud
MBBS MPhil MiBiol CBiol DohNS MRCS
Specialist Registrar in ENT
Head and Neck Surgery
Whipps Cross University Hospital
London, UK

RJ Lowry
Senior Lecturer
School of Dental Sciences
Framlington Place, Newcastle upon
Tyne, NE2 4BW, UK

Robert E Sonnenburg Jr MD

Robert Hong MD
Resident
Department of Radiation Oncology
Loyola University
Health System, Illinois, USA

Robin T Cotton

Robin Youngs MD FRCS

Rodney J Schlosser MD
Department of Otolaryngology
Head and Neck Surgery
Medical University of South Carolina
Charleston, South Carolina, USA

Roger Stupp
Multidisciplinary Oncology Center
University of Lausanne Hospitals
Switzerland

Romaine Johnson MD

Rosemarie A de Souza MD
Department of Internal Medicine
LTM Medical College and General
Hospital, Mumbai, India

Ross A Kerr
Department of Oral Medicine
New York
University College of Dentistry
New York, USA

RP Fernandes MD DDS
Assistant Professor
Department of Oral Maxillofacial
Surgery, University of Florida at
Jacksonville, USA

Ruth Epstein PhD MRCSLT
Head of Speech and Language
Therapy Services
Royal National Throat Nose and Ear
Hospital, London, UK

Sady Selaiman Da Costa
Associate Professor
Department of Ophthalmology and
Otorhinolaryngology
Universidade Federal do Rio Grande
do Sul, Porto Alegre - Rio Grande
do Sul, Brazil

Sameer Khemani MBBS MRCS DOHNS
Specialist Registrar in ENT
Head and Neck Surgery
Whipps Cross University Hospital
London, UK

Samuel M Lam MD FACS
Consultant Facial Plastic Surgeon
Dallas, Texas, USA

Sandrine Faivre MD PhD
Department of Oncology
Hôpital Beaujon, Clichy, France

Sandeep Samant
Department of Otolaryngology
Head and Neck Surgery
University of Tennessee
Memphis, Tennessee, USA

Sandro J Stoeckli MD
Chairman
Department of Otorhinolaryngology
Head and Neck Surgery
Kantonsspital St Gallen
Switzerland

Sarah H Kagan PhD
Consultant Nurse
University of Pennsylvania
School of Nursing Guardian Drive
Philadelphia, USA

Scott Schraff MD
Phoenix Children's Hospital
Phoenix, Arizona

Shankar Sridhar MD
Department of Otolaryngology
Head and Neck Surgery and
Neurological Surgery
Boston University School of
Medicine, Boston
Massachusetts, USA

Shirley SN Pignatari MD PhD
Associate Professor and Head
Division of Pediatric Otolaryngology
Federal University of São Paulo
Division of Pediatric Otolaryngology
Hospital Professor Edmundo
Vasconcelos, São Paulo, Brazil

Shyan Vijayasekaran FRACS

Snehal G Patel MD MS FRCS (GLASG)
Assistant Attending Surgeon
Head and Neck Service, Memorial
Sloan-Kettering Cancer Center
Assistant Professor
Weill-Cornell Medical College
New York, USA

Stephen S Park MD

Steven B Cannady MD

Steven M Feinberg MD
Department of Otolaryngology
Head and Neck Surgery
University of California Irvine School
of Medicine, Orange, California, USA

Steven Pearlman MD FACS
Associate Professor of Clinical
Otolaryngology
Department of Otolaryngology
Head and Neck Surgery, Columbia
University College of Physicians and
Surgeons, New York, USA

Stilianos E Kountakis MD PhD
Professor of Otolaryngology
Medical College of Georgia
Augusta Georgia, USA

Suchir Maitra MBBS
Senior House Officer
Gloucestershire Royal Hospital
Gloucester, UK

Suman Golla MD FACS
Assistant Professor in Otolaryngology
Eye and Ear Institute, School of
Medicine University of Pittsburgh
Pennsylvania, USA

Suresh K Reddy MD FFARCS
Associate Professor and
Director of Education
Dept. of Palliative Care and
Rehabilitation Medicine, UT MD
Anderson Cancer Center
Houston, Texas, USA

Susan D Mccammon MD
Senior Fellow
Head and Neck Service
Memorial Sloan-Kettering
Cancer Center, NY, USA

Sushma Nordemar MD PhD
Department of Otorhinolaryngology
Head and Neck Surgery, Karolinska
Hospital, Stockholm, Sweden

Terry A Day MD
Department of Otolaryngology
Head and Neck Surgery
Medical University of South Carolina,
Charleston, South Carolina, USA

Terry Y Shibuya MD FACS
Assistant Professor
Department of Otolaryngology
Head and Neck Surgery and Chao
Family Comprehensive Cancer
Center University of California Irvine
School of Medicine, Orange
California, USA

Theresa L Whiteside PhD
Professor
Department of Otolaryngology
Head and Neck Surgery and
Pathology
Pittsburgh Cancer Institute
Pittsburgh Pennsylvania, USA

Thom R Loree MD FACS
Professor and Chairman
Department of Head and Neck
Surgery, Roswell Park Cancer
Institute, Buffalo, NY, USA

Thomas Costello MD
Chief Resident
Department of Otolaryngology
Head and Neck Surgery
University of Tennessee Health
Science Center
Memphis, Tennessee, USA

Thomas F Heston MD
Residency Program Director and
Chief, Maxillofacial Surgery Service

Timothy Lian MD
Associate Professor
Department of Otolaryngology
Head and Neck Surgery
Louisiana State University Health
Science Center, Shreveport
Louisiana, USA

Todd T Kingdom MD
Associate Professor and Director
Rhinology and Sinus Surgery
Department of Otolaryngology
University of Colorado, Aurora
Colorado, USA

Tom JB Vauterin
Head and Neck Fellow
The Sydney Head and Neck
Cancer Institute, Sydney, Australia

Ulrike Bockmühl MD PhD
Department of Otorhinolaryngology
Head and Neck Surgery
Klinikum Fulda gAG
Teaching Hospital of the Philipps
University Marburg, Fulda, Germany

Veena A Nagar MD

Vicky Khattar
Senior Resident
Department of ENT and
Head and Neck Surgery
TN Medical College and
BYL Nair Charity Hospital
Mumbai, India

Vijaya Patil MD
Additional Professor
Department of Anesthesia
Critical Care and Pain
Tata Memorial Hospital
Mumbai, India

Vikki L Noonan DMD DMSc
Associate Professor of Oral and
Maxillofacial Pathology, Boston
University School of Dental
Medicine, Boston, USA

Vinaya Chakradeo MD

Wei-Zen Wei PhD
Professor, Department of
Microbiology and Immunology and
Karmanos Cancer Institute, Wayne
State University School of Medicine
Detroit, Michigan, USA

William M Mendenhall MD
Department of Radiation Oncology
University of Florida College of
Medicine, Gainsville, Florida, USA

William Nnuma MD
Senior Resident, Department of
Otolaryngology, Tufts University
School of Medicine, Tufts-New
England Medical Center, Boston
Massachusetts, USA

William W Shockley MD FACS
Professor and Vice Chairman
Department of Otolaryngology
Head and Neck Surgery
University of North Carolina School
of Medicine, Chapel Hill
North Carolina, USA

Wolfgang Draf MD
Department of ENT Diseases
Head, Neck and Facial Plastic Surgery
International Neuroscience Institute
Hanover, Germany

Yolanda YP Lee
Associate Consultant
Department of Diagnostic Radiology
and Organ Imaging
Prince of Wales Hospital
Hong Kong

Zahoor Ahmad MBBS MS FRACS
Vice Chairman
Department of Otolaryngology
Head and Neck Surgery
Counties Manukau Health
Middlemore Hospital and
Manukau Surgery Center
Auckland, New Zealand

Ziv Gil MD PhD

Zvoru GG Makura
MBChB FRCSEd FRCS (ORL-HNS)
Consultant ENT/Head and Neck
Surgeon, Leeds Teaching Hospitals
Hon Senior Lecturer University of
Leeds Medical School, UK

Foreword

It is estimated that over five hundred thousand patients are diagnosed with cancers in the head and neck area annually worldwide. This number is gradually rising. In spite of significant advances in basic sciences to understand the mechanisms of carcinogenesis and molecular profiling, technological advances in imaging and navigational surgery and significant advances in reconstructive surgery, not much progress has taken place in terms of improved outcomes of therapy in head and neck cancer. Clearly, management of these tumors has become quite a complex undertaking and no one specialist is able to provide all the necessary aspects of multidisciplinary care for cancers in the head and neck area. For advanced stage tumors, multidisciplinary involvement is crucial to successful outcome. Increasing emphasis is being laid on minimizing the impact of therapeutic interventions and improving the quality of life while keeping improved survivorship as the focal point of any therapeutic program.

Dr Chris de Souza and his associates are to be congratulated for putting together a unique textbook covering the broad range of various topics in head and neck cancer. Contributors to this extraordinary collection of manuscripts are leaders in the field from all corners of the world. The editors are aware of the high cost of major textbooks in head and neck cancer which is not affordable in the South Asian subcontinent by a majority of physicians and students involved in the management of patients with cancers of the head and neck. The emphasis is placed on producing a low-cost textbook which provides the most up-to-date information on topics and issues of current interest at an affordable price. It is my belief that they have succeeded in doing so.

Advances in the management of head and neck cancer happen on a continuous basis. Clearly, this compendium provides the state-of-the-art-and-science in the field of head and neck surgery and oncology as it is practiced today. The diversity of authorship of topics in this book reflects a global view of leaders in their areas of expertise. The list of contributors also reflects that head and neck cancer is a global disease and should have a common theme of understanding the biology of the disease and its therapeutic interventions. Clearly, the focus would be to improve outcomes and quality of life worldwide such that the wide discrepancies in outcomes in various parts of the world are narrowed in the years to come. I feel that this textbook will provide the reader with the most up-to-date knowledge in the field of head and neck cancer and the information on therapeutic interventions as they are practiced globally. This textbook is essential reading for the trainee in head and neck surgery and should be on the bookshelf of all physicians caring for head and neck cancer and in libraries of cancer institutions and medical schools worldwide.

Jatin P Shah MD FACS
Hon FRCS (Edin) Hon FRACS Hon FDSRCS (Lond)

Professor of Surgery, Weill Medical College of Cornell University
EW Strong Chairman in Head and Neck Oncology
Chief, Head and Neck Service, Memorial Sloan-Kettering Cancer Center
New York, USA

Foreword

The Head and Neck is truly an important intersection not only between vital structures but also between that of many medical and surgical disciplines. This is brought out amply in this compendium. This textbook is a timely reminder that collaboration between multiple disciplines is absolutely necessary if not vital to bring about effective treatment for our patients.

It is a truism that medicine advances rapidly. Some might even say that a textbook might be behind times, especially in the age of the Internet and instant communication. This is not applicable in the case of *Head and Neck Surgery*. Timeless principles still hold true and this book combines the old which still hold true in modern medical practice and that which is modern helps augment our knowledge.

I must compliment the editors who involved an impressive array of authors. The list of chapters is carefully drawn to encompass all aspects of Head Neck Surgery. The Oncology section begins with a beautifully written chapter on the historical perspective of Head Neck Oncology. In words of the great Roman writer and politician Marcus Tulius Cicero: "The causes of events are ever more interesting than the events themselves." The chapters on "Quality of Life in Head and Neck Cancer" and "Outcome Assessment in Head and Neck Cancer" demonstrate increasing emphasis on such issues hitherto less talked about a decade back. The chapter on "Endoscopic Head and Neck Surgery" proves the role of current state-of-art minimal access tools in less disfiguring surgery without jeopardizing safety. Chapters on—Anesthetic Considerations, Nursing Considerations, Palliation, etc. make it one of the most comprehensive Head and Neck books to my knowledge. It is good to see that editors have given due importance to translational research and molecular mechanisms in the Head and Neck Oncology.

I hope the noble purpose of this book, which is the dissemination of knowledge and sharing of ideas is fulfilled and I am sure that a future second edition will validate the purpose of all that is written here.

Rajendra A Badwe
Director, Tata Memorial Center
Mumbai, India

Preface

Head and Neck Surgery is a well-established and important medical specialty the world over. It lies at the intersection of several disciplines. A glance at the table of contents of this book illustrates this.

With advances in technology, there has been a significant increase in the quantum of medical literature now available. For the novice who has just embarked on the study of Head and Neck Surgery, this can be dauntingly enormous, contradictory, and at times, confusing. *Head and Neck Surgery* was written to address this very issue and to present distilled knowledge on this subject in a lucid, comprehensive, and easy-to-understand manner. This book has something for each reader: The beginner can find information about techniques as well as guidance regarding which approach to take. The expert and experienced head and neck surgeon can find discussions on issues regarding controversies and recent advances in the field.

The book has been compiled by experts in the field from all over the world. They are not just outstanding head and neck surgeons, but also excellent teachers, who have graciously and unselfishly contributed to this book, sharing their skills and providing technical inputs, so that others may benefit from their experience. For the editors and authors of this book, this has been a singularly satisfying experience. We are happy that this book will ultimately benefit the people at the center of our medical universe: Our patients.

I am deeply indebted to all the editors of this book who have shown phenomenal commitment by devoting much time and effort to produce this book. We are also very grateful to the authors of individual chapters, who have worked hard to produce chapters of very exacting standards of excellence. We also thank our families for allowing all of us the luxury of time to put together a book of this magnitude and nature.

I thank the publishers for their cooperation, help and time especially since most of the editors and authors are from so many different parts of the world to produce a truly international textbook.

Chris de Souza MS DORL DNB FACS (USA)
Mumbai, India

ACKNOWLEDGEMENT

The Editor-in-Chief is thankful to Springer Science and Business Media for granting the permission to reproduced in part from *Rhinology and Facial Plastic Surgery* (Springer, 2009) Chapter 16: Rhinosinusitis (pages 189-201) (de Souza and de Souza), and Chapter 22: Fungal Rhinosinusitis (pages 255-269) (de Souza and Rodrigues) in my book *Head and Neck Surgery*, 2 vols.

Contents

SECTION 2: FACIAL PLASTICS

SECTION 3: ONCOLOGY

RHINOLOGY

CHAPTER 1

Anatomy of the Lateral Nasal Wall

Renuka A Bradoo

A sound knowledge of the anatomy of the lateral nasal wall is a crucial element in the making of a safe and effective endoscopic sinus surgeon. This anatomy is best understood by studying the sagittal section of a cadaveric head. This specimen should be dissected in a sequential manner starting medially within the nasal cavity and proceeding laterally up to the orbit. We shall study these sections in this chapter.

The cadaveric head when cut in the immediate parasagittal plane reveals the lateral nasal wall. On first impression, this area appears as a series of elevations and depressions. The lateral nasal wall extends from the nasal vestibule to the posterior choana, which is formed by medial surface of the medial pterygoid plate. The nasopharynx extends beyond the posterior choana up to prevertebral muscles. What is striking is that the lateral nasal wall extends up to approximately 50% of the distance of the entire sagittal section of the head (Fig. 1.1).

Anteriorly, the lateral nasal wall is lined by skin and has hair: this is the vestibule (Fig. 1.2). Behind this is the atrium, a plain structureless area lined by nasal mucosa. The atrium shows a bulge anterior to the attachment of the middle turbinate which is formed by the underlying agger nasi cell. Very often, a ridge can be discerned extending from the agger nasi cell to an apex on the superior border of the inferior turbinate. This ridge overlies the nasolacrimal duct.

Behind the atrium are the three scrolls of the inferior, middle and superior turbinates, overlying the respective meatii. Occasionally, there may be a supreme turbinate. Above and behind the superior turbinate is the sphenoethmoidal recess, which gets its name from the fact that this area forms a niche between the posterior ethmoid cells and the sphenoid sinus.

The inferior turbinate is fairly straight and without structure. The eustachian tube opens in the nasopharynx 1 cm behind its posterior attachment. The elevation of the eustachian tube is called the torus tubaris, behind which is a deep cleft called fossa of Rosenmüller. The middle turbinate, unlike the inferior turbinate, is

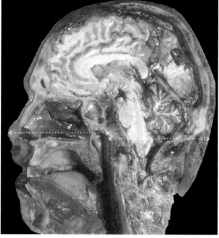

Fig. 1.1: Sagittal section of the head

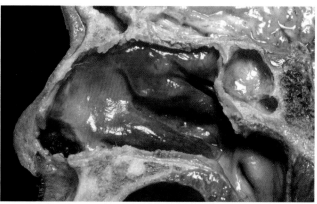

Fig. 1.2: The lateral nasal wall

convoluted and shows many anatomical variations. Its posterior end lies at the level of the roof of the posterior choana.

The skull base in the anterior cranial fossa slopes downwards at an angle of approximately 15° in the anteroposterior direction. The olfactory nerves can be seen perforating the cribriform plate in this area.

The middle turbinate is a convoluted structure bending in different planes similar to a dried leaf. It can be divided into three parts, depending on its attachment and its orientation in the three-dimensional space (Fig. 1.3).

- The anterior one-third is in the sagittal plane and is attached to the cribriform plate at the junction of the medial and lateral lamellae. It also takes a small anterior attachment to the frontonasal process of the maxilla.
- The middle one-third lies in the coronal plane and is attached to the lamina papyracea. It separates the anterior ethmoidal cells from the posterior ethmoidal cells. Since it stabilizes the middle turbinate, it is called the ground lamella or basal lamella.
- The posterior one-third lies in the horizontal plane and is attached to the lamina papyracea and perpendicular plate of the palatine bone extending up to the roof of the posterior choana.

The middle turbinate is trimmed (Fig. 1.4). Its anterior, middle and posterior attachments can now be demarcated. The structures within the middle meatus which form the key area or osteomeatal unit can now be

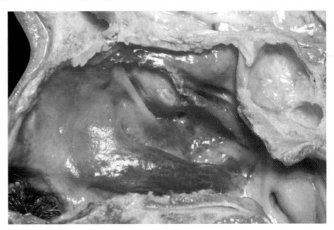

Fig. 1.4: The middle turbinate is trimmed to expose the osteomeatal unit. An accessory ostium is seen in the hiatus semilunaris

visualized. This is the area into which the frontal, maxillary and anterior ethmoidal sinuses drain. Most anteriorly is a curved ridge called the uncinate process. Behind this is the well pneumatized and most constant anterior ethmoidal cell, namely the ethmoidal bulla. These structures are separated from each other by a semilunar groove called the hiatus semilunaris inferioris. The hiatus semilunaris is two-dimensional and leads into a three-dimensional space called the infundibulum.

Rarely (8%), the bulla may be rudimentary or absent. It may be separated posteriorly from the ground lamella of the middle turbinate by a recess called the retrobullar recess (Fig. 1.5). Occasionally, the bulla does not extend up to the base of the skull and is separated from it by the suprabullar recess. The retrobullar and suprabullar recesses together form a semilunar space above and behind the bulla called the sinus lateralis of Grunwald. This space opens into the middle meatus by a semilunar

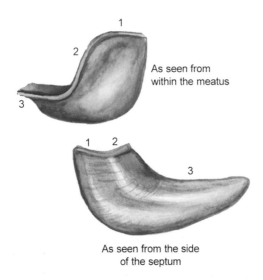

Fig. 1.3: Attachments of middle turbinate: 1: to cribriform plate, 2. to lamina papyracea, 3. to perpendicular plate of palatine bone

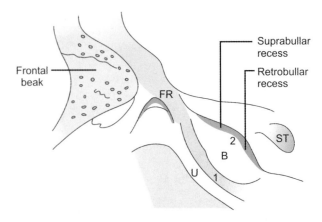

Fig. 1.5: The suprabullar and retrobullar recesses, 1. the hiatus semilunaris inferioris, 2. the hiatus semilunaris superioris

cleft which is opposite in orientation to the hiatus semilunaris inferioris and is called the hiatus semilunaris superioris. Thus, the hiatus semilunaris inferioris leads into the infundibulum and the hiatus semi-lunaris superioris leads into sinus lateralis of Grunwald. The roof of the sinus lateralis is formed by the ethmoid fovea and its floor by the ethmoidal bulla. It is limited posteriorly by the ground lamella of the middle turbinate and anteriorly it opens into the frontal recess. Laterally is the lamina papyracea, and medially is the middle turbinate. The hiatus semilunaris superioris is absent when the bulla is attached either to the skull base superiorly or to the ground lamella posteriorly.

The infundibulum leads directly or indirectly into the frontal recess (Fig. 1.6). The frontal recess can be a surgically challenging area to operate upon as it very often shows variations in anatomy.

- The frontal recess is bounded anteriorly by the agger nasi cell, which is considered to be a part of the frontal recess. Therefore, the anterior wall of the frontal recess is formed by the anterior wall of the agger nasi cell.
- The posterior wall is formed by the bulla ethmoidalis. If there is a suprabullar recess, it will open into the posterior wall of the frontal recess.
- The lateral wall of the frontal recess is formed by the lamina papyracea.
- The medial wall is formed by the middle turbinate.
- Superiorly, the frontal recess opens via the frontal ostium into the frontal sinus. Seen from above, the frontal sinus opening is funnel-shaped and is placed at the posterior and medial end of the floor of the frontal sinus. This funnel-shaped region is called the frontal infundibulum. Thus, in sagittal cross-section, the frontal infundibulum, frontal ostium and the

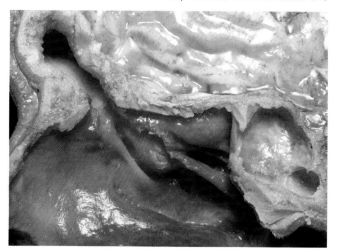

Fig. 1.6: The frontal recess

frontal recess together form the 'hour-glass configuration' so often described.

Thus, the frontal sinus lies much more anterior to the frontal recess when seen endoscopically.

The upper end of the uncinate process lies within the frontal recess. It shows great variation in anatomy. It can:
- extend up to the base skull,
- attach to the middle turbinate,
- turn forwards to be attached to the insertion of the middle turbinate,
- lie free in the middle meatus,
- be pneumatized.

Most commonly (in 80%), it attaches to the lamina papyracea in the form of a dome. This upper-dome-shaped attachment of the uncinate process within the frontal recess has been graphically described by Stammberger as an eggshell in an inverted egg-cup. The recess which is enclosed within this dome, is called the recessus terminalis. In this case, the frontal sinus opens medial to the uncinate process.

The components and contents of the frontal recess are extremely variable:
- The agger nasi cell may be small or large, single or multiple and rarely absent.
- The bulla may be small or large, extending up to the skull base or stopping short at the suprabullar recess.
- The upper end of the attachment of the uncinate process has many variations as already described.
- The anterior ethmoidal cell may migrate antero-superiorly into the frontal recess to produce different types of **frontal cells,** viz.:

Type I → a single cell above the agger nasi cell.

Type II → two or more cells above the agger nasi cell.

Type III → a large cell extending well into the frontal sinus mimicking the frontal sinus itself (the frontal bulla).

Type IV → an isolated **loner cell** lying separately within the frontal sinus.

The uncinate process is cut to expose the infundibulum (Fig. 1.7). The opening of the maxillary sinus lies in the depths of the infundibulum well hidden by the uncinate process. It is usually ovoid, tunnel-like, having three dimensions. Conversely, the accessory ostium is easily seen; it is usually circular and has only two dimensions. The relations of the maxillary ostium are:
- *inferiorly* the inferior turbinate,
- *superiorly* the lamina papyracea and the orbit,
- *posteriorly* the posterior fontanelle,
- *anteriorly* the nasolacrimal duct.

The anterior fontanelle, an area of double layer of mucosa without any underlying bone, is found antero-inferior to the uncinate process. Similarly, the posterior

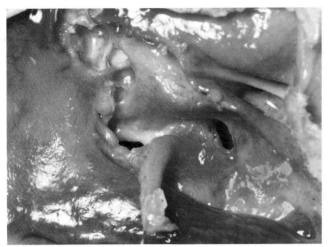

Fig. 1.7: The uncinate process is cut to reveal the infundibulum, maxillary ostium, accessory ostium and the infundibular cells

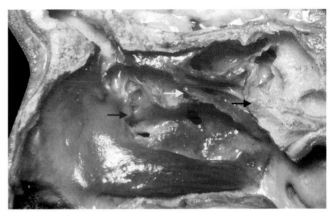

Fig. 1.9: Anterior and posterior ethmoidal cells dissected to show the four lamellae marked by arrows: Uncinate process (blue), anterior wall of bulla (green), ground lamella (yellow), anterior wall of sphenoid (black)

fontanelle lies posterior and a little above the posterior attachment of the uncinate process. The mucosa in these fontanelles may be dehiscent to produce accessory ostia.

The routes of drainage of the different sinuses can be seen (Fig. 1.8). The bulla may drain into the middle meatus, the hiatus semilunaris inferioris or into the sinus lateralis when present. The frontal sinus drains into the frontal recess either medial or lateral to the uncinate process depending on the mode of attachment of the uncinate process. It may also drain into the suprabullar recess when it is present. The maxillary sinus shows no variation in drainage and always drains into the infundibulum. The sphenoid sinus drains into the sphenoethmoidal recess. The ostium is seen high on the anterior wall of the sinus approximately 1 to 1.5 cm above the roof of the posterior choana very often partially hidden by the superior turbinate.

The anterior and posterior ethmoid cells are dissected taking care to leave the intervening ground lamella of the middle turbinate intact. It can now be seen that the

endoscopic surgeon has to traverse four main barriers in the coronal plane as he proceeds in an anteroposterior direction into the nose (Fig. 1.9). These are, from anterior to posterior—the uncinate process, anterior wall of the bulla, the ground lamella and the anterior wall of the sphenoid. The surgeon may also encounter the ground lamella of the superior and if present, the supreme turbinate if he dissects superolaterally.

The relationship of the posterior ethmoidal cells to the sphenoid sinus is an important one and must be understood clearly by the novice surgeon to avoid complications. Consider the following facts: In a sagittal section, the posterior ethmoidal cells can be seen extending for a short distance over the sphenoid sinus. They also lie in the lateral nasal wall compared to the sphenoid, which lies in the midline. The well-pneumatized sphenoid sinus extends posteriorly up to the clivus. Thus, the sphenoid sinus lies posterior, inferior and medial to the posterior ethmoid cells (Fig. 1.10).

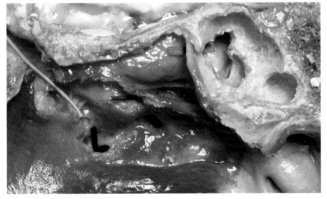

Fig. 1.8: Drainage of maxillary sinus (black), bulla (blue), frontal sinus (light brown), sphenoid sinus (green)

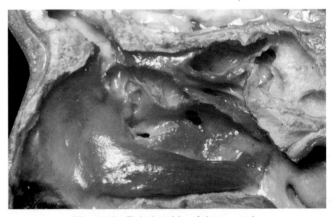

Fig. 1.10: Relationship of the posterior ethmoid cells to the sphenoid sinus

In 10% of cases the posteriormost ethmoidal cell may extend posterolaterally over the sphenoid sinus for a much longer distance. This cell is then called the Onodi cell. Thus, the Onodi cell when present, insinuates itself between the optic nerve and the sphenoid sinus. The optic nerve, therefore, produces a bulge in the Onodi cell instead of in the sphenoid sinus.

Once the ethmoidal cells have been completely cleared, we can see the paper–thin bone which separates the nasal cavity from the orbit (Fig. 1.11). This is the lamina papyracea which appears yellowish due to the underlying orbital fat. The maxillary ostium has been widened to gain a view of the interior of the sinus. It can be seen that the lamina papyracea, and consequently the orbit, is just 2–3 mm above the level of the maxillary ostium.

The inferior turbinate has been trimmed. It overlies a smooth fairly structureless inferior meatus. Although the inferior turbinate is fairly straight, its attachment shows a peak or apex approximately 1 cm behind its anterior end (Fig. 1.12). The nasolacrimal duct opens in the roof of the inferior meatus at this apex, and is guarded by a valve called Hasner's valve. The canal for the naso-lacrimal duct has been dissected. It lies approximately 5 mm anterior to the normal maxillary ostium. The nasolacrimal duct is split open to visualize the lacrimal sac, duct and Hasner's valve.

It is necessary to continue the dissection into areas beyond the lateral nasal wall such as the orbit, nasolacrimal system and lateral wall of the sphenoid for two reasons. Firstly, the surgeon must be aware of the various anatomical relationships in these areas so as to

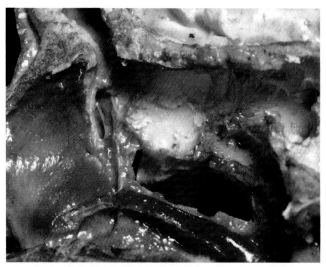

Fig. 1.12: The lacrimal apparatus and its relationship to the maxillary ostium and lamina papyracea

avoid complications and secondly, it may at times be necessary to intervene surgically in these regions.

The lamina papyracea has been removed and the orbital periosteum has been cut to expose the orbital fat (Fig. 1.13). Anteriorly, a pad of fat separates the vital structures of the orbit from the nose. However, posteriorly the medial rectus is in close relation with the lamina papyracea.

The sphenoid sinus is opened widely by removing the intersphenoid septum. There are two bulges in the lateral wall: *Superiorly* is the bulge of the optic nerve, *inferiorly* and *posteriorly* is the internal carotid artery (ICA). The groove between the two is the caroticooptic recess. An extensively pneumatized sphenoid sinus may show

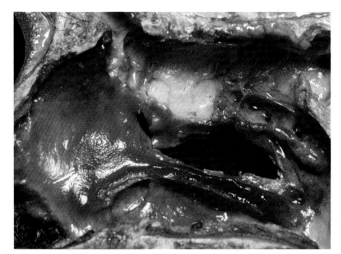

Fig. 1.11: The relationship of the maxillary ostium to the lamina papyracea. The inferior turbinate has been trimmed

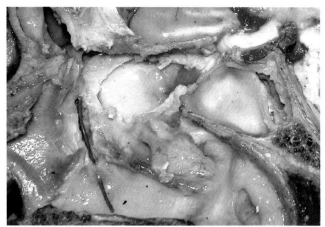

Fig. 1.13: Orbital contents showing orbital fat anteriorly and medial rectus posteriorly. The structures in the lateral wall of the sphenoid are also seen

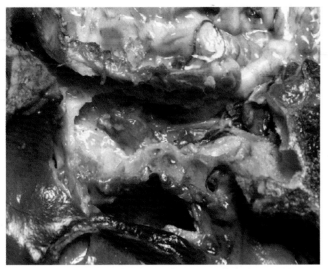

Fig. 1.14: Relationship of the optic nerve, pituitary and internal carotid artery

a lateral recess due to pneumatization of the greater wing between the foramen rotundum and the vidian canal. In such a case, two additional bulges can be seen: the maxillary nerve inferolaterally and the vidian nerve inferomedially.

The lateral wall of the sphenoid sinus has been dissected to expose the siphon of the internal carotid artery and the optic nerve. The relationships between the ICA, the optic nerve and pituitary gland can be seen (Fig. 1.14).

BLOOD SUPPLY OF THE LATERAL NASAL WALL

The lateral nasal wall is mainly supplied by the anterior and posterior ethmoid arteries which are branches of the ophthalmic artery, a part of the internal carotid system and the sphenopalatine artery which is a branch of the maxillary artery, a part of external carotid system.

Anterior Ethmoidal Artery

The anterior ethmoidal artery is given off from the ophthalmic artery in the orbit. It enters the nose, traverses across the roof of the ethmoidal sinus in an anteromedial direction and then leaves the nose at the lateral lamella of the cribriform plate to enter the cranial cavity. Thus, the canal in which it traverses from the orbit to the cranial cavity is called the orbitocranial canal. The lateral end of the canal is at the suture line of the frontal bone and lamina papyracea. Medial end of the canal at the cribriform plate is the thinnest part of the anterior cranial fossa. The canal is oblique and runs at a variable distance below the roof of the ethmoid to which it is attached by a

bony mesentery. The anterior ethmoidal artery lies 1 to 2 mm behind the point where the anterior wall of the bulla meets the skull base. If the bulla does not extend up to the skull base, the artery lies within the suprabullar recess. Another important finding is that the artery is present where the vertical posterior wall of the frontal sinus turns to form the horizontal base of the skull.

On entering the cranial cavity, the artery turns anteriorly along the cribriform plate in a sulcus called the ethmoidal sulcus. It gives off a meningeal branch and then re-enters the nasal cavity on either side of the crista galli. It then passes in a groove along the inner surface of the nasal bone supplying the upper part of the septum and the lateral nasal wall. It appears on the external surface of the nose through a notch between the nasal bone and the upper lateral cartilage.

Posterior Ethmoidal Artery

The posterior ethmoidal artery arises from the ophthalmic artery in the orbit and passes through the fissure between the frontal bone and the lamina papyracea 6 mm in front of the optic foramen to enter the nasal cavity. It usually lies high in the roof of the ethmoid and may not be easily seen. It passes anteromedially to gain entry into the cranial cavity at the level of the cribriform plate. It traverses the cribriform plate in an anterior direction for a short distance and passes through one of its foramina to re-enter the nasal cavity and supply the upper and posterior part of nasal septum.

Sphenopalatine Artery

The sphenopalatine artery is the terminal part of the maxillary artery in the pterygopalatine fossa. It passes medially through the sphenopalatine foramen to enter the nasal cavity above the posterior end of the middle turbinate. It gives off lateral nasal branches, which supply the nasal conchae and meatii. Its medial branch crosses the anterior face of the sphenoid bone to supply the septum.

The sphenopalatine artery along with the terminal branches of the greater palatine artery, the anterior ethmoidal artery and the superior labial branch of the facial artery forms the Keisselbach's Plexus in the Little's area, which is responsible for the anterior epistaxis.

The structures which make up the lateral nasal wall separate the nasal cavity from the orbit laterally and the brain superiorly. It therefore goes without saying that if one is to operate safely in this area without risking the vision or life of the patient, it is necessary to have a complete understanding of the three-dimensional anatomy of this area.

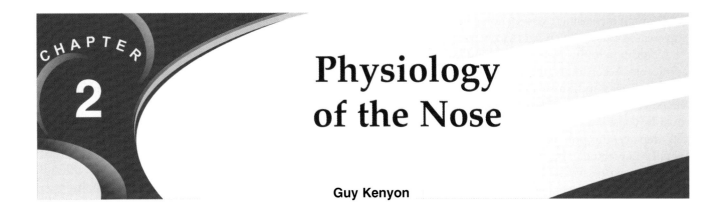

Physiology of the Nose

Guy Kenyon

The purpose of respiration is, in a broad sense, to provide oxygen to the body for metabolic processes and to remove carbon dioxide, and waste products of metabolism, from the body. The majority of this gas exchange takes place in the lower reaches of the lung but prior to this process the air requires to be warmed, humidified and filtered. An adult inspires over 10^4 liters of air a day; this air will contain pollutants, including industrial effluent, diesel particulate and the oxides of nitrogen and sulphur, all of which are irritants. Additionally, dust particles and pollens as well as bacteria and viruses will also be inhaled in copious amounts and all of these act to challenge the competence of the respiratory system. The nose, with remarkable efficiency, conditions the air and provides a defence against outside attack.

Many aspects of the physiology of the nose remain unknown and relatively unexplored, in spite of the considerable morbidity that attends nasal dysfunction and in spite of a long history of nasal surgery.[1] The physiology of the nose and of the paranasal sinuses is, in fact, extremely complex and for various reasons research in these areas has been somewhat neglected in the past, and it is only in the last few years that the mysteries of nasal function are being explored; the intricacies of nasal physiology are still a mystery.

All accounts of nasal physiology document that during these phases of flow, the nose functions to warm, humidify and clean the inspired air as well as cool and remove water vapor from the expired air. However, we know little of how this is actually accomplished. The nose also adds resonance and quality to speech production apart from being the portal for olfaction, the site for much of the added resistance in the respiratory system and the organ that is in the frontline of providing the body's defences. Moreover, nasal neurovascular reflexes are important in initiating such basic mechanisms as sneezing and heat exchange. In this chapter, aspects of form and function that are generally agreed upon, are discussed rather than dwelling on more speculative aspects of pathophysiology. Since many aspects of the detailed physiology and immunology are at present unclear, and since a coherent message has yet to emerge to explain many aspects of nasal homeostasis and of the reactions of the nose to external stimuli, the account of these functions must necessarily be regarded as partial and incomplete.

AIRFLOW

In the normal subject, the respiratory rate is between 10 to 18 cycles a minute in adults at rest. Respiration is biphasic and, the phases are not of equal duration. Inspiration, which lasts approximately 2 seconds, is an active phenomena requiring metabolic effort whereas expiration (which lasts on average 3 seconds) is passive and is largely dependent on the elastic recoil of the lung: as a result, the pressures generated in the airway are dissimilar during inspiration and expiration. The inspiratory linear velocity is maximal at the nasal valve (6 to 18 m/sec), decreases to 2 m/sec in the main part of the nasal airway and increases again in the nasopharynx. During expiration, the air speed is about 1 to 2 m/sec and is evenly distributed in the nasal cavity with an increase to 3 to 6 m/sec at the nasal valve.[2]

The 'ideal' gas is incompressible and has no viscosity.[3] All real gases fall short of these ideals and, as a result, correction factors, which are often based on empirical data, have to be incorporated into any analysis.

For a steady state, the volume flow rate in a structure of uniform diameter is equal to the cross-sectional area multiplied by the velocity. Thus:

$V = a \times u$

where V = the flow rate, a = the cross-sectional area and u = the fluid velocity

Thus, an increasing cross-sectional area will result in a decreased fluid velocity and vice versa.

In addition to this Newton's second law of motion is applicable. Accordingly, the principle of conservation of energy applies and, in relation to the nose, the sum of the potential energy and kinetic energy of gas transport must be constant. For fluid such as air, which has very low density, the potential energy is negligible and is usually neglected. The mathematical relationship is, therefore, expressed by a modification of Bernoulli's principle, which states that:

$P/\rho + u^2/2 = \text{constant}$

where P = fluid pressure, ρ = fluid density and u = fluid velocity

This simple equation plus that which expresses continuity of flow allows some important conclusions to be drawn about flow in cylindrical tubes. However, the nose is not a straight cylinder of uniform diameter and air is not, of course, an 'ideal' gas. In a curved tube, such as the nose, a mass of gas moving along a tube shows a maximal velocity at the center of the flow. Transverse movement of gas with currents of circulation moving at right angles to the main flow are also set up by the forward movement of the gas, a phenomenon known as 'secondary flow'. Moreover, velocity is also lost as fluid moves along the tube due to the viscosity of the material and due to the resistance offered by the surrounding structures.

Viscosity is, perhaps, best envisaged by thinking of a moving column of gas as being composed of successive layers of material. The internal shearing stresses between these layers are proportional to the relative velocity, velocity gradient and coefficient of viscosity. For a fluid flowing through a straight cylindrical structure the layers of fluid particles move along a uniform straight line (laminar flow) and the flow is dominated by the viscous forces: the resistance is therefore proportional to the fluid velocity. At a specific pipe diameter and above a certain velocity the fluid will no longer flow in a laminar fashion but will demonstrate eddy currents or turbulence.

The Reynolds number, named after the Engineering professor who first described the relationship, predicts that this transition from laminar to turbulent flow is dependent on the relative magnitude of inertial to viscous forces.

This number (Re) is expressed algebraically as:

$Re = \rho\,{}^{ud}/_{\mu}$

where ρ = fluid density, u = fluid velocity, μ = fluid viscosity and d = diameter of the structure

With steady flow through smooth pipes of constant diameter, the transition from laminar to turbulent flow occurs at a Reynolds number of about 2000. Any irregularity within the pipe will tend to cause disruption of flow resulting in the lowering of the Reynolds number at which transition occurs.

Such considerations have led to attempts to model nasal airflow on the basis of laminar and turbulent flow in pipes. However, as already inferred, the standard equations are really only valid if the air flows through straight pipes of constant diameter and at a distance from the inlet to the pipe where the flow pattern has become well established. Within the nose, air flows through the vestibule and then the nasal valve area (an area of restriction) and then into the main body of the nose where the walls diverge. Where flow is restricted, the velocity will increase and, as a result, the fluid pressure will decrease. Where the cross-sectional area is increasing, a decreasing velocity flow will be recorded and this decreasing velocity is associated with an increase in fluid pressure. Previous work has shown that the greatest pressure drop does indeed occur across the nasal valve area[4,5] and has shown that the nasal valve area represents the main site of airflow resistance.[6] The airflow can be measured at different pressure differences in the area of the nasal valve and the curves that result are similar to those obtained during rhinomanometry.[7]

Such theoretical considerations allow some insight into the physical principles behind nasal airflow but do not allow for the mechanical properties of the alar cartilages, soft tissues and phasic activity in the alar muscles. All of these structures add dynamics to the nasal airflow which cannot, presently, be quantified accurately. Airflow simulations created either with laboratory models or by computer simulations suffer from the same disadvantages but due to the inaccessibility of the nasal cavity, are all that we currently have as realistic models of normal nasal performance.

The earliest such studies of airflow were, in fact, performed with *in vitro* models of the nasal cavity made either of half heads or of casts from human cadavers in whom the nasal septum was replaced with a transparent plate. More recently, transparent models of the nasal cavity have been manufactured from CT images. The early work suggested that air currents in the nose are largely laminar and showed that air enters the nose and rises almost vertically towards the anterior end of the middle turbinates. The current is then deflected to pass between the middle turbinates and the septum and downwards towards the posterior end of the inferior turbinates. Qualitative visualization of the nasal airflow patterns using smoke in a model without the inferior and middle turbinates confirms that the inspired air takes a sharp turn into the nasopharynx while expiratory flow exhibits a double eddy in the nasal chamber (Fig. 2.1).[8] Such studies demonstrated that air stream patterns during quiet inspiration are almost independent of the flow rate and are concentrated mainly in the middle meatus.

Non-invasive measurements performed with laser Doppler velocimeter during quiet breathing have also shown that airflow in the nose is mostly laminar and have suggested that flow is streamlined by the turbinates with greater velocities in the lower half of the cavity and near the septum.[9] Local measurements with a hot-wire anemometer have reinforced these findings[10] as have measurements with a digital particle image velocimetry, which uses successive images of illuminated micro-particles in the moving field to visualize and analyze the flow field. However, such measurements in two-dimensions almost certainly fall short of explaining the complex nasal airflow patterns that occur during exercise and other physiological challenges.

Computer simulations of inspiratory airflow in the nasal cavity have also been performed using numerical methods for airflow in complex enclosures. Computers render analysis of the geometry of the nasal cavity from anatomical images such as CT scans. This enables analysis of various parameters[11] and the results have again shown that the main flux of air tends to flow through the middle meatus and along the floor of the nose. Such simulations have also suggested that the turbinates determine the paths for airflow. Local turbulence may be generated down-stream of the turbinates but the degree and rate of dissipation of such currents are not yet known.

HUMIDIFICATION

The nasal cavity performs majority of the airconditioning that equilibrates the inspired air with alveolar conditions. The gradient of temperature and humidity between ambient air and the point along the respiratory tract where the core temperature and 100% relative humidity are achieved varies during the breathing cycle. It is also influenced by the temperature and humidity of the inspired air, by whether the patient is breathing nasally or orally and whether there is any pathology within the nose.[25] A healthy human consumes up to 350 kilocalories of heat and 400 milliliters of water in one day to condition the inspired air at moderate environmental conditions (25°C and 50% relative humidity). About one-third of this is recovered during expiration.[12,13] *In vivo* measurements of air temperature within the nose throughout the respiratory cycle acquired with a thermocouple show that the nasal cavity heats the inspired air to about 34°C.[14,15] Inspiration of very cold air reduces the air temperature in the pharynx. While these findings are true for quiet breathing, additional airconditioning must take place in the trachea and main bronchi in order to completely condition the inspired air to alveolar conditions.[13]

The first generation of mathematical models for simulations of heating water vapor exchange were developed as simple channels or axi-symmetrical tubes and assumed a steady state of inspiratory airflow.[16-18] More recent work has assumed a variation in inspiratory flow and has shown that inhaled air is normally warmed and humidified to 90% of alveolar conditions before reaching the nasopharynx.[11] The turbinates increased the rate of local heat and moisture transport by improving mixing and by maintaining thin boundary layers, but the instantaneous heat and water vapor transfer to inspired

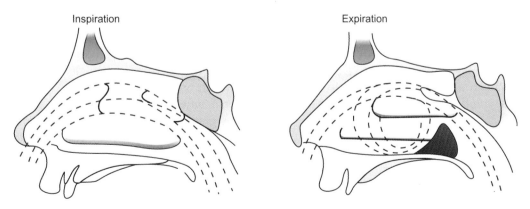

Fig. 2.1: Nasal airflow patterns

air is significantly reduced during periods of increased airflow velocity.

While these studies confirm that there is ample time for heating and humidification in normal noses in normal environments,[19] during exercise the muscle demands for oxygen are elevated and maximum ventilation may increase by up to 30-fold. The general patterns of heat and water vapor transport with exercise are similar to those in normal breathing but the rates of heat and water vapor flux required to maintain near-alveolar conditions clearly increases with moderate exercise.[20]

While exercise is important for modification of nasal anatomy, age too may modify it and affect its air conditioning capacity. A recent study revealed changes in the elderly including a gradual rise in cavity volume, presumably induced by mucosal atrophy.[21] Such changes may hamper the efficiency of heat and water vapor transport, but we do not know by how much or whether such changes are seen universally with age. More importantly, we have no idea how surgery or other trauma affects airconditioning within the nose.

PROTECTION OF THE AIRWAY

Protection of the lower airway is one of the major func-tions of the nose and is accomplished by a combination of mechanical and chemical means. The former largely consists of the protection afforded by the mucociliary escalator and the latter is mostly dependent on the immune system.

Mechanical Protection

The mucociliary system is able to remove particles of 30 μ or more from the inspired air. This includes most common particles including pollens, which are among the smallest particles deposited on the nasal mucosa and which account for the nose being the predominantly affected site in extrinsic allergy. Other characteristics of smaller particles, such as their shape and surface smoothness, may determine whether they are deposited.

The mucociliary system requires active secretion of nasal mucus and an active ciliary system to perform efficiently. These components will be considered in turn.

NASAL SECRETIONS

Mucus Biochemistry

The majority of information on the nature of nasal mucus has been obtained from samples produced from the lower respiratory tract. From such analyses, we can deduce that the mucus in the nose is composed of many elements including water and ions from the serous glands and from transudation through the capillary network, glycoproteins from the mucous glands, enzymes such as lysozyme and lactoferrin and immunoglobulins of all classes. Complement, α-2 macroglobulin and C-reactive protein are also secreted.

Glandular mucus and goblet cells contain large secretory granules which can be seen as lucent areas on electron microscopy. These contain the acidic glycoproteins.[22] Serous cells contain discrete, electron-dense granules which contain material of two different densities: they are thought to contain neutral glycoproteins, enzymes and immunoglobulins of the IgA class.

The glycoproteins form about 80% of the dry weight of mucus[23] and each consists of a single-sugar side chain linked covalently to a polypeptide chain: disulphide linkages polymerize these units. Hydoxyamino acids form up to 70% of the amino acid content of which serine is the most abundant in nasal mucus.[24] The glycoproteins are classified as acidic or neutral. Acidic elements are provided by either sialic acid (to form a sialomucins) or a sulphate group (to form a sulphomucin). Neutral glycoproteins contain fucose and form fucomucins.

Glycoproteins give mucus its two most commonly measured properties, viscosity and elasticity. Other compounds such as immunoglobulins and albumin do not add much to the flow characteristics of the mucus. Most of the protein structures help to defend the host from the environment whereas the water and ions help a role in maintaining respiratory function. The role of mucus in covering the nasal mucosa and in the action of the cilia upon it depend on its elastic properties.[25]

Proteins are derived either from the circulation or could be produced within the mucosa or the surface cells. Comparisons of levels within the plasma or serum with edema fluid or nasal secretions suggest local production. Indeed some compounds such as lactoferrin are present only in nasal secretions, which confirm its origin in the glandular epithelium. It is produced mainly by the serous cells and acts by binding divalent metal ions, as does transferrin within the circulation.

Lysozymes are also produced by secretion from the serous glands in the nose; some also come from tears which enter the nasal secretions through the nasolacrimal duct. These enzymes are also produced from leucocytes (found in nasal secretions), and in the mucosa. The action of lysozymes is non-specific and they only act on bacteria that have no capsular cover. In addition, a small number of different antiproteases have been demonstrated and the secretion of these proteins is increased with infection. They include α1-antitrypsin, α1-antichymotrypsin, α1-macroglobulin and others from leucocytes. Their role is unclear.

All components of complement have been identified in nasal secretions. The liver produces C3 as also locally by macrophages. It is activated both by non-specific and specific immunological responses through the alternative and classical pathways. It has a variety of functions including the lysis of microorganisms and enhancement of neutrophil function as well as leucotaxis. Lipids such as phospholipids and triglycerides are also present, but their exact function is not known.

Evaporation may account for a part of the hyper-osmolality of the Na^+ and Cl^- found in mucus but active ionic transport also contributes.[26] Active secretion takes place mainly within the serous glands, which produce the major proportion of the water in nasal secretions.

All classes of immunoglobulins have been found in nasal secretions. The immunoglobulins involved in mucosal defence, namely IgA and IgE have been found in greatest concentration and their concentrations in nasal secretions is considerably greater than those found in the serum.

Mucus Pathophysiology

The physics of normal airflow has been outlined earlier in this chapter. Air passing at an unvarying speed in a smooth straight tube of constant caliber produces no turbulence and light particles in that air remain air-borne. However, turbulence causes air-borne particles to be deposited on the adjacent nasal walls, not at the point of turbulence but immediately beyond that point. The more abrupt the change in direction of flow, the more likely there is of turbulence and, as a consequence, the greater the deposit of particular matter. This phenomenon has been called the 'impingement effect'. A similar deposit occurs if, instead of being bent, a tube is constricted, as it is in the nose in the region of the nasal valve. In this case, the deposit accumulates distal to the constriction.

Moisture-laden air deposits droplets of water at the impingement points and, conversely, dry air passing through a wet tube will produce localized drying at these points. Ciliary activity requires, above all, a moist medium. Drying is fatal to cilial function and to the ciliated epithelial layer itself. If the situation exists, or is created, in the nose in which local drying occurs, then the protective mucus blanket at that point becomes thick and sticky, the cilia no longer propel it and conditions become favorable for bacterial growth and penetration.

Ciliary Activity

As we have seen the majority of nasal mucus is produced in the nasal cavity. There it is formed in two layers, the upper being the most viscous and the lower, adjacent to the cilia, being more watery. The cilia move freely within the aqueous layer and move the mucus only as the head of the cilium passes the highest arc of its beat.

The cilia in the nose propel mucus backwards towards the nasopharynx. The nasal cilia are relatively short (5 μ) and over 200 are present on each cell. Each has a surface membrane that encloses nine paired outer microtubules that encircle a single inner pair of microtubules. The outer pairs also have inner and outer dynein arms. At the base of the cilia, the microtubules blend into the basal body of the cell with the outer pairs becoming triplets and the inner pair disappearing completely. Each triplet is structurally similar to the centrioles of mitotic cells and it has been suggested that centrioles migrate to the cell surface to form the structures.[27]

The beat frequency of the cilia is between 10 Hz and 20 Hz at normal body temperature. This does not appear to vary over a fairly large temperature range (between 32°C and 40°C). Each beat consists of a rapid propulsive/ followed by a slow recovery phase. During the propulsive phase, the cilium is straightened and the tip in gauges the viscous lair of the mucus blanket. During the recovery phase, the cilium is bent and lies in the aqueous layer. The energy to this movement is produced by the conversion of ATP to ADP by ATPase lying in the dynein arms and the reaction is dependent on an adequate concentration of magnesium ion. ATP is generated by the mitochondria near the cell surface next to the basal bodies of the cilia.

Not only drying but also temperature change pro-duces effects in ciliary beat frequency. Extremes of cold (< 10°C) and heat (> 45°C) cause cessation of activity. Similarly, changes in the ionic composition of the mucus will also affect ciliary function. Isotonic saline allows preservation of normal cilial activity but concentrations above 5% and below 0.2% cause paralysis. Changes in K^+ ion composition have to be non-physiological before effecting movement[28] and, in like manner, changes in acidity and alkalinity have to be very marked before cilial function is impaired. Drugs also affect cilial activity. Neuro-transmitters affect beat frequency: Acetylcholine increases the rate while adrenaline decreases it; the effects of α and β agonists is variable. Propranolol decreases ciliary beat frequency in a dose-dependent manner[28] and it is of interest that cocaine causes immediate paralysis in concentrations above 10%. Following a one-week course of corticosteroids, saccharine clearance is reduced which also implies that these drugs reduce ciliary activity.[29] Perhaps the commonest *in vivo* factor affecting function is, however, infection, which may also cause the surface epithelium to be partly lost.

Immunological Protection

The nasal mucus contains different compounds which are able to neutralize antigens either by innate mechanisms or by acquired immunity. Secretion of the two main surface immunoglobulins IgE and IgA is well known but, in addition, immunoglobulins of the IgM and IgG classes are also activated if the mucosa is breached.

Specific immunity is the responsibility of the lymphoreticular system. The lymphocytes in the nose, as in other areas of the body, can conveniently be thought of as belonging to either of the two groups, namely those associated with the cellular and the humoral systems. T-cells, associated with the cellular system, can be subdivided by surface markers into suppressor, helper and killer cells. Primed lymphocytes in the mucosa as well as macrophages and Langerhans cells present antigen to T-cells; Fokkens et al believe that the Langerhans cells have a particular role to play in this regard in the nasal mucosa.[30]

Responses in the tonsils, adenoids and other aggregations of lymphoid tissue within the respiratory and gastrointestinal tracts (the gut-associated lymphoid tissues) are mainly through production of IgA and IgE. If the wider parts of the lymphoreticular system are involved, such as the lymph nodes or the spleen, then the immunoglobulins IgG and IgM are also produced.

Non-specific immunity is conferred by a number of macromolecules that interact with bacteria, especially those without capsules. These macromolecules include lactoferrin, lysozymes, complement and antiproteases. Alien proteins are then engulfed through the actions of polymorphs and macrophages.

Specific immunity is produced by immunoglobulins and interferon. Viruses and mycobacteria initiated cell-mediated immunity with production of IgA and IgE produced as the first line of defence in the nose. IgA, which produces indissoluble complexes in nasal mucus, combines with immunologically primed surface cells to promote phagocytosis. It is found in-considerable

concentration in nasal mucus and has two subgroups IgA1 and IgA2. IgA2 forms the largest subgroup and accounts for as much as 70% of the total protein in nasal secretions. It is a dimer that is transferred passively through the interstitial fluid and is actively taken up by the seromucinous glands and the surface epithelium. In the epithelium, a secretory piece is attached that makes it stable in mucus. When it reacts with an antigen, it forms an insoluble complex that is swallowed and destroyed by the acid in the stomach. It does not activate complement.

IgE is the main immunoglobulin causing allergic reactions and was first identified by Ishazaki and Ishazaki.[31] It is mainly produced in lymphoid aggregates such as the tonsils and adenoid, but it is also produced in the nasal submucosa. It becomes firmly attached to mast cells and to basophils and, when two molecules of allergen-specific IgE occupy adjacent receptor sites on mast cells, degranulation will ensue. It also does not activate complement.

In addition to its molecular component, mucus also contains cells that are immunologically active. These include epithelial cells, leucocytes, basophils, eosinophils, mast cells and macrophages. Leucocytes and macrophages migrate through the mucosa from the circulation and are important for surface phagocytosis.

NASAL VASCULATURE AND NERVE SUPPLY

The arrangement of the blood vessels in the nose is complex and varies at different sites. Changes in resistance to airflow are produced by alterations in the blood flow in the lining of the nose and by controlled changes in the capacitance and the resistance vessels.

Measurement of the nasal blood flow is difficult because any instrument introduced into the nose alters flow if the mucosa is stimulated. Flow, therefore, has to be inferred, either by looking at changes in the color of the mucosa or by measurement of alterations in temperature or by photoelectric plethysmography.

Subtle changes in arterial blood flow and in arteriovenous shunting and venous pooling allow almost unlimited permutations of mucosal perfusion. However, in clinical practice three main patterns are recognized. These are:

- Hyperemia with both shunting and venous congestion.
- Reduced arterial perfusion with no shunting which results in a bluish venous congestion.
- Ischemia.

Nasal Autonomic Nervous System

The autonomic nervous system controls the vascular reflexes in the nose and the distribution of various parts of the system is well known from textbooks of anatomy.

The sympathetic and parasympathetic nervous systems supply the nose and affect the level of engorgement of the nasal mucosa as well as the production of mucus through control of capacitance vessels and sinuses, airway smooth muscle and the submucosal glands. Throughout the head and neck, the distribution of these nerves, and of the sensory nerves, obey an invariable discipline (Fig. 2.2).[32]

- The first rule is that the local ganglion (in the case of the nose the pterygopalatine) is the point of synapse for pre-ganglionic parasympathetic fibers that originate in the brain. The ganglia also transmit sympathetic and sensory fibers, but these are post-ganglionic and have already synapsed elsewhere: they simply traverse the ganglion en route to their peripheral distribution. The pre-ganglionic fibers from the sensory system have their synapse in the trigeminal ganglion and the sympathetic system synapse in the upper cervical sympathetic chain, and not in the ganglion itself.
- The second rule is that the sympathetic supply runs with the local arterial supply and is distributed with it. Thus, in the case of the nose the pterygopalatine ganglion is the synaptic point for a parasympathetic supply that originates in the superior salivatory nucleus in the pons and exits the brain as the nervus intermedius. Via the greater superficial petrosal nerve, this forms the nerve of the pterygoid canal in conjunction with sympathetic post-ganglionic fibers arising from the superior cervical ganglion which run on the internal carotid artery. This nerve, therefore, carries parasympathetic fibers from the greater superficial petrosal nerve and sympathetic fibers from the deep petrosal nerve en route to innervation of the sinonasal mucosa.

The differing branches of the autonomic system not only regulate the state of the vasculature, they also control and modify nasal secretion. Many texts speak of both the parasympathetic and sympathetic nerve fibers supplying the vasculature as well as the glandular epithelium. However, postganglionic fibers may release more than one neurotransmitter for there certainly seems to be a discrepancy between the expected experimental response and the responses often seen *in vivo*.

What is agreed is that changes in nasal mucosal thickness are predominantly due to alterations in the complex vascular system within the mucosa.[33] Anatomically, the nasal submucosa contains a complex array of arteries, arteriovenous anastomoses and the veins and venous sinusoids in the submucosa and the lamina propria (extending from the basement membrane of the epithelium to the central osseous layer containing venous sinusoids as well as seromucinous glands and lymphocytes and other immunocompetent cells). The largest venous sinusoids form structures termed 'cushion veins' at their distal ends that can expand and contract depending on the degree of sympathetic activity. In addition, there are also radiator vessels near the surface of the nasal mucosa as well as an arteriovenous anastomoses. These structures, along with the large number of mucus glands in the mucosa, ensure efficient humidification and warming of the inspired air.

Experimental evidence shows that the sympathetic system regulates blood flow by regulating resistance vessels with sympathetic stimulation resulting in decongestion of the mucosa with a lowered resistance and a reduced blood flow in the nasal mucosa. The sinusoids become engorged or constricted according to the extent of vasodilatation or constriction in the veins and arteriovenous anastomoses and the sympathetic tone driving these changes is probably influenced by the partial pressure of carbon dioxide (pCO_2) via the carotid and aortic chemoreceptors.[13] In turn, high sympathetic outflow leads to low resistance within the cushion veins with collapse of the venous sinusoids and shrinkage of the nasal mucosa while a reduction in tone causes swelling of the veins, distension of the sinusoids and a corresponding increase in the thickness of the nasal

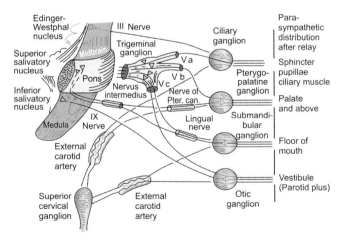

Fig. 2.2: Distribution of the nervous systems supplying the nose

x

mucosa.[33] By contrast parasympathetic stimulation is said to lead to relaxation of capacitance vessels allowing congestion, and even edema formation, in the nasal tissues.

Until recently, it was believed that the autonomic nervous system simply exerted its effect by secretions of adrenaline/noradrenaline and acetylcholine at sympathetic and parasympathetic nerve endings respectively. However, the picture becomes more complicated with the discovery of many other neurotransmitters including vasoactive intestinal polypeptide (VIP) and neuropeptide Y, both of which are associated with sympathetic nerve endings. In addition, stimulation of α- and β-adrenoceptors results in effects on the nasal vasculature with α-receptor stimulation causing constriction.[34]

The role of the autonomic nervous system in regulating nasal secretion has been elucidated by studies examining the effect of interfering with sympathetic and parasympathetic inputs. Division or blockage of sympathetic nerves causes nasal obstruction with rhinorrhea[35] while division of the parasympathetic nerves causes a reduction in nasal secretion in subjects with intractable rhinorrhea.[36]

Autonomic innervation and nasal mucosal inflammation are also inter-related. It is now well-known that autonomic imbalance plays a role in airway hyperactivity in asthma if the balance between the stimulatory effects of α-adrenoceptor and cholinergic receptors and the moderating influence of β-adrenoceptor stimulation are disturbed. Antibodies for β2-adrenoceptors have recently been discovered in asthma patients[37] and animal studies have shown that β-adrenoceptor function is disturbed in experimentally induced nasal hypersensitivity.[38]

The erectile tissue of the nasal mucosa exhibits regular cyclical congestion and decongestion, which is well documented in both humans and animals.[39,40] There is a tendency, therefore, to breathe through one side or the other of the nose at a time. This cycle has a periodicity of 2 to 6 hours but does not, it seem, occur in all individuals and estimates of its presence seem to vary between being seen in as few as 20 to 30%[13] or as many as 80% of the population.[41] Most are unaware of its existence since total nasal resistance remains unchanged. Its purpose remains obscure—although it does appear to be under hypothalamic control and may represent the variation in sympathetic outflow from the brain as a result of some type of cerebral cyclical activity or, alternatively, it may be important in nasal physiology protecting one side of the nose at a time from the damaging effects of inspired air.

Nasal secretion may also in some way interface with changes in airflow and some studies have shown that electrical stimulation of the vasomotor area of the brainstem in cats can produce reciprocal changes in sympathetic tone of the nasal blood vessels.[42]

Nasal Sensation

Sensory receptors in the nose are possibly responsible for the sensation of airflow as well as providing the afferent arm for a number of nasal reflexes, including sneezing. Although this is discussed later in the chapter, it must be said that the distribution of sensory receptors in humans is not well understood. Excluding the olfactory area the nasal mucosa has four main areas histologically: These are the nasal vestibule, the valve area, the nasopharynx and the main part of the nasal mucosa (Fig. 2.3). The nasal vestibule is lined by stratified squamous epithelium and contains thermoreceptors and the nasal valve area is rich with dermal papillae, which may act as thermo- and chemoreceptors.[43] However, the nasopharynx has no receptors described and the main bulk of the mucosa contains only isolated C-fibers.[44]

The nose is also subject to a series of reflexes and it must be presumed that nasal sensation must have an important role in initiating such responses.

Externally, the vessels and nerves pass within the subcutaneous tissues immediately deep to the skin and above the underlying muscles. There are several nasal muscles and no absolute consensus as to how they are disposed, which has led one author to comment that 'a uniform description (of cartilages and muscles) is still lacking'.[45] This perhaps matters little since only two are of any clinical significance and these are the **levator labii**

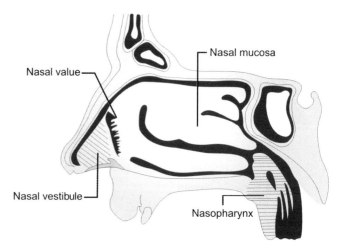

Fig. 2.3: Main histological areas of the nasal mucosa

superioris and **depressor sepi nasi**. The second of these probably matters little in terms of the physiology of nasal responses but the first is attached to the lateral crus of the lower lateral cartilage on each side and stents the alar rim. By so doing it assists in keeping the external nasal valve open. Thus, when the reaction of this muscle is pronounced, the patient demonstrates alar flaring: conversely altered flow–pressure relationships and premature external valve collapse may result if this function is impaired in patients with facial palsy.[5,46,47] That there is a degree of reflex flaring at times of increased oxygen demand is well-known and can be seen in pictures of athletes when they are running. However, the way in which this response is coordinated is unclear and the pathways responsible for its activation are unknown.

External stimuli can also alter the nose in other ways. For example, it is also well known that there are reflex changes in patency as an accompaniment of normal exercise.[48,49] Isotonic exercise up to a weigh work rate of 120 watts causes a gradual reduction in nasal resistance to around 50% of normal values. This is, in turn, thought to be due to an increase in nasal sympathetic tone[49] but it is of interest that a similar degree of isometric exercise has no effect.[50,51]

Resistance is also affected by posture. Moving from an erect to a supine position causes an increase in nasal resistance which is possibly related to increased jugular venous pressure[52] and lying on one side causes nasal resistance to be increased—a change that is mirrored by axillary pressure: this also causes ipsilateral nasal obstruction and contralateral nasal decongestion.[53]

In addition to all this all mammals, including humans, exhibit the diving reflex. Contact with water or with a cold wet cloth may induce apnea and bradycardia with an associated increase in arterial blood pressure. There is evidence to suggest that 'cold' receptors are important in initiating this reflex[54-56] and on exposure to cold air there is a decrease in blood flow and in nasal patency.[57] Conversely, exposure to hot air results in an increased nasal patency with no parallel change in nasal blood flow.[57,58] Changes in humidity do not appear to influence nasal patency.

Chemical irritation of the nose by tobacco smoke, ammonia and sulphur dioxide may produce a similar response and the afferent limb of this reflex is thought to be the trigeminal nerve which, when stimulated, can cause sneezing.[59] Sneezing is thought to be mediated through the vidian nerve but it is uncertain precisely which modalities in the nasal mucosa cause nasal hypersensitivity. Certainly, the nose is sensitive to light touch and it must also contain irritant receptors if the afferent arm of the sneezing reflex is intact.

Airflow appears to be detected by cold receptors near the nasal vestibule.[60,61] However, the exact mechanisms responsible for the detection of flow, and sensation of patency are not yet fully understood. In determining flow it may be that the rate of cooling is somehow important.

It is also well-known that the sensation of patency can be enhanced by inhalation of the L-isomer of menthol whereas the R-isomer has no effect (Fig. 2.4) implying some degree of sophistication in terms of the stereo-chemistry of the receptor responsible.[62] However, neither isomer appears to have any effect on nasal resistance and how the perception of flow is altered by such inhalations is not at all clear.

Finally, the role of hormone receptors in the nose remains unclear. It is, of course, well-known that some, but not all, women suffer rhinitis of pregnancy. Empirically this would seem likely to be hormonally driven since symptoms remit rapidly after parturition as circulating hormone levels drop. There have also been isolated reports of women on high-dose contraceptive pills experiencing rhinitis suggesting that exogenous hormone may stimulate receptors in the nose. However, low level of estrogen receptor activity is found in approximately half of all patients, both male and female, with rhinitis. More importantly progesterone receptor activity, which is found only in women patients, is very low and is found in only a few cases.[63] Therefore, the role of estrogen and of progesterone in the nose is uncertain, and the origin of rhinitis of pregnancy, which can be very distressing in some patients, remains obscure.

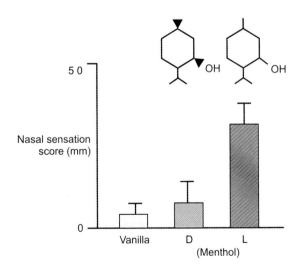

Fig. 2.4: Comparative patency score of menthol

OLFACTION

Odors are a complex mixture of compounds. Studies in olfaction concentrate on single compounds or mixtures with two or three chemicals. For the person to experience a sense of smell the odorant must reach the relevant mucosa and must also be soluble in water and lipid. Humans are able to discriminate between a large number of odorants but the olfactory mucosa and pathway is rapidly fatigued; however, it also recovers quickly.

The maximum exposure of the olfactory area is achieved by sniffing which causes turbulent airflow in the upper part of the nose. Animal studies suggest that the olfactory stimulus is augmented by increasing the velocity of airflow.[64]

Olfactory Epithelium

The area of the olfactory epithelium varies between species. Humans have 200 to 400 mm^2 of sensory epithelium, which is studded with receptor cells with modified cilia, which increase the available surface area and project, like normal cilia, into the surrounding mucus. Odorants are absorbed into the water fraction of the mucus and react with receptor cells at specific sites. This causes leakage of K^+ and Cl^- ions, which acts to depolarize the cells.[65] After a latent period of up to 400 ms, a slow compounds action potential can then be recorded from the olfactory mucosa. This has been called the electro-olfactogram.[64] The speed of the rising phase varies with the intensity of the stimulus and the recovery or falling phase is an exponential decay with a time constant of 0.9 to 1.45 ms.

The olfactory epithelium is situated in the superior aspect of the nose on each side and flows over the cribriform plate, the superior turbinate and the superior parts of the septum and sections of the middle turbinate. It harbors sensory receptors from the olfactory bulbs as well as some free nerve endings from the trigeminal system. It loses its general homogeneity as early as the first few weeks of life when metaplastic islands of epithelium (similar to respiratory epithelium) appear, and it is presumed that this is the result of insults from the environment such as viruses, bacteria and toxins.

There are six distinct cell types within the neuro-epithelium. These include bipolar sensory receptor neurons, supporting cells, microvillar cells, globose basal cells, horizontal basal cells and cells lining the Bowman's glands. There are approximately 6 million bipolar neurons in the adult olfactory neuroepithelium and these are thin dendritic cells with rods containing cilia at one end and long central processes at the other end. The olfactory receptors are located on the ciliated dendritic ends and the 1 million undated axons coalesce into 40 bundles, termed filia, which are ensheathed by Schwann-like cells. In turn, the filia traverse the cribriform plate to enter the anterior cranial fossa as the olfactory nerve. There are microvillar cells near the surface of the neuroepithelium but their exact functions are unknown. Supporting cells join the neurons and the microvillar cells and also project microvilli into the mucus. Their functions include insulating receptor cells from one another, regulating the composition of the mucus, deactivating odorants and protecting the epithelium from foreign agents. The basal cells are located near the basement membrane and are the progenitor cells from which the other cell types arise.

The Bowman's glands are a major source of mucus within the region of the olfactory cleft. The odorant receptors are located on the cilia of the receptor cells. Each receptor cell expresses a single odorant receptor gene.

There are approximately one thousand classes of receptors known and olfaction itself appears to be mediated by specific receptors in the cells which, when stimulated, produce a guanine nucleotide binding protein that interacts with a type 3 adenyl cyclase within neuroepithelium[66] to produce depolarization of the cell membrane and signal propagation. It has been found that adrenergic and muscarinic antagonists block some of the responses in the olfactory receptor neurons whereas glutamine antagonists do not. In turn, this suggests that there is some degree of receptor specificity.[67] However, there is also some evidence to suggest that each cell can also be responsive to a wide range of stimuli. In turn, this implies that a single receptor accepts may recognize a range of molecular entities.

There is no interaction between the individual receptor cells. Each receptor cell is connected to the olfactory bulb by non-myelinated nerve fibers. These fibers terminate and synapse on olfactory glomeruli each of which receives about 25,000 fibers and which acts as an integrator. The conduction time between receptor cells and the glomerulus is just 50 ms and the glomeruli fire with an all-or-none response into the mitral or tufted cells whose axons transport the signal through the lateral olfactory tract. Inhibition is derived from feedback from higher cortical centers.

The higher centers consist of the anterior olfactory nucleus, which sends impulses to the opposite bulb and also to the ipsilateral forebrain through the anterior commissure. The primary olfactory cortex includes the olfactory tubercle and the prepyriform and preamygdaloid areas. There are also projections to the thalamus, where there is a degree of integration with taste fibers, and some connections to the hypothalamus.

There is also some trigeminal input although smell is largely independent of this system as, with high concentrations of odorants, there can be a degree of irritation in the nose. This may be a factor in interpreting the intensity of certain compounds.[68]

Olfactory Responses

The olfactory response exhibits variation in threshold and adaptation. The threshold concentration can vary by up to 10^{10} depending on the chemical nature of the stimulus. The threshold for perception is certainly lower than that for identification. It would seem that smell does not have an absolute threshold but depends, to a large extent, on the level of inhibitory activity generated by higher centers. Adaptation is both a central and peripheral phenomenon, which causes the threshold to increase with ongoing exposure: recovery of the electro-olfactogram is rapid when the stimulus is withdrawn. Changes in the nasal mucus and its pH will alter olfactory adaptation. The threshold decreases with age and is both increased and altered by hormones, particularly the sex hormones. In humans, some genetic variation is present (which is similar to the genetic background for color blindness) and there is also a familial lack of perception to certain odors which is more common in males.

There is no satisfactory classification of odors but it has been suggested that there may be as many as 30 primary odors which are recognized by humans based on the stereochemistry of compounds and variations of anosmia which are present in humans.[69] The human being has difficulty in detecting variations in intensity of more than 17 odors. Further, because humans do not rely on conscious detection of odor, training is necessary for scientific experiments and for occupations such as wine tasting which require a 'good nose'. Humans certainly appear to be better at it kept it the pleasantness of an odor rather than being able to recognise it. The pleasantness is largely cultural and is therefore learned. If two odors are mixed the resulting intensity is always less than the sum of the two individually perceived intensities and is dominated by the stronger component.

Theories about the function of smell recognition remain unproven. Moncrieff[70] suggested that molecular structure was important although no stereospecific olfactory receptors have been demonstrated. It has also been suggested that some cells in the mucosa, which contain carotenoids, could generate a photochemical reaction similar to that which takes place in the eye.[71] The alternative is that certain receptors could have stereospatial configurations so that the receptor only fires when the surface membrane is altered,[72] or that the molecular property of the odorant could account for receptor specificity.[73] Finally, the olfactory mucosa morphology, particularly the siting of receptor cells and their position within the olfactory mucosa may be relevant.[74]

Olfaction is certainly important in regulating behavior in all animals and insects but has a relatively limited role in humans. However, smell is used in four main areas of behavior in animals and these include detection and consumption of food, recognition, territorial marking and sexual behavior. In humans only eating and sexual behavior are important. In the former, olfaction is related to the recognition of different food types and with the initiation of digestion. In turn, this is mediated through the lateral and ventromedial hypothalamus and stimulation causes salivation with the increase in output of gastric acid and enzymes in the small intestine. The degree of involvement of olfaction in human sexual behavior is unknown but the influence of smell is probably underestimated. Certainly, in the animal kingdom, especially insects, olfaction plays a major part in the normal sexual response.

THE NOSE AND THE VOICE

The generator for vocalization is, of course, the larynx, which produces the vowel sounds and also the pitch of the voice. However, modification of the vibrating column of air by the pharynx, tongue, lips and teeth adds the consonants and the nose adds quality. The sound resonates within the nose and mouth, and the nose modifies this by allowing some nasal escape of air. If too little air escapes from the nose during speech then vocalization appears stifled, as patients with large adenoids (rhinolalia clausa). If too much air escapes, then rhinolalia aperta ensues. The nose is most effective when resonating at the laryngeal frequencies. It is doubtful whether the sinuses have any added effect on modifying the voice although they may help in some way with auditory feedback since transmission of sound through the facial skeleton does allow some monitoring of the voice. Many nasal conditions affect the quality of the voice by blocking the passage of air in expiration. Thus, patients with severe allergic rhinitis, common cold and nasal polyps often have an altered vocal quality.

CONCLUSION

Humans can live in tropical or arctic climates and can shift from one extreme environment to another within very short periods of time without injuring the respiratory system. This remarkable adaptation is in no small part due to the extraordinary ability of the nose to provide an environment, which will modify the air, which we breathe in a myriad of ways. We have little clear insight as to how this is accomplished and, as a result, remain largely ignorant of how to treat those with nasal disorders. It is to be hoped that in the years to come an increased interest in this important area of research will rectify our ignorance and allow a more complete picture to emerge of the mechanisms by which the nose contributes to our normal homeostasis.

REFERENCES

1. McKinney P, Cunningham BL. History: In *Rhinoplasty*. London: Churchill Livingstone, 1989; 1–8.
2. Proctor DF. The upper airways: Nasal physiology and defence of the lungs. *Ann Rev Respir Dis* 1977; 115:97–129.
3. Massey BS. In *Mechanics of Fluids*. London:van Nostrand Reinhold, 1970; 87–92.
4. Bridger GP. Physiology of the nasal valve. *Arch Otolaryngol* 1970; 92:543–553.
5. Cole P. The four components of the nasal valve. *J Rhinol* 2003; 172: 107–110.
6. Cole P, Chaban R, Naito K. Simulated septal deviations. *Rhinology suppl* 1988; 1:26.
7. O'Neill G, Tolley NS. The dynamics of airflow. In *Nasal Airway Evaluation Techniques Related to Surgery. Facial Plastic Surgery*. New york: Thieme, 1984; 74:215–221.
8. Proetz AW. Air currents in the upper respiratory tract and their clinical importance. *Ann Otol Rhinol Laryngol* 1951; 60:439–467.
9. Girardin M, Bilgen E, Arbour P. Experimental study of velocity fields in a human nasal fossa by laser anemometry. *Ann Otol Laryngol Laryngol* 1983; 92:231–236.
10. Hahn I, Scherer PW, Mozell MM. Velocity profiles measured for airflow through a large scale model of the human nasal cavity. *J Appl Physiol* 1993; 75:2273–2287.
11. Naftali S, Schroter RC, Shiner RJ, Elad D. Transport phenomena in the human nasal cavity: A computational model. *Ann Biomed Eng.* 1988; 26:831–839.
12. Proctor DF, Swift DL. Temperature and water vapor adjustment. In *Respiratory Defence Mechanisms*, Brain JD, Proctor DJ, Reid LM (Eds) 1977; 95–124. New york: Marcell Dekker.
13. McRae D, Jones AS ,young P, Hamilton JW. Resistance, humidity and temperature of the tracheal airway. *Clin Otolaryngol* 1995; 20:355–356.
14. Primiano FP, SGM, Montague FW, Kruse KL, Green CG, Horowitz JG. Water vapor and temperature dynamics of the upper airway of normal and CF subjects. *Eur Respir J* 1988; 1:407–414.
15. Williams R, Rankin N, Smith T, Galler D, Seakins P. Relationship between the humidity and temperature of the inspired gas and the function of the nasal mucosa. *Crit Care Med* 1996; 24:1920–1929.
16. Farley RD, Patel KR. Comparison of air warming in the human airway with thermodynamic models. *Med Biol Eng Comput* 1988; 26:628–632.
17. Hanna LM, Scherer PW. A theoretical model of localized heat and water vapor transport on the human respiratory tract. *J Biomech Eng* 1986; 108:19–27.
18. Daviskas E, Gonda I, Anderson S D. Mathematical modeling of heat and water transport in the human respiratory tract. *J Appl Physiol* 1990; 69:362–372.
19. Schroter RC, Watkins NV. Respiratory heat exchange in mammals. *Respir Physiol* 1989; 78:357–368.
20. Wolf M, Naftali S, Schroter RC, Elad D. Airconditioning characteristsics of the human nose. *J Laryngol Otol* 2001; 1182:87–92.
21. Muallem–Kalmovich L, Elad D, Zaretsky U, Adonsky A, Chetrit A, Sadetzski S, Segal S, Wolf M. Nasal changes in the elderly—acoustic rhinometry analysis. Proceedings of the 19th Congress of the European Rhinological Society, ulm. *Rhinology Suppl* 2002; 30.
22. Lamb D, Reid L. Histochemical and autoradiographic investigations of the serous cells of the human bronchial glands. *J Pathology* 1970; 100:127–138.
23. Masson PL, Heremans JF. Sputum proteins. In *Sputum: Fundamentals and Clinical Pathology*, Dulfano MJ (Ed). Illinois: Charles C Thomas, 1973; 412–474.
24. Boat TF, Kleineman JI, Carlson DM, Maloney WM, Matthews LW. Human respiratory tract secretions 1. Mucous glycoproteins secreted by cultured nasal polyp epithelium from subjects with allergic rhinitis and cystic fibrosis. *Am Rev Respir Dis* 1974; 110:427–441.
25. Widdicombe JG, Wells UK. Airway secretions. In *The Nose: Upper Airway Physiology and the Atmospheric Environment* Proctor DF, Anderson I Amsterdam (Eds): Elsevier 1982; 215–244.
26. Widdicombe JG, Welsh M. Ion transport by dog tracheal epithelium. Federation Proceedings, 1980; 39:3062–3066.
27. Sleight M. *Cila and flagella*. London: Academic Press, 1974.
28. Robson A, Smallman L, Drake-Lee A. Factors affecting ciliary function *in vitro*: A preliminary study. *Clin Otol* 1992; 17: 125–129.
29. Holmberg K, Pipkorn U. Mucociliary transport in the human nose. The effect of topical glucocorticoid treatment. *Rhinology* 1985; 23:181–186.
30. Fokkens W, Brekhuis-Fluitsma D, Rijntjes E, Vroom T, Hoefsmit E. Langerhans cells in the nasal mucosa of patients with grass pollen allergy. *Immunobiology* 1991; 182:135–142.
31. Ishizaka K, Ishazaki T. Identification of E antibodies as a carrier of reaginic activity. *J Immunol* 1967; 99:1187–1198.
32. Last RJ. *Anatomy: Regional and Applied*. Edinburgh: Churchill Livingstone, 1972.
33. Cauna N, Cauna D. The fine structure and innervation of the cushion veins of the human nasal respiratory mucosa. *Anat Rec* 1975; 181:1–16.
34. Aschan G, Drettner B. An objective investigation of the decongestive effect of xylometazaline. *Eye, Ear, Nose Throat Monthly* 1964; 43:66–74.

35. Moore DC. *Stellate ganglion block.* Illinois: Charles C Thomas 1954.
36. Golding-Wood PH. Observations on petrosal and vidian neurectomy in chronic vasomotor rhinitis. *J Laryngol Otol* 1961; 74:232–247.
37. Wallukat G, Woolenberger A. Autoantibodies to β_2 adrenergic receptors with antiadrenergic activity from patients with allergic asthma. *J Allergy Clin Immunol* 1991; 88(4):581–587.
38. Kubo N, Kamazawa T. Functional disturbances of the autonomic nervous nerves in nasal hyperactivity:an up-to-date review. *Acta Otolaryngol Stockh* 1993; 500 (Suppl):97–108.
39. Eccles R. The domestic pig as an experimental animal for studies on the nasal cycle. *Acta Otolaryngol Stockh* 1978; 85: 431–436.
40. Hasegawa M, Kern EB. The human nasal cycle. *Mayo Clin Proc* 1977; 52:28–34.
41. Heetderks DL. Observations of the reaction of normal nasal mucous membrane. *Am J Med Sci* 1927; 174:231–244.
42. Bamford OS, Eccles R. The central reciprocal control of nasal vasomotor oscillations. *Pflugers Arch* 1982; 394:139–143.
43. Jones AS, Crosher R, Wight RG, Lancer JM, Beckingham E. The effects of local anesthesia of the nasal vestibule on nasal sensation of airflow and nasal resistance. *Clin Otol.* 1987; 12:461–464.
44. Eccles R. Relationship between measured nasal airway resistance and the sensation of airflow. *Facial Plastic Surgery* 1990; 74:278–282.
45. Bruintjes TD, van Olphen AF, Hillen B. Review of the functional anatomy of the cartilages and muscles of the nose. *Rhinology* 1996; 34(2):66–74.
46. Haight J SJ, Cole P. The site and function of the nasal valve. *Laryngoscope* 1983; 93(1):49–55.
47. Bridger GP, Proctor DF. Maximum nasal inspiratory flow and nasal resistance. *Ann Otol* 1970; 79:481–488.
48. Ramos G. On the integration of respiratory movements: The fifth nerve afferents. *Acta Phys Lat Am* 1960; 10:104–111.
49. Dalimore NS, Eccles R. Changes in human nasal resistance associated with exercise, hyperventilation and rebreathing. *Acta Otolaryngol Stockh.* 1977; 84:416–421.
50. Wilde AD, Ahmed K, Cook JA, Jones AS. The nasal response to isometric exercise. *Clin Otol* 1995; 20:345–347.
51. Wilde AD, Cook JA, Jones AS. Nasal airway response to isometric exercise in non-eosinophilic intrinsic rhinitis *Clin Otol* 1996; 21:84–86.
52. Rundercrandtz H. Postural variations of nasal patency. *Acta Otolaryngol Stockh* 1969; 68:435–443.
53. Wilde AD, Cook JA, Jones AS. Nasal airway response to changes in axillary pressure in non-eosinophilic intrinsic rhinitis. *Clin Otolaryngol* 1997; 22(3):219–221.
54. Angell-James JE, Daly M de B. Reflex respiratory and cardiovascular effects of stimulation of receptors in the nose of the dog. *J Physiol.* 1972; 220:3–696.
55. Cook JA, Hamilton JW, Jones AS. The diving reflex in non-eosinophilic non-allergic rhinitis. *Clin Otol* 1996; 21:226–227.
56. Sherman IW, Jones AS. The response of the nasal vasculature to simulated diving. *Clin Otol* 1992; 17:92.
57. Olsson P, Bende M. Influence of environmental temperature on human nasal mucosa. *Ann Otol Rhinol Laryngol* 1985; 94:153–155.
58. Cole P, Forsyth R, Haight JSJ. Effects of cold air and exercise on nasal patency. *Ann Otol Rhinol Laryngol* 1983; 92:196–227.
59. Richardson PS. Reflexes concerned in the defence of the lungs. *Bull Eur Physiopath Respir* 1981; 17:979–1012.
60. Tsubone H. Nasal flow receptors of the rat. *Resp Physiol* 1989; 75:51–64.
61. Clarke R, Jones AS. Nasal airflow receptors: The relative importance of temperature and tactile stimulation. *Clin Otol* 1992; 17:388–392.
62. Eccles R, Griffiths DH, Newton CG, Tolley NS. The effects of menthol isomers on nasal sensation of airflow. *Clin Otol* 1988; 13:25–29.
63. Wilson JA, Hawkins RA, Sangster K, von Haake NP, Tesdale A, Leese AM, Murray JA, Maran AG. Estimation of oestrogen and progesterone receptors in chronic rhinitis. *Clin Otol* 1986; 114:213–218.
64. Ottoson D. Analysis of the electrical activity of the olfactory epithelium. *Acta Physiol Scand Suppl* 1956; 122:1–83.
65. Takagi SF, Wyse GA, Kitamura H, Ito K. The role of sodium and potassium ions in the generation of the electro-olfactogram. *J Gen Physiol* 1968; 1:552–578.
66. Bakalyar H, Reed R. Identification of a specialised adenyl cyclase that may mediate odourant detection. *Science* 1990; 250:1403–1406.
67. Firestein S, Shepherd G. Neurotransmitter antagonists block some odor responses in olfactory receptor neurones. *Neuroreport* 1992; 3:661–664.
68. Cain WS. Contribution of the trigeminal nerve to perceived odour magnitude. *Ann N York Acad Sci* 1974; 237:28–34.
69. Amoore J. A plan to identify most primary odors. In: *Olfaction and Taste* Pfaffman C. (Ed) New york: Rockefeller university Press, 1969; 158–171.
70. Moncrieff R. *The Chemical Senses.* London: Leonard Hill, 1967.
71. Briggs M, Duncan B. Pigment and olfactory mechanisms. *Nature* 1962; 195:1313–1314.
72. Morzell M. Evidence for a chromatographic model of olfaction. *Gen Physiol* 1970; 56:46–63.
73. Laffort P, Patte E, Etcmeto O. Olfactory coding in the basis of physiochemical properties. *Ann NY Acad Sci* 1974; 237: 193–208.
74. Holley A, Doving K. Receptor sensitivity, acceptor distribution, convergence and neural coding in the olfactory system. In *Olfaction and Taste* ed le Magna J and Macleod P. London: np, 1977; 113–128.

Measurement of Nasal Function and Nasal Valve Surgery

Guy Kenyon, John Pickett, Peter Andrew

Measurement of Nasal Function

Guy Kenyon, John Pickett

The nose provides airconditioning and humidification of the inhaled air as well as protects the body through the mucociliary escalator and through filtration and the secretion of lysozyme and immunoglobulins.[1,2] When the flow of air is unimpeded, the nasal airway also allows odorants to interact with the olfactory epithelium, thus providing the subject with a sense of smell. But it is as a resistor that the nose receives most attention in routine clinical practice since patients with obstructive symptoms constitute the majority of referrals and form the bulk of the patients receiving surgery.

Perhaps due to this, much effort has been made to try and measure nasal airway performance. Indeed such measurements are not new. Mirror misting or other assessments of the pattern of exhaled air from the nose as a means of assessing performance were advocated at the end of the nineteenth and at the beginning of the twentieth centuries and Hirschman[3] used a modified cystoscope to examine the sinuses. Unfortunately, as will be shown, in spite of many technical advances our means of accurately assessing patients objectively have not advanced into routine practice in most centers.

This is, perhaps, because efforts to measure nasal airway performance frequently fail to correlate with the pathological processes that are observed within the nose. Empirically, it would seem obvious that the two should be related but they are not. There appear, in fact, to be four possible states. Thus, a patient may have:

- A normal nose and no complaint.
- A complaint of obstruction that appears to have an obvious cause that can be identified and is corrected medically or surgically with apparent relief such as rhinitis, a deviated septum or unilateral polyp.

- A highly congested nose with turbinate hypertrophy or septal deviation but no apparent complaint.
- A complaint of obstruction in the presence of an airway that appears widely patent—the so-called 'empty nose syndrome'.

This lack of synergy between the patient's symptom and the physical findings is also manifest in a lack of correlation between measurements of resistance and the patient's subjective assessment of their own airway.[4]

In the light of this, many clinicians in routine practice do no more than ask the patient how readily they believe they can breathe through the nose. Such an assessment is normally accompanied, at least in a research setting, by measurement on a visual analog scale. But it is a wholly objective analysis that is desirable especially if surgical and medical intervention is to be properly assessed. To that end, much effort has been made to try to devise methods that give a reproducible and objective assessment of nasal airway performance although many of the papers that have been written on the subject have poor power and are level 4 or 5 evidence at best.

The main methods that have been used for airway assessment will be presented here. The first category makes measurements of the ease with which air passes through the nose, either from the subject's own effort or from an externally generated source. The second measures the dimensions of the nasal cavity and the points at which resistance to flow may be abnormally high. In both of these categories there are a number of different individual methods that have been developed to accomplish the measurement, each with their own advantages and disadvantages. Finally, there are a number of other methods that have been used and that will be alluded to. In the discussion that follows each of these processes will be described and the literature surrounding each method outlined.

TECHNIQUES

Rhinomanometry

Rhinomanometry provides a direct measurement of nasal resistance. By measuring the pressure gradient across the nasal cavity and the volume flow through the nose, the hydraulic resistance can be calculated, $R = \Delta P/V$.

Such measurements can be either active or passive with the pressure measured either at the anterior or posterior nares. Passive methods measure pressure changes while externally generated airflow is directed at a known rate through a mouthpiece. Active anterior rhinomanometry has been found to offer better reproducibility than posterior rhinomanometry and the latter measurements do not mimic normal physiological flow. As a result they have been, for all practical purposes, abandoned.

In contrast, active methods, where the pressure gradient across the nose is generated while the patient breathes quietly, have been the subject of many reports in the literature. There are two such methods.[5] In posterior active rhinomanometry the pressure is measured in the mouth (Fig. 3.1) and this measurement is presumed to give a recording which is equal to the pressure in the nasopharynx. The pressure gradient across the whole nose can be assessed at a variety of flow rates to give a measure of resistance. In active anterior rhinomanometry, the pressure gradient is assessed by occluding one nostril either by using a nozzle or by applying adhesive tape and measuring the pressure in the anterior nares (Fig. 3.2). No air can, of course, flow in the occluded side but the pressure measurement made is assumed to equal the pressure in the nasopharynx and, hence, to represent the pressure gradient on the contralateral side. Deriving the pressure in this way is termed anterior rhinomanometry.

The total resistance can then be calculated from the unilateral measurements using the formula:

$$^1/R_{total} = {}^1/R_{right} + {}^1/R_{left}$$

In both posterior and anterior rhinomanometry measurements of flow are usually made using a pneumotachograph connected to a mask covering the nose or nose and mouth. A nozzle can be used to connect this directly to the nostril for anterior rhinomanometry, but this is not commonly done as it is felt to be more likely to distort the nose and disrupt the measurement. A good seal is required, as leaks will cause errors in the

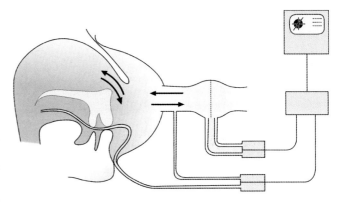

Fig. 3.1: Posterior active rhinomanometry

flow measurement. A further option is to use a head out body box to derive the flow signal. This eliminates the need to use a mask as, during respiratory movements, air is inspired or expired and air surrounding the body is displaced from the box. If the mouth is closed measurements of air flow therefore reflect the flow through the nose.[6]

A graph of the pressure plotted against flow is sigmoid in shape as increasing turbulence at higher flow rates results in higher resistance to flow (Fig. 3.3). Progressively increasing pressures, therefore, result in progressively smaller increases in flow. There is currently no complete mathematical description of the pressure/flow relationship over the whole breathing cycle and, for this reason, it is necessary to present results in a consistent way to enable meaningful comparisons between centers and operators.

A number of schemes for this have been proposed. As resistance varies at different pressures and flows, and

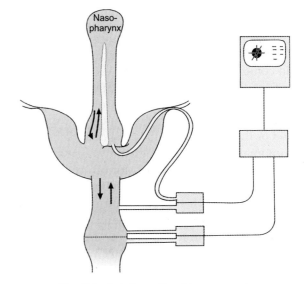

Fig. 3.2: Anterior active rhinomanometry

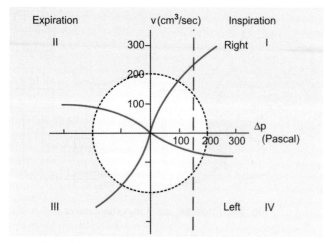

Fig. 3.3: Result of increasing pressures on flow rates

therefore varies across the respiratory cycle, the resistance is often quoted at standard pressure gradients such as 50, 100, 150, calculated using the formula $R = \Delta P/V$.[7] An alternative has been outlined by Broms.[8] If the pressure is plotted against flow during the breathing cycle, such that one Pa on the pressure axis is the same length as one cm^3/s on the flow axis, then the equation $V(r) = V_0 + C_r$ can be used where:

$V(r)$ = the angle between a line from the intercept of the curve with a circle of radius (r) to the origin and the flow axis

V_0 = the angle of the curve to the flow axis at the origin

C_r = a constant (reflects non-linearity, that is, turbulence)

Taking the radius r as 100 (100 Pa and 100 cm^3/s), 200, 300, is thought to give an adequate description of the whole curve.

O'Neill[9] proposed and validated an improved mathematical model using log transforms of the pressure and flow data.[9] However, this has yet to find routine use and in commercial devices the consensus guidelines of the International Committee for Standardization of Rhinomanometry (ICSR) published in 1984 are usually followed.[7] These recommended that either the Broms method or the resistance at 150 Pa should be used.

Rhinomanometry has, over the years, come to be regarded as the 'gold standard' for objective measurement of nasal function but its validity is still open to question. Even with the adoption of standardized operating procedures as recommended by the ICSR, studies on the accuracy and reproducibility of the technique have reported coefficients of variation for their measurements from less than 5% up to 60% even when the ICSR protocols are followed.[10-12] It is difficult to believe that such a wide range could not owe something to differences in experimental technique, but in most reports due to insufficient information about the protocols meaningful comparisons between different studies cannot be made. Carney reported coefficients of variation of up to 60% when performing active anterior rhinomanometry according to ICSR guidelines although this figure was improved to 15% when they used their revised 'Nottingham' protocol.[13] The latter involved greater attention to removing air leaks and repeating measurements when strict acceptance criteria for the curves were not reached. It seems likely that other investigators adopt similar strategies to achieve lower coefficients of variation but often such information is omitted when data is reported.

If the reproducibility is operator- and technique-dependent then it is also true that there will be variability due to the mucosal element of resistance over the medium to long-term. Decongestion before measurement largely removes this source of variability but at the cost of limiting the technique to the study of cartilaginous and bony structural abnormalities rather than the mucosal element of resistance.

Relatively few studies in the last twenty years have addressed the accuracy and repeatability of rhinomanometry and, more importantly, the correlation of the results achieved with the patient's perception of obstruction. Clarke[14] found a significant correlation when short-term changes in rhinomanometric variables following decongestion by xylometazoline were related to changes in sensation of obstruction measured on a visual analog scale.[14] However, a short-term reduction in resistance, which can be related by the subject to an almost immediate change in sensation of nasal patency, is likely to be different from the long-term view that the patient may have of his or her nasal patency. In the longer term the variability of both the patient's symptoms and in the measurements made during rhinomanometry mean that the correlation between the two is likely to be lost. In practice one might anticipate that rhinomanometry would always be capable of detecting large changes in resistance, such as would be expected after surgery. However, in fact the correlation of rhinomanometric changes with the findings following surgery are poor. The situation is confusing. Thus, among many similar papers, one group of authors found that there was a significant improvement in the measurements made on the narrowed side following septal surgery,[15] while others have reported no significant improvement in measurements made on patients having rhinoplasty and functional septoplasty.[16] Rhinomanometry thus, as opposed to a subjective impression of patient satisfaction, has limited value in clinical assessment.

Acoustic Rhinometry

Acoustic rhinometry is a technique that is able to measure the cross-sectional area of the nasal cavity as a function of the distance from the anterior nares. A sound pulse with a frequency content typically from 100 to 10,000 Hz or continuous wide band noise of frequencies up to about 25 kHz is generated by a spark or loudspeaker and is fed into the nose through probe inserted into the nasal vestibule (Fig. 3.4). The reflected sound waves are detected by a microphone mounted within the probe, which consists of a tube of known dimension with the sound source at one end. The other end is applied, using an adapter, to the nostril. The microphone is mounted in the wall of the sound tube between the sound source and the nose.

Changes in acoustic impedance occur where the cross-sectional area changes. These changes in impedance result in reflection of the incident sound waves, the strength of the reflection being dependent on the magnitude of the impedance changes. By analyzing the magnitude and timing of reflected sound pulses the cross-sectional area change and its distance from the microphone detector can be measured (Fig. 3.5). The measured cross-sectional area can be integrated to derive nasal volume.

The method assumes sound is propagated in one direction, that the walls of the nasal cavity are rigid and that there is no loss of sound energy as the sound moves down the nose. It also assumes that the nose is symmetrically bifurcate.

Most recent developments have produced instruments using continuous wide band noise. Comparison of the generated noise and measured noise, which

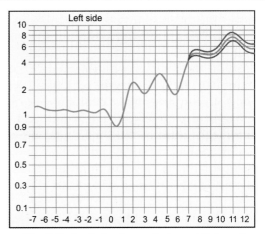

Fig. 3.5: Analysis of magnitude and timing of reflected sound pulses

includes the reflected component, allows the reflections to be extracted and from this information an area–distance curve can be plotted. This continuous analysis as opposed to the pulse response analysis means that the measurement rate can be higher than the 20 per second or so available from the pulse type acoustic rhinometers.

Acoustic rhinometry is quantitative and quick to perform although the accuracy of the technique is very dependent on the positioning of both the probe and the patient. Coefficients of variability of 8 to 12%[17,18] have been reported for repeated measurements with the probe removed and replaced between measurements. Other errors may be introduced due to nasal airflow and movement during measurement, nasal distortion, an imperfect seal between probe and nostril and the presence of ambient noise. Careful measurement techniques such as recommended by the Standardization Committee on Acoustic Rhinometry can reduce some of these errors.[19] These include using an acoustic gel to provide a seal between the probe and the nose, ensuring constant room temperature and humidity, training operators and by rejecting poor quality curves. In addition there must be adequate time for the subject to acclimatize and the patient must be given clear instructions.

Acoustic rhinometry has been validated using physical models (both anatomic and cylindrical tubes), cadavers and by *in vivo* studies. Model studies have correlated cross-sectional areas and volumes against the known or measured dimensions of the model.[20,21] In cadavers the dimensions measured by acoustic rhinometry have been compared to CT, water displacement or estimates made from the areas of dissected nasal cavity.[21,22] *In vivo* comparisons with CT, MRI and water displacement have also been made,[23–29] and comparisons

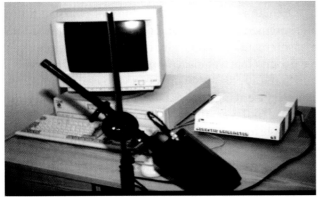

Fig. 3.4: Equipment for acoustic rhinometry

have been made with the result obtained with rhinomanometry, with spirometry and with the patient's subjective symptoms.[30–35]

In general the dimensions measured by acoustic rhinometry have tended to agree reasonably with the 'true' dimensions in these validation studies but a number of potential sources of error have been found. These include air leaks between the sound tube and nostril, distortion of the nasal vestibule and valve[36] and, in the posterior part of the nose, both systematic underestimation and overestimation of nasal dimensions. Underestimation beyond a narrow constriction has been attributed to reflection of the sound impulse at the constriction[37], while the overestimation has been attributed to sound leakage into the sinuses or the contralateral airway.[19,25,38]

Hamilton found considerable systematic errors in the cross-sectional areas of a plastic tube model measured by acoustic rhinometry, which varied with the area of constriction measured.[39] They concluded that the absolute dimensions measured were unreliable, but that the effects of interventions and dynamic changes could be monitored. Other errors in measurements, especially in children, have been found due to a mismatch between the dimensions of the sound tube and the nasal cavity when using adult instruments.[20] Newer instruments with probes designed specifically for infants and children have addressed this issue.[40]

Coefficients of variation of 2 to 15% have been reported for repeated measurements using acoustic rhinometry.[21,41] This variability is thought to be due largely to positional variation of the probe within the nares. However, averaging repeated measurements only marginally improved day-to-day repeatability in a study on decongested noses which perhaps indicates that the method is prone to other, systematic, errors in measurement and assessment.[18]

SPIROMETRIC TECHNIQUES

The use of spirometry and peak flow measurement in respiratory medicine is well established and such methods of measurement are familiar to most clinicians. Traditionally, spirometers operate by measuring directly the displaced air volume during various breathing maneuvers. These devices rely on a moving cylinder or bellows arrangement and they are still considered to be the gold standard for such measurements. However, newer electronic devices generally use a flow sensor, the output of which is integrated to yield volume: These represent a more flexible and convenient measurement

technique and allow inspiratory as well as expiratory measurements.

More popular for nasal assessments have been peak flow rate measurements using a Wright peak flow meter. These small, usually mechanical, meters are frequently used for pulmonary assessment and can be fitted with a nasal mask and used to assess the expiratory phase of respiration. They can also be reversed to give a peak inspiratory measurement. While less accurate than a formal spirometer these devices are inexpensive enough to allow their use for repeated measurements in the consulting room or in the patient's home. As such they have a distinct advantage over other techniques for monitoring relatively slow changes in nasal function.

There has been considerable debate as to which parameters should be routinely measured. The most commonly reported spirometric variables for nasal patency assessment have been nasal peak inspiratory or expiratory flow rates with other variables, such as forced inspiratory or expiratory volume in 1 second and nasal forced vital capacity, being less favored. When a number of variables were compared to resistance measured by rhinomanometry, peak inspiratory flow rate correlated better with resistance values (negatively) than other spirometric variables.[42] However, coefficients of variability reported for peak nasal inspiratory and expiratory flow rates have ranged from < 3 to > 9% with the variability of inspiratory measurements being consistently greater than for those in expiration.[43] Despite this greater variability inspiratory measurements have found greater acceptance perhaps due to the risk of contamination of the meter with mucus during expiration and also because there is a proper perception that inspiratory measurements, with a tendency of the lateral wall of the nose to collapse in this respiratory phase, are frequently more relevant to the investigation of the patient's complaint of obstruction.

Opinion is divided on the utility of peak nasal flow measurements in practice. Some authors endorse such measurements in certain circumstances,[44–47] while others have found that technical problems such as alar distortion due to the applied pressure needed to seal the mask and alar collapse at high flow rates,[43,46] and poor repeatability and diurnal variability,[48] make the technique too unreliable for routine use. The effort of forced inspiratory or expiratory maneuvers has also been shown to act as a mechanical stimulus to the nose in some rhinitic patients, which caused an increase in nasal resistance.[49]

As with other methods of measurement the correlation of peak flow measurements with subjective symptoms is inconsistent. In one study peak nasal inspiratory flow was found to correlate well with symptom scores in perennial allergic rhinitis sufferers after treatment with corticosteroids or placebo.[35] However, other studies have found either no correlation or a poor correlation between peak nasal inspiratory flow and subjective assessment.[46,50,51] Thus, there are doubts not only as to which parameter should be measured but also as to whether the measurements made represent a realistic insight as to the patient's complaint.

Forced Oscillation

The forced oscillation technique involves the superposition of a small amplitude, low frequency (usually < 100 Hz), oscillating signal onto normal tidal breathing. A loudspeaker is used to generate the signal and the resulting pressure and flow variations are recorded using a pneumotachograph. The resistance derived in this manner is of the entire airway. By recording with the nose included in the measurement volume, and then either subtracting the flow recorded at the same pressure with a nasal clip in place and calculating resistance from the resultant nasal-only flow and pressure, or by subtracting the resistance recorded breathing through the mouth only, the nasal resistance can be estimated.

$$|Z_{nasal}| = |Z_{total}| - |Z_{oral}|$$

Relatively few reports on the validity of these measurements are available.[52–54] Potential drawbacks of the technique are that it is complex, time consuming and the data analysis is not straightforward. The assumption that subtraction of the thoracic and oral components from the total resistance derives nasal resistance may not be entirely valid and dynamic changes in nasal or thoracic resistance could introduce errors as the total and oral resistances are not recorded simultaneously.

OTHER TECHNIQUES

Many other techniques have attempted to characterize nasal function. Most notably these have included attempts to add objectivity to the Zwaardermaker technique using liquid crystal thermography but this simple technique has not enjoyed widespread acceptance to date as it was found not to give a clinically useful measure of nasal obstruction.[55] More recently we have also measured the patterns of humidified air exhaled from the nose onto a fixed plate, using a thermal camera (Fig. 3.6).[56] The plate medium chosen was normal copy

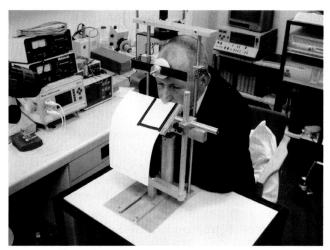

Fig. 3.6: Thermal camera measurement of exhaled humidified air

paper (Xerox 80 g/m^2) as this was found to heat sufficiently quickly to form an image on each consecutive breath. The system was first tested in continuous flow conditions in a temperature controlled laboratory (23°C ± 0.5°C), with an air cylinder and control valve, humidifier and rotameter type flowmeter used to supply a controlled flow of humidified and warmed air.

Figure 3.7 shows the typical image obtained and also shown is an isotherm, which was plotted at a value halfway between the peak temperature and ambient temperature (in this case 27.9°C). The area enclosed by this isotherm can be measured and the value obtained normalized by dividing by the area of the whole plate, measured from the same image. An increase in normalized 50% area is seen with increasing flow and we are currently trying to correlate the measurements

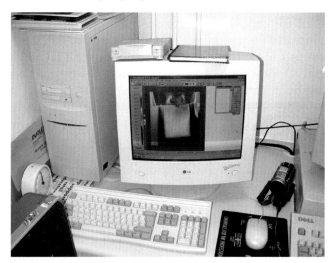

Fig. 3.7: Image of nasal function noted halfway between peak temperature and ambient temperature

made with this technique to the reported sensation of obstruction in normal subjects and patients. We are also currently investigating the use of Schlieren photography to see if we can use the image of the plume of expired air from the nose to make some form of subjective assessment of nasal airflow.

CONCLUSION

Of all the techniques available rhinomanometry is the closest to a 'gold standard' for nasal assessment. Acoustic rhinometry is also widely used and spirometry has enjoyed the support of some authors. Other attempts to measure nasal obstruction have also been mentioned in this chapter and those that have not been mentioned in depth include measurements of the proportion of nasal to oral inspired or expired volume[57,58] and manometric rhinometry which has been used to measure nasal volume.[59] In addition endoscopic measurement of the dimensions of the nasal airway using image-processing techniques have been used.[60] However, as with more established methods, all these techniques have found limited support in practice principally because no technique has, to date, been found to reliably correlate with the reported symptom of obstruction.

To address this we clearly need a greater under-standing of the physiology of normal nasal airflow. In addition the basic methodologies used may also need altering and refining. We have, for instance, tried to ensure greater validity by utilizing mental alerting during measurement, as is done during caloric irrigation, to distract the patient from the task in hand and to try and ensure that subject is unaware of his or her own breathing pattern. We have also favored non-contact techniques, since the very validity of techniques that require facial contact or the insertion of nozzles or pressure tubes into the nose has to be questioned. This is so since it is known that application of a face mark alters the respiratory breathing patterns of neonates[61] and from this it might be adduced that any form of local stimulation is likely to alter the pattern of respiration and, hence, the performance of the nasal airway. Certainly the insertion of probes or applications of masks must, at the very least, cause some minor degree of alteration of function and stenting the ala, as is done in acoustic rhinometry, clearly changes the whole dynamic of the external valve. For these reason measurements of the pattern of exhaled air are empirically attractive but whether it will be possible to demonstrate the clinical utility of such 'no touch' techniques, and whether they have any advantages over more established methods, remains to be proven.

In a world of evidence-based practice and health care commissioning there is certainly a need to demonstrate objective evidence of outcome from treatment. At present, without a reliable system for nasal airway measurement, there is no such evidence base for much of what is done to the nose by medical and surgical intervention. Frequently, the evidence for or against a particular procedure is contradictory. Where results are available there are often methodological flaws and inconsistencies which invalidate the conclusions drawn and make them difficult to substantiate. Furthermore most studies on the performance of the various measurement techniques presently available offer level 4 evidence, at best, and do not follow the recently published STARD guidelines for the reporting of studies of diagnostic accuracy.[62] Thus, in a recent systematic review of all the available literature 942 articles were identified concerning the objective assessment of outcomes from septal surgery. However, only 13 of these papers were found to have any real validity and, in fact, methodological inconsistencies with inadequately specified inclusion criteria ruled out all but three of these for meta-analysis.[63]

An ideal technique would quantify the level of obstruction in such a way as to be able to inform the choice of therapy and would correlate well with the subjective sensation experienced by the patient. Objective measure-ments are also necessary to aid comparisons between treatments. However, the reality is that the inter- and intra-test variation in measurements of nasal obstruction are too variable for any one means of assessment to be reliable currently and, until we have a better under-standing of the basic physiology, the best we can do at present is to use a combination of measurement techniques together with clinical judgement and the reports of the patients own sensation of obstruction.

REFERENCES

1. Glatzel P. Prufung der Luft durgangigkeit der Nase. *Ther Gegenw* 1901; 42:348 apud Hilberg O, Jackson AC, Swift DL, Pedersen O F. Acoustic rhinometry: Evaluation of nasal cavity geometry by acoustic reflection. *J Appl Physiol* 1989;66: 295–303.
2. Zwaardermaker H. Attembeschlag als Hulfsmittel zur Diagnose der Nasalen Stenosen. *Arch Laryngol Rhinol* 1894; 1:174–177.
3. Hirschman A. Über Endoskopie der Nase und deren Nebenhöhlen Eine neue Untersuchungsmethode. *Arch Laryngol* 1903; 143:195–202.
4. Jones AS, Willatt DJ, Durham LM. Nasal airflow: Resistance and sensation. *J Laryngol Otol* 1989; 103(10):909–911.
5. Clement PA. Different typed of rhinomanometers, standardization, pathologic shapes of rhinomanometric recordings, pitfalls, and possible errors. *Facial Plast Surg* 1990; 7(4):230–244.

6. Cole P, Havas T. Nasal resistance to respiratory airflow: A plethysmographic alternative to the face mask. *Rhinology* 1987; 25(3):159–166.

7. Clement PA. Committee report on standardization of rhinomanometry. *Rhinology* 1984; 22(3):151–155.

8. Broms P, Jonson B, Lamm CJ. Rhinomanometry II A system for numerical description of nasal airway resistance. *Acta Oto-Laryngologica* 1982; 94(1–2):157–168.

9. O'Neill G, Tolley NS, Hollis LJ, Hern JD, Almeyda JS. Analysis of rhinomanometric data based upon a model of nasal airflow and logarithmic transformation of the data. *Clin Otolaryngol Allied Sci* 1996; 21(6):524–527.

10. Corrado OJ, Ollier S, Phillips MJ, Thomas JM, Davies RJ. Histamine and allergen induced changes in nasal airways resistance measured by anterior rhinomanometry: Reproducibility of the technique and the effect of topically administered antihistaminic and anti–allergic drugs. *Br J Clin Pharmacol* 1987; 24(3):283–292.

11. Schumacher MJ. Nasal dyspnea: The place of rhino-manometry in its objective assessment [Review] [37 refs], *Am J Rhinol* 2004; 18(1):41–46.

12. Shelton DM, Eiser NM. Evaluation of active anterior and posterior rhinomanometry in normal subjects, *Clin Otolaryngol Allied Sci* 1992; 17(2):178–182.

13. Carney AS, Bateman ND, Jones NS. Reliable and reproducible anterior active rhinomanometry for the assessment of unilateral nasal resistance. *Clin Otolaryngol Allied Sci* 2000; 25(6):499–503.

14. Clarke RW, Cook JA, Jones AS. The effect of nasal mucosal vasoconstriction on nasal airflow sensation, *Clin Otolaryngol Allied Sci* 1995; 20(1):72–73.

15. Jalowayski AA, Yuh YS, Koziol JA, Davidson TM. Surgery for nasal obstruction—evaluation by rhinomanometry, *Laryngoscope* 1983; 93(3):341–345.

16. Courtiss EH, Goldwyn RM. The effects of nasal surgery on airflow. *Plast Reconst Surg* 1983; 72(1):9–21.

17. Fisher EW, Morris DP, Biemans JM, Palmer CR, Lund VJ. Practical aspects of acoustic rhinometry: Problems and solutions. *Rhinology* 1995; 33(4):219–223.

18. Harar RP, Kalan A, Kenyon GS. Improving the reproducibility of acoustic rhinometry in the assessment of nasal function. *Orl J Oto-Rhino-Laryngol Related Spec* 2002; 64(1):22–25.

19. Hilberg O, Pedersen OF. Acoustic rhinometry: Recommen-dations for technical specifications and standard operating procedures [erratum appears in *Rhinology* 2001; 39(2):119], *Rhinology Suppl* 2000; 16:3–17.

20. Buenting JE, Dalston RM, Smith TL, Drake AF. Artifacts associated with acoustic rhinometric assessment of infants and young children: A model study. *J Appl Physiol* 1994; 77(6):2558–2563.

21. Hilberg O, Jackson AC, Swift DL, Pedersen OF. Acoustic rhinometry: Evaluation of nasal cavity geometry by acoustic reflection. *J Appl Physiol* 1989; 66(1):295–303.

22. Mayhew TM, O'Flynn P. Validation of acoustic rhinometry by using the Cavalieri principle to estimate nasal cavity ume in cadavers. *Clin Otolaryngol Allied Sci* 1993; 18(3):220–225.

23. Corey JP, Gungor A, Nelson R, Fredberg J, Lai V. A compari-son of the nasal cross-sectional areas and umes obtained with acoustic rhinometry and magnetic resonance imaging. *Otolaryngology – Head Neck Surg* 1997; 117(4):349–354.

24. Gilain L, Coste A, Ricolfi F, Dahan E, Marliac D, Peynegre R, Harf A, Louis B. Nasal cavity geometry measured by acoustic rhinometry and computed tomography. *Arch Otolaryngology—Head Neck Surg* 1997; 123(4):401–405.

25. Hilberg O, Jensen FT, Pedersen OF. Nasal airway geometry: Comparison between acoustic reflections and magnetic resonance scanning, *J Appl Physiol* 1993; 75(6):2811–2819.

26. Hilberg O, Pedersen OF. Acoustic rhinometry: Influence of paranasal sinuses, *J Appl Physiol* 1996; 80(5):1589–1594.

27. Mamikoglu B, Houser S, Akbar I, Ng B, Corey JP. Acoustic rhinometry and computed tomography scans for the diagnosis of nasal septal deviation, with clinical correlation. *Otolaryngol – Head Neck Surg* 2000; 123(1 Pt 1):61–68.

28. Min YG, Jang YJ. Measurements of cross-sectional area of the nasal cavity by acoustic rhinometry and CT scanning. *Laryngoscope* 1995; 105(7 Pt 1):757–759.

29. Taverner D, Bickford L, Latte J. Validation by fluid volume of acoustic rhinometry before and after decongestant in normal subjects. *Rhinology* 2002; 40(3):135–140.

30. Ahmad RL, Gendeh BS. Evaluation with acoustic rhinometry of patients undergoing sinonasal surgery. *Med J Malaysia* 2003; 58(5):723–728.

31. Austin CE, Foreman JC. Acoustic rhinometry compared with posterior rhinomanometry in the measurement of histamine– and bradykinin-induced changes in nasal airway patency. *Br J Clin Pharmacol* 1994; 37(1):33–37.

32. Kim CS, Moon BK, Jung DH, Min YG. Correlation between nasal obstruction symptoms and objective parameters of acoustic rhinometry and rhinomanometry. *Auris Nasus Larynx* 1998; 25(1):45–48.

33. Porter MJ, Williamson IG, Kerridge DH, Maw AR. A comparison of the sensitivity of manometric rhinometry, acoustic rhinometry, rhinomanometry and nasal peak flow to detect the decongestant effect of xylometazoline. *Clin Otolaryngol Allied Sci* 1996; 21(3):218–221.

34. Roithmann R, Cole P, Chapnik J, Barreto SM, Szalai JP, Zamel N. Acoustic rhinometry, rhinomanometry, and the sensation of nasal patency: A correlative study. *J Otolaryngol* 1994; 23(6):454–458.

35. Wilson AM, Sims EJ, Robb F, Cockburn W, Lipworth BJ. Peak inspiratory flow rate is more sensitive than acoustic rhinometry or rhinomanometry in detecting corticosteroid response with nasal histamine challenge. *Rhinology* 2003; 41(1):16–20.

36. Hamilton JW, McRae RD, Jones AS. The magnitude of random errors in acoustic rhinometry and re–interpretation of the acoustic profile. *Clin Otolaryngol Allied Sci* 1997; 22(5): 408–413.

37. Cankurtaran M, Celik H, Cakmak O, Ozluoglu LN. Effects of the nasal valve on acoustic rhinometry measurements: A model study. *J Appl Physiol* 2003; 94(6):2166–2172.

38. Djupesland PG, Rotnes JS. Accuracy of acoustic rhinometry. *Rhinology* 2001; 39(1):23–27.

39. Hamilton JW, Cook JA, Phillips DE, Jones AS. Limitations of acoustic rhinometry determined by a simple model. *Acta Oto-Laryngologica* 1995; 115(6):811–814.

40. Djupesland P G, Lyholm, B. Nasal airway dimensions in term neonates measured by continuous wide–band noise acoustic rhinometry. *Acta Oto–Laryngologica* 1997; 117(3):424–432.

41. Nurminen M, Hytonen M, Sala E. Modelling the reproducibility of acoustic rhinometry, *Stat Med* 2000; 19(9):1179–1189.

42. Jones AS, Viani L, Phillips D, Charters P. The objective assessment of nasal patency. *Clin Otolaryngol Allied Sci* 1991; 16(2):206–211.

43. Enberg RN, Ownby DR. Peak nasal inspiratory flow and Wright peak flow: A comparison of their reproducibility. *Ann Allergy* 1991; 67(3):371–374.

44. Clarke RW, Jones AS. The limitations of peak nasal flow measurement. *Clin Otolaryngol Allied Sci* 1994; 19(6):502–504.

45. Frolund L, Madsen F, Mygind N, Nielsen NH, Svendsen UG, Weeke B. Comparison between different techniques for measuring nasal patency in a group of unselected patients. *Acta Oto-Laryngologica* 1987; 104(1–2):175–179.

46. Clarke RW, Jones AS, Richardson H. Peak nasal inspiratory flow—the plateau effect. *J Laryngol Otol* 1995; 109(5):399–402.

47. Sims EJ, Wilson AM, White PS, Gardiner Q, Lipworth BJ. Short–term repeatability and correlates of laboratory measures of nasal function in patients with seasonal allergic rhinitis. *Rhinology* 2002; 40(2):66–68.

48. Blomgren K, Simola M, Hytonen M, Pitkaranta A. Peak nasal inspiratory and expiratory flow measurements—practical tools in primary care? *Rhinology* 2003; 41(4):206–210.

49. Braat JP, Fokkens WJ, Mulder PG, Kianmaneshrad N, Rijntjes E, Gerth van WR. Forced expiration through the nose is a stimulus for NANIPER but not for controls. *Rhinology* 2000; 38(4):172–176.

50. Gleeson MJ, Youlten LJ, Shelton DM, Siodlak MZ, Eiser NM, Wengraf CL. Assessment of nasal airway patency: A comparison of four methods. *Clin Otolaryngol Allied Sci* 1986; 11(2):99–107.

51. Morrissey MS, Alun-Jones T, Hill J. The relationship of peak inspiratory airflow to subjective airflow in the nose. *Clin Otolaryngol Allied Sci* 1990; 15(5):447–451.

52. Lemes LN, Melo PL. Simplified oscillation method for assessing nasal obstruction non-invasively and under spontaneous ventilation: A pilot study. *Med Biol Engg Comp* 2003; 41(4):439–444.

53. Shelton DM, Pertuze J, Gleeson MJ, Thompson J, Denman WT, Goff J, Eiser NM, Pride NB. Comparison of oscillation with three other methods for measuring nasal airways resistance. *Respir Med* 1990; 84(2):101–106.

54. Tawfik B, Sullivan KJ, Chang HK. A new method to measure nasal impedance in spontaneously breathing adults. *J Appl Physiol* 1991; 71(1):9–15.

55. Canter RJ. A non-invasive method of demonstrating the nasal cycle using flexible liquid crystal thermography. *Clin Otolaryngol Allied Sci* 1986; 11(5):329–336.

56. Pickett JA, Levine M, Birch M, Kenyon GS. Thermographic measurement of nasal airway function: A modern approach to an old technique. In 20th Congress of the European Rhinologic Society (ERS) 23rd International Symposium on Infection and Allergy of the Nose (ISIAN), Istanbul, p 214.

57. Drake AF, Keall H, Vig PS, Krause CJ. Clinical nasal obstruction and objective respiratory mode determination. *Ann Otol Rhinol Laryngol* 1988; 97(4 Pt 1):397–402.

58. Oluwole M, Gardiner Q, White PS. The naso-oral index: A more valid measure than peak flow rate? *Clin Otolaryngol Allied Sci* 1997; 22(4):346–349.

59. Porter MJ, Maw AR, Kerridge DH, Williamson IM. Manometric rhinometry: A new method of measuring the ume of the air in the nasal cavity. *Acta Oto-Laryngologica* 1997; 117(2):298–301.

60. Bellussi L, Ferrara GA, Mezzedimi C, Passali GC, D'Alesio D, Passali D. A new method for endoscopic evaluation in rhinology: Videocapture. *Rhinology* 2000; 38(1):13–16.

61. Fleming PJ, Levine MR, Goncalves A. Changes in respiratory pattern resulting from the use of a facemask to record respiration in newborn infants. *Ped Res* 1982; 16(12):1031–1034.

62. Bossuyt PM, Reitsma JB, Bruns DE, Gatsonis CA, Glasziou PP, Irwig LM, Moher D, Rennie D, de Vet HC, Lijmer JG. Standards for Reporting of Diagnostic Accuracy: The STARD statement for reporting studies of diagnostic accuracy: Explanation and elaboration. *Clin Chem* 2003; 49(1):7–18.

63. Patel N, Singh, Kenyon GS. 2005, in preparation.

Nasal Valve Surgery

Guy Kenyon, Peter Andrew

INTRODUCTION

The causes of nasal obstruction are often held to be due either to mucosal disease or to anatomical abnormality. In the former group cilial dysfunction and atrophic changes may play a role but the commonest causes of mucosal dysfunction are undoubtedly a group or disorders that are characterised by the generic term "rhinitis". However, if allergic rhinitis is excluded, it has to be admitted that many of the causes of a hypertrophic and hypersecreting mucosa remain ill-defined.

The exact role of the mucosa in the genesis of a patient with a subjective complaint of obstruction remains obscure as does the manner by which an anatomically deviated nasal septum and hypertrophied nasal turbinates many cause some, but not all, patients to complain. Not only is the size of the nasal airway not immediately correlated with the patient's complaint but the role of surgical correction of the septum and turbinates remains controversial and unproven.[1] This being so it is scarcely surprising that a lack of clarity also exists as to the role of the nasal valve – although there can be little doubt that abnormality in the structure which is normally referred to in this context can cause nasal obstruction in some cases. In fact, as will be seen there are in fact, two valves which interact one with another in helping to regulate flow in the lower third of the nose and the pathology relating to derangement of the structure in this area here, while poorly understood, may be the sole cause of a patient's symptoms. Indeed some have suggested that valve dysfunction is the cause of symptoms in the majority of patients presenting with nasal blockage[2] – although such a view may well be skewed due to the fact that these surgeons were reporting a cohort of revision patients seen in a plastic surgery practice who had undergone excessive dorsal hump resection and detachment of the upper lateral cartilages. Certainly, the notion that such findings are more common than septal or turbinate pathology is unproven as well as probably being alien to the majority of otolaryngologists.

THE INTERNAL NASAL VALVE

The structure most commonly referred to as "the nasal valve" lies at the isthmus or narrowest part of the nose in the coronal plane at the head of the inferior turbinate. However, to describe this area as a valve is really a misnomer. A valve regulates flow or, in strict anatomical terms, is a "membranous part of a vessel preventing the flow of liquids in one direction and allowing it another".[3] Such a definition is clearly invalid in the nose where flow is obviously bi-directional and is driven by the phases of the respiratory cycle which, in turn, is driven by the lungs. Nonetheless the name has become hallowed by common usage.

The first description of a nasal valve is normally attributed.[4] He defined the valve as the area of the maximal resistance within the anterior part of the respiratory tract, but there has subsequently been a degree of dispute and contention as to exactly what constitutes this entity anatomically.[5] Undertook a series of radiological studies which suggested that the narrowest area of the nose was at the junction of the lower and upper lateral cartilages whereas cadaver impressions have suggested that the narrowest area is the piriform aperture.[6] More dynamic studies with nasal probes have suggested that the area of highest pressure change is in the plane of the head of the inferior turbinate and the same studies also suggested that this plane actually changes depending on the state of congestion or constriction of the head of the inferior turbinate.[7] The role of the head of the inferior turbinate was also stressed by studies that have shown that decongestants halve nasal resistance.[8] But, while this may be true, it has also to be said that there is a tendency for this area to collapse at high flow rates[9] which implies some a variability in floe imposed by the lateral nasal wall at this site.

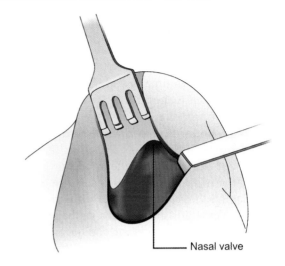

Fig. 3.8: Exposure of the nasal valve

Misnomer or not, what is now agreed is that this area at the nasal isthmus constitutes what has now become known as the internal nasal valve.[2,10] This area offers the greatest resistance to airflow and can be measured in studies using acoustic rhinometry as the point of minimal cross-sectional area. In strict anatomical terms this valve appears to lie in the coronal plane at the head of the inferior turbinate and the "valve" also consists of the caudal part of the upper lateral cartilage and the angle between this structure and the dorsal septum just beyond the plane of the piriform aperture (the isthmus nasi). It is shown in diagrammatic manner in Fig. 3.8 and in anatomical cross-section in Fig. 3.9. The shape of the latter structure differs between Caucasian (leptorrhine) and

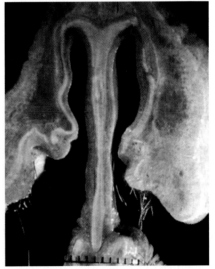

Fig. 3.9: Axial section through cadaveric nostril demonstrating nasal valve

Negroid (platyrrhine) noses,[11] but it is generally agreed that the important anatomy at this site is the retention of the angle between the upper lateral and the dorsal septum—which should be between 10 and 15°. If scarring is produced here by trauma or injudicious trimming of the upper lateral cartilages during routine rhinoplasty nasal obstruction may result.

There is no doubt that the lateral nasal wall at this point also moves in a medial direction with forced inspiration, but this can have little impact on nasal flow – at least in the normal nose. This is so since the part of the lower lateral that can actually exhibit any tendency to inward movement is limited. In a cephalad direction the upper lateral cartilage is, of course, fixed to and slightly under-runs the nasal bones and this must limit movement. In a caudal direction the upper laterals turn back on themselves in the scroll area and are stented by the lower lateral cartilages, which flare during times of maximal inspiratory flow and which thus support the lower margins of the upper laterals through the medium of the inter-cartilaginous ligaments. Movement of the lateral wall in this internal valve area is thus restricted. This argument was supported by experiments in normal subjects which showed that the minimal cross-sectional area of the nose, when measured by acoustic rhinometry, is increased by over 40% when topical vasoconstrictors are applied to the mucosa whereas external nasal splints have relatively little effect at this site.[10]

THE EXTERNAL NASAL VALVE

The external valve is formed by the external nares and its supporting structures. These consist of the columella medially, which is fixed, and by the lateral crura of the lower lateral cartilages, which are mobile. There is no doubt that these parts of the soft tissue structures of the nose display a tendency to collapse at high rates of inspiratory flow, and this tendency is normally resisted by the function of the overlying dilator nares muscles and by the levator labii alaeque nasi muscle which is inserted into the lateral crura on each side. Inward collapse is also resisted by the tensile strength of the cartilages, but if these are traumatised or either weakened or over-resected as part of a rhinoplasty operation, then collapse may follow. Equally, if there is a high abutment of the lateral crus and a cephalad rotation of this cartilages towards the piriform aperture then the soft tissue triangle at the rim of the nose is unsupported and the tissues then tend to collapse at high flow rates—particularly in older patient when the tissues loose their tensile strength. Finally, because of the importance of the overlying facial

muscles in stenting the alae, facial paralysis may also cause an interruption to inspiratory flow and may cause altered flow-pressure relationships as the alae show a tendency to collapse during normal inspiratory efforts.[7,12] What all this clearly demonstrates is the importance of the integrity of the local anatomy in the maintenance of this outer valve. Physiologically, unlike the internal valve where flow is primarily influenced by the state of mucosal engorgement, the peak flow is increased substantially by splinting and stenting of this valve and especially by the insertion of a prosthesis such as a Francis ala dilator: By contrast the effects of vasoconstriction on inspiratory flow, while still marked, are less profound.[10]

Teleologically, it is impossible to ascertain why these areas exist - although they may be important in allowing a sensation of normal resistance to flow. Moreover exactly how these two valvular areas interact in response to differing physiological stimuli is also not understood. Clearly, in times of maximal inspiratory effort the alae flare and the mucosa decongests with abolition of the nasal cycle – allowing flow rates to increase in response to the body's increased oxygen demand. However, the receptors and reflexes initiating and moderating such a response are not clearly identified – either at a local level or more centrally.

VALVE PATHOLOGY

The causes of obstruction at the internal nasal valve may be primary or secondary. Primary causes are most commonly due either to high deviations of the septum into the critical area formed by the internal valve angle or to mucosal edema in the same area. Occasionally, a degree of collapse of the upper lateral cartilage in this region may also contribute. Secondary causes following surgery or other trauma include scarring at the apex as well as structural collapse or over-narrowing at the piriform aperture during rhinoplasty surgery. Structural narrowing of the nose in the internal valve area is also more common in noses with short nasal bones and a long narrow middle third—as this leaves the cartilaginous structures relatively unsupported by the short nasal bones. In secondary cases there is a characteristic deformity seen externally which resembles an inverted V (Fig. 3.10).

Causes of obstruction at the external valve area are also best thought of as being either primary or as being secondary to surgical intervention. In primary cases the lateral crus of the lower lateral cartilage is either weak or malpositioned and the latter category includes patients with a paradoxical inversion or a more cephalid/ caudal

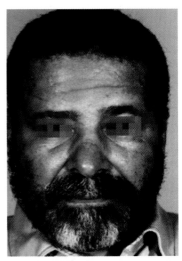

Fig. 3.10: Deformity of nasal valve resembling an inverted V

position of the lateral crus than is normal. As has already been mentioned secondary external valve collapse also follows excessive resection of the lateral crus, with resultant collapse: The latter symptom may present sometime distant from the initial surgery and is particularly difficult to correct.

CLINICAL ASSESSMENT

Cottle was the first to highlight the fact that simple septoplasty and turbinate surgery will not cure all patients with nasal blockage and was the first to demarcate and name differing areas within the septum.[13] He divided the septum into five areas; the nostril and vestibule (external valve), the nasal valve angle (internal valve), the attic area, the mid-turbinate area and the posterior turbinate area (Fig. 3.11).

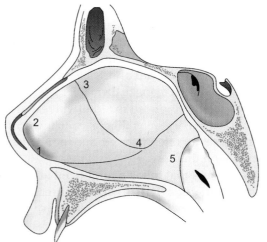

Fig. 3.11: Five areas of the nasal septum. (1) Nostril and vestibule (External valve), (2) Nasal valve angle, (3) Attic area, (4) Mid-turbinate area, (5) Posterior turbinate area

The attic is intimately related to the keystone area of the dorsum where it joins with the caudal part of the nasal bones. This are cannot be defiled during normal septal surgery or a saddle deformity may result. The mid and posterior turbinate areas are, however, amenable to septoplasty. In particular the area of the nasal valve is important and in one series of 500 patients presenting with nasal blockage, 13% had obstruction at the level of the nasal valve.[14] The assessment of the level of septal deviation is thus of paramount importance prior to embarking on a surgical cure for obstructive symptoms.

The clinician must also be aware that pathologies may co-exist. Consider the patient with a marked septal deviation and bilateral alar collapse. Prior to surgery angulation of the dorsal septum may mask the co-existent external valve collapse on the narrowed side, as the ala is stented by the septum. On the contralateral side alar collapse also occurs but passes unnoticed as the cartilage can collapse with impunity into a widely open airway. The patient, who is likely to be complaining of unilateral obstruction, then has successful septal surgery but no surgery to stiffen or reposition the alae. On the previously narrowed side the stenting of the ala is removed by surgery but the ala can now collapse - with the result that, to the patient, the airway remains obstructed on this side. On the contralateral side, which was previously patent, ala movement is not altered but is now clinically manifest as a complaint of obstruction as the centralization of the septum causes a relative narrowing of the airway. To everyone's chagrin the patient, who previously enjoyed a nasal airway on one side, now complains of bilateral obstruction.

HISTORY AND EXAMINATION

A full history and examination are obviously mandatory in all patients with symptoms of obstruction. Great detail is clearly redundant in the context of this chapter but a history of previous rhinoplasty or septal surgery is obviously relevant, as are symptoms that suggest that obstruction is not bi-phasic but is, instead, occurring predominantly during the inspiratory phase of respiration. Equally, the clinician should also record whether blockage is unilateral or bilateral, whether it is constant or intermittent and whether it is relieved in whole or in part by nasal steroids or nasal splints. Frequently patients with external valve collapse will have had recourse to Cottle's maneuver – where pulling on the malar skin is routinely employed to open the external valve to avoid obstruction during inspiration (Fig. 3.12). Sometimes, they will have tried external splints - such as

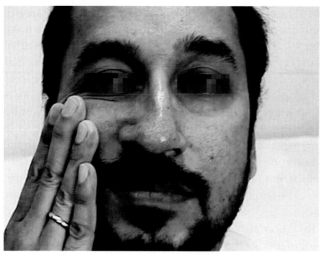

Fig. 3.12: Cottle's maneuver: Pulling on malar skin to open the external valve

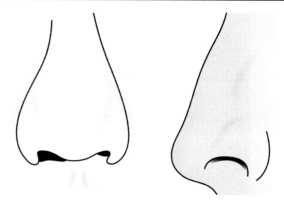

Fig. 3.14: The parenthesis deformity

the proprietary *Breathe right* strips (Fig. 3.13) that are widely available. However, patients may not volunteer such information unless specifically asked.

Clear cut external deformity may be obvious but clues as to the true nature of the patient's pathology may nonetheless be ignored. A characteristic inverted V deformity should raise the suspicion of internal valve pathology. In like manner the patient with a high abutment of the ala frequently exhibits what has been called the parenthesis deformity (Fig. 3.14).[15] Simple observation of the nose may also reveal alar or middle third collapse and patients with internal valve deformity often exhibit a pinched look to the middle third during respiration and a loss of the dorsal aesthetic line in repose. If suspicion of pathology is present the Bachman

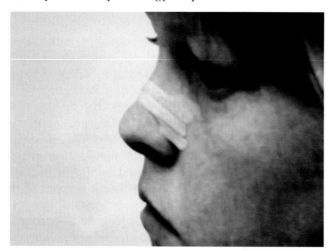

Fig. 3.13: External splint (Breathe right) to keep the external valve open

maneuver may also be helpful. This latter test assesses the inner valve function by applying a small cotton applicator at the apex of the inner valve. The valve angle is thus enlarged, and a positive result gives further credence to the possibility of an inner valve collapse.

Such an examination should also be accompanied by an assessment of the nasal airflow in the resting position during quiet respiration as well as during forced inspiration and expiration. Mirror misting in an out-patient setting is frequently all that is available and is normally sufficient and laboratory confirmation of impaired flow, altered resistance or reduced cross-sectional area, whilst ideal, is not normally necessary.

MANAGEMENT OF NASAL VALVE DEFICIENCY

In many cases of nasal valve incompetence, surgical intervention will be required. However, a conservative approach is also possible – especially in minor cases.

Optimizing medical treatment with regards to underlying rhinitis, if present, is clearly important and may help to reduce nasal resistance at the internal nasal valve angle and abolish the perception of obstruction. For minor cases of internal valve narrowing external paper splintage may also suffice to alleviate the symptoms, or at least to make them tolerable. In patients with major collapse of the external valve a trial of a suitably sized Francis alar dilator is also worthwhile, although these are often rejected due to the discomfort associated with their use.

In the account that follows surgery for abnormalities of the internal and external valves will be presented. Congenital causes of external valve deficiency including the cleft palate nose with resultant vestibular stenosis will not be discussed here although many of the same principles are utilized in their correction.

Internal Valve Surgery

Internal valve surgery relies primarily upon reduction of the head of the inferior turbinate either undertaken alone or in conjunction with maneuvers designed to enlarge the angle between the upper lateral cartilages and the dorsal septum. Turbinate surgery is widely practised and may be simply accomplished by the use of diathermy, cryotherapy, a laser or–more recently–coblation techniques. Such surgery is not specialist and will not be described further here.

To increase the angle between the septum and upper lateral cartilages two main techniques have been promoted. In minor cases of inner valve deficiency the modified Z-plasty technique is frequently preferred.[16] In this technique a flap of mucosa is rotated into the valve area so as to augment the surface area of the valve. Such a technique is useful in cases of simple scarring and adhesion but requires insertion of sialastic splints in the postoperative period so as to reduce the chances of further adhesion formation.

In more complicated cases, and when the angle of the internal valve is severely reduced, the main aim of surgical correction is to augment the angle and this is most readily accomplished by insertion of spreader grafts as advocated by Sheen (Fig. 3.15).[17] These are cartilage grafts, normally prepared from autograft cartilage, which are secured with fine sutures so that they lie in an extramucosal pocket on one or both sides of the nose and open the internal valve angle. The original description of spreader grafts was of an endonasal placement and as an adjunct in primary rhinoplasty, for they also have the secondary effect of re-establishing the dorsal aesthetic lines and hence improving the cosmetic appearance of the nose. They may still, of course, be employed as a means of cosmetic enhancement but they are now more readily used in revision cases where over-resection of the roof of the middle vault has resulted in collapse or

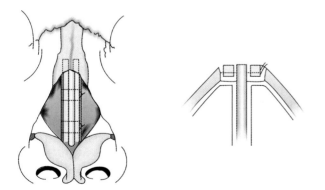

Fig. 3.15: Spreader grafts placed to open the valve angle

pinching of the internal valve. In such patients an external rhinoplasty approach to the dorsum is normally required.

External Nasal Valve Surgery

In patients with external valve collapse it is normally preferable to open the nose by and external rhinoplasty approach as, by so doing, the nature of the pathology can be more readily ascertained and the surgery tailored to the abnormalities revealed. However, there is a role for the internal approach in selected cases.

It seems to the authors that in cases where augmentation is required to strengthen the valve the general principal should be that, where possible, cartilage is placed as an underlay graft rather than as an overlay. This is clearly more correct empirically—as supporting a collapsing structure is clearly more effective if it is bolstered from below. In addition the graft needs to have some degree of robustness in order to be effective: An onlay graft that has strength may be effective but, if it is also readily palpable, will most probably not be acceptable cosmetically —especially in patients with thin skin. Grafts should therefore be fashioned so as they can be inserted in a mucosal pocket as an underlay to existing structures wherever this is practicable.

Of course a graft may not be necessary in some cases. If the lateral crus is well formed but is simply placed in too cephalad a position then such malposition can simply be corrected by transposing the crus to a more favorable site. If the crus is transected at the junction between the intermediate and lateral crura and rotated by 180° and secured it in a more caudal position then this simple maneuver will help to bolster the valve and prevent collapse. Occasionally, such transected crura can be swapped from one side to another—as this may improve apposition during suturing.

Two techniques can be used for transection. One technique involves complete dissection of the whole lateral crus and inversion but this involves dissecting the scroll area and can weaken the attachments between the lower and upper laterals. Therefore, if this technique is used the free or distal end of the lateral crus needs to be re-attached to the scroll area with polydioxanone (PDS) or nylon following the transposition. The other technique involves transecting the middle part (middle part where?) of the lateral crus only and leaving the free edge attached. In both cases the lateral crura can be further supported by the use of a lateral crura spanning suture, which will further increase distal flaring and help prevent collapse.

Obviously in both such approaches it it is important to dissect and preserve the vestibular mucosa. Moreover, it is also important to appreciate that, especially when operating on the lower lateral cartilages through the external approach tip projection can be weakened owing to disruption of the inter-domal ligaments. In such circumstances a columella strut placed between the medial crura will help to preserve projection and will help to maintain the airway.

An alternative approach is to bolster the collapsing lateral crus with a batten graft placed deep to the lateral crus (Fig. 3.16).[18] Such grafts, fashioned either from conchal or from septal cartilage, are ideally placed as caudal as possible to the natural lateral crus and are positioned such that they lie along the supra alar crease and onto the piriform aperture. These grafts should be slightly concave with the convexity facing the nasal vestibule. They have proved to provide good long-term results in follow-up over an eight year period, and are also effective at dealing with problem of alar pinching along the supra alar crease.

When then the lateral crus is weak due to previous over resection then reconstruction is necessary. New cartilages can be fashioned from harvesting the conchal bowl. The two resultant grafts, from the concha cavum and the cymber concha, are almost exactly equal in size and make satisfactory replacement crura. When sutured to the remnant cartilage and are very satisfactory in restoring function and improving the aesthetics in patients with pinched unnatural looking noses following over-resection.

In more severe cases where there is also deficiency of the middle vault restoration of form and function can be achieved using a butterfly graft.[19] These are also harvested from the concha and are rimmed to form a bi-lobed structure, which is then positioned on the dorsum of the middle vault and placed underneath the lateral crura and sutured into position. It is important aspect

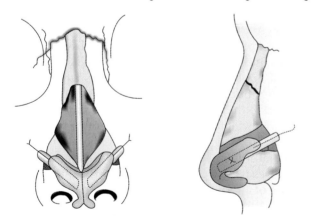

Fig. 3.16: Bolstering the collapsed lateral crus with a batten graft. Note the graft is placed deep to the lateral crus

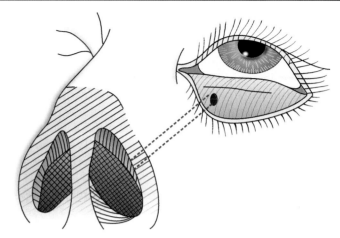

Fig. 3.17: Gortex sling hitching the ala to a titanium screw that is placed below the infraorbital ring

that the graft springs open the lateral crura for, if this does not happen, function may not be restored. Because of this it may be necessary to reverse the graft with concavity superior but, while this allows for increased flaring, such grafs may then produce an adverse cosmetic outcome.

Where a facial nerve palsy causes external valve the structure is, of course, likely to be normal. In such patients a hitching suture placed through a alar crease incision will anchor the alar to the maxillary periostium. Alternatively a *Gortex* sling can be employed whereby the alar is hitched up and anchored to a titanium screw inserted below the infraorbital ring (Fig. 3.17).[20] However, this procedure requires three incisions as sublabial and lower blepharoplasty incisions are required to mobilize subcuticular pockets and insert the screw and an alar crease incision is also required in order to attach the *Gortex* sling.

CONCLUSION

There is no doubt that disturbance of the function of the nasal valves cause obstruction in some patients. How these two valves interact is not fully understood but it appears that the paradoxical movements of the alae are essential to support the caudal upper lateral cartilages during inspiration and that, in turn, the supporting structures and muscles play a vital role in maintaining normal nasal patency. Thus, when routine rhinoplasty surgery is undertaken violation of the scroll area should be shunned wherever possible and aggressive cartilage resection of the alae should not be undertaken if a delayed complaint of nasal obstruction is to be avoided.

Medical measures to deal with valve complaints are unlikely to prove satisfactory for many and surgery is, therefore, often necessary. Such surgery may be difficult – especially in noses where scaring is marked, but the results are often highly gratifying and worthwhile. To some extent what is achieved will depend on the circumstances pertaining at the time. The general principles that result in a successful outcome have been outlined in this chapter but individual ingenuity is often also required if a reasonable outcome is to be achieved. What is important is that the patient is not dismissed and that we move, *en masse*, from the concept of septal and turbinate surgery being the only measures that will suffice in patients presenting to us with symptoms of nasal obstruction. Clearly, there is an emerging consensus to the effect that such an approach is too simplistic and we should be more aware than we are that the causes of surgically correctable obstruction are more complex than we had previously thought. In that regard it is not too extreme to suggest that the nasal valves should be examined and assessed in all our patients on a routine basis.

REFERENCES

1. Roblin DG, Eccles R. W*hat, if any, is the Value of Septal Surgery?* Clinical Otolaryngology 2000; 120(5):580-595.
2. Constantian MB, Clardy RB. *The Relative Importance of Septal and Nasal Valvular Surgery in Correcting Airway Obstruction in Primary and Secondary Rhinoplasty.* Plastic and Reconstructive Surgery 1996;98(1): 38-54.
3. Cassel's New English Dictionary 1999.
4. Mink PJ. *Physiologie der Oberen Luftwege.* Acta Otolaryngologica, Stock 1920; supplement 42.
5. Van Dishoeck HA. *Olfactometry in Children.* Monatsschr Ohrenheilkd Laryngorhinol 1965; 99(10): 460-462.
6. Bachmann W, legler U. *Studies of the Structure and Function of the Anterior Section of the Nose by Means of Luminal Impressions.* Acta. Otolaryngologica 1972; 73: 433-442.
7. Haight J, Cole P. *The Site and Function of the Nasal Valve.* Laryngoscope 1983; 93: 49-55.
8. Jones AS et al. The Nasal Valve: A Physiological and Clinical Study. *Journal of Laryngology and Otology* 1998; 102: 1089-1094.
9. Kasperbauer J, Kern E. *Nasal Valve Physiology. Implication in Nasal Surgery.* Otolaryngol Clin North Amer 1987; 20(4): 699-719.
10. Shaida AM, Kenyon GS. *The Nasal Valves: Changes in Anatomy and Physiology in Normal Subjects.* Rhinology 2000; 38: 7-12.
11. Olaki M, Naito K, Cole P. *Dimensions and Resistances of the Human Nose: Racial Differences.* Laryngoscope 1991; 101(3): 276-278.
12. Bridger G, Proctor DF. *Maximum Nasal Inspiratory Flow and Nasal Resistance.* Annals of Otology, Rhinology and Laryngology 1970; 99:481-488.
13. Cottle MH. Rhino-sphygmo-manometry and Aid in Physical Diagnosis. *International Rhinology* 1968; 6:7.
14. Elwany S, Thabet H. Obstruction of the Nasal Valve. *Journal of Laryngology and Otology* 1996; 110: 221-224.
15. Sheen JH, Sheen AP. *Aesthetic Rhinoplasty.* 2nd ed. 1987; St louis: Mosby.
16. Nolste Trenite GJ. *Rhinoplasty A Practical Guide to Functional and Aesthetic Surgery of the Nose.* 3rd ed, Nolste Trenite G J. 2005, The Hague: Kugler.
17. Sheen JH. Spreader Graft: Amethod of Reconstructing the Roof of the Middle Nasal Vault following Rhinoplasty. *Plastic Reconstructive Surgery* 1984; 73: 230-237.
18. Kalan A, Kenyon GS, Seemungal TA. Treatment of External Nasal Valve (alar rim) Collapse with an Alar Strut. *Journal of Laryngology and Otology* 2001; 115(10): 788-791.
19. Clark JM, Cook TA. The Butterfly Graft in Functional Secondary Rhinoplasty. *Laryngoscope* 2002; 112(11): 1917-1925.
20. Paniello RC. Nasal Valve Suspension. An Effective Treatment for Nasal Valve Collapse. *Arch. Otolaryngology Head and Neck Surgery* 1996; 1342-1346.

The Olfactory System and its Disorders

Letícia Schmidt Rosito, Mariana Magnus Smith
Sady Selaiman Da Costa

ANATOMY AND PHYSIOLOGY

The nasal cavities are formed by an extensive mucosa surface that lines a series of anatomical saliencies and re-entries, and allows inhaled air to come into contact with the covering tissues. The nose performs a series of functions in addition to the passage and regulation of inhaled air: Moisturizing, filtering and heating the air.[1] Perhaps, one of the most important functions of the nasal cavities is the sense of smell.[2]

Over the last few decades, there has been a renewed interest in the study of olfactory function.[3] Phylogenetically, smell is one of the oldest senses,[4] the olfactory cortical areas being older than the primary cortical regions that process other stimuli. The major difference,[5] however, between the primary olfactory system in mammals compared with other sensorial systems, is that there is no thalamic passage between the peripheral receptors and the olfactory cortex.[6] Thus, as with other regions of the sensorial system in which there is powerful feedback between the cortex and thalamic stations, there is greater feedback between the olfactory bulb and piriform cortex.[7,8] This process may help to refine the information processed in the bulb and in turn, influence the nature of the information presented to the piriform cortex.

The neurons that[9] represent the interface between the environment and the nervous system are the first odorant receptor neurons that are located in the olfactory epithelium in the nasal cavity in mammals. The nerve fascicles pass through small communications in the ethmoid bone portion that represents the roof of the nasal cavity, called the cribriform plate.

In rats, millions of odorant[10] receptor neurons that express approximately 1000 odorant receptors are located in the olfactory epithelium and are projected to around 1800 olfactory bulb glomeruli, the specific gromerular target depending on the odorant receptor expressed in each neuron.[11] The receptor neurons form a synapse with the second neurons and interneurons in the glomerulus. The glomeruli are morphologic[12] units composed of the odorant receptor cell terminals, the olfactory bulb projection neurons or second neurons (tufted cells T and mitral cells M) and the interneurons called periglomerular cells. Different subregions of the amygdala receive direct projections from the M/T neurons of the olfactory bulb. In particular, the nucleus of the lateral olfactory tract, the periamygdaloid cortex, anterior cortical nucleus and the amygdaloid nucleus regions. Other areas that receive projections from the olfactory bulb include the perirhinal cortex and entorhinal cortex (containing the third neurons). The third neurons situated in the amygdala and piriform cortex send projections to the entorhinal cortex, which in turn sends information to the dentate gyrus and hippocampal complex.

Neuroanatomy, therefore, suggests that distinct odors are first represented, in part, by the stimulation of distinct odorant receptor neurons, secondly by the activity of the mitral projection and tufted neurons,[13] whose identities may be discovered by their glomerular projections and thirdly, by the distinct synaptic fields activated in the third olfactory neurons.

The greatest scientific discoveries[14] in this area over the last few years, however, are related to the odorant receptors. In 1989, a specific G-protein olfactory neuron[15] was identified, suggesting that the mechanism coupled to the G-protein may be involved in the transduction of olfaction. Since then, Linda Buck, (winner of the Nobel Prize in 2004), has conducted exhaustive research to identify G-protein coupled receptors (GPCR) in the olfactory epithelium. Her experiments revealed sequences of multiple membranes of the family of receptors. In addition to their sharing sequences not seen in other GPCRs, the receptors are highly variable in sequence, consistent with the ability to recognize odorants with different structures. Northern blots and cDNA library screens showed that the receptor families were predominantly or exclusively expressed in the sensitive olfactory neurons. Genomic library screens with a mixed receptor probe revealed over 100 receptors per haploid genome. Given the limited complexity of the probe, this suggests that the family of odorant receptor genes may be composed of, at least, many hundreds of genes. In contrast with the immune system, in which both rearrangement and somatic mutation are involved in the generation of a diversity of antigen receptors, it would seem that each odorant receptor gene codifies a single receptor protein. It is known that mammals have approximately 1000 different types of odorant receptors and that each olfactory sense neuron expresses only one type. It is also known that each receptor recognizes multiple odorants, but that different odorants are detected by different combinations of receptors. Thus, the odorant receptors are used combinatorially to codify odorant entities in a scheme that may generate over a billion different odor codes, and thus allow a virtually unlimited number of chemical odors to be discriminated.

OLFACTORY DYSFUNCTIONS

Classification and Etiology

The assessment and treatment of a patient with complaints related to the sense of smell may be very complex and is frequently frustrating, because of the variety of pathologies that may be manifested in this way and the difficulty of definitive etiologic diagnosis in many cases.

Clinical manifestation of olfactory dysfunction may be classified as follows:[16]

- Anosmia—complete loss of olfaction
- Hyposmia—partial loss of olfaction
- Parosmia—qualitative alteration of olfaction
- Cacosmia—subjective sensation of disagreeable odor

From the etiologic point of view, it is initially possible to classify olfactory dysfunctions as conductive and neurosensorial pathologies. **Conductive** conditions are those in which some anatomic alteration or pathology prevents the inhaled air from reaching the roof of the nasal cavity and, therefore, impedes or diminishes odor perception. In this condition, there are the obstructions

generated by septal deviations, chronic inflammatory and infectious processes and tumors of the nasal cavity. Obstructive conditions in general have a better functional recovery prognosis with specific treatment, whereas **neurosensorial** conditions are caused by pathologies that affect the olfactory neurons or central areas of the olfactory way. In this group, there are the secondary alterations to upper respiratory infections (URI), cranioencephalic traumatism and neurological diseases like multiple sclerosis and Alzheimer's disease. The diagnosis of these situations is more complex and their prognosis is also poorer.

Some physiologic situations may alter olfaction. Thus, it is known for example, that as from the fifth decade of life, humans may present with a gradual process of diminished olfaction (presbiosmia). The sense of smell is also altered during pregnancy, being sharper in the first trimester and gradually decreasing in sensitivity by the end of gestation. Situations such as hunger, nausea and obesity increase olfactory sensitivity, while satiety diminishes it. The most frequent pathologic causes of olfactory alterations and their characteristics are presented as follows. The prevalence of the most frequent causes is listed in Table 4.1.

Mechanical Obstruction

These could be septal deviation in the superior portion of the sept, obstructive hypertrophy of the nasal shells and choanal atresia. Tumors, benign (such as nasosinus polyps or antrochoanal polyps) or malignant, may appear in nasal cavities and cause obstruction.

Inflammatory Processes

Rhinitis conditions[17] (especially allergic) are common causes of olfactory alterations because they generate edema of the mucosa and increased nasal cavity secretion, both of which reduce the inhaled air reaching the odorant receptors.

Infection

Infectious processes are also considered to be frequent causes of hyposmia and even anosmia.[18] The pathophysiologic process may be conductive, secondary to edema and production of secretion by de-aeration of the paranasal cavities. However, situations of respiratory neuroepithelium invasion, especially sensitive to viral action, particularly the influenza virus, also occur. In these

Authors	Infectious inflammatory disease (%)	Post upper airway infection (%)	Idiopathic conditions (%)	Cranial traumatism (%)
Cain et al (441 cases)	30.2	18.6	21	8.6
Temmel et al (278 cases)	21	36	18	17
Miwa et al (345 cases)	21.4	17.1	28.4	17
Seiden et al (428 cases)	14	18	18	18

Table 4.1: Etiologies found in the largest published series

cases of viral infection of the neuron cells, recovery is rare, and the older the patient, the worse it is.

Traumatism

Cranioencephalic traumatism conditions are responsible for olfactory alterations, especially in traumas of sudden deceleration, which may lead to rupture of the nerve filaments at the level of the cribriform plate. Studies have demonstrated that around 5% of patients with cranial traumatism evolve with partial or total olfactory loss. Magnetic resonance imaging studies in these situations indicate diminished olfactory bulb volume.

Tumors

In addition to the tumors of the nasal cavity itself, as already mentioned, there are also central neoplasias that compress the olfactory bulb and cause olfactory alteration, for example, meningiomas and suprasellar tumors. However, the clinical presentation of these pathologies is only rarely hyposmia or anosmia, and diagnosis is suspected by the correlated symptoms. Here it is important to emphasize the possibility of olfactory neuroblastomas or esthesioneuroblastomas, malignant neoplasias that present exactly at the level of the cribriform plate, are intranasal and intracranial in extent, and whose first symptom is usually anosmia.

Endocrinologic Pathologies

Patients with diabetes mellitus present with greater prevalence of olfactory dysfunction than the population in general, probably due to neuropathy. There is no relation between the glycemic level and the degree of olfactory alteration. Other endocrinologic diseases may also run their course with hyposmia.

Neurological Diseases

In persons with multiple sclerosis, Parkinson's disease, Alzheimer's disease and epilepsies, hyposmia or even anosmia may be present concurrent with other disease. However, the most frequent neurological cause in these situations is encephalic vascular accident.

Intoxication

Chemical substances like benzene, formaldehyde, solvents and carbon monoxide, as well as nicotine have been related to olfactory alterations. Several medications may also generate anomalies in this area, such as opiates, anticonvulsants, immunosuppressors, anthelmintics and anerobicide antibiotics.

Iatrogenic Disorders

These are especially related to surgical procedures in the cribriform plate region and to radiotherapy in this area.

Idiopathic Conditions

This category includes all cases in which it is not possible to find a definite cause for the clinical condition. With the evolution of research on olfactory alteration and the development of more precise diagnostic techniques, the conditions considered to be idiopathic have gradually diminished.

INVESTIGATIONS

While specific tests to characterize and quantify olfactory losses, as well as very specific radiological examination for assessment of these have been formulated, no method excels the detailed clinical history and complete regional physical examination for investigating the cause.

In **anamnesis,**[19] it is important to define the initial presentation of the condition, whether gradual or abrupt, and whether the patient relates it to a predisposing factor among those described above. Complete otorhinolaryngological examination must be made, nasal endoscopy being fundamental, with emphasis on visualizing the roof of the nasal fossa. The other cranial pairs must also be carefully tested. In patients with suspected associated dementia, the literature suggests that the Mini Mental State Examination be applied.

There are various **olfactory function tests** available for clinical use. These tests may be classified as **qualitative** (in which the tested individual must differentiate odors) or **quantitative** (which seek to establish the patient's olfactory threshold). Among the specific tests, perhaps the one most used is the UPSIT (The University of Pennsylvania Smell Identification), a commercially available test consisting of 40 microencapsulated odorants in a scratch-and-sniff format (Sensonics, Haddon Heights, NJ).

Radiological studies are carried out in the majority of patients who complain of anosmia or hyposmia without apparent cause. Computerized tomography is the best method for evaluating integrity of the cribriform plate bone. Magnetic resonance imaging provides information about the soft tissues and is very useful for identifying central alterations and for demonstrating the integrity of the dura mater. Functional magnetic nuclear resonance may be performed, in which specific cerebral activity is detected after stimulation with odorants. This exam, however, has up to now, primarily been used in research centers in this area. Several authors discuss the real need for performing image examinations in all patients with isolated hyposmia or anosmia, bearing in mind that in most cases, the exam does not change medical conduct.

TREATMENT

Treatment of olfactory dysfunction depends directly on the cause established. Obstructive anatomic alterations must be managed surgically, as well as cases of tumoral lesions in nasal fossae. Whenever a surgical procedure is proposed to a patient with hyposmia or anosmia for a probable obstructive cause, the real probability of postoperative improvement must be discussed in detail.

In cases of hyposmia due to allergic rhinitis, the use of corticoid spray may be beneficial for reducing the edema of the mucosa and normalizing the production of secretion. But in patients with undefined cause, the use of topical corticosteroids may not provide any benefits. On the contrary, various authors demonstrate clinical improvement with high doses of systemic corticotherapy in these patients.

No treatment has yet been defined for anosmia or hyposmia secondary to upper airway infection. It is estimated that approximately one-third of patients experience improvement in symptoms over a period of six months. The use of topical, systemic and zinc corticoids brought about no benefit.

REFERENCES

1. Buck, LB. The molecular architecture of odor and pheromone sensing in mammals. *Cell 2000*; 100:611–618.
2. Buck, LB. The search for odorant receptors. *Cell 2004*; S116:S117–S118.
3. Buck LB, Axel, R. A novel multigene family may encode odorant receptors: A molecular basis for odor recognition. *Cell 1991*; 65:175–187.
4. Busaba NY. Is imaging necessary in the evaluation of the patient with an isolated complaint of anosmia? *Ear Nose Throat* 2001; 80:892–896.
5. Cain WS, Gent JF, Goodspeed RB. Evaluation of olfactory dysfunction in the Connecticut Chemosensory Clinical Research Center. *Laryngoscope* 1988; 98:83–88.
6. Davis R. Olfactory learning. *Neuron* 2004; 44:31–48.
7. Doty RL, Shaman P, Kimmelman CP. University of Pennsylvania smell Identification Test: A rapid quantitative olfactory function test for the clinic. *Laryngoscope* 1984; 94: 176–178.
8. Holdbrooke E, Leopold D. Anosmia: Diagnosis and management. *Cur Opin Otolaryngol Head Neck Surg* 2003; 11: 54–60.
9. Kern RC, Quinn B, Rousseau G. Post-traumatic olfactory dysfunction. *Laryngoscope* 2000; 110:2106–2109.
10. Kern RC, Conley DB, Haines GK, Robinson AM. Patho-logy of the olfactory mucosa: Implications for the treatment of olfactory dysfunction. *Laryngoscope* 2004; 114: 279–285.
11. Landis BN, Konnerth CG, Hummel, T. A study on the frequency of olfactory dysfunction. *Laryngoscope 2004*; 114:1764–1769.
12. Levy LM. Why should neuroradiologists study patients with smell loss? *Am J Neuroradiol* 2003; 24:556–558.
13. Malnic B, Godfrey PA, Buck LB. The human olfactory receptor gene family. *Proc Natl Acad Sci* 2004; 101:2584–2589.
14. Miwa T, Furukawa M, Tsukatani T. Impact of olfactory impairment on quality of life and disability. *Arch Otolaryngol Head Neck Surg* 2001; 127:497–504.
15. Ranganathan R, Buck LB. Olfactory axon pathfinding: Who is the pied piper? *Neuron* 2002; 35: 599–604.
16. Sam M, Vora S, Malnic B et al. Odorants may arouse instinctive behaviors. *Nature* 2001; 412:142.
17. Santos DV, Reiter ER, Dinardo L, Costanzo R. Hazardous events associated with impaired olfactory function. *Arch Otolaryngol Head Neck Surg* 2004; 130:317–319.
18. Seiden AM, Duncan HJ. The diagnosis of a conductive olfactory loss. *Laryngoscope* 2001; 11:9–14.
19. Yousen DM, Geckle RJ, Bilker WB et al. Posttraumatic olfactory dysfunction: MR and clinical evaluation. *Am J Neuroradiol* 1996; 17:1171–1179.

CHAPTER 5

Juvenile Nasopharyngeal Angiofibroma

Renuka A Bradoo

Juvenile nasopharyngeal angiofibroma (JNA) bears the dubious reputation of being one of the most surgically challenging tumors in the head and neck region. Its propensity to grow through narrow bony crevices along the base skull and its highly vascular nature often make it difficult to achieve complete excision of the tumor, resulting in the frequently reported recurrences. Although Hippocrates may have been the first to recognize the nature of this polypoidal tumor, it was not until 1940 that the term 'angiofibroma' was coined by Friedberg.[1] Martin, Ehrlich and Abels in 1948, described the associated features of JNA and the hormonal theory of its origin. The first successful resection of a probable JNA is credited to Liston in 1841 at University College Hospital in London.

JNA is an uncommon tumor, the reported incidence varying from 1 in 5,000 to 1 in 60,000 ENT patients. It accounts for 0.5% of all head and neck tumors[2] and is considered the most common benign neoplasm of the nasopharynx.

JNA occurs almost exclusively in young males. The most common age group is 10 to 18 years, with an average age of around 14 years.[3,4] The youngest case reported in literature was a newborn infant.[5] Fu et al have reported a case of JNA in a 79-year-old man.[6]

Angiofibromas do rarely occur in females. The highest incidence in female patients was 16% reported by Handousa[3] in Egypt. The author has personal experience of one such case. Chromosomal studies are advisable in these patients.

ETIOPATHOGENESIS—A REVIEW OF LITERATURE

In spite of the numerous theories proposed to explain the origin of JNA, the exact histogenesis of the tumor remains debatable. The tumor is most commonly believed to arise at the site where the sphenoidal process of the palatine bone articulates with the base of the sphenoid and the horizontal ala of the vomer. This area forms the superior border of the sphenopalatine foramen and lies just above the posterior end of the middle turbinate.[7]

Speculations on the tissue's origin were first made in the nineteenth century by Nelaton,[8] Verneuil,[9] and Tillaux,[10] who defined angiofibromas as fibrous neoplasms arising from periosteum or embryonic fibro-cartilage of the skull base. Assuming its nasopharyngeal origin, Coenen,[11] Sebileau,[12] Ringertz[13] and Som and Neffson[14] further speculated that cartilage or periosteum served as a matrix for angiofibromas. Whereas authors such as Martin et al[15] and Dane,[16] focused on a hormonal imbalance as the cause of these tumors, Sternberg,[17] and Hubbard[18] started to discuss angiofibromas as vascular neoplasms similar to hemangiomas. In 1942, Brunner[19] finally described endothelium-lined vascular spaces in the fascia basalis and proposed that angiofibromas originated from this tissue. Similarities to nasal erectile tissue were noted by Osborn.[20] Schiff[21] suggested that angiofibromas were ectopic vascular tissue that grew as a result of alterations in pituitary activity. Maurice and Milad[22] interpreted angiofibromas as hamartomas resulting from misplaced genital erectile tissue. The variety of vascular irregularities associated with angio-fibromas led Beham et al to conclude that they are vascular malformations. In addition to the two main theories of either fibrous or vascular origin, many other hypotheses have been proposed. One such theory proposes that these tumors originate from non-chromaffin paraganglionic cells present at the terminal end of the maxillary artery.[23] All attempts to date have failed to define a widely accepted origin of this rare fibrovascular tumor.

The last decade has seen numerous studies being conducted in an attempt to understand the underlying deranged molecular mechanisms which lead to the formation of this tumor, most commonly in adolescent boys. Immunohistochemical studies, *in vitro* culture of tumor cells and the behavior of tumor tissue in animal models are only some of the methods that have been used. The role of factors such as androgens, transforming growth factor (TGF β1) and vascular endothelial growth factor (VEGF)[24] has been studied. mRNA coding for proto-oncogenes and suppressor genes related to proliferation of tumor has also been undertaken.

Nagaii et al found that transforming growth factor (TGF) B_1 and IGF-II show statistically increased expression in these tumors than in controls suggesting that they may be growth regulators of nasopharyngeal angiofibromas. Platelet derived growth factor (PDGF-B) can contribute, at least in part to neovascularization and fibrosis.[25]

Recent evidence suggests that angiofibromas are extracolonic manifestations of familial adenomatous polyposis.[26,27] JNA has been reported to occur at increased frequency among patients with familial adenomatous polyposis (FAP), suggesting that it is a true neoplasm with alterations of the adenomatous polyposis coli (APC)/ β-catenin pathway.[28]

The immunohistochemical localization of β-catenin only to the nuclei of stromal cells further suggests that the stromal cells, rather than endothelial cells are the neoplastic cells of JNA. However, certain studies suggest that these tumors are predominantly vaso-proliferative malformations because of their tendency to bleed, their striking vascularity and the presence of angiogenic growth factors within the endothelial cells.[29,30] Some other studies have found androgen receptors in both endothelial and stromal cells although the staining was more intense in the latter.[31]

Schick et al studied sex chromosome observations in JNA. They found a significant loss of chromosome Y in combination with a gain of chromosome X.[32]

Even as extensive research to discover the etiological factor(s) in this tumor continues, a widely accepted theory of origin is yet to be established.

PATHOLOGY

On gross examination, the tumor is a firm, lobulated, non-encapsulated mass which is pinkish white. It has a broad, sessile base in the posterior part of the nasal cavity and the nasopharynx. A primary, non-operated tumor has a

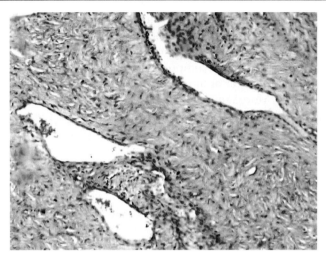

Fig. 5.1: Histological section (H and E stain) of JNA showing thin walled vascular channels within partially collagenized fibrous stroma (*Courtesy*: Department of Pathology, LTM Medical College and General Hospital, Mumbai)

definite pattern of adherence to surrounding structures from which it takes parasitic blood supply.

The consistency and friability of the tumor depends on the relative percentage of vascular to fibrous tissue within it, which may vary in individual tumors. It is generally noted that the fibrous component and nodularity increases with increase in age of the patient.

Microscopically, the tumor is composed of thin walled vessels of varying caliber interspersed in a mature connective tissue stroma. The vessels typically have a single endothelial cell lining without a muscularis layer (Fig. 5.1). This explains the propensity of the tumor to bleed profusely as the vessels do not constrict on being cut. The tumor cells show features of both fibroblasts and smooth muscle cells and are termed as myofibroblasts. The presence of JNA can be evidenced preoperatively by electron micrographs showing dense perichromatin granula distributed irregularly within the nuclei of fibroblasts.[33]

MODE OF SPREAD

The tumor usually originates where the palatine bone articulates with the body of the sphenoid to form the sphenopalatine foramen. Due to its benign nature, it has a propensity to grow through narrow bony crevices along the base skull widening fissures and foramina, but without destroying intervening bone. The tumor grows medially into the nasal cavity. It extends for a variable distance anteriorly but more often extends posteriorly into the nasopharynx. As the nasopharyngeal component enlarges, it begins to block the posterior choana of the opposite nostril and may also cause the soft palate to bulge downwards. Occasionally, a lateral extension of the nasopharyngeal component may grow laterally over the upper border of the superior constrictor through the sinus of Morgagni to attain the parapharyngeal space behind the pterygoid plates. This portion of the tumor is globular in shape and tends to occupy the pterygoid fossa between the two pterygoid plates.

The tumor may also extend into the sphenoid sinus eroding through the floor of the sinus. It tends to remain in the submucosal plane within the sphenoid sinus. Rarely, a very large tumor may erode the lateral wall or roof of the sinus to compress the cavernous sinus or pituitary gland.

From its origin at the sphenopalatine foramen, the tumor very commonly tends to grow laterally through the foramen into the pterygopalatine fossa. Here it lies anterior to the pterygoid plates and behind the postero-lateral wall of the maxillary sinus. It causes widening of the pterygopalatine fossa and anterior bowing of the posterior wall of the maxilla. Involvement of the maxillary sinus itself is fairly infrequent. It may continue to grow further laterally to enter the infratemporal fossa. Here, it usually enlarges to form a large bulky mass. The tumor can extend inferiorly behind the medial pterygoid muscle to enter the parapharyngeal space. It may also extend under the zygoma to produce a swelling in the temporal fossa. Thus, one can have two large masses of the tumor, one in the nose and nasopharynx and the other in the infratemporal fossa with an intervening small pedicle at the pterygopalatine fossa.

From the pterygopalatine fossa the tumor may also grow superiorly to enter and widen the inferior orbital fissure. The tumor always remains outside the orbital periosteum. In the event of involvement of the orbit at the level of the orbital apex, the tumor may extend from the inferior orbital fissure into the superior orbital fissure. It may then extend intracranially through the superior orbital fissure to cause involvement of the cavernous sinus.

The roof of the infratemporal fossa is formed by the greater wing of the sphenoid. The tumor may directly erode the greater wing or widen and pass through the foramen ovale to enter the cranial cavity lateral to the cavernous sinus in an extradural plane (Figs 5.2A and B).

CLASSIFICATION

There are numerous classifications described in literature. However, the Andrew–Fisch classification[34] and Radkowsky (revised Sessions) classification[35] are particularly useful in planning management protocols and predicting prognosis.

Andrew-Fisch Classification

The latest and most widely used classification is the Andrew-Fisch classification (1989):

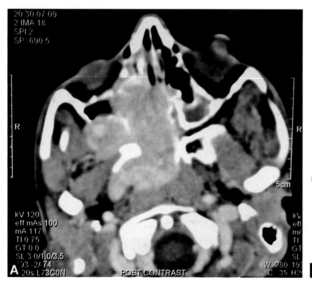 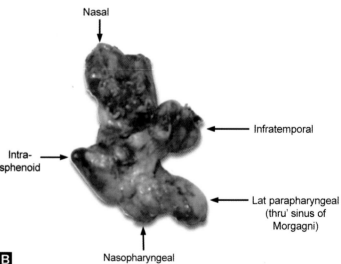

Figs 5.2A and B: (A) Contrast-enhanced axial CT scan showing characteristic mode of spread of tumor. (B) Postoperative tumor specimen of the same patient showing extensions that correlate with the preoperative CT scan

Stage I: Tumor limited to the nasopharynx and nasal cavity; bone destruction is negligible or limited to the sphenopalatine fossa.

Stage II: Tumor involving the pterygopalatine fossa or maxillary, ethmoid or sphenoid sinus with bone destruction.

Stage IIIA: Tumor involving the infratemporal fossa or orbital region without intracranial involvement.

Stage IIIB: Tumor involving the infratemporal fossa or orbital region with intracranial, extradural (parasellar) involvement.

Stage IVA: Intracranial, intradural tumor without infiltration of cavernous sinus, pituitary fossa or optic chiasma.

Stage IVB: Intracranial intradural tumor with infiltration of cavernous sinus, pituitary fossa and/or optic chiasma.

Radkowsky Classification

Stage IA: Tumor limited to posterior nares and/or nasopharyngeal vault.

Stage IB: Tumor involving the posterior nares and/or nasopharyngeal vault with involvement of at least one paranasal sinus.

Stage IIA: Minimal lateral extension into the pterygomaxillary fossa.

Stage IIB: Full occupation of the pterygomaxillary fossa with or without superior erosion of orbital bones.

Stage IIC: Extension into the infratemporal fossa or extension posterior to the pterygoid plates.

Stage IIIA: Erosion of the base skull (middle cranial fossa/base of pterygoids)—minimal intracranial extension.

Stage IIIB: Extensive intracranial extension with or without extension into the cavernous sinus.

MODE OF ADHERENCE

The primary, non-operated JNA shows a predictable and definite mode of adherence to surrounding structures. The tumor almost always has adhesions to the posterior end of the middle turbinate. It often has flimsy adherence to the superior turbinate and is almost never adherent to the inferior turbinate. It is very frequently adherent to the posterior end of the septum. It shows dense adhesions in the nasopharynx, especially the fossa of Rosenmuller, basisphenoid and the roof of the posterior choana. It is almost never attached to the floor of the nasal cavity. The

sphenoid sinus is commonly invaded by the tumor. Fortunately, this extension of the tumor occurs submucosally and there are usually no adhesions to the walls of the sphenoid sinus. A tumor invading the pterygopalatine and infratemporal fossa tends to grow by compressing the surrounding tissues, and hence a plane of cleavage can be easily obtained between the firm tumor tissue and the surrounding soft tissue. This advantage is lost in a previously operated tumor. Hence, the best chance of complete tumor removal is at the first surgery itself. The presence of tumor in the pterygopalatine and infratemporal fossa may cause marked anterior bowing of the posterolateral wall of the maxilla, but surprisingly the sinus itself is not very commonly involved.

A recurrent, previously operated tumor does not show any predictable patterns of adherence. The adhesions are far more dense and it is very often difficult to distinguish normal tissue from the tumor.

BLOOD SUPPLY

The tumor is supplied most commonly by the ipsilateral maxillary artery. Other major feeding vessels are the maxillary artery of the opposite side and the ascending pharyngeal artery. There may also be a feeder from the vidian canal and small vessels from the internal carotid artery which may perforate the body of the sphenoid to supply the tumor directly. The tumor usually has a significant internal carotid artery supply when there is an intracranial component or the external carotid artery has been ligated during the first surgery in a recurrent, previously operated tumor.

CLINICAL FEATURES

Unilateral nasal obstruction and recurrent profuse epistaxis in a young male patient are the hallmarks of this disease. The epistaxis is profuse, recurrent in nature and from one nostril. The patient may present with anemia. The degree of nasal block depends on the size of the tumor. A large nasopharyngeal extension can cause snoring, mouth breathing, adenoid facies, rhinolalia clausa and signs of eustachian tube dysfunction, such as blocking of ears, otalgia and a conductive hearing loss. The patient may also have a sense of heaviness on one side of the face though headache is not very common.

A small tumor extension into the pterygopalatine fossa or infratemporal fossa does not cause any specific symptoms. However, a large mass may present with a bulge in the cheek or proptosis if the orbit is involved (Fig. 5.3). Intracranial involvement is usually extradural, asymptomatic and is usually detected only on

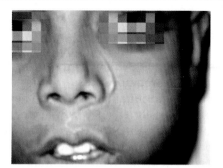

Fig. 5.3: Patient of JNA presenting with a bulge on the cheek and a facial scar from previous surgery

radiological investigation. However, a case of meningitis, diabetes insipidus, proptosis and ptosis due to involvement of the meninges, compression of the pituitary gland and involvement of the cavernous sinus respectively has been seen by the author. Symptoms suggestive of direct neural involvement, such as blindness, are very rare.

It is a matter of clinical coincidence that a number of cases undergo a septoplasty or polypectomy for unilateral nasal blockage in which the ENT surgeon has found the tumor or rather the tumor has found the ENT surgeon! Therefore, it behoves the ENT surgeon to have a high index of suspicion while treating young male patients with unilateral nasal obstruction.

DIAGNOSIS

A preliminary diagnosis can usually be made on the basis of the history and clinical examination of the patient. A careful nasal endoscopy helps confirm the diagnosis. A biopsy is usually not necessary and is advisable only in those cases where the histopathological diagnosis seems doubtful, e.g. in the rare event of a female patient of JNA. Examination should also include otoscopy, tuning fork tests, evaluation of the CNS and an ophthalmological examination.

A CT scan with contrast is the gold standard for diagnosing JNA (Fig. 5.4). It gives information regarding the regions involved, erosion of the base skull and vascularity of the tumor. Both axial and coronal cuts with bony and soft tissue windows are necessary to evaluate the tumor in detail. Sagittal reconstructions may further help in understanding the three-dimensional spread of the tumor along the base skull.

An MRI is essential in case of intracranial extension of the tumor and in case of a significant infratemporal or intraorbital extension. In these cases, the MRI helps distinguish tumor tissue from retained sinus secretions and more importantly, from surrounding soft tissue like the brain or pterygoid muscles (Figs 5.5A and B).

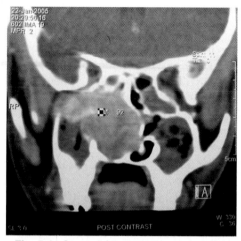

Fig. 5.4: Coronal CT scan showing marked enhancement and the extension of the tumor

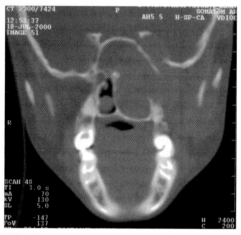

Fig. 5.5A: CT scan (bony window) showing involvement of sphenoid sinus, ITF and intracranial spread

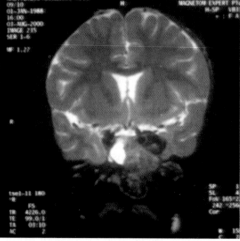

Fig. 5.5B: MRI scan helps (i) differentiate tumor from secretions in sphenoid sinus, (ii) show the relationship of tumor to the ICA and temporal lobe of the brain

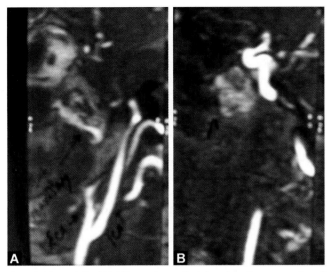

Figs 5.6A and B: (A) MR angiography showing the external and internal carotid artery systems. (B) MR angiography showing the relationship of the tumor to the ICA siphon

An MR angiography is especially useful in intra-cavernous extensions of the tumor. It helps to diagnose compression or encasement of the internal carotid artery by the tumor. Feeder vessels from the ICA system can also be identified (Figs 5.6A and B).

Although MR angiography has the advantage of being a non-invasive procedure, it cannot be substituted for digital subtraction angiography (DSA) which is necessary to embolize vessels feeding the tumor. Highly selective embolization is carried out with a microcatheter using PVA particles (Figs 5.7A and B). This has significantly reduced the complications previously associated with embolization of the proximal larger vessels.

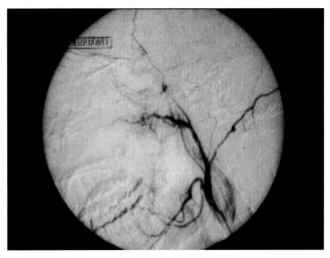

Fig. 5.7B: Postembolization film—complete absence of tumor blush

Intratumoral injection of tissue glue and lipidiol can also be done in tumors which have a significant internal carotid artery supply or recurrent tumors where the external carotid artery has been ligated (Fig. 5.8). The author has attempted surgery after varying intervals of time following embolization. Surgery done 48 to 72 hours after embolization seems to give optimum results.

TREATMENT

Surgery is the primary modality of management of JNA since there is no established medical line of treatment available which has conclusively proved effective against JNA, although hormonal therapy[21,36,37] has been

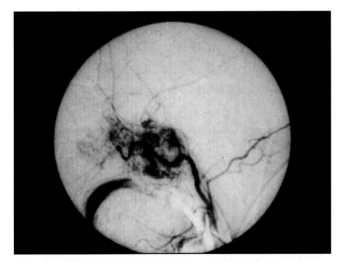

Fig. 5.7A: Digital subtraction angiography—pre-embolization tumor blush

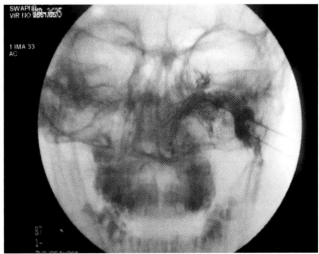

Fig. 5.8: Direct puncture technique of tumor embolization

empirically used. Radiotherapy in the head and neck region for a benign tumor in a young patient is too radical a measure except in those cases of life-threatening, intracranial extension of the tumor.

Principles of Surgery

The basic underlying surgical principles for removal of this tumor are:

1. A wide of the tumor bed including all its extensions by removing intervening bony partitions. The surgeon must have a sound knowledge of the complex anatomy of the base skull in order to do this without causing complications.
2. Subperiosteal dissection of the adhesions of the tumor to surrounding structures so as to avoid breaching tumor parenchyma.
3. Ensure that bleeding is kept to the minimum possible so as to carry out dissection under direct vision in a relatively bloodless field. Various measures such as embolization[38-40] (see box) or ligation of feeding vessels can be done. Besides taking these precautions to reduce blood loss, autotransfusion can also be tried.
4. To try and ensure that the complete tumor is removed preferably in a single piece so that chances of recurrence are reduced.

Preoperative Embolization

- Newer techniques of embolization make use of microcatheters and very fine PVA (polyvinyl alcohol) particles (150 to 250 μ).
- This ensures a more distal and selective embolization of the tumor bed unlike the earlier, more proximal, non-selective and riskier techniques.
- Besides embolization of the main feeder vessels, a direct puncture technique[38] using lipidiol and N-butyl cyanoacrylate (glue) can be done in those tumors with a significant ICA supply or where the external carotid artery has been previously ligated.
- The interval between embolization and surgery can vary from 24 to 72 hours. The author prefers a minimum interval of 48 hours.

Surgical Approaches

A large number of surgical approaches have been described in literature ranging from more limited ones like the lateral rhinotomy and transpalatal approach to the more extensive ones like the Weber Ferguson, maxillary swing and facial translocation approaches.

Most of the open approaches leave a disfiguring scar on the face. The transpalatal and midfacial degloving approaches are exceptions to this. The main disadvantage of limited approaches like the transpalatal and lateral rhinotomy is that they very often fail to expose the entire tumor bed. Semiblind dissection done through these limited approaches can lead to tearing of the tumor and leaving behind tumor extensions which later lead to a recurrence of the tumor. The more extensive approaches provide a wider exposure of the tumor and its extensions, but have the disadvantage of significant postoperative morbidity and a disfiguring scar. The midfacial degloving approach, alone of the open approaches affords a very wide exposure of the tumor bed without leaving behind a facial scar (Fig. 5.9). The last few years have witnessed an increasing number of reports in literature concerning the endoscopic excision of angiofibroma.[41-44] Using the endoscope, it is now possible to break intervening bony septae so as to reach various tumor extensions and operate upon them under direct vision. This naturally results in far better clearance of the tumor than the almost blind probing with fingers which was used earlier. Embolization and meticulous dissection under endoscopic vision have significantly decreased intraoperative blood loss, very often making it possible to complete the surgery without any blood transfusions. Large anterior and postnasal packs can be avoided in most cases which significantly reduces postoperative morbidity. The patient has no external scar but more importantly, since all tumor extensions have been dissected under direct vision, chances of recurrence are significantly lower with endoscopic excision. The disadvantage of endoscopic excision is that torrential hemorrhage would be difficult

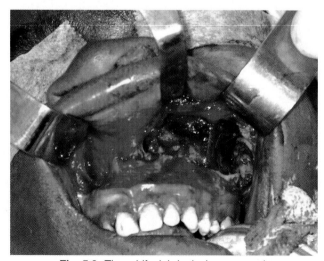

Fig. 5.9: The midfacial degloving approach

to control. Risk of hemorrhage is greater at certain sites, e.g. from the maxillary artery in the infratemporal fossa, the vidian canal, the greater palatine artery, perforating branches of the ICA through the body of the sphenoid and the cavernous sinus. It would be necessary to convert to an open approach if this occurs. In the author's experience, difficult areas to reach endoscopically are the far lateral and lower reaches of the infratemporal fossa, the pterygoid fossa and foramen lacerum (see box).

Surgical Technique for Endoscopic Excision of JNA (Figs 5.10A to D)

- Diagnostic endoscopy to review extensions and adhesions of the tumor.
- Cauterization and dissection of the adhesions to the middle and superior turbinate.
- Partial trimming of the middle turbinate for improved access.
- Opening the maxillary sinus and removing the medial and posterolateral walls to gain access to the infratemporal fossa.
- Cauterization and incision of the infratemporal fossa periosteum to release the tumor.
- Dissection of the infratemporal extension starting at its most lateral boundary.
- Cauterization or clipping of the maxillary artery.
- Clearance of the ethmoid cells and opening the sphenoid by the lateral approach.
- Floor and anterior wall of the sphenoid removed and tumor gradually delivered out of sphenoid sinus.
- Tumor adhesions to septum and nasopharynx cauterized and dissected.
- Tumor delivered transorally once all its extensions have been dissected and it is free of any adhesions.

Advantages

- Meticulous subperiosteal dissection of tumor extensions under direct vision.
- Significantly minimized blood loss.
- None or fewer blood transfusions required.
- No tight nasal packs necessary (Merocel can be kept for 24 to 48 hours). Decreased postoperative morbidity.
- Decreased duration of hospital stay.
- A decrease in the rate of recurrence due to en bloc removal of the entire tumor under direct vision.
- Endoscopic monitoring on follow-up possible.
- No external scar.

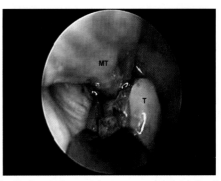

Fig. 5.10A: Endoscopic excision—cauterization of adhesions of the tumor (T) to the middle turbinate (MT) using a crocodile action cautery forceps

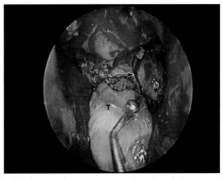

Fig. 5.10B: Medial and posterolateral walls of the maxillary sinus have been removed. The tumor in the nasal cavity (T), with its pterygopalatine and infratemporal fossa extension (*) is seen along with the intervening perpendicular plate of palatine bone (arrow)

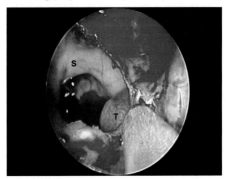

Fig. 5.10C: Dissection of the tumor (T) from the sphenoid sinus (S)

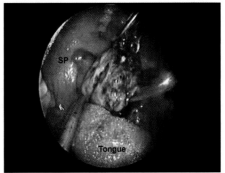

Fig. 5.10D: Transoral delivery of the tumor (SP—soft palate)

Prerequisites and Limitations

- A good preoperative embolization is mandatory for endoscopic surgery.
- Severe intraoperative hemorrhage may make it necessary to either convert to an open procedure or to stage the surgery.
- A very large intranasal mass may not allow adequate access for the endoscope.
- Erosion of the greater wing of the sphenoid, e.g. the foramen lacerum, can be more directly approached through a Weber Ferguson than an endoscopic approach.

Choice of Approach

There is no single approach which is suitable for all types of tumors. The approach one chooses would depend first and foremost upon the stage of the tumor and the regions involved. Other factors such as the experience of the surgeon and the infrastructure available would also play a role. With growing experience, it is now possible to tackle large tumors endoscopically. In fact, the endoscope may give access to hitherto 'blind' areas such as the cavernous sinus and the pterygoid fossa. With increasing experience we have come to realize that a wide open approach may not necessarily give as good an access to deeper hidden crevices as the endoscope would. The endoscope could also be used along with an open approach to maximize the benefits of both. It is also useful for monitoring the patients for follow-up.

Amongst the open approaches, one of the most versatile is the midfacial degloving, which affords wide access to both the nasal cavity as well as the pterygopalatine and infratemporal fossa. It leaves behind no scar. The disadvantage is the significant postoperative morbidity in the form of facial edema. The maxillary swing, mandibular swing and facial translocation approaches are most likely to be used for huge tumors especially recurrent ones where there are dense adhesions obliterating tissue planes which prevent the tumor being delivered out. Intraorbital extensions through the inferior orbital fissure and to a limited extent into the superior orbital fissure can be dealt with endoscopically. Large extensions into the infratemporal fossa are difficult to handle endoscopically. However, the author has devised a 'push-pull' technique whereby a finger is inserted through a small incision in the buccogingival sulcus to 'push' the tumor while a forcep helps 'pull' and deliver the tumor endoscopically.

Intracranial extensions of the tumor continue to remain a dilemma. It is possible to remove an extradural extension through the greater wing of sphenoid. This is better done using an open approach like the midfacial degloving or the Weber Ferguson approach. Minimal involvement of the cavernous sinus can be dealt with endoscopically provided there is a safe plane of cleavage between the tumor and the internal carotid artery and the main nerves in the lateral wall of the cavernous sinus. It may not be possible to deal with greater intracranial involvement surgically. Such cases may be followed up in the hope of spontaneous regression of the tumor.[45] The gamma knife may be used for a small localized intracranial lesion. Hormone therapy has also been tried on the premise that the tumor is hormone-dependent. Radiotherapy should be a last resort and be used in those cases of intracranial tumors which continue to show increase in size.

The principles of management of recurrent tumors remain the same as that for primary tumors. However, it must be said that it is more difficult to achieve a complete en bloc removal of a recurrent tumor. This is because of the dense adhesions which anchor the tumor to the surrounding tissues and the difficulty in identifying tumor tissue from surrounding non-specific fibrous tissue. Recurrent tumors also are notorious for deriving a large component of their blood supply from the internal carotid system especially if the external carotid artery has been ligated previously. The author is not in favor of ligation of the external carotid artery except as an emergency measure and instead prefers selective embolization of the tumor. Thus, in angiofibroma surgery, the first chance at tumor removal is nearly always the best chance.

Differential Diagnosis

JNA can occasionally be mistaken for other benign or malignant tumors of the nose and nasopharynx. Of these, the most common lesion to be mistaken for JNA or vice versa is an infected antrochoanal polyp (Fig. 5.11). Stories abound of surgeons attempting a 'polypectomy' much to their own horror and the patient's detriment.

Other conditions which can commonly be confused with the JNA are an angiomatous polyp, a cavernous hemangioma, nasopharyngeal carcinoma, rhabdomyosarcoma, chordoma, Kaposi sarcoma, lymphoproliferative lesions and inverted papilloma. The age of the patient, history of profuse, spontaneous epistaxis and the characteristic features on contrast-enhanced CT scans can usually differentiate a JNA from the above conditions.

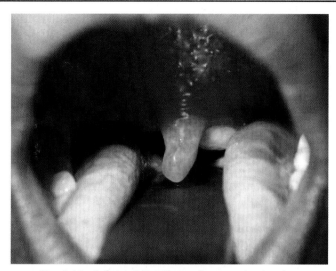

Fig. 5.11: A large JNA with oropharyngeal extension masquerading as an antrochoanal polyp

Prognosis

Recent advances in technology have played a significant role in improving the prognosis of these tumors. High resolution imaging techniques like the CT scan and MRI not only give detailed information about the various extensions of the tumor but have also helped in improving our understanding of the three-dimensional anatomy of the base skull which is critical if one is to remove these tumors safely without any complications. The endoscope gives a magnified, illuminated view and enables us to operate on the extensions of the tumor under direct vision. Newer techniques of embolization have ensured a relatively bloodless field and decreased patient morbidity.

There are various factors which directly impact the long-term prognosis in these patients. A primary tumor has a far better prognosis than a previously operated one. This has already been discussed at length. Recurrence rates of 55% in extensive tumors,[46,47] 25% in moderate size tumors[48] and 15% in small tumors[49] have been quoted. However, in the author's experience, size of the tumor alone is not the only prognostic factor; the actual areas involved are crucial. Certain sites like the superior orbital fissure, interpterygoid fossa, the foramen lacerum and cavernous sinus are more difficult to approach and there is a greater chance of recurrence if these areas are involved. A large intracranial component especially within the cavernous sinus would naturally worsen the prognosis. Very friable tumors and those with a significant post-embolization blush are also difficult to manage. A previous history of early recurrence with rapid regrowth of the tumor suggests an aggressive lesion.

Certain surgical factors also play a role in deciding prognosis. A relatively bloodless surgery where all the extensions of the tumor have been dissected under direct vision and the tumor is delivered either transnasally or transorally in one single piece suggests a good prognosis with a low chance of recurrence. In contrast, the inability to account for certain extensions of the tumor as seen on the CT scan and piecemeal removal of the tumor naturally suggest a more guarded prognosis.

Lastly, but more importantly, good preoperative planning to decide on a customized treatment plan in every individual case goes a long way in improving the prognosis. Reviewing the patient's clinical presentation, his CT, MRI and embolization plates and correlating them with a dry skull significantly increases the chances of complete tumor removal. Thus, the value of a pre-operative brainstorming session cannot be over-emphasized.

Newer Avenues

Future research of JNA would essentially comprise a four-pronged approach.
- To study the various mechanisms which occur at a molecular level that are responsible for the growth of this tumor or hamartoma.
- To device a standard protocol of surgical management on the basis of staging of the tumor. This would need to be based on the collective experience of multiple referral centers which deal with this tumor on a regular basis.
- To assess on a long-term basis, the relative risks and benefits of alternative therapies such as radiotherapy and hormonal therapy. To also assess the role of watchful observation awaiting spontaneous regression of the tumor.
- To assess the role of various factors in deciding the ultimate prognosis of a tumor in any patient.

CONCLUSION

Although JNA is a benign tumor it shows locally aggressive behavior in one of the most complicated anatomical regions of the body, viz. the base skull. It may be difficult to excise completely; this can lead to an unfortunate chain of events which include repeated, extensive and highly morbid surgeries and occasionally even mortality. Those adolescents who receive radio-therapy face a life-time of uncertainty about the development of malignant neoplasms in the head, neck region.

This bleak scenario has been considerably improved upon by the advances in technology, increasing understanding about the behavior of the tumor and the addition of the endoscope to the armamentarium of the surgeon. But the final answers will lie in having a better understanding of the etiopathogenesis of this tumor and its behavior at a molecular level.

REFERENCES

1. Friedberg SA. Nasopharyngeal fibroma. *Arch Otolaryngol* 1940; 31:313–326.
2. Batsakis JG. Vasoformative tumors. In Batsakis JG. (Ed.) *Tumors of the Head and Neck, Clinical and Pathological Considerations*. 2nd ed. Baltimore: Williams & Wilkins Co., 1979; 296–300.
3. Handousa F. Nasopharyngeal Fibroma. *J Laryngol Otol* 1954; 68:647–666.
4. Bensch H, Ewing J. *Neoplastic Diseases*. 4th edn. Philadelphia: WB Saunders and Company, 1941.
5. Chaikovskii VK. Angiofibroma of the nose in a 14-day-old infant girl. *Zh Ushn Nos Gorl Bolezn* 1967; 27:103–104.
6. Fu YS, Perzin KH. Non-epithelial tumors of the nasal cavity, paranasal sinuses, and nasopharynx: A clinicopathologic study. I: General features and vascular tumors. *Cancer* 1974; 33:1275–1288.
7. Neel HB III, Whicker JH, Devine KD et al. Juvenile angiofibroma: Review of 120 cases. *Am J Surg* 126:547–576.
8. Nelaton M. Polype fibreux de la base du crâne: Considerations generales. *Gaz Hop* 1853; 26:22.
9. Verneuil V. Séances de la Societé de Chirurgie de Paris pendant l'année 1860; *Bull Soc Chir* 1861.
10. Tillaux P. *Traité anatomie topographique avec applications á la chirugie*, ed 2. Paris: P Asselin, 1878; 348–349.
11. Coenen H. Das Basalfibroid (typisches Nasenrachenangio-fibrom) ein Skelettumor. *Münch Med Wochenschr* 1923; 70: 829–833.
12. Sebileau P. Considerations sur les fibromes naso–pharyngies. *Annales des Malaides de l'oreille et du larynx* 1923; 38:553–615.
13. Ringertz N. Benign fibromatous tumors in the nasal and paranasal region and maxilla: Juvenile basal fibroma. *Acta Otolaryngol Stock (Suppl)* 1938; 27:158–161.
14. Som ML, Neffson AH. Fibromas of the nasopharynx: Juvenile and cellular types. *Ann Otol* 1940; 49:211–218.
15. Martin H, Ehrlich HE, Abels JC. Juvenile nasopharyngeal angiofibroma. *Ann Surg* 1948; 127:513–536.
16. Dane WH. Juvenile nasopharyngeal fibroma in state of regression. *Ann Otol Rhinol Laryngol* 1954; 63:997–1014.
17. Sternberg SS. Pathology of juvenile nasopharyngeal angio-fibroma: A lesion of adolescent males. *Cancer* 1954; 7:15–28.
18. Hubbard EM. Nasopharyngeal angiofibromas. *AMA Arch Pathol* 1958; 65:192–204.
19. Brunner H. Nasopharyngeal angiofibroma. *Ann Otol Rhinol Laryngol* 1942; 51:29–65.
20. Osborn DA. The so-called juvenile angiofibroma of the nasopharynx. *J Laryngol Otol* 1959; 73:295–316.
21. Schiff M. Juvenile nasopharyngeal angiofibroma: A theory of pathogenesis. *Laryngoscope* 1959; 69:981–1016.
22. Maurice M, Milad M. Pathogenesis of juvenile naso-pharyngeal fibroma. *J Laryngol Otol* 1981; 95:1121–1126.
23. Girgis ICH, Fahmy SA. Nasopharyngeal fibroma: Its histopathological nature. *J Laryngol Otol* 1973; 87:1107–1123.
24. Ferrara N, Houck K, Jakeman L et al. Molecular and biological properties of the vascular endothelial growth factor family of proteins. *Endocr Rev* 1992; 13:18–32.
25. Nagai MA, Butugan O, Logullo A, Brentani MM. Expression of growth factors, proto oncogenes and p–53 in naso-pharyngeal angiofibromas. *Laryngoscope* 1996; 106:190–195.
26. Ferouz AS, Mohr RM, Paul P. Juvenile nasopharyngeal angiofibroma and familial adenomatous polyposis: An association? *Otolaryngol Head Neck Surg* 1995; 113:435–439.
27. Giardiello FM, Hamilton SR, Krush AJ, Offerhaus JA, Booker SV, Peterson GM. Nasopharyngeal angiofibroma in patients with familial adenomatous polyposis. *Gastroenterology* 1993; 105:1550–1552.
28. Abraham SC, Montgomery EA, Giardiello FM, Wu TT. Frequent β-catenin mutations in Juvenile Nasopharyngeal Angiofibromas. *Am J Pathol* 2001; 158:1073–1078.
29. Beham A, Kainz J, Stammberger H, Aubock L, Beham. Schmid C. Immunohistochemical and electron microscopical cauteri-zation of stromal cells in nasopharyngeal angiofibroma. *Eur Arch Otorhinolaryngol* 1997; 254:196–199.
30. Schiff M, Gonzalez AM, Ong M, Baird A. Juvenile naso-pharyngeal angiofibroma contain an angiogenic growth factor: Basic FGF. *Laryngoscope* 1992; 102:940–945.
31. Hwang HC, Mills SE, Patterson K, Gown AM. Expression of androgen receptors in nasopharyngeal angiofibroma: An immunohistochemical study of 24 cases. *Mod Pathol* 1998; 11:1122–1126.
32. Schick B, Rippel C, Brunner C et al. Numerical sex chromo-some aberrations in juvenile angiofibromas: Genetic evidence for an androgen dependant tumor? *Oncology Reports* 2003; 10:1251–1255.
33. Albrecht R, Graffi I, Kuttner K, Graffi A. Zur Kenntnis intra-nuklearer Einschlubkorper beim juvenilen Nasenrachen-fibrom. *Dtsch Gesundh Wes* 1970; 25:1122–1124.
34. Andrews JC, Fisch U, Valvanis A, Aeppli U, Makek MS. The surgical management of extensive nasopharyngeal angio-fibromas with the infratemporal fossa approach. *Laryngoscope* 1989; 99:429–437.
35. Radkowsky D, Mcgill T, Healy GB, Ohlms L, Jones DT. Angio-fibroma: Changes in staging and treatment. *Arch Otolaryngol Head Neck Surg* 1996; 122:122–129.
36. Jafek B et al. Surgical treatment of juvenile angiofibroma. *Laryngoscope* 1973; 83:707–720.
37. Henderson GP Jr, Patterson CN. Further experiences in treatment of juvenile nasopharyngeal angioma. *Laryngoscope* 1969; 79:561–580.
38. Tranbahuy, Borsik M, Herman P et al. Direct intratumoral embolisation of juvenile angiofibroma. *Am J Otolaryngol* 1994; 15(6):429–435.
39. Garcia Cervigon E, Biens, Rufenacht D, Thurel C et al. Pre-operative embolisation of nasopharyngeal angiofibroma. *Neuroradiology* 1988; 30:556–560.
40. Moulin G, Chagnaud C, Gras R et al. Juvenile nasopharyngeal angiofibroma: Comparison of blood loss during removal in embolised group versus non-embolised group. *Cardiovasc Intervent Radiol* 1995; 18:158–161.

41. Bradoo RA, Nerurkar NK, Joshi AA, Muranjan SN. Endoscopic excision of angiofibroma. *Ind J Otolaryngol Head Neck Surg* 2001; 53:51–53.

42. Bradoo RA, Muranjan SN, Nerurkar NK, Joshi AA, Achar P. Endoscopic Excision of Angiofibroma: A comprehensive approach. *Ind J Otolaryngol Head Neck Surg* 2003; 55(4): 255–262.

43. Kamel RH. Transnasal endoscopic surgery in juvenile nasopharyngeal angiofibroma. *J Laryngol Otol* 1996; 110(10): 962–968.

44. Tseng HZ, Chao WY. Transnasal endoscopic approach for juvenile nasopharyngeal angiofibroma. *Am J Otolaryngol* 1997; 18(2):151–154.

45. Weprin LS, Siemers PT. Spontaneous regression of juvenile nasopharyngeal angiofibroma. *Arch Otolaryngol Head Neck Surg* 1991; 117:796–799.

46. Economou TS, Abemayor E, Ward PH. Juvenile nasopharyngeal angiofibroma: An update of the UCLA experience, 1960–1985. *Laryngoscope* 1988; 98:170–175.

47. McCombe A, Lund VJ, Howard DJ. Recurrence in juvenile angiofibroma. *Rhinology* 1990; 28:97–102.

48. Roger G, Tran Ba Huy P, Froelich P et al. Exclusively endoscopic removal of Juvenile Nasopharyngeal Angiofibroma. *Arch Otolaryngol Head Neck Surg* 2002; 128:928–935.

49. Scholtz AW, Appenroth E, Jolly KK, Scholtz LU, Thumfart WF. Juvenile nasopharyngeal angiofibroma: Management and therapy. *Laryngoscope* 2001; 111:681–687.

CHAPTER 6

Congenital Malformations of the Nose and Paranasal Sinuses

Shyan Vijayasekaran, Romaine Johnson
Robin T Cotton, Ravindhra G Elluru

Congenital malformations of the nose and paranasal sinuses are rare. Their presentation ranges from subtle cosmetic deformities to severe ones that may cause life-threatening acute upper airway obstruction in neonates. This chapter will focus on the most commonly seen congenital lesions in the nose and paranasal sinuses. To facilitate a better understanding of these anomalies, we will briefly review the embryogenesis of this anatomic region.

EMBRYOLOGY OF THE NOSE, PARANASAL SINUSES AND ANTERIOR SKULL BASE

Normal nasal development occurs between the fourth and twelfth week of life. During this time, neural crest cells migrate from their origin in the dorsal neural folds around the eye and traverse the frontonasal process. These pluripotent cells undergo rapid proliferation and differentiation into muscle, cartilage and bone, thus creating the facial structure. During this process, facial prominences develop surrounding the stomodeum, which is formed as an invagination of the ectoderm. The stomodeum is surrounded by the frontonasal prominence superiorly, the maxillary processes laterally, and the mandibular processes inferiorly. The nasal placodes, which are two small thickenings in the frontonasal process, begin to burrow, forming nasal pits. The lateral and medial prominences interact with the developing maxillary process, creating multiple paramedian structures (nasal aperture, nasolacrimal ducts and upper lip). Eruption of nasal pits into the choana, fusion of the palatal shelves, and growth of the nasal septum and soft palate coincide with the development of the lateral nasal wall and primitive sinus anatomy. For normal nasal and paranasal growth to occur, all of these rapid changes must occur with complete precision[1] (Fig. 6.1, Table 6.1).

Table 6.1: Structure of the face and the embryological origin

Prominence	Structures
Frontonasal	Nasal dorsum, medial and lateral nasal prominence
Maxillary	Cheeks, lateral portion of upper lip
Medial nasal	Philtrum, collumella, nasal tip
Lateral nasal	Nasal alae
Mandibular	Lower lip

The anterior skull base develops from the frontal, ethmoidal and nasal bones. The foramen cecum forms a defect in the anterior skull base. This structure is closed by its fusion with the fonticulus frontalis, which represents a space between the developing nasal and frontal bones. It is normal for a projection of dura to extend through the foramen cecum, the prenasal space, down to the nasal tip. As the foramen closes, the diverticulum of dura detaches from the overlying ectoderm. Faulty closure may enable persistence of neural tissue in the nasal cavity. If the fonticulus also closes abnormally, there may be persistence of an extranasal path such as seen in encephaloceles and gliomas[2] (Fig. 6.2).

ENCEPHALOCELES

Encephaloceles are extracranial herniations of cranial contents through a defect in the skull. An encephalocele may include meninges only (termed a *meningocele*), or may include both brain and meninges (termed a *meningoencephalocele*). Estimates of the incidence of these lesions vary considerably, ranging from 1 in 3,000 to 1 in 30,000 births in the western world. The incidence in Asian populations is much higher, with a reported incidence of 1 in 6,000 live births. Encephaloceles have no gender

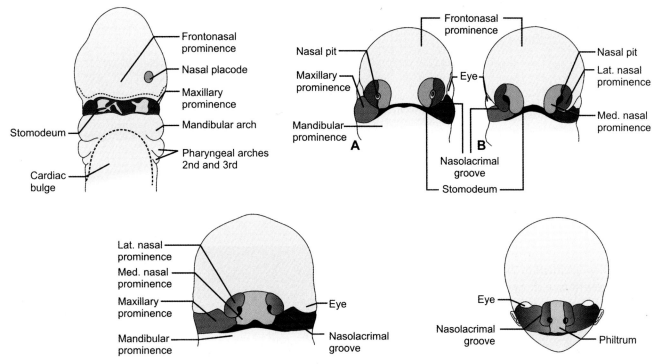

Fig. 6.1: Embryo at 4th, 5th, 6th, 7th and 10th week showing the developing nasal structures
(Sadler TW. Head and Neck Embryology. In Langmans's Medical. Ed 6, Baltimoren 1990, Williams and Wilkins)

predilection and no familial tendency. Approximately, 40% of patients have other associated anomalies.[2-4]

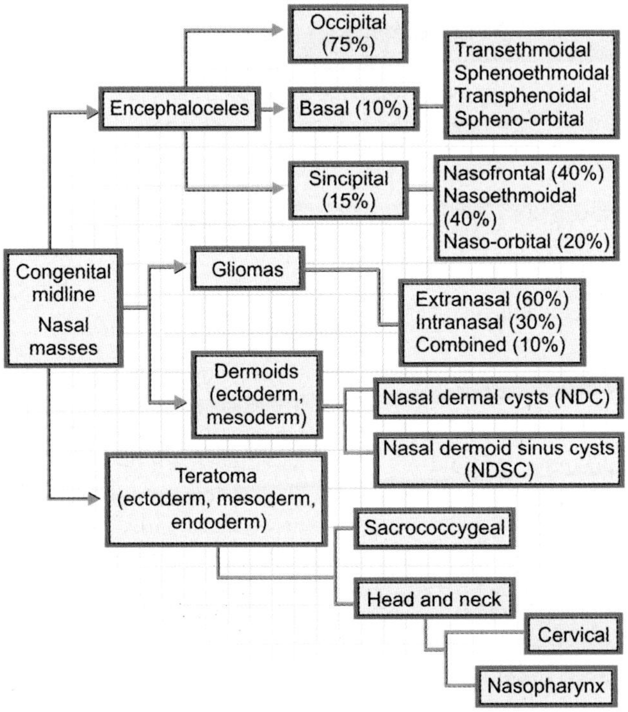

Fig. 6.2: Congenital midline nasal masses

Encephaloceles are divided into occipital, sincipital, and basal types (Tables 6.2 and 6.3). Although in North America and Europe, the majority (75%) of lesions are occipital, their anatomic location excludes them from the scope of the present discussion. Sincipital encephaloceles herniate through a bony defect between the frontal and ethmoid bones anterior to the crista galli, presenting as an external mass over the nose, glabella or forehead (Fig. 6.3). These lesions are further classified according to their location. Nasofrontal sincipital encephaloceles

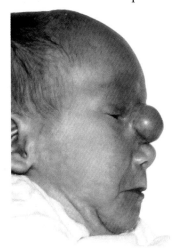

Fig. 6.3: Sincipital encephalocele. A soft bluish compressible mass protruding from the glabellar region

Table 6.2: Sincipital encephaloceles

Type	Course	Clinical features
Nasofrontal	Through bone defect between orbits and forward between nasal and frontal bones to the area superficial to the nasal bones	Glabellar mass Telecanthus Inferior displacement of nasal bones
Nasoethmoidal	Through foramen cecum deep to the nasal bones turning superficially at the cephalic end of the upper lateral cartilage to expand superficial to the upper lateral cartilage	Mass on the nasal dorsum Superior displacement of nasal bones Inferior displacement of the alar cartilages
Naso-orbital	Through the foramen cecum deep to the nasal and frontal bones through a lateral defect in the medial orbital wall	Orbital mass Proptosis Visual changes

present as a glabellar mass, causing telecanthus and inferior displacement of the nasal bones. Nasoethmoidal lesions present as a dorsal nasal mass, causing superior displacement of the nasal bones and inferior displacement of the alar cartilage. Naso-orbital lesions present as an orbital mass, causing proptosis and visual changes.[5] The anatomic course of each of these sincipital encephalocele types is presented in Table 6.2. Basal encephaloceles are less common. They herniate through a bony defect between the cribriform plate and the superior orbital or posterior clinoid fissure, presenting as an intranasal mass (Table 6.3, Fig. 6.4). This mass may not be discovered until later in childhood when it causes nasal obstruction and drainage.

Sincipital and basal encephaloceles appear as soft, bluish, compressible lesions that may transilluminate and pulsate. The classic clinical finding is a positive

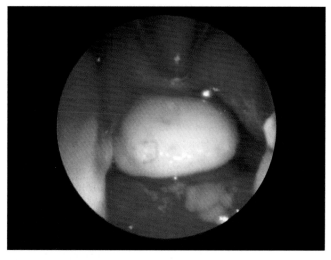

Fig. 6.4: Basal encephalocele seen in nasopharynx with 120° telescope

Table 6.3: Basal encephaloceles

Type	Course	Clinical features
Transethmoidal	Through the cribriform plate into the superior meatus medial to the middle turbinate	Most common type Nasal obstruction Hypertelorism Broad nasal vault Unilateral nasal mass
Sphenothmoidal	Passes through a bony defect between the posterior ethmoid cells and sphenoid	Nasal obstruction Hypertelorism Broad nasal vault Unilateral nasal mass
Transphenoidal	Through a patent craniopharyngeal canal into the nasopharynx	Nasopharyngeal mass Nasal obstruction Associated with cleft palate
Spheno-orbital	Through the superior orbital fissure and out the inferior orbital fissure into the sphenopalatine fossa	Unilateral exophthalmos Visual changes Diplopia

Furstenberg test. Owing to the intracranial connection there is pulsation and expansion of the mass with crying, straining or compression of the jugular veins.

Pathologically, there is a glial component with astrocytes surrounded by collagen, submucosal glands and sometimes nasal septal cartilage. Some lesions exhibit areas of calcification. It is sometimes difficult to differentiate between gliomas and encephaloceles; however, the presence of ependymal tissue is consistent with an encephalocele.[6]

The diagnosis is radiologically confirmed by computed tomography (CT) and/or magnetic resonance imaging (MRI) (Fig. 6.5). The CT evaluation should include high-resolution, thin-section, and contrast-enhanced axial and coronal images, which help delineate the infant's cartilaginous skull base. MRI provides complementary information regarding the fluid and soft tissue characteristics of the mass and is valuable in identifying an intracranial connection. It is also useful in helping to differentiate a meningocele from a meningo-encephalocele. Imaging additionally helps to exclude associated anomalies such as agenesis of the corpus callosum and hydrocephalus.[6]

Encephaloceles are managed surgically. Optimally, there should be multidisciplinary involvement that includes both a neurosurgeon and an otolaryngologist. Most authors advocate intervention in the first few months of life to minimize the risk of meningitis and cosmetic deformities.[2] Additionally, early intervention makes the identification of the intracranial connection technically easier and allows more complete repair of the dural defect.[2] The aim of surgery is complete resection of lesions and meticulous closure of the dural defect so to prevent cerebral spinal fluid (CSF) leakage. Small lesions with minimal skull base defects may be managed endoscopically. Larger lesions require a combined approach with a craniotomy to resect the lesion and subsequent endoscopic removal of the residual nasal tumor. The skull base defect can then be reconstructed using a pericranial flap or split-thickness calvarial bone graft.[6] Neurological function is normal in most patients following surgery. The most commonly encountered postoperative complications are CSF leak, meningitis, and hydrocephalus. Recurrence rates of 4 to 10% have been reported.[7]

GLIOMAS

Whereas encephaloceles maintain a CSF communication to the subarachnoid space, nasal gliomas lack a direct central nervous system attachment. Approximately 5 to 20% of lesions do, however, maintain a fibrous stalk connecting to the subarachnoid space. Gliomas may arise from heterotopic olfactory tissue, neurological tissue within the nasal mucosa, or displaced cells destined to differentiate into neural tissue.[6] It is also possible that these lesions were encephaloceles that were isolated from the CNS as the foramen cecum closed (Fig. 6.6).

These benign masses are extradural collections of glial tissue that present as extranasal (60%), intranasal (30%), or combined (10%) lesions.[8] Extranasal gliomas are smooth, firm, non-compressible masses that occur along the side of the nose, glabella or nasomaxillary suture line.[2] Intranasal gliomas manifest as a pale mass within the

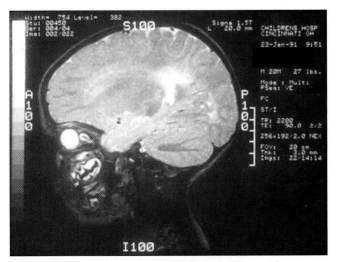

Fig. 6.5: Sagittal MR image of a basal meningoencephalocele protruding into the nasopharynx

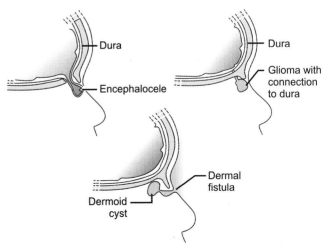

Fig. 6.6: Schematic view of the common midline nasal masses

nasal cavity, with protrusion from the nostril. The nasal fossa on the involved side may be obstructed. The base of the intranasal gliomas most often arises from the lateral nasal wall near the middle turbinate and occasionally from the nasal septum.[8] Although rare, nasal gliomas sometimes extend into the orbit, frontal sinus, oral cavity or nasopharynx. Unlike encephaloceles, gliomas do not change in size with crying or straining and do not transilluminate. They are not familial, though they do have a gender predilection for males (3:2).

The diagnostic evaluation should include a CT scan to assess the bony anatomy of the skull base, an MRI to accurately image soft tissue connections to the CNS, and nasal endoscopy to assess the location, origin and extent of the nasal mass.

Proper management of gliomas requires multidisciplinary approach that includes professionals from otolaryngology, neuroradiology and neurosurgery. Surgical extirpation is required, and delaying this intervention may lead to distortion of the septum or nasal bone, or infection. The surgical approach should allow for excellent exposure and possible exploration of the skull base, and should provide a good cosmetic outcome. The presence of a neurosurgeon at the time of surgery is crucial, should there be an unexpected finding of an intracranial extension. Extranasal gliomas usually require an external incision. Options include lateral rhinotomy, external rhinoplasty, bicoronal incision, and midline nasal incision. The external rhinoplasty approach provides adequate surgical exposure while minimizing facial incisions, and ultimately optimizes the cosmetic outcome. When a fibrous stalk is present that extends deep to the nasal bones toward the base of the skull, a nasal osteotomy is recommended to improve exposure. Following the stalk in its entirety is crucial in determining the possible presence of an intracranial extension. If the nasal mass is large or located in the nasoglabellar region and cannot be safely excised using an external rhinoplasty approach, either a midline nasal incision or a bicoronal approach is required.[6] Due to advancements in surgical instrumentation, image guidance, and surgical techniques, most intranasal gliomas can be treated endoscopically.[9,10] Recurrence rates are between 4 and 10%.[11]

NASAL DERMOIDS

Nasal dermoids are the most common congenital nasal abnormality. They comprise 1 to 3% of all dermoids and approximately 10 to 12% of head and neck dermoids. Unlike teratomas, which contain all three embryonal germ layers, congenital dermoids contain only ectodermal and mesodermal embryonic elements. Mesodermal elements which include hair follicles, sebaceous glands and sweat glands are found in the wall of the cyst and thus differentiate these masses from simple epidermoid cysts. Most dermoid cysts occur sporadically, although familial associations have been reported. Associated abnormalities are seen in 5 to 41% of cases. These include aural atresia, pinna deformity, mental retardation, hydrocephalus, branchial arch sinus, cleft lip and palate, hypertelorism and hemifacial microsomia.[12] Nasal dermoids occur in a sporadic fashion with a slight male preponderance.[12,13]

The etiology of these lesions is controversial and several theories have been proposed to explain nasal dermoid development.[12,13] The most widely accepted theory, known as the **prenasal space theory**, is based on abnormal development of the fonticulus frontalis. This membrane separates the nasal and frontal bones and ossifies to separate the dura and herniating neuroectoderm from the surface epithelium. Normally, the dura separates from the surface epithelium and retracts through the foramen cecum. The retracting dura may drag the surface epithelium inward, causing formation of a sinus tract. In some patients, the sinus tract extends into the intracranial cavity or prenasal space; hence, the dermal sinus or cyst may persist anywhere from the foramen cecum to the nasal tip.[14]

Nasal dermoids manifest as a simple cyst, a cyst with a sinus tract, or a sinus tract alone. Lesions usually present as a firm, lobulated, non-compressible midline mass over the nasal dorsum and may be associated with a sinus opening (Fig. 6.7). They show a negative Furstenberg test and do not transilluminate. There may be intermittent

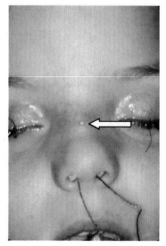

Fig. 6.7: Nasal dermoid presenting as a firm midline nasal swelling associated with a sinus opening

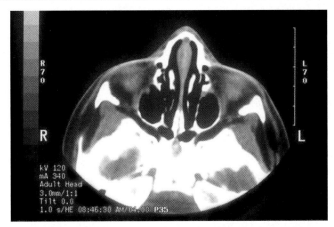

Fig. 6.8: Axial CT of nasal dermoid, evident in the anterior nasal septum as a hypodense lesion

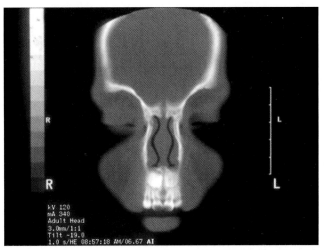

Fig. 6.9: Coronal CT showing a bifid crista galli and an enlarged foramen cecum

discharge or infection. A lesion within the nasal septum will cause nasal obstruction. Although a protruding hair is seen only in a minority of patients, it is pathognomic for a nasal dermoid. Intracranial extension reportedly ranges from 4 to 45%.[12]

CT and MRI provide complementary information. Fine-cut CT (1 to 3 mm) in the axial and coronal planes is best for providing bony anatomy, (Fig. 6.8) whereas MRI is best for assessing soft tissue characteristics. CT scans with intravenous contrast are recommended to differentiate the dermoid from surrounding nasal mucosa. Common findings include a bifid crista galli and an enlarged foramen cecum. Although these findings do not always indicate the presence of an existing intracranial extension, a normal crista galli and foramen cecum may be used to exclude intracranial extension.[15] Multi-planar, thin-section, contrast-enhanced MRI is used to depict the anatomy of the anterior skull base. Contrast is used to differentiate the non-enhancing dermoid from enhancing lesions such as hemangiomas and teratomas. The neonatal crista galli does not contain marrow fat and hence a high-intensity signal on T1-weighted images is suggestive of an intracranial dermoid (Fig. 6.9).

Because aspiration, incision and drainage, curettage and subtotal excision are associated with high recurrence rates, these management approaches are generally not advocated. Assessing the degree of intracranial extension is crucial. In patients in whom the likelihood of intracranial extension is low based on clinical and radiological evaluation, an extracranial operative approach may be planned. In patients with features suggestive of intracranial extension, a combined approach should be prepared for in the event that such extension is confirmed at the time of surgery.

Pollock recommended that any approach to a nasal dermoid should fulfill four criteria:[16]
1. Provide excellent access to the midline.
2. Allow access to the base of the skull.
3. Provide adequate exposure for reconstruction of the nasal dorsum.
4. Result in an acceptable scar.

Several different extracranial approaches have been described. They include lateral rhinotomy, external rhinoplasty, midline vertical incisions and medial paracanthal incisions. The external rhinoplasty incision generally has the best cosmetic result and is thus the most widely used approach. Also, this approach gives access to the skull base and allows for exposure of the nasal dorsum; nevertheless, it provides limited access to lesions in the glabellar region. Alternative approaches include lateral rhinotomy or midline vertical incisions, both of which provide excellent access though with poorer cosmetic outcomes.[12] For lesions in the glabellar area without a sinus opening, a paracanthal incision or a bicoronal approach is recommended. Glabellar lesions with a sinus opening require an elliptical incision to excise the ostium, despite the possibility of a widening scar.

For lesions that extend into the cranial cavity, a craniotomy is sometimes performed; however, its necessity is debatable. Sessions suggested that craniotomy may be avoided and the tract suture ligated if it is devoid of epidermal and adnexal structures at the skull base.[17] This information may be obtained by intraoperative frozen-section biopsy many authors agree with this approach.[12,15] Posnick, however, suggests that epidermal elements may be staggered along the tract and thus postulates that a single biopsy site may provide false-negative information regarding the presence of an intracranial extension of the dermoid tract.[18]

If intracranial extension is seen, a multidisciplinary effort is required for performing a frontal craniotomy. This is usually carried out via a coronal incision using a combined intra- and extracranial approach.

The overall recurrence rate following adequate excision is low. Lesions may, however, recur years after the initial surgery. As such, long-term follow-up is essential.

COMPLETE AGENESIS OF THE NOSE

Congenital absence of the nose, referred to as arrhinia, is extremely rare, with only 29 cases described in the literature (Fig. 6.10). This abnormality is part of the spectrum of holoprosencephaly, the most severe form of which is cyclopia with a single median eye and a single-chambered prosencephalon. Arrhinia includes absence of the external nose and nasal airways, hypoplasia of the maxilla, a small high-arched plate, and hyper-telorism. It is generally sporadic and may occur either as an isolated defect or in association with other facial and cerebral abnormalities.[19] There have also been reports of associations with genetic disorders such as trisomy 10, trisomy 13, and trisomy 21, as well as chromosome 9 inversion and translocation of chromosomes 3 and 12.[3,19,20]

Four theories regarding the embryogenesis of arrhinia have been proposed. These theories respectively involve:

1. Failure of fusion of the medial and lateral nasal processes.
2. Overgrowth and premature fusion of the nasal medial processes.
3. Lack of resorption of the nasal epithelial plugs.
4. Abnormal migration of neural crest cells.[21]

Infants with arrhinia display respiratory distress and cyanosis associated with feeding. Older children may gulp food between breaths, which is referred to as 'canine eating'. Speech is characteristically hypernasal and there are complaints of hyposmia. On physical examination there is an absence of the external nose, nasal septum and sinuses. There may also be associated abnormalities of the eye, including anophthalmia or hypoplasia of the orbits.

Early management is with a cleft palate feeder or a gastrostomy tube. A prosthetic nose may be used until the child is older and can undergo definitive surgical repair. Surgery requires removing incisor teeth, creating an airway through the maxilla, and releasing the high-arched palate. The nasal passage is then lined with split-thickness skin grafts and maintained with long-term stenting. Restenosis is common and serial dilatations are thus required. Reconstruction of the external nose is a multistage procedure that requires the use of tissue expanders, bone, cartilage or prosthetic grafts, and local or regional skin flaps. A dacryocystorhinostomy may be required to prevent recurrent conjunctivitis resulting from the absence of nasolacrimal ducts.[22]

CRANIOFACIAL CLEFTS

Craniofacial clefts are exceedingly rare and generally not seen in routine clinical practice. The hallmarks of this disorder are: ocular hypertelorism, a broad nasal root, lack of formation of the nasal tip, widow's peak scalp bone anomaly, anterior cranium bifidum occultum, median clefting of the nose, lip, and palate, and unilateral orbital clefting or notching of the nasal ala.[1,23] DeMyer and colleagues noted an association between hyper-telorism, cephalic anomalies, and mental deficiency.[24] These authors also noted that the degree of hypertelorism and extent of extracephalic anomalies were associated with the increased likelihood of mental deficiency.

The term 'holoprosencephaly' was coined by DeMyer et al to describe median facial anomalies and the brain morphology associated with these anomalies.[25] Holo-prosencephaly is a failure of the embryonic forebrain to cleave sagittally into cerebral hemispheres, transversely into a diencephalon, and horizontally into olfactory and

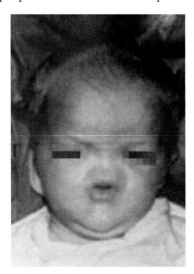

Fig. 6.10: Congenital Arhinia (from Brown K, Rodriguez K, Brown OE. Congenital malformations of the nose. Cummings otolaryngology Head and Neck Surgery. 4th ed. Cummings et al. (Eds) 2005)

optic bulbs. This failure results in a spectrum of facial anomalies that includes:

1. Cyclopia (single eye and single orbit with arrhinia and proboscis).
2. Ethmocephaly (extreme hypertelorism, separate orbits arhinia).
3. Cebocephaly (hypertelorism, proboscis-like nose without cleft lip).
4. Median cleft lip (orbital hypertelorism and flat nose).
5. Median philtrum-premaxilla anlage (hypertelorism, bilateral cleft lip and a median process representing the philtrum maxilla anlage).

The first gene to be associated with holoprosencephaly in humans was the Sonic Hedgehog (SHH) gene. Testing for this gene allows identification of familial forms of holoprosencephaly and evaluation of malformations considered minor variants of the disorder.[23]

The Tessier classification of cranial clefts is the most widely used.[26] This classification is based on specific axes (0 to 14) along the face and cranium. Since the orbit is common to the face and cranium, it distinguishes cranial clefts (9 to 14) from facial clefts (0 to 8). For example, a patient with a median nasal cleft would be considered a 0/14 on the Tessier classification.

MEDIAN NASAL CLEFTS

There is a large degree of variability in the severity of median nasal clefts. This deformity, which is also known as bifid nose and internasal dysplasia, can range from a simple median scar at the cephalic end of the nasal dorsum to a completely split nose, forming separate halves, with independent medial nasal walls. A median cleft lip is a frequently seen associated anomaly.[27] The airway is usually adequate despite the cosmetic appearance. Prior to surgical reconstruction, it is important to rule out a possible dermoid cyst or encephalocele within the nasal-septal area. Surgical reconstruction requires the cooperative efforts of a multidisciplinary team.

LATERAL NASAL CLEFTS

Lateral nasal clefts are rare anomalies that involve defects of the lateral nasal wall or ala. They range from scar-like lines in the ala to triangle-like defects extending into the inner canthal fold and affecting the nasal lacrimal duct system. As with median nasal clefts, lateral nasal clefts require surgical reconstruction using a multidisciplinary approach.

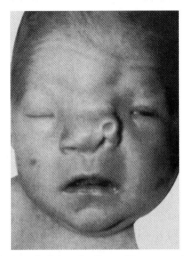

Fig. 6.11: Proboscis lateralis (from Hengerer AS, Wein RO. Congenital abnormalities of the nose and paranasal sinuses. Pediatric Otolaryngology. Bluestone et al (Eds) 4th ed. Saunders. Philadelphia 2003)

PROBOSCIS LATERALIS

Proboscis lateralis is an extremely rare disorder that presents as a tubular sleeve of skin attached to the inner canthus of the orbit and complete agenesis of the paranasal sinuses on the affected side (Fig. 6.11). This lesion is commonly associated with other central nervous system abnormalities.

The most commonly accepted embryologic theory of this disorder is that imperfect mesodermal proliferation occurs in the frontonasal and maxillary processes after formation of the olfactory pits. Epidermal breakdown then occurs, leaving the lateral nasal process sequestered as a tube arising in the frontonasal region. Also, because of this breakdown, the nasolacrimal duct is not formed.[1] The diagnosis is made by physical examination, nasal endoscopy and CT scanning. Treatment is delayed until facial growth is complete, and a prosthetic device is worn until reconstructive efforts begin. Reconstruction involves the use of bone and cartilage grafts and surrounding skin, including the tube of anomalous lateral nasal skin. Restenosis is common and serial dilatations and stenting are often required.[2]

POLYRHINIA AND SUPERNUMERARY NOSTRIL

Polyrhinia (double nose) and supernumerary nostril (accessory nostril) are extremely rare anomalies, with only four reported cases of each.[28] These deformities are associated with pseudohypertelorism, but also have been reported as isolated anomalies. Although there are a number of embryologic theories,[1,28,29] the event thought to be responsible for this anomaly is the incomplete development of the frontonasal process, which results in separation of the developing lateral portions of the nose. The medial nasal processes and the septum are duplicated, thus forming double noses.[1,2,11,26]

Patients with polyrrhinia generally present with a clinical picture similar to that seen in patients with bilateral choanal atresia, and they require the same initial management. The primary step in surgical management is the correction of the choanal atresia. The nasal deformity is later corrected by removing the medial portions of each nose and anastomozing the lateral portions in the midline.[2] The result is a broad flat nose with a depression in the midline which can be corrected by medial infracture of the nasal bones. Supernumerary nostril presents with the external appearance of a small accessory nasal orifice with surrounding redundant soft tissue. The orifice may be lateral, medial or superior to the nose. When there is a true fistula, a discharge from this orifice may occur. Treatment entails excision of the supernumerary nostril and primary closure of the defect or closure with the assistance of local flaps.[28]

CLEFT LIP NASAL DEFORMITY

Children with cleft lip and palate usually have a coexistent nasal deformity. The most severe defects are those associated with a bilateral complete cleft. Children with a bilateral deformity have a flattened nasal tip and a shortened columella 1 to 2 mm in length. They may also have bilateral maxillary hypoplasia and relative prognathism. Less severe deformity is seen in children with unilateral clefts. In these children, the nasal ala on the side of the cleft is more laterally based, giving the appearance of a flat nostril. The caudal septum is also displaced to the cleft side. The maxilla on the cleft side is hypoplastic and the nasal tip has a bifid appearance.

Treatment options include both primary and secondary rhinoplasty. The former approach, performed at the time of cleft repair, is the technique of choice for many surgeons. This option allows for the possibility of future revision should the functional and cosmetic results of primary repair be suboptimal. Both open and closed rhinoplasty techniques have been used. Given the size of the patient's nasal anatomy, the open approach is generally preferred. Secondary rhinoplasty may either be definitive or intermediate. The latter requires two stages of repair. Stage 1, performed between 4 and 6 years of age, aims at providing cosmetic improvement.

Stage 2, performed between ages 8 and 12 years of age, follows orthodontic correction, thus making available an optimal skeletal framework. More definitive rhinoplasty is delayed until skeletal growth is completed. As such, it is performed at between 16 and 18 years of age.[30]

CHOANAL ATRESIA

Choanal atresia occurs when the posterior nasal cavity fails to communicate with the nasopharynx.[5] The anatomic deformity comprises:
1. A narrow nasal cavity.
2. Lateral bony obstruction by the pterygoid plate.
3. Medial obstruction caused by thickening of the vomer.
4. Membranous obstruction.[31-33]

In a study conducted by Brown et al,[31] the incidence of pure bony atresia was found to be 29%, whereas that of mixed bony-membranous atresia was 71%. No patients were found to have a purely membranous atresia.

Choanal atresia has a reported incidence ranging from 1 in 5,000 to 1 in 8,000 live births.[34] Fifty percent of patients with choanal atresia have other associated congenital anomalies. Up to two-thirds of cases are unilateral, with atresia most commonly occurring on the right side.[5] Up to 75% of patients affected bilaterally have other associated anomalies[2] such as CHARGE syndrome (coloboma, heart defects, atretic choana, retardation of growth and development, genitourinary disorders and ear abnormalities). Other anomalies include polydactyly, nasal, auricular and palatal deformities, Crouzon syndrome, craniosynostosis, microcephaly, hypoplasia of the orbit and midface, cleft palate and hypertelorism.[35,36]

There are several theories of embryogenesis. It is generally thought that choanal atresia is related to persistence of the nasobuccal membrane. This membrane forms at the posterior end of the nasal pits, which have burrowed into the midface mesoderm. It usually ruptures between the fifth and sixth week of gestation to produce choanae. Failure of this membrane to rupture is thought to cause choanal atresia.[2] An alternative theory suggests that abnormal migration of neural crest cells results in choanal atresia. This theory is supported by the high incidence of choanal atresia in patients with mandibulofacial dysostosis, which is associated with abnormal neural crest migration.

Patients with unilateral disease present later in life with rhinorrhea and nasal obstruction. On anterior rhinoscopy, the occluded nasal cavity is typically filled with thick, tenacious secretions. Patients with bilateral choanal atresia present as newborns with cyclical

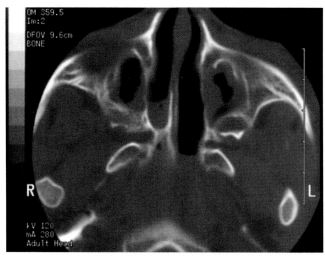

Fig. 6.12: Axial CT scan of unilateral choanal atresia with a complete bony atretic plate and associated soft tissue

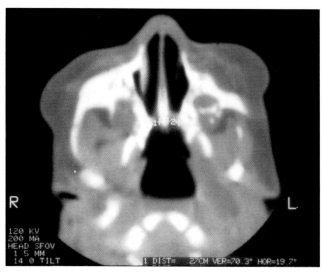

Fig. 6.13: Bilateral choanal stenosis with narrowed yet patent choanae

cyanosis relieved by crying. The event begins with increasing efforts to breathe, tight mouth closure and chest retractions followed by cyanosis. The cycle is broken by crying. A variant of bilateral choanal stenosis presents later in life with mouth breathing, recurrent sinusitis, chronic rhinorrhea, otitis media, malnourishment and speech defects.

The diagnosis of choanal atresia is made clinically by failure to pass a 6 Fr catheter through the nose into the nasopharynx. This is supported by endoscopic examination. CT is used to confirm the diagnosis and reveal the nature and thickness of the atresia.[37] Suctioning and vasoconstriction prior to imaging improve resolution (Fig. 6.12). A diagnosis of choanal stenosis is made when there is a narrowed, yet patent choana. Derkay et al more specifically define this as a choanal space less than 6 mm and the inability to pass a 6F catheter more than 32 mm.[38] This diagnosis should be confirmed by endoscopic evaluation (Fig. 6.13).

Unilateral atresia is not an emergency. Treatment is delayed, allowing for growth of the nose, which enhances the ease of surgery and reduces the risk of postoperative complications and restenosis. Bilateral atresia requires an initial intervention to establish an oropharyngeal or orotracheal airway and nasogastric feeding prior to definitive surgery. In some cases, a tracheostomy is indicated for other airway or cardiopulmonary issues. In these cases, definitive surgery is often delayed, allowing for facial growth.

The timing of surgery is variable. Because of the small size of the face in preterm infants, it may be preferable to wait until adequate growth has occurred. Though

controversial, some surgeons have advocated the 'rule of tens' (the child must weigh 10 lb, have hemoglobin of 10 g/dl, and be 10 weeks old prior to repair).

There has been a shift in the surgical philosophy over the last few decades away from transpalatal (Fig. 6.14) and towards transnasal surgery. The rationale for this change has been the lower risk of dental and facial growth abnormalities associated with the latter approach. The most commonly used approach involves a blunt puncture of the central thin area using a urethral sound or suction instrument. This is carried out under endoscopic guidance using a 0° transnasal telescope or a 120° nasopharyngoscope (Fig. 6.15). Subsequently, backbiting forceps, microdebrider cutters, and/or lasers or drills are

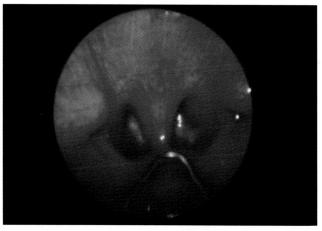

Fig. 6.14: Axial CT scan showing bilateral choanal atresia and a view of the choanal atresia using a 120° nasopharyngoscope

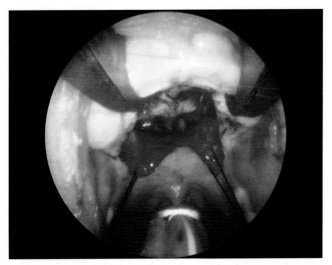

Fig. 6.15: Transpalatal approach to choanal atresia repair; elevation of a pedicled hard palate mucoperiosteal flap based on the greater palatine artery to expose the choanae

used to remove choanal soft tissue and bone. The posterior tip of the middle turbinate is a useful anatomic landmark. Remaining inferior to this structure reduces the risk of intracranial injury.[39]

There are several controversial issues regarding atresia surgery. These include the use of stenting, fibroblast inhibitors (mitomycin C), and the preservation of mucosal flaps. Most studies report significant recurrence rates requiring revision surgery.[40,41] The literature indicates greater success with older children (unilateral atresia), non-syndromic patients, and with surgical procedures that minimise mucosal trauma.

CONGENITAL NASAL PYRIFORM APERTURE STENOSIS (CNPAS)

Congenital nasal pyriform aperture stenosis (CNPAS) is an anomaly that occurs secondary to bony overgrowth of the nasal process of the maxilla and typically presents in the first few months of life. The pyriform aperture is the narrowest part of the nasal cavity, and small changes in cross-sectional area significantly affect airflow by increasing nasal airway resistance. CNPAS most commonly occurs as an isolated anomaly, although it may occur in association with holoprosencephaly.

One theory of embryogenesis maintains that deficient development of the primary palate and bony overgrowth of the nasal process of the maxilla are responsible for this anomaly.[42] A developmental deficiency of the os incisivum could explain the occurrence of a triangular plate, the narrow inferior portion of the nasal cavity, and the associated central maxillary mega-incisor, which is seen in 60% of cases[43] (Fig. 6.16).

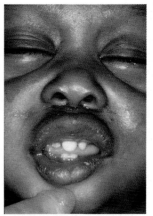

Fig. 6.16: Maxillary mega incisor in association with CNPAS

Newborns present with symptoms similar to those of choanal atresia and failure to pass a nasopharyngeal catheter may result in a misdiagnosis of choanal atresia. These symptoms may be triggered by an upper respiratory infection, which further compromises the already narrow airway. The diagnosis of CNPAS is established by physical evaluation and is best confirmed by CT, which shows that the width of the pyriform aperture, the cross-sectional area of the nasal cavity, and the width of the choana are all reduced. In contrast, the height of the nasal cavity and cross-sectional area of the choana are not altered (Figs 6.17 and 6.18). CNPAS is thus an anomaly that results in narrowing of the entire nasal cavity; this narrowing is most severely manifested anteriorly. In a study describing the CT features that facilitate an accurate diagnosis of CNPAS, Belden and colleagues found the most helpful CT measurement to be the width of the pyriform aperture, defined as the distance between the medial aspects of the maxillae at the level of the inferior meatus on images in the axial plane.[44] These authors reported that the width was never greater than 8 mm in their CNPAS group and never less than 11 mm in their control group. They thus concluded

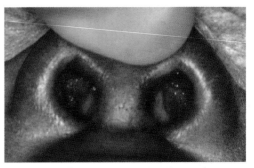

Fig. 6.17: Congenital nasal pyriform aperture stenosis as seen on anterior rhinoscopy

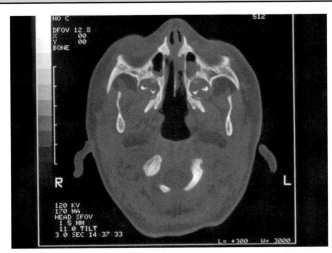

Fig. 6.18: Axial CT scan showing pyriform aperture stenosis secondary to overgrowth of the nasal process of the maxilla causing reduction in the width of the piriform aperture

that width is the singlemost useful measurement for making the radiological diagnosis.

The central maxillary incisor is associated with subtypes of holoprosencephaly. Hypertelorism and a flat nasal bridge are clinical features of the premaxillary dysgenesis associated with holoprosencephaly. Pituitary disorders and dental and facial anomalies are also part of this spectrum, and it is prudent for patients with a central maxillary incisor to undergo a number of investigations, including CT scanning for evaluation of CNS malformations, chromosomal analysis and pituitary function testing.[45]

The prognosis is usually good and surgery is rarely required. Non-operative management with nasal tubes and topical vasoconstrictive drops may be all that is required until growth results in increased nasal airway size. In patients who require surgery, this is best accomplished through the sublabial approach (Fig. 6.19).

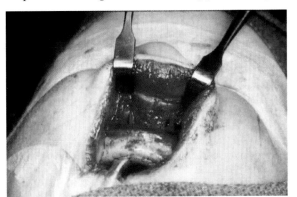

Fig. 6.19: Sub-labial approach to the pyriform aperture; a gingivobuccal sulcus incision is made and a mucoperiosteal flap is raised to expose the pyriform aperture

A gingival buccal sulcus incision is made through to the periosteum so to expose the lateral aspect of the pyriform aperture. The bony lateral margins can then be widened by an otologic drill or curette. Brown et al recommend the use of nasal stents for up to 4 weeks.[42]

NASOLACRIMAL DUCT CYSTS

Nasolacrimal duct cysts are uncommon abnormalities that may lead to nasal obstruction, respiratory distress and epiphora. Because infants are obligate nasal breathers, the presence of a nasolacrimal duct cyst also makes them susceptible to aspiration and feeding difficulties.

Nasolacrimal duct development begins as a thickening of the ectoderm that becomes buried in the mesoderm that is between the lateral nasal process and the maxillary process. The duct begins canalization at its lacrimal end and progresses inferiorly. At birth, approximately 30% of all neonates have distal nasolacrimal duct obstruction, although only about 6% have epiphora. When both the superior and inferior aspects of the duct are obstructed, either unilateral or bilateral cyst formation occurs.[46]

Symptoms are most marked in patients with bilateral cysts. In most children, however, obstruction spontaneously resolves by nine months of age. The diagnosis is made by anterior rhinoscopy or nasal endoscopy, which demonstrate a cystic mass in the inferior meatus (Fig. 6.20). This can be confirmed on a CT scan. The classic features evident on imaging are a dilated nasal lacrimal duct, an intranasal cyst, and cystic dilatation of the lacrimal sac.[46]

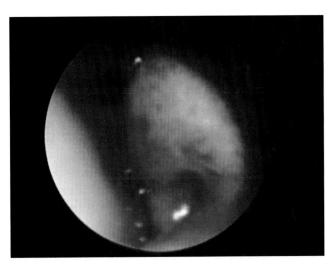

Fig. 6.20: Left nasolacrimal duct cyst in the inferior meatus as seen on anterior rhinoscopy

Surgery is indicated for infants who have feeding problems, infection, and/or respiratory obstruction. The cyst is marsupialized endoscopically. This is best accomplished by a multidisciplinary team that includes an ophthalmologist who may need to perform naso-lacrimal duct probing and possible placement of nasolacrimal duct stents.

NASOPHARYNGEAL TERATOMAS

Teratomas are the most common germ cell tumors of childhood and are almost always benign. These lesions comprise representative tissues from each of three germ layers of the embryonic disk (ectoderm, endoderm and mesoderm) and generally contain tissues foreign to the anatomic site of origin. It is thought that teratomas of the head and neck develop from foci of tissue that fail to follow normal embryonic development. These foci may be remnants of normal embryologic structures that break off or do not migrate along well-defined pathways to their normal destination.[47]

Teratomas occurring in infancy and early childhood are generally extragonadal, whereas those presenting in older children more commonly occur in the ovary or testis.[48] These neoplasms are most commonly located in the sacrococcygeal region, followed by the ovaries, testes, anterior mediastinum, retroperitoneum, and the head and neck, which accounts for less than 5% of all neonatal teratomas. These rare neoplasms, which reportedly occur in 1 of 20,000 to 40,000 live births, may be located in the brain, orbit, oropharynx, nasopharynx, or cervical region. The nasopharynx is the second most common site in the head.

Nasopharyngeal teratomas may be sessile or pedunculated and often protrude through the mouth. Anencephaly, hemicrania, and palatal fissures are associated with these lesions. Maternal clinical charac-teristics may include polyhydramnios due to impaired swallowing and elevated fetoprotein levels. Larger lesions are often diagnosed by prenatal ultrasound. This enables planning for an EXIT (*ex utero* intrapartum treatment) procedure to secure an infant's airway prior to division of the maternal–fetal circulation. The newborn usually presents with severe acute respiratory distress requiring endotracheal intubation or tracheostomy. In patients with smaller lesions, feeding difficulties may be the only presenting symptom.[49]

Fine needle aspiration may be used to assist in establishing the diagnosis and imaging can confirm the diagnosis.[49] Lesions present as cystic and solid areas of

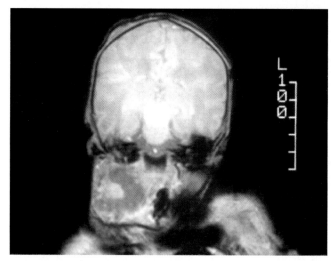

Fig. 6.21: Nasopharyngeal teratoma on coronal MR imaging with characteristic heterogeneous signal intensity

fat density on CT and MRI (Fig. 6.21). There may be areas of bone and tooth formation. Most nasopharyngeal teratomas usually have no intracranial connections and are well-encapsulated. They can be excised through a transoral approach with or without endoscopic assistance. This approach may require splitting of the soft palate or palatal resection. Endoscopic assistance may obviate the need for palatal division or resection.[47] External approaches using a Weber-Ferguson incision or a transcervical incision are also used. If an intracranial component exists, a craniofacial approach is necessary. Outcomes are generally successful and fetoprotein levels are periodically measured to monitor reoccurrence.

REFERENCES

1. Hengerer ASWR. *Congenital abnormalities of the nose and paranasal sinuses*, 4th edn. Philadelphia: Saunders, 2002; 4099–4115.
2. Brown K RK, Brown OE. *Congenital malformations of the nose*, 4th edn. Philadelphia: Elsevier Mosby, 2005; 4099–4109.
3. Keeling JW, Hansen BF, Kjaer I. Pattern of malformations in the axial skeleton in human trisomy 21 fetuses. *Am J Med Genet* 1997; 68:466–471.
4. Sedano HO, Cohen MM, Jr., Jirasek J, Gorlin RJ. Frontonasal dysplasia. *J Pediatr* 1970; 76:906–913.
5. Silva A SJ. *Congenital malformations of the nose and paranasal sinuses*, 1 edn. San Diego: Singular, 1999; 381–391.
6. Rahbar R, Resto VA, Robson CD, et al. Nasal glioma and encephalocele: diagnosis and management. *Laryngoscope* 2003; 113:2069–2077.
7. Puppala B, Mangurten HH, McFadden J, Lygizos N, Taxy J, Pellettiere E. Nasal glioma. Presenting as neonatal respiratory distress. Definition of the tumor mass by MRI. *Clin Pediatr (Phila)* 1990; 29:49–52.

8. Bradley PJ, Singh SD. Nasal glioma. *J Laryngol Otol* 1985; 99:247–252.
9. Burckhardt W, Tobon D. Endoscopic approach to nasal glioma. *Otolaryngol Head Neck Surg* 1999; 120:747–748.
10. Yokoyama M, Inouye N, Mizuno F. Endoscopic management of nasal glioma in infancy. *Int J Pediatr Otorhinolaryngol* 1999; 51:51–54.
11. Van Den Abbeele T, Elmaleh M, Herman P, Francois M, Narcy P. Transnasal endoscopic repair of congenital defects of the skull base in children. *Arch Otolaryngol Head Neck Surg* 1999; 125:580–584.
12. Rahbar R, Shah P, Mulliken JB, et al. The presentation and management of nasal dermoid: A 30-year experience. *Arch Otolaryngol Head Neck Surg* 2003; 129:464–471.
13. Pratt LW. Midline cysts of the nasal dorsum: Embryologic origin and treatment. *Laryngoscope* 1965; 75:968–980.
14. Bradley PJ. The complex nasal dermoid. *Head Neck Surg* 1983; 5:469–473.
15. Pensler JM, Bauer BS, Naidich TP. Craniofacial dermoids. *Plast Reconstr Surg* 1988; 82:953–958.
16. Pollock RA. Surgical approaches to the nasal dermoid cyst. *Ann Plast Surg* 1983; 10:498–501.
17. Sessions RB. Nasal dermal sinuses—new concepts and explanations. *Laryngoscope* 1982; 92:1–28.
18. Posnick JC, Bortoluzzi P, Armstrong DC, Drake JM. Intracranial nasal dermoid sinus cysts: Computed tomographic scan findings and surgical results. *Plast Reconstr Surg* 1994; 93:745–754. discussion 755–764.
19. Shino M, Chikamatsu K, Yasuoka Y, Nagai K, Furuya N. Congenital arhinia: A case report and functional evaluation. *Laryngoscope* 2005; 115:1118–1123.
20. Kjaer I, Keeling JW, Fischer Hansen B. Pattern of malformations in the axial skeleton in human trisomy 13 fetuses. *Am J Med Genet* 1997; 70:421–426.
21. Albernaz VS, Castillo M, Mukherji SK, Ihmeidan IH. Congenital arhinia. *AJHR Am J Neuroradiol* 1996; 17:1312–1314.
22. Ozek C, Gundogan H, Bilkay U et al. A case of total nasal agenesis accompanied by Tessier no. 30 cleft. *Ann Plast Surg* 2001; 46:663–664.
23. Ming JE, Muenke M. Holoprosencephaly: From Homer to Hedgehog. *Clin Genet* 1998; 53:155–163.
24. DeMyer W. The median cleft face syndrome. Differential diagnosis of cranium bifidum occultum, hypertelorism, and median cleft nose, lip, and palate. *Neurology* 1967; 17:961–971.
25. Demyer W, Zeman W, Palmer CD. Familial alobar holoprosencephaly (arhinencephaly) with median cleft lip and palate.report of patient with 46 chromosomes. *Neurology* 1963; 13:913–918.
26. Tessier P. Anatomical classification facial, craniofacial and laterofacial clefts. *J Maxillofac Surg* 1976; 4:69–92.
27. van der Meulen JC, Mazzola R, Vermey-Keers C, Stricker M, Raphael B. A morphogenetic classification of craniofacial malformations. *Plast Reconstr Surg* 1983; 71:560–572.
28. Williams A, Pizzuto M, Brodsky L, Perry R. Supernumerary nostril: A rare congenital deformity. *Int J Pediatr Otorhinolaryngol* 1998; 44:161–167.
29. Nakamura K, Onizuka T. A case of supernumerary nostril. *Plast Reconstr Surg* 1987; 80:436–441.
30. Madorsky SJ, Wang TD. Unilateral cleft rhinoplasty: A review. *Otolaryngol Clin North Am* 1999; 32:669–682.
31. Brown OE, Pownell P, Manning SC. Choanal atresia: A new anatomic classification and clinical management applications. *Laryngoscope* 1996; 106:97–101.
32. Harner SG, McDonald TJ, Reese DF. The anatomy of congenital choanal atresia. *Otolaryngol Head Neck Surg* 1981; 89:7–9.
33. Brown OE, Smith T, Armstrong E, Grundfast K. The evaluation of choanal atresia by computed tomography. *Int J Pediatr Otorhinolaryngol* 1986; 12:85–98.
34. Pirsig W. Surgery of choanal atresia in infants and children: Historical notes and updated review. *Int J Pediatr Otorhinolaryngol* 1986; 11:153–170.
35. Samadi DS, Shah UK, Handler SD. Choanal atresia: A twenty-year review of medical comorbidities and surgical outcomes. *Laryngoscope* 2003; 113:254–258.
36. Leclerc JE, Fearon B. Choanal atresia and associated anomalies. *Int J Pediatr Otorhinolaryngol* 1987; 13:265–272.
37. Crockett DM, Healy GB, McGill TJ, Friedman EM. Computed tomography in the evaluation of choanal atresia in infants and children. *Laryngoscope* 1987; 97:174–183.
38. Derkay CS, Grundfast KM. Airway compromise from nasal obstruction in neonates and infants. *Int J Pediatr Otorhinolaryngol* 1990; 19:241–249.
39. Ey EH, Han BK, Towbin RB, Jaun WK. Bony inlet stenosis as a cause of nasal airway obstruction. *Radiology* 1988; 168:477–479.
40. Manning SC, Bloom DC, Perkins JA, Gruss JS, Inglis A. Diagnostic and surgical challenges in the pediatric skull base. *Otolaryngol Clin North Am* 2005; 38:773–794.
41. Kubba H, Bennett A, Bailey CM. An update on choanal atresia surgery at Great Ormond Street Hospital for Children: Preliminary results with Mitomycin C and the KTP laser. *Int J Pediatr Otorhinolaryngol* 2004; 68:939–945.
42. Brown OE, Myer CM, 3rd, Manning SC. Congenital nasal pyriform aperture stenosis. *Laryngoscope* 1989; 99:86–91.
43. Van Den Abbeele T, Triglia JM, Francois M, Narcy P. Congenital nasal pyriform aperture stenosis: Diagnosis and management of 20 cases. *Ann Otol Rhinol Laryngol* 2001; 110:70–75.
44. Belden CJ, Mancuso AA, Schmalfuss IM. CT features of congenital nasal piriform aperture stenosis: Initial experience. *Radiology* 1999; 213:495–501.
45. Arlis H, Ward RF. Congenital nasal pyriform aperture stenosis. Isolated abnormality vs developmental field defect. *Arch Otolaryngol Head Neck Surg* 1992; 118:989–991.
46. Tabor MH, Desai KR, Respler DS. Symptomatic bilateral nasolacrimal duct cysts in a newborn. *Ear Nose Throat J* 2003; 82:90–92.
47. Kountakis SE, Minotti AM, Maillard A, Stiernberg CM. Teratomas of the head and neck. *Am J Otolaryngol* 1994; 15:292–296.
48. Azizkhan RG, Caty MG. Teratomas in childhood. *Curr Opin Pediatr* 1996; 8:287–292.
49. April MM, Ward RF, Garelick JM. Diagnosis, management, and follow-up of congenital head and neck teratomas. *Laryngoscope* 1998; 108:1398–1401.

Common Cysts and Tumors of the Jaws

Pushkar Mehra, Vikki L Noonan

CYSTS OF THE JAWS

Cystic lesions, defined as pathological cavities remarkable for the presence of an epithelial lining, are commonly encountered in the oral cavity. The epithelial lining of oral cystic lesions may be derived from a variety of sources including residua of epithelium persisting following odontogenesis, from glandular tissue such as salivary and seromucous glands, from the sinonasal tract, and from dermal epithelial tissue. Although the pathogenesis of cysts of the oral cavity is incompletely understood, appropriate clinicopathologic correlation typically makes it possible to render a definitive diagnosis.

The classification of oral cystic lesions is somewhat controversial. In the text that follows, the classification of odontogenic cysts will be divided into cysts of either odontogenic or non-odontogenic origin. Additionally, lesions of a 'pseudocystic' nature are described, remarkable for the absence of a true epithelial lining. The following discussion is written with an aim to delineate the characteristic clinical and histologic features of some common cysts of the oral cavity, and to provide pertinent information for the clinician to render an appropriate diagnosis and provide optimal treatment for these cystic lesions.

ODONTOGENIC CYSTS

An odontogenic cyst develops from remnants of odontogenic epithelium that may persist in the oral cavity following tooth development.[1] Although the pathogenesis of odontogenic cysts is incompletely understood, stimulation and proliferation of these odontogenic epithelial residua are thought to result in cyst development.[2-5] Bone resorption associated with expansion of a cystic lesion gives rise to a radiolucent bony defect.

Frequently, a thin radiopaque border is appreciated at the periphery of a cystic radiolucency. This sclerotic border may represent the capacity for reparative bone to develop at a faster rate than the rate of bone resorption secondary to cystic growth.

Developmental Odontogenic Cysts

Dentigerous Cyst

In the final stages of tooth development, the outer and inner enamel epithelial tissues merge to form the reduced enamel epithelium. Proliferation of this epithelial lining and subsequent expansion of the subjacent follicular space leads to cyst formation. Although the exact pathogenesis is uncertain, differing theories suggest methods whereby accumulation of luminal fluid leads to dentigerous cyst formation and expansion. One possibility suggests that follicular tissue venous flow is obstructed by pressure of the impacted tooth as it moves towards eruption. This yields extrusion of serum through capillary vascular channels and subsequent fluid accumulation.[6,7] Another theory suggests dentigerous cysts develop secondary to degeneration of follicular tissue when eruption is impeded. Subsequent increase in osmotic pressure from these degenerating cells causes cyst formation.[8] Further cyst expansion occurs as lining epithelial cells slough into the lumen and increase fluid osmolality. Although the dentigerous cyst is thought to be developmental in nature, some appear to arise secondary to an inflammatory stimulus.[9] Here, the cystic lesion involves the crown of an unerupted tooth with an overlying nonvital deciduous predecessor exhibiting extensive carious involvement.

By definition, a dentigerous cyst is associated with the crown of an unerupted tooth and is adherent to the cemento-enamel junction. Dentigerous cysts comprise approximately 20% of all cystic lesions of the jaws, [10,11] and are found in highest frequency associated with the most commonly impacted teeth: Third molars and canines. Most dentigerous cysts are asymptomatic and discovered on routine radiographic examination presenting as a well circumscribed unilocular to multilocular radiolucency around the crown of an unerupted tooth (Fig. 7.1A). Large cystic lesions may compromise the integrity of the mandible. Since many other odontogenic cysts and tumors can present in a dentigerous configuration, histologic evaluation is required in order to make a definitive diagnosis.

Histopathologic examination shows stratified squamous epithelium and fibromyxomatous connective tissue in cystic configuration. The cystic epithelial lining is thin and may occasionally contain Rushton bodies. Foci of lining cells exhibiting mucous differentiation or a ciliated luminal surface can be observed. When inflammation is present, the epithelial lining is typically hyperplastic with a complicated, anastomosing rete ridge architecture. Occasional discrete odontogenic epithelial rests and dystrophic calcifications may be found in the cyst wall. Rare cases of muco-epidermoid carcinoma and clonal transformation of the cystic epithelial lining to squamous cell carcinoma have been reported.[12]

Diagnostic work-up and treatment: Dentigerous cysts can vary in size; if allowed to enlarge, they may, overtime, cause significant bony expansion and destruction of large portions of the jaws. A panoramic radiograph is usually sufficient for treatment planning of most cases, but CT scans are of immense value for large cysts.

For large lesions, especially cysts with an aggressive behavior, an incisional biopsy may be indicated to rule out other cysts and tumors. Aspiration of all lesions is recommended to rule out vascular lesions. This can easily be accomplished with a 14- or 16-guage needle under local anesthesia. If the aspirate contains straw-colored fluid, a diagnosis of a cystic lesion is more likely, versus a situation with a lack of aspirate, which may lead the practitioner to think in terms of a solid lesions like ameloblastomas, which can have very similar radiographic and clinical appearances (Fig. 7.1B).

The preferred treatment for dentigerous cysts is complete removal of the lesion via enucleation. Surgery is usually performed through an intraoral approach. A full thickness mucoperiosteal flap is raised, and if required, bone is removed to access the cyst. The round back edge of a surgical curette is then used to lift the thick-walled cyst from its bony cavity. Even if the cyst is in close proximity to the inferior alveolar neurovascular bundle, it can generally be separated from the bundle with careful dissection. The associated tooth is extracted concurrently. Adjacent teeth do not need to be extracted unless a specific indication for tooth sacrifice exists (e.g. inability to remove the complete cyst because of lack of surgical access, or severe external root resorption). Figures 7.1C and D show a maxillary dentigerous cyst with extension into the maxillary sinus. The patient was treated with enucleation and removal of associated impacted tooth via an intraoral approach.

Marsupalization of large dentigerous cysts can be performed, but is not generally popular as it involves prolonged treatment time and also carries the risk of

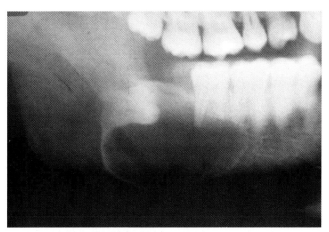

Fig. 7.1A: A well-defined, unilocular, radiolucent pericoronal lesion of the mandible related to an impacted mandibular third molar tooth. This lesion was a dentigerous cyst

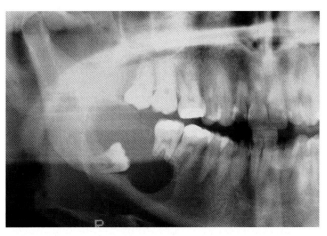

Fig. 7.1B: Another well-defined, unilocular, radiolucent pericoronal lesion related to an impacted mandibular third molar tooth. This lesion was a unicystic ameloblastoma. Note that the lesion has caused resorption of adjacent teeth roots

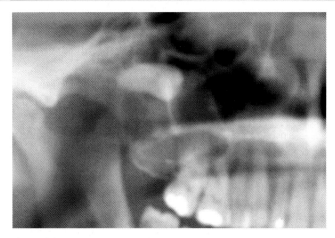

Fig. 7.1C: Preoperative panoramic radiograph showing a large dentigerous of the right maxilla causing displacement of the impacted third molar superiorly towards the orbital floor

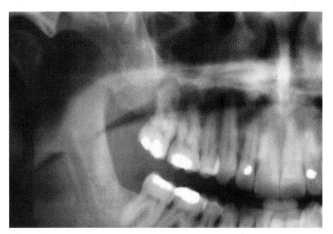

Fig. 7.1D: Postoperative radiograph of the patient in Fig. 7.1C after intraoral surgery for removal of cyst via enucleation and extraction of third molar

neoplastic transformation. It does not decrease the chance of pathological fracture or infection. In certain selected cases of large cysts, additional treatment including intermaxillary fixation and bone grafting may be indicated. Recurrence is extremely rare unless incomplete removal of the cyst was performed during initial surgery.

Eruption Cyst

Representing a soft-tissue counterpart to the dentigerous cyst, an eruption cyst occurs within the alveolar mucosa and arises following formation of a cleft between the crown of an erupting tooth and its associated dental follicle. This cystic lesion presents clinically as a flesh-colored to translucent swelling of the alveolar mucosa superficial to an erupting tooth. Frequently, hemorrhage into the cystic cavity may impart a bluish color to the lesion.

Eruption cysts are typically seen in young children, generally between the ages of five and nine, and are commonly found in the permanent dentition with the first molars and maxillary anterior teeth most frequently affected.[13] Occasionally, patients with multiple eruption cysts are encountered. One recent report in the literature documents the development of an eruption cyst in a young patient taking cyclosporin A. Here, medication-induced fibrous hyperplasia of the overlying alveolar mucosa may have predisposed the patient to eruption cyst formation.[14] At least one other case of a similar nature has been reported in a child with kinky hair disease receiving anticonvulsant therapy with diphenyl-hydantoin.[15]

Histologically, the eruption cyst is located within the connective tissue in close approximation to the surface mucosa and is lined by unremarkable stratified squamous epithelium.

Treatment: Typically, eruption cysts do not require surgery, and almost always resolve without intervention. Occasionally, an eruption cyst may prevent eruption of the underlying tooth, and in these cases, 'de-roofing' of the cyst may be indicated to allow for eruption. If an infected eruption cyst is seen, treatment may require a localized incision and drainage procedure with antibiotic treatment. Care should be taken during any surgery as overzealous instrumentation may cause damage the underlying erupting tooth.

Lateral Periodontal Cyst

The lateral periodontal cyst is presumed to originate from residual remnants of dental lamina retained within the alveolar bone following tooth development.[16] Presenting clinically as a well-circumscribed solitary 'teardrop-shaped' radiolucency in between the roots of vital teeth (Fig. 7.2), the lateral periodontal cyst attains a size that is on average no greater than one centimeter in the largest dimension.[17,18] These lesions have a predilection for occurring in the mandible, anterior to the first molar, and are most frequently encountered in the premolar region.[16-18] A variant of the lateral periodontal cyst called the botryoid (resembling a cluster of grapes) odontogenic cyst typically presents in a multilocular configuration. A higher recurrence rate has been reported for the botryoid variant, which may be related to difficulties encountered in completely removing the multilocular lesion in its entirety.

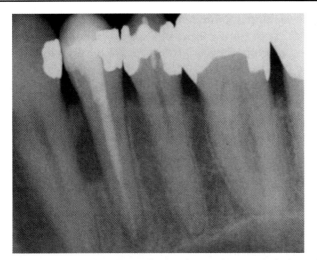

Fig. 7.2: Periapical radiograph showing a characteristic lateral periodontal cyst between the canine and 1st premolar teeth. Note that many odontogenic keratocysts can also present at his location with a similar radiographic appearance

Histopathological examination of the lateral periodontal cyst reveals a stratified squamous epithelial lined cavity remarkable for focal areas of nodular intraluminal proliferation. Glycogenated clear cells are commonly dispersed throughout the lining epithelium and may comprise a significant component of the nodular epithelial foci. Hyalinization of unknown significance is frequently appreciated within the cyst wall proximal to the epithelial lining.[17] In contrast to the conventional lateral periodontal cyst, the botryoid variant typically shows multiple independent epithelial-lined cavities, however, the epithelial linings of the cystic spaces are histologically identical to the conventional counterpart. Both the solitary and multilocular lesion lack remarkable significant inflammation, unless secondarily infected. One rare case of squamous cell carcinoma arising from the lining of a lateral periodontal cyst has been documented in the literature.[19,20]

Treatment: Enucleation of the lesion is the treatment of choice for a true lateral periodontal cyst. Bone regeneration within the surgical defect will occur spontaneously. A broad-based full-thickness mucoperiosteal flap is recommended as it allows for adequate coverage of the bony defect and minimizes the chances of postoperative periodontal disease. Most lesions are accessed via a labial or buccal approach. Recurrence is very rare, and most often related to incomplete removal of the original cyst. Root divergence, if present, will become reduced or become normalized even without orthodontic treatment. Multilocular lesions should also be treated with enucleation, but as the epithelial lining is thin, potential for incomplete removal, and thus recurrence is greater. Follow-up for approximately 10 years is recommended for multilocular lesions because of the limited number of reported cases and lack of complete understanding of its behavior.

Odontogenic Keratocyst

The odontogenic keratocyst is believed to arise from remnants of the dental lamina retained within the alveolar bone following tooth development. Remarkable for an aggressive infiltrative growth pattern and a high rate of recurrence, the odontogenic keratocyst is thought by some to be best regarded as a benign cystic neoplasm.[21] Odontogenic keratocysts occur both in a sporadic fashion and as a component of the nevoid basal cell carcinoma syndrome, in which patients may develop multiple lesions. Recently, the gene for nevoid basal cell carcinoma syndrome was mapped to chromosome 9q22.3 and shown to be the human homologue to the Drosophila segment polarity gene *ptc* patched (PTCH).[22,23] This tumor suppressor gene functions as a component of the Hedgehog signaling pathway and has been isolated in both sporadic and syndrome-associated odontogenic keratocysts.[24]

The odontogenic keratocyst presents over a wide age range with the average age at presentation approximately 30 years.[25] Depending on the treatment modality employed to extirpate the lesion, a wide recurrence rate has been reported, ranging from 1 to 56%.[26] The odontogenic keratocyst most often presents in the posterior mandible and is frequently found in a dentigerous configuration associated with the crown of an unerupted tooth. Our experience has shown a significant number of odontogenic keratocysts presenting in the mandibular canine and first premolar regions mimicking the lateral periodontal cyst. Still, many odontogenic keratocysts are found within the alveolar bone unassociated with tooth structure. Occasionally, these lesions present in the maxilla, most frequently in the incisor-canine region.[25] Given the proclivity for this lesion to tunnel through the bone, odontogenic keratocysts may reach a large size prior to detection, and may show either a unilocular or multilocular radiographic appearance (Figs 7.3A and B). It is not uncommon for patients to present with pain and expansion in the region of the lesion.[25,27]

Histopathologically, the odontogenic keratocyst is remarkable for a uniformly thin stratified squamous cystic epithelial lining, approximately six to eight cell

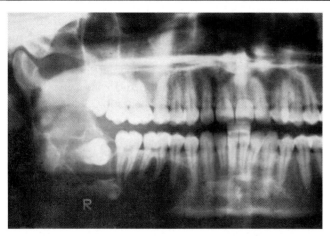

Fig. 7.3A: Large multilocular odontogenic keratocyst of the right mandible associated with an impacted third molar tooth. The lesion involves the condylar and coronoid processes of the mandible

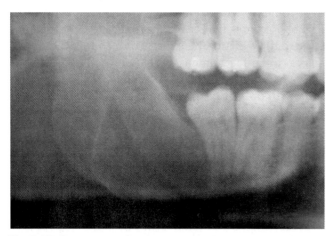

Fig. 7.3B: Recurrent, unilocular odontogenic keratocyst of the right posterior mandible. An impacted third molar tooth had been extracted many years previously by another surgeon, and the patient gave a history of a small cystic lesion that was enucleated, but not sent for histopathologic examination

layers in thickness. The luminal surface exhibits parakeratosis with focal surface corrugations akin to corrugated cardboard when viewed on end. Parakeratotic debris may be appreciated within the cystic lumen. The basal epithelial layer of the cystic lining exhibits nuclear palisading and hyperchromaticity. In the presence of inflammation, the cystic epithelial lining often loses these characteristic features and demonstrates a more hyperplastic appearance with transformation to a non-keratinizing stratified squamous morphology. Cell proliferation markers and cytokeratin expression patterns are altered in odontogenic keratocysts in the context of inflammation.[28,29] This alteration has been demonstrated

in cysts undergoing decompression and irrigation prior to surgical removal. In this context, the alteration in composition suggests a transformation to a lesion that is less proliferative and less amenable to recurrence.[29]

Treatment: The odontogenic keratocyst remains an enigma for clinicians and researchers, although gains in knowledge in recent years have improved the understanding of this lesion. Goals of treatment include the lowest rate of recurrence with least degree of morbidity to the patient, and ruling out the presence of Nevoid Basal Cell Carcinoma Syndrome. Enucleation of the lesion, by itself, is not an acceptable form of treatment. The cystic lining of these lesions is very friable, and will tend to fragment during enucleation, thereby leading to an increased incidence of incomplete removal of lesions. Root canal therapy is not required for teeth that test negative to pulp vitality testing, but these teeth should be monitored closely. If the lesion invaginates around teeth roots, it should be curetted out completely. The teeth that are instrumented in their radicular portions may become deinnervated but are not devitalized, and most regain responsiveness to pulp testing within one to two years.

The general approach for treating these lesions is enucleation and curettage. The most commonly employed method of curettage after enucleation is 'mechanical curettage' in the form of a 'peripheral ostectomy' using hand or rotary instruments. Some authors recommend use of additional 'chemical curettage' using Carnoy solution. This is a chemical fixative that is applied to the bony cavity following enucleation and curettage, and it has been demonstrated that after a 5 minute application, the chemical penetrates bone up to a depth of 1.54 mm.[30,31] Thermal curettage with cryotherapy has also been shown to be effective, but is not very popular.[32] Many clinicians have adopted the practice of removal of a rim of keratinized gingival tissue (especially on the lingual aspect) as it is believed that recurrences may arise from the residual odontogenic tissue (epithelial rests) in this area.

Alternative therapies for treatment include marsupalization and resection. Marsupalization of large lesions has been shown to be effective, but most surgeons agree that it has limited indications. Proponents of marsupalization claim that the cystic lining becomes thicker and easier to remove after prolonged irrigations, and a significant reduction in the size of the lesion (including complete elimination of cysts) can be attained; in contrast, others contend that it may lead to a higher rate of recurrence, especially in multilocular cases, and that the treatment has the disadvantages of a long-protracted course which does not decrease the incidence of pathological fracture or infection.

Resection may be indicated in two instances: (1) multiple recurrences after enucleation and curettage procedures, and/or (2) large multilocular keratocysts in which an enucleation and curettage procedure would result in near continuity loss by itself. Initial resection margins should be approximately 1.0 to 1.5 cm based on panoramic radiographs. Intraoperative radiographs of a resected specimen can be invaluable tools as they can help the clinician with intraoperative clinical decision making for deciding final surgical margins. Figures 7.4A to E show treatment of a large OKC of the mandible treated by one-stage mandibular resection and reconstruction. Traditionally, resection has often performed in enbloc fashion, with sacrifice of the inferior alveolar neurovascular bundle. However, certain new modifications to this surgery have recently been proposed in an attempt to preserve the inferior alveolar nerve.

Location of an odontogenic keratocyst also influences treatment philosophies. Some surgeons recommend more aggressive treatment for maxillary odontogenic keratocysts as compared to mandibular lesions. This philosophy is based on the fact that there is a lack of thick cortical boundaries in the maxilla, and large lesions can rapidly extend into soft tissues and 'dangerous' areas like the orbit and infratemporal fossa. However, for small lesions, enucleation and curettage is very effective. In this area, a sinus communication will often result, but this will readily heal with good primary closure. The presence of the maxillary sinus should not intimidate the clinician

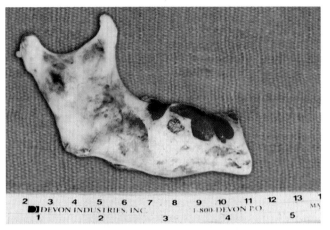

Fig. 7.4B: The mandible has been resected. The lingual aspect of the mandible and medial aspect of the ramus show cortical perforations

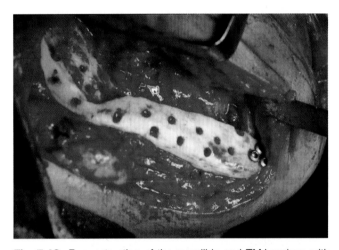

Fig. 7.4C: Reconstruction of the mandible and TMJ regions with cancellous marrow grafts (not cortical block grafts) harvested from the iliac crest. A freeze-dried cadaveric mandible has been used as a tray for placement of the cancellous bone grafts

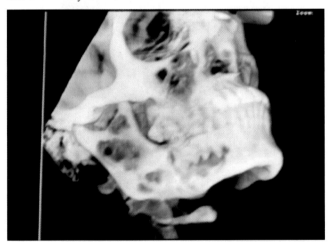

Fig. 7.4A: 3-D CT scan reconstruction showing a large odontogenic keratocyst of the right mandible. Note extracortical extension of the lesion as evidenced by bony perforations in the ascending ramus area

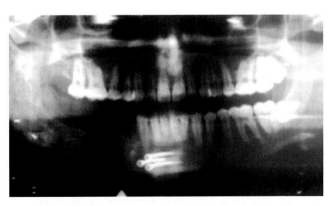

Fig. 7.4D: Postoperative panoramic radiograph showing reconstructed right mandible

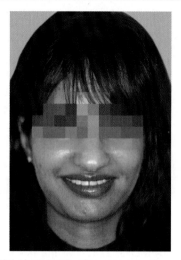

Fig. 7.4E: Facial photograph after reconstruction with cancellous marrow bone grafts demonstrating effective recreation of facial contour and balance

into being less thorough in this location and thereby invite recurrence.

The authors of this chapter have used all the above treatment modalities (excepting cryotherapy, which they have not used) with excellent success. Each case must be individually assessed, and treatment rendered with the aims of performing the least morbid surgery with the lowest rate of recurrence.

Prognosis: A wide variance in recurrence rates has been reported in the literature. However, a critical analysis of the literature reveals a wide array of treatment methods with limited scientific stratification of data regarding size, location, origin, and recurrence. Many reasons for recurrence have been proposed including:[33,34] (a) collagenase production, (b) daughter or satellite cysts, (c) budding, (d) incomplete removal, and, (e) increased mitotic activity.

Nevoid Basal Cell Carcinoma Syndrome

Nevoid basal cell carcinoma syndrome represents a condition of autosomal dominant inheritance remarkable for marked variability in expressivity. Recently, the gene for this syndrome was mapped to chromosome 9q22.3, the human homologue to the Drosophila segment polarity gene *ptc* patched (PTCH).[22,23] Litanies of stigmata are associated with nevoid basal cell carcinoma syndrome with widespread involvement affecting the jaws, extensive areas of the skin, the axial skeleton, and central nervous system.[35] Although a diverse array of clinical features may be seen in association with the syndrome including enlarged occipitofrontal circumference, calcification of the falx cerebri, rib anomalies, spina bifida, and mild ocular hypertelorism, the most serious manifestation of the syndrome with potential life threatening consequence is the proclivity to develop multiple basal cell carcinomas.[36] Additional skin lesions associated with nevoid basal cell carcinoma syndrome include epidermal cysts of the skin and palmar/plantar pits. With regard to the oral cavity, patients with nevoid basal cell carcinoma syndrome may develop multiple odontogenic keratocysts. Differing from sporadic cases of odontogenic keratocysts, syndrome-associated odontogenic keratocysts typically present in a younger patient population.

Diagnostic work-up: Plain X-rays should include: (a) skull films including an A-P and panoramic X-rays to visualize intracerebral calcifications and keratocysts respectively, (b) chest X-rays to assess rib abnormalities, and, (c) lumbosacral views to evaluate for spina bifida. Skin examination with biopsy of suspicious lesions should be performed. Palmar and plantar pits can be easily seen if they are coated with an iodine solution. Measurements of the occipitofrontal circumference and intercanthal distance are also important. Figures 7.5A to E show a patient with nevoid basal cell carcinoma syndrome. The maxillary odontogenic keratocysts were treated with enucleation and curettage, and the large mandibular

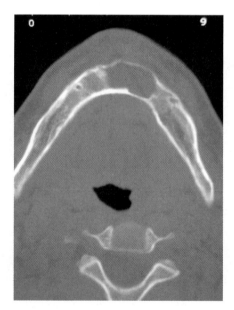

Fig. 7.5A: Axial CT scan of a patient with Gorlin's syndrome showing radiolucent lesions (odontogenic keratocysts) of the mandible

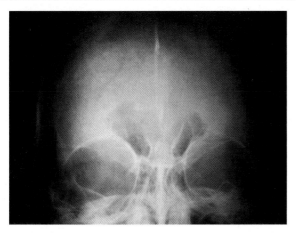

Fig. 7.5B: Plain film of the skull showing a calcified falx cerebri

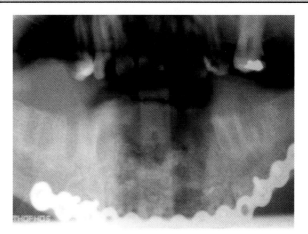

Fig. 7.5E: Postoperative panoramic radiograph showing reconstructed anterior mandible

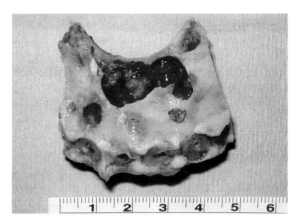

Fig. 7.5C: Resected mandible with multiple odontogenic keratocysts

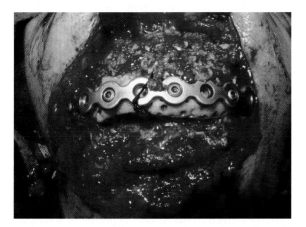

Fig. 7.5D: Reconstruction of the mandible with a bone plate and cancellous marrow cellular grafts harvested from the iliac crest and platelet-rich plasma. Advantages of cancellous bone grafts harvested from the iliac crest include the ability to obtain excellent height and width of bone, and perform the surgery with minimal morbidity. Most patients ambulate the same day and leave the hospital within 1–2 days after surgery

keratocysts necessitated mandibular resection. Simultaneous mandibular reconstruction was performed with iliac crest bone grafts and platelet rich plasma.

Treatment: Genetic counseling is recommended for all patients since the inheritance pattern is autosomal dominant. However, approximately 40% of cases are new mutations. Treatment should follow the same general principles that are used for treating isolated odontogenic keratocysts. Although multiple cysts are the characteristic finding, some patients may only have solitary lesions. Most patients are young in age, and thus, most odontogenic follicles may have functionally usable teeth; thus, marsupialization and orthodontics to guide eruption may be options for treatment. Skin lesions are usually basal cell carcinomas, but the type of lesions seen in these patients is not as aggressive as the ones seen from actinic damage. Thus, observation before radical removal may be indicated. It has been suggested that only those lesions with ulceration, rapid growth, bleeding, or encrustment be removed, and all others be observed. Long-term follow-up of these patients affected with this syndrome is recommended.

Orthokeratinizing Odontogenic Cyst

Not all keratinizing odontogenic cysts behave equally. Although historically the orthokeratinizing odontogenic cyst was thought to represent a variant of the odontogenic keratocyst, the orthokeratinizing odontogenic cyst is now understood to simply represent an odontogenic cyst that exhibits orthokeratosis. Typically, discovered on routine radiographic examination, orthokeratinizing odontogenic cysts present as solitary well-circumscribed radiolucencies. Most frequently presenting in the posterior mandible and often found in a dentigerous configuration around the crown of an unerupted tooth, orthokeratinizing odontogenic cysts have a predilection for occurring in males and present over a wide age range.[37] Unlike the parakeratinized odontogenic keratocyst, orthokeratotic odontogenic cysts do not exhibit an aggressive character and seldom recur. Differences in expression patterns of cytokeratins, tenascin, and extracellular matrix proteins between orthokeratinizing odontogenic cysts and the odontogenic keratocyst further support the distinction between the two entities and the differences in biologic behavior.[38] Differences in expression levels of these cellular constituents are suggestive of a decreased capacity for cell migration and a more mature keratinization pattern in the orthokeratinized variant.

Histopathological examination of an orthokeratinizing odontogenic cyst shows a cystic cavity lined by orthokeratinized stratified squamous epithelium. Orthokeratotic debris may be appreciated within the cystic lumen. A prominent keratohyaline granular cell layer is present just below the orthokeratotic surface. The epithelium is uniformly thin; approximately, six to eight cell layers in total thickness. The basal epithelial cell layer is typically flattened cuboidal, and lacks the characteristic nuclear palisading observed in parakeratinized odontogenic keratocysts.

Treatment

Simple enucleation is recommended and recurrence is not expected following complete removal of the lesion.

Glandular Odontogenic Cyst

Originally coined by Gardner,[39] the term glandular odontogenic cyst denotes a recently described developmental odontogenic cyst remarkable for an often-aggressive biologic behavior. Clinically, the glandular odontogenic cyst most frequently presents in the anterior mandible, occasionally crossing the midline. Although the glandular odontogenic cyst has been reported over a wide age range the lesion is typically encountered in adults over the age of 20 years, with pain and expansion commonly encountered.[40] This cystic lesion typically presents distinctly apical to teeth which respond positively to vitality testing. Rarely, the glandular odontogenic cyst may assume a dentigerous configuration;[41] however, unilocular, multilocular, and even multicentric lesions have been reported unassociated with tooth structure.[40] Recurrence is not uncommon and has been reported to be greater than 21%.[40,42]

Histopathologically, the glandular odontogenic cyst is lined by stratified squamous epithelium. The luminal aspect of the epithelial lining is remarkable for the presence of eosinophilic cuboidal to columnar cells that may assume an irregular subtle papillary configuration. Surface cilia, scattered mucous cells, and cells with clear cytoplasm are often noted. Foci of epithelial proliferation are frequently encountered and pools of mucicarmine positive material surrounded by cuboidal eosinophilic cells are seen yielding a duct-like appearance. The basal epithelial cell layer is often hyperchromatic, and the epithelial-connective tissue interface is flat without demonstrable rete ridge architecture.

Treatment

Controversy continues to surround this lesion, and until more clear cut data from longer follow-up studies is available, in the authors' opinion, enucleation and curettage is the recommended treatment. Recurrence has been reported if enucleation alone is performed. It may be prudent to get a second opinion from an experienced oral and maxillofacial pathologist, who could study serial sections of the specimen. There have been some reports of low-grade mucoepidermoid carcinomas arising in patients approximately 3 to 5 years after the lesions were originally diagnosed as glandular odontogenic cysts. Controversy exists as to the validity of these reports since they may have represented initially underdiagnosed muco-epidermoid carcinomas. All patients with this diagnosis should be closely monitored.

Calcifying Odontogenic Cyst

The calcifying odontogenic cyst represents an uncommonly encountered developmental odontogenic cyst occurring with equal frequency in the maxilla and mandible. Unique in its proclivity to occur in association with other odontogenic tumors, the calcifying odontogenic cyst has been shown to present as a 'hybrid' lesion together with odontoma, ameloblastic fibroma, adenomatoid odontogenic tumor, and ameloblastoma.[43-46]

The calcifying odontogenic cyst may present exclusively within bone or peripherally as a soft tissue mass within the alveolar mucosa. Additionally, a solid neoplasm exists often referred to as the *dentinogenic ghost cell tumor* that shares many histologic features with the cystic lesion and may behave in an aggressive fashion. The varied presentation of the calcifying odontogenic cyst has historically made the classification scheme for this entity cumbersome. Many authors support the idea that the calcifying odontogenic cyst exists in two clinical-pathologic forms: One as a cystic lesion, the other as a neoplastic lesion.[47,48] Others suggest the lesion simply represents a neoplasm with the potential for cyst formation.

The intraosseous calcifying odontogenic cyst typically presents in patients in their second decade of life,[49] while the peripheral and neoplastic solid lesions are typically reported to have a later onset.[50] The intraosseous lesions have a propensity for occurring anterior to the first molar and are well-circumscribed with either a unilocular or multilocular configuration on radiographic examination. Occasionally, the lesions contain radiodensities consistent with foci of calcification (Fig. 7.6). Peripheral lesions present on the alveolar mucosa and show a nodular proliferation clinically indistinguishable from other common benign gingival nodules, and with occasional erosion of the subjacent alveolar bone.[51] If the lesion is located proximal to the apices of teeth, divergence of roots and marked root resorption are not uncommon.[52]

The calcifying odontogenic cyst histopathologically resembles craniopharyngioma and pilomatirixoma of the skin. Interestingly, each of these lesions has been shown to harbor a somatic β-catenin mutation. This mutation is thought to disrupt the differentiation process coordinated by the WNT signaling pathway with subsequent lesional formation.[53] Histologically, the cystic lesions consist of a cavity lined by epithelial cells showing a columnar basal epithelial cell layer exhibiting reversed nuclear polarity with overlying stellate reticulum-like epithelium yielding

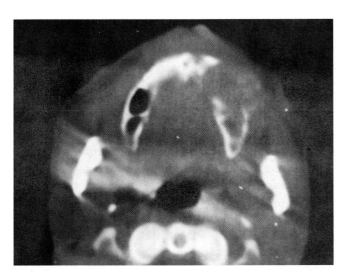

Fig. 7.6: Axial CT scan showing a calcifying odontogenic cyst of the maxillary alveolus

a distinct resemblance to the ameloblastoma. So-called 'ghost cells' characteristic of the lesion are present in variable amounts and consist of polygonal eosinophilic cells with central pale-staining regions representing absence of nuclei. These ghost cells, which may consist of aberrantly differentiated keratinocytes[54] or foci of coagulative necrosis,[55] form a syncytial appearance and often calcify. Dysplastic dentin may be seen and is thought to result from induction by proximal odontogenic epithelium. The neoplastic solid form of the calcifying odontogenic cyst shows a mature fibrous stroma with islands of odontogenic epithelium exhibiting columnar peripheral cells with reversed nuclear polarity surrounding a stellate reticulum like core. The epithelial islands contain sheets of ghost cells, variable foci of calcification, and dentinoid formation. An invasive growth pattern, atypical mitotic figures, necrosis, and cellular pleomorphism may suggest transformation to an aggressive or malignant variant.[56]

Treatment

There is no consensus regarding the biologic behavior of these lesions. While most researchers believe that these lesions have limited biologic behavior, some feel that many variants of these lesions exist, and that some of these variants have neoplastic potential.[55] When one reads contemporary oral and maxillofacial surgery literature, recommendations for treatment of calcifying odontogenic cysts are generally confined to either enucleation or enucleation with curettage for central cystic lesions, and simple excision for peripheral variants.[55,57]

Inflammatory Odontogenic Cysts

Buccal Bifurcation Cyst

Eruption of the mandibular first molar teeth begins with emergence of the mesiobuccal cusp into the oral cavity. It is hypothesized that at the time of initial eruption, a focus of inflammation just apical to the epithelial attachment stimulates epithelial proliferation.[58] This epithelial proliferation serves as the epithelial lining of the buccal bifurcation cyst. Although an inflammatory etiology is the likely explanation in most cases, in some instances a genetic predisposition to development of the lesion may also play a role as the lesion has also been reported in identical twins.[59] The buccal bifurcation cyst is an uncommon lesion presenting in children typically preceding eruption of the mandibular first molar.

Clinically, many features proposed by Stoneman and Worth[58] are characteristic of the lesion. First, the cystic lesion is associated with vital teeth having a radiographically normal periodontal ligament and lamina dura. Further, expansion of the cystic lesion on the buccal surface of the tooth causes tipping of the root apices toward the lingual cortical plate making the apices visible lingual to the crown when viewed on an occlusal radiograph. This tilting often increases the prominence of the lingual cusp.[60] Buccal swelling and a periosteal reaction are not uncommon.[59]

Histologically, the buccal bifurcation cyst is characterized by a cystic cavity lined by hyperplastic, stratified squamous epithelium. A prominent chronic inflammatory cell infiltrate is found within the cyst wall and marked exocytosis of inflammatory cells can be appreciated within the epithelial lining. Treatment usually involves simple enucleation similar to dentigerous cysts. It is recommended that teeth in association with these lesions be preserved.

Periapical Cyst

The periapical cyst typically develops secondary to sustained antigenic stimulation from the root canal of a non-vital tooth. Keratinocyte growth factor produced by connective tissue fibroblasts is thought to stimulate transformation of odontogenic epithelial rests of Malassez within the alveolar bone from a quiescent epithelial rest into a cystic epithelial lining.[61] Various cytokines then act to stimulate peripheral bone resorption and promote cyst enlargement in conjunction with expansion secondary to increased osmotic pressure.[62] Unless secondarily infected, the periapical cyst presents clinically as an asymptomatic lesion that is discovered on routine radiographic examination. Associated with the apex of a tooth containing necrotic pulpal tissue, the periapical cyst presents as a well-circumscribed radiolucency indistinguishable from a periapical granuloma (Fig. 7.7A). If associated with an accessory root canal, the periapical cyst often presents laterally along the root surface and is often referred to as a *lateral radicular cyst*. Elimination of the inciting inflammatory stimulus by treatment of the infected tooth with either a root canal procedure or extraction typically leads to resolution. If lesional tissue persists within the alveolar bone following extraction of the affected tooth, a residual cyst may result. Overtime, these residual lesions may regress secondary to lack of an inflammatory stimulus.

Histopathologically, the periapical cyst consists of a cystic cavity lined by hyperplastic, stratified squamous

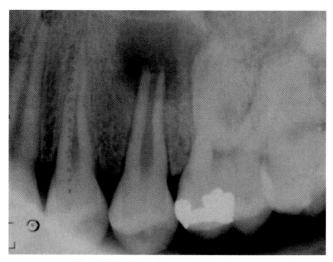

Fig. 7.7A: Periapical cysts are present at the apex of non-vital teeth

epithelium. A mixed inflammatory infiltrate is noted within the cyst wall with inflammatory cell exocytosis appreciated throughout the epithelium. Rushton bodies may often be appreciated characterized by intraepithelial lamellar concretions. These calcified bodies are thought to result from single epithelial cell apoptosis and necrosis with subsequent dystrophic calcification.[63] Cholesterol cleft formation and dystrophic calcification may be observed within the cyst wall. Additionally, the cyst wall may also contain amorphous eosinophilic hyaline rings that represent fibrosed inflammatory exudate. These hyaline bodies are often seen in association with multinucleated giant cells.

Treatment: Treatment of most periapical (radicular) cysts involves removal of the offending cause, i.e. tooth pulp infection. In general, every effort should be made to preserve the tooth. If the tooth can be salvaged, endodontic therapy (root canal therapy) is indicated; conversely, if the tooth is non-salvageable, then extraction of the tooth is recom-mended. If the endodontic treatment is not adequately performed or if the root canals are not optimally sealed, the inflammatory process perpetuates, and the cyst may continue to enlarge. Surgical curettage with apicoectomy and retrofill may be indicated in these cases. In cases where extraction of the tooth is performed, but the cyst is not removed, one should expect cyst involution with time. If spontaneous involution does not occur within a reasonable period of time, further treatment may be indicated. Occasionally, untreated periapical cysts can increase significantly in size and cause extensive bone destruction (Fig. 7.7B).

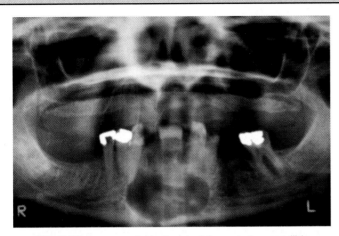

Fig. 7.7B: Large periapical cyst of the anterior mandible

Cysts of the Jaws of Nonodontogenic Origin

Nasopalatine Duct Cyst

Representing the most common intraoral nonodontogenic cyst,[64] the nasopalatine duct cyst is believed to be derived from residua of embryonic ductal structures that persist within the incisive canal. The specific inciting event that causes the quiescent epithelial rest to experience cystic degeneration is unknown, however, local trauma, focal inflammatory events such as infection, and spontaneous proliferation have been hypothesized to initiate the process of cyst development.[65-67]

Although reported over a wide age range, and occasionally reported in children,[68,69] nasopalatine duct cysts typically present in patients in the fifth to seventh decade of life.[66] Common presenting symptoms include pain and swelling in the anterior palate posterior to the maxillary central incisors (Fig. 7.8A). Secondary infection may yield intermittent drainage of purulent exudate from the lesion with associated waxing and waning of symptoms. Radiographic examination reveals a well-circumscribed radiolucency between the apices of the maxillary central incisors. Occasionally, the radiolucency is remarkable for a heart shape, which may result from superimposition of the nasal spine on radiographic imaging or a true invagination of the cystic lesion by the nasal septum. Pure soft tissue lesions that do not involve the underlying bone occasionally occur and are referred to as cysts of the incisive papilla.

Histopathological examination of the lesion reveals an epithelial-lined cystic cavity. The composition of the epithelial lining is variable most typically showing pseudostratified ciliated columnar and/or stratified squamous differentiation. Mucous cells are frequently noted within the cystic epithelial lining. The cyst wall generally contains contents of the incisive canal including numerous neurovascular bundles, mature hyaline cartilage, and minor salivary gland lobules. The cyst wall may contain variable numbers of inflammatory cells.

Treatment: Simple enucleation is the recommended treatment for these cysts. The maxillary anterior teeth must be pulp tested to rule out the possibility of odontogenic origin, but clinicians must be aware that there may be false negative results. If bone erosion is seen labially on CT scanning, access via a labial approach is recommended. However, some large lesions may require a palatal approach. A posteriorly based full-thickness flap is raised, and the lesion enucleated (Fig. 7.8B). Care should be taken while performing surgery on large lesions, as the cyst is frequently found to be adherent to the palatal mucoperiosteum. These areas may require careful and often sharp dissection to avoid palatal tissue tears during surgery.

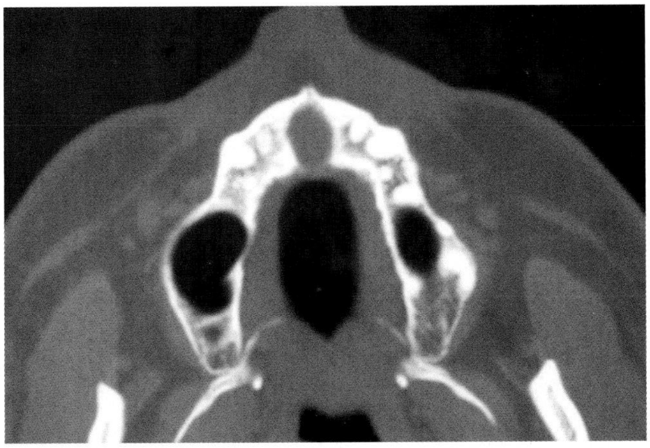

Fig. 7.8A: "Heart-shaped" radiolucency in the anterior palate, which is characteristic of a nasopalatine duct cyst

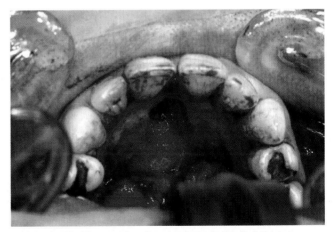

Fig. 7.8B: The cyst has been exposed via a full-thickness palatal mucoperiosteal flap

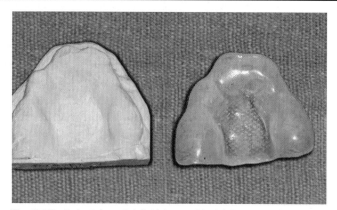

Fig. 7.8C: A dental model (left) is used to fabricate a soft-thermoplastic splint (right), which is used postoperatively as a "bandage"

The authors recommend the use a soft thermoplastic splint (Fig. 7.8C) if a palatal surgical approach is used. The splint can be secured with screws, wires, or sutures, and has the following advantages: (a) increased patient comfort, (b) provides protection to those areas with iatrogenic tears that have been repaired, and (c) provides support to palatal soft tissue which can otherwise dehisce from hematoma formation in the bony cavity. In the authors' experience, bone grafting is not usually needed as the bony cavity will spontaneously generate bone. Recurrence is not expected after complete removal of these lesions.

Nasolabial Cyst

The nasolabial cyst is a developmental cyst thought to either be derived from rests of epithelium persisting after incomplete degeneration of the embryonic nasolacrimal duct or from epithelium entrapped during fusion of the medial and lateral nasal processes.[70,71] The lesion presents as a swelling of the upper lip lateral to the ala of the nose with intraoral obliteration of the maxillary labial vestibule. Occasionally, a cup-shaped defect secondary to pressure erosion of the subjacent bone may be appreciated.[70] With an apparent propensity for occurring in females, the nasolabial cyst has occasionally been reported to occur bilaterally.[71]

Histopathological examination of the nasolabial cyst shows a cystic cavity typically lined by pseudostratified ciliated columnar epithelium containing scattered mucous cells, however squamous, cuboidal and columnar differentiation may be appreciated.[72,73] A variable inflammatory infiltrate may be observed within the cyst wall.

Treatment: A true nasolabial cyst should not have any bony involvement, and is non-odontogenic in origin.

However, large cysts can result in some bony erosion due to pressure (nasoalveolar cysts). Pulp testing of the maxillary anterior teeth should be performed to rule out odontogenic infection as the source of the swelling. Treatment involves simple excision, and recurrence is not expected. Perforation into the nasal cavity should be expected in approximately half the cases.[74]

Gingival Cysts of the Adult

The gingival cyst of the adult is thought to be derived from residua of dental lamina persisting within the alveolar mucosa following tooth development. Typically, presenting on the buccal surface of the alveolar mucos in the mandibular premolar and canine region, the gingival cyst of the adult commonly occurs in patients 40 to 60 years of age. The lesion represents a swelling that may exhibit a slight blue to gray coloration. A resorptive defect of the alveolar bone may be appreciated subjacent to the soft tissue lesion. Treatment involves simple excision and primary closure. Recurrence is not seen.

Palatal Cysts of the Newborn

Palatal cysts of the newborn are thought to derive from either entrapment of epithelium along embryonic lines of fusion or from embryonic epithelial residua of developing minor salivary gland lobules. Common lesions discovered in neonates, palatal cysts present as small yellow-white nodules on the palate often in the midline at or near the junction of the hard and soft palate. Although occasionally solitary, these cystic lesions often present in small clusters.[75]

Histopathological examination of a palatal cyst of the newborn shows an epithelial lined cavity, which often contains keratinaceous debris. The cystic epithelial lining shows a stratified squamous differentiation and may communicate with the surface mucosa.

No treatment except parental reassurance is needed. Typically, palatal cysts spontaneously involute or rupture into the oral cavity by 3 to 4 months of age.

Dermoid Cyst

The dermoid cyst represents a developmental non-odontogenic cystic lesion thought to derive from pleuripotential cells entrapped within the formative oral tissues. These pleuripotential cells possess the capacity to develop into tissues from each representative germ layer. A complex nomenclature exists for these cystic lesions. The term 'dermoid' cyst is an inclusive term with further sub-classification of cystic variants into three categories defined by the constituent germ layers represented within the cystic lesion. First, the term 'epidermoid' cyst is used for simple cystic lesions comprised of an epithelial lining and surrounded by an unremarkable fibrous connective tissue wall. When the cystic lesion consists of both an epithelial lining and contains dermal adnexa in the cyst wall such as sebaceous glands and hair appendages, it is considered compound in nature and the term 'dermoid' cyst is applied. Lastly, the name 'teratoid' cyst is reserved for complex lesions comprised of an epithelial-lined cavity with both epithelial and non-epithelial elements within the cyst wall such as bone, muscle, and gastrointestinal tissue.[76,77] Despite attempts at sub-classification, the term 'dermoid' is typically understood to represent all developmental cysts arising in this locale.[78]

Clinically, the dermoid cyst typically presents as a fluctuant midline swelling of the floor of the mouth (Fig. 7.9A), however, lateral presentations have been reported, and lesions that may represent dermoid cysts presenting at other intraoral sites such as the tongue and in the mandible have also been described.[79-82] If the lesion develops above the geniohyoid muscle, dyspnea and dysphagia may develop. Lesions occurring below the geniohyoid muscle yield a characteristic 'double chin' appearance. Although these lesions typically present in patients in the second and third decade of life, occasional congenital lesions are reported.[77,83]

Histopathological examination of a dermoid cyst shows a cystic epithelial lining that may show pseudostratified ciliated columnar or orthokeratinized stratified squamous epithelial differentiation. The contents of the cystic cavity often contain abundant keratinaceous debris. Variable apocrine and eccrine dermal appendages and pilosebaceous structures may be found within the cyst wall. In addition to dermal adnexal structures, complex teratoid cystic lesions may contain variable amounts of mesenchymal tissue including muscle, gastrointestinal, respiratory epithelium and bone within the cyst wall.

Treatment: These lesions can vary tremendously in size and location. Aspiration will usually show return of straw colored fluid with keratin-like material. Small lesions in easily accessible surgical sites may be excised in an office setting under local anesthesia or intravenous sedation. However, larger and deeper lesions and those in surgically 'difficult' areas will require wider access, possible transcutaneous incisions, and general anesthesia in a hospital setting. CT scan or MRI examination may be useful in treatment planning of large lesions (Figs 7.9B, C). A thick-walled cyst with a fluid-filled center is appreciated on these radiographs.

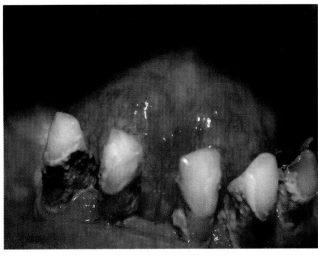

Fig. 7.9A: Intraoral photograph showing a large dermoid cyst causing a raised swelling in the midline of the floor of mouth region

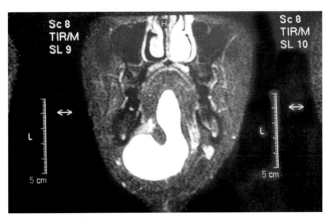

Fig. 7.9B: MRI examination shows a fluid-filled lesion extending below the mylohyoid muscle

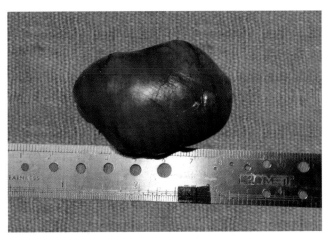

Fig. 7.9C: The excised dermoid cyst after removal via an intraoral approach

Dermoid cysts are common in the floor of the mouth, and care should be taken to preserve the submandibular ducts and lingual nerves during surgery in this area. Treatment usually involves excision of the lesion from surrounding tissue via a transoral and/or transcutaneous approach. The cysts may, at times, be adherent to the adjacent tissues, and this may necessitate a combination of blunt and sharp dissection for optimal removal. If the cyst is large, removal will often leave a significant defect with large dead space; thus, layered closure of the wound with drain placement is recommended. Even if the surgery was performed transorally, in many instances of large lesions, it may be a good idea to place a drain through a transcutaneous stab incision in the submental crease as this allows for dependent drainage.

PSEUDOCYSTS OF THE JAWS

Simple Bone Cyst

The simple bone cyst represents a non-neoplastic intrabony cavity devoid of an epithelial lining. Although the cause for each lesion may be different, the simple bone cyst is currently thought to represent a focal vasodynamic abnormality. This vascular irregularity may result from increased regional blood flow at the site of bone remodeling giving rise to a hydrodynamic anomaly with secondary venous obstruction and bone cyst formation.[84,85] Representing approximately 1% of all cyst-like lesions of the jaws, the simple bone cyst most frequently presents in the anterior mandible in patients under the age of 20 years.[86,87] Radiographically, the simple bone cyst traditionally presents as a unilocular radiolucent lesion that is remarkable for interdental 'scalloping' between the roots of vital teeth without cortical expansion, however multilocular lesions, lesions presenting in a dentigerous configuration, and multiple lesions occurring in the same patient have been reported.[88] Additionally, simple bone cysts are often seen in association with fibro-osseous lesions.[89-93] Here, it has been suggested that irregular vascularity in the fibro-osseous lesion leads to obstruction of lymphatic drainage with subsequent cystic degeneration.[93]

Histopathological examination of tissue removed from a simple bone cyst cavity consists of fragments of fibrous connective tissue and extravasated erythrocytes, granulation tissue and spicules of vital bone from the cavity wall. Since this lesion does not represent a true cyst, no epithelial lining is appreciated.

Treatment

Most lesions are diagnosed only after surgical exploration. Aspiration of these cavities will often show some initial air bubbles, followed by some straw-colored fluid, and then by blood. The continued negative pressure of aspiration disturbs the medullary capillaries, and initiates bleeding from them. In cases of a positive bloody aspirate, it is important to rule out vascular lesions. An idiopathic bony cavity can be differentiated from a vascular lesion by first removing the syringe, but leaving the needle in place. The bleeding should cease in cases of an idiopathic bony cavity, but will continue in cases of large vascular lesions. As in any surgical procedure of this kind, after aspiration, a bony window should be removed, and the area accessed. A thorough examination should be performed for any cystic lining. On surgical exploration, an empty bony cavity is observed. Sometimes, a fibrinous mass may be encountered within the cavity. The bony walls should be curetted, and usually this is all that is required. The exploration surgery stimulates bony fill and remodeling within the lesion in most cases.

ANEURYSMAL BONE CYST

The aneursymal bone cyst is a central osteolytic lesion that occurs in either a solitary fashion as a primary lesion or in association with a pre-existing neoplasm such as a central giant cell granuloma, benign fibro-osseous lesion, osteosarcoma, or osteoblastoma.[94,95] Uncommon in the jaws, the aneurysmal bone cyst typically presents in patients younger than 20 years, has a predilection for occurring in the posterior mandible and a propensity for recurrence.[96-98] The cause of this lesion is incompletely understood. Recent studies have shown the primary subset of aneurysmal bone cysts represent a true neoplastic process with chromosomal translocation $t(16;17)(q22;p13)$ and transcriptional upregulation of the ubiquitin protease gene (USP6).[99-101] So-called 'secondary' aneurysmal bone cyst-like areas described in association with other benign and malignant neoplasms may represent a morphologically similar non-specific growth pattern that can occur in many primary bone lesions secondary to disrupted vascular supply.

Clinically, pain and swelling of recent onset are typically reported in patients with an aneurysmal bone cyst. Radiographic findings include a unilocular to multilocular soap-bubble or honeycomb radiolucency with bony expansion and occasional cortical perforation.

Histopathologic examination of lesional tissue reveals multiple sinusoidal spaces filled with erythrocytes and surrounded by a cellular fibrous connective tissue stroma. Multinucleated osteoclast-type giant cells,[102] osteoid, woven bone, and fine, reticular calcifications are often found at the periphery of the blood-filled spaces.

Treatment

Complete thorough curettage of the lesion and bony cavity is the conventional treatment. Many surgeons also advocate the use of cryotherapy or cauterization of the bony cavity following curettage. This is based on the fact that there is a high recurrence rate in the literature for aneurysmal bone cysts in the general skeleton. Recurrent or large lesions that risk pathological fracture may require en bloc resection with 0.5 to 1.0 cm margins, followed by jaw reconstruction. The surgeon can expect significant hemorrhage until the pathologic tissue is entirely removed, especially in large lesions. Although recurrence has been reported, it is rare if adequate curettage is performed during initial surgery. The solid lesions are virtually indistinguishable with central giant cell 'lesions'.

Many non-surgical treatments are gaining in popularity for the treatment of many giant cell lesions of the jaws. These include treatment with corticosteroids, calcitonin hormone, and more recently anti-angiogenic pharmaceutical therapy.[103-105]

TUMORS OF THE JAWS[a]

ODONTOGENIC TUMORS

Inductive interaction between odontogenic epithelial and ectomesenchymal tissues plays a critical role in the development of odontogenic tumors. Conventionally, the classification follows histogenesis with the neoplastic component of an odontogenic tumor dictating placement in the classification scheme. Traditionally, odontogenic tumors are divided into three categories: epithelial, ectomesenchymal, or mixed odontogenic tumors. First, epithelial odontogenic tumors represent those tumors in which the neoplastic component consists of odontogenic epithelium without ectomesenchymal proliferation. Conversely, ectomesenchymal odontogenic tumors are those tumors that derive from ectomesenchymal elements. Although odontogenic epithelium may be appreciated in tumors of ectomesenchymal odontogenic origin, odontogenic epithelium does not participate in the neoplastic process. Lastly, odontogenic tumors in which both odontogenic epithelial and ectomesenchymal elements contribute to the neoplastic proliferation are classified as 'mixed' odontogenic tumors.

Given the complexity of odontogenic tumors, biological behavior and proliferative capacity interact to determine clinical outcome and prognosis. Treatment philosophy, therefore, serves to eradicate lesional tissue with least morbidity and maximum preservation or restoration of function.

EPITHELIAL ODONTOGENIC TUMORS

Adenomatoid Odontogenic Tumor

The adenomatoid odontogenic tumor is thought to originate from neoplastic transformation of dental lamina residua that persist within the alveolar bone following tooth development.[106] Incompletely understood events stimulate these odontogenic epithelial rests to proliferate with subsequent tumor formation. The adenomatoid odontogenic tumor most commonly presents in the anterior maxilla in female patients under the age of 20 years.[107] Lesions located centrally within bone are frequently seen in a dentigerous configuration, most often in association with the crown of an impacted canine.[108] Other lesions present in an extrafollicular location, independent of an unerupted tooth and occasionally mimicking periapical pathology.[109-111] Peripheral lesions have been reported that are exclusively confined to soft tissue and are clinically indistinguishable from other benign gingival nodules.[109]

Often noted on routine radiographic examination or when investigating the chief complaint of delayed eruption, the adenomatoid odontogenic tumor most commonly presents as a radiolucent lesion with a distinct radiopaque border[112] surrounding the crown of an unerupted tooth and extending beyond the cemento-enamel junction (Fig. 7.10). Small radiopaque foci,

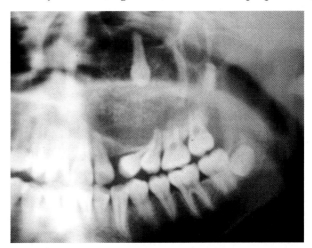

Fig. 7.10: Plain film showing a radiolucent lesion surrounding the entire tooth, a feature which is characteristic of an adenomatoid odontogenic tumor

so-called 'snowflake' calcifications, are frequently appreciated within the cystic lesion. Extrafollicular lesions are also well-circumscribed, many of which show displacement of vital teeth.[110,111]

Histopathologic examination of the adenomatoid odontogenic tumor shows an encapsulated proliferation of spindled epithelial cells oriented in sheets and whorls. The presence of amelogenin and enamelin has been shown within the tumor cell population, which suggests a pre-ameloblastic nature.[113] Although, no true glandular tissue is present within the lesion, the adenomatoid odontogenic tumor is remarkable for variable numbers of duct-like structures. Columnar odontogenic epithelial cells exhibiting nuclear polarization away from the pseudo-lumina line the duct-like structures. Rosette-like structures containing amyloid-positive material may also be appreciated. Abortive enamel and dentin formation within the tumor generates small foci of calcification that may be apparent on radiographic examination.

Treatment

Adenomatoid odontogenic tumors usually occur in the anterior maxilla of young individuals and commonly present as a unilocular radiolucency. Based on the location and radiographic appearance, differential diagnosis includes lesions such as dentigerous cyst, calcifying odontogenic cyst, calcifying epithelial odontogenic tumor, and desmoplastic ameloblastoma. An incisional biopsy may be indicated to establish a definitive diagnosis prior to treatment.

Aspiration will usually draw out straw-colored fluid. Surgical enucleation is the recommended treatment. A full-thickness mucoperiosteal flap is raised, and a bony window is made through the thinned-out cortex to access the lesion. The thick walled nature of the AOT lends itself to easy removal from its bony crypt. Recurrence is very rare. The impacted tooth is generally present within the cyst lumen, and is removed with the cyst.

Squamous Odontogenic Tumor

The squamous odontogenic tumor is an infrequently encountered benign odontogenic neoplasm remarkable for a locally infiltrative growth pattern. Central lesions most likely arise from neoplastic transformation of odontogenic epithelial rests of Malassez retained within the periodontal ligament space following tooth root development.[114] Rare peripheral lesions are thought to originate from rests of dental lamina that persist within the gingival tissues.[115,116]

Remarkable for a random distribution throughout the maxilla and mandible, the squamous odontogenic tumor presents over a wide age range and is most commonly encountered in the third decade of life.[117] Typically, presenting as a wedge-shaped radiolucency within the inter-radicular alveolar bone, the slow-growing neoplasm often presents asymptomatically with discovery on routine radiographic examination. In other instances, swelling, periodontal defects, tooth mobility and pain are reported.[117] Peripheral lesions confined exclusively to the soft tissue are impossible to distinguish clinically from other benign gingival nodules. Pressure resorption of the underlying alveolar bone in the peripheral variant may create a saucer-shaped radiolucent defect subjacent to the soft tissue neoplasm. Rare examples of the squamous odontogenic tumor involving multiple quadrants have been reported, and multifocal lesions occurring within individuals of the same family have also been described.[118,119]

Histopathologic examination of the squamous odontogenic tumor shows squamous epithelial islands of irregular size and shape within a mature fibrous connective tissue stroma. The epithelial islands are characterized by smooth, rounded borders with fluid lines, the peripheral cells of which are generally cuboidal or markedly flattened. Within the epithelial islands single cell dyskeratosis and central cystic degeneration are often noted. Additionally, foci of dystrophic calcific material and laminated calcifications are frequently appreciated.

Treatment

The squamous odontogenic tumor is a rare tumor, and there are few known characteristic signs to suggest its occurrence. Because most squamous odontogenic tumors present as well-circumscribed, unilocular radiolucencies, serious consideration must be given to the thought that the lesion may represent a more common cyst or tumor such as an odontogenic keratocyst, lateral periodontal cyst, ameloblastoma, or odontogenic myxoma. An incisional biopsy is indicated to confirm the diagnosis. It is important that the specimen be submitted for histologic diagnosis to an experienced oral pathologist, since the histopathologic presentation can resemble an ameloblastoma or squamous cell carcinoma to an individual unfamiliar with the lesion.[120]

Recommended surgical treatment usually involves enucleation and curettage. Because the lesion is benign but infiltrative, the surgical approach must be individualized. If the presence of tooth roots interferes with through curettage, tooth removal may be required.

Occasionally, resection of the alveolus without creating a continuity defect may be needed to permit complete removal of the tumor. If the lesion perforates bony cortices, removal of the overlying soft tissue should be considered. Recurrence is rare after complete removal.

Calcifying Epithelial Odontogenic Tumor (CEOT)[b]

The calcifying epithelial odontogenic tumor represents a rarely encountered odontogenic neoplasm of controversial origin. While some authors contend the neoplasm is derived from reduced enamel epithelium,[121] recent investigation suggests the lesion originates from neoplastic transformation of dental lamina residua persisting within the alveolar bone following tooth formation.[122] The calcifying epithelial odontogenic tumor most commonly presents in the posterior mandible of patients in the third to fifth decade of life,[103] however, the lesion has been reported to occur over a broad age range involving various sites throughout the maxilla and mandible. Typically, the calcifying epithelial odontogenic tumor arises centrally within bone, often presenting as a slow-growing, expansile, painless mass located in a dentigerous configuration surrounding the crown of an unerupted tooth. A peripheral variant of the calcifying epithelial odontogenic tumor confined exclusively to the soft tissue has been reported,[123] and is clinically indistinguishable from other benign gingival nodules. Radiographically, the central calcifying epithelial odontogenic tumor presents as a unilocular or multilocular radiolucent lesion with scalloped margins and variable foci of radiopacity (Fig. 7.11). Lesions

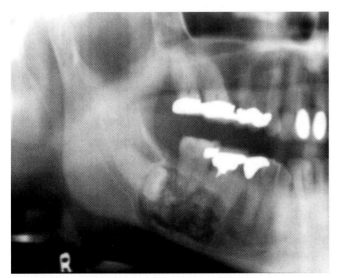

Fig. 7.11: The calcifying epithelial odontogenic tumor often presents as a radiolucent lesion with variable degree of radiopacities, and an associated impacted tooth

presenting in a dentigerous configuration often show foci of calcification in close proximity to the crown of the involved tooth. Peripheral lesions may occasionally produce a pressure resorptive defect of the alveolar bone subjacent to the soft tissue neoplasm.

Histological examination of the calcifying epithelial odontogenic tumor reveals sheets of polyhedral epithelial cells remarkable for deeply eosinophilic cytoplasm and conspicuous intercellular bridges in a mature fibrous connective tissue stroma. Nuclear pleomorphism is often appreciated within the epithelial component of the lesion; however, this variability in nuclear morphology does not suggest malignant biologic behavior. Additionally, the epithelial component may contain variable numbers of glycogen-rich clear cells of unknown biologic significance.[124] Foci of amorphous extracellular eosinophilic product exhibiting the tinctorial and ultrastructural features of amyloid are appreciated throughout the lesion. Although the matter of much debate, current concepts support the idea that this eosinophilic product represents a form of amyloid derived from a novel protein encoded by the FLJ20513 gene.[125] Calcific foci are appreciated in varying abundance throughout the lesion. The small, droplet-like calcific foci frequently unite to form large syncytial conglomerations.

Treatment

CEOT may present as either a radiolucency or more commonly, as a mixed radiolucent-radiopaque lesion. With the former presentation, the differential diagnosis must include common odontogenic lesions such as a dentigerous cyst, odontogenic keratocyst, ameloblastoma, or an odontogenic myxoma. For mixed density lesions, the differential diagnosis should include such entities as the calcifying odontogenic cyst, ameloblastic fibro-odontoma, desmoplastic ameloblastoma, and fibro-osseous lesions.

Once a diagnosis has been established, CT should be obtained to accurately delineate the exact location and extension of the tumor. Surgical treatment should be advised on a case-specific basis. Although the 1992, World Health Organization conference describes the CEOT as a benign, locally invasive neoplasm without a recurrence pattern, there are reports of up to 30% recurrence within 2 to 3 years.[126] A review of the recurrent cases shows that most were originally treated by enucleation and curettage. Based on the paucity of reported cases and the high rate of recurrence with conservative management, it is generally agreed that this tumor should be resected with 1 to 2 cm margins. Immediate or delayed bone reconstruction can be performed as per the surgeon's preference.

AMELOBLASTOMA[c]

The ameloblastoma represents a benign yet locally aggressive odontogenic tumor remarkable for the capacity to insinuate itself into surrounding tissues and recur with high frequency. Although the pathogenesis is uncertain, it is likely the ameloblastoma arises from neoplastic transformation of dental lamina residua persisting within the alveolar bone following tooth development.[127,128] Three variants of ameloblastoma are recognized and are notable for differing clinical characteristics and biologic behavior: The conventional 'solid' variant, the unicystic variant, and the peripheral variant confined exclusively to the soft tissue.

The conventional ameloblastoma rarely presents in patients under the age of twenty years and has a predilection for occurring in the posterior mandible. Typically, presenting as a slow-growing, painless, expansile mass, the conventional ameloblastoma is known for a remarkably high rate of recurrence. Frequently, arising in a dentigerous configuration associated with the crown of an unerupted tooth, the conventional ameloblastoma classically presents as a multilocular radiolucency remarkable for a 'soap bubble' or honeycomb appearance (Fig. 7.12A), however unilocular lesions are occasionally encountered (Fig. 7.12B). One distinctive variant termed the *desmoplastic ameloblastoma* is remarkable for a mixed radiolucent-radiopaque appearance and has a predilection for occurring in the anterior maxilla. Histopathologically, the conventional follicular ameloblastoma shows infiltrative

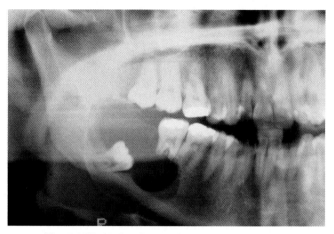

Fig. 7.12B: Unilocular ameloblastoma resembling a dentigerous cyst

islands of odontogenic epithelium on a mature fibrous connective tissue stroma. The epithelial islands consist of a central stellate reticulum-like core rimmed by columnar epithelial cells exhibiting palisading and reversed nuclear polarity with cytoplasmic vacuolization proximal to the basement membrane. Histologic variants in which the stellate-reticulum like areas are composed of either squamous epithelium or granular cells are seen. Other histologic variants include the plexiform pattern in which the proliferating odontogenic epithelium forms anastomosing cords rimmed by peripheral cuboidal to columnar ameloblast-like cells. The desmoplastic ameloblastoma shows a densely collagenized fibrous connective tissue stroma with condensed islands and cords of odontogenic epithelium. Peripheral columnar cells with characteristic palisading and reversed nuclear are not easily seen. A rarely encountered basal cell pattern has also been described, however the biologic behavior of the variant patterns is indistinguishable.

The unicystic ameloblastoma most commonly develops in the posterior mandible during the second and third decades of life.[129] Possessing a more favorable prognosis than its conventional counterpart, the unicystic ameloblastoma most frequently presents as a unilocular radiolucency surrounding the crown of an unerupted tooth. Based on this proclivity to occur in a pericoronal configuration, the unicystic ameloblastoma is often diagnosed clinically as a dentigerous cyst with the definitive diagnosis made only after submission of lesional tissue for histologic examination. Rare extra-follicular lesions are occasionally encountered. Histologic examination shows a cystic epithelial lining remarkable for features defined by Vickers and Gorlin[130] including a hyperchromatic columnar basal epithelial cell layer

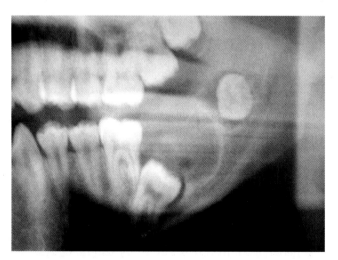

Fig. 7.12A: Multilocular presentation of an ameloblastoma

exhibiting palisading and reversed nuclear polarity with cytoplasmic vacuolization proximal to the basement membrane. The overlying epithelium is typically dis-cohesive resembling the stellate reticulum. A plexiform histologic variant remarkable for a cyst lining comprised anastomosing cords of odontogenic epithelium lined by cuboidal to columnar ameloblast-like cells is appreciated, however, the biologic behavior of this variant does not significantly differ from the traditional unicystic pattern. Occasionally, mural extension of the process into the cyst wall is appreciated. Here, isolated islands of odontogenic epithelium with the histopathologic features of the conventional follicular ameloblastoma are seen infiltrating the surrounding fibrous connective tissue stroma. The biologic behavior of a unicystic amelo-blastoma with mural involvement is similar to that of the conventional ameloblastoma.[131] Clearly, the capacity to distinguish between a unicystic ameloblastoma with or without mural involvement is critical. Specimens with histologic features suspicious for unicystic amelo-blastoma should be thoroughly evaluated for mural involvement by an experienced oral pathologist.

Predominantly located in the posterior mandible, the peripheral variant of ameloblastoma is confined exclusively to the alveolar mucosa and is clinically indistinguishable from other benign gingival nodules. Like the conventional variant, the peripheral amelo-blastoma is thought to arise from rests of dental lamina; however, the possibility that some lesions may arise from oral mucosal epithelium cannot be excluded.[132,133] Peripheral lesions may occasionally produce a pressure resorptive defect of the alveolar bone subjacent to the soft tissue neoplasm.[132] Histologic examination of the peripheral ameloblastoma shows unremarkable oral mucosa overlying a mature fibrous connective tissue stroma. Within the fibrous connective tissue, infiltrative islands of odontogenic epithelium are seen remarkable for a central stellate-reticulum-like core surrounded by columnar epithelial cells exhibiting hyperchromaticity, reversed nuclear polarity, and cytoplasmic vacuolization. Occasionally, the stellate-reticulum like areas are replaced by stratified squamous epithelium. A plexiform pattern showing anastomosing cords of odontogenic epithelium rimmed by peripheral cuboidal to columnar epithelial ameloblast-like cells is also seen. A rare basal cell pattern has been reported, however no significant difference in biologic behavior is appreciated amongst the histologic variants.

AMELOBLASTIC CARCINOMA AND MALIGNANT AMELOBLASTOMA

Ameloblastic carcinoma is a rarely encountered malignancy characterized by overt cytologic atypia within a lesion that is otherwise histologically indistin-guishable from ameloblastoma. Although occasional mitotic activity is noted in benign lesions, abundant atypical mitotic figures in conjunction with nuclear pleomorphism, calcific foci, necrosis and robust cellularity are features of malignant transformation. Figures 7.13A to G show a 16-year-old male with ameloblastic carcinoma of the mandible. This patient was treated with mandibular resection and reconstruction, neck dissection, and radiation treatment. At the time of publication of this chapter, the patient has undergone hyperbaric oxygen treatment and functional rehabili-tation with endosseous dental implants. The so-called malignant ameloblastoma represents an unusual situation in which a cytologically benign ameloblastoma metastasizes to distant locale. The incidence of malignant ameloblastoma is rare and the pathogenesis is poorly understood.

Treatment

Conventional Ameloblastoma

Resection using 1.0 to 1.5 cm margins and removal of one uninvolved anatomic barrier is indicated. If enucleation and curettage is employed as the treatment modality, one should expect a recurrence of 70 to 85%, but it may take up to 5 years for the recurrences to become apparent. Ameloblastomas treated by resection do not usually recur. Figures 7.14A to D show a 42-year-old woman with an ameloblastoma of the anterior mandible. As the tumor had perforated beyond the bony cortices, a staged treatment plan was used. Initially, the tumor was resected and a reconstruction plate applied for bone stabilization. The mandible was reconstructed three months later with iliac crest bone grafts. Functional rehabilitation was achieved with implant supported dental restorations.

Unicystic Ameloblastoma

Involvement limited exclusively to luminal epithelium without mural extension: These tumors should be treated more conservatively with enucleation and thorough curettage. Figures 7.15A to D show a patient with

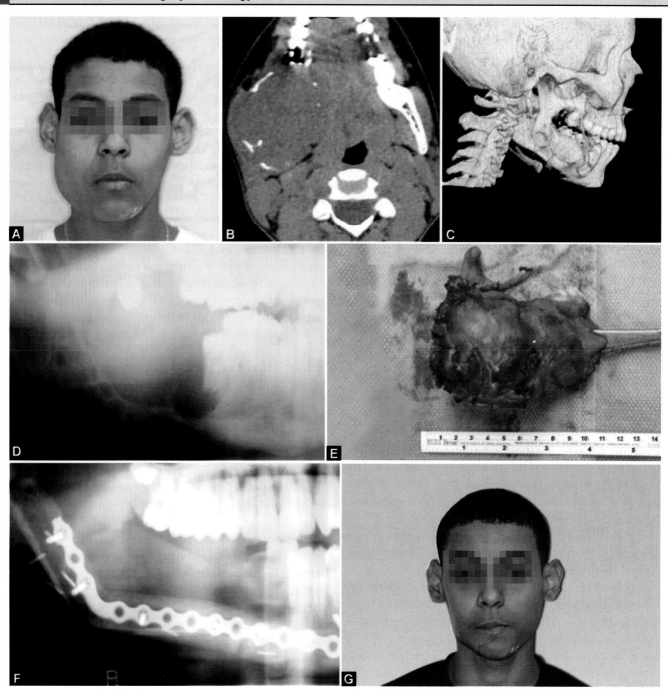

Figs 7.13A to G: (A) Facial photograph of a 16-year-old male with severe facial asymmetry. (B) CT scan showing large mass in the right mandible with extension into surrounding areas. (C) 3-D reconstruction of CT scan demonstrating extensive bone destruction in the right mandibular body, angle, and ramus regions. (D) Plain film radiograph showing significant osteolysis of the mandible. (E) The carcinoma has been resected as an en bloc specimen. Simultaneous bilateral modified neck dissections were performed. (F) Mandibular reconstruction with a fibular free flap using microvascular techniques. Note lack of adequate bone height and volume as compared to the contralateral mandible. This often occurs with fibular free flaps since the fibula is a long tubular bone, which is much smaller than a human mandible. A fibular free flap technique was preferred in this case because of the malignant nature of disease and need for immediate postoperative radiation. (G) Postoperative photograph showing aesthetic results after free flap mandibular reconstruction. Although this is an acceptable result considering the extensive resection, the postoperative facial contour is not optimal

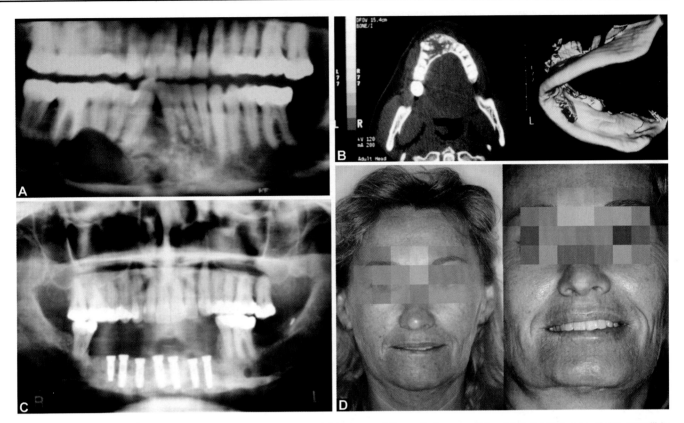

Figs 7.14A to D: (A) Panoramic radiograph showing an ameloblastoma of the anterior mandible. (B) Axial CT scan of the mandible showing the bone expansion and destruction associated with the lesion. (C) The tumor has been removed, and the mandible reconstructed with cancellous marrow grafts and dental implants. (D) Facial photograph showing achievement of adequate esthetics using cancellous bone marrow grafts. These grafts allow molding of the bone into the normal facial contour and alveolar arch forms and should be used as first choice in benign tumor reconstructive surgery. (*Courtesy*: Figs A to C Dr David Cottrell, Boston, MA, USA)

unicystic ameloblastoma who was treated with enucleation and curettage of the lesion, bone grafting of the defect, and placement of dental implants.

Peripheral Ameloblastoma

These tumors lack the aggressiveness and biological behavior of a central conventional ameloblastoma. They can usually be treated by excision of the soft tissue lesion with a rim of soft tissue tumor-free margins. The exact margin of soft tissue to be excised beyond the tumor is controversial, but generally, 1.0 to 1.5 cm margins are considered adequate. Recurrence after adequate treatment is rare.

Recurrent Ameloblastoma

Most recurrent tumors arise as a result of inadequate treatment during initial surgery. On an average,

recurrence usually occurs 5 to 10 years after treatment, and is best managed by resection. Although arguable, it is recommended that the resection should be based on initial radiographs; 1.5 cm margins are recommended based on the extent of the original tumor. Basing the resection margin on the 'new' recurrent tumor radiograph treats only the isolated recurrent lesion. This approach risks further recurrences in the original tumor area which is still left untreated.

CLEAR CELL ODONTOGENIC CARCINOMA

The clear cell odontogenic carcinoma represents an uncommon malignant odontogenic tumor with the propensity for locally aggressive behavior, frequent recurrence, and locoregional and distant metastasis. Although the pathogenesis is incompletely understood, immunohistochemical studies support an odontogenic origin for the neoplasm.[134] Clinically, the clear cell

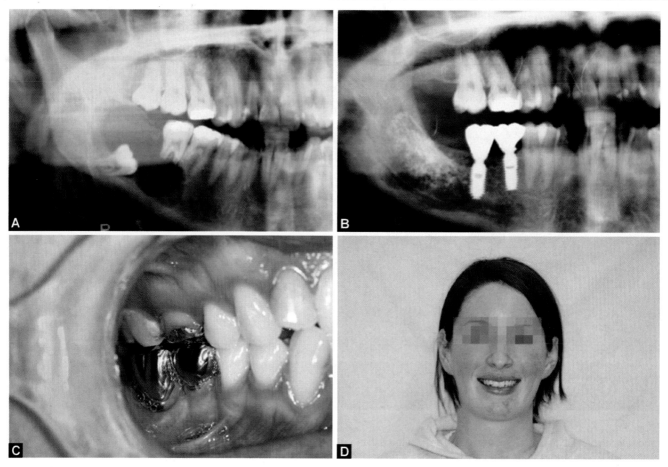

Figs 7.15A to D: (A) Unicystic ameloblastoma without mural involvement of the right posterior mandible. Note that this radiographic appearance is virtually indistinguishable from many other common odontogenic cysts and tumors. (B) The lesion has been removed via an intraoral approach with enucleation and curettage with peripheral ostectomy, and the bone defect reconstructed with particulate bone. Delayed placement of implants is performed approximately 5 months after bony reconstruction of the jaw. (C) Intraoral photograph demonstrating result of functional dental rehabilitation with fixed, implant-supported restorations. (D) Postoperative facial photograph showing excellent facial form and esthetics demonstrating the benefits of an intraoral approach for removal of the tumor and reconstruction of jaw bone

odontogenic carcinoma has a propensity for occurring in the mandible of females in the ninth decade of life. When the lesion presents in males it occurs significantly earlier, most commonly presenting during the fourth and fifth decades.[135] Occasionally pain, expansion, and tooth mobility are encountered, however, lesions may be asymptomatic and discovered on routine radiographic examination.[136] Radiographically, the clear cell odontogenic carcinoma may possess either a multilocular or unilocular appearance remarkable for indistinct irregular borders and frequent resorption of adjacent tooth structure.[137]

Histopathologic examination reveals three predominant patterns: A monophasic pattern, a biphasic pattern, and a pattern remarkable for subtle ameloblastic differentiation.[138] The monophasic pattern shows sheets and cords of glycogen-rich clear cells occasionally divided into a lobular configuration by fine, fibrous septae. This histologic variant can be challenging to distinguish from intraosseous salivary gland tumors such as mucoepidermoid carcinoma and from metastatic renal cell carcinoma. The biphasic pattern consists of infiltrating nests of polygonal eosinophilic cells associated with variable numbers of glycogen-rich clear cells. The third histologic variant is remarkable for subtle ameloblastic differentiation consisting of nests of clear cells rimmed peripherally by columnar cells exhibiting palisading and reversed nuclear polarity. Each histologic variant may contain foci of dystrophic calcification. Immunohistochemical stains for low-molecular weight cytokeratins and epithelial membrane antigen are positive within the tumor cells, as well as periodic acid-Schiff (PAS) positive, diastase labile cytoplasmic staining consistent with the presence of glycogen.

Treatment

This is a rare malignant odontogenic neoplasm, which is capable of regional and distant metastasis. Eversole et al[139] reported on 14 cases, out of which 4 patients died within 7 to 21 years of diagnosis. The following protocol has been suggested in managing these tumors.[b]
1. Confirm histopathological diagnosis. Do not assess malignancy-based on the absence or presence of mitoses.
2. Rule out metastatic disease.
3. Resection should be guided by preoperative CT and/or MR imaging and by intraoperative frozen section samples. The tumor cell nests 'wander' distant from the main tumor mass of the lesion.
4. All neural structures in close proximity to the tumor should be sacrificed. Soft tissue overlying perforated cortical bone should be excised.
5. Bone and soft tissue resection must maintain at least 2 to 2.5 cm tumor free margins in all dimensions.
6. Follow-up and periodic visits should be scheduled every 3 months for the first year, every 6 months for the next 5 years, and yearly thereafter.

Figures 7.16A to E show a 70-year-old female with clear cell odontogenic carcinoma of the anterior mandible. The patient underwent mandibular resection and

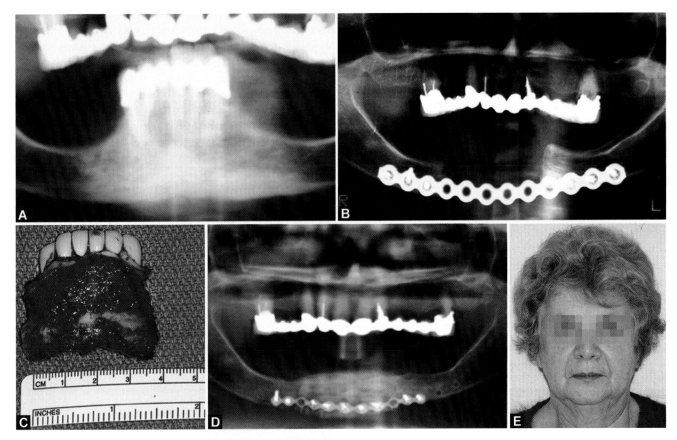

Figs 7.16A to E: (A) Periapical radiograph showing a small radiolucent lesion in the anterior mandible (Clear Cell Odontogenic Carcinoma). (B) Initially, a bone plate was used to reconstruct and stabilize the jaw. This staged technique allows for postoperative radiation therapy, when required. (C) The mandible has been resected with 2.0 cm margins. (D) Reconstruction of the anterior mandible has been achieved with cancellous marrow grafts harvested from the iliac crest. Note the height and volume of bone that has been created using this technique of bone reconstruction and bone regeneration. (E) Postoperative frontal view of the patient after jaw bone reconstruction. Again, note that selective placement of cancellous bone grafts harvested from the iliac crest allows for reconstruction of optimal facial form and contour

reconstruction with iliac crest bone grafts. At the time of publication of this chapter, the patient is two years post-surgery and remains recurrence-free.

ECTOMESENCHYMAL ODONTOGENIC TUMORS[d]

Odontogenic Fibroma

The central odontogenic fibroma represents a benign mesenchymal odontogenic neoplasm presenting clinically as a painless expansile mass exhibiting slow growth and pronounced cortical expansion. Remarkable for a slight female predilection, the central odontogenic fibroma presents with equal frequency in the maxilla and mandible, with the anterior maxilla and posterior mandible being the most commonly involved sites.[140] Radiographically, the central odontogenic fibroma shows either a unilocular or multilocular radiolucency often presenting in a dentigerous configuration around the crown of an unerupted tooth.[140,141] Resorption of adjacent tooth structure is frequently described.[140] Peripheral lesions confined exclusively to the soft tissue are occasionally encountered and are clinically indistinguishable from other benign gingival nodules. In some instances, the peripheral odontogenic fibroma may contain calcific foci that are evident on radiographic imaging.

Histologic examination of the odontogenic fibroma shows a proliferation of mature fibrous connective tissue of variable cellularity. Additionally, foci of inactive odontogenic epithelium may be appreciated in variable amounts throughout the lesion. Some authors support the idea of two distinct histologic variants, the simple type and World Health Organization (WHO) type.[142] The simple type shows a delicate collagenous stroma with scattered stellate-shaped fibroblasts, nests of odontogenic epithelium in variable amounts, and foci of dystrophic calcification. The WHO pattern consists of a densely cellular fibrous connective tissue stroma with abundant foci of odontogenic epithelium oriented in nests or cords. Dysplastic dentin or cementum-like calcification may be appreciated. Although the existence of the distinct histologic variants is debated extensively in the literature, the discussion is essentially academic as the biologic behavior between the histologic variants is indistinguishable.

Treatment

Incisional biopsy is required as the clinical presentation may be suggestive of more aggressive lesions. Although they are believed to be benign lesions with finite growth potential, recurrences or re-growth of residual lesions has been reported.[143,144] Although very rare, there are some reports that show a markedly aggressive and infiltrative behavior similar to a fibrosarcoma.[143]

Generally speaking, these lesions should be treated with enucleation and curettage. The lesions readily separate from their bony cavity, and should not show any evidence of bony infiltration. The inferior alveolar nerve bundle should be preserved, whenever possible. It has been recommended that teeth in the lesional area be removed. Recurrence is not expected, and if occurs, a review of the histopathological examination of the original specimen should be done.

Peripheral odontogenic fibromas should be excised down to bone with a 3 to 5 mm rim of soft tissue margin. Recurrence is not expected if excision is adequately performed.

Cementoblastoma

The cementoblastoma represents a benign ectomesenchymal odontogenic tumor derived from neoplastic cementoblasts. This slow-growing lesion is remarkable for originating from and insinuating itself within the tooth root apparatus. Clinically, the cementoblastoma demonstrates dramatic growth potential and the capacity to over-run the root structure of adjacent teeth as the lesion expands. Although rare cases involving the deciduous dentition have been reported,[145] the cementoblastoma typically involves the erupted mandibular permanent molar or bicuspid teeth of patients in their second and third decades of life.[146] Frequently pain, expansion of the cortical plates, and displacement of teeth are described. Radiographically, the cementoblastoma typically presents as a well-circumscribed radiopacity intimately fused to and obscuring tooth root structure (Fig. 7.17). A radiolucent rim frequently surrounds the

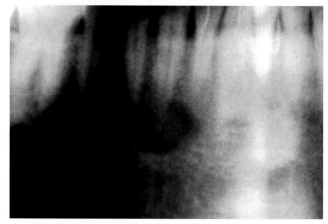

Fig. 7.17: A cementoblastoma frequently presents as a radiopaque mass attached to the root of a tooth. There may also be a radiolucent rim surrounding the radiopacity

lesion. Purely radiolucent lesions are rare but have been reported.[146,147]

Histopathologic examination of the cementoblastoma shows a proliferation of plump cementoblasts embedded in a stroma of haphazardly arranged calcified matrix exhibiting prominent basophilic reversal lines and disorderly lacunae. A fibrovascular connective tissue stroma and variable numbers of multinucleated osteoclast-type giant cells are also appreciated. Poorly mineralized trabeculae of eosinophilic matrix arranged in radiating cords are often noted at the periphery of the lesion.

Treatment

The cementoblastoma is a slow growing, benign lesion of odontogenic origin, and thus, the primary recommended treatment is enucleation with curettage. The lesion has a distinct fibrous connective tissue wall, and is usually easy to separate from bone. The offending tooth is generally extracted with the lesion attached. However, there are some reports where the lesion was removed with tooth root amputation and the tooth was preserved with endodontic treatment. In the author's experience, an unfavorable crown-root ratio would most likely result with such treatment.

Odontogenic Myxoma

The odontogenic myxoma is a benign ectomesenchymal odontogenic tumor characterized by the replacement of bone with a grossly gelatinous tissue composed of delicate collagen fibers and abundant glycosaminoglycans. Perhaps derived from the mesenchymal tissue of either a developing tooth or the periodontal ligament, the odontogenic myxoma may gain its capacity to proliferate and progress from disregulation of antiapoptotic proteins and the secretion of matrix metalloproteinases.[148] Typically, presenting in the posterior mandible of patients in the second to fourth decade of life,[149] the odontogenic myxoma is a slow-growing neoplasm remarkable for tooth displacement, pain, expansion, perforation of the bony cortex and the capacity to insinuate itself into the surrounding soft tissue. The lesion presents as either a unilocular or multilocular radiolucency remarkable for a 'soap bubble' or 'honeycomb' appearance. Residual bony trabeculae persisting within the lesion are oriented at right angles to each other and may yield an appearance akin to the strings of a tennis racket.

Histopathologic examination shows a background of myxomatous connective tissue and finely dispersed stellate and spindle-shaped cells. The myxomatous stroma is predominantly composed of glycosamino-glycans. Occasional foci of odontogenic epithelium may be appreciated within the lesion, however, the epithelium is not always encountered and is uninvolved with the neoplastic process. Immunohistochemical stains are positive for vimentin and focally positive for muscle specific actin within the tumor cell population.[150]

Treatment

Definitive treatment involves resection with 1.0 to 1.5 cm tumor-free bony margins, and one uninvolved anatomic barrier. Primary or secondary jaw reconstruction can be performed as per surgeon preference. Some surgeons advocate enucleation with curettage for small (1 to 2 cm), unilocular lesions; However, a review of most recurrent cases shows that they were initially treated by this modality. Recurrences may not be evident until 5 years or more after such surgery. The authors of this chapter do not recommend enucleation and curettage as a form of treatment for odontogenic myxomas. This 'conservative' treatment should be reserved for those individuals who specifically prefer or request palliative correction over curative resection, or for those individuals whose general anesthetic risk is too great to undergo curative surgery.

MIXED ODONTOGENIC TUMORS

Odontoma

One of the most commonly encountered odontogenic tumors, the odontoma may actually represent a developmental hamartoma rather than a true neoplastic process. Regardless of classification as either an odontogenic neoplasm or developmental anomaly, the odontoma represents a so-called 'mixed' lesion exhibiting a proliferation of both odontogenic epithelium and mesenchymal tissue. Classified into two distinct types: The compound variant and the complex variant, the odontoma is comprised of a proliferation of odontogenic tissues in variable amounts and arrangements.

The compound odontoma most commonly presents in the first or second decade of life with a predilection for occurring in the anterior maxilla (Figs 7.18A, B).[151,152] Compound lesions are characterized by a proliferation of odontogenic tissues in appropriate odontogenic configuration. Often associated with the crown of an unerupted permanent tooth or supernumerary tooth, compound odontomas present as multiple small crudely-formed tooth-like structures circumscribed by a

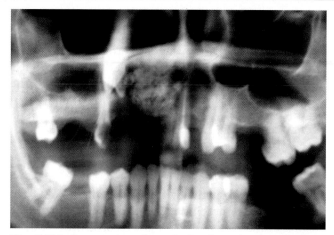

Fig. 7.18A: Panoramic radiograph showing a large, radiopaque mass (complex odontoma) in the anterior maxilla, lateral to the nasal region

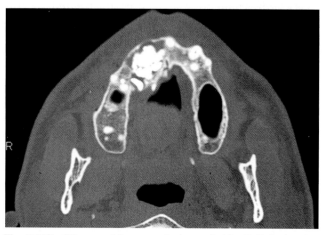

Fig. 7.18B: CT scan of the same lesion as in Fig. 7.18 A showing multiple small radiopaque masses within the lesion

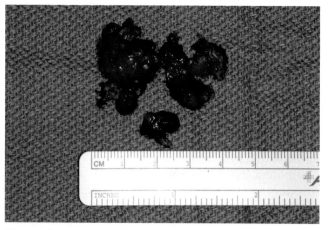

Fig. 7.18C: The odontoma has been excised and as expected, the lesion consists of multiple small tooth-like structures

radiolucent rim and typically noted either on routine radiographic examination or when investigating the chief complaint of delayed eruption. Occasional lesions are reported at the site of a missing tooth, within the interradicular area, or associated with deciduous teeth.[153] Histopathologically, the compound odontoma consists of multiple small, crudely formed, single-rooted 'toothlets'[151] comprised of overlying enamel matrix with underlying dentin and a central pulp chamber.

The complex odontoma typically presents in the posterior mandible of patients in the first or second decade of life (Fig. 7.18C).[151,152] Characterized by a proliferation of odontogenic tissues oriented in a haphazard arrangement, the complex odontoma often presents in association with an unerupted permanent tooth and may exhibit bony expansion. Occasional cases are reported in which the lesion is located in the interradicular area, presents at the site of a missing tooth, or is associated with deciduous teeth.[151,154] Radiographically, the complex odontoma presents as a well-demarcated focus of radiopacity surrounded by a peripheral radiolucent rim. The radiodensity of the radiopaque mass is consistent with that of tooth structure. Histologic examination of a complex odontoma shows a proliferation of odontogenic tissues oriented in a haphazard configuration. Typically, variable amounts of dentin, enamel matrix, pulpal tissues, and cementum are seen juxtaposed with each other in an indiscriminate fashion. Primitive lesions may show multiple foci of early odonotogenesis.

Treatment

Excision of the lesion with enucleation and curettage is curative. These lesions are usually removed via an intraoral approach. A full-thickness flap is made, and bone is removed to expose the lesion. The calcified masses are not adherent to bone, and are often easily removed with usual exodontia instruments or hand curettes. If the lesions are extremely large, they may need to be cut into smaller sections to permit adequate removal without jaw fracture. Spontaneous bone formation is generally sufficient to avoid bone grafting in most cases, but is dependent on the extent of surgery, age and systemic health of the patient. Corticocancellous marrow grafts may be needed if dental implants are planned in the area of surgery, or if the mandible is atrophic and requires bone augmentation for strengthening. Significantly, large lesions may also benefit from intermaxillary fixation or rarely, placement of a bone plate to prevent mandibular fracture.

Ameloblastic Fibroma

The ameloblastic fibroma represents a rarely encountered benign odontogenic tumor composed of a neoplastic proliferation of both odontogenic epithelial and mesenchymal tissues. Although documented to occur over a wide age range, the ameloblastic fibroma typically presents in the posterior mandible of patients in the first or second decade of life.[155] Occurring with slightly greater frequency in males and typically associated with the crown of an unerupted permanent tooth, the ameloblastic fibroma often presents as a painless expansile mass, however asymptomatic lesions are encountered that either present on routine radiographic examination or when investigating disturbances in tooth eruption. Radiographically, the ameloblastic fibroma presents as either a unilocular or multilocular radiolucency with well-defined margins.

Histopathologic examination of the ameloblastic fibroma shows a proliferation of primitive cell-rich mesenchymal tissue with interspersed islands and anastomosing cords of odontogenic epithelium lined by columnar cells exhibiting reversed nuclear polarity and cytoplasmic vacuolization. Frequently, a rim of hyalinization cuffs the epithelial islands. The primitive cell-rich stroma shares a resemblance to the dental papilla, and its presence aids to distinguish the lesion from the ameloblastoma in which a mature fibrous connective tissue stroma is noted.

Occasionally lesions are seen that are clinically indistinguishable from ameloblastic fibroma except for a mixed radiolucent-radiopaque appearance; the radiopaque component possessing the radiodensity of tooth structure. Histologic examination reveals features of an ameloblastic fibroma with variable amounts of calcified tissue comprised of dentin and enamel matrix. Occasionally, crudely formed tooth structures are appreciated. Referred to as the *ameloblastic fibro-odontoma*, this lesion is considered a variant of the ameloblastic fibroma by some and a variant of odontoma by others. Recent studies suggest the mesenchymal component of the lesion promotes the formation of dentin and enamel matrix through inductive effects on the epithelial foci within the lesion.[156]

Malignant transformation of an ameloblastic fibroma or *de novo* malignant lesions sharing features of the ameloblastic fibroma are referred to as *ameloblastic fibrosarcoma*. Often encountered as a recurrent lesion at the site of a pre-existing benign ameloblastic fibroma, the ameloblastic fibrosarcoma presents as a destructive expansile mass with ill-defined radiographic boundaries.

Histopathologically, these lesions are characterized by atypia within the mesenchymal component of the lesion remarkable for dense cellularity, nuclear pleomorphism, hyperchromaticity, and abundant atypical mitotic figures. Interestingly, only the mesenchymal component of the lesion shows features of malignancy with the associated epithelial component demonstrating nondescript cytomorphology.

Treatment

Simple enucleation and curettage is considered curative for ameloblastic fibromas as most lesions tend to be encapsulated and unilocular. The tumor does not invade the inferior alveolar canal or the neurovascular bundle, so nerve preservation is readily achieved. Most recurrences usually result from incomplete removal. Extensive lesions may require mandibular resection with or without continuity defects. Since most patients are very young, bone grafting may not be required if spontaneous bone regeneration is sufficient. Some studies have shown that approximately 45% of fibrosarcomas evolve from ameloblastic fibromas. Thus, recurrent lesions, especially in adults, should be closely examined. Long-term clinical and radiographic follow-up is recommended.

Most cases of ameloblastic sarcomas are considered to be low-grade malignancies, and treatment recommended is resection of bone with 1.5 to 2.0 cm tumor-free margins, and removal of one uninvolved anatomic barrier. Mandibular defects can usually be reconstructed with bone grafts, and maxillary defects are usually covered by custom-made obturators. Radiation treatment is considered to be of limited value, but some clinicians recommend chemotherapy as adjunctive treatment. Long-term follow-up is required because of slow growth rate, and recurrences may not be seen until several years after treatment.

NON-ODONTOGENIC TUMORS

Giant Cell Granuloma

The giant cell granuloma represents a proliferative vascular lesion[157] characterized by the replacement of normal bone with cellular fibrous connective tissue containing numerous multinucleated giant cells, extravasated erythrocytes, hemosiderin-laden macrophages, and trabeculae of reactive bone. Although the pathogenesis is incompletely understood, genetic abnormalities may be the causative factor in at least some lesions.[158] The giant cell granuloma presents centrally within bone; however, histologically identical lesions are frequently seen that arise peripherally in the alveolar mucosa confined exclusively to the soft tissue. The central giant cell granuloma occurs over a wide age range typically presenting in the first three decades of life.[159] Current literature supports the division of central giant cell granulomas into either non-aggressive, intermediate, or aggressive categories based on biologic behavior using features such as: size greater than 5 cm, cortical perforation or thinning, root resorption, pain, marked growth rate, and recurrence after conservative treatment to indicate aggressive tendencies.[160] The central giant cell granuloma has a predilection for occurring in the mandible, frequently presenting in the anterior region and often crossing the midline. Peripheral lesions are clinically indistinguishable from other benign gingival nodules and are not known for aggressive behavior (Figs 7.19A and B). Although recurrence is occasionally reported in peripheral giant cell granulomas, the lesion may represent a focal reactive process and recurrence is probably related to persistence of local inciting factors and/or incomplete removal. Radiographically, the central giant cell granuloma presents as a well delineated unilocular to multilocular radiolucency (Fig. 7.19C). Peripheral lesions often show a saucer-shaped resorptive defect in the alveolar bone subjacent to the soft-tissue neoplasm.

Histopathologically, the giant cell granuloma consists of multinucleated giant cells on a cellular fibrovascular stroma of ovoid mesenchymal cells. Extravasated erythrocytes, hemosiderin-laden macrophages, and trabeculae of reactive bone are appreciated in varying amounts. Although a point of some controversy, the multinucleated giant cells within the giant cell granuloma are most likely osteoclastic in nature and derived from cells of the monocyte/macrophage lineage.[161] The mesenchymal cellular component of the lesion represents the proliferative constituent of the process serving to recruit monocytes and subsequently encourage their differentiation into osteoclast-type giant cells.[162] A correlation between the presence of large multinucleated giant cells and marked stromal cellularity with the tendency for aggressive biologic behavior has been suggested. It is important to note that the histological features of the giant cell granuloma and the so-called brown tumors of hyperparathyroidism are indistinguishable, and that this condition should be considered in the differential diagnosis of all giant cell lesions.

Treatment

Given that the histological features of this lesion are indistinguishable from the so-called brown tumor of hyperparathyroidism, evaluation of serum calcium, phosphate, and parathyroid hormone levels is essential prior to treatment. The most commonly used treatment modality is aggressive curettage. Large lesions that risk pathological fracture may require resection (Fig. 7.19D). If surgery is contemplated, the surgeon must be prepared to encounter significant intraoperative hemorrhage until the entire lesion has been curetted. Figures 7.19 E and F show a 26-year-old man with a large central giant cell granuloma causing pathological fracture of the mandible. This patient was successfully treated by mandibular resection and reconstruction. Intralesional corticosteroid therapy, calcitonin therapy, and more recently anti-angiogeneic therapy have also been shown to be effective in treating these lesions effectively.[103-105]

Benign Fibro-osseous Lesions

Benign fibro-osseous lesions represent those lesions characterized by the replacement of normal bone by fibrovascular connective tissue and woven bone or cementum-like calcification. Three major categories of benign fibro-osseous lesions involve the maxillofacial bones: fibrous dysplasia, cemento-ossifying fibroma, and cemento-osseous dysplasia. Based on histologic similarities amongst the fibro-osseous lesions, clinical, radiographic, and histologic features must be correlated to arrive at a definitive diagnosis.

Fibrous dysplasia represents a benign fibro-osseous lesion characterized by a mutation in the guanine nucleotide-binding protein, α-stimulating activity polypeptide 1 (GNAS 1) gene.[163,164] Divided into forms involving only one bone (monostotic), multiple bones (polyostotic) (Figs 7.20A and B), and forms associated with McCune-Albright syndrome, fibrous dysplasia is a typically slow-growing process that causes painless expansion and deformity. Radiographically, fibrous dysplasia is remarkable for a so-called 'ground glass' mixed radiolucent-radiopaque appearance. The process possesses the tendency to insinuate itself into peripheral normal bone such that the radiographic margins of the lesion are poorly defined. One distinctive feature of fibrous dysplasia involving the mandible is a tendency for superior displacement of the inferior alveolar canal.

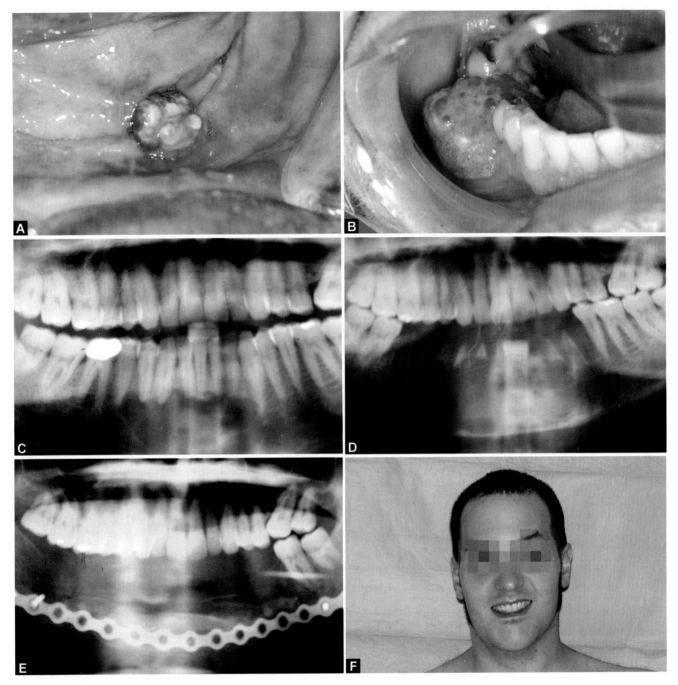

Figs 7.19A to F: (A) Peripheral giant cell granulomas are confined to the gingiva and present as variable colored gingival nodules or masses in the anterior mandible. (B) Posterior mandible. (C) A central giant cell granuloma of the mandible in an 18-year-old male presenting as a well-circumscribed radiolucency in the anterior mandible. (D) The same lesion as in Fig. 7.19 C one year after initial presentation. Note that the lesion has increased in size and exfoliated many teeth. (E) The tumor has been resected and mandible reconstructed with conventional bone grafting techniques. (F) Facial photograph of the patient 3 years after reconstructive surgery

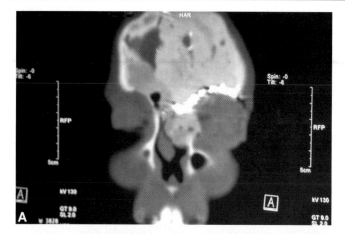

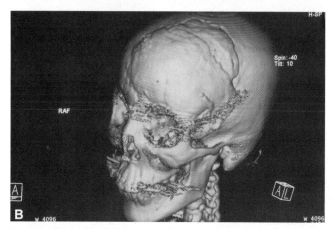

Figs 7.20A and B: (A) Coronal CT scan of a patient affected with craniofacial fibrous dysplasia; note diffuse involvement of the frontal, nasal, and ethnocide bones. (B) 3-D reconstruction of the same patient

Cemento-ossifying fibroma represents a rarely encountered neoplasm the origins of which are incompletely understood. Occurring over a wide age range, the cemento-ossifying fibroma typically presents as a painless expansile mass in the posterior mandible with a proclivity for occurring in female patients. Radiographically, the cemento-ossifying fibroma is a well-demarcated, mixed, radiolucent-radiopaque lesion (Fig. 7.21A) that frequently produces a bowing defect of the mandibular inferior cortical bone and marked tooth displacement. An aggressive variant of the cemento-ossifying fibroma is occasionally seen and is termed the *active ossifying fibroma* or *juvenile ossifying fibroma* (Figs 7.21B, C). Remarkable for an aggressive biologic behavior including a tendency to invade local structures, the lesion typically presents in the first to second decade of life with a predilection for maxillary involvement.

Cemento-osseous dysplasia is a commonly encountered entity with three distinct clinical subtypes: Periapical, focal, and florid cemento-osseous dysplasia. *Periapical cemento-osseous dysplasia* presents clinically as an asymptomatic lesion typically discovered on routine radiographic examination (Fig. 7.22). Remarkable for a propensity to occur in middle-aged black females, periapical cemento-osseous dysplasia commonly presents as a multifocal process involving the apices of vital mandibular anterior teeth. As the lesion matures, a spectrum of radiographic changes ranging from early lesions that are entirely radiolucent to lesions of longstanding duration that are purely radiopaque can be appreciated. In the absence of expansion or other changes in the character of the process, periapical cemento-osseous dysplasia typically requires intervention limited to periodic radiographic observation.

Focal cemento-osseous dysplasia presents clinically as an asymptomatic lesion typically discovered on routine radiographic examination (Fig. 7.23).

Remarkable for a propensity to occur in Caucasian females, focal periapical cemento-osseous dysplasia presents as a solitary lesion at the apex of a vital tooth

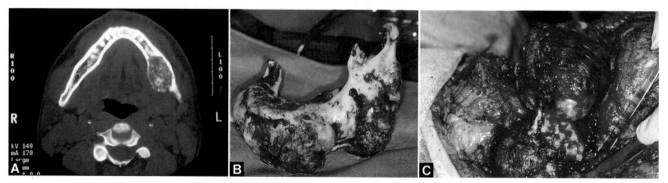

Figs 7.21A to C: (A) CT scan showing a mixed, radiolucent-radiopaque lesion with well-defined borders (ossifying fibro). (B) The juvenile ossifying fibroma is a rare, aggressive variant of an ossifying fibroma. Intraoperative view showing extensive involvement of the tumor. (C) Resected specimen showing near-total complete mandibular resection

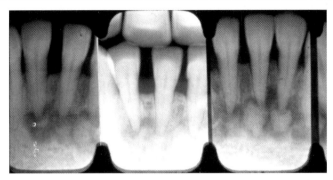

Fig. 7.22: Multiple radiolucent/mixed lesions in the anterior mandible associated with vital teeth is characteristic of periapical cemento-osseous dysplasia

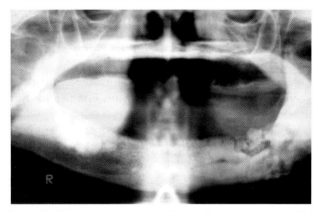

Fig. 7.24: Florid osseous dysplasia usually presents as multiple mixed lesions bilaterally in the posterior mandible

most commonly located in the posterior mandible. Occasionally, lesions are encountered in edentulous regions of the alveolar bone. As the focal process undergoes maturation, a spectrum of radiographic changes ranging from early lesions that are entirely radiolucent to lesions of long standing duration that are purely radiopaque may be appreciated. A peripheral rim of radiolucency is typically noted to circumscribe the lesion. In the absence of clinical expansion or a change in character of the lesion, periodic radiographic observation is the limit of requisite intervention. *Florid cemento-osseous dysplasia* presents clinically as a multifocal process involving more than one quadrant of the maxilla and/or mandible. Remarkable for a propensity to occur in middle-aged black females, florid cemento-osseous dysplasia typically presents as an asymptomatic process noted only on routine radiographic examination.

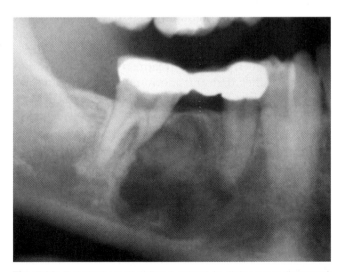

Fig. 7.23: Relatively well-defined, mixed (radiolucent-radiopaque) lesion of the posterior mandible (focal cemento-osseous dysplasia)

Radiographic examination reveals multiple foci of mixed radiolucencies that are often bilateral and symmetric (Fig. 7.24). Florid cemento-osseous lesions exhibit a spectrum of radiographic changes ranging from early lesions that are entirely radiolucent to lesions of long standing duration that are purely radiopaque, and must be clinically differentiated from chronic diffuse sclerosing osteomyelitis. Of note, simple bone cysts are occasionally encountered in association with florid lesions. In the absence of clinical expansion, cystic degeneration, or a change in character of the lesion, periodic radiographic observation is the limit of requisite intervention.

Histopathologic examination of benign fibro-osseous lesions shows replacement of normal bone with fibro-vascular connective tissue and variable amounts of woven bone or cementum-like calcification. Subtle distinctions between the individual entities may suggest a specific histologic diagnosis; however, clinical-pathologic correlation is essential for a conclusive identification.

Treatment

Treatment of each of these lesions is specific, and is beyond the scope of this chapter.

SURGICAL MANAGEMENT OF ODONTOGENIC TUMORS

General Considerations

Odontogenic tumors are relatively rare. However, they vary greatly in their biological behavior. While some lesions are extremely slow-growing, certain others can be extremely destructive. Thus, correlation of clinical, radiographic, and histopathological analysis is essential to prevent over- or undertreatment.

Clinical signs and symptoms are often related to the size and location of the tumor. Age and sex predilections are known for many tumors, but this information must be used in conjunction with other diagnostic information. Most tumors arise from the jaws, thus bone imaging is essential. The panoramic radiograph is a useful initial film since it may be obtained in an office setting and aids in the development of an initial working differential diagnosis. This radiograph shows some general characteristics of the lesion (size, shape, radiolucent versus radiopaque versus mixed, relation to specific anatomic structures). For larger lesions requiring complex treatment planning, a CT scan is recommended. Though MRI examination is not routine, it may be indicated in specific instances, especially for soft tissue imaging.

Histopathological examination is essential to make a definitive diagnosis. An incisional biopsy is usually performed for most lesions. However, excisional biopsies may be indicated in some circumstances such as completely radiopaque lesions (radiographic appearance of teeth or cementum-like tissue) or for lesions less than 1.0 to 1.5 cm size. Multiple biopsy specimens may be needed in some cases to make a definitive diagnosis, particularly if the lesion shows unusual characteristics (e.g. slow growing cystic lesion with root resorption). The specimens should be appropriately labeled, oriented, and sent to a pathologist experienced in odontogenic pathology. It is well established that odontogenic tumors can be very complex; most head and neck tumor surgeons agree that if there is any question, it may be prudent to consult with an oral pathologist before embarking on definitive surgical treatment.

Basic Surgical Principles

Odontogenic tumors encompass a wide spectrum of biologies ranging from aberrant attempts at tooth formation that may represent a hamartoma (e.g. odontoma) to true neoplasms (e.g. ameloblastoma). It is the responsibility of the surgeon to diagnose the specific lesion, and provide appropriate treatment.

Unfortunately, even today, when our understanding of most tumors has significantly increased, many surgeons continue to perform inappropriate surgical procedures. The authors frequently encounter patients treated with over-aggressive surgical approaches, which result in major radical surgery for relatively small, benign lesions which did not require such treatment (e.g. removal of many adjacent teeth and alveolus for a lateral periodontal cyst misdiagnosed to be a keratocyst); conversely, it is not uncommon to see recurrent lesions that may have fared better with a more aggressive initial approach. Almost invariably, when one analyzes the history of these recurrent tumors, he/she finds that they were inappropriately managed initially (e.g. ameloblastoma managed by enucleation and curettage).

Based on the known biology of benign odontogenic tumors, only ameloblastoma, odontogenic myxoma and calcifying epithelial odontogenic tumor require resection-type surgery as these tumors have continued growth potential and invasive properties. Marx has recommended resection for another tumor, the odonto-ameloblastoma. However, both the existence of this tumor as a separate entity and its treatment are, at present, very controversial. All other benign odontogenic tumors are amenable to enucleation and curettage. Rare odontogenic malignancies should be treated using basic principles of malignant tumor surgery including resection, neck dissection and additional treatment as indicated.

The reader should note that at present, there are no absolute guidelines for management of many odontogenic tumors, and treatment of some lesions continues to be controversial. Some of the common surgical terms used in the treatment of odontogenic cysts and tumors are given below:

Enucleation: Removal of soft and hard tissue of the lesion from its bony cavity.

Curettage: Removal of soft and hard tissue of the lesion from its bony cavity, and additionally, removal of some thickness of the wall itself (approximately 1 to 5 mm). This curettage can be accomplished physically (hand or rotary instruments), thermally (cryotherapy), or chemically (Carnoy solution). It should be remembered that while appropriate for most odontogenic cysts, curettage violates basic surgical principles of tumor management. It refers to treatment within the tumor margins rather than outside tumor margins, and also caries the risk of seeding tumor cells (especially physical curettage).

Marginal/peripheral resection: Removal of tumor en bloc within bone without creating a continuity defect. It usually is performed to preserve the inferior border of the mandible, maxillary sinus or nasal structures.

Continuity resection: Resection of tumor en bloc within bone, which creates a continuity defect. This refers to resection of the mandible inclusive of the inferior border and resections of maxilla extending into the sinus or nasal cavities.

Both types of resections may require removal of teeth, mucosa, periosteum with them dependent on tumor invasion. If the temporomandibular joint (TMJ)/condyle is resected with the mandible, it is known as **disarticulation resection.**

Primary versus Secondary Reconstruction

Most odontogenic tumors requiring major surgery (resections) are usually found in the mandible. It should be noted that almost no benign odontogenic neoplasm requires surgery as extensive and debilitating as microvascular reconstruction. These patients are not cancer patients, and the rule of cure with least morbid surgery must be followed. The choice to reconstruct the mandible primarily immediately following resection in the same surgery (primary reconstruction) or secondarily (usually after 8 to 12 weeks as a separate surgery) is often dependent on the numerous factors including but not limited to the tumor (size, perforations), patient (length of surgery, patient preference), and surgeon (expertise and preference). If primary reconstruction with corticocancellous grafts is planned, it is recommended that the practitioner remove adequate teeth (as dictated by the expected resection margins) in the office approximately 12 to 16 weeks prior to surgery. This allows for adequate mucosal healing at the extraction socket site and will prevent inadvertent perforation of the mucosa during bone grafting. If secondary reconstruction is planned, the teeth are usually removed along with the surgical specimen.

SURGICAL TREATMENT OF BENIGN MANDIBULAR ODONTOGENIC NEOPLASMS

Continuity Resection

In general, resection principles require a resection with 1.0 to 1.5 cm margins, removal of one uninvolved anatomic barrier, and frozen sections demonstrating tumor free margins. These resections can be approached via a transoral or transcutaneous approach depending on surgical access and surgeon experience. If the mandible is being reconstructed primarily using corticocancellous bone grafts, then extraoral access should be used.

Intermaxillary fixation should be applied to maintain the relationship of the jaws to each other. The mandible is approached extraorally via a neck incision. The usual dissection plane is deep to the superficial layer of deep cervical fascia, deep to the common facial vein, and deep to the marginal mandibular nerve. It is superficial to the submandibular gland, digastric muscles, and the sternocleidomastoid. If the CT scan shows no cortical perforation, then the periosteum is lifted off the bone in sub-periosteal fashion; if cortical perforation is noted on the CT scan, then supraperiosteal dissection is performed as the periosteum becomes the uninvolved anatomic barrier that is removed with the tumor specimen (Fig. 7.25A).

The tumor is identified via an intraoral (Fig. 7.25A) or an extraoral approach. A mandibular reconstruction plate (locking or non-locking rigid plate) (Fig. 7.25B) is adapted to mimic the normal mandibular contour. It should preferably extend at least 3 holes beyond the anticipated tumor margins on either side of the resected specimen. The plate is temporarily fixed to the mandible prior to resection in order to maintain control of the proximal and distal segments. If the mandibular condyle is to be resected with the specimen, a condyle replacement must be used. Common options include TMJ reconstruction with autogenous tissues like costochondral grafts (Fig. 7.25C) and sternoclavicular grafts in primary reconstruction. For delayed reconstruction cases, one can use temporary metal condylar prostheses that screw onto the plate itself (Fig. 7.25D). If these metal prosthetic condyles are used for temporary purposes in between surgeries, the surgeon must ensure that native TMJ disk is present, since articulation of the metal head on the bony glenoid fossa would otherwise invite complications such as erosion, fracture, pain, and displacement.

As mentioned above, the reconstruction plate is usually stabilized to the mandible first with bicortical screws, unless significant buccal expansion precludes this. The reconstruction plate can either be removed after initial stabilization to allow for mandibular resection or the resection can often be performed with the rigid plate in place. The resection should be planned so that adequate bone (3 to 5 mm) remains in between the mandibular margin and the adjacent tooth. This will prevent bone resorption, periodontal disease, and infection. If delayed reconstruction is planned, layered meticulous closure is performed. Drains are usually placed since significant dead space exists.

In cases of primary reconstruction, the surgeon must remove teeth (as dictated by the expected resection margins) in the office approximately 12 to 16 weeks prior to surgery. This time delay allows for adequate mucosal healing at the extraction socket site and will prevent inadvertent perforation of the mucosa during bone grafting. Since benign odontogenic tumors are slow growing, the rapid turnover oral mucosa is able to close the extraction sockets completely with this time period.

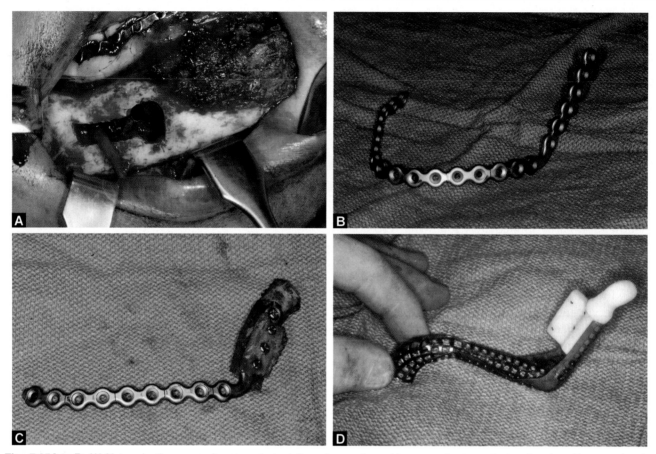

Figs 7.25A to D: (A) Note selective areas of supraperiosteal dissection performed in areas of extracortical perforation. Also note that the mental nerve has been lateralized from its foramen, thereby allowing for nerve preservation. (B) A mandibular reconstruction plate has been contoured to fit the large continuity defect. (C) A costochondral graft harvested from the patient's 5th rib has been adapted to the pre-bent reconstruction plate for TMJ articulation reconstruction. (D) An alloplastic tray with attached condylar prosthesis, which is intended to serve as a temporary mandibular condyle replacement

Extraction of teeth does not seed tumor cells since the periodontal ligament is an anatomic barrier. Three to four months after teeth removal, a similar transcutaneous approach is used for access. Following exposure, mandibular resection and reconstruction are performed concomitantly during the same surgical visit.

Peripheral Resection

This procedure may be performed when resection is indicated, but removal of tumor with the 1.0 to 1.5 cm margins will leave at least 1 cm of native inferior border of the mandible. Leaving less than 1 cm of inferior border carries a higher risk of postsurgical fracture. The resection is usually approached intraorally, and should not be in the form of a rectangle with sharp 90° angles as this increases the likelihood of fracture during mastication and mandibular function. Instead, a gentle rounded curve shape should be employed as this will distribute biting

forces more evenly. Figures 7.26A to E show a patient with an odontogenic myxoma of the mandible treated with a peripheral resection.

Mandibular Reconstruction

There has been significant advancement in mandibular reconstruction techniques over the last few years. While microvascular reconstructive surgery is the most common procedure performed for reconstruction of cancer patients, corticocancellous bone graft reconstruction remains the workhorse and procedure of choice for reconstruction following resection of benign odontogenic neoplasms.

The following terms describe the three common *bone formation mechanisms* in humans:

Osteogenesis: Refers to the formation of bone from osteoprogenitor cells. It can be of two types: *Spontaneous osteogenesis*, which is the formation of bone from cells

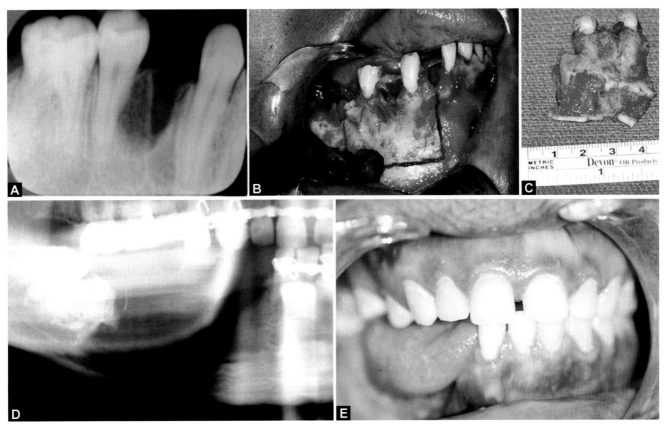

Figs 7.26A to E: (A) Periapical radiograph showing a localized ameloblastoma of the mandibular body region. (B) Surgical osteotomies outlining a marginal madibulectomy procedure (peripheral resection) with 1.5 cm margins for treatment of an odontogenic myxoma. (C) Resected mandibular specimen. Note that the inferior border of the mandible has been spared. (D) Postoperative panoramic radiograph showing very thin segment of inferior mandibular border remains. Leaving less than 1 cm of bone height in this area can increase the risk of mandibular fracture during jaw function. (E) Large soft- and hard-tissue alveolar defect seen after peripheral resection. This defect was not reconstructed with bone due to the patient's preference, and instead, a removable partial denture was fabricated

within the defect, and *transplanted osteogenesis*, which refers to bone formation within the defect from transplanted bone cells (bone grafts). Spontaneous osteogenesis is seen in patients up to approximately 12 years of age, and there are reported cases of regeneration of segments of the mandibles in patients of this age group. However, as the number of osteoprogenitor cells decreases with advancing age, spontaneous osteogenesis becomes unpredictable, and thus bony regeneration is dependent on bone grafting.

Osteoinduction: Refers to formation of new bone by the guided differentiation of stem-cell precursors into secretory osteoblasts by bone inductive proteins. Bone morphogenetic protein (BMP) is a group of well-known inductive proteins. The paucity of BMPs can be appreciated by the fact that only 20 micrograms of BMP are derived from 10 kilograms of bone.

Osteoconduction: Refers to formation of bone from host-derived or transplanted osteoprogenitor cells across a biological (e.g. cadaveric mandibular crib) (Fig. 7.27A) or alloplastic framework (reconstruction plate or tray) (Fig. 7.27B).

Today's reconstructive surgeons must understand bone physiology and bone formation adequately. Modern-day techniques allow the surgeon to manipulate and maximize bone formation by using these three principles for optimal results in mandibular reconstruction techniques.

HEALING OF CANCELLOUS CELLULAR MARROW BONE GRAFTS

The surgical wound consists of a bone clot, which is hypoxic, and creates a steep oxygen gradient from the wound center to the periphery of the tissue bed. When

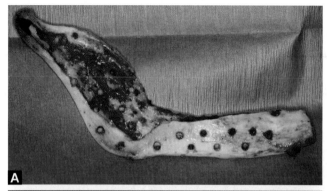

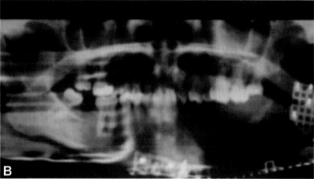

Figs 7.27A and B: (A) A biological mandibular tray/crib (cadaveric mandible) obtained form a tissue bank. Note perforations have been made to promote in-growth of blood vessels. (B) An alloplastic mandibular tray/crib functions as an osteoconductive framework

cancellous bone grafts harvested from the iliac crest are placed into this surgical site, there is transfer of viable osteogenic cells into the wound. The bone graft is initially dependent on this tissue gradient for diffusion of nutrients and survival. Platelets aggregated in the blood clot secrete bone growth factors that additionally attract other cells into the site. Continued hypoxia and lactic acidosis within the surgical wound are potent physio-chemotactic agents that recruit macrophages into the area, and these macrophages secrete angiogeneic factors. This results in revascularization of the bone graft, which although initiated immediately within hours of bone grafting, takes approximately 14 days to be complete. Once revascularization is complete, the bone graft is ready for independent survival.

The surviving endosteal cells of the cancellous bone graft initially form woven bone on each trabeculae. This initial woven bone is laid down randomly and is referred to as *phase 1 bone*. This woven bone bridges the continuity defect, and is gradually replaced by more mineralized, mature, lamellar, *phase 2 bone*, with the replacement process starting at about 4 weeks postoperatively. The amount of phase 1 bone formed is directly dependent on the number of osteoprogenitor cells transplanted. This,

it is advisable to compact bone as much as possible as a denser graft would most likely have more osteo-progenitor cells transferred. Syringes are often used intraoperative to compact bone grafts. Ultimately, all phase 1 bone is completely resorbed by osteoclasts. The osteoclasts release BMP during the resorption process, and this BMP release induces stem cells within the graft (transplanted osteogenesis) and in the surrounding tissues (periosteum, muscles, etc.) to form phase 2 bone (osteoinduction) across the biologic or alloplastic framework (osteoconduction).

Bone grafts for maxillofacial reconstruction are usually harvested from the iliac crest via an anterior or posterior approach as the iliac crest yields the maximum volume of osteoprogenitor cells in an adult human patient. Approximately, 10 cc of non-compacted bone is required for reconstruction of each 1 cm continuity defect of the mandible. While the anterior iliac crest yields approximately 50 cc of bone, a posterior approach may yield three times that amount.

SURGICAL TREATMENT OF BENIGN MAXILLARY ODONTOGENIC NEOPLASMS

Indications for resection of the maxilla remain the same as for the mandible. The surgery usually involves a subtotal or partial maxillectomy depending upon the tumor extent. Generally, 1.0 to 1.5 cm margins are used for most tumors as in mandibular tumors.

Most odontogenic tumors are approached transorally. Unlike cancer surgery, mucosa is only removed if it is infiltrated by the tumor. Thus, generally buccal/labial and palatal sulcular incisions are made, and dissection performed in either a subperiosteal or supraperiosteal plane (dependent on whether the tumor perforates the bony cortices). The maxilla is separated from the pterygoid plates, nasal septum, lateral nasal walls, and zygomatic buttress in standard fashion (Figs 7.28A and B). The infraorbital nerve can usually be preserved for most tumors. It is advisable to avoid performing the osteotomy in the midline as it leaves one central incisor; this situation creates complexity for the prosthodontist to esthetically match the remaining central incisor. Thus, if a hemimaxillectomy if required, it may be advisable to either preserve or extract both central incisors. In the authors' experience, extensive bone grafting should not be performed primarily as most maxillary defects are easily closed by custom-made obturators (Fig. 7.28C). A defect that requires or warrants bone grafting is best repaired approximately 4 to 6 months after resection. Large tumors, especially those with extension into the pterygomaxillary fossa and ethmoidal sinus areas may

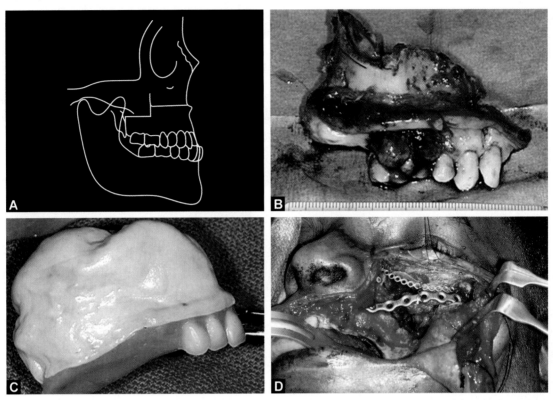

Figs 7.28A to D: (A) Schematic outline of an inferior maxillectomy procedure. (B) Resected maxillary specimen (hemimaxillectomy) for treatment of a melanoma of the maxilla. (C) Customized maxillofacial obturator prosthesis lined by acellular human dermis graft. (D) Intraoperative photograph showing exposure of the right maxilla and infratemporal regions with a modified Weber-Ferguson approach

require wider exposure, and transcutaneous access via a standard Weber Ferguson (Fig. 7.28D) or alternative approach.

RECENT ADVANCES IN MAXILLOFACIAL RECONSTRUCTION

Distraction Osteogenesis

Originally popularized by Ilizarov, distraction osteogenesis has been used in the maxillofacial surgery since the 1970s. However, it is only recently that it has gained a lot of attention, and a lot of progress has been made over the last few years. The technique refers to 'formation of bone via one's own natural mechanisms', and is a biologic process of new bone formation between the surfaces of bone segments that are gradually separated by incremental traction. The traction generates tension that stimulates new bone formation parallel to the vector of distraction. One advantage of the technique is that it simultaneously regenerates soft and hard tissues. It has been used for augmentation of maxillary and mandibular alveoli (prior to dental implant placement) (Figs 7.29A

to F) as well as reconstruction of continuity defects of the mandible (Transport distraction) (Fig. 7.30). Stereolithographic three-dimensional models fabricated using computer aided design-computer aided manufacture (CAD-CAM) technology can be very helpful in treatment planning of complex cases (Fig. 7.31).

Inferior Alveolar Nerve Considerations

Nerve Preservation

Nerve pullout technique: This is a recent technique, which has been popularized at the University of Miami by Robert Marx. It aims at preserving the inferior alveolar nerve during mandibular resections. The rationale behind the approach is that most odontogenic tumors do not invade the epineurium, and thus sacrifice of the nerve is not essential. The surgical approach involves a lateral decortication of the mandible posterior to the posterior resection margin to identify the nerve. Anteriorly, the nerve is transected at the mental foramen. The resection is performed, and then the nerve is pulled out of the specimen posteriorly. If there are attachments from the

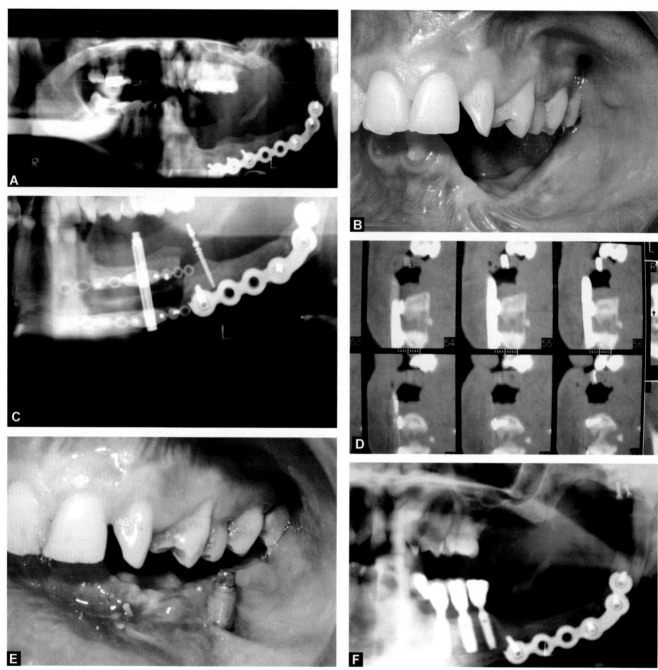

Figs 7.29A to F: (A) Panoramic radiograph showing atrophic mandible after tumor surgery. (B) Intraoral photograph showing significant hard and soft tissue defects. Note loss of height and width of bone. (C) Alveolar distraction osteogenesis has been performed for augmentation of alveolar ridge height. (D) CT scan showing distraction regenerate and proper vector of distraction. (E) Intraoral photograph showing distraction rod with regenerated bone and soft tissue height as compared to Fig. 7.29B. (F) Reconstruction of the distracted segment using endosseous dental implants and fixed dental prosthetics

bundle to the roots of teeth, these may need to be transected to permit pullout of the nerve. Once the nerve is pulled out of the specimen, it is reanastomosed in standard fashion using epineural sutures. Marx claims that the return of sensation in these patients is superior to those that receive a nerve graft, and varies between 80 and 95%. No long-term data is available. In the authors' experience with 14 cases where this technique has been utilized, an average return of sensation of approximately 85% has been seen (Fig. 7.32).

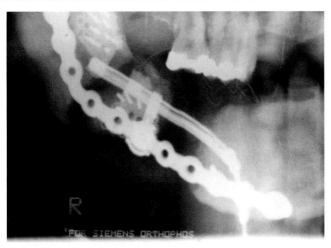

Fig. 7.30: Mandibular transport distraction using an intraoral distraction device

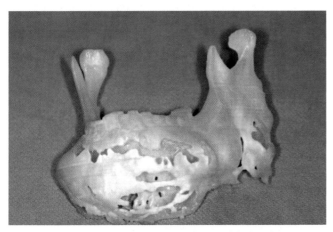

Fig. 7.31: 3-D stereolithographic model showing extensive mandibular tumor

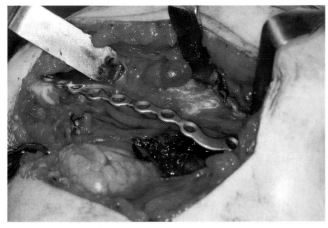

Fig. 7.32: Inferior alveolar nerve preservation techniques allow for maintenance of the sensory sensation to the lower lip

Nerve grafting: Odontogenic cysts and tumors occur most commonly in the mandible. One devastating sequela of mandibular surgery is iatrogenic damage to the inferior alveolar nerve. Historically, it has been noted that most patients will tolerate lower lip anesthesia quite well; however, one must agree that inferior alveolar nerve injury does to some extent, and at least for sometime, cause problems like drooling of saliva, and possible functional problems during speech and mastication. Thus, many surgeons are now offering microsurgical nerve repair as an option to the patient, and this should be discussed in the preoperative treatment planning.

If the inferior alveolar nerve is accidentally injured during surgery, the best time to repair is immediately with direct anastomoses as long as the surgical repair is without tension. In cases of mandibular resection where the nerve is sacrificed, nerve grafting is recommended. The donor graft is usually harvested from the greater auricular nerve or the sural nerve.

Bone Growth Factors

During the last few years, extensive literature is available showing the usefulness of bone growth manipulation using bone growth factors like platelet rich plasma (PRP) and bone morphogenetic proteins (BMPs). Addition of these bone-stimulating substances has been shown to increase bone formation and also decrease the time needed for such bone formation. PRP is abundant in platelet-derived growth factors (PDGFaa, PDGFab, PDGFbb), which induce cellular proliferation and capillary angiogenesis. It also contains transforming growth factor-betas (TGF-betas), which have similar actions as above besides inducing connective tissue differentiation. As research continues and clinical application of these substances increases, it is to be expected that our understanding of bone growth factors will further improve.

Bone and Tissue Engineering

Research is continuing to look for means of possibly eliminating the need for bone graft harvesting. While still in its early infancy, there are some early promising signs. One of the authors (PM) has participated in two surgical cases involving reconstruction of isolated small areas of the jaws (one maxilla and one mandible) using novel techniques being developed at the Boston University School of Dental Medicine. In both of these cases, bone was harvested as a biopsy specimen from the retromolar pad as a quick in-office procedure under local anesthesia.

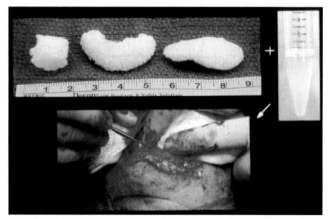

Fig. 7.33: Bone and tissue engineering using customized tissue scaffolds for jaw reconstruction. (*Courtesy*: David Cottrell and Laisheng Chou, Boston, MA)

Osteoblasts isolated from these bone biopsies were cultured in a special laboratory. The patient's own bone cells were regenerated in the lab from these osteoblasts, and then customized osteogenic scaffolds (Fig. 7.33) impregnated with these bone cells were implanted into the patient's jaw in an attempt to regenerate bone. Long-term follow-up including actual biopsy specimens revealed positive bone formation.

Implant-Supported Prosthodontics

Techniques of maxillofacial prosthodontics have also advanced exponentially over the last few years. It is a well-known fact that loss of teeth leads to progressive atrophy of alveolar bone, and denture wear can accelerate this resorptive process. Dental implants can minimize this bone resorption, and are very successful in the maxilla and mandible. Recently, dental restorations supported by zygomatic implants have been used for maxillary dental rehabilitation in patients with atrophic upper jaws; this allows for implant-supported restorations without the need for bone grafting. Dental restorations supported by implants are extremely esthetic, maintain alveolar height and width, and give patients long-term predictable service. Preoperative and postoperative hyperbaric oxygen therapy is recommended for dental implant patients who have a history of radiation therapy to the jaws.

REFERENCES

Textbook

a. Marx RE, Stern D. In: *Oral and Maxillofacial Pathology*: A rationale for diagnosis and treatment. 1st edition. Quintessence Publishing Company, Illinois, 2003.

b. Williams TP, Stewart JCB (Eds). In, Fonseca: *Oral and Maxillofacial Surgery - Surgical Pathology*, Vol 5. 1st edition, W.B. Saunders Company, Philadelphia, 2000.

c. Neville BW, Damm DD, Allen CM, Bouquot JE. *Oral and Maxillofacial Pathology*. 2nd edition. WB. Saunders Company, Philadelphia, 2002.

d. Barnes L. *Surgical Pathology of the Head and Neck*. 2nd edition. Marcel Dekker, Inc., New York, 2001.

Journal

1. Williams TP, Stewart JCB (Eds). In, Fonseca *Oral and Maxillofacial Surgery - Surgical Pathology*, Vol 5. 1st edition, Philadelphia: WB Saunders, 2000.
2. Toller PA. Newer concepts of odontogenic cysts. *Int J Oral Surg* 1972; 1:3–16.
3. Ten Cate AR. The epithelial rests of Malassez and the genesis of the dental cyst. *J Oral Surg* 1972; 34:956–964.
4. Toller PA. Permeability of cyst walls *in vivo*. Investigations with radioactive tracers. *Proc Roy Soc Med* 1966; 59:724–729.
5. Toller PA. Protein substances in odontogenic cyst fluids. *Br Dent J* 1970; 128: 317–322.
6. Main DMG. The enlargement of epithelial jaw cysts. *Odontol Rev* 1970; 21:29–49.
7. Browne RM. The pathogenesis of odontogenic cysts: A review. *J Oral Pathol* 1975; 4(1):31–46.
8. Toller PA. The osmolality of fluids from cysts of the jaws. *Br Dent J* 1970; 129:275–278.
9. Benn A, Altini M. Dentigerous cysts of inflammatory origin: A clinicopathologic study. *Oral Surg Oral Med Oral Pathol Oral Radiol Endo* 1996; 81(2):203–209.
10. Mourshed F. A roentgenographic study of dentigerous cysts: I. Incidence in a population sample. *Oral Surg Oral Med Oral Pathol* 1964; 18:47–53.
11. Dreidler JF, Raubenheimer EJ, van Heerden WF. A retrospective analysis of 367 cystic lesions of the jaw—the Ulm experience. *J Craniomaxillofac Surg* 1993; 21:339–341.
12. Yasuoka T, Yonemoto K, Kato Y, Tatematsu N. Squamous cell carcinoma arising in a dentigerous cyst. *J Oral Maxillofac Surg* 2000; 58:900–905.
13. Aguilo L, Cibrian R, Bagan JV, Gandia JL. Eruption cysts: Retrospective clinical study of 36 cases. *ASDC J Dent Child* 1998; 65(2):102–106.
14. Kuczek A, Beikler T, Herbst H, Flemmig TF. Eruption cyst formation associated with cyclosporin A. A case report. *J Clin Periodontol* 2003; 30:462–466.
15. Nomura J, Tagawa T, Seki Y, Mori A, Nakagawa T, Sugatani T. Kinky hair disease with multiple eruption cysts: A case report. *Oral Surg Oral Med Oral Pathol Oral Radiol Endod* 1996; 82(5):537–540.
16. Wysocki G, Brannon R, Gardner D, Sapp P. Histogenesis of the lateral periodontal cyst and the gingival cyst of the adult. *Oral Surg Oral Med Oral Pathol* 1980; 50:327–334.
17. Cohen D, Neville B, Damm D, White D. The lateral periodontal cyst: A report of 37 cases. *J Periodontol* 1984; 55: 230–234.
18. Carter LC, Carney YL, Perez-Pedlewski D. Lateral periodontal cyst: Multifactorial analysis of a previously unreported series. *Oral Surg Oral Med Oral Radiol Endod* 1996; 81(2):210-216.

19. Baker RD, D'Onofrio ED, Corio RL. Squamous cell carcinoma arising in a lateral periodontal cyst. *Oral Surg Oral Med Oral Pathol* 1979; 47:495–499.

20. Buchner A, David R, Carpenter W, Leider A. Pigmented lateral periodontal cyst and other pigmented oral lesions. *Oral Dis* 1996; 2:229–302.

21. Ahlfors E, Larsson A, Sjogren S. The odontogenic keratocyst: A benign cystic tumor? *J Oral Maxillofac Surg* 1991; 20: 362–365.

22. Wicking C, Bale AE. Molecular basis of the nevoid basal cell carcinoma syndrome. *Curr Opin Pediatr* 1997; 9(6):630–635.

23. Cohen MM Jr. Nevoid basal cell carcinoma syndrome: Molecular biology and new hypotheses. *Int J Oral Maxillofac Surg* 1999; 28(3):216–223.

24. Barreto DC, Gomez RS, Bale AE, Boson WL, De Marco L. PTCH gene mutations in odontogenic keratocysts. *J Dent Res* 2000; 79(6):1418–1422.

25. Myoung H, Hong SP, Hong SD, Lee JI, Lim CY, Choung PH, Lee JH, et al. Odontogenic keratocyst: Review of 256 cases for recurrence and clinicopathologic parameters. *Oral Surg Oral Med Oral Pathol Oral Radiol Endod* 2001; 91(3):328–333.

26. Blanas N, Freund B, Schwartz M, Furst I. Systematic review of the treatment and prognosis of the odontogenic keratocyst. *Oral Surg Oral Med Oral Pathol Oral Radiol Endod* 2000; 90(5):553–558.

27. Brannon RB. The odontogenic keratocyst. A clinicopathologic study of 312 cases. Part I. Clinical features. *Oral Surg Oral Med Oral Pathol* 1976; 42(1):54–72.

28. de Paula AMB, Carvalhais JN, Domingues MG, Barreto DC, Mesquita RA. Cell proliferation markers in the odontogenic keratocyst: Effect of inflammation. *J Oral Pathol Med* 2000; 29:477–482.

29. August M, Faquin WC, Troulis MJ, Kaban LB. Dedifferentiation of odontogenic keratocyst epithelium after cyst decompression. *J Oral Maxillofac Surg* 2003; 61:678–683.

30. Voorsmit RACA. The incredible keratocyst. Thesis, University of Nijmegan, The Netherlands. 1984.

31. Voorsmit RACA, Stoelinga PJ, Van Haelst UJGM. The management of keratocysts. *J Maxillofac Surg* 1981; 9:228–235.

32. Schmidt BL, Pogrel MA. The use of enucleation and liquid nitrogen cryotherapy in the management of odontogenic keratocysts. *J Oral Maxillofac Surg* 2001; 59:720–725.

33. Browne RM. The odontogenic keratocyst: Histological features and their correlation with clinical behavior. *Br Dent J* 1971; 131:249–259.

34. Rud J, Pindborg JJ. Odontogenic keratocysts: A follow-up study of 21 cases. *J Oral Surg* 1969; 27:323–330.

35. Gorlin RJ, Cohen MM, Levin LS. Nevoid basal cell carcinoma syndrome. In *Syndrome of the Head and Neck*, 3rd ed. New York: Oxford University Press, 1990; 372–379.

36. Gorlin RJ. Nevoid basal cell carcinoma syndrome. *Medicine* 1987; 66:96.

37. Wright JM. The odontogenic keratocyst: Orthokeratinized variant. *Oral Surg Oral Med Oral Pathol* 1981; 51(6):609–618.

38. da Silva MJA, de Sousa SO, Correa L, Carvalhosa AA, de Araujo VC. Immunohistochemical study of the orthokeratinized odontogenic cyst: A comparison with the odontogenic keratocyst. *Oral Surg Oral Med Oral Pathol Oral Radiol Endod* 2002; 94:732–737.

39. Gardner DG, Kessler HP, Morency R, Schaffner DL. The glandular odontogenic cyst: An apparent entity. *J Oral Pathol* 1988; 17:359–366.

40. Koppang HS, Johannessen S, Haugen LK, Haanaes HR, Solheim T, Donath K. Glandular odontogenic cyst (sialo-odontogenic cyst): Report of two cases and literature review of 45 previously reported cases. *J Oral Pathol Med* 1998; 27: 455–462.

41. Ide F, Shimoyama T, Horie N. Glandular odontogenic cyst with hyaline bodies: An unusual dentigerous presentation. *J Oral Pathol Med* 1996; 25:401–404.

42. Ramer M, Montazem A, Lane SL, Lumerman H. Glandular odontogenic cyst: Report of a case and review of the literature. *Oral Surg Oral Med Oral Pathol Oral Radiol Endod* 1997; 84(1): 54–57.

43. Toida M, Ishimaru JI, Tatematsu N. Calcifying odontogenic cyst associated with compound odontoma: Report of a case. *J Oral Maxillofac Surg* 1990; 48:77–81.

44. Tajima Y, Yokose S, Sakamoto E, Yamamoto Y, Utsumi N. Ameloblastoma arising in calcifying odontogenic cyst. *Oral Surg Oral Med Oral Pathol* 1992; 74:776–779.

45. Zeitoun IM, Dhanrajani PJ, Mosadomi HA. Adenomatoid odontogenic tumor arising in a calcifying odontogenic cyst. *J Oral Maxillofac Surg* 1996; 54:634–637.

46. Yoon JH, Kim HJ, Yook JI, Cha IH, Ellis GL, Kim J. Hybrid odontogenic tumor of calcifying odontogenic cyst and ameloblastic fibroma. *Oral Surg Oral Med Oral Pathol Oral Radiol Endod* 2004; 98:80–84.

47. Toida M. So-called calcifying odontogenic cyst: Review and discussion on the terminology and classification. *J Oral Pathol Med* 1998; 27:49–52.

48. Praetorius F, Hjorting–Hansen E, Gorlin RJ, Vickers RA. Calcifying odontogenic cyst. Range, variations and neoplastic potential. *Acta Odontol Scand.* 1981; 39:227–240.

49. Buchner A. The central (intraosseous) calcifying odontogenic cyst: An analysis of 215 cases. *J Oral Maxillofac Surg* 1991; 49:330–339.

50. Shamaskin RG, Svirsky JA, Kaugars GE. Intraosseous and extraosseous calcifying odontogenic cyst (Gorlin Cyst). *J Oral Maxillofac Surg* 1989; 47:562–565.

51. Orsini G, Fioroni M, Rubini C, Piattelli A. Peripheral calcifying odontogenic cyst. *J Clin Periodontol* 2002; 29:83–86.

52. Tanimoto K, Tomita S, Aoyama M, Furuki Y, Fujita M, Wada T. Radiographic characteristics of calcifying odontogenic cyst. *Int J Oral Maxillofac Surg* 1988; 17:29–32.

53. Sekine S, Sato S, Takata T, Fukuda Y, Ishida T, Kishio M et al. β-catenin mutations are frequent in calcifying odontogenic cysts, but rare in ameloblastomas. *Am J Pathol* 2003; 163: 1701–1712.

54. Gunhan O, Celasun B, Can C, Finci R. The nature of ghost cells in calcifying odontogenic cyst: An immunohistochemical study. *Ann Dent* 1993; 52(1):30–33.

55. Hong SP, Ellis GL, Hartman KS. Calcifying odontogenic cyst. A review of ninety-two cases with re-evaluation of their nature as cysts or neoplasms, the nature of ghost cells, and subclassification. *Oral Surg Oral Med Oral Pathol* 1991; 72: 56–64.

56. Lu Y, Mock D, Takata T, Jordan RC. Odontogenic ghost cell carcinoma: Report of four new cases and review of the literature. *J Oral Pathol Med* 1999; 28:323–329.

57. Buchner A, Merrel PW, Hansen LS, Leider AS. Peripheral (extraosseous) calcifying odontogenic cyst. A review of forty-five cases. *Oral Surg Oral Med Oral Pathol* 1991; 72:65–70.

58. Stoneman DW, Worth HM. The mandibular infected buccal cyst—molar area. *Dent Radiogr Photogr* 1983; 56:1–14.

59. Shohat I, Buchner A, Taicher S. Mandibular buccal bifurcation cyst. Enucleation without extraction. *J Oral Maxillorfac Surg* 2003; 32:610–613.

60. Pompura JR, Sandor GKB, Stoneman DW. The buccal bifurcation cyst: A prospective study of treatment outcomes in 44 sites. *Oral Surg Oral Med Oral Pathol Oral Radiol Endod* 1997; 83:215–221.

61. Gao Z, Flaitz CM, Madckenzie IC. Expression of keratinocyte growth factor in periapical lesions. *J Dent Res* 1996; 75:1658–1653.

62. Gervasio AM, Silva DAO, Taketomi EA, Souza CJA, Sung S-J, Loyola AM. Levels of GM-SF, IL-, and IL- in fluid and tissue from human radicular cysts. *J Dent Res* 2002; 81:64–68.

63. Pesce C, Ferloni M. Optosis and Rushton body formation. *Histopathology* 2002; 40:109–111.

64. Daley TD, Wysocki GP, Pringle GA. Relative incidence of odontogenic tumors and oral and jaw cysts in a Canadian population. *Oral Surg Oral Med Oral Pathol* 1994; 77:276–280.

65. Allard RHB, Van Der Karast WAM, Van Der Waal I. Nasopalatine duct cyst. Review of the literature and report of 22 cases. *Int J Oral Surg* 1981; 10:447–461.

66. Abrams AM, Howell FU, Bullock WK. Nasopalatine cyst. *Oral Surg Oral Med Oral Pathol* 1963; 16:306–332.

67. Mealey BL, Braun JC, Rasch MS, Fowler CB. Incisive canal cysts related to periodontal osseous defects. *J Perio* 1993; 64:571–574.

68. Ely N, Sheehy EC, McDonald F. Nasopalatine duct cyst: A case report. *Int J Paediatr Dent* 2001; 11:135–137.

69. Elliott, KA, Franzese CB, Pitman KT. Diagnosis and surgical management of nasopalatine duct cysts. *Laryngoscope* 2004; 114(8):1336–1340.

70. Precious DS. Chronic nasolabial cyst. *J Canad Dent Assoc* 1987; 53:307–308.

71. Allard RH. Nasolabial cyst. Review of the literature and report of 7 cases. *Int J Oral Surg* 1982; 11(6):351–359.

72. Nixdorf DR, Peters E, Lung KE. Clinical presentation and differential diagnosis of nasolabial cyst. *J Canad Dent Assoc* 2003; 69:146–149.

73. Pereira Filho VA, Silva AC, Moraes M, Moreira RWF, Villalba H. Nasolabial cyst: Case report. *Braz Dent J* 2002; 13(3):212–214.

74. Roed-Petersen B. Nasolabial cysts. A presentation of five cases with a review of the literature. *Br J Oral Surg* 1969; 7:84–95.

75. Neville BW, Damm DD, Allen CM, Bouquot JE. *Oral and Maxillofacial Pathology.* 2nd edition. Philadelphia: WB Saunders, 2002.

76. Faerber TH, Hiatt WR, Dunlap C. Congenital teratoid cyst of the floor of the mouth. *J Oral Maxillofac Surg* 1988; 46:487–490.

77. Bonilla JA, Szeremeta W, Yellon RF, Nazif MM. Teratoid cyst of the floor of the mouth. *Int J Pediatr Otorhinolaryngol* 1996; 38:71–75.

78. Meyer I. Dermoid cysts of the floor of mouth. *J Oral Surg* 1955; 8:1149–1154.

79. Mandel L, Surattanont F. Lateral dermoid cyst. *J Oral Maxillofac Surg* 2005; 63:140–144.

80. Halfpenny W, Odell EW, Robinson PD. Cystic and glial mixed hamartoma of the tongue. *J Oral Pathol Med* 2001; 30:368–371.

81. Mahmood S, Moody H. Dermoid, teratoma or choristoma? A rare lesion of the tongue in an adult. *Br J Oral Maxillofac Surg* 2003; 41:117–119.

82. Komiyama K, Miki Y, Oda Y, Tachibana T, Okaue M, Tanaka H, et al. Uncommon dermoid cyst presented in the mandible possibly originating from embryonic epithelial remnants. *J Oral Pathol Med* 2002; 31:184–187.

83. Zachariades N, Skoura-Kafoussia C. A life threatening epidermoid cyst of the floor of the mouth. *J Oral Maxillofac Surg* 1990; 48(4):400–403.

84. Watanabe H, Arita S, Chigira M. Aetiology of a simple bone cyst. A case report. *Int Orthop* 1994; 18(1):16–19.

85. Abdel-Wanis ME, Tsuchiya H. Simple bone cyst is not a single entity: Point of view based on a literature review. *Med Hypotheses* 2002; 58(1):87–91.

86. Kreidler JF, Raubenheimer EJ, van Heerden WF. A retrospective analysis of 367 cystic lesions of the jaw–the Ulm experience. *J Craniomaxillofac Surg* 1993; 21(8):339–341.

87. Kaugars GE, Cale AE. Traumatic bone cyst. *Oral Surg Oral Med Oral Pathol* 1987; 63:318–324.

88. Tong AC, Ng IO, Yan BS. Variations in clinical presentations of the simple bone cyst: Report of cases. *J Oral Maxillofac Surg* 2003; 61:1487–1491.

89. Horner K, Forman GH. Atypical simple bone cysts of the jaws. II: A possible association with benign fibro-osseous (cemental) lesions of the jaws. *Clin Radiol* 1988; 39:59–63.

90. Moule I. Unilateral multiple solitary bone cysts. *J Oral Maxillofac Surg* 1988; 46(4):320–323.

91. Fisher AD. Bone cavity in fibro-osseous lesions. *Br J Oral Surg* 1976; 14(2):120–127.

92. Melrose RJ, Abrams AM, Mills BG. Florid osseous dysplasia: A clinical pathologic study of thirty-four cases. *Oral Surg Oral Med Oral Pathol* 1976; 41(1):62–82.

93. Wakasa T, Kawai N, Aiga H, Kishi K. Management of florid emento-osseous dysplasia of the mandible producing solitary bone cyst: Report of a case. *J Oral Maxillofac Surg* 2002; 60(7):832–835.

94. Levy WM, Miller AS, Bonakdarpour A, Aegerter E. Aneurysmal bone cyst secondary to osseous lesions: Report of 57 cases. *Am J Clin Pathol* 1975; 63:1–8.

95. Martinez V, Sissons HA. Aneurysmal bone cyst: A review of 123 cases including primary lesions and those secondary to other bone pathology. *Cancer* 1988; 61:2291–2304.

96. Vergel De Dios AM, Bond JR, Shives TC, McLeod RA Unni KK. Aneurysmal bone cyst: A clinicopathologic study of 238 cases. *Cancer* 1992; 69:2921–2931.

97. Rapidis AD, Vallianatou D, Apostolidis C, Lagogiannis G. Large lytic lesion of the ascending ramus, the condyle, and the infratemporal region. *J Oral Maxillofac Surg* 2004; 62:996–1001.

98. De Silva MVC, Raby N, Reid R. Fibromyxoid areas and immature osteoid are associated with recurrence of primary aneurysmal bone cysts. *Histopathology* 2003; 43:180–188.

99. Panoutsakopoulos G, Pandis N, Kyriazoglou I, Gustafson P, Mertens F, Mandahl N. Recurrent t(16. 17)(q22. p13) in aneurysmal bone cysts. *Genes Chromosomes Cancer* 1999; 26:265–266.

100. Oliveria AM, Perez-Atayde AR, Inwards CY, Medeiros F, Derr V, Hsi BL, et al. USP6 and CDH11 oncogenes identify the neoplastic cell in primary aneurysmal bone cysts and are absent in so-called secondary aneurysmal bone cysts. *Am J Pathol* 2004; 165(5):1773–1780.

101. Oliveria AM, Hsi BL, Weremowicz S, Rosenberg AE, Dal Cin P, Joseph N et al. USP6 (Tre2) fusion oncongenes in aneurysmal bone cyst. *Cancer Res* 2004; 64:1920–1923.

102. Liu B, Yu SF, Li TJ. Multinucleated giant cells in various forms of giant cell containing lesions of the jaws express features of osteoclasts. *J Oral Pathol Med* 2003; 32:367–375.

103. Carlos R, Sedano HO. Intralesional corticosteroids as an alternative treatment for central giant cell granuloma. *Oral Surg Oral Med Oral Pathol* 2002; 93:161–166.

104. Pogrel MA. Calcitonin therapy for central giant cell granuloma. *J Oral Maxillofac Surg* 2003; 61(6):649–653.

105. Kaban LB, Troulis MJ, Ebb D, August M et al. Antiangiogenic therapy with interferon alpha for giant cell lesions of the jaws. *J Oral Maxillofac Surg* 2002; 60(10):1103–1111.

106. Philipsen HP, Samman N, Ormiston IW, Reichart PA. Variants of the adenomatoid odontogenic tumor with a note on tumor origin. *J Oral Pathol Med* 1992; 21:348–352.

107. Giansanti JS, Someren A, Waldron CA. Odontogenic adenomatoid tumor (adenoameloblastoma). *Oral Surg Oral Med Oral Pathol* 1970; 30:69–86.

108. Philipsen HP, Reichart PA, Zhang KH. Adenomatoid odontogenic tumor: Biologic profile based on 499 cases. *J Oral Pathol Med* 1991; 20:149–158.

109. Philipsen HP, Birn H. The adenomatoid odontogenic tumor. Ameloblastic adenomatoid tumor or adeno-ameloblastoma. *Acta Pathol Microbiol Scand* 1969; 75(3):375–398.

110. Curran AE, Miller EJ, Murrah VA. Adenomatoid odontogenic tumor presenting as periapical disease. *Oral Surg Oral Med Oral Pathol Oral Radiol Endod* 1997; 84(5):557–560.

111. Philipsen HP, Srisuwan T, Reichart PA. Adenomatoid odontogenic tumor mimicking a periapical (radicular) cyst: A case report. *Oral Surg Oral Med Oral Pathol Oral Radiol Endod* 2002; 94:246–248.

112. Philipsen HP, Reichart PA. Adenomatoid odontogenic tumor: Facts and figures. *Oral Oncol* 1998; 35:1–7.

113. Murata M, Cheng J, Horino K, Hara K, Shimokawa H, Saku T. Enamel proteins and extracellular matrix molecules are co-localized in the pseudocystic stromal space of adenomatoid odontogenic tumor. *J Oral Pathol Med* 2000; 29:483–490.

114. Cataldo E, Leww WC, Giunta JL. Squamous odontogenic tumor. A lesion of the periodontium. *J Periodontol* 1983; 54(12):731–735.

115. Saxby MS, Rippin JW, Sheron JE. Case report: Squamous odontogenic tumor of the gingiva. *J Periodontol* 1993; 64:1250–1252.

116. Baden E, Doyle J, Mesa M, Fabie M, Lederman D, Eichen M. Squamous odontogenic tumor. Report of three cases including the first extraosseous case. *Oral Surg Oral Med Oral Pathol* 1993; 75(6):733–738.

117. Philipsen HP, Reichart PA. Squamous odontogenic tumor (SOT): A benign neoplasm of the periodontium: A review of 36 reported cases. *J Clin Periodontol* 1996; 23(10):922–926.

118. Mills WP, Davilla MA, Beattenmuller EA, Koudelka BM. Squamous odontogenic tumor: Report of a case with lesions in three quadrants. *Oral Surg Oral Med Oral Pathol* 1986; 61:557–563.

119. Leider AS, Jonker AL, Cook HE. Multicentric familial squamous odontogenic tumor. *Oral Surg Oral Med Oral Pathol* 1989; 68:175–181.

120. Ruskin JD, Cohen DM, Davis LF. Primary intraosseous carcinoma: Report of two cases. *J Oral Maxillofac Surg* 1988; 46:425.

121. Pindborg JJ. A calcifying epithelial odontogenic tumor. *Cancer* 1958; 11:838–843.

122. Philipsen HP, Reichart PA. Calcifying epithelial odontogenic tumor: Biological profile based on 181 cases from the literature. *Oral Oncol* 2000; 36:17–26.

123. Houston GD, Fowler CB. Extraosseous calcifying epithelial odontogenic tumor: Report of two cases and review of the literature. *Oral Surg Oral Med Oral Pathol Oral Radiol Endod* 1997; 83(5):577–583.

124. Anavi Y, Kapla I, Citir M, Calderon S. Clear-cell variant of calcifying epithelial odontogenic tumor: Clinical and radiographic characteristics. *Oral Surg Oral Med Oral Pathol Oral Radiol Endod* 2003; 95:332–339.

125. Sololmon A, Murphy CL, Weaver K, Weiss DT, Hrncic R, Eulitz M et al. Calcifying epithelial odontogenic (Pinborg) tumor-associated amyloid consists of a novel human protein. *J Lab Clin Med* 2003; 142:348–355.

126. Hicks MJ, Flaitz CM, Wong ME. Clear cell variant of the calcifying epithelial odontogenic tumor: Case report and review of literature. *Head Neck* 1994; 16:272–274.

127. McClatchey KD. Tumors of the dental lamina: A selective review. *Semin Diagn Pathol* 1987; 4(3):200–204.

128. Crivelini MM, de Araujo VC, de Sousa SO, de Araujo NS. Cytokeratins in epithelia of odontogenic neoplasms. *Oral Dis* 2003; 9(1):1–6.

129. Robinson L, Martinez MG. Unicystic ameloblastoma: A prognostically distinct entity. *Cancer* 1977; 40:2278–2285.

130. Vickers RA, Gorlin RJ. Ameloblastoma: Delineation of early histopathologic features of neoplasia. *Cancer* 1970; 26:699–710.

131. Gardner DG. Some current concepts on the pathology of ameloblastomas. *Oral Surg Oral Med Oral Pathol Oral Radiol Endod* 1996; 82(6):660–669.

132. Philipsen HP, Reichart PA, Nikai H, Takata T, Kudo Y. Peripheral ameloblastoma: Biological profile based of 160 cases from the literature. *Oral Oncol* 2001; 37:17–32.

133. Anneroth G, Johansson B. Peripheral ameloblastoma. *Int J Oral Surg* 1985; 14:295–299.

134. Kumamoto H, Kawamura H, Ooya K. Clear cell odontogenic tumor in the mandible: Report of a case with an immuno-histochemical study of epithelial cell markers. *Pathol Int* 1998; 48:618–622.

135. Brandwein M, Al-Naief N, Gordon R, Urken M. Clear cell odontogenic carcinoma: Report of a case and review of the literature. *Arch Otolaryngol Head Neck Surg* 2002; 128(9):1089–1095.

136. August M, Faquin W, Troulis M, Kaban L. Clear cell odontogenic carcinoma: Evaluation of reported cases. *J Oral Maxillofac Surg* 2003; 61:580–586.

137. Siriwardena BSMS, Tilakaratne WM, Rajapaksha RMSK. Clear cell odontogenic carcinoma—a case report and review of literature. *Int J Oral Maxillofac Surg* 2004; 33:512–514.

138. Eversole LR. Malignant epithelial odontogenic tumors. *Semin Diagn Pathol* 1999; 16(4):317–324.

139. Eversole LR, Duffey DC, Powell NB. Clear cell odontogenic carcinoma: A clinicopathologic analysis. *Arch Otolaryngol Head Neck Surg* 1995; 121:685–688.

140. Daniels JSM. Central odontogenic fibroma of mandible: A case report and review of the literature. *Oral Surg Oral Med Oral Pathol Oral Radiol Endod* 2004; 98:295.

141. Wesley RK, Wysocki GP, Mintz SM. The central odontogenic fibroma. Clincial and morphological studies. *Oral Surg Oral Med Oral Pathol* 1975; 40:235–245.

142. Gardner DG. The central odontogenic fibroma: An attempt at clarification. *Oral Surg Oral Med Oral Pathol* 1980; 5: 425–432.

143. Doyle JL, Lamster IB, Baden E. Odontogenic fibroma of the complex (WHO) type: Report of six cases. *J Oral Maxillofac Surg* 1985; 43:666–668.

144. Daley TD, Wysocki GP. Peripheral odontogenic fibroma. *Oral Surg Oral Med Oral Pathol* 1994; 78:329.

145. Herzog S. Benign cementoblastoma associated with the primary dentition. *J Oral Med* 1987; 42:106–108.

146. Brannon RB, Fowler CB, Carpenter WM, Corio RL. Cementoblastoma: An innocuous neoplasm? A clinicopathologic study of 44 cases and review of the literature with special emphasis on recurrence. *Oral Surg Oral Med Oral Pathol Oral Radiol Endod* 2002; 93:311–320.

147. Eversole LR, Sabes Wr, Dauchess VG. Benign cementoblastoma. *Oral Surg Oral Med Oral Pathol* 1973; 36:824–830.

148. Bast BT, Pogrel A, Regezi JA. The expression of apoptotic proteins and matrix metalloproteinases in odontogenic myxomas. *J Oral Maxillofac Surg* 2003; 61:1463–1466.

149. Simon ENM, Merkx MAW, Vuhahula E, Ngassapa D, Stoelinga PJW. Odontogenic myxoma: A clinicopathological study of 33 cases. *Int J Oral Maxillofac Surg* 2004; 33:333–337.

150. Lo Muzio L, Nocini P, Gianfranco F, Procaccini M, Mignogna MD. Odontogenic myxoma of the jaws: A clinical, radiologic, immunohistochemical, and ultrastructural study. *Oral Surg Oral Med Oral Pathol Oral Radiol Endod* 1996; 82(4):426–433.

151. Hisatomi M, Asaumi J-I, Konouchi H, Honda Y, Wakasa T, Kishi K. A case of complex odontoma associated with an impacted lower deciduous second molar and analysis of the 107 odontomas. *Oral Dis* 2002; 8:100–105.

152. Philipsen HP, Reichart PA, Praetorius F. Mixed odontogenic tumors and odontomas. Considerations on interrelationship. Review of the literature and presentation of 134 new cases of odontomas. *Oral Oncol* 1997; 33:86–99.

153. Haishima K, Haishima H, Yamada Y, Tomizawa M, Noda T, Suzuki M. Compound odontomes associated with impacted maxillary deciduous central incisors: Report of two cases. *Int J Paediatr Dent* 1994; 4:251–256.

154. Piatelli A, Perfetti G, Carraro A. Complex odontoma as a periapical and interradicular radiopacity in a deciduous molar. *J Endod* 1996; 22:561–563.

155. Trodahl JN. Ameloblastic fibroma: A survey of cases from the Armed Forces Institute of Pathology. *Oral Surg Oral Med Oral Pathol* 1972; 33(4):547–558.

156. Yagishita H, Taya Y, Kanri Y, Matsuo A, Nonaka H, Fuhita H et al. The secretion of amelogenins is associated with the induction of enamel and dentinoid in an ameloblastic fibro-odontoma. *J Oral Pathol Med* 2001; 30:499–503.

157. Kaban LB, Troulis MJ, Ebb D, August M, Hornicek FJ, Dodson TB. Antiangiogenic therapy with interferon alpha for giant cell lesions of the jaws. *J Oral Maxillofac Surg* 2002; 60: 1103–1111.

158. Buresh CJ, Seemayer TA, Nelson M, Neff JR, Dorfman HD, Bridge J. t(X. 4)(q22. q31.3) in giant cell reparative granuloma. *Cancer Genet Cytogenet* 1999; 115:80–81.

159. Kaffe I, Ardekian L, Taicher S, Littner MM, Buchner A. Radiographic features of central giant cell granuloma of the jaws. *Oral Surg Oral Med Oral Pathol Oral Radiol Endod* 1996; 81(6):720–726.

160. Chuong R, Kaban LB, Kozakewich H. Central giant cell lesions of the jaws: A clinicopathologic study. *J Oral Maxillofac Surg* 1986; 44:708–713.

161. Itonaga I, Hussein I, Kudo O, Sabokbar a, Watt-Smith S, Ferguson D et al. Cellular mechanisms of osteoclast formation and lacunar resorption in giant cell granuloma of the jaw. *J Oral Pathol Med* 2003; 32:224–231.

162. Regezi JA, Pogrel MA. Comments on the pathogenesis and medical treatment of central giant cell granulomas. *J Oral Maxillofac Surg* 2004; 62(1):116–118.

163. Cohen MM Jr, Howell RE. Etiology of fibrous dysplasia and McCune–Albright syndrome. *Int J Oral Maxillofac Surg* 1999; 28:366–371.

164. Cohen MM Jr. Fibrous dysplasia is a neoplasm. *Am J Med Gen* 2001; 290–293.

Fungal Rhinosinusitis

Chris de Souza, J Peter Rodrigues

Fungi include several thousand species of eukaryotic spore bearing organisms that obtain simple organic compounds by absorption. Fungi have no chlorophyll and reproduce by both sexual and asexual means. The fungi are usually filamentous and their walls have chitin. Two major groups of organisms make up fungi. The filamentous fungi are called moulds while the unicellular fungi are called yeasts. Ten characteristics of true fungi are as listed below.

1. All are eukaryotic. They possess membrane bound nuclei (containing chromosomes) and a range of membrane bound cytoplasmic organelles (mitochondria, vacuoles, endoplasmic reticulum).
2. Most are filamentous. They are composed of individual microscopic filaments called hyphae which exhibit apical growth and which branch to form a network of hyphae called mycelium.
3. Some are unicellular, i.e. yeasts.
4. Protoplasm of a hypha or cell is surrounded by a rigid wall. They are composed primarily of chitin and glucans. Sometimes the walls of some species contain cellulose.
5. Many reproduce both sexually and a sexually and this often results in the production of spores (Fig. 8.1).
6. Fungal nuclei are typically haploid and hyphal compartments are often multinucleate. The exception are Oomycota and some yeasts which possess diploid nuclei.
7. All are achlorophyllous and are incapable of photosynthesis.
8. All are chemoheterotrophic (chemo-organotrophic), that is to say fungi use pre-existing organic substances of carbon in their environment and the energy from chemical reactions to synthesise the organic compounds they require for growth and energy.
9. Fungi possess a characteristic range of storage compounds like trehalose, glycogen, sugar, alcohols and lipids.

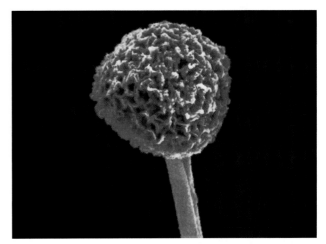

Fig. 8.1: Electron microscopy of aspergillosis

10. They may be free living, parasitic or mutualistic (symbiotic).

Over 60,000 species of fungi are known. Fungal diseases have emerged as major challenges for physicians, microbiologists and basic scientists. The incidence of mycotic infections and the number and diversity of pathogenic fungi have increased recently. It has now been discovered that immunocompetent as well as immunoincompetent individuals can be at risk. Prognosis and therapy depend on the proper identification of the fungus causing infection as well as the treatment modalities given taking into account that the patient's immune system can be made competent if it is not. Fungi are ubiquitous organisms. They are commonly found in the respiratory tract including the nose and paranasal sinuses *(Menezes RA, de Souza CE and desa Souza S, 1987)*. Microscopic colonization of the nose and paranasal sinuses can be found in the normal and in the diseased state as well. Fungi are eukaryotic organisms and they may exist as yeast or as moulds. Yeast is unicellular and reproduce by budding while moulds coalesce as colonies of intertwined hyphae referred to as myceliae.

Of the greater than 60,000 fungal species only about 300 have been documented as playing a role in causing disease in humans. Potential fungal pathogens are confined to 3 major groups. They are (1) Zygomycetes, (2) Aspergillus species and (3) Various dematiaceous genera.

There are two basic types of manifestations that comprise the entity "fungal rhinosinusitis". They are: Invasive and noninvasive manifestations. These may be divided further into five distinct entities. They are:

1. Acute invasive.
2. Chronic invasive (granulomatous and nongranulomatous forms).
3. Fungal balls (mycetomas).
4. Saprophytic colonization.
5. Allergic fungal rhinosinusitis.

These manifestations may overlap or progress from a noninvasive form to an invasive form if the immunologic status of the host changes.

The term acute invasive fungal rhinosinusitis is used when vascular invasion is the predominant histopathological feature and the duration of the disease is less than 4 weeks *(Ferguson, 2000)*. Usually such patients who present with acute invasive rhinosinusitis are immunologically compromised or immunoincompetent. Chronic disease exists when the disease progresses gradually over 4 weeks. Some authors *(de Shazo et al, 1997)* have divided the chronic form to be divided into granulomatous and nongranulomatous forms.

Diagnosis of Invasive Fungal Rhinosinusitis

Potassium hydroxide (KOH) preps or calcoflour white stains should be obtained of material suspected top contain fungus. Fungal cultures themselves may take weeks to identify the fungus (Figs 8.2 and 8.3A and B). Furthermore fungal cultures may be positive in patients without invasive fungal infections being present. Necrotic material or biopsy samples should be evaluated through frozen section. Histologic evidence of fungal invasion is the gold standard for the diagnosis of invasive fungal rhinosinusitis. It is important that a fungal culture be obtained as well so as to help identify the likely antifungal agents that can be used to treat the fungal infection.

Principles of Treatment of Fungal Infections

1. Reversal of the cause of immunocompromise.
2. Administration of systemic antifungal agents.
3. Surgical debridement. Multiple attempts may be necessary.

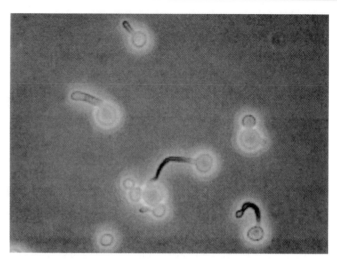

Fig. 8.2: Germ tubes of *Candida albicans*

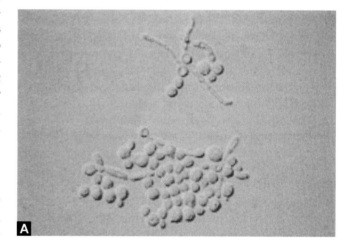

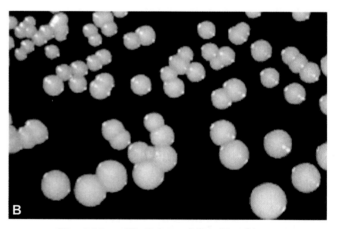

Figs 8.3A and B: Culture of *Candida albicans*

How do Fungi Cause Disease?

To cause an infection the fungus has to first gain access to the host. This necessarily entails a portal of entry, attachment to host cells / host tissues and the capacity to grow within the host. This implies the ability to replicate at 37°C, obtain nutrients and evade the hosts natural defense mechanisms *(Mitchell TG, 2000)*. For dimorphic fungi this also means a conversion an initial morphologic conversion to a tissue form of growth.

Some fungi are capable of colonizing surfaces of epithelial tissues without penetrating and invading the surface. Often fungal rhinosinusitis is characterized by colonization rather than invasion. This produces profound inflammatory and immune responses that can be damaging for the host.

On occasion some fungi can produce potent toxins and mutagens that can cause serious human disease. Less potent irritant and enzymes from fungi attack host cells leading to inflammation or at times immunopathology. Another mechanism is induced when the fungal cell wall antigens stimulate an allergic response in the host *(Ferguson, 1998)*.

The outcome of inhaling fungal spores depends upon the following factors:
1. The number of spores inhaled
2. The size of the fungal particles
3. The integrity of the nonspecific and specific host defenses
4. The pathobiologic potential or virulence of the particular fungus.

The status of the hosts immunity will ultimately determine whether the individual at risk will develop invasive or noninvasive fungal rhinosinusitis. Conditions like diabetic ketoacidosis serve to promote invasion by fungi.

Diagnosing Fungal (Mycotic) Infections

To diagnose accurately the type of fungi present the following are recommended:
1. Microscopic examination of fresh clinical specimens or histopathologic specimens
2. Culture testing of the etiologic agent
3. Serology and skin testing
4. Radiographic imaging
5. Polymerase chain reaction (PCR) methods to detect specific fungal DNA.

Prevention and Prophylaxis in the Immunocompromised Patient

Prevention measures include:
1. Minimizing exposure to fungi most likely to cause rhinosinusitis.
2. Using prophylactic antifungal agents to diminish the risk of tissue invasion by infecting organisms.

Risk Factors

Patients with hematologic disease during the neutropenic phase are at risk. The duration of neutropenia is the most important risk factor in leukemic patients. Other factors that increase the risk further are the concomitant use of corticosteroids, broad spectrum antibiotics and the choice of chemotherapeutic agents.

Bone marrow transplant recipients are at greatest risk in the immediate post-transplant period before engraftment and in the graft versus host disease (GVHD). Chronic GVHD is associated with increased risk of invasive aspergillosis *(Jantunen et al, 1997)*. Patients suffering from GVHD who are also on corticosteroids usually have a poor outcome.

Prevention

Inhalation of fungal spores sets in motion the train of events that could lead to invasive fungal rhinosinusitis. Thus prevention seeks to decrease exposure to fungi. Patients especially those with GVHD are usually hospitalized for long periods of time and usually develop nosocomial fungal infections. Hospital outbreaks are associated with direct contamination of the ventilation system. Demolition or constructive projects near the hospital can contaminate the ventilation system *(Arnow et al, 1991)*. Other sources are potted plants, food, fireproofing or insulation materials.

Potted plants and flowers should not be allowed and ground pepper should not be allowed as seasoning. Air ducts should be cleaned regularly. Birds should be discouraged from nesting on sills and on roofs.

Most outbreaks are related to hospital renovations. Dry wall barriers should be used rather than plastic drapes sealing windows. Frequent vacuuming should be carried out.

Prevention with Prophylactic Antifungal Medications

Principles for starting antifungal mediations are:
1. Target pathogens most likely to cause infection.
2. Identify subsets of patients at risk for fungal rhino-sinusitis.

3. Limiting prophylaxis to the period of time when risk is greatest.
4. Choose a safe well tolerated drug with minimal side effects.
5. Monitor drug related side effects and resistance.
6. Evaluate the cost of a regimen in relation to its efficacy.

Prophylaxis should be limited to patients likely to develop infection and should be given only during period of maximum risk.

Aspergillosis species is the most common pathogen and medication should be directed at this pathogen *(De Carpentier et al, 1994)*. The major target groups based on risk of development of infection should be patients with hematologic malignancies and prolonged neutropenia and those who undergo bone marrow transplantation. The most significant advance against fungal infections has been the use of fluconazole to prevent invasive candidiasis in bone marrow transplant recipients.

Secondary Prophylaxis to Prevent Recurrent Aspergillosis

Secondary prophylaxis against aspergillosis is important in those patients who have suffered a previous attack of aspergillosis in the past and are now undergoing intense chemotherapy or bone marrow transplantation. These patients are at heightened risk of developing a recurrence of an aspergillosis infection *(Viollier et al 1986)*. Even with secondary prophylaxis it has been noted that one third of patients develop a relapse of aspergillosis infection (Figs 8.4A and B).

Recommendations for Preventive Measures

General infection control precautions to ensure that hospital ventilation systems do not transmit filamentous fungi should be routine in all units caring for immuno-suppressed patients. HEPA filtration is recommended but laminar airflow is not.

Diagnosis and Management of Rhinosinusitis before Scheduled Immunosuppression

It is important to identify, diagnose and treat pre-existing rhinosinusitis before starting immunosuppressive therapy.

A careful exam with radiological imaging helps detect patients who may harbor a potentially life threatening infection but who are as yet asymptomatic. Other conditions *(Drakos et al, 1993)* that could lead to rhinosinusitis following immunosuppressive therapy are long-term antibiotic use, indwelling catheters, nasal intubation, steroids, metabolic abnormalities and chronic rhinosinusitis.

Mucormycosis of the Nose and Paranasal Sinuses

Mucormycosis rarely affects a healthy individual. It commonly affects patients suffering from diabetes. It can however occur in any immunocompromised individual. The mainstay of therapy lies in the following:
1. Reversal of immunocompromise
2. Systemic high dose of Amphotericin B
3. Surgical debridement of nonviable tissue.

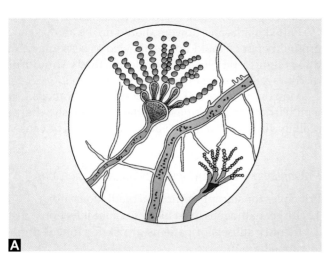 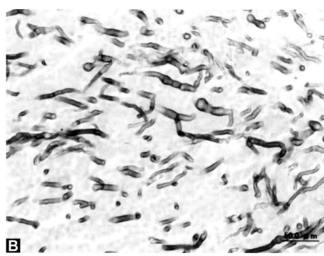

Figs 8.4A and B: (A) Schematic represents the aspergillus, (B) HP section showing aspergillosis

In diabetic patients survivorship ranges from 60 to 90%. When the source of immunocompromise is not quickly reversible survivorship drops down to 20 to 50%.

Mucormycosis is a term used to refer to any fungal infections of the order Mucorales which belong to the class of Zygomycetes. Rhizopus oryzae is the predominant pathogen and accounts for 60% of all forms of Mucormycosis. It accounts for 90% of rhinocerebral Mucormycosis. All fungi of the order Mucorales reproduce sexually as well as asexually. Members of the family Mucoracea have characterized sporangia which envelops numerous asexual spores.

Diabetics presenting with ketoacidosis are disproportionately affected (*Blitzer et al, 1980*). Rhizopus organisms have an active ketone reductase system and thrive in high glucose acidotic conditions. Diabetics also have decreased phagocytic activity because of impaired glutathione pathway. Normal serum inhibits the growth of rhizopus whereas diabetic ketoacidosis stimulates growth (*Gale and Welch, 1961*). Patients on dialysis treated with deferoxamine B (DFO) an iron and aluminium chelator are more susceptible to Mucormycosis.

Other risk factors are prolonged neutropenia, long-term systemic steroid therapy, protein calorie malnutrition, bone marrow transplantation, immunodeficiency, leukemia and intravenous drug users. The relative infrequency of Mucormycosis in AIDS reflects the ability of neutrophils to prevent growth of the fungus. Mucormycosis may have an acute fulminant course or a slower indolent invasive course. When immunocompromise is not easily reversible then the course of the disease is aggressive and rapid.

Signs and Symptoms of Mucormycosis

The leading symptom is fever. This is quickly followed by ulceration in the nose followed by necrosis, periorbital, facial swelling or decreased vision. Ultimately approximately 80% develop a necrotic lesion on the nasal mucosa. Facial numbness is also present in some patients. The importance of anesthesia of the affected facial areas is an early sign of invasive mucormycosis.

Histopathology

A diagnosis of Mucormycosis can be made on histological examination of specimens from a diseased patient. Broad band ribbon like hyphae 10 to 20 microns branched haphazardly along with the absence of septations. Mucor stains easily with hemotoxylin and eosin stains. It can also be seen on histopathology that the organism has a distinct predilection for vascular invasion, predominantly arterial invasion.

Core Message

The treatment is:
1. Reversal of immunocompromise
2. Systemic Amphotericin B
3. Surgical debridement.

Surgery alone is not curative. Hyperbaric oxygen has also been reported to be a useful adjunct in treatment. It reverses ischemic acidotic conditions that cause fungal infections to perpetuate. Hyperbaric oxygen is usually given at two atmospheres for 1 hour on a daily basis for up to 30 sessions. Hyperbaric oxygen does not have a significant impact on mortality. It does however limit the area of deformity by decreasing the required area of debridement.

Aspergillosis

Aspergillosis refers to several forms of disease caused by a fungus in the genus Aspergillus. Aspergillus fungal infections can occur in the ear, eyes, nose, paranasal sinuses and lungs.

Aspergillosis is primarily a disease of the lungs and is caused by the inhalation of airborne spores of the fungus. It does not have distinctive symptoms aspergillosis is thought to be underdiagnosed and underreported. The advanced ability to perform tissue and organ transplants have increased the number of patients vulnerable to fungal infections. Transplant recipients, particularly those receiving bone marrow and heart transplants are highly susceptible to suffering from aspergillosis.

Aspergillosis spores enter the body primarily through inhalation but can also lodge in the eye and ear. The presence of aspergillus is so common that even in asthmatics a positive culture alone is insufficient for a diagnosis.

Treatment of aspergillosis will depend upon the form of aspergillosis present. In case of a mycetoma surgery is indicated. Amphotericin B is the first line of treatment.

The prognosis of recovery from aspergillosis will depend upon the underlying medical condition. If the problem is based upon an allergic response then the patient will likely respond to steroids. The prognosis of invasive aspergillosis is quite poor. Mortality rates have ranged from 50% in some studies to 95% for bone marrow recipients and patients with AIDS.

Chronic Invasive Fungal Rhinosinusitis

Chronic invasive fungal rhinosinusitis usually occurs in healthy individuals who are immunologically intact.

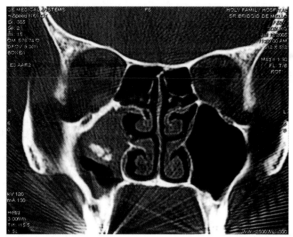

Fig. 8.5: CT scan of the nose and paranasal sinuses showing opacification of the right maxillary sinus with an area of hyper-attenuation. The area of hyper-attenuation is the fungal ball caused by aspergillosis

Usually such patients present with a history of chronic rhinosinusitis symptoms, respiratory tract allergies or nasal polyposis. Some patients who are diabetic even though they are not ketoacidotic present with the granulomatous form of the disease.

Symptoms may take months even years to present. Nasal examination reveals severe nasal congestion and polypoid mucosa. A soft tissue mass can be seen. This is usually covered with debris or thick inspissated nasal secretions.

Imaging modality of choice is CT scanning in the initial stages. Focal or diffuse areas of hyperattenuation (Figs 8.5 and 8.6) within a sinus are a clue to fungal colonization. Often bone erosion or expansion can be seen. This is usually a sign that an invasive process is about to be initiated.

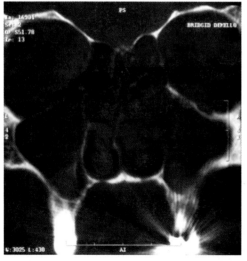

Fig. 8.6: CT scan showing invasive fungal rhinosinusitis

MR imaging is useful to determine if dural invasion or dural involvement has taken place. Differentiation between a malignant neoplasm and chronic fungal rhinosinusitis may be difficult and is best made on histopathology.

Patients suffering from chronic invasive rhinosinusitis are usually immunocompetent. Some workers performed extensive tests to uncover any hidden immunological abnormality. No specific immunological defects were detected. Instead it was discovered that these immunocompetent individuals were suffering from allergic fungal rhinosinusitis (AFRS). Those patients who had the granulomatous type of disease had a cutaneous type 4 hypersensitivity (delayed skin reaction) to aspergillus antigen. None of the nongranulomatous patients showed type 4 reactions, *(De Shazo, 1998)* emphasized that in his report all patients suffering from nongranulomatous chronic invasive fungal rhinosinusitis occurred in patients with diabetes. The formation of a granuloma requires an indigestible organism and cell mediated immunity to be directed towards the inciting agent. It is not clear why certain nonimmunocompromised individuals develop invasive disease. Some speculate that a hot dry, climate in individuals with nasal obstruction predisposes to Aspergillus infections. Still some others believe that anaerobic conditions in the sinus caused by repeated inflammation predispose the patient to invasive fungal disease. Most authors agree that Aspergillus is often a secondary invader of a diseased sinus.

Pathology

Periarterial invasion without direct involvement of fungal elements and no true vascular invasion is a typical feature. Three variants are described.

They are (1) Proliferative (granulomatous pseudotubercles in a fibrous stroma), (2) Exudative-necrotizing (with prominent foci of necrosis), (3) A mixed form.

(De Shazo, 1998) described granulomatous chronic invasive fungal rhinosinusitis as granulomas composed of eosinophilic material surrounded by fungus, giant cells, variable lymphocytes and plasma cells. Nongranulomatous chronic invasive fungal rhinosinusitis is characterized by tissue necrosis, dense fungal hyphae and scanty inflammatory infiltrate. The fungi in this form may breach mucosal barriers to invade blood vessels or just cause arteritis without vascular invasion. Ultimately both granulomatous and nongranulomatous forms can result in tissue necrosis.

Core Message

There is no general agreement on the extent of surgery necessary to arrest or eradicate chronic invasive rhinosinusitis. Neither is it clear at this time if the granulomatous form be treated differently from the nongranulomatous form.

(Washburn, 1994; Washburn et al, 1988) feels that the nongranulomatous form be treated by an aggressive surgical approach, while the granulomatous form responds well to surgery. Current recommendations for both forms are surgery to remove all disease where feasible. This is to be followed by prolonged courses of Amphotericin B and Itraconazole.

Invasive Fungal Rhinosinusitis in the Acquired Immunodeficiency Syndrome (AIDS)

The increasing prevalence of AIDS have left patients suffering from this problem at great risk from suffering from fungal infections. Since by definition these patients are immunocompromised the infections that they suffer are usually serious and have poor outcomes. Aspergillosis is the most common pathogen in AIDS patients. It usually causes arterial invasion, thrombosis and subsequent necrosis of tissue. A. Fumigatus is the most common pathogen isolate in the AIDS population.

Infection by HIV causes selective depletion of CD4 (T helper) lymphocytes. Although impaired cellular immunity predisposes to fungal and intracellular bacterial infections, phagocytic polymorphoneuclear cells and macrophages are the primary defenses against fungal infections, killing the mycelial and conidial forms of the fungus. AIDS patients demonstrate neutrophil and macrophage dysfunction. *(Minamoto, 1992)* cite neutropenia as the single greatest factor predisposing to the development of invasive fungal sinusitis in patients suffering from AIDS. It was also noted that fungal rhinosinusitis was associated with advanced AIDS and low CD4 cell counts.

Core Message

Treatment outcomes of immunocompromised patients suffering from AIDS and invasive aspergillosis infections improves when the infection is diagnosed, identified and treated at the earliest.

Fungal Balls (Mycetomas)

Fungal balls of the nose and paranasal sinuses are composed of matted fungal hyphae. Diagnosis is based on the characteristic histopathology of tangled fungal hyphae. Fungal balls are usually found in one sinus. The maxillary sinus is commonly affected followed by the sphenoid sinus. The host is immunocompetent *(Grosjean and Weber, 2007)*. If immunocompromise occurs then the fungal infection may become invasive and become life threatening. The clinical symptoms may mimic bacterial sinusitis. The treatment is surgical removal and recurrence is rare. In earlier literature the term aspergilloma was used. Now the preferred term is fungal ball.

Older individuals are more commonly affected. No pediatric cases have been reported. A female preponderance has been reported. The incidence of fungal balls may be geographic. It is felt that this may reflect the infrequency of allergic fungal rhinosinusitis.

Clinical Presentation

Symptoms of fungal balls are identical to that of bacterial rhinosinusitis. Symptoms include nasal obstructions, purulent nasal discharge, cacosmia and facial pain. Other unusual symptoms include epistaxis, fever, cough. Ten percent of patients present with nasal polyps.

Radiological Imaging

CT scanning is the imaging modality of choice. A heterogenous opacity is commonly seen. Often radiodensities within the central portion of the soft tissue mass is seen. Occasionally bony destruction is seen. Occasionally a mucocele, foreign body or antrochoanal polyp is seen. Air fluid levels common in bacterial sinusitis is uncommon in fungal balls. Usually only a single sinus is involved.

Histopathology

Fungal balls are extramucosal manifestations. They are noninvasive. Granulomatous reaction is absent. A tangled mat of fungal hyphae is present. The commonest fungus found is aspergillosis. If inmunosuppression develops then the patient is at risk of developing invasive rhinosinusitis.

The most likely cause of fungal balls is the persistence of fungal spores within the nasal cavity and paranasal sinuses. If the fungal spores do not get cleared out by mucocilliary clearance then they can germinate and can cause a fungal ball.

Dental paste as the result of endodontic treatment have been postulated to cause fungal balls. Increased availability of ferritin and zinc can contribute to fungal growth.

Treatment

The treatment of fungal balls is surgical removal. The endoscopic approach is usually sufficient to remove the fungus. Irrigation of the sinus can be done at the same time to ensure totally removal. Once removed adequately by surgery they usually do not recur.

Should an asymptomatic patient undergo surgery for an opacified sinus even though there is no evidence of bony erosion? There are many reports for and against. However if the patient is asthmatic then surgery can be performed. The rational for this is the following. There is a possibility that the "opacified" sinus could be contributing to aggravating attacks of asthma. Furthermore the surgery could provide clues as to why the sinus is opacifed and quiescent disease removed before it does further damage. Surgery serves to remove pathology and provide ventilation and drainage. Symptomatic patients need to undergo surgery.

Those patients who have a fungal ball and are immunocompromised or who will need to be immunosuppressed will need to have surgery to clear out the diseased sinus. This is necessary, for if the fungal ball is allowed to reside in the sinus such patients run the risk of the fungal ball evolving into invasive sinusitis.

Allergic Fungal Rhinosinusitis (AFRS) or Eosinophillic Fungal Rhinosinusitis

Allergic fungal rhinosinusitis (AFRS) is a term introduced by *(Robson et al, 1989)* to describe a constellation of unusual findings in a unique group of patients suffering from chronic rhinosinusitis.

AFRS is believed to have an etiology similar to that of allergic bronchopulmonary aspergillosis (ABPA) *(Houser and Corey, 2000)*. ABPA is felt to be mediated by both type 1 (IgE) and type III (IgG- antigen immune complexes) Gell and Coombs reactions. The Th2 CD4+ subpopulation of T cells, which are prominent in atopic IgE mediated disease are felt to cause the escalation of inflammation seen in ABPA. Interleukins 4, 5, 10 and 13 are released by these cells IL-10 suppresses the alternative Th1 response IL-4 and IL-13 increase class switching of B cells to produce IgE molecules and IL-3 and IL-5 function in eosinophil maturation and activation.

AFRS Clinical Findings

Most patients suffering from AFRS are young, atopic and immunocompetent *(Schubert and Goetz, 1998)*.

Criteria to determine if the rhinosinusitis is AFRS are 5 typical major characteristics:
1. Gross production of eosinophilic mucin containing noninvasive fungal hyphae
2. Nasal polyposis
3. Characteristic radiographic (CT Scan) findings
4. Positive fungal stain or culture
5. Type 1 hypersensitivity.

Six other minor characteristics are:
1. The presence of asthma
2. Unilateral disease
3. Radiographic evidence of bone erosion
4. Fungal culture
5. Charcot Leyden crystals
6. Serum eosinophilia.

AFRS is initiated when an atopic individual is exposed to inhaled fungi. This provides the initial antigenic stimulus. A Gell and Coombs type 1 (IgE) and 111 (immune complex) mediated reaction takes place. An intense eosinophilic inflammatory response occurs. This results in mucosal edema, stasis of secretions and inflammatory exudates which in combination cause obstruction of the sinus ostia. This process may be made worse if other factors like septal deviations and turbinate hypertrophy are also present. The process may then spread to involve adjacent sinuses and produce sinus expansion and erosion. This in turn create an ideal environment for fungi to proliferate. This further increases' antigenic exposure. At some point this cycle becomes self-perpetuating. This results in the production of allergic mucin. Accumulation of allergic mucin causes further obstruction of the involved sinuses which in turn further propagate the allergic process. Secondary bacterial infection may also occur. Invasion of the underlying mucosa is not a characteristic of AFRs.

The aspergillosis organism itself impairs the hosts mucosal defenses. They are capable of altering the host immune response through macrophage and T cell suppression. They reduce the hosts defenses by:
1. Reducing ciliary beat frequency
2. Impairing the function of the host fungicidal proteins within the mucus blanket
3. Fungal allergens are able to deactivate the complement system
4. Interferes with phagocytosis
5. Releases proteolytic enzymes which can destroy the host basement membrane.

Epidemiology

The prevalence of AFRS is approximately between 5 to 10%. AFRS is noted in young age groups from 23 years to

42 years. Pediatric patients present in the same fashion as adults with AFRS. One-third of to one-half of patients suffering from AFRS also suffer from asthma *(Manning and Holman, 1998)*. *(Cody et al, 1994)* described an incidence of 27% of patients who also show sensitivity to aspirin. Patients with AFRS are by definition atopic.

Signs and Symptoms

The incidence of nasal polyposis is almost 100%. Nasal polyposis is a nonspecific indicator of chronic nasal inflammation.

AFRS have typical findings on CT scanning. The central high attenuation can at times be described as "Starry sky", "ground glass" or "serpiginous" pattern. Almost half of patients suffering AFRS have unilateral disease.

Fungal species of the dematiaceous species are most commonly the cause of AFRS. Examination of the mucin retrieved demonstrates eosinophils. Charcot Leyden crystals and fungal hyphae within a background of eosinophilic material is typical of AFRS. Almost half of AFRS patients have only unilateral disease.

Tests to Confirm a Diagnosis of AFRS

1. Total eosinophil count
2. Total serum IgE
3. Antigen specific IgE (both fungal and other inhalant allergens either by *in vitro* testing or by skin testing)
4. Fungal antigen specific IgG
5. Precipitating antibodies
6. Microscopic evaluation of the mucin that was evacuated during surgery
7. Fungal culture of the material evacuated during surgery.

Treatment of AFRS

The traditional treatment of AFRS is surgical clearance of nasal polyposis. Endoscopic clearance is now the widely accepted treatment modality. The gradual accumulation of allergic fungal mucin gives AFRS a predictable characteristic pattern. As the mucus accumulates the involved paranasal sinus begins to resemble a mucocele. The principle of surgery in AFRS is to provide ventilation and drainage while accepting the reality that surgery may not totally eradicate disease. Multiple surgeries may be necessary. Furthermore the treatment lies in combining surgery with aggressive prolonged medication. Despite all this recurrences may still occur.

Core Message

Thus it can be said that the goals of surgery are: (1) Removal of all mucin and fungal debris, (2) Permanent drainage and ventilation of the affected sinuses while preserving the integrity of the underlying mucosa, (3) Surgery should provide postoperative access to previously diseased areas. This is necessary to facilitate removal of debris and mucin in the clinic and allow inspection of areas of the nasal cavity in the clinic which would not have been possible to visualize under normal circumstances.

Systemic Steroids

Waxman et al (1987) suggested the use of systemic steroids in the postoperative period. It should be mentioned that steroids should not be given in the preoperative period as this can cause confusion in the diagnosis. Many studies have provided compelling evidence that the recurrence of AFRS is significantly reduced with the use of systemic steroids. *(Schubert and Goetz, 1998)* reviewed 67 patients suffering from AFRS and reported that oral corticosteroid therapy significantly delayed the need for revision surgery. Steroids can cause a reduction or even a total resolution of the eosinophilic mucin that is required to make a diagnosis. It should also be mentioned that steroids are not without their attendant problems.

Immunotherapy

Fungal immunotherapy was proposed as a possible adjuvant therapy to surgical removal of polypoidal tissue and mucin debris. Initial studies addressed the concerns of provoking a Gell and Cooms type 111 reaction caused by immunotherapy. This was extrapolated from warnings regarding the use of immunotherapy in ABPA. A rise in IgE and IgG4 was reported. However studies *(Quinn et al, 1995)* revealed that not only was immunotherapy safe but that it also produced clinical improvements. A longitudinal study of a cohort of patients treated with immunotherapy followed up for three years showed a significant decrease in disease recurrence. Dependence on systemic and topical steroids was less in this study. Furthermore it was discovered that once surgical removal of mucin and polyps was accompanied by immunotherapy post-surgery then there was a significant decline in the incidence of revision surgery.

(Mabry et al, 1997) have made a considerable effort investigating immunotherapy for AFRS.

They injected allergic individuals subcutaneously with small graded doses of allergens against which they are reactive. The effectiveness of therapy and he level of increased IgG obtained dose dependent. The initial Mabry et al study did not have a control group for comparison. A more recent follow-up study with a control group showed that immunotherapy reduced reliance on systemic and nasal steroid therapy to control disease when compared with patients not receiving immunotherapy after both groups had been treated with surgery followed by systemic steroid therapy. Thus it may seem that immunotherapy may be a promising new direction in which to develop a supplemental treatment option for surgery and steroid therapy.

A lack of availability of the specific fungal antigens would appear to be a major obstacle to forming a treatment protocol. Precise fungal identification is necessary if the treatment is to work. Thus crossover from one fungal antigen to another, if proven, might be useful in solving this problem.

Core Message

All patients suffering from AFRS appear to need surgical debridement with removal of the fungi and nasal polyps. This is necessary to help initiate mucociliary clearance. At present AFRS is thought to be mucosal hypersensitivity directed at fungal antigens that are deposited on the mucosa of the upper respiratory tract.

Removing the allergen would reduce the allergic response. This in turn would reduce the subsequent resulting edema. This would in turn help in the rapid clearance of the fungi by mucociliary clearance. This would then be the ultimate goal of treatment of AFRS.

Antifungals

(Bent and Kuhn, 1996) studied topical and systemic antifungal therapy for AFRS with mixed results. They demonstrated that ketoconazole and amphotericin B were the most effective agents *in vitro*.

Topical Antifungals

It has been hypothesized that once fungi were eliminated locally then the disease process could be halted. *(Ponikau, 1999)* and colleagues treated 51 patients who had CRS that was refractory to all other treatment. These patients were treated with nasal lavages of Amphotericin B every alternate day for 3 months. Their findings revealed a decrease in symptoms and improvement in findings on CT scans and endoscopy in 75% of patients. The flaw of Ponikau's study was that it had no control group. This defect was corrected when a follow-up, randomized, placebo controlled, double blinded trial *(Ponikau, 2005)* found excellent results. There was significant statistical improvement in the CT scan parameters and endoscopic exam in patients treated with amphotericin B nasal lavages as compared to the placebo group.

To eliminate the role of nasal lavages (the effect of saline) *(Weschetta, 2004)* treated 60 patients who had CRS and nasal polyps refractory to standard medical therapy. This study excluded AFRS. Their study was double blinded and randomized controlled. Their study showed that Amphotericin B nasal lavages' was not effective in the treatment of CRS when AFRS was absent.

(Richetti, 2002) evaluated the effectiveness of Amphotericin B nasal lavages that nasal polyposis in 39% of patients resolved.

It can thus be seen that while nasal lavages with Amphotericin B appear promising they need further studying to determine in which situation they will be most effective.

(Bent and Kuhn, 1996) found that the most common pathogens in AFRS were the dematiaceous species (Curvularia, Bipolaris, Alternia) and that these species were sensitive to itraconazole, amphotericin B, nystatin and ketoconazole. They recommended the topical application of ketoconazole dissolved in an acetic acid solution (0.125% or 1 mg/ml) postoperatively. Alternatively suspensions of amphotericin B at a dosage of 50 mg in 10 ml of water (not saline or dextrose) irrigated into the nostrils two to four times a day have been used with good results.

In conclusion it should be said that even the use of the local application of these medications is not conclusively proven. Much work needs to be done before they can be used on a regular basis.

AGENTS FOR TREATMENT OF INVASIVE FUNGAL INFECTIONS

Antifungal treatment principles are the following:
1. Correct identification of the fungus causing the infection.
2. Correct and appropriate use of standard antifungal regimens.
3. The treating clinician should consider initial therapy as an induction phase with optimization in both dose and duration of antifungal medication. The medication should preferable be fungicidal. Combination therapy may be considered.
4. Reversal or control of immunocompromization.
5. Possible drug interactions should be kept in mind.

6. Once the patient has stabilized with treatment, the clinician must consider a treatment regimen both in terms of dose as well as choice of medication to complete a defined course of therapy.
7. Follow-up to prevent and control relapses as extremely important.

Amphotericin B Deoxycholate

Amphotericin B deoxycholate is a polyene macrolide. It has a broad spectrum of activity. It is fungicidal. Its fungicidal activity is caused by its ability to bind preferably to ergosterol which is a major component of the fungal cell membrane. Cell membrane permeability is then increased following attachment of this lipophilic structure to the cell wall. This leads to leakage of intracellular components and ultimately results in fungal cell death. Unfortunately amphotericin B also binds to cholesterol in mammalian cell membranes, resulting in toxicity. Amphotericin B interacts with host cell macrophages and has a positive effect on them through an oxidation dependent process. It is also postulated that Amphotericin B may have an immunomodulating effect.

Amphotericin B has an apparent volume distribution of 4L/kg. Distribution following intravenous administration follows a three compartment model with high concentrations reaching the liver, spleen, lungs, kidneys, muscle and skin. It's protein binding capacity is approximately 91 to 95%. Metabolism of Amphotericin B is not clearly understood. Less than half the dose is accounted for by either biliary or renal clearances. Metabolites have not been identified and blood levels are boy affected by either hepatic or renal failure. Following a biphasic elimination pattern, the initial half life ranges from 24 to 48 hours with a subsequent terminal half life of upto 5 days. Only 5% of Amphotericin B is absorbed when administered orally.

Intravenous doses ranging fro 0.25 to 1.0 mg/kg/d in 5% dextrose are recommended. Doses in adults are 1.2 mg/kg/d while in children the recommended dose is 1.5 mg/kg/d. Some recommend a test dose.

Strategies to enhance tolerability to the infusion include the use of hydrocortisone (25 mg added directly to the infusion) has resulted in dramatic reduction in febrile reactions. Thrombophelibitis is a common problem associated with the administration of Amphotericin B. To avoid this small amounts of heparin to the infusion, using a central line, rotating the infusion site and avoiding highly concentrated preparations. Nephrotoxicity may occur in up to 80% of patients. Azotemia, electrolyte wasting (K^+ and Mg^+) and a decrease in urine concentrating ability are known to occur. To prevent these attendant problems and minimize the risk of nephrotoxicity sodium supplementation can be given. Avoidance of concomitant nephrotoxic drugs should also be carried out.

Amphotericin B possesses activity *in vitro* against most pathogenic fungi found in most humans *(Luna et al, 2000)*. They are *Blastomyces dermatitidis, Cryptococcus neoformans, Coccidioides immitis, Histoplasma capsulatum, Paracoccidioides brasiliensis* and *Sporothrix schenckii*. Variable *in vitro* activity is seen against Aspergillus and the zygomycetes.

The combination of Amphotericin B and flucytosine has demonstrated synergistic fungicidal activity *in vitro* against Candida species, *C. neoformans*, certain fungi causing chromomycosis and Aspergillus spp. Amphotericin B plus is the drug combination of choice for the treatment of cryptococcal meningitis. Amphotericin B in combination with the triazole compounds, fluconazole and itraconazole has demonstrated antagonistic effects with itraconazole more consistently exhibiting antagonism than fluconazole. Triple drug therapy in cryptococcal meningitis has been reported to achieve excellent results. Intraperitoneal administration of Amphotericin B has been reported to be effective for management of fungal peritonitis.

Amphotericin B administered empirically has become the gold standard in patients with persistent fever and neutropenia. Amphotericin B remains the treatment of choice for most progressive life threatening fungal infections including invasive aspergillosis, zygomycosis and severe infections of blastomycosis, coccidioidomycosis, sporotrichosis and histoplasmosis.

Lipid based Formulations of Amphotericin B

Amphotericin B lipid complex (ABLC, Abelcet), Amphotericin B cholesteryl sulfate complex (ABCD Amphotec) and liposomal Amphotericin B (ambisome) use a variety of lipid carriers. The pharmacokinetics of lipid based formulations of Amphotericin B differ significantly from that of Amphotericin B deoxycholate. Lipid based formulations are preferentially delivered into the reticuloendothelial tissues such as the liver and spleen. Doses for these preparations are 1 to 5 mg/kg (liposomal Amphotericin B) 5 mg/kg/d (ABLC) and 3 to 5 mg/kg (ABCD) *(Luna et al, 2000)*.

Core Message

The use of lipid based Amphotericin B may be a wise alternative for individuals unable to tolerate the nephrotoxicity associated with Amphotericin B deoxycholate.

Azoles

The azoles offer an alternative to Amphotericin B without the attendant problems associated with its use.

The azoles are the Imidazoles (clotrimazole, ketoconazole and miconazole) and the triazoles (fluconazole and itraconazole). They have been found to be effective against systemic fungal infections.

Mechanism of Action

The azoles work by primarily inhibiting the cytochrome P450 dependent enzyme lanosterol 14alpha demethylase which is necessary for the conversion of lanosterol to ergosterol. Ergosterol is a vital component of the cellular membrane of fungi and disruptions in the biosynthesis of ergosterol cause significant damage to the cell membrane by increasing its permeability and ultimately causing cell lysis and cell death.

The triazoles, itraconazole and fluconazole have significant pharmacokinetic differences.

Fluconazole is available in the oral and intravenous formulations. It is highly water soluble and in the oral formulation it is absorbed almost completely. A single dose is widely distributed in body fluids. Fluconazole is found in the CSF.

Itraconazole on the other hand is not as well absorbed as fluconazole. The suspension is better absorbed on an empty stomach. Coadministration of acidic beverages such as cranberry juice may enhance absorption. Itraconazole is highly protein bound and achieves relatively low concentrations in the CSF. Metabolism takes place in the liver and is excreted in the urine and the feces.

Daily doses of 200 to 800 mg of Fluconazole have been used. If serum are concentrations used then it is recommended that the measured therapeutic concentration be at least equal to or greater than 1ug/ml.

The metabolism of triazoles takes place in the liver through the cytochrome P450 enzyme system specifically the 3A4 pathways. There is potential for interactions with other medications that use the same pathway. Fatal interactions have been reported between cisapride, terfenadine and astemizole. Thus, concomitant use of these medications along with the triazoles is contraindicated.

Flucytosine

Flucytosine is a cytosine analogue originally formulated for use as an antineoplastic agent. It acts directly on the RNA and DNA of yeast cells. Flucytosine is available as an oral medication. Side effects are usually seen when it is given in combination with Amphotericin B. Myelo-

suppression associated with flucytosine is reversible. The recommended dosage is 10 mg/kg/day in divided doses. Flucytosine has demonstrated antifungal activity *in vitro* against *Cryptococcus neoformans* and Candida species. Resistance to flucytosine occurs because of a single mutation. Thus flucytosine should not be administered as a single agent. It should be given in combination with Amphotericin B and this combination is the treatment of choice for cryptococcal meningitis.

Terbinafine

Terbinafine is an allylamine compound for oral use. Its fungicidal activity is caused by the inhibition of the enzyme squalene epoxidase which results in the depletion of ergosterol which results in cell death. It is now available in the form of topical formulations and tablets. Terbinafine is highly lipophilic and displays a triphasic distribution pattern in humans which consists of a short initial half life followed by an intermediate half life of 11 to 15 hours. Terbinafine is indicated for the treatment of various fungal infections of the nails and skin.

Target sites foor fungal infections include the fungal cell wall and cell membrane, DNA protein synthesis and alterations in metabolism characteristics.

Voriconazole is a new triazole and is a derivative of fluconazole. Stuidies evaluating the pharmokinetics of voriconazole demonstrate a bioavailability of 90% and a mean half life of 6 hours. Clinical trials indicate that Voriconazole is effective against oral and esophageal candidiasis.

Echinocandins are a new class of antifungal agents. They exert antifungal activity by inhibiting 1,3B glucan synthesis for the fungal cell wall. These agents demonstrate antifungal activity against Candida species, Aspergillus species and against *Pneumocystis carinii*. Dual therapy with an azole and even triple therapy in combination with Amphotericin B is currently under study.

As our understanding of fungi improves so will the evolution of antifungal agents. The future holds many promising agents and clinical trials are underway.

BIBLIOGRAPHY

1. Arnow PM, Sadigh M, Costas C et al. Endemic and epidemic aspergillosis associated with in hospital replication of Aspergillosis organisms. *Journal of Infectious diseases* 1991;164: 998–1000.
2. Bent JP and Kuhn FA. Antifungal activity against allergic fungal sinusitis organisms. *Laryngoscope* 1996; 106:1331–1334.
3. Blitzer A, Lawson W, Meyers BR et al. Patient survival factors in paranasal sinus Mucormycosis. *Laryngoscope* 1980;90: 635–648.

4. Cody DT, Neel HB, Ferreiro JA et al. Allergic fungal sinusitis. *Laryngoscope* 1994;104:1074–1079.

5. De Carpentier JP, Ramamurthy L, Denning DW et al. An alogorithmic approach to aspergillus sinusitis. *Journal of Laryngology and Otology* 1994;108:314–316.

6. De Shazo. Fungal sinusitis. *American Journal of Medical Sciences* 1998;316:39–45.

7. De Shazo RD, O'Brien N, Chapin K et al; A new classification and diagnostic criteria for invasive fungal sinusitis. *Archives of Otolaryngolgy Head and Neck Surgery* 1997;123:1181–1188.

8. Drakos PE, Nagler A, Naparstek E et al. Invasive fungal sinusitis in patients undergoing bone marrow transplantation. *Bone Marrow Transplant* 1993;12:203–208.

9. Ferguson BJ. Definitions of fungal rhinosinusitis. *Otolaryngologic clinics of North America* 2000;33:227–235.

10. Ferguson BJ. What role do systemic corticosteroids, immuno-therapy and antifungal drugs play in the therapy of allergic fungal rhinosinusitis? *Archives of Otolaryngology Head and Neck Surgery* 1998;124:1174–1178.

11. Gale GR Welch A. Studies of opportunistic fungi. 1. Inhibition of R oryzae by human serum. *American Journal of Medicine* 1961; 45:604–612.

12. Grosjean P, Weber R. Fungus balls of the paranasal sinuses: A review. *Eur Arch Otorhinolaryngol* 2007;264:461–470.

13. Houser SM and Corey JP. Allergic fungal rhinosinusitis. *Otolaryngologic Clinics of North America* 2000;33:399–408. Review with four illustrated cases. *American Journal of Rhinology* 8:13–18.

14. Janntunen E, Ruutu P, Niskanen L et al. Incidence and risk factors for invasive fungal infections in allogenic BMT recipients. *Bone Marrow Transplant* 1997; 19:801–803.FA: Prognosis for allergic fungal sinusitis. *Otolaryngology, Head and Neck Surgery* 1997;117:35–41.

15. Luna B, Drew RH, Perfect JR. Agents for the treatment of invasive fungal infections. *Otolaryngologic Clinics of North America* 2000;33:277–299.

16. Mabry RL, Mabry CS. Immunotherapy for allergic fungal sinusitis. The second year. *Otolaryngology Head and Neck Surgery* 1997;117: 367–371.

17. Mabry RL, Manning SC Mabry CS. Immunotherapy in the treatment of allergic fungal sinusitis. *Otolaryngology Head and Neck Surgery* 1997;116:31–35.

18. Manning SC, Holman M. Further evidence for allergic pathphysiology in allergic fungal sinusitis. *Laryngoscope.* 1998;108:1485–1496.

19. Menezes RA, de Souza CE, de sa Souza S. Blastomycosis of the paranasal sinuses. *Orbit* 1987; 7:3–6.

20. Minamoto GY, Barlam TF, Vander Els NJ. Invasive aspergillosis in patients with AIDS. *Clinical Infectious diseases* 1992;14:66–74.

21. Mitchell TG. Overview of basic medical mycology. *Otolaryngologic Clinics of North America* 2000;33:237–249.

22. Ponikau JU, Sherris DA, Kern EB. The diagnosis and incidence of allergic fungal sinusitis. *Mayo Clinic Proceedings* 1999;74(9) 877–884.

23. Ponikau JU, Sherris DA, Weaver A. Treatment of chronic rhinosinusitis with intranasal amphotericin B: A randomized placebo controlled double blind pilot trial. *Journal of Allergy and Clinical Immunology* 2005;115(1):125–131.

24. Quinn, J, Wickern G, Whisman B et al. Immunotherapy in allergic Bipolaris sinusitis: A case report. *Journal of Allergy and Clinical Immunology* 1995;95:201–202

25. Robson JMB, Benn RAV, Hogan PG et al. Allergic fungal sinusitis presenting as a paranasal sinus tumor. *Australia and New Zealand Journal of Medicine* 1989;19:351–353.

26. Ricchetti A, Landis BN, Mafoli A. Effect of antifungal nasal lavage with Amphotericin B on nasal polyposis. *Journal of Laryngology and Otology* 2002;116:261–263.

27. Schubert MS, Goetz DW. Evaluation and treatment of allergic fungal sinusitis. 1. Demographics and diagnosis. *Journal of Allergy and Clinical Immunology* 1998;102:387–394.

28. Viollier A F, Peterson DE, De Jongh CA et al. Aspergillus sinusitis in cancer patients. *Cancer* 1986;58:366–368.

29. Washburn RG, Kennedy DW, Begley MG et al. Chronic fungal sinusitis in apparently normal hosts. *Medicine* 1988;67: 231–247.

30. Washburn RG . Fungal sinusitis. *Current Clinical Topical Infectious diseases* 1998;18:60–74.

31. Waxman JE, Spector JG, Sale SR et al. Allergic aspergillus sinusitis. Concepts in diagnosis and treatment of a new clinical entity. *Laryngoscope* 1987; 97:261–266.

32. Weschetta M, Rimek D, Formanek M. Topical antifungal treatment of chronic rhinosinusitis with nasal polyps: A randomized double blind clinical trial. *Journal on Allergy and Clinical Immunology* 2004;113:1122–1128.

Endoscopic Sinus Surgery

Amir Minovi, Wolfgang Draf, Ulrike Bockmühl, Aldo C Stamm
Shirley SN Pignatari, Hugo Canhete Lopes, Hannes Braun
Heinz Stammberger, B Schick, Marc Bassim, Brent A Senior

Principles of Endoscopic Sinus Surgery

Amir Minovi, Wolfgang Draf

The new era in sinus surgery began in the early 1970s with the development of different angled endoscopes based on the new Hopkins rod lens technology and its use in the evaluation of the paranasal sinuses.[1,2] Unlike Messerklinger, who investigated the anatomy and pathophysiology of the nose and its relationship to chronic sinusitis, Draf examined the different sinuses systematically and directly. He was the first person to perform endoscopy of the frontal and the sphenoid sinus. Primarily his goal was to come to more solid indications for sinus surgery, thereby avoiding unnecessary, radical surgeries, especially because at that time the imaging techniques were still poor offering only plain X-ray and sometimes conventional tomography. Soon after, he began (like Messerklinger) to perform endoscopic treatment of inflammatory diseases too. Nasal endoscopy with rigid instruments and computer tomography (CT) of the paranasal sinuses enabled the surgeon to approach the osteomeatal complex (OMC) more precisely. On the basis of Messerklinger's studies, Stammberger and later Kennedy introduced a conservative type of sinus surgery which they named functional endoscopic sinus surgery (FESS).[3,4] The main aim of this surgery is to restore normal mucociliary flow in the region of OMC. Parallel to this, the use of the binocular operating microscope was introduced in sinus surgery as an additional instrument, and was named microendoscopic sinus surgery.[5–8]

ANESTHESIA FOR FESS

Endonasal sinus surgery today is performed usually under general anesthesia in combination with local vasoconstrictor medications. As a local anesthetic, a combination of lidocaine 1% and 1/100,000 to 1/200,000 epinephrine is injected into the agger nasi and uncinate process area. Furthermore better vasoconstriction is achieved by additional placing of cotton swabs soaked in naphazolinhydrochlorid and cocaine 10% (maximal single-dose rate 2 ml) in the nasal cavity for 10 minutes. Bleeding is a major concern during endonasal sinus surgery. In many cases, bleeding can be minimized with the support of anesthetic techniques. The anesthesiologist should be informed continuously about the actual bleeding condition, and should follow surgery on a monitor if available. Intraoperative communication between the ENT surgeon and the anesthesiologist is essential.

If the comorbidities of the patients provide no contraindication, the anesthesiologist should intra-operatively aim at a mean arterial pressure of 60 mmHg and a heart rate of 50 to 60 mmHg. Arterial hypotension will minimize hemodynamic causes for bleeding and, if required, can be achieved by intravenous administration of β-blockade or arterial vasodilators. The influence of various anesthetics on bleeding is under discussion. A total intravenous technique may have advantages with regard to bleeding on the microcirculatory level. If anesthetic techniques fail to provide a clear view of the surgical field, temporary application of cotton plugs soaked with adrenaline 1:1000 is useful. The risk of adrenaline-induced cardiac arrhythmias nowadays is almost negligible, when a total intravenous technique is used and the volatile anesthetic halothane is avoided.

GENERAL ASPECTS AND INSTRUMENTATION

As mentioned above, FESS was developed after the pioneering work of Messerklinger in understanding the pathophysiology of chronic sinusitis. FESS is a philosophy as much as a surgical technique. The philosophy is that with removal of obstructing tissue from a target area, especially in the OMC, normal mucociliary flow is achieved and inflammation in the dependent sinuses resolves. Therefore, it is not necessary to perform extended sinus surgery with the potential of additionally damaging the mucosa. The only aim in FESS is to remove the obstructing tissue while preserving normal non-obstructive anatomy and mucous membrane.[9,10] The development of newer trough-cutting instrumentation has allowed precise removal of diseased tissue, with less chance of mucosal damage. Powered instruments like microdebriders (soft tissue shavers) help enormously to resect the pathology while preserving normal mucosa.[11,12]

The entire surgery is performed endoscopically. The rigid fiberoptic nasal telescope provides superb visualization of the operative field. The 0° rigid telescope is used for most of the surgery. As the angle of the telescope rises, so does the risk of disorientation. Therefore, the 30°, 45° and 70° telescopes are only used for work in areas 'around the corner' like the frontal recess and the maxillary sinus. A camera is usually attached to the eyepiece of the endoscope and the endoscopic view is transmitted to a monitor. The surgeon has the option of performing the surgery while looking through the endoscope or at the monitor, or a combination of both.

INDICATIONS AND CONTRAINDICATIONS

The development of FESS has brought many advantages when compared to common external approaches. The most important are:
- No external incisions and visible scars.
- Minimal intranasal and intrasinus trauma.
- Preservation of the bony framework and mucous membrane needed for restoration of normal mucociliary clearance.

The most common indications for FESS are:
- Chronic and/or recurrent sinusitis unresponsive to prior medical treatment or previous surgery.
- Recurrent chronic sinusitis combined with obstructive nasal polyposis.
- Closure of dural defects.
- Mucocele.
- Orbital and endocranial complications of acute sinusitis especially subperiostal abscess.

- Control of epistaxis.
- Resection of selected tumors.
- Endoscopic intranasal dacryocystorhinostomy (EIDCR).

FESS does not seem to be appropriate for extensive, invasive extraintradural disease involving the paranasal sinuses or the skull base, particularly malignant tumors grown to a major degree through the skull base intradurally.

TECHNIQUE OF FUNCTIONAL ENDOSCOPIC SINUS SURGERY

FESS can be performed under general or local anesthesia depending on the patient's condition, extent of disease and experience of the surgeon. Although for many years experienced surgeons recommended local anesthesia, due to less bleeding and the patient's pain as warning sign if the periorbit or dura are touched, currently almost all surgeons prefer general anesthesia, which has improved remarkably. Most patients enjoy greater comfort and surgeons prefer flexibility in case pathology is more extended than expected. Throat packing is recommended and both eyes should be visible to both the surgeon and the operating nurse during the whole surgery. Two classic endoscopic approaches are used in FESS.[2,13]
- Anterior-to-posterior dissection (Messerklinger)
- Posterior-to-anterior dissection (Wigand)

The surgical steps in FESS will be discussed in the order that structures are encountered, describing the Messerklinger technique in detail. Complete endoscopic sphenoethmoidectomy is indicated for extensive sinus disease. The extent of the surgery depends on the involved area. Satisfactory visualization of the operative field is mandatory for successful dissection. Therefore, it is extremely important to avoid trauma to the mucosa of the anterior portion of the nose. Even minimal bleeding in this area may fog the endoscope and impair visualization. The tip of the endoscope should not be brought too close to the area to be dissected.

The first step consists of an infundibulotomy or uncinectomy, by resection of the uncinate process and exposure of the ethmoid bulla (Figs 9.1A and B). The uncinectomy can be performed in a posterior-to-anterior direction with a backbiter or in an anterior-to-posterior direction with a sickle knife or Freer elevator. The next step depends on the preference and experience of the surgeon. Usually the ethmoid bulla is opened (Fig. 9.2) and anterior ethmoid cells are removed until the basal lamella of the middle turbinate is identified. The basal

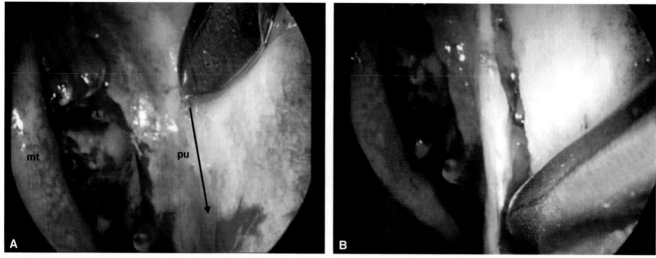

Figs 9.1A and B: Endoscopic view with a 45° angled telescope on the left side. Resection of the uncinate process (pu) with a sickle knife in anterior to posterior technique; mt: middle turbinate

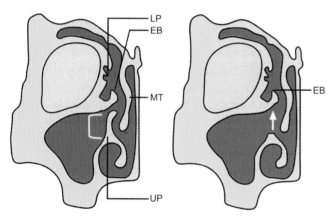

Fig. 9.2: Resection of the uncinate process (UP) and exposure of the ethmoid bulla (EB). After removal of ethmoid bulla, anatomic orientiation by identification of middle turbinate (MT) and lamina papyracea (LP)

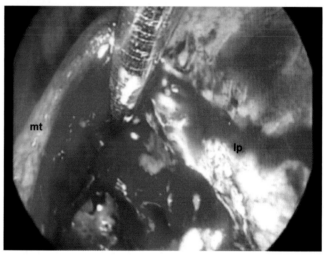

Fig. 9.3: Gentle probing of a left frontal sinus using the 45° angled endoscope. mt: middle turbinate; lp: lamina papyracea

lamella is the lateral vertical attachment of the middle turbinate and is also named ground lamella.

It is mandatory that the surgeon works step-by-step strictly following well-defined anatomic structures. In this stage of surgery, four important landmarks should be identified: medially the middle turbinate; laterally, the lamina papyracea; superiorly, the roof of the ethmoid; and, posteriorly the vertical portion of the ground lamella of the middle turbinate. By perforation of the basal lamella the posterior ethmoid cells are exposed and resected when needed. The frontal recess is explored stepwise by opening the anterior ethmoidal cells and examining the access to the frontal sinus (Fig. 9.3). In the classic Messerklinger technique, the entrance of the frontal sinus is touched as minimally as possible to avoid

scarring and possible secondary obstruction of the frontal recess if pathology allows. At this time the anterior and posterior ethmoid vessels and nerves should be identified along the base of the skull as far they are existing (Fig. 9.4). The anterior ethmoid artery typically runs just anterior to the vertical portion of the basal lamella and posterior to the frontal recess. The more the pneumatization is developed, the larger is the distance of the anterior ethmoidal artery to the skull base.

The maxillary sinus ostium can usually be visualized after the uncinate process has been removed or after the frontal recess work. Enlargement of the natural ostium is performed posteriorly and inferiorly by extending its border to the posterior fontanel (Fig. 9.5). The 45°

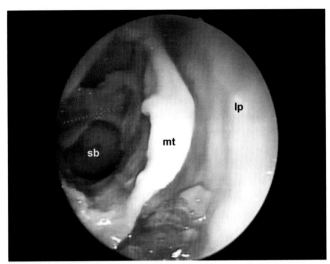

Fig. 9.4: Identification of the right anterior ethmoid artery (dotted red line) along the skull base (sb). mt: middle turbinate; lp: lamina papyracea

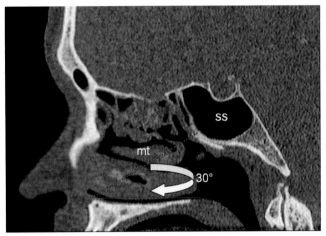

Fig. 9.6: Identification of the anterior wall of the sphenoid sinus: 30° angle from the hard palate and 7 cm posterior to the anterior nasal spine. mt: middle turbinate; ss: sphenoid sinus

telescope is preferred for this step. Extensive dissection too far anterior should be avoided as this may cause damage to the nasolacrimal duct. Although its advantage has not been established, surgical connection of accessory ostia with the natural ostium is routinely performed to prevent circular transportation of secretions. With the help of the 45° and 70° telescope the maxillary sinus is examined and treated, when necessary.

The last step of the surgery is opening of the sphenoid sinus if there are signs of sinusitis. The anterior wall of the sphenoid sinus is located during surgery by identifying the posterior attachment of the middle turbinate, the arch of the posterior choana, and the posterior part

of the nasal septum. The anterior wall is about 7 cm posterior to the anterior nasal spine and may be measured with a marked probe (Figs 9.6 and 9.7).

There are two ways of opening of the sphenoid sinus:

1. Transethmoidally, by identifying the sphenoid ostium lateral the superior turbinate in the sphenoethmoid recess.
2. Transnasally, by perforating the anterior wall about 1.5 cm above the choana at the level of the posterior end of the middle turbinate next to the nasal septum in the midline.

Usually, the anterior wall is very thin and entrance into the sinus, using light pressure of the small nose suction, may be possible. Using a diamond burr may be

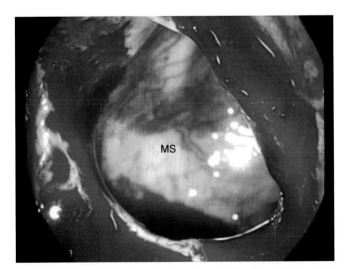

Fig. 9.5: View into the left maxillary sinus (MS) with a 45°- angled endoscope after uncinectomy and enlargement of the natural ostium

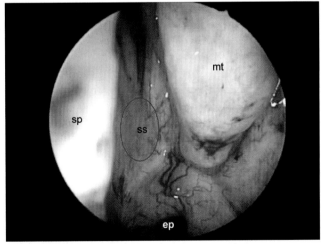

Fig. 9.7: Location of the left sphenoid sinus seen with a 45° endoscope. ss: sphenoid sinus; mt: middle turbinate; ep: epiphayrnx; sp: nasal septum

even safer. Before opening the sphenoid sinus one must study the axial CT to look for a protruding internal carotid artery. The frontal wall is removed working medially with down-biting and up-biting forceps. The lateral parts of the anterior wall need to be handled carefully, because the optic nerve and the carotid artery are located there. The sphenopalatine artery runs inferior and slightly anterior to the anterior wall of the sphenoid sinus. This vessel can be protected by elevating mucosa from the bone inferiorly. An injury of the sphenoplatine artery can be managed mostly with electrical coagulation.

The middle turbinate should be preserved as much as possible. Partial resection is performed only in cases where the middle turbinate prevents access to the middle meatus, or in cases of massive polyposis involving the middle turbinate to prevent recurrent polyposis. Total resection of the middle turbinate has to be avoided in inflammatory diseases since it is an important landmark and plays an essential role in sinunasal physiology. There is evidence that surgery of the middle turbinate can increase the risk of adhesion and scar tissue leading to postoperative frontal sinusitis.[14] The need for packing of the nose depends on the extent of surgery, especially if parts of the middle turbinate were resected. In most cases, packing for 24 hours should be sufficient. Sometimes packing for 1 to 3 days may be necessary.

The posterior-to-anterior technique developed by Wigand starts with a partial resection of the posterior portion of the middle turbinate and the sphenoidotomy. This is followed by removal of the posterior ethmoid cells, identification of the skull base and complete ethmoidectomy from posterior-to-anterior.

Four-Handed Endoscopic Sinus Surgery

This technique was developed by Mark May (1990) and popularized recently by several authors.[15] Sinus surgery is carried out by the surgeon and an assistant. The rigid telescope is held by the assistant thereby enabling the surgeon to work with both hands. The surgeon is able to control the suction with one hand and perform dissection with the other hand. Hence, he/she will be able to reach a good visualization when there is excess bleeding. A detailed description of this technique is given by Simmen and Jones.[16]

High-risk Areas and Complications

The paranasal sinuses present a complex anatomy surrounded by important structures. Despite strong surgical experience, complications may still occur. Major

complications in sinus surgery can lead to a catastrophic outcome for the patient thus making sinus surgery one of the most dangerous surgical treatments in otorhinolaryngology. May et al proposed classifying complications into minor or major categories.[17,18] What follows is a modified, classification scheme as proposed by May:

Minor complications (incidence about 5%) present little morbidity without any significant sequelae for the patient:
- Periorbital subcutaneous emphysema
- Periorbital ecchymosis
- Bronchospasm
- Epistaxis requiring nasal packing
- Dental or lip pain or numbness
- Adhesions requiring treatment.

Major complications (incidence about 0.5%) present significant morbidity, requiring urgent treatment with possible catastrophic outcome for the patient:
- Epiphora requiring surgery
- Hyposmia
- Cerebrospinal fluid leak
- Diplopia
- Impairment or loss of vision
- Meningitis
- Brain hemorrhage or abscess
- Hemorrhage requiring blood transfusion
- Orbital hematoma
- Injury to the carotid artery
- Death.

For prevention of disastrous complications the surgeon should follow certain guidelines and be aware of high-risk areas. A comprehensive summary of surgical recommendations to reduce complications follows:
- Early identification of lamina papyracea and middle turbinate as the most important anatomic landmarks.
- Control of the eye bulb during whole surgery by the surgeon and the operating nurse.
- Bulb pressing test after Draf and Stankiewicz,[19,20] (Fig. 9.8) can be helpful when there is suspicion of injury to the lamina papyracea.
- Always dissecting laterally to the middle turbinate, never medially and superiorly.
- The middle meatal antrostomy should be performed just above inferior turbinate and should not go further anteriorly than the anterior end of the middle turbinate.
- If middle turbinate surgery is needed, the superior part should be preserved as anatomic landmark.
- The anterior wall of the sphenoid sinus is about 7 cm from the nasal opening and the natural ostium lies about 1.5 cm above the choanal bridge.

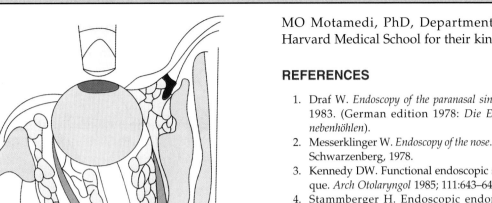

Fig. 9.8: Bulb-pressing test: Gentle pressure of the eye and simultaneous endonasal observation can be helpful to identify the lamina papyracea and possible injuries. In this case orbital fat (arrow) can be identified intranasally by bulb pressing maneuver[19,20]

- Careful surgery in the sphenoid sinus after detailed study of CT scans.
- The septum sinuum sphenoidalium may be posteriorly attached to a thin carotid artery canal, hence removal of the septum with cutting instruments or a diamond drill. Do not fracture the septum!

POSTOPERATIVE CARE AND TREATMENT

No uniform recommendations concerning postoperative care exist in the literature. We would like to offer some general recommendations for postoperative treatment.

Local aftercare of the surgical area by the ENT surgeon:
- Daily, in the first postoperative days and with continuously expanding interval based on each individual patient for about three months.
- Local aftercare should consist of:
  – Removal of fibrin clots and crusts.
  – Separation of synechiae and adhesions.
  – Suction of secretion from the nasal cavity.

Daily local care of the operative area by the patient:
- Minimum of three months.
- Application of topical steroids.
- Inhalation and irrigation of the nose.
- Application of ointments.

ACKNOWLEDGMENT

The authors would like to thank Professor Greim, Director Clinic of Anesthesiology, Fulda Hospital and MO Motamedi, PhD, Department of Cell Biology, Harvard Medical School for their kind cooperation.

REFERENCES

1. Draf W. *Endoscopy of the paranasal sinuses*. Berlin: Springer, 1983. (German edition 1978: *Die Endoskopie der Nasennebenhöhlen*).
2. Messerklinger W. *Endoscopy of the nose*. Baltimore: Urban und Schwarzenberg, 1978.
3. Kennedy DW. Functional endoscopic sinus surgery: Technique. *Arch Otolaryngol* 1985; 111:643–649.
4. Stammberger H. Endoscopic endonasal surgery—New concepts and treatment of recurring rhinosinusitis. I. Anatomic and pathophysiologic considerations. II. Surgical technique. *Otolaryngol Head Neck Surg* 1986; 94:143–156.
5. Heermann H. Ueber endonasale Chirurgie unter Verwendung des binocularen Mikroskopes. *Arch Ohren-Nasen-Kehlkopfheilkd* 1958; 171:295–297.
6. Draf W. Operating microscope for endonasal sinus surgery. First International Symposium: *Contemporary Sinus Surgery*. Pittsburgh, November 1990.
7. Draf W. Endonasal microendoscopic frontal sinus surgery: The Fulda concept. *Op Tech Otolaryngol Head Neck Surg* 1991; 2:234–240.
8. Weber R, Draf W, Keerl R, Schick B, Mosler P, Saha A. Microendoscopic endonasal pansinus operation in chronic sinusitis. Results and complications. *Am J Otolaryngol* 1997; 18:247–253.
9. Kennedy DW, Zinreich SJ, Rosenbaum A et al. Functional endoscopic sinus surgery: Theory and diagnosis. *Arch Otolaryngol Head Neck Surg* 1985; 111:576–582.
10. Stammberger H. *Functional endoscopic sinus surgery*. Philadelphia: BC Decker, 1991.
11. Hawke WM, McCombe AW. How I do it: Nasal polypectomy with an arthroscopic bone shaver. The Stryker 'Hummer'. *J Otolaryngol* 1995; 24:57–59.
12. Setliff RC, Parsons DS. The 'Hummer': New instrumentation for functional endoscopic sinus surgery. *Am J Rhinol* 1994; 8:275–278.
13. Wigand ME. Endoscopic surgery of the paranasal sinuses and anterior skull base. New York: Thieme, 1990.
14. Swanson PB, Lanza DC, Vining EM, et al. The effect of middle turbinate resection upon the frontal sinus. *Am J Rhinol* 1995; 9:191–195.
15. May M, Hoffmann DF, Sobol SM. Video endoscopic sinus surgery: A two–handed technique. *Laryngoscope* 1990; 100: 430–432.
16. Simmen D, Jones N. Surgery of the paranasal sinuses and the frontal skull base. New York: Thieme, 2005.
17. May M, Levine HL, Schatkin B, Mester SJ. Complications of endoscopic sinus surgery. In *Endoscopic Sinus Surgery*, Levine HL, May M (Eds). New York: Thieme, 1993.
18. Keerl R, Stankiewicz JA, Weber R, Hosemann W, Draf W. Surgical experience and complications during endonasal sinus surgery. *Laryngoscope* 1999; 109:546–550.
19. Draf W. Kurs endonasale mikro-endoskopische Chirurgie der Nasennebenhöhlen. Academic Teaching Hospital Fulda, 1986.
20. Stankiewicz JA. Complications of endoscopic sinus surgery. *Otolaryngol Clin North Am* 1989; 22:749–758.

Endoscopic Intranasal Dacryocystorhinostomy

Amir Minovi, Wolfgang Draf

The lacrimal drainage system had been investigated throughout history. During the nineteenth century exstirpation of the lacrimal gland was introduced as the main treatment of suppurative dacryocystitis. In 1893, Caldwell published the first report of endonasal lacrimal duct surgery. He performed a partial resection of the inferior turbinate and followed the nasolacrimal duct from inferior up to the lacrimal sac.[1] In the beginning of the twentieth century, a new era in lacrimal duct surgery began, as Toti introduced the external dacryocystorhinostomy (DCR) and West presented the best known paper of the classic endonasal DCR by fenestration of the lacrimal sac.[2,3] In 1901, a German rhinologist by the name Passow recommended an endonasal approach for surgery of the lacrimal sac.[4]

With rapid development of the new high quality Hopkins rigid nasal endoscopes, rhinologists could achieve a better visualization of the nasal cavity. This led to an advanced endonasal approach and has allowed better controlled access and surgery of the lacrimal drainage system. Rice reported in 1988, a cadaver dissection, demonstrating the feasibility of endoscopic intranasal DCR (EIDCR).[5] The first clinical study of EIDCR was published by McDonogh and Meiring in 1989.[6] In 1958, Heermann presented the use of the operating microscope for surgery of the lacrimal sac. Several authors reported their experience with the endonasal microscopic DCR.[7,8]

ANATOMY

Tear production occurs in the lacrimal gland and is dispersed onto the conjunctival surface. About 25% of the tear fluid evaporates. The internal canthal tendon and the surrounding sophisticated spiral muscle system works as a pump by pressing the lacrimal sac toward the nose. The tears pass four important stations on their way to the nasal cavity (Fig. 9.9):
- Upper or lower lacrimal canaliculi (0.1 to 0.4 mm in diameter)
- Common lacrimal duct
- Lacrimal sac
- Nasolacrimal duct

Most of the tears are transported through the inferior lacrimal canaliculus. The common lacrimal duct is about 1 to 3 mm long and ends in the lacrimal sac, which is located beneath the orbicular tendon. The nasolacrimal duct is about 18 mm long and empties into the inferior meatus.

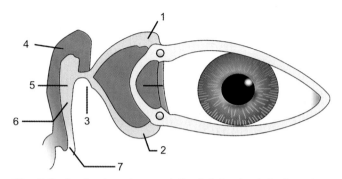

Fig. 9.9: Anatomic scheme of the left lacrimal duct system. (1) superior lacrimal canaliculus, (2) inferior lacrimal canaliculus, (3) common duct, (4) lacrimal sac, (5) Krause's valve, (6) nasolacrimal duct, (7) Hasner's valve

Throughout the lacrimal system, there are a series of valves. The most important are the Krause's valve, between the sac and nasolacrimal duct and the Hasner's valve, at the lower nasal outlet. This latter presents the greatest resistance in the nasolacrimal duct system. The lacrimal fossa surrounds the lacrimal sac. A very helpful anatomic landmark is the head of the middle turbinate. The lacrimal fossa is bounded by the anterior lacrimal crest which is part of the frontal process of the maxillary bone. The posterior lacrimal crest is made up of the lacrimal bone itself.

PATHOLOGY

The most common symptom of dacryostenosis is epiphora. The most common causes of an interrupted lacrimal fluid drainge from the lacrimal sac into the nose are:
- Congenital
- Inflammation: Allergy, rhinosinusitis
- Infection: Herpes simplex, leprosy, syphilis, fungi
- Trauma
- Postoperative: Caldwell-Luc, middle and inferior meatal antrostomy
- Tumors
- Granulomas: Sarcoidosis, Wegener's granulomatosis
- Radiotherapy

DIAGNOSTIC PROCEDURES

Diagnosis of the nasolacrimal pathology begins with a precise clinical history and examination. Most patients report a permanent epiphora and several episodes of dacryocystitis presenting as intermittent swelling of the lacrimal sac with purulent discharge from the lacrimal canaliculi. Prior to surgery an ophthalmologic consultation is recommended.

The clinical examination begins with investigation of the lacrimal puncta. The inferior canaliculus should be probed and the nasolacrimal duct should be evaluated by further irrigation (isotonic saline solution) of the canaliculus with a syringe. The patients should be asked if they can taste the saline solution.

Several diagnostic studies exist for the evaluation of the lacrimal drainage system: [9]

Fluorescein Test

With the Jones test one can examine the patency of the naslocrimal system. Two or three drops of 2% fluorescein are placed in the conjunctival sac after the application of nasal anesthetic and a vasonconstrictor. A dry applicator is placed at the inferior meatus and is removed after 5 minutes. It is then seen whether or not the fluorescein can be determined. This test cannot locate the site of stenosis and is contraindicated in acute dacryocystitis.

Dacryocystography (Fig. 9.10)

A contrast medium is applied into the nasolacrimal duct by probing the inferior canaliculus. Then an anterior-posterior X-ray is performed. With this technique one can localize the site of stenosis.

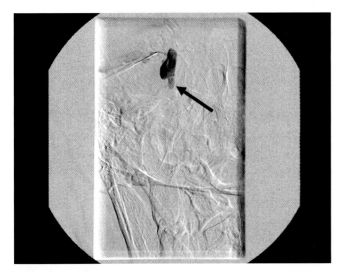

Fig. 9.10: Dacryocystogram in A-P projection after irrigation of the inferior lacrimal canaliculus with contrast medium; dacryocele and postsaccal stenosis (arrow) at the Krause's valve

Dacryocystogammagraphy

Technetium[99] is injected into the conjunctival sac and the flow of this marked fluid is observed under a gamma camera. With this technique one can determine the rate of travel and the level of obstruction.

INDICATIONS

EIDCR is indicated in almost all pathologies causing a postsaccal stenosis. Furthermore, it is indicated if there is a traumatic interruption of the lacrimal canaliculi. The indications for EIDCR are:
- Acute dacryocystitis with empyema
- Dacryocele
- Postsaccal stenosis
- Relapsing dacryocystitis
- Traumatic lesion, especially transection of the lacrimal canaliculi
- In combination with paranasal sinus surgery especially osteoplastic maxillary sinus surgery.

SURGICAL TECHNIQUE

Surgery is usually performed under general anesthesia and application of a local anesthetic and a decongestive agent. Sometimes a septoplasty is necessary in order to achieve an adequate visualization of the lacrimal fossa. In the first stage a mucosal window is created anterior to the head of the middle turbinate and cranial frontal process of the maxilla. The exposed bone is removed with a diamond bur and the lacrimal sac clearly identified (Figs 9.11A to D). The sac should be exposed relatively widely and extended as far as the fundus. In some cases one need to resect some parts of the anterior middle turbinate or open some anterior ethmoid cells. In the next step, a lacrimal duct intubation probe is inserted into the inferior canaliculus and the medial mucosa of the lamical sac is stretched endonasally. With a sickle knife the sac is opened and the medial part of it is completely resected. Biopsies with histological examination for sarcoidosis are often recommended. Finally, the second probe is inserted through the other canaliculus and the ends of the two tubes are knotted intranasally. Unilateral nasal packing is recommended overnight. The silicon tubes can be removed six to eight weeks postoperatively on an outpatient basis under endoscopic control. In the case of primary surgery some authors do not perform an intubation. In contrast intubation for at least six months is recommended in revision surgery.[10,11]

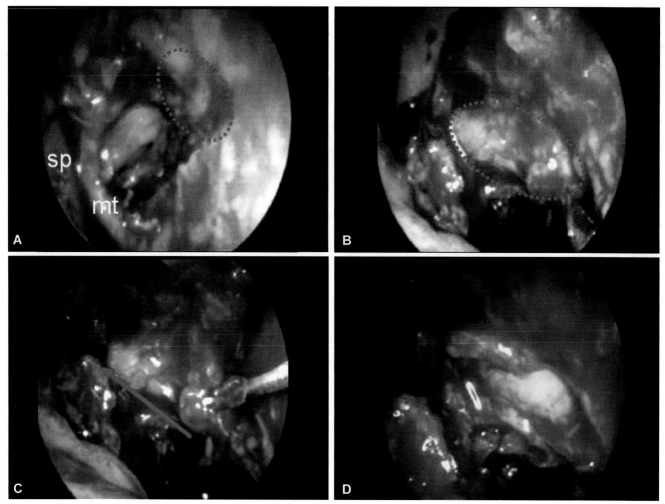

Figs 9.11A to D: Major surgical steps in endoscopic intranasal dacryocystorhinostomy. (A) Exposure of the lacrimal bone by removing of the ethmoid bulla; dotted red lines mark area of the lacrimal sac. (B) Total exposure of the lacrimal sac. (C) Incision of the sac after stretching the medial portion with a probe. (D) Condition after removal of the medial portion

There are certain advantages of the EIDCR:
- No external scar
- Lacrimal pump system remains intact
- Any intranasal concurrent pathology can be addressed at the same time, including adhesions, septal deviation and enlarged middle turbinate
- No contraindication in acute dycryocystitis.

There are certain complications to an endoscopic DCR:
- Sac not found
- Hematoma of the cheek
- Emphysema
- Bleeding
- Reclosure
- CSF leak

The results after EIDCR are very satisfactory. Most authors define success as maintenance of patency after a period anywhere between three months and one year. Rice reported a success rate of 100% in four patients.[12] Sperkelsen treated 152 patients and had a success rate of 96%. The overall success rate is about 85%.[13] The results of endonasal DCR are comparable to external DCR. Hartikainen analyzed prospectively the success rate of 64 patients who were treated either through an external or endonasal DCR. He found a patency rate of 75% in the endoscopic cases versus 91% externally. This did not, however, reach a statistically significant difference. After revision surgery there was a success rate of 97% in both groups.[14]

In 1991, Metson showed that for revision DCR, the endoscopic approach is especially superior to the external approach.[15]

In conclusion, an endoscopic DCR has been shown to be a minimally invasive and safe alternative to the external approach. Its effectiveness has been especially established in revision cases. The results of EIDCR are comparable to those reached by external DCR, and the satisfactory aesthetic advantages (no visible scars) are clear.

ACKNOWLEDGMENT

The authors would like to thank Farhan Taghizadeh, MD, Assistant Professor, Universiy of New Mexico Health Sciences Center, Albuquerque, USA for his kind cooperation.

REFERENCES

1. Caldwell GW. A new operation for the radical cure of obstruction of the nasal duct. *NY Med* 1893; 58: 476.
2. Toti A. Nuovo metodo conservatore di cura radicalle delle suppurazioni cronicle del sacco lacrimale. *Clin Mon Firenze* 1904; 10:385–389.
3. West JM. Eine Fensterresektion des Ductus nasolacrimalis in Faellen von Stenose. *Arch Laryngol Rhinol* 1911; 24:62–64.
4. Passow A. Zur chirurgischen Behandlung des Tränenkanals. *Munch Med Wochenschr* 1901; 48:1403–1404.
5. Rice DH. Endoscopic intranasal dacryocystorhinostomy: A cadaver study. *Am J Rhinol* 1988; 2:127–128.
6. McDonogh M, Meiring H. Endoscopic transnasal dacryocystorhinostomy. *J Laryngol Otol* 1989; 103:585–587.
7. Heermann H. Endonasal surgery with the use of the binocular operating microscope. *Arch Klin Exp Ohren Nasen Kehlkopfheilk* 1958; 171:295–297.
8. Ptok A, Draf W. Operative Behandlung der Tränenwege. *Head Neck Oncol* 1987; 35:188–194.
9. Riveros-Castillo GA, Campos A. Endoscopic transnasal dacryocystorhinostomy. In: *Microendoscopic surgery of the paranasal sinuses and the skull base,* Stamm A, Draf W (Eds). New York: Springer Press, 2000; 415–424.
10. Metson R. Endoscopic surgery for lacrimal obstruction. *Otolaryngol Head Neck* 1991; 104: 473–479.
11. Schauss F, Weber R, Draf W, Keerl R. Surgery of the lacrimal system. *Acta Oto-Rhino-Laryngol Belg* 1996; 50:143–146.
12. Rice D. Endoscopic intranasal dacryocystorhinostomy results in four patients. *Arch Otolaryngol Head Neck Surg* 1990; 116:1061.
13. Sprekelsen MB, Barberan MT. Endoscopic dacryocystorhinostomy: Surgical technique and results. *Laryngoscope* 1996; 106:187–189.
14. Hartikainen J, Antila J, Varpula M, Puuka P, Seppa H, Grenman R. Prospective randomized comparison of endonasal endoscopic dacryocystorhinostomy and external dacryocystorhinostomy. *Larnygoscope* 1998; 108:1861–1866.
15. Metson R. The endoscopic approach for revision dacryocystorhinostomy. *Laryngoscope* 1990; 100:1344–1347.

Endonasal Frontal Sinus Surgery

Wolfgang Draf

- The endonasal type I to III drainages allow to adapt the frontal sinus surgery to the underlying pathology.
- From type I to III upwards surgery is increasingly invasive.
- The type III median drainage[1] is identical with the endoscopic modified Lothrop procedure.[2]
- The concept of endonasal drainages of the frontal sinus implicates preservation of bony boundaries of frontal sinus outlet in contrary to the classic external fronto-orbital procedure.[3-6] This means less danger of shrinking and reclosure with development of mucocele. It is a surgical strategy not just a technique. The fronto-orbital external operation should not anymore be used for treatment of inflammatory diseases.
- In case the type III drainage is technically not possible (A-P diameter of the frontal sinus less than 0.8 cm) or failed the osteoplastic frontal sinus obliteration must be considered.

INDICATIONS

Endonasal surgery of the paranasal sinuses began, apart from a couple of earlier reports, some hundred years ago.[7-11] Only a few skilled surgeons have been able to perform endonasal ethmoidectomy and adequate drainage of the frontal sinus using just headlight and the naked eye, whereas others created serious complications such as CSF leak, meningitis, brain abscess and encephalitis ending in the pre-antibiotic era mostly with the death of the patient. This was the reason why for decades until the 1970s endonasal sinus surgery was not accepted in most of the leading institutions.

The renaissance of endonasal surgery was due to several facts:

- New optical aids such as the microscope and endoscope.
- Improved understanding of physiology and pathophysiology of nasal and paranasal sinus mucosa.

• Patients no longer accepting the sometimes serious sequelae of external operations in addition to an unsatisfactory outcome.
• Remarkable progress in anesthesiology providing the endonasal surgeon with an almost bloodless field.

Between 1980 and 1984 an endonasal surgical concept with different degrees of frontal sinus opening has been worked out and intensively tested before being published.[1]

With increasing experience and referrals of difficult frontal sinus cases, it became obvious that not all problems can be solved via an endonasal route. Therefore, the osteoplastic obliterative frontal sinus operation[12] was included in the concept, in order to deal with all different kinds of frontal sinus problems. In difficult revision cases sometimes the endonasal operation has to be combined with the osteoplastic, mostly obliterative procedure.[1,14]

OPERATIVE TECHNIQUE AND INDICATIONS OF THE ENDONASAL FRONTAL SINUS DRAINAGE ACCORDING TO DRAF

For endonasal frontal sinus operation of any type general anesthesia is required. In addition topical decongestion helps to provide a dry field.

The most important instruments for this surgery are 0° and 45° telescopes, and for special situations, the operating microscope and different blunt and through-cutting forceps. The shaver is very useful for gentle tissue removal and also for drilling in the frontal sinus.

Surgery on the frontal recess is usually preceded at least by an anterior, more often than not by a complete ethmoidectomy. Exceptions are those cases where a complete ethmoidectomy has already been performed. It is important to remove agger nasi cells and to visualize the attachment of the middle turbinate medially, the lamina papyracea laterally, and the anterior skull base with the anterior ethmoidal artery superiorly.

Type I: Simple Drainage

The type I drainage (Fig. 9.12A) is established by ethmoidectomy including the cell septa in the region of the frontal recess.[13] The inferior part of Killian's infundibulum and its mucosa is not touched. This approach is indicated when there is only minor pathology in the frontal sinus and the patient does not suffer from 'prognostic risk factors' like aspirin intolerance and asthma, which are associated with poor quality of mucosa and possible problems in outcome (Table 9.1). In the majority of cases the frontal sinus heals because of the improved drainage via the ethmoid cavity.

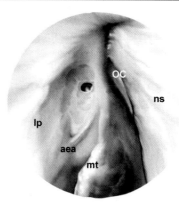

Fig. 9.12A: Type I drainage (simple drainage, right side). aea = anterior ethmoidal artery; lp = lamina papyracea; mt = middle turbinate; ns = nasal septum; oc = olfactory cleft

Type II A and B: Extended Drainage

Extended drainage is achieved after ethmoidectomy by resecting the floor of the frontal sinus between the lamina papyracea and the middle turbinate (type IIA) or the nasal septum (type IIB) anterior to the ventral margin of the olfactory fossa (Figs 9.12B to D).

Hosemann et al showed in a detailed anatomical study that the maximum diameter of a neo-ostium of the

Table 9.1: Indications for endonasal frontal sinus drainage types I to III	
A. Indications type I drainage	
Acute sinusitis	Failure of conservative surgery orbital and endocranial complications
Chronic sinusitis	First time surgery no risk factors (aspirin intolerance, asthma, triad) revision after incomplete ethmoidectomy
B. Indications type IIA drainage	
	Serious complications of acute sinusitis medial mucopyocele tumor surgery (benign tumors) good quality mucosa
Indications type IIB drainage: All indications of type IIA, if the resulting IIA is smaller than 5 × 7 mm. For type IIB, drill necessary.	
C. Indications type III drainage	
	Difficult revision surgery primarily in patients with prognostic risk factors and severe polyposis, particularly patients with triad, mucoviscidosis Kartagener's syndrome ciliary immotility syndrome benign and malignant tumors

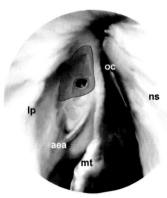

Fig. 9.12B: Type II A drainage (enlarged drainage a, right side); opening of frontal sinus between lamina papyracea and middle turbinate; usually possible without drill

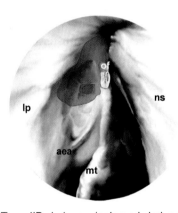

Fig. 9.12C: Type IIB drainage (enlarged drainage B, right side); drainage of the frontal sinus between lamina papyracea and nasal septum; usually medially drill necessary

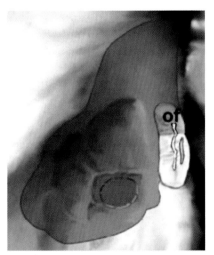

Fig. 9.12D: Type IIB drainage detail with identification of the first olfactory fiber of = olfactory fiber

frontal sinus (type IIA), which could be gained using a spoon or a curette, was 11 mm with an average of 5.6 mm. They also presented an excellent critical evaluation and results.[15-17]

If one needs to achieve a larger drainage opening like type IIB, one has to use a drill because of the increasing thickness of the bone going more medially towards the nasal septum. During drilling with the diamond bur in a classic drill hand piece, bone dust may fog the endoscope demanding repeated cleaning. At this point the microscope is useful in allowing one to work with two hands, while an assistant holds a simple self-retracting speculum according to Cholewa.[18] The endoscopic four-hand technique, introduced by May, is also a useful alternative, allowing the surgeon to work with both hands while an assistant holds the endoscope.[19] The working situation for both surgeons is optimal if the cold light cable is connected *superiorly* with the endoscope, so it is not in the way of the other surgeon.

A great help for drilling in the frontal sinus are new straight and differently curved drills used with the shaver providing simultaneous suction and irrigation thus reducing fogging of the telescopes (Fig. 9.12E).

As soon the frontal recess is identified using the middle turbinate and where identifiable, the anterior ethmoidal artery as landmarks, the frontal infundibulum is exposed and the anterior ethmoidal cells are resected. During surgery repeated considerations of the CT will establish the presence of so-called frontal cells (Fig. 9.12F),[20] which can develop far into the frontal sinus giving the surgeon the erroneous impression, that the frontal sinus has been properly opened. Sagittal CT slices and navigation may be helpful in difficult situations. In the case of frontal cells a procedure called by Stamm-

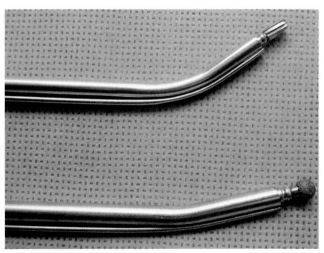

Fig. 9.12E: Shaver drills with suction and irrigation device

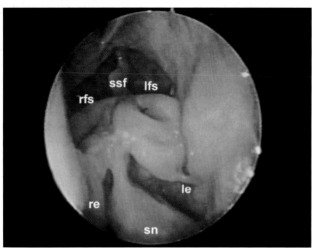

Fig. 9.12F: Type III drainage 1 year postoperatively. Abbreviations: ssf = septum sinuum frontalium; rfs = right frontal sinus; lfs = left frontal sinus; sn = septum nasale; re = right ethmoid; le = left ethmoid)

berger 'uncapping the egg' using a 45° telescope may be necessary, resulting in a type IIA drainage.[21]

If, after a type IIA drainage has been performed, further widening to produce a type IIB is required, the diamond burr is introduced into the clearly visible gap in the infundibulum and drawn across the bone into a medial direction. Care is taken to ensure that the frontal sinus opening is bordered by bone on all sides and that the mucosa is preserved at least on one part of the circumference. To create medially (and safely) the widest possible opening of the frontal sinus floor one should identify the ipsilateral first olfactory fiber (see type III drainage, Fig. 9.12G). At the end a rubber finger stall can be introduced into the frontal sinus for about 5 days.

The indications for one or the other type II drainage in general are listed in Table 8.1. In case one feels the type IIA drainage is too small in regard to the underlying pathology, it is better to perform the type IIB drainage.

Type III: Endonasal Median Drainage

Endonasal median drainage or type III: The extended IIB opening is enlarged by resecting portions of the superior nasal septum in the neighborhood of the frontal sinus floor. The diameter of this opening should be about 1.5 cm. This is followed by resection of the frontal sinus septum or septa, if there are more than one. Starting on one side of the patient one crosses the midline until the contralateral lamina papyracea is reached.

To achieve the maximum possible opening of the frontal sinus it is very helpful to identify the first olfactory fibers on both sides: The middle turbinate is exposed and mm by mm cut from anterior to posterior along its origin at the skull base. After about 5 mm one will see the first olfactory fiber coming out of a little bony hole, slightly medially the origin of the middle turbinate. The same is done on the contralateral side. Finally, the so-called 'Frontal T' results (Fig. 9.13).[22] Its long crus is represented by the posterior border of the perpendicular ethmoid lamina resection, the shorter wings on both sides are provided by the posterior margins of the frontal sinus floor resection.

After that, the ethmoidectomy on the left side is completed the same way as on the right.

Performing the type III drainage in the technically most efficient way, it is helpful to change between the use of endoscope and microscope. Alternatively, this

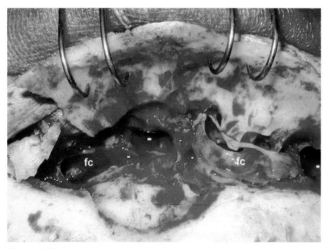

Fig. 9.12G: Frontal sinus view from above after coronal osteoplastic revision. Several frontal cells of different sizes narrow the drainage into the nose (fc = frontal cell)

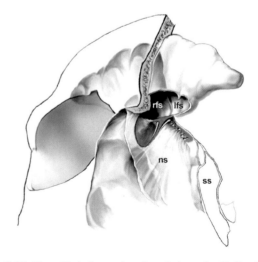

Fig. 9.13: Type III drainage (median drainage) with 'frontal T' (red) and first olfactory fiber on both sides (View from left inferior)

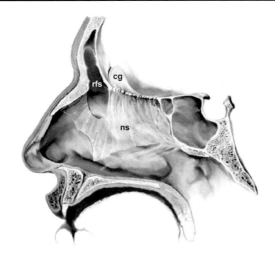

Fig. 9.14: Type III drainage (median drainage) sagittal view: removal of the frontal sinus floor in front of the olfactory cleft

procedure can be done with the endoscope alone, though it is more time-consuming. Curved drills of different angles used with the shaver motor are helpful. They allow more superior movement with the resection of the interfrontal sinus septum and are more complete, offering the removal of an eventual frontal cell. These measures help to create excellent landmarks for the anterior border of the olfactory fossa on both sides which makes the completion of frontal sinus floor resection to its maximum until the first olfactory fiber easier and safer (Fig. 9.14).

Finally, a rubber finger stall is placed into each frontal sinus and two more are put in the ethmoid cavity and the inferior nasal meatus on one and the other side. This packing is left for 7 days under prophylactic antibiotic treatment. The rubber finger stalls do not stick to the surrounding tissue and are therefore easily and painlessly removed. In the interim, a major part of the surgical cavity re-epithelialized, which simplifies the postoperative treatment.

In difficult revision cases one can begin the type III drainage primarily from two starting points, either from the lateral side as already described or medially. The primary lateral approach is recommended if the previous ethmoidal work was incomplete and the middle turbinate is still present as a landmark. One should adopt the primary medial approach, if the ethmoid has been cleared and/or if the middle turbinate is absent.

The medial approach begins with the partial resection of the perpendicular plate of the nasal septum, followed by identification of the first olfactory fiber on each side as already described.

The endonasal median drainage is identical with the NFA IV and the 'modified Lothrop procedure'.[2,19]

Lothrop himself warned against using the endonasal route, since it was still dangerous during his time,[23,24] and performed the median drainage via an external approach. Halle in 1906, created a large drainage from the frontal sinus directly to the nose using the endonasal approach with no more aids than headlight and naked eye.

The principal difference between the endonasal median frontal sinus drainage and the classic external Jansen, Lothrop, Ritter, Lynch and Howarth operation is that the bony borders around the frontal sinus drainage are preserved. This makes it more stable in the long-term, avoids an external scar, and reduces the likelihood of reclosure by scarring, which may lead to recurrent frontal sinusitis or a mucocele.

The endonasal median drainage (type III) is indicated (Table 9.1) after one or several previous sinus operations have not resolved the frontal sinus problem including an external frontoethmoidectomy. It is also justified as primary procedure in patients with severe polyposis and other prognostic 'risk factors' affecting outcome, such as aspirin intolerance, asthma, Samter's triad (aspirin hypersensitivity, asthma and allergy), Kartagener syndrome, mucoviscidosis and ciliary dyskinesia syndrome. Its use in patients with severe polyposis without these risk factors is undetermined and needs to be evaluated. It seems that patients with generalized polyposis but who still show in the periphery of the sinuses along the skull base air on coronal CT (halo sign) have a comparatively better prognosis than those without, and can be managed by a more conservative technique. It is useful also for removal of benign tumors in the frontal sinus and the ethmoid as long the main part of the tumor in the frontal sinus is medial a postoperative vertical line through the lamina papyracea. In addition the use of the type III drainage makes the removal of malignant tumors which are just reaching the frontal sinus safer.

RESULTS OF ENDONASAL FRONTAL SINUS SURGERY

Judging *results* of endonasal frontal sinus surgery requires a postoperative follow-up of ten or more years.[25,26] The failure rate of Neel et al with a modified Lynch procedure grew from 7% at a mean follow-up of 3.7 years to 30% at 7 years.[25]

Weber et al[27] carried out in 1995 and 1996 two studies. In the first retrospective study, patients who underwent endonasal frontal sinus drainage (471 type I drainages, 125 type II drainages, and 52 type III drainages) between 1979 and 1992 were evaluated. From these groups,

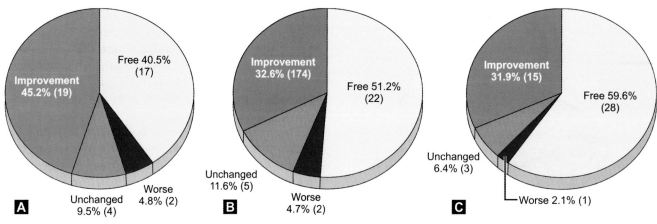

Figs 9.15A to C: Subjective judgment of results of frontal sinus surgery 1 to 12 years after surgery;
(A) Type I drainage. (B) Type II drainage. (C) Type III drainage

random patients were examined: 42 patients with type I drainage, 43 with type II drainage, and 47 with type III drainage have been included in the study. In each patient the indication was chronic polypoid rhinosinusitis, except in 5 cases with type III drainage in which an orbital complication presented associated with acute sinusitis. The follow-up period was between 1 year and 12 years with a median of 5 years. The subjective estimation of operative results by the patients is shown in Figs 9.15A to C. Applying subjective and objective criteria to evaluate the success of endonasal frontal sinus drainage (grade 1 = endoscopically normal mucosa, independent of the subjective complaints; grade 2 = subjectively free of symptoms, but with endoscopically visible inflammatory mucosal changes; grade 3 = no subjective improvement and pathologic mucosa = failure) it was possible to achieve a success rate of 85.7% with type I drainage, 83.8% with type II drainage and 91.5% with type III drainage. This means that, despite the choice of prognostically unfavorable cases, type III drainages appeared to show the best results though this was not statistically significant among the three groups.

In a second study, endoscopic and CT examinations were systematically carried out (Figs 9.16 and 9.17).[27,28] After 12 to 98 months follow-up of patients with type II drainage, 58% of 83 frontal sinuses were ventilated and normal. A ventilated frontal sinus with hyperplastic mucosa was seen in 12%. Scar tissue occlusion with total opacification on CT was evident in 14%. In 16% total opacification was due to recurrent polyposis. Patients were free of symptoms or had only minor problems in 79%.

Twelve to 89 months following type III drainage, 59% of 81 frontal sinuses were ventilated and normal. A ventilated frontal sinus with hyperplastic mucosa was

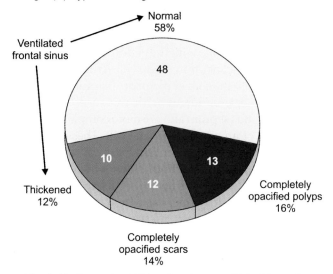

Fig. 9.16: Synopsis of CT and endoscopy 12 to 98 months following Type II drainage (from Weber et al 2000)[28]

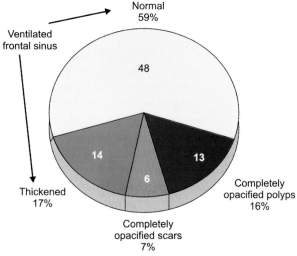

Fig. 9.17: Synopsis of CT and endoscopy 12 to 98 months following Type III drainage (from Weber et al 2000)[28]

seen in 17%. Scar tissue occlusion with total opacification on CT was obvious in 7% and, in 16%, there was total opacification due to recurrent polyposis. The patients were free of symptoms or had only minor problems in 95%. Already this first series of re-evaluation of long-term results demonstrates the value of the endonasal frontal sinus surgery.

In a retrospective study Mertens et al compared the results of 236 patients operated on between 1985 and 1993 using different techniques.[29] After follow-up of 3 to 10 years only 8% of patients needed revision. The lowest revision rate was seen after endonasal technique according Draf's classification (5.9%) compared to the osteoclastic techniques according to Jansen-Ritter (Lynch) and Riedel (10.6%).

POSTOPERATIVE CARE

There are different ways of *postoperative care*. Overtime the following standards have proved to be efficient:

Packing

Rubber finger stalls (Rhinotamp; Vostra Aachen) filled with sponge have stood the test of time as safe hemostasis, stimulator of re-epithelialization of bare bone, painless to remove and cost-effective. In case of type I to type IIB drainage the packing is left for 2 to 5 days without antibiotic prophylaxis. It is of utmost importance to fix the rubber finger stalls with threads at the nasal dorsum to avoid aspiration. The more stabile the middle turbinate at the end of operation, the shorter the time of uncomfortable packing can be. The risk of adhesions and synchiae is low because this type of packing suppresses the development of granulations.

After a type III drainage we leave the packing in place for 7 days postoperatively as already recommended by Toffel for another type of tamponade.[30] He removes then the packing under general anesthesia. Leaving rubber finger stalls for one week carries the following advantages:

1. The fibrinoid phase of wound healing is somehow overcome. Reclosure of the large drainage by scars is remarkably reduced, since bare bone is re-epithelialized almost completely.
2. For removal of packing there is no need for sedation or general anesthesia. Rubber finger packs are not binding to the wound. Removal of the tamponade does not lead to renewed tissue trauma. The patients are prepared preoperatively for a somewhat uncomfortable postoperative time. This is by far compensated by the optimal wound healing and easy postoperative care with less crusting.

Local Postoperative Therapy

The question whether intensive mechanical cleansing should be done postoperatively or the wound cavity is self-cleaning without external measures is very controversial. In an obstructed nose or sinus, when the patient has complaints that can be explained with occlusion of the osteal region by crusts, mechanical cleaning must be done. However, since each cleaning leads to injury, freshly granulating tissue and partial removal of new epithelium, a rather controlled and conservative approach to instrument cleaning seems appropriate.

The following measures can be performed by the patient on their own:

1. Irrigation with saline solution at least once a day, sometimes more frequently.
2. 1 to 3 times/day application of one of the corticosteroid sprays. One hour after the corticosteroid spray the use of peanut oil for general care of the mucosa is recommended.

In patients with extreme crusting one should ask for medication which is accompanied as side effect by desiccation of the mucosa as for example psychopharmaca or beta-blocker. After changing the medication spectacular improvement is possible.

General Postoperative Medication

Antibiotics: They are indicated in the postoperative period for 1 to 2 weeks in case of acute or purulent sinusitis. In type III drainage patients antibiotics should be applied as prophylaxis as long the tamponade is in place.

Antiallergic medical therapy: This may be recommended for 6 weeks postoperatively if by history or specific tests allergy is proven. Presence of a large number of eosinophilic leukocytes in the inflamed tissue may additionally help decision-making. In less severe cases we prescribe day antihistamines, in severe allergy patients (e.g. Samter's triad) the combination of antihistamines with low-dose corticosteroid medication for 6 weeks is helpful to prevent early recurrence of polyps. In about 50% of triad patients a leukotriene antagonist is of significant effect to prevent recurrence of polyposis.

COMPLICATIONS

In principle the complication rate of endonasal frontal sinus drainage procedures is low and well corresponding to the frequency of complications in endonasal pansinus operations.

An evaluation with special respect to endonasal frontal sinus surgery has not been performed. The operation even with identification of the first olfactory fibers can be classified as very safe when optical aids such as micro-scope and/or endoscope are used following the techniques described.

We have analyzed the complications of our endonasal microendoscopic pansinus operations in two studies.[31,32] The significant complications were:

1. Injury to the periorbit in 14%. This had no further consequences except one patient, who developed periorbital hematoma. No cases of blindness or other orbital lesions like muscle injury with double vision or lacrimal drainage obstruction occurred.
2. Dural injury occurred in 2.3%. The subsequent course was uneventful and free of complications after immediate plastic closure of the defect with preserved fascia and fibrin glue. Persistent CSF leakage or meningitis was not observed.
3. In only one patient a postoperative disturbance of the sense of smell was confirmed by a smell test. Even, if a type III drainage was performed using the 'frontal T' technique with identification of the first olfactory fiber on each side, the sense of smell was mostly improved due to reopening of the olfactory cleft rather than decreased because of surgical irritation of olfactory fibers.

CONCLUSION

The endonasal frontal sinus drainages type I to III and as ultimate procedure in case the endonasal solution is not possible or unsuccessful, the osteoplastic flap procedure mostly with obliteration, provide a surgical concept suitable for treatment of any type of frontal sinus inflammatory diseases.

Since the endonasal frontal sinus operations respect the outer osseous borders of the newly created frontal sinus drainage the chance of complete re-epithelialization of eventually bare bone is very likely. Therefore, the danger of frontal sinus outlet shrinking leading to a mucocele is minimized.

This concept has revolutionized frontal sinus surgery, whereas the classic external fronto-orbital frontal sinus operation according to Jansen-Ritter or Lynch or Howarth must be estimated as obsolete for treatment of chronic inflammatory diseases of the frontal sinus.

REFERENCES

1. Draf W. Endonasal micro-endoscopic frontal sinus surgery. The Fulda concept. *Op Tech Otolaryngol Head Neck Surg* 1991; 2:234–240.
2. Gross WE, Gross CW, Becker D, Moore D, Phillips D. Modified transnasal endoscopic Lothrop procedure as an alternative to frontal sinus obliteration. *Otolaryngol Head Neck Surg* 1995; 113:427–434.
3. Jansen A. Eroeffnung der Nebenhoehlen der Nase bei chronischer Eiterung. *Arch Laryngol Rhinol (Berl)* 1894; 135–157.
4. Ritter G. Eine neue Methode zur Erhaltung der vorderen Stirnhoehlenwand bei Radikaloperationen chronischer Stirnhoehleneiterungen. *Dtsch Med Wochenschr* 1906; 32:1294–1296.
5. Howarth WG. Operations on the frontal sinus. *J Laryngol Otol* 1921; 36:417–421.
6. Lynch RC. The technique of a radical frontal sinus operation which has given me the best results. *Laryngoscope* 1921; 31:1–5.
7. Schaeffer M. Zur Diagnose und Therapie der Erkrankungen der Nebenhoehlen der Nase mit Ausnahme des Sinus maxillaris. *Dtsch Med Wschr* 1890; 19:905–907.
8. Spiess G. Die endonasale Chirurgie des Sinus frontalis. *Arch Laryngol* 1899; 9:285–291.
9. Ingals EF. New operation and instruments for draining the frontal sinus. *Ann Otol Rhinol Laryngol* 1905; 14:513–519.
10. Halle M. Externe und interne Operation der Nebenhoehleneiterungen. *Berl klin Wschr* 1906; 43:1369–1372,1404–1407.
11. Halle M. Die intranasalen Operationen bei eitrigen Erkrankungen der Nebenhoehlen der Nase. *Arch Laryngol Rhinol* 1915; 29:73–112.
12. Tato JM, Bergaglio OE. Surgery of frontal sinus. Fat grafts: New technique. *Otolaryngologica* 1949; 3:1.
13. Lang J. *Clinical Anatomy of the Nose Nasal Cavity and Paranasal Sinuses.* Stuttgart: Thieme, 1989.
14. Keerl R, Constantinidis J, Schick B, Saha A. Endonasal and External Micro–Endoscopic Surgery of the Frontal Sinus. In *Micro-endoscopic Surgery of the Paranasal Sinuses and the Skull Base*, Stamm A, Draf W (Eds). New York: Springer, 2000; 257–278.
15. Hosemann WG, Weber RK, Keerl RE, Lund VJ. *Minimally Invasive Endonasal Sinus Surgery.* New York: Thieme, 2000; 54–59.
16. Hosemann W, Gross R, Goede U, Kuehnel T. Clinical anatomy of the nasal process of the frontal bone (spina nasalis interna). *Otolaryngol Head Neck Surg* 2001; 125:60–65.
17. Hosemann W, Kuehnel T, Held P, Wagner W, Felderhoff A. Endonasal frontal sinusotomy in surgical management of chronic sinusitis: A critical evaluation. *Am J Rhinol* 1997; 11:1–9.
18. Cholewa ER. 1888 cited after Tange RA, Pirsig W. Het neusspeculum. Door de eeuwen heen. Universiteitsmuseum van de Universiteit van Utrecht. Glaxo BV 1990.
19. May M, Schaitkin B. Frontal sinus surgery: Endonasal drainage instead of an external osteoplastic approach. *Op Tech Otolaryngol Head Neck Surg* 1995; 6:184–192.
20. Lang J. Clinical anatomy of the nose, nasal cavity and paranasal sinuses. New York: Thieme, 1989; 58–59.
21. Stammberger H. FESS: 'Uncapping the egg'. The endoscopic approach to frontal recess and sinuses. np: Storz Company Prints, 2000.
22. Draf W. Frontal sinus fractures. In *The frontal sinus*, Kountakis S, Senior B, Draf W. Berlin: Springer (Eds), 2005.
23. Lothrop HA. The anatomy and surgery of the frontal sinus and anterior ethmoidal cells. *Ann Surg* 1899; 29:175–215.
24. Lothrop HA. Frontal sinus suppuration. *Ann Surg* 1914; 59:937–957.

25. Neel HB, McDonald TJ, Facer GW. Modified Lynch procedure for chronic frontal sinus diseases: Rationale, technique, and long-term results. *Laryngoscope* 1987; 97:1274.
26. Orlandi RR, Kennedy DW. Revision endoscopic frontal sinus surgery. *Otolaryngol Clin North Am* 2001; 34:77–90.
27. Weber R, Draf W, Keerl R, Schick B, Saha A. Micro-endoscopic pansinus operation in chronic sinusitis: Results and complications. *Am J Otolaryngol* 1997; 18:247–253.
28. Weber R, Keerl R, Huppmann A, Draf W, Saha A. Wound healing after endonasal sinus surgery in time-lapse video: A new way of continuous *in vivo* observation and documentation in rhinology. In *Micro-endoscopic Surgery of the Paranasal Sinuses and Skull Base*, Stamm A, Draf W. (Eds) New York: Springer, 2000; 329–345.
29. Mertens J, Eggers S, Maune S. Langzeitergebnisse nach Stirnhoehlenoperationen: Vergleich extranasaler und endonasaler Operationstechniken. *Laryngorhinootol* 2000; 79:396–399.
30. Toffel PH. Secure endoscopic sinus surgery with middle meatal stenting. *Op Tech Otolaryngol Head Neck Surg* 1995; 6:157–162.
31. Weber R, Draf W. Komplikationen der endonasalen mikro-endoskopischen Siebbeinoperation. *Head Neck Oncol* 1992a; 40:170–175.
32. Weber R, Draf W. Die endonasale mikroendoskopische Pansinusoperation bei chronischer Sinusitis. II. Ergebnisse und Komplikationen. *Otorhinolaryngologia Nova* 1992b; 2: 63–69.

Preoperative Diagnosis in Functional Endoscopic Sinus Surgery

Amir Minovi, Wolfgang Draf

The most important aim of any surgical procedure is to relieve the patients' symptoms. Not all symptoms of chronic sinusitis can be eliminated with surgical treatment. It is, therefore, vital to take the time to listen to the patient and to establish their main problems. A discussion is then required to make clear to the patient what can be achieved with surgery and which symptoms are likely to be improved. It is also necessary to remember that sinus surgery is not about treating a CT scan, but is part of the management of a well-informed patient.

HISTORY

In general, the history taken should include the following aspects:

Symptoms of the Present Illness

Patients frequently present to the surgeon with their diagnosis, instead of describing their signs and symptoms. Detailed questioning about the patients symptoms is required concentrating on the duration, time of onset and any symptom-free intervals. The patient should also be asked for the most common symptoms of chronic sinusitis. These include:
- Nasal obstruction
- Postnasal drip
- Headache and location
- Recurrent swelling
- Facial pressure
- Hyposmia

Past Medical and Surgical History

Most patients who are referred for sinus surgery have been treated medically in the past. Many of them have had several courses of antibiotics in conjunction with systemic and/or topical corticosteroids. It is mandatory to ask all patients about any previous sinus surgery. The following questions require particular attention:
- Episodes of antiobiotic therapy
- Duration of local/systemic corticosteroid treatment
- Previous surgery
- Success of previous surgery and symptom-free intervals after surgery
- Any other medication, particularly agents which can cause mucosal swelling as a side effect such as antihypertensive drugs
- Presence of Samter's triad (polyps, asthma, aspirin intolerance).

PHYSICAL EXAMINATION AND ENDOSCOPY

Routine physical examination includes anterior rhinoscopy and rigid/flexible endoscopy. The anterior rhinoscopy gives the surgeon a first impression of the sinonasal condition. The following features should be noted from this examination:
- Septal deviation
- Color, texture and turgor of the mucosa
- Size and shape of the turbinates

Endoscopic examination of the nasal cavity with rigid and flexible endoscopes is now the gold standard in the preoperative evaluation of chronic sinusitis.[1,2] In our hospital we prefer the flexible endoscope as it is well-tolerated, even in children, and most patients do not even require local anesthesia. A 0° or 30° angled rigid endoscope can also be used to examine the nasal cavity. Before using a rigid endoscope a mixture of topical anesthetic and a vasoconstrictor should be applied to the nasal mucosa. By displaying the endoscopic image on a TV monitor, it is possible to demonstrate any pathology to the patient. The following anatomical structures should be evaluated routinely:

- Relationship between the middle turbinate and the nasal septum
- Paradoxical middle turbinate (a medially rather than laterally concave middle turbinate)
- The extent of resection of a previously trimmed middle turbinate
- The presence of a concha bullosa (an air-filled, pneumatized middle turbinate)
- The extent and size of any polyps.

Olfactory Testing

The evaluation of olfaction preoperatively is mandatory. Up to 45% of patients with chronic sinusitis complain of olfactory dysfunction.[3] Olfactory tests can be performed either objectively or subjectively. In objective olfactometry the patient is given a flow of air with constant humidity and temperature. Then an olfactory stimulus (vanillin) is added to the air flow. Then olfactory evoked potentials are recorded. In subjective olfactometry the patient sniffs a series of sample odors and is asked to identify them. However, some patients may have difficulties in the identification of the odors. Three different kinds of odors can be distinguished: Pure olfactory odors (e.g. vanilla, cinnamon, lavender), odors with a trigeminal component (acetic acid, ammonia) and odors with smell components (chloroform).[4,5]

ACOUSTIC RHINOMETRY AND RHINOMANOMETRY

Acoustic rhinometry is a non-invasive technique to measure the cross-sectional area of regions of the nasal airway. It has become more and more popular since it is rapid, non-invasive and requires minimal cooperation from the subject. In acoustic rhinometry a sound pulse reflected from the airway is measured and is converted mathematically into a map of the cross-sectional area of the airway versus the distance from the site of introduction of the pulse.[6,7] In this technique a short-duration sound pulse is directed into the nasal airway with the help of a wave tube. The sound pulse travels through the airway and is partially reflected when there is a change in the cross-sectional area. The reflected signals are recorded and analyzed to produce a rhinogram. Adults with subjectively normal nasal airflow have a characteristic rhinogram. In case the patient does not feel improvement of airflow postoperatively this investigation may be repeated as objective documentation. It is interesting to note that a patients' subjective feeling about nasal airflow and the objective measurement do not always correlate.

Rhinomanometry is an objective technique, in which changes in air pressure and the speed of air flow through the nasal cavities are measured during breathing. This allows the nasal resistance to airflow to be calculated. In anterior rhinomanometry the transnasal pressure at the anterior end of the nose is measured. This technique does have some limitations. Measurements are unreliable in patients with septal perforations. Also, resistance can only be measured in one nostril at a time. In posterior rhinomanometry the air pressure is measured in the nasopharynx by placing a catheter in the mouth. This technique does not require closure of either nostril making it possible to measure air resistance bilaterally. Nasal resistance should be measured before and after decongestion of the nose and the data compared. In general, two major types of nasal obstruction can be distinguished:

- Mucosal hypertrophy which should be corrected by topical decongestion leading to a decrease of resistance on rhinomanometry.
- Structural abnormalities such as a septal deviation which cannot be improved with decongestion resulting in no change in nasal resistance.

A nasal resistance greater than $0.3\,\mathrm{Pa/cm^3}$ per second usually causes symptomatic nasal obstruction.

IMAGING

Computerized tomography (CT) is absolutely essential in planning endoscopic sinus surgery. In the event of a postoperative complication, a surgeon has little medicolegal defence if a preoperative CT scan was not performed. Scanning is best performed in the axial plane with additional coronal and sagittal reconstructed images. This minimizes any artefacts caused by dental fillings. Sagittal planes are very helpful to determine the extension of the frontal and sphenoid sinuses. Ideally, a CT should be done when the disease is quiescent and there is no acute inflammation of the sinuses. The extent of mucosal disease found at the time of surgery may differ from what is shown on the CT scan. In the majority of the cases the findings are underestimated in the CT.[8] With the help of the CT the surgeon should evaluate extension and distribution of the disease and analyze important anatomical landmarks, variants and any surgically hazardous anatomy. CT scans should be shown to the patients preoperatively to explain the proposed surgery. The CT scans must be present in the operating room for the surgeon to review during surgery. Several authors suggested a preoperative checklist for CT evaluation in functional endoscopic sinus surgery.[9,10] We recommend the following CT work-up, ideally done with the radiologist on the day of surgery:

First step: (Fig. 9.18)
- General overview of the paranasal sinuses in the coronal planes.
- Are the sides (right and left) correctly labelled?
- Assess the ostiomeatal complex.
- Degree of pneumatization in the ethmoid cells.

Second step: (Figs 9.19 and 9.20)
- Evaluation of important anatomical landmarks (axial and coronal planes).
- *Uncinate process*: Shape, course and side of insertion.
- *Lamina papyracea*: Possible dehiscent areas.
- *Middle turbinate*: Degree of pneumatization, presence of a concha bullosa, extension of resection in previous surgery.

Third step: (Figs 9.21 and 9.22)
- Evaluation of the frontal sinus (axial planes).
- Size and location of the frontal recess.

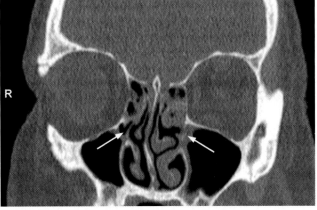

Fig. 9.18: Coronal CT scan allowing assessment of the ostiomeatal complex (arrows), extent of sinusitis and degree of pneumatization in the ethmoid region

- Anterior-posterior diameter of the frontal sinus.
- Presence of frontal cells.
- Shape of the septum sinuum frontalium, there may be more than one.

Fourth step: (Fig. 9.23A to C)
- Evaluation of the skull base (axial and coronal planes).
- Shape of the skull base and orbit.
- Relationship of the olfactory fossa and ethmoid roof.
- Thickness of the skull base and possible bony dehiscence along skull base.
- Position of anterior ethmoidal neurovascular bundles.

Fifth step
- Evaluation of the sphenoid sinus (axial planes).
- Shape and extension of the sphenoid sinus.

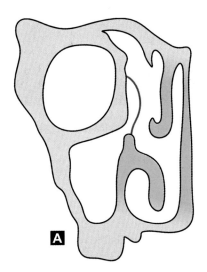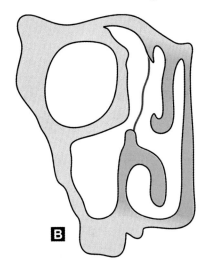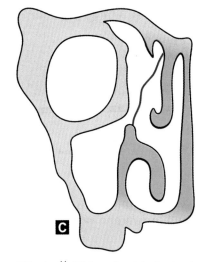

Figs 9.19A to C: Anatomical variations of the uncinate process according to Stammberger and Hawke;[11] (A) Insertion into the lamina papyracea. The frontal sinus drains medially into the middle meatus. (B) Insertion to the skull base. (C) Insertion to the middle turbinate. In both these cases the frontal sinus drains laterally into the ethmoidal infundibulum

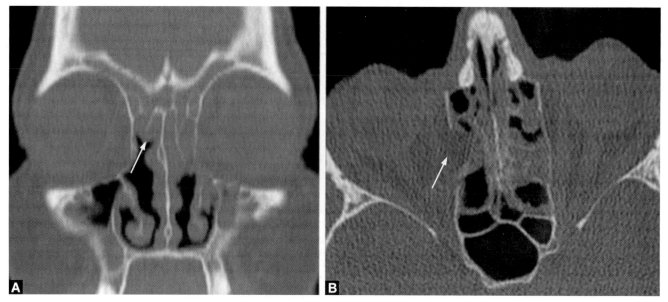

Figs 9.20A and B: (A) Coronal CT in a patient with previous sinus surgery showing a partially resected middle turbinate. (B) Axial CT of a different patient showing partial dehiscence of the lamina papyracea

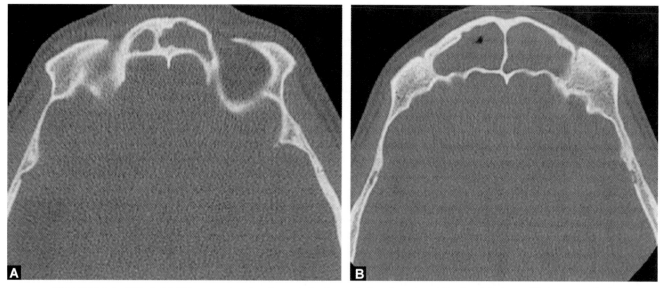

Figs 9.21A and B: Axial CT scans showing the anterior to posterior diameter of the frontal sinus. (A) Asymmetrical small frontal sinuses. (B) Symmetrical frontal sinuses with lateral extension

- Course of the septum sinuum sphenoidalium and side of insertion.
- Presence of an Onodi-cell.
- Protrusion and possible bony dehiscence of the internal carotid artery and optic nerve.

INFORMED PATIENT CONSENT

Before surgery the patient should be informed about the advantages and possible complications of the surgery. It is mandatory to mention possible catastrophic complications. The following points should be included in the preoperative conversation with the patient:

- Failure, revision surgery.
- Alternative forms of treatment.
- Bleeding, infection, wound healing disturbances.
- Injury to the optic nerve with possible reduced vision and blindness.
- Injury to the ocular muscles with possible permanent double vision.
- Injury of the dura with cerebrospinal fluid leaks, meningitis, encephalitis.

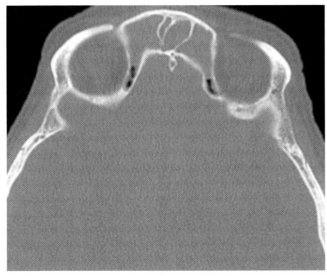

Fig. 9.22: Axial CT showing multiple frontal cells

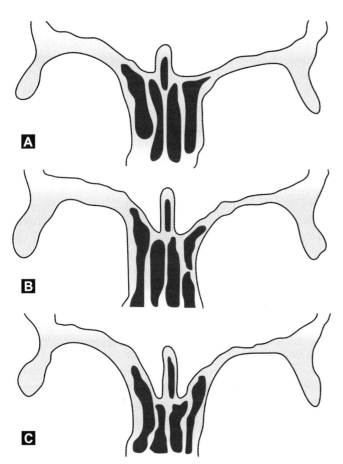

Figs 9.23A to C: Configuration of the ethmoid roof according to the olfactory groove depth as described by Keros[12]
(A) Type I: 1–3 mm. (B) Type II: 4–7 mm. (C) Type III: 8–16 mm

- Epiphora.
- Olfactory disturbances.
- Hypesthesia in the palate, teeth, or face.
- Burns to the upper lip in case of contact with a hot drill, although extremely rare.

It has been shown that the better the patient is informed regarding the necessary surgical steps, limitations, possible failures and complications the more he will trust the surgeon even if the result is below his expectations. Meticulous postoperative care adds to this significantly.

ACKNOWLEDGMENTS

The authors would like to thank Professor Hofmann, Director, Department of neuroradiology and Ben Hunter, BSc, MBBS, MRCS, Department of Otorhinolaryngology and Head and Neck Surgery, Torbay Hospital, Devon, United Kingdom for their kind cooperation.

REFERENCES

1. Draf W. *Endoscopy of the Paranasal Sinuses*. Berlin: Springer, 1983. (German edition 1978: *Die Endoskopie der Nasennebenhöhlen*).
2. Messerklinger W. *Endoscopy of the Nose*. Baltimore: Urban und Schwarzenberg, 1978.
3. Levine HL, May M. *Endoscopic Sinus Surgery*. New York: Thieme, 1993.
4. Duty RL. *Handbook of Olfaction and Gustation*. New York: Decker, 1995.
5. Seiden AM. *Taste and Smell Disorders*. New York: Thieme, 1997.
6. Jackson AC, Butler JP, Miller EJ et al. Airway geometry by analysis of acoustic pulse response measurements. *J Appl Physiol* 1977; 43:523–536.
7. Hilberg O, Jackson AC, Swift DL et al. Acoustic rhinometry: Evaluation of nasal cavity geometry by acoustic reflection. *J Appl Physiol* 1989; 66:295–303.
8. Mann WJ, Amedee RG, Iemma M. An assessment of radiologic discrepancies in patients with paranasal sinus disease. *Am J Rhinol* 1992; 6:211–213.
9. Haetinger RG. Imaging of the nose and paranasal sinuses. In *Micro-endoscopic Surgery of the Paranasal Sinuses and the Skull Base*, Stamm AC, Draf W (Eds). New York: Springer, 2000; 53–81.
10. Mason JDT, Jones NS, Hughes RJ, Holland IM. A systematic approach to the interpretation of computed tomography scans prior to endoscopic sinus surgery. *J Laryngol Otol* 1998; 112:986–990.
11. Stammberger H, Hawke M. *Essentials of Functional Endoscopic Sinus Surgery*. St.Louis: Mosby, 1993.
12. Keros P. Ueber die praktische Bedeutung der Niveauunterschiede der Lamina cribrosa des Ethmoids. *Laryngorhinootol* 1962; 41:808–813.

Endonasal Microendoscopic Sinus Surgery for Tumors

Ulrike Bockmühl

While the frequency of benign tumors of the nose, the paranasal sinuses and the anterior skull-base is not known, malignant sinonasal tumors account for approximately 3% of all head and neck malignancies.[43] The signs and symptoms of the sinonasal tumors are non-specific for long periods of time and depend mostly on their location and size. Nasal obstruction, hyposmia, blood-stained nasal discharge or a vague feeling of pressure or headache may be predominant symptoms. If they occur unilaterally, it might be the first suspicion of a tumor. Symptoms like visual disturbance (i.e. reduction of vision, double vision), meningitis, CSF leak, external swelling of the cheek or forehead, epiphora, irritation of the first or second branch of the trigeminal nerve (hyperesthesia and pain) are signs of extensive tumor growth beyond the limits of the nose or sinuses.

The diagnostic investigation should always include endoscopy, and imaging studies, such as computed tomography (CT) and magnetic resonance imaging (MRI). They are important for evaluation of the location and extent of the lesion, surgical planning and postoperative follow-up. To get the optimum information we recommend performing both CT and MR imaging. The vascularity of a lesion can be evaluated with digital subtraction angiography. If the tumor has reached or involved the internal carotid artery a balloon occlusion test should be performed together with perfusion scintigraphy of the brain. In cases with suspected CSF leak a CT or MR cisternography might be a helpful investigation.

Depending on the type and extent of the tumor, surgical, radiotherapeutic and/or chemotherapeutic strategies are appropriate measures. While for the majority of tumors the accepted treatment of choice is complete wide local resection, controversy surrounds the surgical approach that should be used. Traditionally, in the last century most sinonasal tumors were removed en bloc via transfacial approaches like lateral rhinotomy or midfacial degloving or as anterior craniofacial resection which is carried out by a combination of frontal craniotomy and one of the transfacial approaches. However, recent refinements in endoscopic and microscopic techniques together with the development of related surgical instruments have led to expanded endonasal surgery beyond for chronic sinusitis to complete resection of tumors in the nasal cavity, paranasal sinuses as well as at the anterior and central skull base showing comparable rates of recurrence to an external approach.[3,17,34,39,45,55,64] Moreover, when properly indicated and planned, for the majority of benign but also malignant tumors endonasal procedures are superior to the traditional external techniques. This is due to the following advantages:

1. Via the endonasal approach one gets the optimal overview over almost the entire paranasal sinus system.
2. Dura defects from the lower third of the frontal sinus posterior wall down to the sphenoid roof can be reliably closed exclusively endonasally.
3. The bony boundaries of the surgical field can be preserved. This means less danger for cele formation and reduced disturbance for the growing midfacial skeleton in children.
4. It is the most minimal invasive way avoiding visible scars and facial distorsion.

In this chapter, our experience with the endonasal endoscopic and/or microscopic approach to anterior skull base lesions is described.

GENERAL PRINCIPLES

Although the endonasal approach is the least traumatic the following preconditions should be realized for successful removal of the pathology and consideration of functional and aesthetic aspects:

1. The surgeon must have an extensive and reliable knowledge of the anatomy.
2. The surgeon must have vast experience in endonasal surgery of inflammatory diseases, traumatology and endonasal duraplasty, and must be thoroughly familiar with the surgical technique of type III frontal sinus drainage according to Draf.[16]
3. The surgeon must be familiar with the prevention and management of possible complications (intra-orbital hematoma, damage to the lacrimal system, CSF leaks, major bleeding).
4. Since both the microscope and endoscope have advantages and disadvantages, the surgeon should be able to use both in order to optimize his work.
5. Navigation is highly recommended.

6. The surgeon should also have expertise in head and neck surgery including the different external approaches in this area, i.e. he must be able to switch intraoperatively from an endonasal to external approach and to perform an appropriate reconstruction of soft tissue or bone.
7. Intracranial extension by itself is not a contraindication to the endonasal approach. Rather it depends on the degree and the experience of the surgeon. However, those cases should be carefully discussed with the neuroradiologist and the neurosurgeon.
8. If the surgeon lacks neurosurgical training close cooperation with neurosurgeons (not only in major intra-extracranial cases) is mandatory.
9. The surgical procedures should be performed under general anesthesia.
10. In general, we achieve vasoconstriction by placing cotton swabs soaked in naphazolin hydrochloride in the nasal cavity for 10 minutes followed by subsequent injection of lidocain with 1:200.000 adrenaline at the lateral nasal wall as well as the septum.
11. Intraoperatively frozen sections should be obtained to ensure complete tumor removal.

A criticism of the endonasal approach is the impossibility to obtain en bloc resection. Certainly, en bloc removal of tumors is the ideal choice and it is often achieved in smaller lesions, but radical extirpation of the disease does not depend on it as shown by our long-term results of inverted papilloma and malignant tumors. Instead, the primary purpose is to identify and widely remove the tumor origin as well as the infiltrated structures, in most malignancies including anterior skull-base and dura and lamina papyracea. Therefore, it is acceptable to resect larger tumors segmentally.[3,34,39,48,68,72,76]

In our experience there are two major limitations to the use of the endonasal microendoscopic approach, first is extensive involvement of the frontal sinus.[34,68,76] We believe that an exclusive endonasal approach is contraindicated if the disease largely involves the frontal sinus mucosa, especially in hyperpneumatized sinuses, because it is difficult to remove the diseased mucosa in the supraorbital region and to at least drill the underlying bone (Fig. 9.24). The second major limitation is a tumor originating from the posterolateral, anterior or inferior wall of the maxillary sinus. Other limitations that are managed better with external procedures such as the subcranial approach according to Raveh[53] or the midfacial

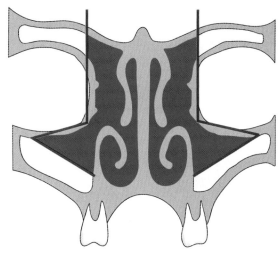

Fig. 9.24. Tumor locations in which endonasal surgery is indicated (blue area): Lesions not exceeding more laterally than a vertical plane through the lamina papyracea (black line) and lesions that do not originate from the posterolateral, anterior or inferior wall of the maxillary sinus

degloving[10] are extensive intracranial and intraorbital infiltration, respectively and in recurrent lesions associated with massive scar tissue.

BENIGN TUMORS

Benign sinonasal tumors represent a large collection of diverse lesions. They are divided histopathologically into tumors and pseudotumors, and on their histogenesis they are classified as epithelial, mesenchymal or neural. Table 9.2 summarizes the authors' experience with common benign tumors.[3] Between 1993 and 2003 we have treated 215 benign tumors surgically. Of these, 118 (54%) tumors were removed exclusively endonasally.[3] Osteomas, inverted papillomas and juvenile angifibromas were the most prevalent tumor types and therefore will be explained in more specific details and by representative examples.

Osteoma

The most frequent location of craniofacial osteomas is the frontal sinus, followed by the ethmoid, maxillary sinus and sphenoid sinus respectively.[47] They originate on the sinus wall, but their cause is still uncertain. The age of presentation is most commonly the second to fifth decade, with a male-to-female ratio of approximately 3:1. Osteomas most frequently are discovered incidentally on radiographs or may enlarge, producing symptoms like swelling or rare complications such as visual impairment

Table 9.2: Most frequent benign sinonasal tumor entities

Pseudotumors
  Polyps
  Mucoceles
  Mucus retention cysts
  Aneurysmal bone cysts
  Meningoencephaloceles

Tumors
Epithelial
  Adenoma
Inverted papilloma
  Papilloma
Mesenchymal
  Chondroma
  Fibroma
  Fibrous dysplasia
  Hemangioma
Juvenile angiofibroma
  Ossifying fibroma
Osteoma
  Paraganglioma
Neural
  Neurinoma

and intracranial neurological complications as meningitis or pneumen-cephalus with seizure, referable to their location near the orbit or anterior cranial base.[56,61]

In our own hands approximately 68% of the osteomas can be resected exclusively endonasally.[55] During the endonasal procedure mucosa should be preserved as much as possible. Small osteomas with a small origin may be removed in one piece. If the neoplasm has a wide base, attaches to the skull base, particularly next to the olfactory fossa or is of a larger size, it should preferably removed by piecemeal resection. The drill plays an important role, allowing either debulking the lesion from inside until the shell is thin enough to be gently fractured and removed under direct vision avoiding damage of the dura, olfactory fibers or orbital contents. This needs to be done as long as the tumor is still immobile which eases the procedure remarkably allowing larger tumors to be removed through the small nostrils. It depends on the size of the frontal sinus and of the tumor as to whether a type II or a type III drainage of the frontal sinus results. If endonasal removal is not possible, the osteoplastic flap procedure via a coronal incision is the alternative allowing complete tumor resection with the best aesthetic result. It depends on how far the mucosa has been preserved during tumor removal whether the sinus may be left alone or obliteration is needed.

Inverted Papilloma (IP)

In 1991, the World Health Organization classified sinonasal papillomas into three different histopathologic types: Exophytic or fungiform papilloma, columnar cell papilloma and inverted papilloma.[58] IP is the most common type and accounts for approximately 70% of all sinonasal papillomas and from 0.5 to 4% of all neoplasms of the sinonasal tract.[27] They are characterized by a high recurrence rate, a tendency for malignant transformation and multicentric involvement. Recurrence rates up to 50% are reported, with almost all tumors recurring at the site of the previous surgery.[2,7,27,41,52] Malignant transformation occurs in about 11% of cases with IP.[2] IP occur mostly in the fifth and sixth decades with a male to female distribution of 5:1.[27,52] Although the cause of IP is still unknown, it has been demonstrated by molecular-biologic analysis that human papilloma virus is involved in IP formation being detected in up to 86% of these tumors. In particular, viral subtypes 6, 11, 16 and 18 were most frequently found.[22]

The invasive capacity to surrounding structures and the propensity to be associated with squamous cell carcinoma, make the treatment of IP particularly challenging for the surgeon. IP usually arise from the lateral nasal wall, in the middle meatus, often extending to the ethmoid and maxillary sinuses. In advanced cases, extension into all of the ipsilateral paranasal sinuses may occur, whereas intracranial growth and dura penetration are rare.[44]

To choose the best surgical approach, i.e. to assess the endonasal resectability preoperative imaging is inalienable. Patients' symptoms are more or less aspecific, and it is almost impossible to distinguish IP from inflammatory polyps at the time of clinical examination, even in unilateral distribution of nasal polyps. In the assessment of sinonasal expansile lesions CT scan with contrast medium is generally considered the examination of choice. However, CT cannot differentiate between retained secretion and inflamed mucosa from IP. This limitation can be overcome by using MRI, which, apart from differentiating neoplastic tissue from inflammatory changes, identifies a convoluted cerebriform pattern suggestive for IP on T2-weighted or enhanced T1-weighted sequences in about 80% of cases.[49] An example is shown in Figs 9.25A and B. Because involvement of IP in the frontal and maxillary sinus may be limited to the region around the ostium, MRI is especially important for preoperative determination of the tumors' origin. For better comparison of treatment results tumors should be classified according to the Krouse staging system for IP.[35]

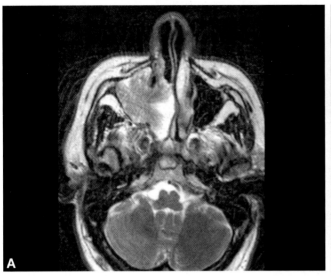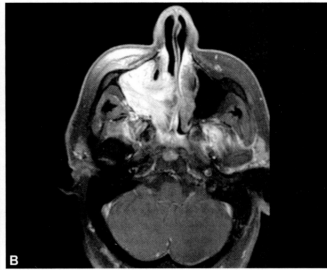

Figs 9.25A and B: MRI showing typical convoluted cerebriform pattern suggestive for inverted papilloma (IP) on enhanced. (A) T1-weighted. (B) T2 sequences

The analysis of our patient material revealed that we removed 70% of IP exclusively via an endonasal micro-endoscopic procedure.[45] Figures 9.26A and B show a typical example. In 23% of the cases a combined approach and in 6.9% an osteoplastic maxillary sinus operation were performed. All T1 (n = 11) and T2 (n = 37) tumors but only 35% of the T3 lesions were resected exclusively endonasally. In primary tumors an endonasal approach was chosen in 74% of the cases in contrast to 58% in revision cases. There were no major complications in our series.

As radical surgery is the primary purpose the tumor origin has to be identified and IP has to be widely removed along the subperiosteal plane including drilling the underlying bone! The success is judged mainly by the recurrence rate and the treatment morbidity. Incomplete tumor resection is regarded as the source of recurrent IP growth. Supportive evidence for this is that recurrent lesions appear at the primary site within a short follow-up period.[36] In our series, we have found an overall recurrence rate of 10.3% within the mean observation interval of 73.9 months. Related to the

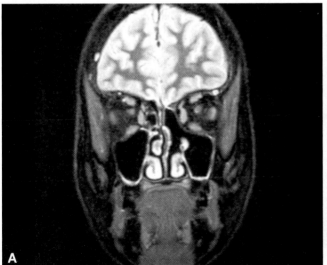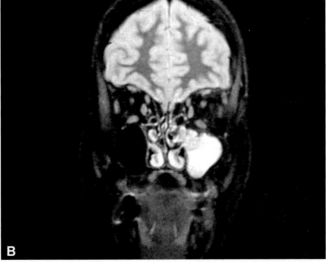

Figs 9.26A and B: T1-weighted coronal magnetic resonance images enhanced with contrast medium showing an inverted papilloma (IP) arising from the left middle meatus. (A) Preoperative scan. (B) Postoperative appearance three years after resection by performing a Draf's type IIa drainage

endonasal approach the incidence of recurrent tumors was 10% compared to 15% after combined approaches.[45] The recurrence rates of the most recent reports on endoscopic surgery of IP varied between 0%[31,68] and 27%.[34,38,41,69,71,73,75]

Juvenile Angiofibroma (JA)

This is a highly vascularized tumor composed of connective tissue intertwined with blood vessels that occur almost exclusively in adolescent adults. Although, these tumors are benign, they are locally aggressive eroding adjacent bone and growing through natural foramina and fissures. They account for approximately 0.5% of all head and neck tumors.[25] JA usually arises from the posterolateral wall of the nasal cavity, where the sphenoid process of the palatine bone meets the sagittal wing of the vomer and the pterygoid process of the sphenoid bone. More specifically, it originates at the sphenopalatine foramen and the posterior end of the middle turbinate, from which the angiofibroma can extend into the nasal cavity and nasopharynx, the paranasal sinuses, the pterygomaxillary, zygomatic and infratemporal spaces and the cranial base. Based on the tumor extension JA should be classified according to Fisch.[20]

The maxillary artery is the main blood supplier, but the JA may receive blood from secondary branches of the internal carotid artery. Other sources of blood include the pharyngeal, palatine and recurrent meningeal arteries. When the JA extends into the infratemporal fossa, there may be additional vascularization from the temporal and facial arteries.[13,63]

Diagnosis of JA is essentially clinical and requires weighting of the clinical findings and the CT and MR imaging results. The major symptoms in our series of 43 patients were nasal obstruction and epistaxis. A bulge in the soft palate, proptosis, diplopia, epiphora, irritation of the second branch of the trigeminal nerve and facial deformity are prevailing signs of more extensive tumors.

The efficacy of bleeding control and the localization and size of the tumor are crucial factors in treatment choice. Thereby, the most common and effective method of treatment is surgical removal after hyperselective intratumoral embolization.[63,70] Radiation may reduce the tumor size[19] but malignant change of JA has been reported.[74] Chemotherapy has been advocated for treatment of extensive JA considered to be inoperable using protocols similar to those for malignant tumors.[24] Hormone administration has failed to demonstrate any arteriographic changes in the vascular pattern of JA.[63]

The surgical techniques we use to resect JA include the endonasal approach as well as midfacial degloving and, rarely, the infratemporal approach or combinations of these procedures. Of the 43 JA we have treated 14 tumors (32%) were removed exclusively endonasally after hyperselective intratumoral embolization.[3] Among them, 11 tumors were classified as type II, one JA as type I and two tumors as type III according to Fisch. Figures 9.27A to G show a typical example. In general, all JA of type I and II are suitable for endonasal microendoscopic resection, which however are only a third of all JA.[60] In the majority of cases endonasal resection itself consists of a sphenoethmoidectomy, the removal of the medial and posterior maxillary sinus wall to get enough overview and access to the maxillary artery which will be clipped within the pterygoid fossa independent of embolization. Sometimes, it may be necessary to partly cut or mobilize the nasal septum. Since the JA has a pseudocapsule the principle should be to surround the tumor removing it in one piece which eases complete resection especially from the soft tissue of the pterygoid or infratemporal fossa. To prevent recurrences it is most important to cut the soft tissue tumor roots within the area of the sphenopalatine foramen. Finally to ensure entire tumor removal it is necessary to drill the surrounding bony borders and to take frozen sections. Even after complete embolization there can be plenty of blood loss during surgery. That is why we routinely use the cell saver system for immediate retransfusion of the patient's blood after filtration and washing.[54] Additionally, we request all patients with JA to donate their own blood 8 to 4 weeks before operation. There were no major complications in our series. During a mean follow-up period of 65 months we have seen 1 recurrence four years after initial surgery.[3] It was also resected endonasally, and the patient is without signs of tumor now.

MALIGNANT TUMORS

Management of sinonasal malignancies requires at first an understanding of the pathology of skull-base lesions and the formulation of a treatment plan with a multidisciplinary oncological team. Treatment decisions should be made individualized on the basis of histology, tumor stage, feasibility of complete resection, reconstructive options for restoration of form and function, treatment risks and morbidity and patient's medical condition. Therefore, it is mandatory to stage the

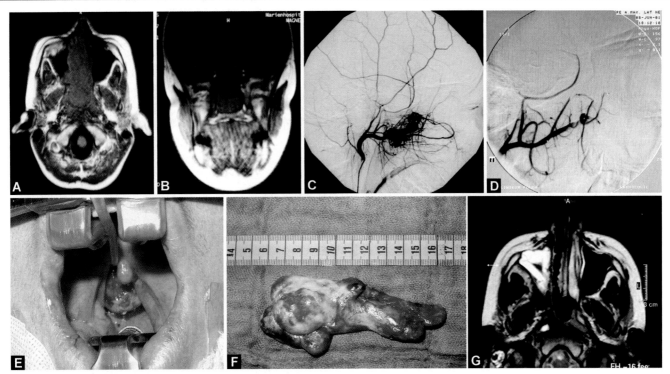

Figs 9.27A to G: Typical example of a juvenile angiofibroma (JA) type II according to Fisch that was removed exclusively endonasally. (A and B) Preoperative T1-weighted axial and coronal MR scans showing a JA in the right nasal cavity and nasopharynx originating from the sphenopalatine foramen. (C and D) Angiogram of the right external carotid artery before and after hyperselective intratumoral embolization. (E) Tumor extension in the nasopharynx. (F) Tumor specimen after endonasal en bloc resection. (G) T2-weighted axial MR scan 2 years postoperatively without evidence of recurrence

malignancies according to the UICC classification system.[50] In general, the mainstay of treatment is surgery followed by postoperative radiation. When incurable, palliation of symptoms becomes a primary goal, often achieved by adjuvant chemoradiation.

At present, the endonasal microendoscopic surgery of malignant anterior skull base tumors is discussed controversially, and craniofacial en bloc resection is still considered the gold standard.[5,8,11,21,23,26,57] However, recently we could demonstrate favorable prognosis of our patients with endonasally resected tumors. Generally, 5-year disease-specific survival rates of sinonasal malignant tumors are reported between 40 and 60%.[23,57,62,66] Histology, T stage (especially brain and deep soft tissue involvement, involvement of the sphenoid sinus), previous treatment and positive surgical margins have been described to be predictive factors for poor prognosis.[57,62,66] Out of 135 malignant tumors that we have primarily treated by surgery between 1993 and 2003, 54 (41%) were removed exclusively via the endonasal approach.[3] In particular, patients with endonasally removed adenocarcinomas, squamous cell carcinomas and esthesioneuroblastomas (n = 29) showed a 5-year

disease-specific survival rate of 78.4% compared to 66.4% of the patients (n = 51) who underwent conventional external approaches.[3] Thus, we feel the endonasal approach should be used in any case of smaller tumors, where a margin of resection is possible. It is then of vital importance that the complete removal, i.e. the extent of surgery, is not compromised by the micro-endoscopic technique.

Even in endonasal microendoscopic surgery the en bloc resection of malignant tumors is usually the surgeon's main goal. In this regard, our philosophy is to dissect around the tumor body from all sides along normal anatomical structures as demonstrated in Figs 9.28A and B. In many cases it means to start anteriorly with a frontal sinus drainage type III according to Draf[16] then resecting the upper nasal septum and explore the anterior skull base dissecting the tumor down to the sphenoid sinus. This includes in many cases the removal of the cribriform plate, the crista galli and the surrounding dura. Laterally, the margin of dissection is the periorbit and medially usually the nasal septum or the opposite nasal cavity and in large lesions the opposite periorbit. In case of periorbital infiltration the periorbit can be

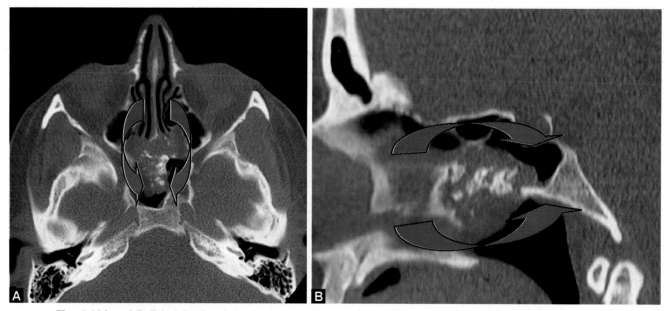

Figs 9.28A and B: Principle of endonasal microendoscopic tumor surgery: To dissect around the tumor body along normal anatomical structures preferable to achieve the en bloc tumor resection

removed and reconstructed with Tutoplast Fascia Lata® of the Tutogen Medical Company. If the anterior skull base including the dura needs to be removed we prefer to dissect from lateral to medial, but it is possible too going the other way round.[32] Duraplasty generally is performed as described by Schick in the previous chapter. However, it is not always possible to achieve en bloc resection. Instead, it is also suitable to perform a piece meal resection. No evidence exists, as yet, that supports a danger of tumor spread because of debulking. In some circumstances it will be necessary to combine the endonasal approach with an external procedure (i.e. a midfacial degloving[10] or a subcranial approach according to Raveh[53]) to achieve clear margins. Then, the surgeon must have the expertise to proceed. Under the circumstances that incomplete tumor removal is expected (tumor abutting the internal carotid artery, the optic nerve or the cavernous sinus, i.e. in adenoid cystic carcinoma or chordoma or in metastases) endonasal palliative surgery may be indicated, not for the purpose of cure but as an attempt to achieve considerable improvement in quality of life. Finally, it is important to recognize when endonasal resection is not in the patient's interest, e.g. tumor infiltration of the frontal lobe, the cavernous sinus or the orbit. While more recently endonasal endoscopic techniques[32,33] have extended what can be resected there is no evidence yet that these increase life expectancy or reduce morbidity and one not experienced should be very careful adopting advanced procedures.[29]

Table 9.3: Common malignant sinonasal tumor histologies (in descending order of frequency). Most prevalent tumor entities of the authors' patient series are marked in italics.

Squamous cell carcinoma
Adenocarcinoma
Adenoid cystic carcinoma
Mucosal melanoma
Esthesioneuroblastoma
Sinonasal neuroendocrine carcinoma
Sinonasal undifferentiated carcinoma
Lymphoma
Sarcoma
Metastases from other sites

Table 9.3 shows the most common malignant sinonasal tumor histologies. In our own patient series adenocarcinoma (n = 30), squamous cell carcinoma (n = 27) and esthesioneuroblastoma (n = 23) have been the most prevalent tumor types that were primarily operated between 1993 and 2003. They will be explained in more specific details and by representative examples.

Squamous Cell Carcinoma (SCC)

This is the most common malignancy of the sinonasal tract. There is a strong association between sinonasal SCC and nickel exposure.[51] Occupational exposure to soft tissue wood[15] or asbestos[40] has also been linked to development of sinonasal SCC. Although tobacco and alcohol are major risk factors for SCC of the upper

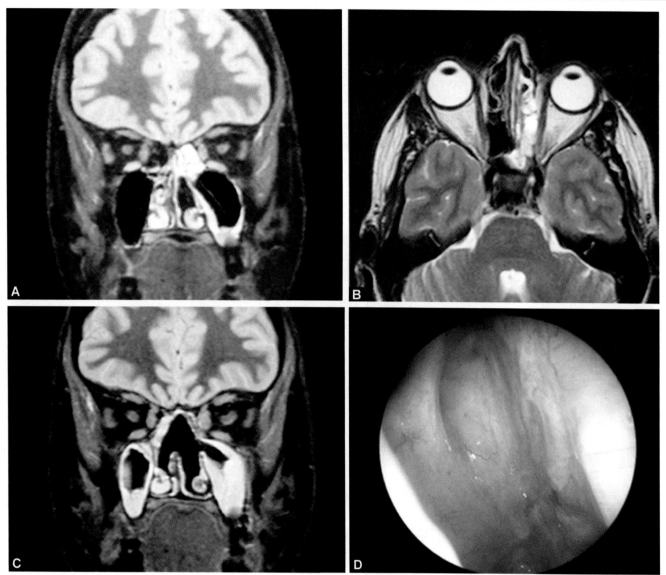

Figs 9.29A to D: Squamous cell carcinoma (SCC) of the left ethmoid sinus (T2 stage). (A) Preoperative T1-weighted coronal. (B) T2-weighted axial MR scans showing the contrast enhanced tumor in the left ethmoid. (C) T1-weighted coronal MR scan without signs of recurrency 2 years after complete endonasal microendoscopic tumor resection. (D) Postoperative appearance in the nasal airway and olfactory cleft

aerodigestive tract, they have not been shown to be causative in sinonasal carcinogenesis. The most frequent site of origin for SCC is the maxillary sinus, followed by the nasal cavity, ethmoid sinuses and sphenoid sinus.[62] Within the nasal cavity, SCC most commonly arises from the lateral wall.[1] The degree of differentiation does not carry as much prognostic significance as the stage of disease. In general, the 5-year disease-specific survival rate is around 55%.[3,43,57,66]

Endonasal microendoscopic resection of SCC we recommend only for T2 staged tumors that are located in the nasal cavity and the ethmoid sinus, respectively. One typical example is shown in Figs 9.29A to D. Possibly T3 tumors too might be removable by the endonasal approach if they only superficially infiltrate lamina papyracea and periorbit or the cribriforme plate, respectively. That applies to T4a tumors too if they only have grown into the sphenoid or frontal sinus. Maxillary sinus tumors should be removed unvariably via a trans-antral approach if necessary with maxillectomy.[5,43,57]

Adenocarcinoma (AC)

This is the second most common malignancy of the sinonasal cavities,[43] although in ours and some other

European series this tumor entity occurs more commonly than SCC.[3,66] They most commonly involve the ethmoid sinuses. There is a significantly higher incidence of AC in workers exposed to hard wood dust particles.[65] A variety of morphological forms have been described, which can be divided into well-differentiated types (solid, glandular and papillary) and further as intestinal types (papillary-tubular, alveolar-mucoid, signet ring and mixed).[1] Unlike SCC, the tumor grade has prognostic significance; high-grade neoplasms have a dismal prognosis, with approximately 20% 3-year survival.[1] All intestinal-type AC are considered high-grade; however, the papillary variant behaves more indolently.

Interestingly, all primary intestinal-type AC are reactive for CK20 and positive for CK7. Coordinate analyses of CK7 and CK20 reactivity may aid the differential diagnosis of AC in the sinonasal tract.[14]

The reported 5-year disease-specific survival rate vary widely between 30 and 80%.[3,43,57,66] Concerning endonasal microendoscopic tumor resection we follow the same principle as described for SCC, only T2 staged AC of the nasal cavity and the ethmoid sinus, respectively are suitable to be safely removed by this technique. T3 and T4 tumors are subject to the same restrictions as SCC. Figures 9.30A to D demonstrates a typical example.

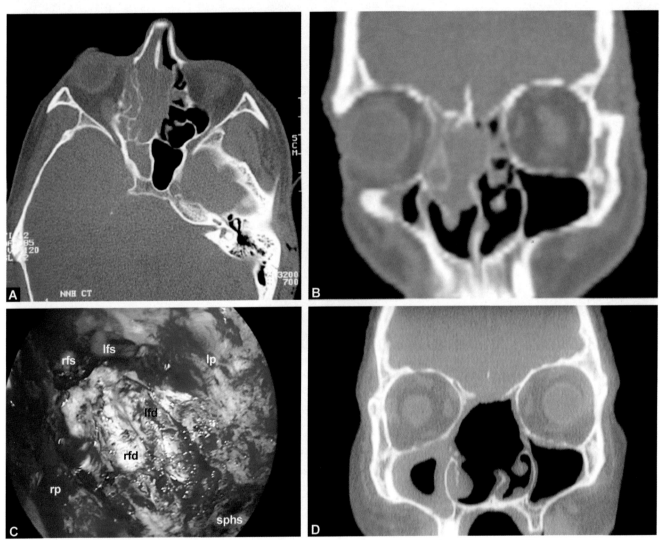

Figs 9.30A to D: Adenocarcinoma (AC) of the right ethmoid sinus extending into the sphenoid sinus and the nasal cavity as well as infiltrating the nasal septum (T4a stage according to the UICC because of the sphenoid sinus involvement. (A and B) Preoperative axial and coronal CT scans showing the space-occupying lesion. (C) View at the anterior skull-base at the end of the endonasal tumor resection: rfs = right frontal sinus, lfs = left frontal sinus, lp = left periorbit, rp = right periorbit, lfd = left frontal lobe dura, rfd = right frontal lobe dura, sphs = sphenoid sinus. (D) Postoperative coronal CT scan without signs of recurrence 4 years after primary endonasal surgery

Esthesioneuroblastoma (ENB)

ENB Also known as olfactory neuroblastoma, it is a rare neuroectodermal tumor originating from the olfactory epithelium. It accounts for about 3% of all intranasal tumors.[6] These tumors have no gender predilection and have a bimodal age distribution; one peak occurs in the second decade of life and the second peak in the sixth decade. ENB belongs to the category of 'small round cell tumors' (SRCT) such as primitive neuroectodermal tumors (PNET), rhabdomyosarcomas, neuroblastomas, small cell carcinomas, neuroendocrine carcinomas or malignant lymphomas.[67] Hyams proposed a histological grading system for ENB in which grade 1 tumors have an excellent prognosis and grade 4 tumors are uniformly fatal and histologically difficult to distinguish from other SRCT.[28] These tumors should be classified by the Morita staging system which is an extended Kadish categorization.[30,46] Nodal metastases is common, e.g. in patients with metastases in cervical lymph nodes survival was reported to be 29% compared to 64% for patients with N0 disease.[18] However, of most of the malignant sinonasal tumors invading the skull base, ENB have the most favorable prognosis with possible 5-year disease-specific survival rates of up to 90%.[3,37,42] Most authors favor a combination of surgery and radiotherapy achieving the highest cure rates.[4,18,42,57,66]

Endonasal microendoscopic resection of ENB can be advocated for tumors of Morita/Kadish stage A or B (no evidence of intracranial extension). Thereby, it is possible to resect the cribriform plate, the crista galli, the olfactory bulbs, and their surrounding dura along with the top of the septum and the middle turbinates where they are attached to the skull base.[3,9,12,60,72] Interestingly, compared to SCC many ENB also infiltrate the dura but less frequently the brain resulting in a much higher resectability. Figures 9.31A to D demonstrate a typical

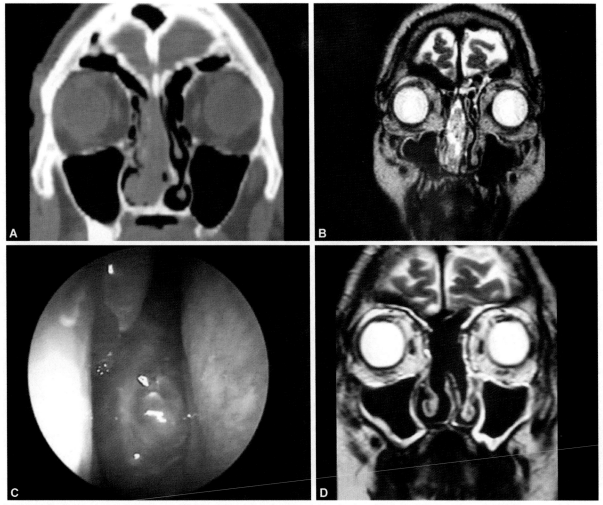

Figs 9.31A to D: Esthesioneuroblastoma (ENB) of the right nasal cavity and ethmoid sinus (Morita stage A). (A) Preoperative coronal CT scan. (B) Preoperative coronal T1-weighted contrast enhanced MR scan. (C) Tumor appearance in the right nasal cavity exhibiting a blue-red color. (D) Postoperative coronal T1-weighted MR scan without signs of recurrence 5 years after endonasal surgery

example of an ENB that can be resected via the endonasal routes. Although the series of tumors removed endonasally in conjunction with radiotherapy are few and limited they have not shown an increase in local recurrence rates or poorer prognosis.[3,12]

POSTOPERATIVE MANAGEMENT

Postoperative Course

In all cases with anterior skull-base resection (both cribriform plates and crista galli) and duraplasty or dura strengthening as well as in all cases with a large common nasal cavity it will be packed by a continuous ointment tamponade on a silicon sheet that is placed directly on the duraplasty. The silicon film helps re-epithelialization creating a moist chamber. If the tumor could be resected by an onesided paranasal sinus operation the nose will be packed with rubber finger stalls (Rhinotamp® from the Vostra Company). These will be removed 3 to 7 days postoperatively. In all expanded endonasal resections the silicon film and the ointment tamponade will be taken out after 10 days. Usually, the patients are hospitalized for 3 to 10 days, depending on the severity. At the time of nasal package the patients are given antibiotics (usually cephalosporin of the second generation).

After removal of the nasal package the patients have to nurse their noses, i.e. use greasy ointment several times a day and if necessary get gentle debridement at an outpatient visit. In all cases without duraplasty we recommend ample douching with a physiological salt solution at least twice a day. In this regard, the patients have to know that if there was full-thickness mucosal excision it may take up to one year for normalization and a possible restart of cilia function.[59] With superficial mucosal damage it may take only several weeks.[59] Figures 9.32A to D demonstrate the postoperative wound healing after anterior skull-base resection.

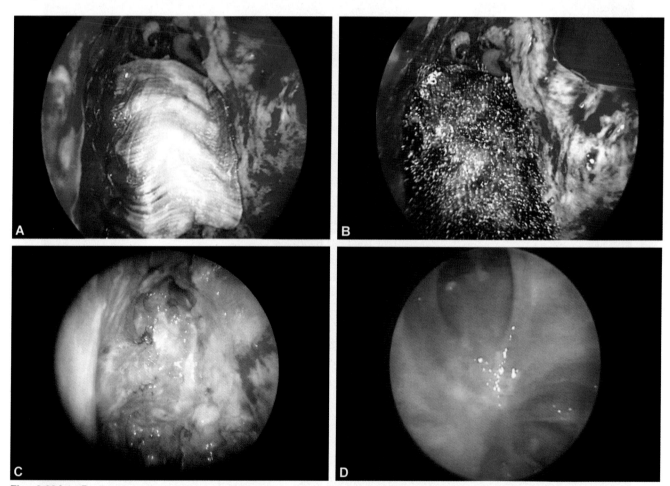

Figs 9.32A to D: Postoperative appearance of the nasal airway and anterior skull base in the same patient (from Fig. 9.30); (A) At the end of the operation when the dura was covered with Tutoplast Fascia Lata® of the Tutogen Medical Company. (B) with surgical on top for stabilization. (C) Condition after 6 months still showing granulation. (D) Condition 1,5 years after primary treatment presenting normal mucosa

Follow-up

Generally, follow-up consisted of endoscopic examination of the nasal cavity and MR imaging. In all malignant tumors we perform regular clinical controls quarterly in the first and second year after operation, in the third year twice an year and thereafter only annually. Three months after surgery we usually perform an MRI scan of the paranasal sinuses and the skull-base, respectively, as well as of the neck to exclude lymph node metastases. Afterwards MRI is repeated once an year. Importantly, preoperative staging includes thoracic CT, which postoperatively will also be repeated yearly, since solitary metastases are respectable. This regimen was recommend by the authors for inverted papilloma and juvenile angiofibroma too, except in neck and thoracic imaging. In fibrous dysplasia, ossifying fibroma, paraganglioma and mucoceles we follow our patients quarterly only in the first year and then simply yearly. Patients with other benign tumors will have the first postoperative control 3 months after surgery including a CT (in osteomas) or an MRI; thereafter they will only have endoscopic examination yearly.

CONCLUSION

The concept of endonasal microendoscopic surgery is no longer an alternative but a very valid treatment modality in tumor surgery of the nasal cavity, paranasal sinuses and the anterior and central skull-base. Therefore, it is always essential to check whether the endonasal approach is possible. In principle, surgery in this field should be as extensive as necessary, but as minimally traumatic as possible but to do this requires a lot of experience. In our hands following a stepladder of four surgical techniques: (Endonasal, Midfacial degloving[10], Osteoplastic frontal sinus approach, Subcranial approach according to Raveh[53] has proved to be very efficient), the advantage of all these approaches is avoidance of visible scars, a fact very much appreciated by the patients. The lateral rhinotomy is generally reserved if exenteration of the orbit is needed simultaneously.[16] However, individual anatomy and pathology and the personal experience of the surgeon ultimately lead to the choice of approach and operative treatment.

The key to success in endonasal microendoscopic surgery is locating the origin of the tumor, defining its extent, and completely removing all diseased tissue including the surrounding normal mucosa. So far, results achieved by this approach are comparable to those of external procedures. The following preconditions should be realized for successful removal of the disease and consideration of functional and aesthetic aspects:

1. Extensive experience in endonasal surgery (sinusitis, traumatology, duraplasty).
2. Vast experience in head and neck tumor surgery.
3. Optimized technical equipment (both microscope and endoscope, navigation).
4. Experience in control of complications.
5. Strict follow-up of the patients using endoscope and CT or MR imaging is mandatory.
6. Interdisciplinary working with neurosurgeons and neuroradiologists is important.

ACKNOWLEDGMENTS

To Professor W Draf for surgical teaching and his comments on the manuscript.

To Professor E Hofmann, Head of the Neuroradiology Department at the Klinikum Fulda gAG, for imaging and embolization.

REFERENCES

1. Batsakis J. Pathology of tumors of the nasal cavity and paranasal sinuses. In *Comprehensive management of head and neck tumors,* Thawley SE (Ed) Philadelphia: WB Saunders, 1999; 522–539.
2. Bielamowicz S, Calcaterra TC, Watson D. Inverting papilloma of the head and neck: the UCLA update. *Otolaryngol Head Neck Surg* 1993; 109:71–76.
3. Bockmühl U, Minovi A, Kratzsch B, Hendus J, Draf W. Stellenwert der endonasalen mikro-endoskopischen Tumorchirurgie. *Laryngol Rhinol Otol* 2005; 84:884–891.
4. Bradley PJ, Jones NS, Robertson I. Diagnosis and management of esthesioneuroblastoma. *Curr Opin Otolaryngol Head Neck Surg* 2003; 11:112–118.
5. Bridger GP, Kwok B, Baldwin M, Williams JR, Smee RI. Craniofacial resection for paranasal sinus cancers. *Head Neck* 2000; 22:772–780.
6. Broich G, Pagliari A, Ottaviani F. Esthesioneuroblastoma: a general review of the cases published since the discovery of the tumour in 1924. *Anticancer Res* 1997; 17:2683–2706.
7. Calcaterra TC, Thompson JW, Paglia DE. Inverting papillomas of the nose and paranasal sinuses. *Laryngoscope* 1980; 90: 53–60.
8. Cantu G, Solero CL, Mariani L, Salvatori P, Mattavelli F, Pizzi N, Riggio E. Anterior craniofacial resection for malignant ethmoid tumors—a series of 91 patients. *Head Neck* 1999; 21:185–191.
9. Casiano RR, Numa WA, Falquez AM. Endoscopic resection of olfactory neuroblastoma. *Am J Rhinol* 2000; 15:271–279.

10. Casson PR, Bonnano PC, Converse JM. The midfacial degloving procedure. *Plast Reconstr Surg* 1974; 53:102–113.

11. Castelnuovo P, Belli E, Bignami M, Battaglia P, Sberze F, Tomei G. Endoscopic nasal and anterior craniotomy resection for malignant nasoethmoid tumors involving the anterior skull-base. *Skull Base Surg* 2006; 16(1):25–30.

12. Chandler JR, Goulding R, Moskowitz L. Nasopharyngeal angiofibroma: staging and management. Ann Otol Rhinol Laryngol 1984; 93:322–329.

13. Choi HR, Sturgis EM, Rashid A. Sinonasal adenocarcinoma: evidence for histogenetic divergence of the enteric and non-enteric phenotypes. *Hum Pathol* 2003; 34:1101–1107.

14. Demers PA, Kogevinas M, Bofetta P. Wood dust and sinonasal cancer: pooled re-analysis of twelve case–control studies. *Am J Ind Med* 1995; 28:151–166.

15. Draf W. Endonasal frontal sinus drainage type I–III according to Draf. In *The frontal sinus*, Kountakis S, Senior B, Draf W (Eds) Berlin: Springer, 2005; 219–232.

16. Draf W, Schick B, Weber R, Keerl R, Saha A. Endonasal micro-endoscopic surgery of nasal and paranasal sinus tumors. In *Micro-endoscopic surgery of the paranasal sinuses and the skull-base*, Stamm AC, Draf W (Eds) New York: Springer, 2000; 481–488.

17. Dulguerov P, Allal AS, Calcaterra TC. Esthesioneuroblastoma: A meta-analysis and review. *Lancet Oncol* 2001; 2:683–690.

18. Fagan JJ, Snyderman CH, Carrau RL, Janecka IP. Nasopharyngeal angiofibromas: selecting a surgical approach. *Head Neck* 1997; 19:391–399.

19. Fisch U. The infratemporal fossa approach for nasopharyngeal tumors. *Laryngoscope* 1983; 93:36–44.

20. Fliss DM, Zucker G, Cohen A, Amir A, Sagi A, Rosenberg L, Leiberman A, Gatot A, Reichenthal E. Early outcome and complications of the extended subcranial approach to the anterior skull-base. *Laryngoscope* 1999; 109:153–160.

21. Gaffey MJ, Frierson HF, Weiss LM, Barber CM, Baber GB, Stoler MH. Human papillomavirus and Epstein–Barr virus in sinonasal Schneiderian papillomas. An *in situ* hybridization and polymerase chain reaction study. *Am J Clin Pathol* 1996; 106:475–482.

22. Ganly I, Patel SG, Singh B, Kraus DH, Bridger PG, Cantu G, Cheesman A, De Sa G, Donald P, Fliss DM, Gullane P, Janecka I, Kamata SE, Kowalski LP, Levine PA, Medina Dos Santos LR, Pradhan S, Schramm V, Snyderman C, Wei WI, Shah JP. Craniofacial resection for malignant paranasal sinus tumors: Report of an International Collaborative Study. *Head Neck* 2005; 27:575–584.

23. Goepfert H, Cangir A, Lee YY. Chemotherapy for aggressive juvenile nasopharyngeal angiofibroma. *Arch Otolaryngol* 1985; 111:285–289.

24. Gullane PJ, Davidson J, O'Dwyer T, Forte V. Juvenile angiofibroma: a review of the literature and a case series report. *Laryngoscope* 1992; 102:928–933.

25. Howard D, Lund VJ. Surgical options in the management of nose and sinus neoplasia. In *Tumours of the upper jaw* Harrison DF, Lund VJ (eds). Edinburgh: Churchill Livingstone, 1993; 329–336.

26. Hyams VJ. Papillomas of the nasal cavity and paranasal sinuses. A clinicopathological study of 315 cases. *Ann Otol Rhinol Laryngol* 1971; 80:192–206.

27. Hyams VJ, Batsakis JG, Michaels L. Olfactory neuroblastoma. In *Tumors of the upper respiratory tract and ear*, (Eds) Hyams VJ, Batsakis BJ, Michaels L. (Eds) Washington: Armed Forces Institute of Pathology, 1988; 240–248.

28. Janecka IP, Sen C, Sekhar LN, Ramasastry S, Curtin HD, Barnes EL, D'Amico F. Cranial base surgery: Results in 183 patients. *Otolaryngol Head Neck Surg* 1994; 110:539–546.

29. Kadish S, Goodman M, Wang CC. Olfactory neuroblastoma. A clinical analysis of 17 cases. *Cancer* 1976; 37:1571–1576.

30. Kamal SA. Inverted papilloma of the nose. *J Laryngol Otol* 1981; 95:1069–1079.

31. Kassam A, Snyderman CH, Mintz A, Gardner P, Carrau RL. Expanded endonasal approach: The rostrocaudal axis. Part I. Crista galli to the sella turcica. *Neurosurg Focus* 2005; 19:E3.

32. Kassam A, Snyderman CH, Mintz A, Gardner P, Carrau RL. Expanded endonasal approach: The rostrocaudal axis. Part II. Posterior clinoids to the foramen magnum. *Neurosurg Focus* 2005; 19:E4.

33. Kraft M, Simmen D, Kaufmann T, Holzmann D. Long–term results of endonasal sinus surgery in sinonasal papillomas. *Laryngoscope* 2003; 113:1541–1547.

34. Krouse JH. Development of a staging system for inverted papilloma. *Laryngoscope* 2000; 110:965–968.

35. Lawson W, Kaufman MR, Biller HF. Treatment outcomes in the management of inverted papilloma: an analysis of 160 cases. *Laryngoscope* 2003; 113:1548–1556.

36. Levine PA, Debo RF, Meredith SD, Jane JA, Constable WC, Cantrell RW. Craniofacial resection at the University of Virginia (1976–1992): Survival analysis. *Head Neck* 1994; 16:574–577.

37. Llorente JL, Deleyiannis F, Rodrigo JP, Nunez F, Ablanedo P, Melon S, Suarez C. Minimally invasive treatment of the nasal inverted papilloma. *Am J Rhinol* 2003; 17:335–341.

38. London SD, Schlosser RJ, Gross CW. Endoscopic management of benign sinonasal tumors: A decade of experience. *Am J Rhinol* 2002; 16:221–227.

39. Luce D, Leclerc A, Begin D. Sinonasal cancer and occupational exposures: a pooled analysis of 12 case-control studies. *Cancer Causes Control* 2002; 13:147–157.

40. Lund VJ. Optimum management of inverted papilloma. *J Laryngol Otol* 2000; 114:194–197.

41. Lund VJ, Howard D, Wei WI. Olfactory neuroblastoma: past, present and future? *Laryngoscope* 2003; 113:502–507.

42. Maghami E, Kraus DH. Cancer of the nasal cavity and paranasal sinuses. *Expert Rev Anticancer Ther* 2004; 4:411–424.

43. Miller PJ, Jacobs J, Roland JT, Cooper J, Mizrachi HH. Intracranial inverting papilloma. *Head Neck* 1996; 18:450–454.

44. Minovi A, Kollert M, Draf W, Bockmühl U. Inverted papilloma: Feasibility of endonasal surgery and long-term results of 87 cases. *Rhinology* 2006; 44:205–210.

45. Morita AEM, Olsen KD, Foote RL, Lewis JE, Quast LM. Esthesioneuroblastoma: prognosis and management. *Neurosurgery* 1993; 32:706–715.

46. Namdar I, Edelstein DR, Hup J, Lazar A, Kimmelmann CP, Soletic R. Management of osteomas of the paranasal sinuses. *Am J Rhinol* 1998; 12:393–398.

47. Nicolai P, Berlucchi M, Tomenzoli D, Cappiello J, Trimarchi M, Maroldi R, Battaglia G, Antonelli AR. Endoscopic surgery for juvenile angiofibroma: when and how. *Laryngoscope* 2003; 113:775–782.

48. Ojiri H, Ujita M, Tada S, Fukuda K. Potentially distinctive features of sinonasal inverted papilloma on MR imaging. *Am J Roentgenol* 2000; 175:465–468.

49. O'Sullivan B, Shah JP. New TNM staging criteria for head and neck tumors. *Semin Surg Oncol* 2003; 21:30–42.

50. Pedersen E, Hogetveit AC, Andersen A. Cancer of respiratory organs among workers at a nickel refinery in Norway. *Int J Cancer* 1973; 12:32–41.

51. Phillips PP, Gustafson RO, Facer GW. The clinical behavior of inverting papilloma of the nose and paranasal sinuses: report of 112 cases and review of the literature. *Laryngoscope* 1990; 100:463–469.

52. Raveh J, Turk JB, Ladrach K, Seiler R, Godoy N, Chen J, Paladino J, Virag M, Leibinger K. Extended anterior subcranial approach for skull-base tumors: long–term results. *J Neurosurg* 1995; 82:1002–1010.

53. Schick B, El Tahan AER, Brors D, Kahle G, Draf W. Experiences with endonasal surgery in angiofibroma. *Rhinology* 1999; 37:80–85.

54. Schick B, Steigerwald C, El Tahan AER, Draf W. The role of endonasal surgery in the management of frontoethmoidal osteomas. *Rhinology* 2001; 39:66–70.

55. Shady JA, Bland LI, Kazee AM, Pilcher WH. Osteoma of the frontoethmoidal sinus with secondary abscess and intracranial mucocele: Case report. *Neurosurgery* 1994; 34:920–923.

56. Shah JP, Kraus DH, Bilsky MH, Gutin PH, Harrison LH, Strong EW. Craniofacial resection for malignant tumors involving the anterior skull-base. *Arch Otolaryngol Head Neck Surg* 1997; 123:1312–1317.

57. Shanmugaratnam KSL. Histological typing of tumours of the upper respiratory tract and ear. World Health Organization. Berlin: Springer-Verlag, 1991.

58. Shaw CK, Cowin A, Wormald PJ. A study of the normal temporal healing pattern and the mucociliary transport after endoscopic partial and full-thickness removal of nasal mucosa in sheep. *Immunol Cell Biol* 2001; 79:145–148.

59. Simmen D, Jones NS. Manual of endoscopic sinus surgery and its extended applications. Stuttgart: Thieme, 2005.

60. Smith ME, Calcaterra TC. Frontal sinus osteoma. *Ann Otol Rhinol Laryngol* 1989; 98:896–900.

61. Spiro JD, Soo KC, Spiro RH. Squamous cell carcinoma of the nasal cavity and paranasal sinuses. *Am J Surg* 1989; 158: 328–332.

62. Stamm AC, Watashi CH, Malheiros PF, Harker LA, Pignatari SSN. Micro-endoscopic surgery of benign sino-nasal tumors. In *Micro-endoscopic surgery of the paranasal sinuses and the skull base*, Stamm AC, Draf W. (Eds) New York: Springer, 2000; 489–514.

63. Stammberger H, Anderhuber W, Walch C, Papaefthymiou G. Possibilities and limitations of endoscopic management of nasal and paranasal sinus malignancies. *Acta Otorhino-laryngol Belg* 1999; 53:199–205.

64. Stern S, Hanna E. Cancer of the nasal cavity and paranasal sinuses. In *Cancer of the head and neck* Myers EN (ed). Philadelphia: WB Saunders, 1996; 205–233.

65. Suarez C, Llorente JL, Fernandez De Leon R, Maseda E, Lopez A. Prognostic factors in sinonasal tumors involving the anterior skull-base. *Head Neck* 2004; 26:136–144.

66. Tarkkanen M, Knuutila S. The diagnostic use of cytogenetic and molecular genetic techniques in the assessment of small round cell tumors. *Curr Diagn Pathol* 2002; 8:338–348.

67. Tomenzoli D, Castelnuovo P, Pagella F, Berlucchi M, Pianta L, Delù G, Maroldi R, Nicolai P. Different endoscopic surgical strategies in the management of inverted papilloma of the sinonasal tract: experience with 47 patients. *Laryngoscope* 2004; 114:193–200.

68. Tufano RP, Thaler ER, Lanza DC, Goldberg AN, Kennedy DW. Endoscopic management of sinonasal inverted papilloma. *Am J Rhinol* 1999; 13:423–426.

69. Ungkanont K, Byers RM, Weber RS, Callender DL, Wolf PF, Goepfert H. Juvenile nasopharyngeal angiofibroma: An update of therapeutic management. *Head Neck* 1996; 18: 60–66.

70. Von Buchwald C, Larsen AS. Endoscopic surgery of inverted papillomas under image guidance: A prospective study of 42 consecutive cases at a Danish University Clinic. *Otolaryngol Head Neck Surg* 2005; 132:602–607.

71. Walch C, Stammberger H, Anderhuber W, Unger F, Kole W, Feichtinger K. The minimally invasive approach to olfactory neuroblastoma: Combined endoscopic and stereotactic treatment. *Laryngoscope* 2000; 110:635–640.

72. Winter M, Rauer RA, Gode U, Waitz G, Wigand ME. Invertierte Papillome der Nase und der Nasennebenhöhlen. Langzeiterge-bnisse nach endoskopischer endonasaler Resektion. *Head Neck Oncol* 2000; 48:568–572.

73. Witt TR, Shah JP, Sternberg SS. Juvenile nasopharyngeal angiofibroma: a 30-year clinical review. *Am J Surg* 1983; 146:521–525.

74. Wolfe SG, Schlosser RJ, Bolger WE, Lanza DC, Kennedy DW. Endoscopic and endoscope-assisted resections of inverted sinonasal papillomas. *Otolaryngol Head Neck Surg* 2004; 131:174–179.

75. Wormald PJ, Ooi E, van Hasselt CA, Nair S. Endoscopic removal of sinonasal inverted papilloma including endoscopic medial maxillectomy. *Laryngoscope* 2003; 113:867–873.

Management of Complications in Endonasal Microendoscopic Surgery

Ulrike Bockmühl, Wolfgang Draf

The paranasal sinuses present a complex anatomy surrounded by important structures, such as the anterior and middle cranial fossae, the orbit and its contents, vascular structures (including the internal carotid arteries, the anterior and posterior ethmoid arteries, the maxillary arteries and their branches), the cavernous sinus and cranial nerves I–VI. The risk of damaging these structures during microendoscopic sinus surgery must be always considered. The possible complications can be classified according to severity as *minor* and *major* and according to the time of appearance as *immediate* or *delayed*.

Minor complications are those that present little morbidity and do not compromise the life of the patient. They occur in 2–21% of patients who undergo endonasal sinus surgery.[3,11,12] and include synechias, crusts, minor bleeding, nasal-septum perforation, headache, facial pain, alteration of dental sensitivity, edema, local infection, periorbital ecchymosis, palpebral edema, subcutaneous emphysema or paraffin granuloma due to ointment packages (Figs 9.33A and B), stenosis of sinus ostia, postoperative sinusitis, epiphora, hyposmia and exacerbation of bronchial asthma. In cases of frontal sinus dranage type III scarring at the upper lip caused by the burr (Figs 9.34A and B) or a dimple in the lateral nasal wall due to a through and through resection of the frontal process of the maxilla (Figs 9.35A and B).

Major complications present significant morbidity and a possibility of mortality. They comprise:

1. Orbital injuries, i.e. damage of the optical nerve or the extraocular muscles resulting in orbital hematoma, diplopia, proptosis, decrease of visual acuity or blindness.
2. Intracranial damage, i.e. cerebrospinal fluid (CSF) leak, intracranial hemorrhage and hematoma, damage to the brain itself, meningitis, cerebral abscess, damage to the olfactory nerve, injury to cranial nerves III–VI, pneumocephalus or stroke.
3. Bleeding (including intracranial bleeding) due to injury of the internal carotid, ethmoidal and maxillary arteries and the cavernous sinus.

The reported incidence of major complications due to endonasal sinus surgery varies between 0.75 and 8%.[3,4,10,14,16] The most frequent immediate complications are CSF leakage, intraoperative bleeding and orbital hematoma. Delayed complications include meningitis, progressive loss of vision or smell, bleeding, synechia and infection.[3,9,14]

There are several risk factors that may increase the possibility of complications: previous sinus surgery leading to the absence of anatomical landmarks, bleeding, infection, extensive disease and inexperience of the surgeon.

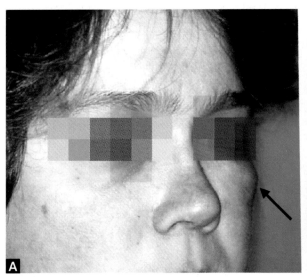
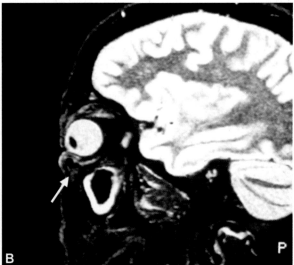

Figs 9.33A and B: (A) Patient 4 weeks after sinus surgery showing paraffin granuloma within the left lower lid due to ointment packages. (B) T1-weighted sagittal MRI presenting a hypodense lesion within the lower lid corresponding to the paraffin granuloma

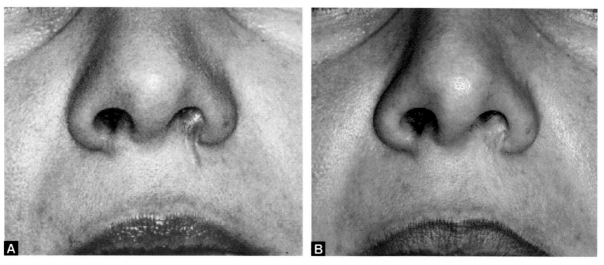

Figs 9.34A and B: (A) Scarring at the upper lip caused by a hot burr during frontal sinus drainage type III after 4 weeks. (B) and after six months

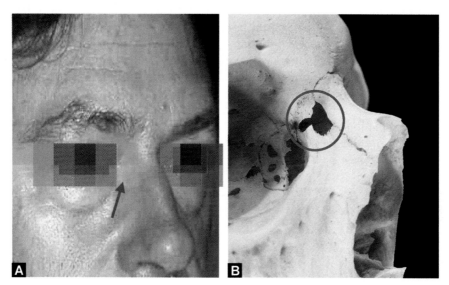

Figs 9.35A and B: (A) Patient showing a dimple in the right lateral nasal wall due to a through and through resection of the frontal process of the maxilla. (B) Cadaver dissection demonstrating a similar defect

To avoid complications of endonasal microendoscopic sinus surgery adequate preoperative examination of the patient is the first step. This mainly includes clinical history as well as sinonasal endoscopy and imaging studies. The latter principally consists of high resolution axial computed tomography (CT) with coronal and sagittal reconstructions. They are mandatory in paranasal sinus surgery. In addition, magnetic resonance imaging (MRI) should always be considered in malignancies and in cases of unilateral lesions, e.g. to look for a possible inverted papilloma.

ORBITAL COMPLICATIONS

The greatest danger of injury to the orbital cavity occurs during ethmoidectomy and sphenoethmoidectomy, respectively. This is due to the extensive and intimate anatomic relationship between the ethmoid cells and the orbit and because of the run of the optic nerve along or through the sphenoid sinus. Occasionally middle meatal antrostomy may prove dangerous, usually when the maxillary sinus is small and the inferior turbinate has a high bony insertion. Therefore, when operating in the paranasal sinuses, it is best to have the eyes exposed and kept moist with simple eye ointment and to ask the assistant to look for any eye movement and for pupil differences.

Violation of the Orbit with Fat Herniation

If the lamina papyracea is cracked or a segment is removed during the procedure, this may cause a minor ecchymosis. This will settle spontaneously in 3-4 days. In case of a defect of the orbital wall, with disruption of the periorbit, the orbital contents protrude into the nasal airway. Although fat has a yellow hue, it can look remarkably like nasal polyps. Palpation of the closed eye by the assistant, or the surgeon, will tell whether it is orbital fat as it will move abruptly with this maneuver. If it is fat, do not panic; there is a temptation to push it back into the orbit (this will fail), to pull it out (this will make the damage to the orbit worse), or to cauterize it. None of these is necessary and they may cause more harm. If powered instrumentation is being used, this should be stopped because the suction can easily remove the fat, which is then sheared off, and this makes matters worse. If the surgeon is experienced enough to continue, placing a moist neurosurgical patte over the fat can protect this area while the rest of the procedure is completed. As long as the only damage done is opening the periosteum, the only problem will be some periorbital ecchymosis or hematoma (Fig. 9.36).

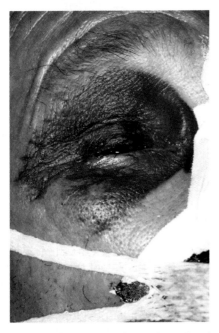

Fig. 9.36: Periorbital hematoma due to damaging the lamina papyracea and opening the periosteum

The patient should be advised to avoid blowing the nose or stifling any sneezes for 8 days in order to prevent periorbital emphysema. It is best to give prophylactic antibiotics to avoid the theoretical risk of orbital cellulites. The tension within the orbit should be monitored by gently comparing it with the other eye to ensure there is no bleeding or pressure building up in the posterior compartment. If the globe is tense and proptosed then decompression may be required. Moreover, the axis of the pupils should also be checked. If it is altered, this may indicate that a considerable amount of the orbital contents has been removed or proptosed into the airway, or the medial rectus muscle has been damaged. Under these circumstances, an urgent ophthalmological opinion should be sought.

Retro-orbital Hemorrhage

In the majority of patients the anterior ethmoid artery is dehiscent at some point.[5] The surgeon should avoid damaging it. If the artery is simply opened gentle bipolar diathermy will arrest bleeding. While tearing it can cause marked bleeding, the main concern is that if it is transacted and it retracts back into the orbit, this can cause considerable increase of the pressure in the posterior compartment of the eye and place the retinal artery and its supply to the retina at risk. If there is significant bleeding into the posterior compartment of the orbit, the eye will proptose, the orbit will become very firm, and the pupil will dilatate. After a few minutes the flashlight test will reveal an afferent defect, i.e. there will be no constriction of the pupil by light stimulation. A patient who is awake will mention a reduction or loss of vision. In this situation treatment must be undertaken as quickly as possible in order to avoid secondary damage to the optic nerve.[13] Some evidence suggests that the optic nerve can withstand ischemia for up to one hour.[2] Therefore, one should not wait for an ophthalmologist to arrive unless they will do so well within one hour. Assessing the vascular supply of the retinal vessels with an ophthalmoscope is inadequate and should not be relied upon. To diminish the ocular pressure large doses of steroids can be additionally administered. To decompress the orbit in the fastest way we recommend performing a lateral canthotomy and cantholysis of the lower lid as this is both quick and efficient and is associated with minimum morbidity.

Figures 9.37A to C show an example of a lateral canthotomy and inferior cantholysis. After local anesthesia a straight scissors should be used to divide

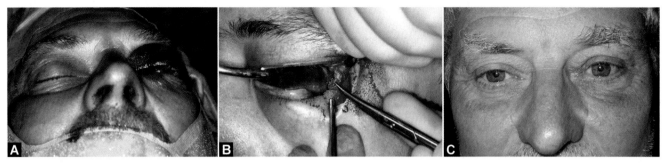

Figs 9.37A to C: (A) Example of a left side retro-orbital hemorrhage due to endonasal sinus surgery. (B) Technique of a lateral canthotomy and an inferior cantholysis. Cut of the left lateral canthus down to the bone of the orbital rim and to the depth of the lateral sulcus of the conjunctiva. (C) Patient six months after lateral canthotomy with imperceptible aesthetic and functional result

the lateral canthus down to the bone of the orbital rim and to the depth of the lateral sulcus of the conjunctiva. It is important to protect the globe in order to avoid corneal abrasion or conjunctival damage. The lower lid is then retracted downward to subsequently divide the lateral ligament and the septum orbitale using the scissors. This makes the globe as well as the contents of the orbit prolapsing forward. Only little blood-stained exudates will come out, but do not expect much bleeding and do not probe into the posterior compartment of the orbit. Usually suturing is not required. Immediately after this procedure the pupil reflexes, the pressure of the orbit and the vision will recover. Over the next 2–3 days, the orbit will retract to its normal position and the incision will normally be almost imperceptible as it fades into the crow's foot of the eye (Figs 9.37A to C).

Damage of the Medial Rectus Muscle

In the anterior half of the orbit the external eye muscles are well protected by a major layer of orbital fat. This decreases the more one is going backwards. Medial rectus damage occurs usually through deeper penetration into the orbit as a result of inattention, particularly in the posterior compartment: If the orbital periosteum is traversed, the assistant should notice movement of the globe. The surgeon has to be very cautious while operating on the lateral nasal wall in this area. Unfortunately, even if it is recognized at the time, it is very difficult to prevent scarring and diplopia that are likely to result. To investigate the possibility of reparative surgery, persistent diplopia needs to be evaluated by CT and by an ophthalmologist. Figures 9.38A and B presents a coronal CT and MR image, respectively, showing damage to the left medial rectus muscle.

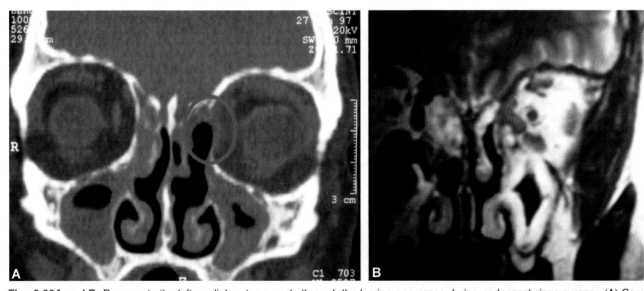

Figs 9.38A and B: Damage to the left medial rectus muscle through the lamina papyracea during endonasal sinus surgery. (A) Coronal CT scan showing the bony defect of the lamina papyracea. (B) T2-weighted coronal MRI showing the deformed medial rectus muscle (red)

Optic Nerve Lesion

Direct or indirect damage to the optic nerve usually occurs from the use of forceps or electrocautery on the superior-lateral sphenoid sinus wall or in the posterior ethmoid cells, especially the Onodi cell. The optic nerve can be prominent in 20% of patients in the upper half of the lateral wall of the sphenoid sinus, but is rarely dehiscent.[8] Figure 9.39 shows an axial CT scan of a patient with dehiscent right optic nerve. Another cause of blindness during sinus surgery can be penetration of the orbit through the lamina papyracea. In these situations, loss of vision can be partial or total. When there is no direct injury of the optic nerve, vision can recover; nasal packing should then be removed, large doses of steroids should be administered to decompress the nerve. However, if the assistant looks out for the eye movement when the surgeon is operating on the lateral wall, it is unlikely that the nerve could be damaged before it was noted that the orbit had been entered.

Bleeding

Intraoperative or postoperative bleeding resulting from paranasal sinus operations originates from the internal carotid artery system via the anterior or posterior ethmoid arteries, which are branches of the ophthalmic artery. Bleeding can also originate from the external carotid artery via the maxillary artery and its terminal branches. In general, there is an increased risk for bleeding in patients who have undergone previous surgery because of the formation of new vessels in the operated area.

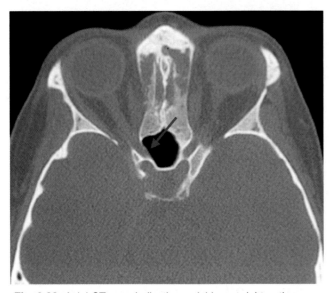

Fig. 9.39: Axial CT scan indication a dehiscent right optic nerve

If there is excessive bleeding, check that the patient is 20° body-up and that the arterial mean pressure is maintained at 65–74 mmHg and the heart rate below 60 beats per minute. Use copped swabs soaked in naphazoline hydrochloride or neurosurgical patte soaked in epinephrine (1:10000) on the side with the bleeding and move on to work on the other side while bleeding abates. It is possible to work from side to side, transferring the pack periodically. If in spite of these measures there is still bleeding that cannot be controlled by diathermy and cleared with a larger sucker, then stop operating and have a further trial of medical treatment. The patient's safety is the primary concern.

Sphenopalatine Artery

There are several branches of the sphenopalatine artery that can be damaged during sinus surgery. The anterior branches come through the lateral nasal wall directly above the attachment of the inferior turbinate. If the middle meatal antrostomy is opened widely up to the posterior wall of the maxillary antrum, a branch of the sphenopalatine artery will often be cut and require cautery. Another branch comes through the middle turbinate, and if more than half of the anterior part of the middle turbinate is removed, this artery often bleeds. The septal branch from the posterior tributary of the sphenopalatine artery runs across the anterior wall of the sphenoid sinus. If the sphenoid ostium is opened lower to the floor of the sinus, this branch will be found and it can bleed substantially.

If electrocoagulation or dry drilling with the diamond burr is not sufficient to stop bleeding the maxillary artery should be clipped within the pterygopalatine fossa after removing the posterior wall of the maxillary sinus. In case this also fails embolization via digital substraction angiography is indicated.

Ethmoid Arteries

Damage of the anterior and posterior ethmoid arteries can have serious consequences like retro-orbital hemorrhage (see above). To stop bleeding from these vessels, one can use either bipolar forceps or unipolar suction diathermy (Figs 9.40A and B). Some of the bipolar suction forceps now available help to remove the blood and smoke at the same time. One has to be careful not to introduce the electrocautery forceps into the arterial canal, which has been described to may result in a CSF leak.[9] When cautery is performed at the level of the posterior ethmoid artery, propagation of heat can damage the optic

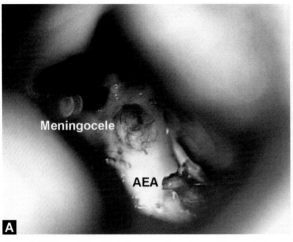 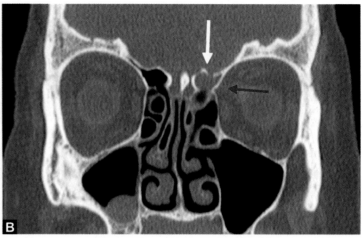

Figs 9.40A and B: (A) Intraoperative situs after exploring a spontaneous meningocele at the anterior ethmoid roof in front of the anterior ethmoid artery (AEA) which was electrocoagulated. (B) CT scan in axial reconstruction showing a bony defect (white arrow) at the left anterior ethmoid roof in front of the anterior ethmoid artery (red arrow)

nerve. In revision cases there is an increased risk of bleeding, and due to retraction of the ethmoid arteries into their canal, bleeding from these arteries can be difficult to identify when it occurs at the point where it leaves the canal.

If it is impossible to control bleeding that originates from the ethmoid arteries via the endonasal route, an external approach through the orbit is preferable, electrocoagulating or clipping the anterior and posterior ethmoid artery with bipolar cautery under microscopic view.

Internal Carotid Artery and Cavernous Sinus

Injury to the internal carotid artery (ICA) and the cavernous sinus produce severe bleeding that puts the life of the patient at risk. These injuries are occasionally seen in sphenoid-sinus surgery and should be avoided by good preoperative image evaluation since the prevalence of anatomical variations is well documented. Usually, the septum sinuum sphenoidalium is going straight to one of the carotid arteries; sometimes, it is split going to both sides. The internal carotid arteries can be exposed and dehiscent within the sphenoid sinus (Fig. 9.41). Depending on the extent of the injury, control of bleeding originating from the ICA can be accomplished trying to close the defect with Tutoplast Fascia Lata® of the Tutogen Medical Company and packing the sphenoid sinus with surgical (and fibrine glue), compressing the carotid artery in the neck, hypotensive anesthesia and blood transfusion. If the bleeding persists, digital subtraction angiography using a detachable intravascular balloon is indicated.[1] However, even if the bleeding from

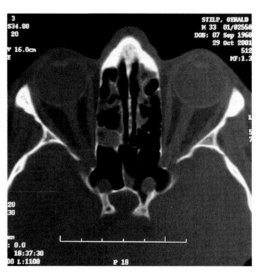

Fig. 9.41: Anatomical variation of the carotid arteries being both exposed and dehiscent within the sphenoid sinus and implicating also dehiscent optic nerves

the ICA could be stopped by packing a digital subtraction angiography should be performed in any case to exclude intracerebral bleeding and to search for possible aneurysmata or a dissection of the ICA. Figures 9.42A to D show a patient whose left ICA was damaged during sinus surgery. Immediate postoperative angiography explained an aneurysma spurium of the ICA which could be successfully coiled.

Injuries to the walls of the cavernous sinus are repaired by packing with surgical, fat or muscle and fibrin glue.

Injury to the roof of the ethmoid cells, with penetration into the region of the frontal lobe, can also disrupt the

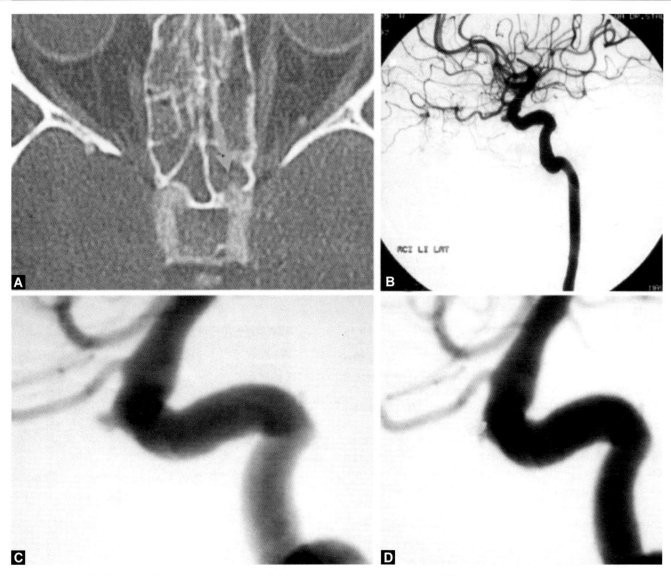

Figs 9.42A to D: (A) Axial CT scan after damaging the left internal carotid artery (ICA) during endonasal sinus surgery (arrow). (B and C) After packaging immediate postoperative angiography explained an aneurysma spurium of the left ICA which. (D) Could be successfully embolized

frontopolar branch of the anterior cerebral artery, requiring immediate imaging evaluation (CT and MRI, possibly also angiography). This type of damage produces ischemia, vascular spasms and focal neurologic deficits.[9] Although, the management is described to be primarily medical[9], severe intracranial bleeding may require craniotomy (Figs 9.43A and B).

Intracranial Lesions

Damage of the anterior skull base can produce leakage of cerebrospinal fluid (CSF), meningitis, tension pneumocephalus, brain hemorrhage, neurologic deficit, brain abscess or death.[6,9]

CSF Leak

One of the most frequent complications that can occur during sinus surgery is CSF leakage. The thinnest area of the skull base is adjacent to where the anterior ethmoid artery enters the anterior skull base at the lateral lamella of the cribriform plate. The next most common area of possible CSF leakage is where the middle third of the middle turbinate starts to attach more laterally from the skull base to the lateral nasal wall. It is here that it can inadvertently be grasped, twisted, or pulled and a defect created, since the skull base tends to angle inferiorly as the surgeon works posteriorly, and the height of the posterior ethmoid sinuses varies. In order to prevent CSF

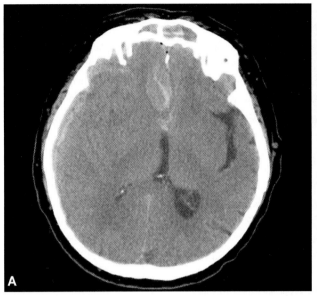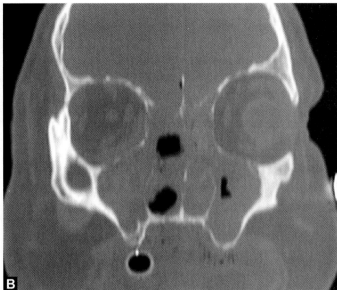

Figs 9.43A and B: (A) Axial and (B) coronal CT scan of a patient in whom the surgical instrument entered the brain and caused severe intracranial bleeding from the frontopolar branch of the anterior cerebral artery. This complication required neurosurgical intervention to stop bleeding

leakage there are some key points that need to be observed:

1. One should not fiddle around the attachment of the middle turbinate to the roof of the anterior skull base unless one is familiar with this area.
2. It is safest to open the posterior ethmoid cells once you have found the height of the roof of the sphenoid sinus: if one stays below this level there is only minimal danger to go through the skull base.
3. Do not angle your instruments medially toward the lateral lamella as the skull base is extremely thin in this area and you are more prone to cause a leak.

In case of a CSF leak clear fluid may be seen emanating from a skull base defect. It looks like a clear stream in a pool of blood and it often pulsates. When the leakage is identified, it must be repaired during the same operation. The edges of the bony defect should therefore be defined. Many graft materials have been described, ranging from a 'bath plug' fat graft for small leaks[17] to a free turbinate or conchal cartilage gaft for larger defects.[7] In general, in small dura lesions we use Tutoplast Fascia Lata® of the Tutogen Medical Company and for large defects abdominal fat and fascia lata from the patient. Whenever possible we recommend performing an underlay dura plasty as described by Schick in the previous chapter. To exclude further complications like we recommend a control CT immediately after operation. We have found that a lumbar drain is unnecessary. The graft is usually supported by some layer of surgicel, and the nose will be packed for 7 to 10 days depending on the size of the defect. During this time prophylactic antibiotics are given to avoid the potential risk of developing meningitis.

If the skull base has been traversed there may also be a risk of developing tension pneumocephalus. This means the presence of air in the intradural space. The patient may complain of headache and neurological deficits within the direct postoperative period. CT or MR imaging will help confirm the site. Pneumocephalus drainage is advisable when there is brain compression, due to hypertensive pneumocephalus. Importantly, in those cases the closure of the defect has to be revised and fixed.

Brain Injury

Inadvertent intradural penetration may cause direct damage to cerebral tissue and is a potentially fatal complication. Simple penetration with a forceps, without removal of brain tissue, may only cause cerebral edema. However, damage of small blood vessels can result in subarachnoid hemorrhage, which may not always must be visible during operation. Then the most important but unspecific postoperative symptom is headache or unconsciousness. In any suspect case postoperative imaging controls should be performed. If a skull base lesion was identified and closed during surgery post-operative imaging is mandatory. In the patient shown in

Fig. 9.43, the surgical instrument entered the brain and caused not only subarachnoid hemorrhage but severe intracranial bleeding from the frontopolar branch of the anterior cerebral artery. This complication required neurosurgical intervention to stop bleeding.

In general, secondary to direct injury of cerebral tissue a brain abscess can occur. The main symptoms are fever, headache and neurologic manifestations developing 2 to 4 weeks after sinus surgery. Although the abscess can be treated medically we recommend a surgical drainage depending on the location either by the ENT surgeon or the neurosurgeon.

Cranial Nerve Injuries

The most frequent injury to a cranial nerve is damage to the terminal branches of the olfactory nerves, usually accompanied by a CSF fistula. Involvement of the III, IV and VI nerves is secondary to an injury of the cavernous sinus.

GENERAL CONSIDERATIONS

- Complications of endonasal microendoscopic surgery of the paranasal sinuses are related to multiple factors, principally their complex anatomy, the type and extent of the disease, the history of previous sinus surgery and, above all, the experience of the surgeon. On the other hand, it has been proven that fatal complications are not rarely created by experienced surgeons as they perform most extended surgery.[15]
- Complications have decreased, mainly because of diagnostic advances in imaging (CT and MR), use of microscope and endoscope, modern anesthesia techniques and improved use of instruments, clinical resources and therapies.
- Reduction of complications begins with preventive measures that include meticulous preoperative evaluation with endoscopes and careful scrutiny of the imaging studies.
  The surgeon performing the surgery should have attended several courses, should have performed at least 10 cadaver dissections, should have assisted in many operations and should insist on an optimal supervision for at least the first 20 cases.
- The surgeon should always orientate on anatomical landmarks. In difficult revision cases navigation can be very helpful.

- The main reasons for complications are poor visibility due to bleeding or blood on the lens. It is important not to operate, probe, remove, or grasp anything that one cannot see!
- Keeping the patient's eyes uncovered in the surgical field facilitates the surgeon's orientation in relation to the orbit, possibly allowing earlier identification of any injuries to the orbital cavity.
- In case of complications one should immediately inform the patient and his relatives giving true and intensive explanation. This is the best strategy to avoid medicolegal problems.
- The surgeon must always keep in mind that the surgical procedure should be as extended as necessary but as small as possible!

ACKNOWLEDGMENT

To Professor E Hofmann, Head of the Neuroradiology Department at the Klinikum Fulda gAG, for imaging.

REFERENCES

1. Hollis LJ, Walsh RM, Bowdlere DA. Radiology in focus: *Massive epistaxis following sphenoid sinus exploration.* J Laryngol Otol 1994; 108:171–174.
2. Jones NS. Visual evoked potentials in endoscopic and anterior skull base surgery. J Laryngol Otol 1997; 111:513–516.
3. Keerl R, Stankiewicz J, Weber R, Hosemann W, Draf W. Surgical experience and complications during endonasal sinus surgery. *Laryngoscope* 1999; 109:546–550.
4. Kinsella JB, Calhoun KH, Bradfield JJ, Hokanson JA, Bailey BJ. Complications of endoscopic sinus surgery in a residency training program. *Laryngoscope* 1995; 105:1029–1032.
5. Lang J. Clinical anatomy of the nose, nasal cavity and paranasal sinuses. *Stuttgart*: Thieme, 1989.
6. Maniglia AJ. Fatal and other major complications of sinus surgery: Analysis of 2108 patients – incidence and prevention. *Laryngoscope* 1991; 101:349–354.
7. Marshall A, Jones NS, Robertson I. CSF rhinorrhea: A multi-disciplinary approach to minimise patient morbidity. *Br J Neurosurg* 2001; 15:8–13.
8. Simmen D, Jones NS. *Manual of Endoscopic Sinus Surgery and Its Extended Applications.* New York: Thieme, 2005.
9. Stamm AC. Complications of micro-endoscopic sinus surgery. In *Micro-endoscopic Surgery of the Paranasal Sinuses and the Skull Base,* Stamm AC, Draf W (Eds). New York: Springer, 2000; 581–593.
10. Stammberger H. *Functional Endoscopic Sinus Surgery.* St. Louis: Mosby, 1991.
11. Stankiewicz JA. Complications of endoscopic sinus surgery. *Otolaryngol Clin North Am* 1989; 22:749–758.

12. Stankiewicz JA. Cerebrospinal fluid fistula and endoscopic sinus surgery. *Laryngoscope* 1991; 101:250–256.

13. Thompson RF, Gluckman JL, Kulwin D. Orbital hemorrhage during ethmoid sinus surgery. *Otolaryngol Head Neck Surg* 1990; 102:45–50.

14. Weber R, Draf W, Keerl R, Schick B, Saha A. Endonasal microendoscopic pansinus operation in chronic sinusitis. II. Results and complications. *Am J Otolaryngol* 1997; 18: 247–253.

15. Weber R, Keerl R, Hosemann W, Schauss F, Leuwer R, Draf W. Complications with permanent damage in endonasal paranasal sinus operations—more frequent in experienced surgeons? *Laryngorhinootologie* 1998; 77:398–401.

16. Wigand ME. Endoscopic surgery of the paranasal sinus and anterior skull base. New York: *Thieme*, 1990.

17. Wormald PJ, McDonagh M. Bath plug technique for the endoscopic management of cerebrospinal fluid leaks. *J Laryngol Otol* 1997; 111:1042–1046.

Revision Surgery

Amir Minovi, Wolfgang Draf

The decision for revision surgery is not easy for the patient or for the surgeon particularly, if the surgeon also performed the previous surgery. Sometimes colleagues use the term 'iatrogenic' sinusitis suggesting possible mistakes of the previous surgeon. The term 'post-operative' sinusitis seems to be clear and neutral in regard to the reason of a failure.

If the patient complains about persistent or recurrent symptoms endoscopy of the nose, MRI and in case of likelihood of revision surgery computerized tomography may be indicated. Sagittal reformation gives excellent information on the situation in the frontal recess area (Fig. 9.44).[1] Whenever possible the updated images should be compared with the previous ones.

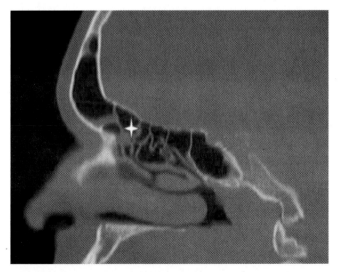

Fig. 9.44: Sagittal reformatted paranasal sinus CT gives the best possible information about the relation of the anterior ethmoidal cells and frontal sinus infundibulum

WHAT MAKES REVISION SURGERY NECESSARY?

View of the Patient

The patient goes back to a surgeon since his expectations in regard to the relief of his preoperative symptoms have not been fulfilled or improvement was temporarily only. This might be more likely, if the surgeon having been in charge has not been moderate and promised too much. It is by far better to keep the expectations of the patient low. This is particularly true for symptoms of headache and reduced smelling. There is no doubt that only headache caused by inflammatory sinus disease, generally a pyocele, can be improved by a sinus revision. Percussing the anterior frontal sinus wall and pressing the floor of the frontal sinus and thus creating pain is a very reliable sign of a frontal sinus inflammation. Sometimes, consultation with a neurologist is important, particularly if the patient reports migraine in the family. Several useless revisions in those patients are not too rare. After the 'classic' external frontoethmoidectomy via an infra-eyebrow incision severe neuralgic headache is due to irritation of the supraorbital or the supratrochlear nerves. Revision surgery must be avoided.

In general the surgeon should keep in mind that all he can do is to improve the drainage of the sinuses in question. The mucosa cannot be changed to a completely normal one. In addition it is difficult to predict any improvement in smell.

Analysis of the Surgeon

According to history, clinical examination and imaging the following questions need to be answered:

1. Was the previous diagnosis correct or is another diagnosis more likely?

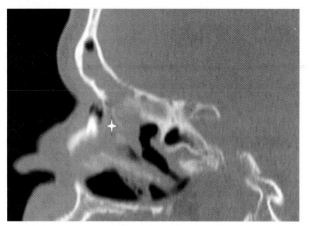

Fig. 9.45: Incomplete ethmoidectomy. Anterior ethmoid cells are blocking the frontal sinus drainage (+)

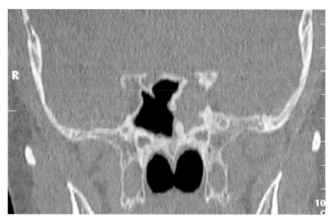

Fig. 9.46: Situation after four surgeries due to chronic sphenoidal sinusitis. Defect of the lateral sphenoidal sinus wall with protruding internal carotid artery (+). Dangerous situation for revision surgery

2. If the patient brings his images with him they must be of a quality that the questions in discussion can be answered.
3. A detailed analysis of the situation is necessary for clearing up another question: Why did previous surgery fail? There are different reasons for that: Most commonly the anterior ethmoidectomy was not extended enough to provide sufficient drainage of the maxillary and frontal sinus (Fig. 9.45). Sometimes unnecessary weakening of the ground lamella of the middle turbinate may be the cause of lateralization of the middle concha blocking the drainage of the ethmoid and the frontal sinus.
4. In triad patients with severe polyposis latest at the first revision the maximum operation is indicated including type III drainage of the frontal and also type III drainage of the sphenoid sinus (removal of the whole anterior wall, the septum sinuum sphenoidalium and part of the posterior nasal septum).
5. It is of utmost importance to analyze the images for dangerous anatomical findings like skull base and lamina papyracea defects or a very deep cribriform plate. It is also necessary to check whether the optic nerve and the internal carotid artery are in a safe position for the surgeon or protruding far into the lumen of the sphenoid sinus covered by a thin bony lamella only (Fig. 9.46).

PRINCIPLES AND TECHNIQUES

Once revision surgery is indicated careful planning is essential. The decision has to be made if the endonasal technique is still suitable for the individual case or an external procedure needs to be preferred.

Endonasal endoscopic revision is possible as long there is no serious problem in the frontal sinus. Sometimes, the use of the operating microscope can be helpful, for example in the case of severe bleeding.

The osteoplastic obliterative frontal sinus operation is the gold standard of surgical treatment of a chronic inflammatory disease, if a frontal sinus problem cannot be solved via the endonasal route. The older and for many decades 'classic external frontoethmoidectomy' according to Jansen (1894), Ritter (1906), Lynch (1921) or Howarth (1921) via an infra-eyebrow incision, is now regarded as 'obsolete' since the frequency of postoperative mucoceles rises with the duration of postoperative follow-up (up to 40%).[2-5] This is partly due to the resection of the bony borders of the newly created frontal sinus drainage, which means that about 50% of the drainage are lined by soft tissue, with a much higher tendency for shrinkage. The strategy of the osteoplastic obliterative operation is to remove with microscope and with the endoscope very meticulously in all the mucosa the narrow parts of the sinus to create a reliable barrier between nose and ethmoid on one side and the frontal sinus on the other and to fill the frontal sinus with freshly harvested autogenic fat. This way the frontal sinus is excluded from the paranasal sinus system. The rate of postoperative mucocele does not exceed 10% in experienced hands.

Endonasal Revision

In general the surgeon should expect more difficulties in surgical revision than in a virgin case. Orientation on landmarks is even more essential. In endonasal revision one has to take in account that the problem is located mainly in the frontal sinus not in the ethmoid. In this situation the medial approach to the frontal sinus for a type III drainage starting with partial resection of the nasal septum at the frontal sinus floor is recommendable to avoid repeated traumatization of the ethmoidal mucosa.

In revision cases after incomplete ethmoidectomy it is recommended that a wide approach to the ethmoid is created using a drill or punch when possible. Punches and through-cutting instruments help to preserve the mucosa, whereas the drill is more destructive in this respect.[15] The wide approach to the ethmoid is obtained by exposing the lacrimal bone and thinning it out as well as parts of the agger nasi and part of the frontal process of the maxilla until the lamina papyracea is clearly to be seen. This facilitates better visualization of the frontal recess to allow further work on the frontal sinus floor, but also makes the postoperative treatment less painful.

Identification of anterior skull base as an important landmark is essential for performing a really complete ethmoidectomy which is the prerequisite of an efficient revision. Due to scars and massive bone reaction as sequelae of previous surgery and also as consequence of continuing inflammatory disease, this may be difficult to identify.

Bleeding sometimes increases the difficulties. Local application of adrenaline 1:2000 for a few minutes using neurosurgical pads is recommended and does not cause major cardiovascular side effect.[6]

For identification of the skull base the 'posterior-anterior technique' after removal of the anterior sphenoid sinus wall offers some advantages if the 'anterior-posterior approach' seems risky.[7] The identification of the anterior ethmoid artery is of great help for finding the infundibulum of the frontal sinus and to decide on the necessary opening of it. It is important to provide good frontal sinus drainage by opening the remaining agger nasi cells and the so-called frontal cells. Sagittal CT reformations are helpful for the analysis of individual anatomy. The relation of the anterior ethmoidal artery and the anterior skull base is identified by means of high-resolution coronal sections. The anterior ethmoidal artery runs the deeper to the anterior skull base the better the pneumatization is on the other hand this vessel is sometimes located within the skull base: In that case it cannot be identified without exposing the dura mater.

For details of the classification and indications of the differently wide frontal sinus drainage as type I–III (see *Endonasal Frontal Sinus Surgery*).[8–10]

External Revision

With increasing experience and referrals of difficult frontal sinus cases, it became obvious that not all difficulties can be solved via an endonasal route. Therefore, the osteoplastic obliterative frontal sinus operation[11] was included in the concept, in order to deal with the different kinds of frontal sinus problems. In some patients the endonasal operation has to be combined with the osteoplastic, mostly obliterative procedure.[8–10] The indications of the osteoplastic frontal sinus obliteration are listed in Table 9.4.

Table 9.4: Indications of the osteoplastic frontal sinus obliterative procedure
1. Endonasal type III drainage not possible (frontal sinus less than 8 mm anterior-posterior diameter)
2. Frontal sinus too small (less than 8 mm anterior-posterior diameter)
3. Major destruction of the posterior wall
4. Lateral mucopyocele
5. Inflammatory complication after trauma (alloplastic material). Frequently without obliteration because of good quality mucosa.
6. Large osteoma
7. Aesthetic correction of pneumatosinus frontalis dilatans

Surgery requires general anesthesia. In cases of acute inflammatory complications antibiotic therapy should precede the operation.

The incision for a uni- or bilateral osteoplastic frontal sinus operation is selected individually, taking into consideration aesthetic aspects, prevention of complications and prevailing anatomical and pathological conditions (Fig. 9.47). We use the bitemporal coronal incision for large frontal sinuses, in unilateral operations and in patients with normal hair growth (Fig. 9.48A). Young men must always be asked about the hair growth patterns of their father and brothers, because the coronal incision leaves a visible scar in bald persons.

The incision is made beginning at the attachment of the helix (or slightly ventral to it) on one side and is carried over the vertex approximately 5 cm behind the hairline to the corresponding point on the opposite side. A tightly stretched silk thread may be helpful as a marker. In the frontotemporal region, care should be taken not to damage the superficial temporal vessels. We inject a local anesthetic with adrenaline (suprarenin) to lessen the bleeding from the scalp incision. The remaining bleeders are controlled by bipolar coagulation and the use of special scalp clamps on the edges. These clamps are left in place, covered by moist gauze till the end of the operation. Bleeding is usually minor after the clamps are removed. The residual bleeding can be stopped by bipolar coagulation.

In case of large frontal sinuses and the risk of significant hair loss, a frontal crease for the incision may be preferred (Fig. 9.47).[12]

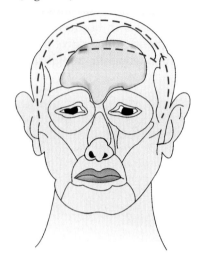

Fig. 9.47: Different incisions for osteoplastic frontal sinus surgery[14]

In cases secondary to a trauma, soft tissue injuries could provide an approach and, if necessary, they should be widened in the relaxed skin tension lines or skin folds (Fig. 9.47). The incision is extended to the periosteum without injuring it. Using partly blunt, partly sharp dissection extending to the supraorbital ridge and over the root of the nose, we pull the scalp flap caudally on both sides, leaving behind the periosteum and the bone. In this way, the entire frontal bone is exposed on both sides, thus preserving the supraorbital nerve.

Next, the template of the frontal sinus that was excised from the occipitofrontal X-ray is placed correctly with respect to the side and orientation on the roof of the nose so that the borders of the frontal sinus can be marked on the periosteum with a marker pen (Fig. 9.48A). The periosteum is then incised approximately 1.5 cm outside the template and is elevated slightly past the marking in the bone from which the periosteum has been elevated, a few millimeters inside the marked line. The oscillating saw is excellent for this and is directed at an acute angle towards the frontal sinus (Figs 9.48B and C). In this way, a cutting surface that is as wide as possible is created so the bony lid replaced later is stable. The bone incision reaches the supraorbital ridge on both sides. When opening the frontal sinus bilaterally, the intersinus septum must be separated from the anterior sinus wall with the help of a chisel curved over the surface. The fracture and the elevation of the bony lid are done with a wide osteotome (Fig. 9.48D). During caudal fracture, the supraorbital ridge is preserved. The bony lid is fashioned so that it hinges on the periosteal flap. The diseased tissue is then removed according to the pathological-anatomical findings (Fig. 9.48E). Fractures must be exposed to their full extent, repositioned and, if necessary, a dural lesion has to be treated with duraplasty. In cases secondary to trauma or osteoma removal, where is healthy frontal sinus mucosa, it must be decided whether the mucosa especially that of the infundibulum is healthy enough to preserve the frontal sinus as part of the paranasal sinus sytem or whether an obliteration should be carried out. A type III median drainage technique can be performed easily with the optimum exposure described above. If obliteration is indicated, the frontal sinus mucosa has to be removed meticulously using microscope and endoscope drilling away the inner layer with a burr, similar to the technique of cholesteatoma removal in the middle ear (Fig. 9.48F). This is the only way to remove the mucosa completely and to avoid earlier or later mucocele. The mucosa in the region of the frontal sinus infundibulum is everted nasally, and the drainage opening is obturated with bone or cartilage splints fixed with fibrin glue. The cavum conchae is an ideal donor site for cartilage perichondral graft taking. The graft is tightly sealed either with the overlapping perichondrium and as a second layer with an autogenic galea-periosteal graft or solution-dried fascia. The fascial piece and the bone or cartilage graft should securely seal the frontonasal contact area, but must not cover a large area of the drilled bone of the frontal sinus because, if they do, no nourishing blood vessels can grow out of the bone into the fat used for obliteration (Fig. 9.48G). Through this three-layered closure, the frontal sinus is securely isolated from the nasal cavity, and re-entry and growth of mucosa into the sinus with the associated risk of mucocele formation is prevented.

Next, abdominal fat is freshly harvested. If the patient has undergone appendectomy, the fat is taken from the mostly right-sided scar. Otherwise, we place the incision around the navel in order to prevent confusion between an appendectomy scar and that of the incision for harvesting fat. Precise hemostasis and the insertion of a drain for about 3 days are necessary. The risk of hematoma formation is relatively high. The abdominal fat is temporarily preserved in isotonic saline solution and is placed into the frontal sinus as larger pieces held together by fibrin glue, until the sinus cavity is completely filled (Figs 9.48G and H). Finally, the periosteum bone lid is replaced and wedged closed with a tap of the mallet, and the periosteum is sutured. Since the periosteal incision lies approximately 15 mm away from the bone

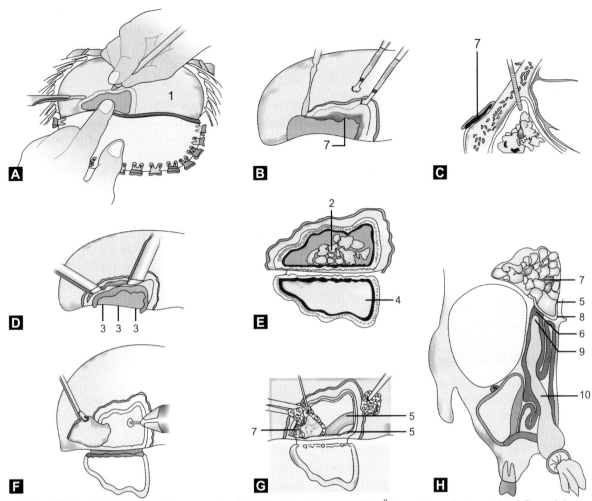

Figs 9.48A to H: Technical details of the osteoplastic obliterative sinus operation.[8] 1 = galeaperiosteum, 2 = inflamed tissue, 3 = burr holes, 4 = frontal bone inner table, 5 = overlapping perichondrium, 6 = cavum conchae cartilage, 7 = fat cubes, 8 = fibrin glue (blue), 9 = nasal mucosa, 10 = rubber finger stall packing

incision, the sutures now lie away from the edges of the incision in the bone, so they are covered by periosteum. If the bone lid fractures during elevation, these bony fragments should be fixed together with absorbable thread or with miniplates to repositioning of the whole lid. To the end of the operation, the scalp flap is flipped back into place, two tube drains are inserted, and the coronal incision is closed in one layer with interrupted 'O' sutures. A light pressure bandage suffices for better placement of the scalp. The tube drains are removed after 2 days. Later removal causes pain.

If there is an extensive defect in the posterior frontal sinus after clearance of the frontal sinus particularly following a severe head injury, it must be decided whether obliteration or a cranialization with complete removal of the posterior wall fragments is the better choice.[13] Even in this situation precise debridement of all mucosa particles is necessary, otherwise 20–30 years later even intradural mucoceles may develop (Fig. 9.49).

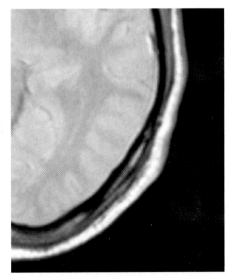

Fig. 9.49: Situation 20 years after trauma. Intradural mucocele

SPECIFIC FAILURES DEMANDING REVISION SURGERY

Postoperative Frontal Sinusitis after Type I and Type II Drainage

Sometimes, after ethmoidectomy and type I or type II drainage, patients may develop more problems in the frontal sinus than before surgery. The CT control will confirm if a postoperative frontal sinusitis has developed.

Remnant ethmoidal cells may have caused a recurrent sinusitis or repeated mechanical irritation of the mucosa in the frontal recess may cause a severe scar around Killian's infundibulum. Both pathologies may block the frontal sinus drainage.

This can be avoided by performing at least a complete anterior ethmoidectomy and extremely atraumatic handling of the frontal recess mucosa. For treatment a type IIa drainage after previous type Ia type IIb drainage after a previous type IIa and type III drainage after a previous type IIb is recommended.

Reclosure after Type III Drainage

Several technical issues can lead to this problem:

1. The 'chimney' between the anterior ethmoid and the frontal sinus has not been opened wide enough. It is important after identification of the anterior ethmoidal artery to go along the skull base medially the lamina papyracea into the frontal sinus.
2. The anteroposterior opening of the frontal sinus floor particularly in the midline is very small. The identification of the first olfactory fibre bilaterally and the creation of the 'frontal T' will help avoid this problem.
3. The resection of the septum/a sinuum frontalium has been missed or was not performed to a satisfying degree. The new curved drills with 15° and 60° angle are ideal for this purpose.
4. The resection of the superior nasal septum was very small. The diameter of resection must be 1.5 cm just in front of the 'frontal T' and below the frontal sinus floor.
5. The packing between the ethmoid and the frontal sinus was not left long enough. Seven days proved to be the best using rubber finger packings.

II a/b is indicated, in case of Samter's triad and other prognostic risk factors type III drainage is the best choice. If the patient had numerous operations before and this was to be his 'last' sinus operation, one has to choose between type III drainage and the osteoplastic flap procedure with obliteration. If the frontal sinus is large enough and has an anterior-posterior diameter of at least 0.8 mm, type III drainage may be tried. If the frontal sinus has a smaller diameter, the frontal sinus fat obliteration is the safer though more extensive technique.

FOLLOW-UP

After revision surgery patients need to be followed-up to judge the result of recent measures and to detect problems early. Most important is the clinical examination including endoscopy. A patient who is free of complaints and with satisfying endoscopic findings does not usually need additional imaging. If there was a mucocele along the skull base, quite laterally in the frontal sinus or in lateral recess of the sphenoid sinus near to the optic nerve with some potential of nerve compression it is recommendable to ask for a magnetic resonance imaging 3 months after surgery. Depending on the finding another one may be planned an year later. Whenever possible CT control examination should be avoided as long there is no indication for further surgery due to the X-ray exposure.

BACKGROUND

1. Instead of the term 'iatrogenic' sinusitis it is better to talk about 'postoperative' sinusitis, which does not give a reason of prejudice in regard to the previous surgeon.
2. The decision for revision surgery is difficult. It needs vast experience.
3. There must be a reasonable correlation between complaints and radiologic findings. It should not be forgotten that the surgeon operates patients and not on the images derived on CT or MRI.
4. It can be very difficult to differentiate between headache caused by inflammatory sinus disease and neurologic headache. Family history for migraine needs to be evaluated.
5. Highly suspicious for frontal sinus headache is pain during percussion of the anterior wall and during pressure at the floor of the frontal sinus.
6. Potential compression of the optic nerve by a mucocele justifies revision surgery without major complaints.
7. In most of the cases revision is necessary due to incomplete anterior ethmoidectomy blocking the frontal sinus drainage.
8. In the majority of patients revision can be managed successfully via the endonasal route.
9. In triad patients with severe polyposis latest at the first revision the maximum operation is indicated including type III drainage of the frontal and also type III drainage of the sphenoid sinus.

10. The external osteoplastic, mostly obliterative frontal sinus operation must be part of the armamentarium of the experienced sinus surgeon for solution of exceptionally difficult frontal sinus problems.

REFERENCES

1. Hofmann E. Anatomy of nose and paranasal sinuses in sagittal computed tomography. *Klinische Neuroradiologie* 2005 (in print).
2. Jansen A. Eroeffnung der Nebenhoehlen der Nase bei chronischer Eiterung. *Arch Laryng Rhinol (Berl)* 1894; 135–157.
3. Ritter G. Eine neue Methode zur Erhaltung der vorderen Stirnhoehlenwand bei Radikaloperationen chronischer Stirnhoehleneiterungen. *Dtsch Med Wochenschr* 1906; 32: 1294–1296.
4. Howarth WG. Operations on the frontal sinus. *J Laryngol Otol* 1921; 36:417–421.
5. Lynch RC. The technique of a radical frontal sinus operation which has given me the best results. *Laryngoscope* 1921; 31: 1–5.
6. Stammberger H. *Functional endoscopic sinus surgery*. Philadelphia: BC Decker, 1991.
7. Wigand ME. Endoskopische Chirurgie der Nasennebenhöhlen uund der vorderen Schädelbasis. Stuttgart: Thieme, 1989.
8. Draf W. Surgical treatment of inflammatory diseases of the paranasal sinuses. Indication, surgical technique, risks, mismanagement and complications, revision surgery. *Arch Otorhinolaryngol* 1982; 235:131–305.
9. Draf W. Endonasal micro-endoscopic frontal sinus surgery. The Fulda concept. *Op Tech Otolaryngol Head Neck Surg* 1991; 2:234–240.
10. Draf W. Endonasal Frontal Sinus Drainage Type I–III according to Draf. In *The Frontal Sinus*, Kountakis St, Senior B, Draf W (Eds) New York: Springer, 2005.
11. Tato JM, Bergaglio OE. Surgery of frontal sinus. Fat grafts: New technique. *Otolaryngologica* 1949; 3:1.
12. Bosley WR. Osteoplastic obliteration of the frontal sinuses. A review of 100 patients. *Laryngoscope* 1972; 82:1463–1476.
13. Donald PJ, Ettin M. The safety of frontal sinus fat obliteration when sinus walls are missing. *Laryngoscope* 1986; 96(2):190–193.
14. Draf W, Weber R, Keerl R, Constantinidis J, Schick B, Saha A. Endonasal and external micro-endoscopic Surgery of the frontal sinus. In *Micro-endoscopic surgery of the paranasal sinuses and skull base*, eds Stamm A, Draf W. New York: Springer, 2000; 257–278.
15. Moriyama H, Fukami M, Yanagi K, Ohtori N, Kaneta K. Endoscopic endonasal treatment of ostium of the frontal sinus and the results of endoscopic surgery. *Am J Rhinol* 1994; 8:67–70.

Sinonasal Polyposis: Surgical Aspects

Amir Minovi, Wolfgang Draf

Sinonasal polyposis has been described as an immunologic mediated chronic inflammatory disease of the paranasal sinuses. Its cause has been extensively discussed in the literature.[1-3] Nasal polyps are pale yellow pedunculated benign nasal masses with a smooth surface. They are filled with an edematous stroma and inflammatory cells (Fig. 9.50). In this chapter we would like to discuss how to clinically approach patients with a nasal polyposis and how to manage nasal polyposis surgically.

PREOPERATIVE EVALUATION

Patients with sinonasal polyposis typically suffer progressive nasal obstruction, rhinorrhea, facial pressure or headache, hyposmia and loss of smell. Polyps mainly causes an obstruction of the ostiomeatal complex with recurrent or chronic rhinosinusitis. Sinonasal polyposis can be found associated with several diseases:
- Bronchial asthma
- Aspirin intolerance
- Samter's triad (concurrent aspirin sensitivity, asthma, nasal polyposis)
- Ciliary dysfunction syndrome (Kartagener's)
- Mucoviscidosis
- Allergic eosinophilic fungal sinusitis.

The main medical treatment in patients with sinonasal polyposis is anti-inflammatory medications like local or systemic glucocorticoids. Surgical intervention is indicated when polyposis is not clearly reduced and the

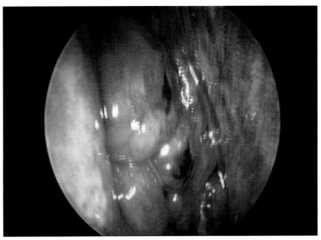

Fig. 9.50: Extended sinonasal polyposis in a patient with Samter's triad

patient still has symptoms of chronic sinusitis. Inverted papillomas, meningoceles, and sinonasal neoplasms, such as esthesioneuroblastoma can resemble polypoid tissue. Therefore, we recommend performing an MRI prior to surgery when there is a unilateral polyposis. In children, an antrochoanal polyp is one of the most common pathologies of unilateral polyposis Figs 9.51A to D.

To our knowledge the success of surgical treatment in nasal polyposis depends on the possible presence of prognostic factors. The goals of the treatment should include:

- Decrease in the size of nasal polyps
- Relieve of nasal obstruction and facial pressure
- Reestablishment of mucociliary flow
- Improvement of olfactory function
- Refraining from smoking.

It is mandatory to have a detailed preoperative conversation with the patient and emphasize the fact that given certain comorbid factors like asthma, aspirin intolerance or allergic rhinitis, they should not expect a permanent success rate with surgery. The patient should be informed that revision surgery may be needed during the course of the disease. Senior et al. demonstrated that

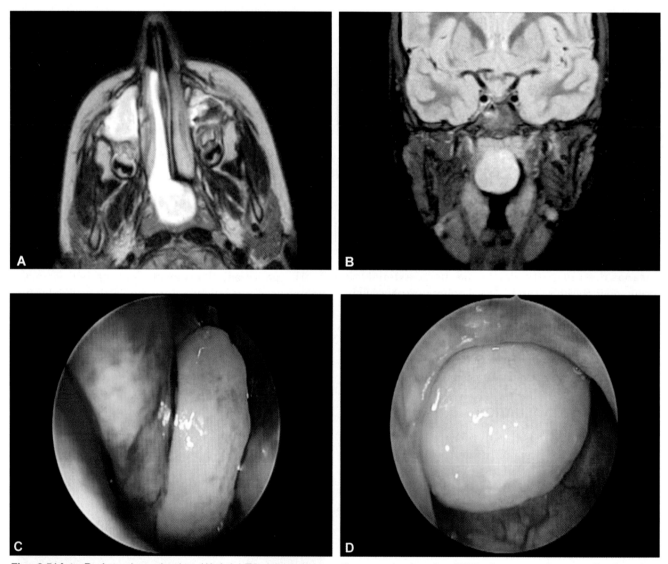

Figs 9.51A to D: Antrochoanal polyp. (A) Axial T2-weighted magnetic resonance imaging (MRI) shows complete opacification of the right maxillary sinus the middle meatus. (B) Extension into the nasopharynx seen on coronal planes. The polyp is hyperintense on T2-weighted MR images. (C) Endoscopic view of an antrochoanal polyp as a single large polyp in the middle meatus. (D) With extension into the nasopharyx as seen transorally

smokers with polyps and advanced chronic sinusitis will require a revision surgery.[4] The surgical management is to re-establish normal anatomy but not to heal the diseased mucosa. In our experience the following patient groups can be distinguished with decreasing prognosis:
- Antrochoanal polyp (best prognosis)
- Simple polyposis
- Polyposis with allergy and asthma
- Samter's triad
- Mucoviscidosis
- Kartagener syndrome (worst prognosis).

Surgical Management

Treatment of nasal polyposis started 2000 years ago with a simple polypectomy by pulling a sponge through the nose. This method was first described by Hippocrates.[5] The surgical treatment of nasal polyposis changed dramatically with the new revolutionary era of sinus surgery, which started in the 1970s with the development of optical aids such as endoscope and the operating microscope. Nowadays a simple polypectomy is rarely carried out. The standard treatment in chronic polypoid sinusitis is endonasal sinus surgery. Furthermore the development of powered instruments like the soft-tissue shaver[6] and angled diamond burrs has clearly helped to manage varying degrees of chronic polypoid sinusitis. In cases of massive polyposis, the soft tissue shaver (Fig. 9.52) has proven very helpful in removing the polyps with relative ease and minimal bleeding.

The extent of surgery should be discussed with the patient. Figure 9.53 shows algorithm in the surgical management of sinonasal polyposis irresponsive to conservative treatment. In simple nasal polyposis we do not recommend a simple polypectomy. Prior to the surgical procedure the patient should receive a systemic corticosteroid therapy for five days (20 mg of prednisone). Instead of a conservative endonasal surgery an uncinectomy with a complete ethmoidectomy and frontal sinus type I drainage after Draf (See *Endonasal Frontal Sinus Surgery*) should be performed. Patients with a 'halo sign' on the CT scan (Fig. 9.54) are also candidates for

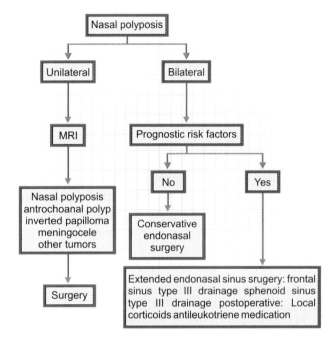

Fig. 9.53: Management of nasal polyposis

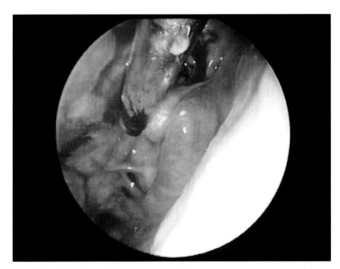

Fig. 9.52: Removal of polypoid tissue in severe sinonasal polyposis with the soft tissue shaver

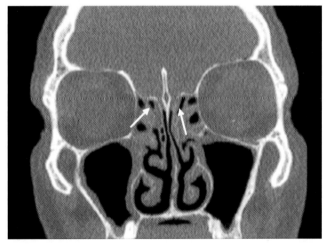

Fig. 9.54: Coronal CT scan in a patient with chronic rhinosinusitis with polyposis shows air (arrows) along the skull base (halo sign) as a good prognostic factor

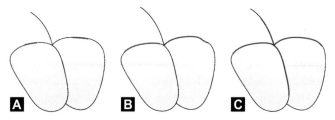

Figs 9.55A to C: Endonasal sphenoid sinus drainage according to Draf.[7] (Axial view). (A) Enlargement of natural opening of the sphenoid sinus as sphenoid sinus type I drainage. (B) Removal of the frontal wall of the sphenoid sinus resulting in sphenoid sinus type II drainage. (C) Resection of both anterior walls, the septum sinuum sphenoidalium and about 5–8 mm of the posterior margin of the nasal septum achieving a wide sphenoid sinus type III drainage

not too extended surgical treatment since they have a better prognosis. In cases of unilateral sinonasal polyposis the extent of surgery depends on the pathology. An antrochoanal polyp should be removed totally with its stalk to avoid a recurrence. In cases of an inverted papilloma the surgical approach depends on the extent of sinus involvement. Patients with prognostic risk factors like a Samter's triad are primarily treated in our department with extensive endonasal sinus surgery. This surgery includes:

- Uncinectomy
- Complete ethmoidectomy
- Frontal sinus type III drainage according to Draf
- Sphenoid sinus type III drainage according to Draf (Figs 9.55A to C).[7]

Our experience has been that in most patients who come for a revision surgery, the anterior ethmoid is not completely removed. Hence, it is very important to perform a complete ethmoidectomy with special care on the anterior ethmoid cells in primary surgical treatment.

Postoperative aftercare by patient is similar to those patients with chronic sinusitis without polyposis as described in the *Principles of Endoscopic Sinus Surgery*. We recommend during the first weeks after surgery consequent local aftercare with removal of mobile fibrin and blood clots. The patients should perform local irrigation of the nose with isotonic saline solution and application of topical corticoids for at least three months. If tissue eosinophilia is detected we recommend placing the patients on systemic corticoids and an antihistamine preparation for six weeks.[8] In patients with prognostic risk factors like Samter's triad we recommend long-term use of topical corticoids and if effective oral antileukotriene medications.[9]

ACKNOWLEDGMENTS

The authors would like to thank Farhan Taghizadeh MD, Assistant Professor, Universiy of New Mexico Health Sciences Center, Albuquerque, USA for his kind cooperation.

We also thank sincerely Professor Erich Hofmann, Director, Department of Neuroradiology and his co-workers for the permanent excellent cooperation and allowing us the publication of the radiologic images.

REFERENCES

1. Kaliner MA, Osguthorpe JD, Fireman P, Anon J, Georgitis J, Davis ML, Naclerio R, Kennedy D. Sinusitis: Bench to bedside. Current findings, future directions. *Otolaryngol Head Neck Surg* 1997; 117: S1–S7.
2. Ponikau JU, Sherris DA, Kern EB, Homburger HA, Frigas E, Gaffey TA, Roberts GD. The diagnosis and incidence of allergic fungal sinusitis. *Mayo Clin Proc* 1999; 74:877–884.
3. Braun H, Stammberger H, Buzina W, Freudenschuss K, Lackner A, Beham A. Incidence and detection of fungi and eosinophilic granulocytes in chronic rhinosinusitis. *Laryngo-Rhino-Otol* 2003; 82:330–340.
4. Senior BA, Kennedy DW, Tanabodee J, Kroger H, Hassab M, Lanza D. Long-term results of functional endoscopic sinus surgery. *Laryngoscope* 1998; 108:151–157.
5. Vancil ME. A historical survey of treatments for nasal polyposis. *Laryngoscope* 1969; 79:435–445.
6. Hawke WM, McCombe AW. How I do it: Nasal polypectomy with an arthroscopic bone shaver: The Stryker 'Hummer'. *J Otolaryngol* 1995; 24:57–59.
7. Draf W. Advanced course on endonasal micro-endoscopic surgery of the paranasal sinuses, Fulda Hospital, 1991.
8. Draf W, Weber R. Endonasal microendoscopic pansinusoperation in chronic sinusitis. I. Indications and operation technique. *Am J Otolaryngol* 1993; 14:394–398.
9. Ulualp SO, Sterman BM, Toohil RJ. Antileukotriene therapy for the relief of sinus symptoms in aspirin triad disease. *Ear Nose Throat J* 1999; 78:604–616.

Transsphenoidal Pituitary Surgery

Aldo C Stamm, Shirley SN Pignatari, Hugo Canhete Lopes

Pituitary tumors account for approximately 11% of intracranial tumors. Although they are sometimes treated medically, surgery is the principal therapeutic modality.[1]

The complex anatomy of the skull base, along with the proximity of the optic nerves, internal carotid arteries and the cavernous sinus, make the access to pituitary tumors challenging.[2,3,5,7,8]

The first operation for a pituitary tumor was performed in the late nineteenth century through a frontal craniotomy. Transsphenoidal approaches to the sella were developed soon afterwards, but their morbidity and mortality were very high.[5]

These approaches are still in use today because technological advances have made them much safer. Mortality declined with the introduction of antibiotics, and the use of the operating microscope combined with fluoroscopy allowed more precise management of the sella. In the past two decades transsphenoidal pituitary surgery has undergone a revolution with the introduction of endoscopes. Endoscopes provide better illumination and magnification; this reduces the likelihood of injury to structures near the sella, and allows better management of complications such as cerebrospinal fluid leakage and nasal bleeding. This improved visualization resulted in further refinements and new goals for this surgery. Rather than simply trying to avoid complications and decompress the optic chiasm, surgeons now try to preserve nasal function and precisely resect the tumors, and achieve endocrinologic cure.[2-4,6-10]

ANATOMY

The sphenoid bone is located at the base of the skull, anterior to the temporal and basilar portions of occipital bone. The body of the sphenoid bone contains the sphenoid sinuses, separated from each other by an intersinus septum that is usually displaced to one side. Other parasagittal minor septae inside sphenoid sinuses are not uncommon, and often the posterior edge of one of these minor septae marks the carotid bulge. The sphenoid sinuses are extremely variable in size and shape, and in their relationship to the sella. The sphenoid sinus may be classified by the extent to which it is pneumatized as postsellar, presellar, or conchal; the postsellar type is the most pneumatized in which the sellar floor bulges into the well-pneumatized sinus. Posterior to the

sphenoid sinus, the basi-sphenoid articulates with the occipital bone through a synostosis to form the clivus. The anterior surface of the sinus contains its natural ostium, which empties into the sphenoethmoidal recess behind the superior and/or supreme nasal turbinates. The natural sphenoid ostium lies about 15 mm above the upper margin of the choana, and is slightly oblique in the endoscopic view. Directly lateral to the sphenoid sinus lies the cavernous sinus and its contents. Depending on the extent of pneumatization, some adjacent structures (e.g. the internal carotid artery, optic chiasm and nerve, maxillary and mandibular divisions of trigeminal nerve, and the vidian nerve) may bulge into its walls, and form identifiable protuberances (carotid prominence, optic prominence). The groove between the optic and carotid prominences is the optic-carotid recess, which varies in depth and represents pneumatization of the anterior clinoid processes. Some posterior ethmoid cells may pneumatize above the sphenoid sinus forming an anatomic variation known as Onodi's cell.[5,8-10]

The sella turcica contains the anterior and posterior lobes of the pituitary gland and the distal portion of pituitary stalk. The sella turcica is covered by a reflection of dura mater, the diaphragma sella, which attaches to the clinoid processes, and has a small dehiscence allowing transmission of the pituitary infundibulum and its surrounding arachnoid. The cavernous sinuses are immediately lateral to the sella in the parasellar space and contain the carotid artery and cranial nerves III,IV and most medially, VI. The paired cavernous sinuses are joined by an intercavernous sinus, forming the circular venous sinus. Laterally, posteroinferiorly and adjacent to the inferior aspect of the cavernous sinus lies Meckel's cave with the trigeminal ganglion.[5,8-10]

SURGICAL TECHNIQUE

Surgery is performed under general anesthesia. The patient is positioned supine on the operating table with his dorsum elevated about 30 degrees. In addition to the face, the anterolateral aspect of one of the patient's thighs must be surgically prepared in order to take the fascia lata and subcutaneous fat if necessary. The nasal cavity is decongested with vasoconstrictor moistened cotton, and the nasal septum infiltrated with lidocaine/vasoconstrictor solution. We use lidocaine 2% with epinephrine 1:2000 in the topical solution, and lidocaine 2% with epinephrine 1:100.000 for submucosal infiltration of the septum. The endoscope is attached to a 3-chip camera.

Surgical access to the sphenoid sinus may be achieved through three different approaches:
- Direct transnasal
- Transseptal
- Resection of posterior nasal septum.

DIRECT TRANSNASAL ACCESS

The nasal cavity is inspected with a 4 mm 0° endoscope. The sphenoid sinus may be directly accessed, or some adjuvant procedures, such as septoplasty, partial resection of middle turbinate or nasal polypectomy may be required to improve access. The middle turbinate is laterally displaced and the superior turbinate partially resected. The sphenoid ostium is then identified and the sphenoid sinus is probed with a seeker/palpator. Electrocoagulation of sphenoethmoidal recess inferior to the sphenoid ostium is carried out in order to prevent bleeding from septal or nasopalatine arteries. The anterior wall of the sphenoid sinus is then resected with a micro-Kerrison punch or a microdrill. Care must be taken not to remove excessive bone inferolaterally where arteries enter the nasal cavity through the sphenopalatine foramen. Some posterior ethmoid cells may be removed in order to improve access. This approach is preferred when the lesion is unilateral and when there has been previous surgery (Fig. 9.56).

TRANSSEPTAL ACCESS

After nasal septal infiltration, an anterior septal incision extending to the nasal floor is performed. For most cases we prefer incisions on the right side of the septum. A subperichondral and subperiosteal dissection of the nasal septum is carried out with a suction elevator; then the posterior portion of the nasal septum is resected with Jansen-Middleton forceps, allowing identification of sphenoid rostrum and the sphenoid ostia on the anterior wall of sphenoid sinus with 0° endoscopes.

The anterior wall of sphenoid sinus may be removed with a micro-Kerrison punch, small osteotomes, or a microdrill. Care must be taken not to pull out the mucosa of sphenoid sinus, and not to injure the nasopalatine artery, in order to avoid unfavorable scarring and unnecessary bleeding. The inferior bony wall of the sphenoid sinus is often a site of bleeding at this stage, and such bleeding is ideally controlled with a diamond burr or monopolar electrocoagulation. The sphenoidotomies are enlarged, and the median septum is resected with strong cutting forceps (Fig. 9.57). At this stage, the structures within the sphenoid sinus, including the sella turcica, carotid prominences and optic prominences, can be identified. In conchal-type sphenoid sinuses, access to the floor of the sella turcica may be improved with the use of a microdrill in the clivus region. Paramedian septae may be removed with cutting forceps.

The removal of the sellar floor is carefully begun in the midline with small osteotomes or a microdrill, and continued with a micro-Kerrison punch enlarging the opening superiorly to the planum sphenoidale, inferiorly to the clivus, and laterally to the carotid prominences.

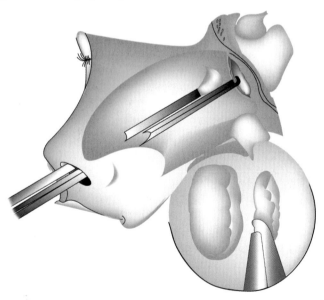

Fig. 9.56: Direct transnasal approach to the sphenoid sinus

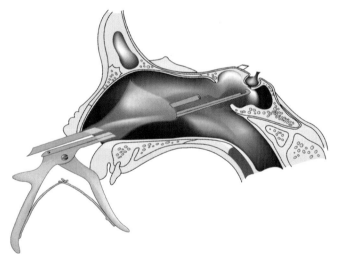

Fig. 9.57: Endoscopic transseptal approach to the sphenoid sinus

Bipolar electrocautery is used on the intended incision line of the dura mater, and the incision made with a scalpel. Most commonly we use a rectangular incision with resection of the incised dura mater, but cross-shaped and x-shaped incisions may also be used. The incision must not be extended far superiorly, in order to avoid bleeding from intercavernous sinus or a cerebrospinal fluid leak. The pituitary tumor may be soft and easily removed with aspiration, or hard, necessitating removal with curettes and cupped-tip forceps. The use of 30 and 45° angled endoscopes provides wide-angle vision to all the recesses. Bleeding at this stage is controlled with pieces of surgicel®. Potential cerebrospinal fluid leaks may be repaired with grafts of fat or fascia lata from the thigh, and fibrin glue. In these cases, a lumbar drain is placed and maintained for about five days.

No reconstruction of the sella is required in most cases, but it may be necessary after removal of large macroadenomas to prevent the descent of the optic chiasm into the sellar cavity.[2]

After hemostasis of the surgical cavity with surgicel® and gelfoam®, the middle turbinate is returned to its original position, the septal incision is sutured and the nasal cavity is packed.

This is the most conservative access to the sella, and leaves the anatomy of nasal cavity intact.

RESECTION OF POSTERIOR NASAL SEPTUM

After septal infiltration, monopolar electrocautery is used to make the incisions on the nasal septum. A vertical incision is made about 2 cm anterior to the sphenoid ostium, joining a horizontal incision made about 1.5 cm above the floor of the nasal cavity. The mucoperiosteum may be reflected laterally and used as a flap, or resected and used as a graft. The cartilaginous portion of the nasal septum is then transected with a Freer elevator or a suction elevator, and resected with a strong cutting forceps or a Jansen-Middleton forceps. The contralateral muco-periosteum of the septum is then resected or reflected in the same way, and the nasopalatine artery carefully electrocoagulated. The removal of the anterior sphenoid wall and the sellar floor, and the sellar tumor resection are performed in a manner very similar to that described for the transseptal approach. The posterior nasal resection provides wide access to the sphenoid sinus, allowing four hands of two surgeons to work through the two nares at the same time (Fig. 9.58). This capability is especially helpful when dealing with a hard tumor, tumors with parasellar extension, or when there

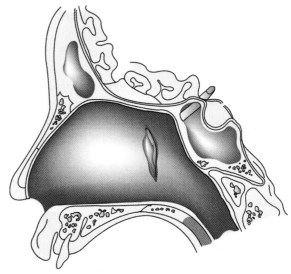

Fig. 9.58: Incision of the posterior region of the nasal septum, which will be followed by its removal, initiating the surgical access to the sphenoid sinus

is troublesome bleeding. This approach is also advantageous in a previously operated nasal cavity, avoiding the mani-pulation of a scarred nasal septum.

REFERENCES

1. Butler AB, Netsky MG. Classification and biology of brain tumors. In *Neurological surgery*, Vol.3, ed Youmans JR. Philadelphia: WB Saunders, 1973; 1297–1339.
2. Cappabianca P, Cavallo LM, Divitiis E. Endoscopic endonasal transsphenoidal surgery. *Neurosurgery* 2004; 55:933–941.
3. Elias WJ, Laws ER Jr. Transphenoidal approach to lesions to the sella. In *Operative neuro-surgical techniques: Indications, methods and results*, 4th edn, Schmidek HH (Ed). Philadelphia: WB Saunders, 2000; 373–384.
4. Har-El G. Endoscopic transnasal trassphenoidal pituitary surgery – Comparison with the traditional sublabial transseptal approach. *Otolaryngol Clin N Am* 2005; 38:723–735.
5. Isaacs RS, Donald PJ. Sphenoid and sellar tumors. *Otolaryngol Clin North Am* 1995; 28:1191–1229.
6. Jankowski R, Auque I, Simon C. Endoscopic pituitary tumor surgery. *Laryngoscope* 1992; 102:198–202.
7. Sethi DS, Pillay PK. Endoscopic surgery for pituitary tumors. *Oper Tech Otolaryngol Head Neck Surg* 1995; 7:264–268.
8. Stamm A, Pignatari SSN. Transnasal endoscopic-assisted surgery of the skull base. In *Otolaryngology Head Neck Surgery*. 4th edn, Cummings CW, Flint PW, Harker LA (Ed). Philadelphia: Elsevier Mosby, 2005; 3855–3876.
9. Stamm A, Bordasch A, Vellutini E, Pahl F. Transnasal micro-endoscopic surgery for pituitary tumors. Proceedings of the ERS and ISIAN Bologna, Monduzzi (Ed) 1998; 341–347.
10. Stamm A, Bordasch A, Vellutini E, Pahl F. Transnasal endoscopic surgery of the sella and parasellar regions. In *Micro-endoscopic surgery of the paranasal sinuses and the skull base*, eds Stamm AC, Draf W. Berlin: Springer-Verlag, 2000; 555–567.

Endoscopic Optic Nerve and Orbital Decompression

Hannes Braun, Heinz Stammberger

Traditional surgical approaches to decompress the optic nerve as well as the orbit include: craniotomy by the neurosurgeon, extranasal transethmoidal, transorbital, transantral and intranasal microscopic approaches.

Endonasal endoscopic optic nerve decompression (OND) offers some advantages over the more traditional approaches: Excellent visualization of the area, 180° medial decompression of the optic nerve canal, relatively short operative time, decreased morbidity, no disruption of olfactory tract fibers with preservation of olfaction, rapid recovery time, no external scars, no injury to the developing teeth in children and less stress in a patient who may have multisystemic traumata.[1] Potential disadvantages and limitations are:

- The superior and lateral aspect of the optic canal cannot be reached via this approach. Decompression is limited to the inferior and medial portion of the optic canal.
- When opening the optic nerve sheath a cerebrospinal fluid (CSF) fistula could possibly result from opening the subarachnoidal space. Additional damage to the optic nerve may be caused by iatrogenic injury to the nerve fascicle itself or a medially arising ophthalmic artery.

Orbital decompression can reverse optic neuropathy, elevated intraorbital pressure, exposure keratitis and cosmetic changes produced by Graves orbitopathy.[4] Endoscopic transnasal decompression of optic nerve and orbit can be performed simultaneously in one session, if required.

INDICATIONS

Indications and contraindications for optic nerve decompression, orbital decompression (OD) or both are listed in Tables 9.5 and 9.6:

The most common indication for OND is (post-) traumatic blindness.

Injuries of the optic nerve may result from direct or indirect trauma to the optic nerve or as a result of both. The most common form of traumatic optic neuropathy is indirect, as a result of concussive force to the head, particularly the forehead.[5] Indirect trauma occurs when force is transmitted via the bones or by displacement of the globe.[2] Various mechanisms of injury may play a role, resulting in intraneural edema, hematoma, injury to the microvasculature as well as direct fractures of the optic

Table 9.5: Indications for optic nerve decompression (OND), orbital decompression (OD), or both

- Trauma with immediate unilateral blindness
- Trauma with progressive loss of vision
- Mucoceles
- Ischemic optic neuropathy
- Fibrous dysplasia and tumors (palliative)
- Endocrine orbitopathy (Graves disease)
- Acute optic neuropathy associated with acute retinal necrosis syndrome
- Optic nerve meningeoma
- Intraorbital bleeding, hematoma
- Inflammation
- Mycotic processes with progressive loss of vision
- Foreign body
- Cosmesis

Table 9.6: Contraindications for optic nerve decompression (OND), orbital decompression (OD), or both

- Complete disruption, discontinuity of the optic nerve or optic chiasm
- Complete atrophy of the optic nerve
- Carotid cavernous sinus fistulae
- (Pseudo-)aneurysm of the internal carotid artery
- Massive damage of brain substance (hematoma, pressure)
- Other life-threatening problems making any surgical procedure hazardous
- Inexperienced surgeon

canal with moderate bony compression, bony fragments injuring or even transecting the optic nerve. A completely transected/disrupted optic nerve clearly is a contraindication for an OND.[1]

Preoperatively, a (pseudo-)aneurysm of the internal carotid artery and/or an internal carotid artery-cavernous sinus fistula must be excluded.

Other indications for OND with or without orbital decompression are mucoceles, pseudotumor orbitae, ischemic optic neuropathy, fibrous dysplasia, endocrine orbitopathy, acute optic neuropathy associated with acute retinal necrosis syndrome, optic nerve meningioma.[1] Beside these a clear indication for OD of course is an intraorbital bleeding resulting in decreasing or complete loss of vision, refractant to appropriate medical therapy.

PREOPERATIVE INVESTIGATIONS

Patients with injury to the orbit and/or optic nerve are usually victims of blunt (poly-)trauma, e.g. car or bike accidents, and others.[1,3] Therefore, all these patients should be seen by a trauma team to evaluate if multisystemic injuries occured and to establish a treatment plan. Frequently, because of the severity of the other injuries, an adequate history and eye examination are difficult to obtain. An ophthalmologist should always be consulted immediately to examine the patient, as it is the ophthalmologist who would give the indication for an OND. Typically, the retina and optic disc initially appear normal, and the only objective finding is the presence of a relative afferent pupillary defect. Optic atrophy does not become apparent until 3–4 weeks after trauma.

Visual fields should be tested to help identify injury to the optic chiasm or to the orbital vasculature.[1]

Fundoscopic examination may provide helpful information and avoid unnecessary surgery. If total atrophy of the optic nerve is displayed, there is no reason for OND, because restoration of vision is impossible.[1]

Radiographic evaluation should include: Coronal computed tomography cuts, especially to rule out or confirm other lesions of the anterior skull base and to depict the anatomical situation for the approach to the optic nerve and orbit (e.g. is there an Onodi cell, herniation of orbital fat blocking the way back to sphenoid sinus).[1]

Radiographic evaluation must include axial computed tomography cuts with thin slices in order to evaluate the orbital content as well as the course of the optic nerve and if depicted the damage to the bony canal of the optic nerve (Figs 9.59A and B). The absence of a radiologically evident fracture does not exclude the possible presence of a fracture. Interpretation of such 'false negative' CT findings may lead to under-treatment of the patient who might otherwise benefit from surgical decompression.[4]

If available, computer assisted navigation-systems help in addition.

(MR-) Angiography should be considered if an internal carotid artery–cavernous sinus fistula or an aneurysm of the internal carotid artery is suspected.[1]

SURGICAL ANATOMY

The bony optic canal carries the optic nerve and the ophthalmic artery, which comes from the internal carotid artery. The optic nerve is a direct continuation of brain and therefore shows all meningeal layers (pia, arachnoidea, dura). Due to its anatomical course the optic nerve is divided into three topographical segments: the intraorbital, the intracanalicular and the intracranial one.

The intraorbital optic nerve is about 25 mm long and extends from the back of the eyeball to the orbital apex. At the apex of the orbit the intracanalicular portion of the optic nerve enters the optic canal for a distance of 9 mm. The intracranial portion of the optic nerve stretches from the posterior optic canal to the optic chiasm with a variable length (3 to 16 mm).[5]

The intracanalicular portion of the optic nerve is the site most frequently involved in indirect lesions such as blunt trauma. If an injury occurs in this segment of the nerve, OND may be most beneficial.[1]

The dural covering of the optic nerve consists of two layers: The outer layer, arising from the orbital apex, where the dura from the central nervous system splits to form the periorbit as well as the optic nerve sheath, and

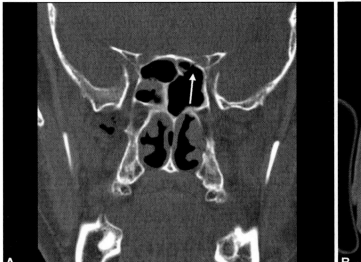
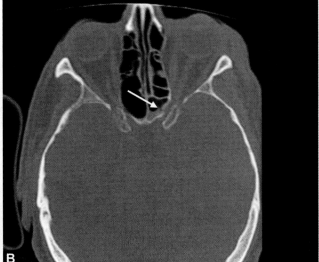

Figs 9.59A and B: (A) Coronal CT demonstrating a fracture (arrow) of the bony canal of the left optic nerve. (B) Axial cut from the CT in Fig. (A) demonstrating a fracture (arrow) of the bony canal of the left optic nerve

the arachnoid attached to the inner portion of the dural sheath. If in OND this subarachnoid space is opened a potential CSF leak occurs.[1]

In endoscopic OND the approach is from anterior and medially. Posterior ethmoidal cells, which have pneumatized considerably laterally to and/or superiorly of the sphenoid sinus are called Onodi cells, or sphenoethmoidal cells.[1] In 12% or more the optic nerve will be running through such a posterior ethmoidal cell (Figs 9.60 and 9.61). The optic nerve tubercle or even the

optic nerve canal can be prominent in its lateral wall, before entering sphenoid sinus proper.

If not recognized preoperatively on the scans or during posterior ethmoidectomy the surgeon may traumatize the optic nerve, misjudging its actual position.

The ophthalmic artery typically enters the nerve sheath from inferolateral and thus would not be in the surgical field of an endoscopic endonasal approach (Fig. 9.62).

In more than 15% of patients the ophthalmic artery enters from the medial side of the orbital aperture of the optic canal and than could be injured in endoscopic OND (Fig. 9.63).[1,6] Attempts to pack or cauterize a bleeding

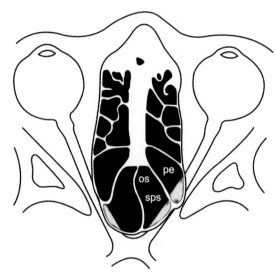

Fig. 9.60: Schematic drawing, axial view from above: Close relationship between the optic nerve and a posterior ethmoid air cell (pe = posterior ethmoid air cell, sps = sphenoid sinus, os = natural ostium of sphenoid sinus) (Modified after Stammberger[1])

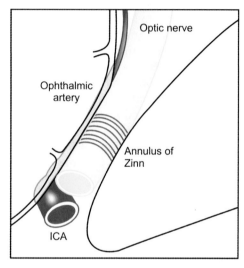

Fig. 9.62: Normal course of the ophthalmic artery. After leaving the right internal carotid artery (ICA) it swings inferolateral to the optic nerve (Modified after Stammberger[1])

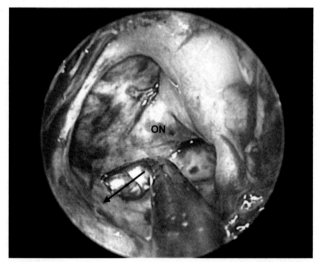

Fig. 9.61: Endoscopic view of the relationship of a left posterior ethmoidal cell and left optic nerve (ON). Moving the instrument (curette) further posterior could damage the optic nerve. The way into sphenoid sinus proper would be medial and down, as indicated by the tip of the curette (arrow)

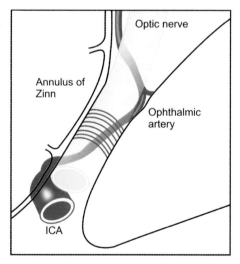

Fig. 9.63: The right ophthalmic artery remains on the medial side of the optic canal internal carotid artery (ICA) (Modified after Stammberger[1])

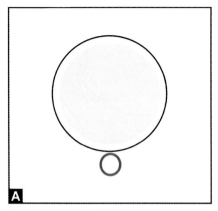 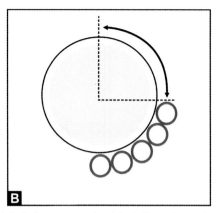 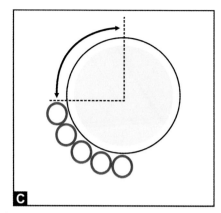

Figs 9.64A to C: (A) Normal course of the ophthalmic artery at six o'clock (frontal cut; view from anterior onto the optic nerve) (Modified after Stammberger[1]. (B and C) Potential variations of the course of the ophthalmic artery on both sides (view from anterior onto the optic nerve, as one would encounter during surgery). A "safe" slitting of the optic nerve sheath would be above the equator on both sides (arrows) (Modified after Stammberger[1])

ophthalmic artery in these cases would be counter-productive regarding optic nerve function (Figs 9.64A to C).

Another important structure is the fibrous annulus of Zinn at the orbital apex, where the muscles of the eye insert. In this area too, the pia and arachnoid fuse and is usually located at the entrance to the most narrow portion of the optic canal. Therefore this is a likely site for compression of the optic nerve. In OND one must be certain, that this annulus is incised during slitting of the optic nerve sheath in order to achieve adequate decompression, as this is the least expandable portion of fibrous tissue around the optic nerve.

SURGICAL TECHNIQUE

Endoscopic Optic Nerve Decompression

A transnasal endoscopic sphenoethmoidectomy is performed with preservation of the middle turbinate, if possible. Initially, the papyraceous lamina as well as the periorbit must not be damaged, as this could lead to a herniation of orbital fat and subsequently would make the way back to sphenoid sinus proper more difficult. After identifying the sphenoid sinus the opening should be enlarged to get a clear overview about the anatomical situation. This can be done very gently and safely with circular cutting punches. The bulging of the internal carotid artery and optic nerve can be identified as they course through the lateral wall and/or roof of sphenoid sinus. Then, at a distance of about 10 mm anterior to the optic tubercle, the papyraceous lamina is removed without violating the periorbit, as this might lead to a herniation of orbital fat and obstruct the surgeon's view.

Sometimes it is necessary to thin out the bony covering of the optic canal from the orbital apex posteriorly (Figs 9.65A and B). Therefore, we use a specially designed diamond burr. The rotating burr can be retracted into a protective sheath until it is in the right position for drilling, thus preventing entanglement of the soft tissues in the drill burr. An irrigation system is built into the drill, too. A dissector modified from the Fisch ear instruments is used to elevate the thinned bone from over the optic nerve (Fig. 9.65C). Extreme care should be taken not to exert pressure on the optic nerve, i.e. towards laterally, with the instruments. The removal of bone over the optic nerve should be extended about 2 to 4 mm beyond the fracture line. The procedure leads to a bony decompression, resulting in a nearly 180° liberation of the optic nerve on its medial and inferior aspects. In addition the optic nerve sheath and the annulus of Zinn potentially contribute to pressure on the optic nerve. The incision of the optic nerve sheath and the fibrous annulus of Zinn is accomplished with a delicate sickle knife (Fig. 9.65D). Slitting the optic nerve sheath is a procedure controversially discussed in literature. We would open the nerve sheath in certain cases: Patients with an intra-sheath hematoma, fracture of the intracanalicular portion of the optic nerve canal, or lateral displacement of the bony optic canal with impingement on the optic nerve, papillary edema and/or bleeding. Also in cases where the impression of a bulging optic nerve is obtained, the sheath would be opened. By opening the optic nerve sheath we potentially create a cerebrospinal fluid leak.

If necessary optic nerve decompression can be combined with an orbital decompression, which would be performed after the decompression of the optic nerve.

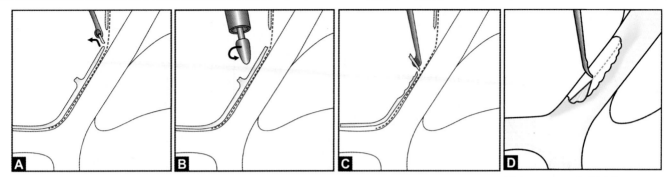

Figs 9.65A to D: (A) Delicate removal of lamina papyracea 1 cm anterior to the optic nerve tubercle. (B) In cases with thick bone over the optic nerve tubercle, it can be thinned out with a diamond burr. (C) The thinned bone layers are carefully removed medially. (D) If necessary, the optic nerve sheath can be incised with a sickle knife, exposing the optic fascicle. This should be done above the equator, as shown in Figs 9.64B and C (Modified after Stammberger[1])

Endoscopic Orbital Decompression

After complete ethmoidectomy, with preservation of middle and superior turbinate, at a distance of about 10 mm anterior to the optic tubercle, the papyraceous lamina is removed without violating the periorbit initially. Care must be taken not to injure the anterior ethmoidal artery, as this might lead to bleeding and the need for cauterization. If the bleeding artery slips back into the orbit, this also might lead to a rapid exophthalmos and consecutively, an increase of pressure on the optic nerve and its vessels. An orbital decompression must be done immediately. It is not recommended that the surgeon search for the artery within the orbit, or cauterize the artery within the orbit, as this could lead to an iatrogenic damage to the optic nerve. If necessary (e.g. decompression of the orbit in endocrine orbitopathy) the floor of the orbit can be removed endoscopically, too. The border for this procedure is the canal of the infraorbital nerve, which must not be injured. After preparation of the periorbit, it is incised from posterior to anterior with a sickle knife. Only the tip of the knife should cut through the periorbit in order not to damage the orbital content (medial rectus muscle, vessels or the optic nerve itself). Care must be taken, that the protruding orbital fat does not block the drainage pathways out of the frontal and maxillary sinuses. If so, the natural ostium of maxillary sinus should be enlarged and part of the medial wall of the maxillary sinus should be resected.

Postoperatively, the patient is advised not to blow the nose for a few days, as this could lead to orbital emphysema and may cause an infection of the orbital content.

CONSERVATIVE TREATMENT WITH CORTICOSTEROIDS

The two options available for the treatment of traumatic optic neuropathy are surgical decompression and corticosteroids. Medical therapy includes intravenous administration of methyl prednisolone 30 mg/kg body weight as a loading dose (~ 2 gm per 70 kg in an adult). This dose should be halved every 6 hours over a period of 24 hours. Like other authors we would recommend both treating options (surgery and corticosteroids) simultaneously.[7]

Patients with no initial light perception seem to have a worse prognosis for visual improvement. The International Optic Nerve Trauma Study showed that the prognosis for visual recovery is poor when the initial visual acuity was "no light perception".[3] The authors also demonstrated no significant differences in final visual acuity, after correction for baseline visual acuity, between surgical decompression of the optic canal, treatment with corticosteroids, and observation alone. They also stated, that there is no clear indication that optic canal decompression produces better results than corticosteroid treatment and there is also no evidence that dose of corticosteroids and the timing of the beginning of corticosteroid therapy and surgery are key factors.[3]

Authors' Results

From 1990 till 2005, we operated 51 patients with indirect trauma to the optic nerve. 37 (72.5%) showed no light perception, 10 (19.7%) had a visual loss < 0.2, an afferent defect or prolonged visual evoked potentials (VEP). Preoperative ophthalmologic data of 4 patients were not available any more for evaluation. In 8 patients retrospective follow-up data were not available.

Follow-up of 43 patients demonstrated the following results: postoperatively 20 patients (46.5%) showed no improvement of blindness 6 patients (14%) recovered full vision; In 17 patients (39.5%) vision recovered up to 0.5, but showed a persisting impairment of the visual field.

GENERAL GUIDELINES AND CONCLUSIONS

- Endonasal endoscopic optic nerve decompression is an elegant and non-traumatizing surgical technique.
- This procedure should only be performed by most experienced endoscopic surgeons. Knowledge of anatomy is crucial.
- OND does not affect the primary contusion necrosis of the optic nerve but might help to reduce factors responsible for secondary axonal loss, like pressure upon the optic nerve caused by edema, hematoma or displaced bony fragments of the optic nerve canal.
- However, clear indications for OND are yet to be established.
- We agree with the authors of the International Optic Nerve Trauma Study that it is clinically reasonable to decide whether or not to treat on an individual basis.[3]
- If necessary optic nerve decompression can be combined with an orbital decompression, which would be performed after the decompression of the optic nerve.
- Surgeons undertaking sinus surgery must be able to perform an orbital decompression, as this procedure would be necessary, if orbital complications occur (e.g. intraorbital bleeding).

REFERENCES

1. Luxenberger W, Stammberger H, Jebeles JA, Walch C. Endoscopic optic nerve decompression: The Graz experience. *Laryngoscope* 1998; 108:873–882.
2. Siracuse-Lee DE, Kazim M. Orbital decompression: Current concepts. *Curr Opin Ophthalmol* 2002; 13:310–316.
3. Levin LA, Beck RW, Joseph MP et al. The treatment of traumatic optic neuropathy: The International Optic Nerve Trauma Study. *Ophthalmology* 1999; 106:1268–1277.
4. Wohlrab TM, Maas S, De Carpentier JP. Surgical decompression in traumatic optic neuropathy. *Acta Ophthalmol Scand* 2002; 80:287–293.
5. Bhatti MT, Stankiewicz JA. Ophthalmic complications of endoscopic sinus surgery. *Surv Ophthalmol* 2003; 48:389–402.
6. Lang J. Anatomy of optic nerve decompression and anatomy of the orbit and adjacent skull base in surgical anatomy of the skull base. In *Surgery of the Skull Base. An Interdisciplinary Approach,* Samii M, Draf W, eds. Berlin: Springer, 1989; 16–19.
7. Rajinganth MG, Gupta AK, Gupta A, Bapuraj JR. Traumatic optic neuropathy. *Arch Otolaryngol Head Neck Surg* 2003; 129:1203–1206.

Endonasal Duraplasty

B Schik, Wolfgang Draf

Cerebrospinal fluid fistulas of the anterior skull base could be due to various causes. Most commonly they are observed after a trauma (major or minor head injuries), occur due to dura opening in paranasal sinus surgery or are of congenital origin. While congenital CSF fistulas have been regarded to be very rare for a long time, they have been detected in recent years more frequently using modern imaging techniques. Therefore, congenital skull base defects have to be taken into account in case of a possible dural defect.

Recurrent meningitis, meningitis caused by upper airway pathogens, and/or CSF rhinorrhea are highly suspicious of the presence of a CSF fistula and demand a careful investigation to detect a possible CSF fistula. One should especially keep in mind that CSF fistulas, independent of their cause, may remain unnoticed for a long time. In our own series we have detected several dural defects years or even decades after their presumed time of onset with the longest time period being 48 years.[1]

Independent of their cause a tight dura closure is required in frontobasal CSF fistulas as the patients are at risk of developing endocranial complications, mainly meningitis, until a sufficient dura repair has been accomplished. Meningitis is expected in case of an unrepaired traumatic dura lesion in 3 to 50%.[1] Therefore, knowledge of the various causes, diagnostic concepts and surgical techniques for endonasal dura repair are of utmost importance to the rhinologist.

HISTORY

After the first duraplasty has been performed successfully by Dandy via an intracranial approach, Dohlman described in 1948, the external, extracranial approach for dura repair.[2,3] Already in 1952, Hirsch reported the first endonasal repair of a sphenoidal CSF fistula.[4] But like the description of the endonasal closure of a CSF fistula at the cribriform plate by Vrabec and Hallberg the possibility of an endonasal frontobasal dura repair did not gain attention for a long time.[5] Due to the experience of a possible excellent endonasal anterior skull base exposure using modern optical aids such as endoscope and microscope, a large number of frontobasal CSF fistulas have been managed in the recent years endonasally with high success rates.[6,7] The endonasal approach is currently the preferred approach to close CSF fistulas of the anterior skull base with high success rate (more than 90%), low morbidity and frequent preservation of the sense of smell.[8] Thus, the rhinologist should provide the option of endonasal duraplasty for management of frontobasal CSF fistulas.

SITE OF CSF FISTULAS

CSF fistulas occurring in paranasal sinus surgery are most commonly located at the conjunction of the olfactory groove and the ethmoidal roof in the anterior part of the ethmoid. Especially if the olfactory groove is very deep in relation to the ethmoidal roof (type III according to Keros) there might be only a very thin bony border separating the olfactory groove from the ethmoidal cavity (Fig. 9.66A). Injury of the skull base during paranasal sinus surgery may furthermore occur at the posterior ethmoidal roof. Due to embryological development the conjunction between the posterior ethmoidal roof and the sphenoidal plane can be built up by a thinner bone than is found at the anterior ethmoidal roof and the sphenoidal plane. Furthermore, the surgeon has always to consider that the skull base is deeper at the posterior than at the anterior ethmoidal roof not representing a strictly horizontal plane. Thus in case the ethmoidectomy is performed from the anterior to posterior direction the skull base may be injured at the posterior ethmoidal roof in front of the sphenoidal plane (Fig. 9.66B).

Skull base formation in embryology starts by fusion of cartilaginous precursors that will be followed by an enchondral ossification. A disturbance of the fusion of these cartilaginous precursors can result in a congenital skull base defect and a CSF fistula. Thus, the fusion areas of the cartilaginous precursors have to be considered as areas of predilection for possible CSF fistulas. They are located at the prenasal space (anterior fusion area of the cribriform plate), along the fusion area of the cribriform plate with the ethmoidal roof, in front of the sphenoidal plane and in case of a well pneumatized sphenoid sinus at its posterior lateral border as a parasellar bony defect[9] representing a persistent lateral craniopharyngeal canal (Fig. 9.67). In case one or more of the cartilaginous precursors are not arising during embryological development a corresponding huge frontobasal skull base defect is observed (Fig. 9.68). Dealing with congenital skull base defects one should be aware that due to the complexity of embryological development more than one skull base defect might be present.[10,11] Thus, even if one skull base defect has been detected in preoperative imaging one should not miss to evaluate the whole skull base in order to detect a possible second CSF fistula.

DIAGNOSIS

In regard to the importance of closing a frontobasal CSF fistula diagnostic schedules have to be defined in the responsibility that a CSF fistula must not remain unnoticed. The possible difficulties in defining presence and localization of a CSF fistula demand a close cooperation with the laboratory and the neuroradiologist.

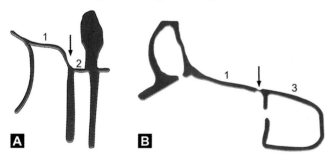

Figs 9.66A and B: In case of a significantly different level of the ethmoid roof and the cribriform plate. (A) the bony junction between both (arrow, lateral lamella of the cribriform plate) is an area of predilection for dura injury during paranasal sinus surgery. If the ethmoidectomy is performed in an anterior to posterior direction a dura opening may occur in front of the sphenoid plane. (B) (arrow) due to the down sloping skull base representing an oblique plane and a thinner bone in this area

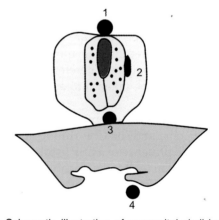

Fig. 9.67: Schematic illustration of congenital skull base defects that might be located at the prenasal space (1), at the junction of the cribriform plate and the ethmoid roof (2), in front of the sphenoidal plane (3) or at the parasellar region (4)

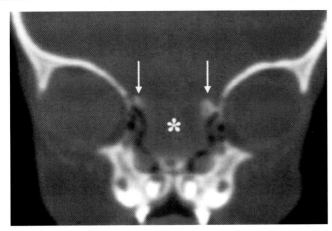

Fig. 9.68: The computed tomography imaging shows the finding of a huge encephalocele (*) reaching down to the nasal floor. This congenital skull base defect is the result of a failure in development of the cribriform plates. Only rudimental ethmoidal roofs (arrows) have been developed

Only a continuing team work in this field will succeed in providing the best possible diagnostic work-up for the patients.

In the diagnosis of a CSF fistula one must prove the existence of a CSF fistula (by analyzing the nasal discharge) and identify the precise localization of the site of a CSF fistula. The nasal discharge can be analyzed through different techniques. The determination of β2-transferrin,[12] albumin/prealbumin ratio,[13] and β-trace protein[14] use the principle of comparing the specific protein content in the nasal discharge and the serum as the target proteins have a different concentration in the cerebrospinal fluid and the serum. For the β-trace protein this ratio is the highest with 33 and analysis can be done rapidly. Though testing for β-trace protein has been recommended in recent years, the other methods are also well-established that have been used very successfully at the centers that have focused on them.

The four most important tools for localization of a CSF fistula are computed tomography, magnetic resonance imaging, cisternography (MR or CT) and fluorescein nasal endoscopy. High-resolution computed tomography is a very valuable tool to detect bony defects or fractures.[15] If not 1 mm slices but 2 mm or 4 mm slices are taken, computed tomography may fail to detect a small dehiscence. While coronal sections are best suited to analyze the ethmoidal roof, cribriform plate and sphenoidal plane (Fig. 9.69A), axial sections are superior means for the evaluation of the posterior frontal sinus wall as well as the lateral and posterior sphenoid sinus walls. As a lateral skull base CSF fistula communicating with the middle ear can cause nasal discharge or posterior nasal drip via the eustachian tube, imaging should include evaluation of the lateral skull base. With MRI the skull base can be examined in multiple planes without radiation exposure. Encephaloceles and meningoceles can be excellently visualized by this technique. Even more, magnetic resonance imaging may localize precisely an active CSF fistula by CISS sequences[16] or T2-weighted images in case of well aerated paranasal sinuses (Fig. 9.69B). If computed tomography and magnetic resonance imaging have failed to detect the CSF fistula despite of a highly suspicious laboratory result indicating

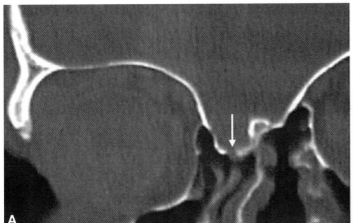
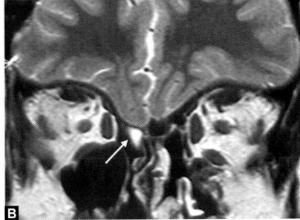

Figs 9.69A and B: This congenital bony defect at the junction of the ethmoid roof to the cribriform plate (arrow) had been detected only by the presented section of a 1 mm high-resolution coronal computed tomography. (A) While the previous and following sections did not show a bony defect. T2-weighted magnetic resonance imaging. (B) Of the same patient was even able to visualize cerebrospinal fluid just below the CSF fistula in an ethmoidal cell (arrow)

cerebrospinal fluid in the nasal discharge, a CT- or MR-cisternography is a further diagnostic option.[17,18] After lumbar application of an appropriate contrast medium an active CSF fistula can be visualized with high success rates. But in case of an inactive CSF leak at the time of investigation the success rate drops significantly. Success rates for cisternography were reported to be 92% in active CSF fistulas, but only 40% in inactive CSF fistulas.[19]

Fluorescein nasal endoscopy is a diagnostic tool which can be used to answer the question if a CSF fistula is present or not as well as to localize a CSF fistula intraoperatively. In addition, fluorescein allows to detect a thin scar at the skull base which is not sufficient to prevent inflammatory endocranial complications but is the reason for absence of an active CSF-leakage at the time of investigation. In this case endonasal exploration of the skull base enables the surgeon to detect the thin scar by fluorescein impregnation requesting to accomplish a tight duraplasty. By nasal endoscopy using the appropriate filters a dilution of the fluorescein until 1:10,000,000 is detectable in the nose and paranasal sinuses. Thus, fluorescein nasal endoscopy is highly sensitive and offers additional informations that cannot be obtained by the other diagnostic techniques. In order to avoid side-effects by use of the fluorescein nasal endoscopy, lumbar application of a 5% fluorescein solution without any stabilization additives (0.05–0.1 ml of the 5% fluorescein solution/10 kg body weight, but never more than 1 ml) is recommended. Seizures, dysesthesia, opisthotonus or cranial nerve palsies are possible complications of lumbar fluorescein application, but large series have demonstrated excellent experiences consi-dering avoidance of wrong fluorescein solutions, too high fluorescein concentrations and too large amounts of the fluorescein solution.[20,21]

AREAS OF ENDONASAL SKULL BASE ACCESS

Most rhinobasal dural defects can be managed endonasally. One of the prerequisites for selection of the endonasal approach for dura repair is that the defect can be exposed completely via the endonasal approach; insufficient exposure of the defect is one reason for possible failure of endonasal duraplasty. The size of the dura defect is of less importance if the defect can be completely visualized. It has been found in endonasal tumor resections with the need of extended dura resection that the dura of the ethmoid roof, the cribriform plate, and the sphenoidal plane can be reconstructed endonasally. Nevertheless a surgeon might define a

personal size limit of dural defects for endonasal closure in regard of his own experiences.

The areas of the ethmoid roof and the cribriform plate are accessible endonasally. In case a CSF fistula is located within the confines of the cribriform plate and the smell function is preserved it has to be weighed up if the endonasal or an intradural approach with insertion of grafts between the olfactory fibers is best suited to preserve olfaction. Dural defects of the sphenoid sinus are an ideal indication to be managed endonasally. Especially cerebrospinal fluid fistulas placed at the lateral or posterior border of the sphenoid sinus cannot be closed easily by an external approach. Dural repair at these sites can be an excellent opportunity to initiate inter-disciplinary co-operation with neurosurgeons. In case the anterior skull base has been covered after a severe trauma with a galea-periosteal flap via an external approach, the rhinologist can be asked to close the unreachable dural defects at the lateral or posterior confines of the sphenoid sinus. Dural defects of the posterior frontal sinus wall can be closed endonasally in selected cases if they are located in the inferior part and medial to a vertical plane through the lamina papyracea. One has to answer the question if at least an extended endonasal frontal sinus access (type III according to Draf) allows sufficient exposure of the dural defect. Otherwise an endonasal approach cannot be recommended.

GRAFT MATERIALS

Many graft materials have been used for dura repair. In general, one can distinguish between autologous, allogenic and synthetic grafts. Nowadays autologous grafts are preferred since one can avoid a transfection arising from an allogenic graft. For autologous grafts the rhinologist can harvest mucosal or mucosal/periosteal transplants from the turbinates. From more distant sites temporalis fascia, fascia lata, periost, perichondrium, cartilage, muscle, or fat tissue may be harvested as further autologous grafts. If fat tissue is used for duraplasty one should avoid a direct contact of the fat tissue with the intracranial cerebrospinal fluid as fat necrosis risks an aseptic lipoid meningitis postoperatively.[22]

If allogenic grafts are desired, allogenic fascia, allogenic pericardium or acellular dermis should be preferred instead of allogenic dura due to their lower risk of causing a transfection. Furthermore the preparation of the allogenic grafts by the various procedures before they are offered commercially should not result in a cross-linked collagen graft as they cannot be broken down in the wound healing process and would act similar to a synthetic graft. The general advantage of an allogenic graft is its availability without any donor site morbidity. In addition, these materials do not shrink and are usually more stiff being therefore easier to handle during surgery.

In principle the inserted graft acts as a scaffold in the wound healing process and is replaced by connective tissue. The mostly collagenic extracellular matrix of the different cellular or acellular grafts is broken down by enzymatic and cellular processes and replaced by connective tissue. In children the osteogenic capacity can be the reason for a bony closure of the defect. Additionally a cellular component arising from the dura at the defect margins has to be considered. This cellular outgrowth is of benefit for graft stabilization and contributes to a tight defect closure. We found in own studies of culturing grafts that collagen surfaces are highly attractive for the migration of dural fibroblasts onto the graft surface. No migration of cells was found onto bony or cartilaginous surfaces and only few cells migrated onto poly-p-dioxanon sheets (PDS-sheets) as a representative of a synthetic graft material.[23] Thus, collagen grafts are grafts of first choice for dura repair. In case bone or cartilage is intended to be used they should be harvested as composite grafts. At the contact site to the dura they should be covered by periosteum or peri-chondrium to be attractive for cell migration from the dura borders.

SURGICAL TECHNIQUES

The main principle of endonasal duraplasty is to place a graft at the site of the defect. The graft can be placed through the defect intracranially on the dura (intradural underlay, Fig. 9.70A), inserted between the elevated dura margins and the bone (extradural underlay, Fig. 9.70B), or fixed onto the bone from below (onlay, Fig. 9.70C). A combination of these methods may also be used to ensure safe dura repair. The combination of an underlay and onlay grafting has been termed *sandwich technique*. Such a combination is advisable in larger defects and in case of persistent CSF fistulas where increased CSF production is expected. Some surgeons routinely use lumbar drainage to reduce the CSF pressure weighting on the grafts, but this has been found unnecessary in most cases.[6]

A special situation in graft placement has to be considered in case of dura repair close to the cribriform plate as dura elevation at the defect margins may injure olfactory fibers. However, one has to take into account that even if an endonasal duraplasty is performed in the area of the cribriform plate olfaction is preserved to a

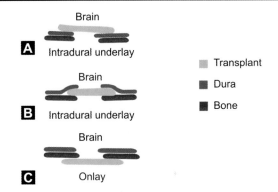

Figs 9.70A to C: In general three different modalities of graft placement in endonasal duraplasty should be distinguished. The graft can be placed on the dura (intracranial underlay technique), between the elevated dura margins and the bony skull base (extradural underlay technique) or onto the bony skull base from below (onlay technique)

certain extent. Olfactory fibers at the site of repair and all olfactory fibers on the opposite site are intended to be preserved in endonasal duraplasty. Aiming to preserve olfaction completely, an intradural approach without brain elevation enabling the surgeon to place grafts between the exposed olfactory fibers is a possible alternative to the endonasal approach.

The technique of graft placement to close a cerebrospinal fluid fistula at the cribriform plate depends on the olfactory function. If preoperative testing proves a loss of olfaction grafts can be placed in the underlay or onlay technique at the cribriform plate. In case olfactory function has been lost on one side the graft is placed laterally at the ethmoidal roof in an underlay technique and in the midline in a created pouch between the septal bone and septal mucosa (Fig. 9.71A). In case of intact olfaction dural defects at the conjunction of the ethmoidal roof and cribriform plate the graft should be placed at the lateral border in the underlay technique while it is placed medially in the onlay technique (Fig. 9.71B). This specific graft placement may fail to cover the posterior and anterior border of the defect sufficiently; a second graft (onlay graft) should be placed. As an alternative to the combined underlay/onlay graft placements an onlay graft can be chosen as the primary graft.

In the sphenoid sinus various specific aspects have to be considered in intended endonasal duraplasty. Due to the basal cisterns high CSF pressure might weigh down on the duraplasty. The optic nerves, internal carotid arteries, and the cavernous sinus might prohibit elevating the dura borders for an extradural underlay graft placement. Removal of bone fragments in case of a traumatic CSF fistula is a challenge in regard to the

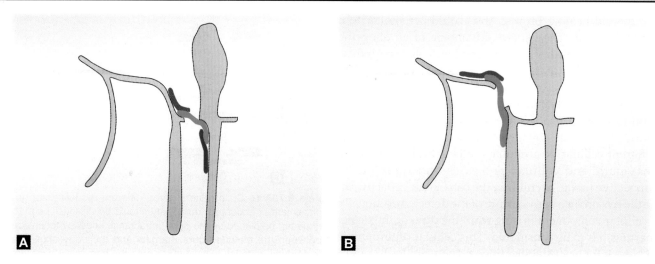

Figs 9.71A and B: (A) If olfaction has been lost only unilaterally at the side of the CSF fistula the graft can be placed laterally in the underlay technique and medially in a pouch between the bony septum and the mucosa. (B) In case of preserved olfaction and a CSF fistula being located at the junction of the ethmoid roof and the cribriform plate the graft can be placed laterally in the underlay technique and medially in the onlay technique. An alternative would be in both cases to place the graft in the onlay technique

important neurovascular structures in close relation to the dural defect. Furthermore a lateral recess can be difficult to visualize prohibiting complete exposure of a dural defect. In such cases, in addition to the above techniques (onlay, underlay) two further techniques have been developed for sphenoidal dura repair: the tobacco pouch technique according to Kley and the fat obliteration of the sphenoid sinus.[24,25] For both techniques the mucosa of the sphenoid sinus should be removed completely. For the tobacco pouch technique a sufficient piece of fascia lata is formed into a tobacco pouch by a suture and filled with gelatine sponge. The pouch is introduced into the sphenoid sinus filled by the dry sponge. The fascia lata is pressed against the bony borders of the sphenoid sinus by removal of the suture and moistening of the sponge. This technique is especially valuable in case of multiple sphenoidal dural defects. In case of the fat obliteration technique a collagen transplant is wedged into the dural defect and the sinus totally obliterated by fat tissue pieces. Finally the sphenoid sinus opening is closed by insertion of grafts at the anterior sinus border.

IMPORTANT CONSIDERATIONS TO AVOID FAILURES

The two most common reasons for failure of endonasal dura repair are insufficient size of the transplant and unstable placement. If an autologous graft is used for dura repair one has to consider that these grafts (in contrast to allogenic grafts) have a shrinkage rate of up to 30%. Thus, a graft covering the defect only slightly at the end of surgery may not be covering the defect sufficiently during the wound healing process (Fig. 9.72A). Only an

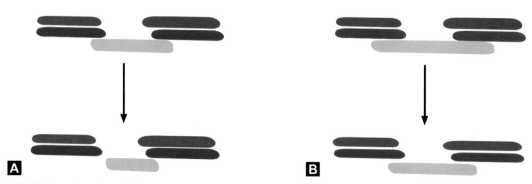

Figs 9.72A and B: Failure of endonasal dura repair due to shrinkage. (A) Graft covering the defect only slightly at the end of surgery may not cover it sufficiently during the wound healing process. (B) An autologous graft that covers the defect sufficiently even after shrinkage will provide safe dura repair

autologous graft that covers the defect sufficiently even after shrinkage will provide a safe dura repair (Fig. 9.72B). From animal experiments evidence is given that the wound healing process will fix the graft one week after placement to the necessary extent so that a displacement will not occur.[26] Therefore, the surgeon has to ensure stable graft placement for one week. To achieve stable graft placement fibrin glue, cellulose sponge, mucosal flaps and different nasal packings have been suggested. Fibrin glue is not found to be necessary by all surgeons and is discussed in the context of possible transfections. Nevertheless fibrin glue is used nowadays frequently. In experimental studies we found that fibrin glue provides an attractive extracellular matrix that accelerates cellular migration into the site of the defect.[27] In addition the different fibrin glues offered today contain to various degrees growth factors which also stimulate the wound healing process. In the light of these two aspects fibrin glue is attractive for graft stabilization.

ACKNOWLEDGMENTS

We would like to acknowledge the cooperation of and to express our profound thanks to Professor JP Haas and Dr G Kahle (Institute of Radiology, Klinikum Fulda).

REFERENCES

1. Schick B, Weber R, Kahle G, Draf W, Lackmann GM. Late manifestations of traumatic lesions of the anterior skull base. *Skull Base* 1997a; 7:77–83.
2. Dandy WD. Pneumocephalus. intracranial pneumocele or aerocele. *Arch Surg* 1926; 12:949–982.
3. Dohlman G. Spontaneous cerebrospinal rhinorrhea. *Acta Otolaryngol Suppl* 1948; 67:20–23.
4. Hirsch O. Successful closure of cerebrospinal fluid rhinorrhea by endonasal surgery. *Arch Otolaryngol* 1952; 56:1–13.
5. Vrabec DP, Hallberg OE. Cerebrospinal fluid rhinorrhea by endonasal surgery. *Arch Otolarnygol* 1964; 80:218–229.
6. Schick B, Ibing R, Brors D, Draf W. Long-term study of endonasal duraplasty and review of the literature. *Ann Otol Laryngol Rhinol* 2001; 114:142–147.
7. Kirtane MV, Gautham K, Upadyaya SR. Endoscopic CSF rhinorrhea closure:our experience in 267 cases. *Otolaryngol Head Neck Surg* 2005; 132:208–212.
8. Lund V. Endoscopic management of cerebrospinal fluid leaks. *Am J Rhinol* 2002; 16:17–23.
9. Schick B, Brors D, Prescher A. Sternberg´s canal – cause of congenital sphenoidal meningocele. *Eur Arch Otorhinolaryngol* 2000; 257:430–432.
10. Schick B, Draf W, Kahle G, Weber R, Wallenfang T. Occult malformations of the skull base. *Arch Otolaryngol Head Neck Surg* 1997b; 123:77–80.
11. Schick B, Prescher A, Hofmann E, Steigerwald C, Draf W. Two occult skull base malformations causing recurrent meningitis in a child – a case report. *Eur Arch Otorhinolaryngol* 2003a; 260:518–521.
12. Oberascher G. Otoliquorrhoe–Rhinoliquorrhoe, Salzburger Konzept zur Liquordiagnostik. *Laryngol Rhinol Otol* 1988; 67:375–381.
13. Bohner J, Hesse W. Albumin/Präalbumin–Quotient zur Diagnostik der Liquorrhoe. *Lab Med* 1989; 13:193.
14. Bachmann G, Petereit H. Beta-trace protein as sensitive marker for liquorrhea. *Acta Neurol Scand* 2004; 110:339–341.
15. Lloyd MN, Kimber PM, Burrows EH. Post-traumatic cerebrospinal fluid rhinorrhea:modern high-definition computed tomography is all that is required for the effective demonstration of the site of leakage. *Clin Radiol* 1994; 49:100–103.
16. Klein S, Woischnek D, Firsching R, Heinrichs T. Magnetic resonance imaging diagnosis of craniobasal cerebrospinal fluid fistulas by 3D-CISS sequence. *Zentralbl Neurochir* 2000; 61:150–154.
17. Colquhoun IR. CT cisternography in the investigation of cerebrospinal fluid rhinorrhea. *Clin Radiol* 1993; 47:403–408.
18. Reiche W, Komenda Y, Schick B, Grunwald I, Steudel WI, Reith W. MR cisternography after intrathecal Gd–DPTA application. *Eur Radiol* 2002; 12:2943–2949.
19. Eljamel MS, Pidgeon CN, Toland J, Philips JB, O'Dwyer AA. MRI cisternography, and the localization of CSF fistulae. *Br J Neurosurg* 1994; 8:433–437.
20. Wolf G, Greistorfer K, Stammberger H. Endoscopic detection of cerebrospinal fluid fistulas with a fluorescence technique. Report of experiences with over 925 cases. *Laryngorhinootologie* 1997; 76:588–594.
21. Keerl R, Weber RK, Draf W, Wienke A, Schaefer SD. Use of sodium fluorescein solution for detection of cerebrospinal fluid fistulas: An analysis of 420 administrations and repeated complications in Europe and the United States. *Laryngoscope* 2004; 114:266–272.
22. Hwang PH, Jackler RK. Lipoid meningitis due to aseptic necrosis of a free fat graft placed during neurootologic surgery. *Laryngoscope* 1996; 106:1482–1486.
23. Schick B, Wolf G, Romeike BF, Mestres P, Praetorius M, Plinkert PK. Dural cell culture. A new approach to study duraplasty. *Cells Tissues Organs* 2003b; 173:129–137.
24. Kley W. Diagnose und operative Versorgung von Keilbeinhöhlenfrakturen. *Z Laryng Rhinol* 1967; 46:469–475.
25. Samii M, Draf W. *Surgery of the skull base: An interdisciplinary approach.* Berlin: Springer, 1989; 135–138.
26. Wolf G, Plinkert PK, Schick B. Cell transplantation for a CSF fistula. Experience with fibrin glue and fibroblasts. *Head Neck Oncol* 2005; 53:439–445.
27. Gjuric M, Goede U, Keimer H, Wigand ME. Endonasal endoscopic closure of cerebrospinal fluid fistulas at the anterior cranial base. *Ann Otol Rhinol Laryngol* 1996; 105:620–623.

Minimally Invasive Pituitary Surgery

Marc Bassim, Brent A Senior

The first successful removal of a pituitary tumor was performed in 1889 by Horsley via a transcranial approach. In 1907, Schlofer introduced the transsphenoidal approach by following a transethmoidal route using a lateral rhinotomy incision. The first endonasal approach was described by Hirsch two years later in 1909. In 1910, Cushing introduced the use of the sublabial-transseptal approach that has been in favor since then. The introduction of the operating microscope by Hardy and of intraoperative fluoroscopy by Guiot in the 1950s and 1960s allowed further refinement of this technique. It was not until 1987 that Griffith and Veraapen reintroduced the endonasal approach using microscopy as an alternative to the sublabial approach. Finally in 1992, Jankowski et al reported the first successful endoscopic resection of a pituitary tumor via the transsphenoidal approach.[1–5]

Since then, many authors have reported on their experience using an endoscopic approach to the sella and surrounding structures. The reported rate of complications has been at least comparable to the traditional sublabial approach, with a generally shorter hospital stay and overall morbidity.[1,2,5,6] With its brighter illumination, proximity to the operative field and different angulations available, the endoscope provides a significantly improved exposure and visualization, especially around corners not generally accessible with the traditional microscopic approach.

Using an endoscopic approach requires a surgeon who is well aware of the sinonasal anatomy and is experienced in the use of such instruments. Typically, the neurosurgical curriculum does not include such training; otolaryngologists, on the other hand, have extensive endoscopic training and routinely operate on the sinonasal cavities for different conditions. Close cooperation and communication between the two teams therefore allows a safe, and rapid approach in which each surgeon performs that part with which he is the most comfortable.

The following is an overview of the evaluation, and surgical management of patients with various pituitary tumors. The use of this approach, almost exclusively over the last six years, has allowed us to refine our technique and bring forth new developments, which facilitate a more complete tumor removal and more comfortable patient recovery while minimizing the rate of complications.

ANATOMY

Pituitary Gland

The pituitary gland is a reddish-gray body, measuring approximately 1 cm in diameter, attached to the brain through the infundibulum and resting in the hypophyseal fossa. The gland is composed of two lobes from different embryological origin. The anterior lobe derives from the ectoderm, and starts developing around the fourth week of gestation when an evagination of the stomodeum enlarges dorsally, forming Rathke's pouch. This then is gradually sealed off from the aerodigestive tract, forming a cyst that is then invaded by some mesodermal tissue to form the anterior lobe of the pituitary. A diverticulum arising from the floor of the third ventricle then abuts this lobe and eventually develops into the infundibulum and posterior lobe of the pituitary.[7]

The anterior lobe of the pituitary is composed of epithelial cells surrounded by vascular sinusoids. Three distinct cell types are identified on hematoxylin and eosin staining. Acidophils include somatotropes and lactotropes; basophils include thyrotropes, gonadotropes, and corticotropes; while chromophobes are essentially non-secretory. The hormonally active substances secreted by each cell type are presented in Table 9.7.

The posterior lobe is composed largely of unmyelinated axons whose cell bodies are located in hypothalamic nuclei. These neurons secrete antidiuretic hormone (ADH) and oxcytocin.

Table 9.7: Different cell types in the anterior pituitary and their products[7]

Cell type	Hormone
Somatotropes	Growth hormone (GH)
Lactotropes	Prolactin
Thyrotropes	Thyroid stimulating hormone (TSH)
Gonadotropes	Luteinizing hormone (LH) and follicle stimulating hormone (FSH)
Corticotropes	Adrenocorticotrophic hormone (ACTH)

Sella Turcica

The pituitary gland sits in the sella turcica, a deep depression on the superior aspect of the body of the sphenoid bone. It is located behind the tuberculum sellae,

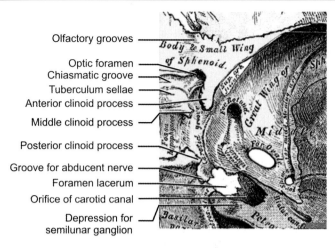

Olfactory grooves

Optic foramen
Chiasmatic groove
Tuberculum sellae
Anterior clinoid process

Middle clinoid process

Posterior clinoid process

Groove for abducent nerve
Foramen lacerum
Orifice of carotid canal

Depression for
semilunar ganglion

Fig. 9.73: Anatomy of the sella turcica,
adapted from Gray's Anatomy

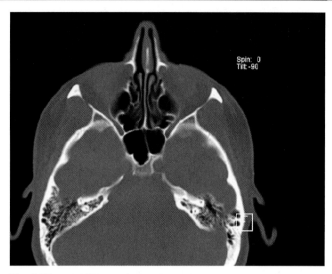

Fig. 9.74: Axial CT scan image illustrating the asymmetric sphenoid sinus with the intersinus septum traveling toward the patient's left carotid

which itself is just posterior to the optic chiasm. The posterior boundary of the sella is defined by the dorsum sellae and the posterior clinoid processes. Below the dorsum sellae is the clivus, which slopes inferiorly and is continuous with the occipital bone (Fig. 9.73).[8] The lateral extensions of the tuberculum sellae form the anterior clinoid processes.

The roof of the fossa is formed by the diaphragm, which is a dural fold traversed by the pituitary stalk. An arachnoid invagination separates the diaphragm and the pituitary capsule. The lateral extension of the diaphragm forms the roof of the cavernous sinus.

The pituitary gland therefore lies in close proximity to multiple vital structures including the optic chiasm and nerves, the carotid arteries, the third, fourth fifth, and sixth cranial nerves in the cavernous sinus, as well as the basilar artery and brainstem posteriorly. Proper knowledge of this anatomy is therefore essential during these approaches.

Sphenoid Sinus and Sinonasal Anatomy

The sphenoid sinus starts developing at about the twelfth week of gestation by posterior evagination of the sphenoethmoid recess. The sinus is not present at birth, but pneumatization starts at about 5 to 7 years of age, and adult size is usually reached by 15 to 18 years.[8]

The sphenoid sinus is variably pneumatized into the sphenoid bone. Three types of sphenoid sinuses are described according to the relation to the sella. A conchal sphenoid is one which has pneumatized only to a small degree with thick bone still over the face of the sella. Sellar pneumatization occurs when pneumatization has

occurred to the face of the sella, while post-sellar describes a sinus that has pneumatized beyond the face of the sella. The majority of adult sinuses are of the sellar type and post-sellar type.

The two sphenoid sinuses are separated by a septum that is off the midline in 60 to 70% of cases; the two cavities are therefore rarely symmetrical (Fig. 9.74).

The roof of the sinus is formed by the planum sphenoidale anteriorly, and the sella posteriorly. The posterior wall corresponds to the clivus. The lateral walls of the sinuses form the medial wall of the cavernous sinus on each side. Intercavernous sinuses connect the two sides and usually run inferior to the gland but can run anteriorly. These connections can be a source of annoying bleeding intraoperatively when the dura is incised.

Multiple structures can be seen running along the walls of the sphenoid sinuses. The canal of the Vidian nerve runs laterally along the floor. The carotid arteries run along the lateral walls, at approximately 5 and 7 o'clock. The optic nerves run more superiorly along the lateral walls, at approximately 2 and 11 o'clock. The optico-carotid recess is located between the bulges of these two structures and may extend into the anterior clinoid process (Fig. 9.75).[2]

The sphenoid ostium is located along the superior aspect of the anterior wall. Different methods have been described for intraoperative localization of the ostium, as discussed in the surgical technique section.

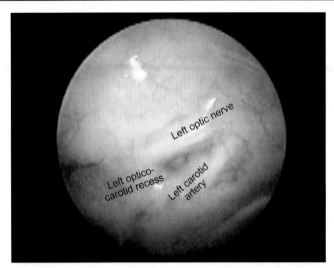

Fig. 9.75: Left optic carotid recess. The optic nerve and carotid artery are clearly visible

SURGICAL INDICATIONS

Indications for excision of hormonally inactive adenomas include compressive symptoms such as hypopituitarism and visual changes, pituitary apoplexy (hemorrhage into the tumor) or severe headaches. Patients with hormonally active prolactinomas are referred for surgery after failure of medical management. Patients with acromegaly, hyperthyroidism, or Cushing's disease are offered

surgery as a primary therapy. The same is true for patients with Rathke's cleft cysts, chordomas and arachnoid cysts.

Preoperative Evaluation

Patients with pituitary adenomas are best evaluated by a multidisciplinary team including an endocrinologist, a neurosurgeon, an otolaryngologist, an ophthalmologist and a radiation oncologist.

During the preoperative visit with the otolaryngologist, a complete history and head and neck examination is performed. Flexible endoscopy is essential for evaluating the sinonasal anatomy and ruling out any concurrent infectious process that may mandate a delay in surgery. The CT scan is reviewed for further anatomic details such as the presence of Onodi cells, asymmetry of the sphenoid cavity, or possible dehiscence of the carotid arteries (Fig. 9.76). The operative plan and potential variations is discussed by the two operative teams. At our institution, all patients obtain a fine cut CT scan for use with the computer-guided navigational system. Occasionally, the preoperative MRI and CT are fused together on the navigational system, allowing for improved intraoperative orientation and visualization of critical structures such as the carotid artery (Fig. 9.77). The risks and benefits of the procedure are discussed at

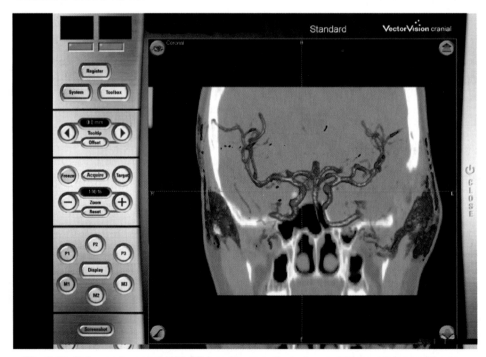

Fig. 9.76: Enhanced coronal MRI-CT fused image, illustrating a dehiscent left carotid artery

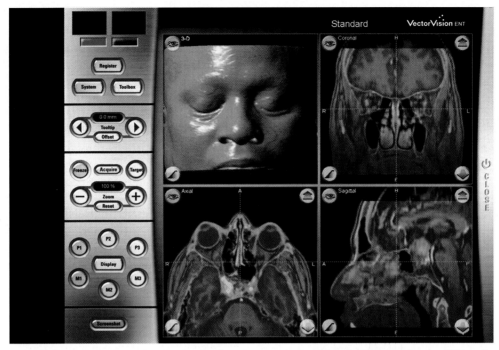

Fig. 9.77: Screenshot illustrating the enhanced anatomic detail obtained with fusing the MRI and CT scan images on the computer guidance system

length and all questions are answered. The expected postoperative course and potential complications are also explained to the patient and family.

Preoperative evaluation by an ophthalmologist is essential. This includes visual acuity and visual fields as well as retinal exam, and serves as a baseline for postoperative comparisons to determine improvement, or possibly degeneration in vision.

A significant number of patients with pituitary tumors will usually present to the surgical team referred by an endocrinologist, sometimes after unsuccessful conservative medical management. These preoperative medications are usually continued; hyperthyroidism is ideally well controlled, and stress doses of steroids are given preoperatively as necessary.

Surgical Technique

The surgical instruments used in the endoscopic endonasal approach are essentially the same as those used by otolaryngologists in the regular endoscopic sinus surgery approach. The regular 4 mm endoscope with different angulations is used; for the major part of the procedure, the straight endoscope provides the best illumination and visualization. Angled scopes are usually used later in the procedure after the sella is entered and

the tumor removed. The use of stereoscopic endoscopes has been described to allow for a three-dimensional view. These reports, however, remain mostly anecdotal.

The patient is positioned in the 'beach-chair' position, with the torso elevated at approximately 30° and the knees slightly bent for comfort. The head is rotated approximately 15° towards the surgeon. In the earlier cases, we used a three-point pin holder, such as a Mayfield head holder, but we have found this to be unnecessary and time consuming. Instead, the patient's head rests on a foam donut, which allows the degree of flexion and rotation to be optimized for exposure during different parts of the procedure.

We routinely use a computer-guided navigation system; this facilitates identification of sellar landmarks and orientation in relation to the tumor while negating the need for fluoroscopy. The latest navigation systems allow for rapid, simple registration in addition to easy integration and tracking of the surgeon's own instrumentation (Fig. 9.78).

The patient's face is not prepared in a sterile fashion in our endonasal approaches, as the instruments will be passing through a contaminated nasal cavity. The abdomen is always prepared, in case a decision is made to use a fat graft at the end of the procedure for CSF leak repair. Care is taken to maintain sterility of the abdominal

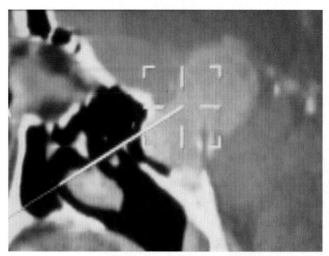

Fig. 9.78: Sagittal CT screen shot from the computer guidance system showing the probe inside the tumor

region with the nasal field being kept distinct throughout the procedure.

Hemostasis is aided by performing greater palatine blocks by injecting approximately 1.5 ml of a solution of 1% lidocaine with 1/100,000 epinephrine transorally into the greater palatine canal bilaterally. The nasal cavities are decongested with pledgets soaked in a solution of 0.05% oxymetazoline hydrochloride. Under endoscopic guidance, more lidocaine with epinephrine is injected at the junction of the horizontal portion of the basal lamella and lateral nasal wall in the region of the sphenopalatine foramen to obtain a sphenopalatine artery block.

Most neurosurgeons are trained to perform pituitary surgery via the midline, trans-septal route. The endoscopic transnasal approach, however, is an extra-axial approach and will result in a slightly different perspective for sellar visualization. The side of approach to the tumor is determined by several factors including, most notably, the degree of obstruction of the nasal cavity. Is the septum markedly obstructing on one side versus the other? Is one side simply smaller than the other? The preoperative endoscopic exam following maximal decongesting of the nose along with review of preoperative CT aids in this assessment. For smaller pituitary lesions that are off the midline, and for those larger tumors extending laterally into the cavernous sinus, the contralateral nasal cavity presents a better angle of approach. Indeed, since the endonasal approach is a few degrees off the midline, it allows better exposure of the contralateral sphenoid and cavernous sinus. Rarely, an approach using both nasal cavities has been used, with the endoscope in one side and the instruments in the other. This can be the case in patients with unusually narrow nasal cavities and is usually reserved for the tumor resection part of the procedure where more than one instrument has to be inserted in addition to the endoscope.

The approach to the anterior face of the sphenoid follows the paraseptal corridor, medial to the middle turbinate. This approach allows the remaining sinuses lateral to the middle turbinate to be left undisturbed, minimizing the risk of postoperative sinusitis. When necessary, gentle lateralization of the middle turbinate is done with the soft end of a Hurd tonsil retractor. Occasionally, a concha bullosa is encountered which may need to be resected to provide good access.

Key to the identification of the sphenoid sinus ostium is the identification of the superior turbinate and the region of the sphenoethmoid recess. The recess is bounded by the skull base superiorly, the superior turbinate laterally and the septum medially and always contains the ostium of the sphenoid sinus. The ostium can be well seen after decongesting the superior turbinate with local anesthesia and conservatively resecting its posterior-inferior third using the powered shaver. The ostium is always located medial to the turbinate, just posterior to its inferior edge in the sphenoethmoid recess (Fig. 9.79). Jho has described using the inferior edge of the middle turbinate as a landmark for orientation to the floor of the sella. This margin leads to the clival indentation, about 1 cm below the level of the sellar floor.[2]

The posterior septal branch of the sphenopalatine artery crosses the inferior aspect of the sphenoethmoidal recess on its way to supply the mucosa of the septum.

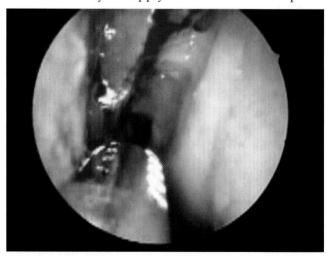

Fig. 9.79: Right sphenoethmoid recess after resection of the posterior inferior third of the superior turbinate. This allows clear identification of the sphenoid ostium

Transection of this artery while performing the sphenoidotomy can lead to annoying intraoperative bleeding but can usually be well-controlled with bipolar cautery or topical decongestant packing. Vasoconstriction may be further obtained by injection of lidocaine/epinephrine solution along the posterior septum, prior to any incision in the face of the sphenoid.

Once the sphenoid sinus ostium is identified, the sinus is entered and the ostium enlarged in an inferior and medial direction, away from structures along the lateral wall of the sinus until the ostium has been enlarged to a point where the endoscope can be inserted into the sinus in order to visualize the lateral extent of the sinus. The bone of the sphenoid rostrum is resected using a combination of Kerrison rongeurs and punches until the nasal septum is encountered; occasionally a high-speed drill is used for resection of this relatively thick bone. A partial posterior septectomy is then performed using backbiting forceps. This allows exposure of the contralateral face of the sphenoid. The intersinus septum is resected, allowing exposure of the sella. Great care is taken in resection of the intersinus septum, as it frequently attaches posteriorly over the carotid.

The various surface landmarks of the sella are illustrated in Fig. 9.80. Medially, the sella is bordered by the tubercle rostrally, and the clivus caudally. As discussed earlier, the optic nerves are seen at 11 and 1 o'clock, while the cavernous portions of the internal carotid arteries are located at 5 and 7 o'clock. The carotid arteries are C-shaped with the concavity oriented laterally. Again, great caution must be exercised, especially around the arteries, as these can be dehiscent in approximately 10% of the cases.

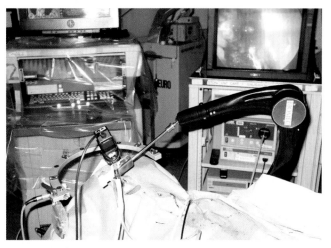

Fig. 9.81: Operating room setup, showing the pneumatic holder

At this point, the endoscope is attached to a fixed holder, freeing up the surgeon's second hand. We have used a pneumatic holder with a custom-designed end-piece (Fig. 9.81). The mucosa on the posterior wall of the sphenoid sinus is coagulated with a bipolar cautery. The sella is then entered with a 4 mm chisel or high-speed drill depending on the thickness of the sellar face and the opening enlarged with a Kerrison rongeur. Occasionally, bleeding can be encountered from anterior intercavernous connections described above; this can usually be readily controlled with microfibrillar collagen and temporary pressure. The dura is then cauterized and opened with a sickle knife and rotating scissors (Fig. 9.82). The tumor mass typically bulges through the dural opening. Samples are taken and sent for frozen section

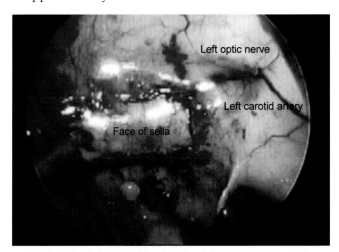

Fig. 9.80: Endoscopic view of the anterior wall of the sella with the different surface landmarks labeled

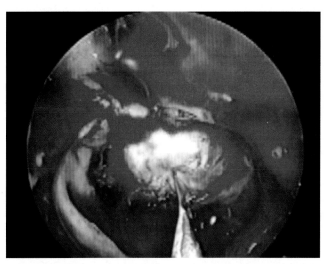

Fig. 9.82: Sickle knife used to incise the dura after resection of the bone of the anterior face of the sella

and permanent pathology before any suction is used, especially when dealing with microadenomas and smaller lesions. The tumor is then removed with a combination of suction and neurosurgical ring curettes with different angulations. Tumor tissue is usually easily differentiated from normal yellow pituitary tissue.

Once the bulk of the tumor is removed, the scope may be detached from the scope holder and inserted into the sella to facilitate more detailed exploration for residual tumor. Angled scopes may be used in order to examine the crevices of the sella. Frequently, however, as more tumor is removed, the diaphragm of the sella and normal pituitary tissue will tend to descend into the void thus created. This can obscure visualization, especially in the lateral recesses of the cavity. In order to improve visualization in this setting, we have developed the technique of 'hydroscopy.' This technique uses normal saline irrigation under pressure attached to either the straight or angled endoscopes. The pressure of the saline flooding the field serves to expand the soft tissue boundaries of the sella including the diaphragm while also improving visualization by washing away small amounts of blood and clot. With improved visualization, this technique allows inspection of the cavity and ensures as complete a removal of tumor tissue as possible. Similarly, the pressure of the irrigation helps to wash out small bits of residual tumor otherwise poorly accessible in recesses of the sella.

At the end of the procedure, hemostasis is obtained using a hemostatic substance such as microfibrillar collagen in thrombin. This is allowed to sit for a few minutes in the sella and is then irrigated out.

Reconstruction of the sella, we have found is not necessary in the vast majority of cases. The only indication for reconstruction in our current practice is the intra-operative suspicion of a CSF leak. In a review of our first 28 cases without sellar reconstruction, only one case of CSF leak was found, comparable with reported rates of 0.8 to 6.4%. No cases of empty sella syndrome have been identified.[4] A larger review including our first one hundred cases is in process and results appear to be very similar.

Postoperative Management

Postoperatively, the patient is admitted to a regular floor bed for 24 hours allowing for routine neurological monitoring. An MRI is obtained on the first postoperative day to evaluate completeness of resection. Patients are generally discharged home on antibiotics, and hormonal replacement as necessary. Patients are instructed to avoid

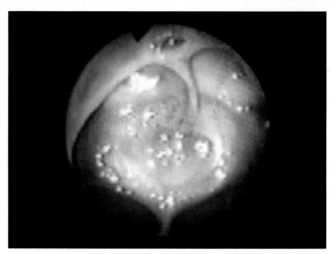

Fig. 9.83: Endoscopic view of the posterior wall of the sphenoid on the first postoperative visit. The defect is very well mucosalized with no evidence of herniation or CSF leaks

nose blowing or sneezing through the nose in order to avoid displacement of mucus into the open sellar cavity.

At the first postoperative visit approximately three weeks later, sinonasal endoscopy is performed to confirm appropriate healing; typically, the posterior sphenoido-tomy is usually covered by a healthy mucosal layer (Fig. 9.83) and patients may resume gentle nose blowing. Patients are closely followed by the neurosurgery and the endocrinology teams; visits to the otolaryngologists beyond that are on an as-needed-basis only.

Complications

Compared to the traditional sublabial transseptal (SLTS) approach, the endoscopic approach provides improved complication rates. Indeed, in a comparison of our first 50 cases of MIPS as compared to our last 50 cases of SLTS, the total complication rate per patient, in addition to postoperative epistaxis, lip anesthesia, and septal per-foration rates were significantly lower in the endoscopic approach.[5,9] The reported rates of major complications are low: meningitis (0.4–2%), intracranial hemorrhage (0.4–3%), ophthalmoplegia (0.5–4.6%), carotid injury (0–1.1%).[5] Postoperative diabetes insipidus (DI) is usually transient, and can be seen in up to 60% of patients. The rate of permanent DI is reported to be between 0.4–3%.[5] Patients with Cushing's disease are usually discharged home on a regimen of hydrocortisone (20 mg in the morning and 10 mg in the evening). This is then adjusted on subsequent visits to the endocrinologist.

CSF leak is the most common serious complication of pituitary surgery. Intraoperative CSF leaks are managed with packing of the sella and sphenoid sinus. We usually

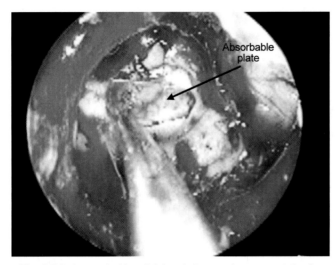

Fig. 9.84: A resorbable miniplate is inserted to support the fat graft inserted in the sella after detection of a CSF leak

use an abdominal fat graft, supported by an absorbable miniplate inserted subdurally (Fig. 9.84). The sphenoid sinus is then packed with an absorbable material such as microfibrillar collagen.

Postoperative CSF leaks usually occur within the first 72 hours and manifest as clear rhinorrhea or salty taste. Initial management is conservative with strict bedrest, head of bed elevation, and stool softeners. Insertion of a lumbar drain may be necessary if the leak persists after 48 hours or patients may be taken back to the operating room and the leak repaired as described above. We have occasionally used a free mucosal graft, harvested from the contralateral septum to allow faster mucosalization and healing. Rarely, with recurrent leaks, patients may require lumboperitoneal shunting.

CONCLUSION

In summary, the endoscopic approach to pituitary tumors provides improved patient comfort and a low rate of morbidity compared to a sublabial transseptal approach. It provides improved illumination and visualization, and, as such, may improve completeness of tumor removal. It does not require the learning of new skills when a team approach is used coordinating the abilities of the otolaryngologist and neurosurgeon. It may be rapidly, effectively and safely incorporated into their practice with a very flat learning curve. Further advances in endoscopic equipment and techniques will likely allow for improved results and the extension of such results beyond the confines of the sella and surrounding structures to other areas of the skull base.

REFERENCES

1. Carrau RL, Jho HD, Ko Y. Transnasal-transsphenoidal endoscopic surgery of the pituitary gland. *Laryngoscope* 1996; 106:914–918.
2. Jho HD. Endoscopic pituitary surgery. *Pituitary* 1999; 2: 139–154.
3. Senior BA, Dubin MG, Sonnenburg RE, Melroy CT, Ewend MG. Increased role of the otolaryngologist in endoscopic pituitary surgery: endoscopic hydroscopy of the sella. *Am J Rhinol* 2005; 19:181–184.
4. Sonnenburg RE, White D, Ewend MG, Senior BA. Sellar reconstruction: is it necessary? *Am J Rhinol* 2003; 17:343–346.
5. White DR, Sonnenburg RE, Ewend MG, Senior BA. Safety of minimally invasive pituitary surgery (MIPS) compared with a traditional approach. *Laryngoscope* 2004; 114:1945–1948.
6. Jho HD, Carrau RL, Ko Y, Daly MA. Endoscopic pituitary surgery: an early experience. *Surg Neurol* 1997; 47:213–222; discussion 222–213.
7. Anatomy and histology of the pituitary gland: Colorado State University, 2003. http://arbl.cvmbs.colostate.edu/hbooks/pathphys/endocrine/hypopit/histo.html
8. Gray H. The sphenoid bone. In *Gray's Anatomy*, 20th edn, Lewis WH (Ed). Philadelphia: Lea and Febiger, 1918.
9. Sonnenburg RE, White D, Ewend MG, Senior B. The learning curve in minimally invasive pituitary surgery. *Am J Rhinol* 2004; 18:259–263.

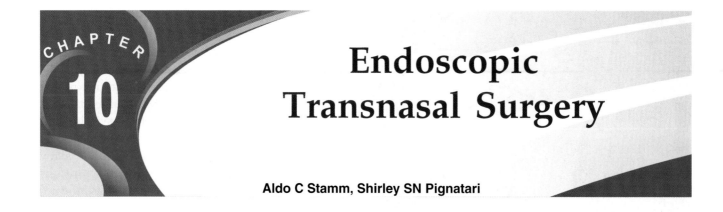

CHAPTER 10

Endoscopic Transnasal Surgery

Aldo C Stamm, Shirley SN Pignatari

Despite the improvement of the management of the lesions involving the paranasal sinuses and skull base since the introduction of transnasal microscopic and endoscopic techniques, along with advanced new surgical instrumentation, effective and safe treatment of lesions involving the skull base is still a challenge. Several approaches using microscopic surgical techniques have been proposed, seeking to optimize the exposure and minimize the risk of complications. All such microscopic anterior skull base approaches aimed at avoiding nerve and brain retraction have been developed along two basic anterior midline routes, the transoral and the transnasal.[1,2] Surgical approaches are more straight and are quicker, avoid extensive cerebral retraction, and have a lower rate of morbidity when compared to classic approaches. The traditional boundaries of the paranasal sinus surgical approach may be expanded to include other regions such as the anterior and medial cranial base, clivus and posterior fossa, orbit and optic nerve, and also the craniocervical junction.

Nevertheless, despite lower morbidity and fewer complications, the problems of infection, cerebrospinal fluid leakage, difficulty in controlling intradural bleeding, and lack of appropriate surgical instruments still exist. One of the most challenging surgical step remains the difficulty of repairing large dural defects.[5]

The main endoscopic gateway to approach the skull base is through the sphenoid sinus. However, the transnasal and transethmoidal accesses may be used for other purposes, besides serving as a door to the sphenoid sinus, for example, in lesions involving orbit and anterior skull base such as CSF, and tumors of the ethmoid sinuses.

CLASSIFICATION

- The Extended transnasal surgical approaches are:
- Transnasal direct
- Transethmoidal
- Transseptal
- Transplanum
- Transsphenoidal–transpterygoid
- Transsphenoidal–transclival
- Transnasal–transpharyngeal (cranial cervical junction)
- Combined

Transnasal Direct Approach

The operation is carried out through one nostril. If the nasal cavity is very narrow and if the passage for the endoscope and operating instruments is limited due to a septal deviation, septoplasty is done first. After identification of the middle and superior turbinates, the posterior region of the nasal septum and the choanal arch, the ostium of the sphenoid sinus is probed with the seeker/palpator. To improve access the superior turbinate is identified and removed with a through-cutting forceps. When the surgical access is very narrow, the posterior portion of the middle turbinate can also be removed by using microscissors or shaver. The sphenoid sinus is initially opened with a delicate curette or with an atraumatic aspirator medially and inferiorly. The aperture is then enlarged with a micro-Kerrison punch, incorporating the natural ostium into the opening, carefully avoiding or cauterizing the septal artery which crosses the anterior wall of the sphenoid sinus in that region. The 4 mm 0° endoscope is used for this step of the surgery. This approach can be particularly useful for the following clivus lesions: CSF, clivus meningocele, clivus mucocele and Infection (bacterial, fungus) with erosion of the sphenoid sinus and concomitant involvement of the clivus.

Transethmoidal Approach

Transethmoidal approach may be necessary in conjunction with the direct transnasal, in cases when a larger field is warranted. In such situations, most of the time, the middle turbinate is removed as part of the procedure. This combined approach is particularly useful for lesions that involve the anterior skull base such as malignant tumors, anterior skull base dural defects, and it is also useful as part of the surgical access for clivus chordoma, petrous apex lesions, and lesions that extend to the lateral recess of the sphenoid sinus.

First, an ethmoidectomy is performed beginning with the resection of the uncinate process and followed by resection of the ethmoid bulla and the remaining ethmoid cells. During the resection of the posterior ethmoid cells, the surgeon must correlate direct observation and intraoperative review of the CT scan to determine whether an Onodi cell is present, and, if so, to understand its relationship to the optic-nerve canal and the internal carotid artery. Identification of the medial orbit wall, as much of the roof of the fovea ethmoidalis, including observation of the posterior and anterior ethmoidal bundle can be helpful, since they are good landmarks.

The initial opening of the sphenoid sinus is made with a delicate curette or with an atraumatic aspirator medially and inferiorly. The sphenoidotomy is then enlarged with a micro-Kerrison punch, incorporating the natural ostium into the opening.

Removal of the middle turbinate is usually necessary in order to create a single cavity between the nasal septum and the medial wall of the orbit. When an even larger surgical field is needed, bilateral ethmoidectomy as well as resection of both middle turbinates are performed. The middle turbinate mucoperiosteum can be used as a free graft to repair dural defects that were created by the lesion or its removal.[5] Figures 10.1A and B show the pre- and postoperative CT of a patient with esthesioneuroblastoma. The tumor was removed through transnasal–transethmoidal approach with dural resection.

Transseptal Approach

The transseptal approach (anterior, posterior, and with removal of the posterior nasal septum–bi-nostril approach) was conceived to provide a midline access to the sphenoid sinus region through the nasal septum, avoiding damage to the structures in the nasal cavity and avoiding the lateral wall of the sphenoid sinus and the nearby carotid artery and optic nerve. The transeptal approach has been particularly useful to access the clivus, sella and parasellar regions since they are midline structures.

The surgeon first performs a submucoperichondrial and submucoperiosteal infiltration with lidocaine (2%) and epinephrine (1:100,000) producing a hydraulic dissection that facilitates surgical elevation. A vertical hemi-transfixion incision is made at the caudal edge of the septal cartilage and septal flaps are elevated as in performing a septoplasty. Disarticulation of the osseo-cartilaginous junction (septal cartilage, ethmoid plate and vomer) is performed with the suction elevator, preserving

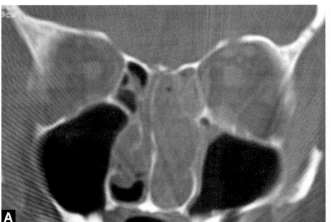
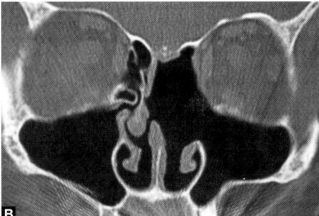

Figs 10.1A and B: Coronal CT of a 55-year-old patient with esthesioneuroblastoma, submitted to a transnasal-transethmoidal endoscopic resection with dural removal and reconstruction. Pre- and postoperative aspects

the uppermost part of the osseocartilaginous junction to avoid postoperative dorsal nasal saddling. The posterior attachment of the septum to the perpendicular plate of the ethmoid is fractured. The posterior part of the septal bone, which obstructs access to the sphenoid rostrum, is resected with a Jansen-Middleton forceps. The muco-periosteum of the anterior wall of the sphenoid sinus is elevated until the sinus ostia on both sides are visualized. At this point, the anterior wall of the sphenoid sinus is entirely exposed. The sphenoid rostrum and the anterior wall is then opened with a chisel, and is enlarged with a micro-Kerrison punch or a high-speed drill. The sphe-noidotomy is made large enough to allow easy simul-taneous introduction of a 4 mm endoscope and a surgical instrument.

Posterior Septal Incision

Although the caudal hemitransfixion incision described above is useful when a simultaneous correction of a septal deviation is necessary, it is often advantageous to make the initial septal incision more posteriorly, closer to the rostrum of the sphenoid sinus. Pituitary tumors and inverted papillomas occasionally recur in the sphenoid sinus, and in these situations a more posterior incision avoids repeated dissection of scarred septal flaps. In these situations, a vertical transfixion incision is made 1.5 cm anterior to the sphenoid sinus ostium, joining a second horizontal incision 1.0 cm below the superior edge of the nasal septum. The mucoperiosteum of both sides can be removed or just retracted laterally, and the bony nasal septum is then removed. If there is a dural defect at the end of the procedure, the mucoperiosteal flap can be used in the dural repair.

The transseptal approach to the sphenoid sinus can be extended to access the sella, parasellar regions, petrous apex, the clivus, and the cavernous sinus.[5]

Transnasal Approach with Removal of the Posterior Part of the Nasal Septum (Bi-nostril Approach)

The posterior part of the nasal septum is removed to enlarge the operative field. The septal mucosa can be elevated and retracted on one or both sides and then replaced or resected at the end of the procedure. This modification permits two surgeons to work simul-taneously, one through each nostril. For example, one can hold a suction in one nostril, while the surgeon works with the endoscope and a surgical instrument in the other. The use of three or four instruments including the

endoscope, facilitates tumor removal, and it is essential in cases with intradural extension, particularly helping to control intradural bleedings. It is also very helpful when removing large lesions in the posterior third of the nasal cavity, sphenoid sinus, clivus, sella and parasellar regions, especially highly vascularized, and solid tumors.

Transsphenoidal–transplanum Approach

The surgical access to the *planum sphenoidal* may be obtained through the sphenoid sinus or through the anterior skull base. It can be useful to treat several lesions, particularly the suprasellar and infrachiasmatic ones.

Transsphenoidal–transpterygoidal Approach

The transsphenoidal–transpterygoidal approach is usually combined with removal of the medial and posterior wall of the maxillary sinus. This surgical access is mostly used to treat lesions located on the lateral extent of the sphenoid sinus (pterygoid compartment), larger lesions in the pterygopalatine or zygomatic fossae such as angiofibromas, CSF fistulas and meningoencephalo-celes/encephaloceles in the middle fossae. This approach can also be extended to gain exposure to the cavernous sinus.[6]

Transsphenoidal–transclival Approach

Approach to the Clivus and Cavernous Sinus

Despite the fact that anterior approaches offer a more direct anatomical approach to the structures beyond the clivus, the risks of cerebrospinal fluid leakage and infection limit most of the above-mentioned approaches to extradural lesions, especially those that work through the non-sterile operative field.[3] The major advantage of the midline transfacial approaches is the direct anterior surgical access through the large spaces of the nasal cavity, nasopharynx, and oral cavity and paranasal sinuses. However, these midlines routes are restricted by critical neurovascular structures such as the internal carotid artery, optic nerve, cavernous sinus, cranial nerves and the orbital contents.[4] Figure 10.2 shows the trans-sphenoidal transclival surgical access.

Combined Approaches

Unfortunately, many lesions do not respect the anatomic boundaries for which the approaches outlined above are ideal. In many instances it is necessary to combine some

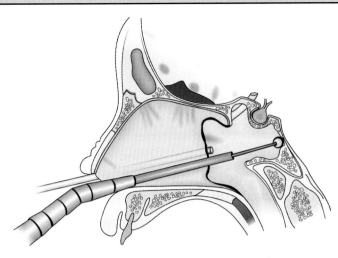

Fig. 10.2: Schematic drawing showing a bi-nostril surgical approach with resection of the posterior part of the nasal septum. A diamond burr is being used to remove the bone of the clivus

of the above approaches, for example, the transnasal direct with the transethmoidal, or the transsphenoidal–transpterygoidal with the transethmoidal, etc.

Extended applications of transnasal endoscopic assisted techniques can be safe and effective. However, problems such as infection, cerebrospinal fluid leakage, and difficulty controlling intradural bleeding still remain.

It is always important to keep in mind that, while technology (in the form of endoscopes, image guided system, image studies and advanced anesthetic drugs) is essential for the development and improvement of a such a surgical procedures, the success of this kind of surgery, will principally depend on the perfect knowledge of the anatomy, intense endoscopic surgery training, and partnership with a multidisciplinary team.

REFERENCES

1. Archer DJ, Young S, Uttley D. Basilar aneurysms: A new trasclival approach via maxillotomy. *J Neurosurg* 1987; 67: 54–58.
2. Bouche J, Guiot G, Rougerie J, Freche C. The transsphenoidal route in the surgical approach to chordoma of the clivus. *Ann Otolaryngol Chir Cervicofac* 1966; 83:817–834.
3. Gibbons M, Sillers MJ. Minimally invasive approaches to the sphenoid sinus. *Otolaryngol Head Neck Surg* 2002; 126:635–641.
4. Janecka IP, Nuss DW, Sen CN. Facial translocation approach to the cranial base. *Acta Neurochir Suppl (Wien)* 1991; 53:193.
5. Stamm A, Pignatari SN. Transnasal endoscopic-assisted surgery of the skull base. In: *Otolaryngology Head Neck Surgery*, Cummings CW, Flint PW, Harker LA, (Eds) 4th edn. Philadelphia: Elsevier Mosby, 2005; 3855–3876.
6. Zhou D, Patil AA, Rodriguez-Sierra J. Endoscopic neuroanatomy through the sphenoid sinus. *Minim Invas Neurosurg* 2005; 48:19–24.

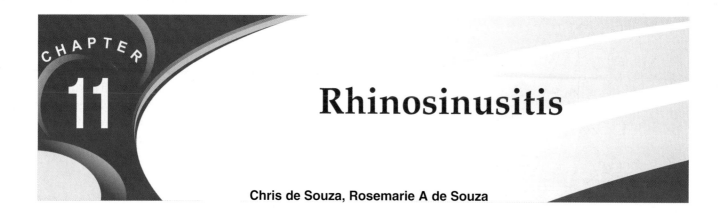

Rhinosinusitis

Chris de Souza, Rosemarie A de Souza

Rhinosinusitis is a group of disorders characterized by inflammation of the mucosa of the nose and the paranasal sinuses.[1] This definition was accepted by the task force convened by the American Academy of Allergy, Asthma and Immunology, The American Academy of Otolaryngology—Head and Neck Surgery, The American Rhinologic Society and the American College of Allergy, Asthma and Immunology who had convened a task force of 30 physicians to formulate definitions by consensus.

This group by consensus decided to use the term rhinosinusitis instead of sinusitis because sinusitis is almost always accompanied by concurrent nasal airway inflammation and in many cases sinusitis is always preceded by symptoms of rhinitis.

Furthermore, it was previously believed that all of chronic rhinosinusitis is caused by sinus ostial obstruction. Ostial obstruction is the result of chronic rhino-sinusitis. While ostial obstruction may be the end result, the causes of ostial obstruction are many and diverse. It is now appreciated that rhinosinusitis, especially chronic rhinosinusitis, may be caused by multiple factors such as:

- Persistent infection caused by biofilms and osteitis.
- Allergy and other disorders of immunity.
- Intrinsic factors of the upper airway.
- Superantigens from *Staphylococcus aureus* in chronic rhinosinusitis (CRS) with nasal polyps.
- Colonizing fungi that induce and sustain eosinophilic inflammation.
- Metabolic disorders including aspirin sensitivity.

Each mechanism may act in concert with other mechanisms or individually for a given patient. This task force by consensus also classified rhinosinusitis in the following way:

- Acute presumed bacterial rhinosinusitis
- CRS without polyps

- CRS with polyps
- Allergic fungal rhinosinusitis (AFRS).

DIAGNOSIS

Rhinosinusitis is a clinical diagnosis based largely on history, clinical examination and imaging modalities. The physical symptoms needed to make a diagnosis of rhinosinusitis are classified as major and minor symptoms.

Major Symptoms

- Nasal obstruction/blockage
- Nasal discharge/purulence/discolored postnasal discharge
- Hyposmia/anosmia
- Facial congestion/fullness
- Facial pain/pressure (facial pain must be accompanied by another major factor to qualify for CRS).

Minor Symptoms

- Fever
- Halitosis
- Headache
- Cough
- Fatigue
- Dental pain
- Ear pain/ear pressure or fullness

To qualify for a diagnosis of CRS the patient must have at least two major symptoms, or one major symptom with two or more minor symptoms, or nasal purulence on examination.[2] Facial pain is not considered a symptom of CRS without other nasal signs and symptoms. The signs and symptoms should persist for at least 12 weeks to qualify as CRS. A separate subcategory for acute exacerbations of CRS was also described. In this category symptoms worsen but return to baseline following treatment.

ACUTE (PRESUMED BACTERIAL) RHINOSINUSITIS

Acute rhinosinusitis is caused by the presence of bacteria within the sinus cavity whose ostium is obstructed. Acute rhinosinusitis is usually infectious in nature while the causes of CRS are varied.

All sinus infections enter the sinus via the nasal cavity. During a cold, nasal fluid containing bacteria, viruses and inflammatory mediators are blown into the sinuses where they produce inflammation. Mucosal edema, cellular infiltration and mucus thickened by exocytosis of mucin from the numerous goblet cells in the sinus epithelium are the results. It is estimated that of the viral infections only 0.5 to 2% are complicated by secondary bacterial infections.[3]

In the immunocompetent person living in the general community acute rhinosinusitis is typically believed to be induced by viruses and usually does not require antibiotics for the first 10 to 15 days. Beyond this time-frame if the symptoms persist then bacteria are presumed to be present and antibiotics could and should be given.[1] Patients presenting with acute rhinosinusitis usually present with anterior and/or purulent nasal discharge, nasal obstruction, facial pain and hyposmia.

The duration of acute sinusitis is less than or equal to 4 weeks. The patient's history must include two or more major factors to be diagnosed as 'acute rhinosinusitis'.

Most physicians need to resolve the following issues:
- Is an antibiotic necessary?
- Those against prescribing an antibiotic argue that most infections are viral and will resolve spontaneously. The medication that can be given are those which provide relief from symptoms. These medications are usually in the form of antipyretic and systemic decongestants.

  Furthermore, antibiotics given in the presence of a viral infection may result in bacterial resistance and colonization of these bacteria thus complicating a viral infection.

  However, if the symptoms are present for more than two weeks, bacteria can then be presumed to be present and antibiotics can and should be given. However, all efforts should be made to correctly identify the pathogen causing acute rhinosinusitis. This will help choose the appropriate antibiotic.

- How should the samples of pus be retrieved that will accurately reflect the pathogen causing the infection? Most procedures add to costs, are time-consuming and require expertise that may not be available to the primary physician who is invariably the family physician. Thus, in the presence of an acute infection, most physicians prefer to use standardized treatment protocols and reserve retrieval of pus samples for special circumstances such as an immuno-compromised individual, refractory infections that have not responded to first line treatment in their treatment protocols and situations where fungal and unusual infections may be suspected. Infections that have been complicated is another situation where retrieval of the actual bacteria is crucial to effective treatment.
- Is radiological imaging necessary?

  Plain X-rays of the nasal cavity and paranasal sinuses have been replaced by CT scans and MRI. Plain sinus X-ray films might be adequate in situations where acute rhinosinusitis is suspected.[1] Plain X-ray films, although less costly are generally less reliable than CT and MRI scans. In most situations of acute rhinosinusitis physicians prefer to base the diagnosis on history and clinical findings. Imaging modalities such as CT scans and MRI are reserved for situations where an acute infection becomes complicated, usually in a situation where the infection has extended beyond the boundaries of the nasal cavity and paranasal sinuses.
- What is the role of surgery in acute (presumed bacterial) rhinosinusitis?

The role of surgery is limited. It lies in:
- Encouraging adequate drainage in a sinus that does not drain even though adequate and appropriate medication is given.
- Retrieval of representative samples of pus from the sinus cavity.
- Surgery is indicated when complications are present; drainage of the sinus, retrieval of samples of pus and decompression of the orbit by draining the abscess.

In summary, the criteria for the diagnosis of acute (presumed bacterial) rhinosinusitis should have symptoms that persist for up to ten days until a maximum of 24 days. Fever should be present. Symptoms for diagnosis should include anterior and/or posterior nasal discharge, nasal obstruction and facial pain.

Objective documentation should include the following:

Nasal airway examination for purulent discharge. Radiographic evidence of acute rhinosinusitis.

CHRONIC RHINOSINUSITIS (CRS)

Statistics from the Center for Disease Control (CDC) indicate that 32 million adults in the USA (16% of the adult population) suffer from rhinosinusitis with 73 million restricted activity days, 13 million yearly physician visits and a cost of six billion dollars every year.[4] Patients with CRS usually suffer from significant lowering in the quality of life.

The diagnosis of CRS can be made when the parameters of several criteria are met. Appropriate symptoms of CRS should be present for a period of twelve weeks. Findings on CT scanning and nasal endoscopy should be documented and should be indicative of chronic ongoing disease. It should be understood that various forms of CRS exist. Various forms of CRS exist because the causes of CRS are varied.

Pathological changes of CRS are edema (Figs 11.1A to C), loss of submucosal glands, ulceration, loss of cilia, fibroplasias, bone remodeling and later changes of goblet cell formation.

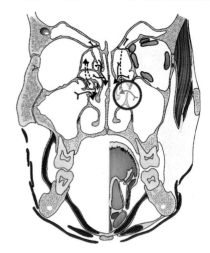

Fig. 11.1A: Edema at the ostium (circle) of the maxillary sinus

Physical Findings in CRS

External

Erythema and swelling over the maxillary, ocular, orbital and frontal areas.

Anterior Rhinoscopy

- Hyperemia
- Edema
- Crusts
- Pus
- Polyps

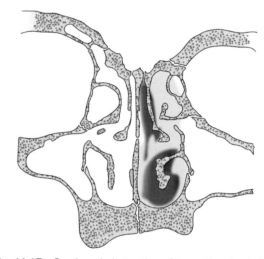

Fig. 11.1B: Continued obstruction of the ostium leads to mucosal hypertrophy and tetention of fluid

Nasal Endoscopy

- Discoloration of the turbinates
- Pus in the region of the ostiomeatal complex
- Polyp formation

The specificity of endoscopy is 85% while that of rhinoscopy is 75%.[5] With the possible exception of deviated nasal septa, anatomic variants do not seem to be significantly associated with CRS.[6] Endoscopic examination by an ENT surgeon is very useful in CRS. There is a high correlation between the findings on endoscopic examination and those on CT scan findings.[7] Prospective studies of endoscopy demonstrate sensitivity of 74% and a specificity of 84% when correlated with CT scanning for CRS. Stankiewicz and Chow in their study

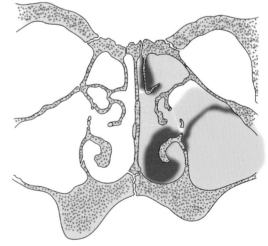

Fig. 11.1C: Edema becomes more pronounced. The fluid has become purulent. The patient now has fully developed CRS

found that nasal endoscopy had a positive predictive value of 74% and a negative predictive value of 64% in CRS.[8]

RADIOLOGICAL DIAGNOSIS

CT scanning is now the gold standard for imaging of the paranasal sinuses. MRI has better soft tissue detail than CT scanning. MRI is not associated with exposure to ionizing radiation. However, CT scanning is still the preferred imaging method of choice because of the speed of acquisition and the bony detail which is unavailable with MRI.

However, radiographic findings of CRS are also seen in 27 to 42% of asymptomatic individuals.[9]

CT Scan Staging

The modified Lund Mackay system is used for staging sinus disease. Scores are based on radiographic findings of the sinuses and the ostiomeatal complex.

Sinuses	Scores for	
	Left	Right
• Maxillary		
• Anterior ethmoid		
• Posterior ethmoid		
• Sphenoid		
• Frontal		
• Ostiomeatal complex		

Scores range from 0 (no abnormality) to 1 for partial opacification, or 2 for total opacification. The ostiomeatal complex is scored as 0 (not opacified) or 2 (occluded). These scores are added to give a total for each side.

Many studies have challenged the guidelines for diagnosing CRS. Studies are being conducted on seeking correlations between objective findings and subjective criteria.

CT Correlation with CRS Symptoms

When a patient presents with symptoms of CRS but has no findings on CT scanning, alternative diagnoses should be sought. Similarly, if a patient has no symptoms of CRS but has findings of CRS such a patient is followed up without intervention.

Several studies have shown that CT scans and symptoms do not necessarily correlate. In the general population there is evidence of findings of disease on CT scanning even though the person is asymptomatic. A prospective study of patients without symptoms of CRS found that 27% had mucosal changes suggestive of CRS on CT scanning.[9] Another retrospective study

demonstrated that symptomatic patients who had CT scans for non-sinus disease were found to have Lund scores as high as 5.[10] These studies demonstrate that CT alone cannot be used as the only indicator for CRS and that a baseline of mucosal change should be expected in the asymptomatic population. One retrospective study identified no significant correlation between mucosal abnormalities on CT scan and patient's symptoms.[11] Many authors recommend using CT scans for surgical preparation but not for determining the need for surgical intervention. Some prospective studies have investigated the discrepancy between symptoms and CT findings. CT scans as the sole modality for identifying CRS is not 100% accurate.

Nasal Endoscopy in Correlation with CRS Symptoms

Nasal endoscopy can be useful in establishing the diagnosis of CRS. In one report 240 patients who met the criteria of CRS and CT findings were examined using nasal endoscopy.[12] There was a high degree of correlation (75% specificity and 84% sensitivity).

To avoid the problems of a pre-selected and clearly surgical population, a prospective study examined the findings of nasal endoscopy, CT scan and CRS symptoms.[8] In this group the sensitivity of endoscopy with CT scan was 46% and the specificity of nasal endoscopy with that of CT scan was 86%. Positive and negative predictive values of nasal endoscopy with that of CT scan was 74% and 64% respectively. This study concluded that nasal endoscopy that was negative for disease correlated well with a negative CT scanning.

Thus, both nasal endoscopy and CT scanning are objective measures that can increase accuracy of CRS diagnosis. Nasal endoscopic observation of pus, polyps or other disease can help confirm a diagnosis of CRS. For areas that cannot be observed with nasal endoscopy, CT scanning can prove useful in diagnosing disease. It may be concluded that the use of combining symptoms, findings on nasal endoscopy with the findings on CT scans can all be used reliably and accurately for the diagnosis and treatment of CRS.

Pathogenesis

The exact mechanism causing chronic sinusitis is unclear. Many mechanisms are postulated.
- Osteitis
- Biofilms
- Fungi

- Superantigens
- Allergy

Chronic rhinosinusitis is due to inflammation. The causes of which are many, while acute rhinosinusitis is usually the result of infection.

Osteitis

Norlander et al identified a periosteal reaction of fibrosis, bone degradation and neo-osteogenesis in sinusitis in rabbits.[13] Perloff et al demonstrated that inflammation could spread to non-involved non-infected sinus bone in an animal model.[14] Despite the lack of direct infection, inflammation was seen on the bone of the control side that was normal prior to the infection. The infection typically spreads through the haversian canals resulting in widening of the spaces through osteoclastic resorption and increased vascularity.

Osteomyelitis versus osteitis: The bones of the paranasal sinuses lack marrow spaces seen in the long bones of the body.

Furthermore, in osteomyelitis, bacteria invade the marrow spaces. But in osteitis of the paranasal sinuses no bacteria have been identified. Bolger et al have found bacteria in the sinus lumen, on the surface of the sinus mucosa but not in the deep submucosa or in the actual bone.[15] While the exact mechanism is not clear at this time it is postulated that bacteria could cause bony pathology by increasing the inflammatory mediators, prostaglandins and leucotrienes that stimulate osteoblasts and so bring about bony remodeling.

Kennedy et al postulate that just debridement of overlying mucosal disease frequently does not result in resolution of disease.[16] Instead debridement of the underlying bone results in resolution of disease.

Those who advocate minimally invasive sinus surgery state that the goal of minimally invasive surgery is to establish ventilation and drainage.[17] Once this objective has been achieved, they state that rhinosinusitis will resolve and normal drainage will soon be established. However this is not universally true. Endoscopic sinus surgery should require removal of all bony partitions, especially in the ethmoid sinus. Removal of all the bony partitions serves to remove osteitic bone, bone that might act as a biofilm. This would not only perpetuate an infection but it would also impede drainage. Furthermore, such patients will need prolonged antibiotic treatment. Some authors recommend the use of nebulized steroids, topical antifungal agents and oral leukotrienes and low-dose macrolide therapy.[18] Further research is

needed to answer many of the questions that surround osteitis as the cause of CRS. Only then would a clear strategy on treatment evolve.

Biofilms

A biofilm is a structured community of organisms enclosed in a self-produced polymatrix which is adherent to a living or inert surface. It may be made up of fungi or bacteria that communicate with each other in a co-operative manner. The matrix is slime-like and includes polysaccharides, nucleic acids and proteins.

Bacterial biofilms are complex organizations of bacteria that are anchored to a living or inert surface. They often originate as a collection of independent free floating planktonic bacteria that attach to a surface and form microcolonies.

The bacteria accumulate in a community till a 'critical point' is reached. At this point a phenomenon known as 'quorum sensing' occurs. This means that a cascade of protein expression occurs which leads to a biofilm phenotype. This phenotype is marked by the formation of towers, layers and water channels.

Thus, bacteria living in a phenotype can evade host defences and become less susceptible to systemic or local antibiotics. These biofilms can break off releasing bacteria in their planktonic form to cause new acute infections and form more biofilms.

Biofilms resist antibiotic therapy through the following mechanisms:
1. The polysaccharide coat causes slow or incomplete penetration of antibiotics.
2. Once inside a biofilm antibiotics may be deactivated or neutralized when positively charged antibiotics interact with negatively charged polymers of the biofilm.
3. Accumulation of inhibitive waste products or depletion of a needed substrate may put bacteria into a non-growing (suspended animation) state. This confers relative resistance to antibiotics. Thus, when the antibiotic is stopped the bacteria can start regrowing and cause infections once more.
4. Changing nutrient gradients could also lead to osmotic forces that could cause a stress response which could result in fewer porins in each bacterial cell wall. This in turn leads to less efficient diffusion of antibiotics into the bacterial cytoplasm.
5. Biofilm development passes through five stages:
    a. *Attachment*: Bacteria attach to a surface. This leads to a cascade of gene expression.

b. *Adherence*: Bacteria adhere tightly to the surface on which that are attached, otherwise biofilm will be impossible.

c. *Aggregation*: The bacteria aggregate into colonies.

d. *Maturation*: The biofilm matures and differentiates into complex mushroom-shaped towers.

e. *Detachment*: The bacteria break off from the original biofilm, embolize and cause acute infections elsewhere and form a new biofilm elsewhere.

Superantigens (SAgs)

Superantigens (SAgs) are toxins of microbial or viral origin that target the immune system triggering massive polyclonal T-cell proliferation and activation. In genetically susceptible hosts with pre-existing immuno-pathology and bacterial infections SAgs production may be responsible for the induction of disease and its persistence. SAgs are powerful T-cell mitogens with concentrations of less than 0.1 pg/ml sufficient to result in immense uncontrolled systemic release of proinflammatory cytokines. SAgs have the unique ability to bypass conventional major histocompatibility complexes (MHC) of the immune systems, activating CD4+ and CD8+ T-cells in a major MHC II-dependent but not restricted pattern.

Conventional antigens are typically internalized and processed into smaller peptides by antigen presenting cells (APCs). These are then packaged on the membrane surface in conjunction with MHC molecules for presentation to T-cells.

In contrast unprocessed SAgs bind as intact molecules to a region outside the peptide binding groove on the class II MHC molecule, then sequentially bind the T-cell receptor (TCR) by means of the variable region of the TCR B chain. This binding effectively crosslinks the TCR and MHC II molecule and results in activation of up to 20 to 30% of the host T-cell population. This is in contrast to the conventional antigen response which activates only 0.001 to 0.0001% of all T-cells. This is the mechanism that some pathogens use to thwart the immune response. The end result of the superantigens leads to corruption of the immune response which greatly encourages the transmission and virulence of the organism.[19]

There is supporting evidence that SAgs greatly influence immunomodulatory and proinflammatory cells and an association exists between SAgs and allergic rhinitis and CRS with nasal polyposis (CRS/NP). The SAg hypothesis of CRS with nasal polyposis is supported by the following observations:

1. A high rate of toxin-secreting staphylococcus cultured from the nasal cavity of patients who suffer from CRS/ NP.
2. A high prevalence of SAg-specific IgE in polyp tissue.
3. VB skewing present in polyp lymphocytes.
4. Correlation between lymphocyte skewing and serum IgE to SAg in individual patients who have CRS/NP suggesting a systemic and local response to the same SAg.
5. SAg has been detected in the nasal cavity of patients who suffer from CRS/NP.

Data in support of the SAg hypothesis only accounts for 50% of patients who suffer from CRS/NP. Since staphyloccocal strains are very ubiquitous this explanation for this observation remains unclear. The complex interaction between SAgs and the genetics (MHC II alleles) of the host is one likely explanation. The ability of the SAgs to access the host immune system by transcytosis may be highly variable. The genetic susceptibility to mucosal damage may be a major factor in developing CRS with or without nasal polyposis. The most significant area of research would be the demonstration of clinical efficiency of SAg-directed therapy.

The Role of Bacteria in CRS

Potential pathogens can relocate during a viral respiratory tract infection. They can shift from the nasopharynx into the sinus cavity causing rhinosinusitis. Although bacteria can be found in the sinuses of most patients who have CRS, the exact cause of the inflammation associated with this condition is uncertain. The role of bacteria in CRS associated with nasal polyposis is uncertain. However, many clinicians believe that bacteria play a major role in the cause of CRS and therefore use antimicrobials in the treatment of CRS. The chief difficulty lies in correctly isolating and identifying the causative organism. The difficulties are reflected in the available medical literature and are listed below.

1. Various methods are used to sample the sinus cavity. This leads to lack of standardization and unreliability.
2. The area through which the trocar or endoscope was passed was not sterilized.
3. Differences in microbiological culture technique.
4. Failure to evaluate cultures for anaerobes.
5. Lack of assessment of the inflammatory response.
6. Lack of quantification of bacteria.

Studies have described significant differences in the microbial pathogens present in CRS as compared to those found in acute rhinosinusitis. *Staphylococcus aureus*,

S. epidermidis, anerobes and Gram-negative bacteria predominate in CRS. The pathophysiology of CRS differs from acute rhinosinusitis. The exact events leading to CRS have been difficult to identify or prove. It is postulated that CRS is an extension of unresolved acute rhino-sinusitis.[20] It is also postulated that anerobes play a considerable role in CRS. Adequate and appropriate antibiotics help eradicate disease. Sometimes, surgical drainage is needed to make medical treatment effective.

Medical Management of CRS

Recently there has been increased interest in macrolides in the treatment of CRS. The immunomodulating properties of the macrolides has generated deep interest.

It has been found that there is extensive tissue uptake and intracellular accumulation as far as macrolides are concerned.[21] Macrolides accumulate in inflammatory cells at concentrations several hundred times than found in extracellular fluid. It has been found that cytokines stimulate the accumulation of macrolides antibiotics in macrophages *in vitro*. This suggests that at sites where inflammation occurs cells may accumulate more macrolides than under normal circumstances. Macrolides are essentially bacteriostatic and bind to the 50S subunit of the ribosome, thus inhibiting protein synthesis. Macrolides are effective against gram-positive cocci and anerobes. They have very limited gram-negative activity. Macrolides reduce the virulence of certain organisms. Macrolides also alter the architecture and structure of bacterial biofilms. Macrolides decrease interleukin 8 (IL8) synthesis. By decreasing IL8 synthesis neutrophil recruitment is reduced. This blocks the vicious cycle of IL8 production and neutrophil exudation.

Apoptosis (programmed cell death) of inflammatory cells is accompanied by an attenuation of the activity of these cells. Therapeutic induction of apoptosis provides an opportunity by which the inflammatory response can be modulated. Macrolides accelerate apoptosis in human neutrophils. Phagocytic cells can produce toxic reactive oxygen which destroys bacteria that have been phagocytosed. This oxygen while harmful to bacteria can also be harmful to the host tissue especially if it is generated in excess. Macrolides produce a dose-dependent reduction in superoxide that is produced by neutrophils. Recruitment of inflammatory cells to a site of inflammation involves the cells adhering to the vascular endothelium before transmigration. Macrolides downregulate the expression of cell surface adhesion molecules on neutrophils. Inhibition of molecule expression therefore seems to be another possible mechanism by which macrolides exert anti-inflammatory activity. Macrolides have also been found to have beneficial effects on mucus production as well in improving mucociliary clearance.

Macrolides are not very effective in situations where the serum IgE is elevated or in situations of allergic fungal CRS. Macrolides have been found to be effective in persistent purulent rhinorrhea, when no allergy is present and when the patient has not experienced relief with local nasal steroids. Nasal cultures need to be taken and they need to be taken periodically as long as the patient is taking the macrolides. All the macrolides have been found to have a beneficial effecting CRS.

NASAL POLYPOSIS

Nasal polyposis is believed to affect 1 to 4% of the general population in the USA. However, the incidental findings at autopsy show that the figure may be much higher. The incidence of allergy is not higher in patients who have polyps as compared to the population as a whole. Patients suffering from nasal polyposis do not have higher rates of positive allergy skin tests. Nasal polyposis is associated with a number of systemic disorders like aspirin intolerance, intrinsic asthma, primary ciliary dyskinesia and cystic fibrosis. They are frequently observed in chronic rhinosinusitis, allergic CRS and chronic sinonasal inflammation. Nasal polyposis is now known to have many causes; these are discussed in Chapter 9 (Sinonasal Polyposis: Surgical Aspects).

Treatment of Chronic Rhinosinusitis

There is no defintive protocol for the treatment of CRS. Most clinicians have their own protocols that have varying degrees of success.

The key to successful treatment lies in careful history taking, detailed comprehensive physical examination, including nasal endoscopy followed by high-resolution CT scans of the nose and paranasal sinuses. Based on the understanding of the cause of CRS, the clinician can choose the line of treatment. First-line treatment includes administration of systemic and topical corticosteroids.[22] These may be contraindicated in the presence of fulminant infection or in patients who are immuno-compromised and especially in diabetics.

Appropriate antibiotics can be given. Effectiveness of the macrolides in CRS make them the antibiotics of choice.

Decongestants and sinus drainage procedures did not prove to be superior to saline in the treatment of maxillary rhinosinusitis. The use of bacterial lysates was found to be beneficial, but antihistamines were not found to be beneficial. Randomized control trials found nasal douching to be effective in reducing systems, improving the quality of life as well as reversing changes seen on CT scanning and nasal endoscopy.

The role of surgery is effective but needs to be accompanied by appropriate medication. Endoscopic sinus surgery has evolved significantly. So much so that disease processes that previously needed major surgeries that were accompanied by significantly morbidity and external incisions can now be safely carried out with great expertise with dramatic improvement in results.
The principles of endoscopic sinus surgery are:
• Provide adequate drainage by widening the obstructed ostia so that they now drain naturally, freely and physiologically.
• Provide adequate ventilation of the paranasal sinuses.
• Provide adequate inspection of areas that could not be visualized earlier.
Details of Endoscopic Sinus Surgery are discussed in chapter 9.

CRS VERSUS NASAL SEPTAL DEVIATIONS

Bhattacharya notes that traditionally patients with CRS have been treated differently from NSD.[23] Patients suffering from CRS reported more symptoms in the nasal symptom domain versus patients who only had NSD. Patients with NSD reported higher mean nasal obstruction scores but lower rhinorrhea and dysosmia symptom severity scores. He notes the higher severity of oropharyngeal symptoms in patients suffering from CRS. Patients suffering from CRS often complain of cough, dental pain and otalgia as compared to those who have a NSD. Patients suffering from CRS tend to have more extranasal symptoms which usually result in higher symptom scores. It was noted by Bhattacharya that patients with CRS incur a higher economic burden that those who have NSD. Also, the number of workdays lost is far higher in those with CRS than in those with NSD.

Yasan et al reported that mild to moderate NSD were not a risk factor for CRS.[24] Only gross NSD present a genuine risk for developing CRS. The greater the septal deviation the greater the risk of developing CRS. Three pathophysiological hypotheses explain how NSD cause CRS.
• Mechanical obstruction
• Aerodynamic changes
• Alterations in sinusal ventilation and antral pressures.
NSD when very significant can cause dysfunction in the above three dynamics which ultimately affect

mucociliary clearance of the sinus and its ostium which then results in CRS. Unfortunately there are no further studies which evaluate if CRS resolves with the surgical straightening of the nasal septum.

Complications of Rhinosinusitis

Complications of rhinosinusitis are divided into orbital and intracranial complications.

Orbital complications: Most orbital complications occur in children. Ethmoiditis commonly results in orbital cellulitis. This is because the lamina papyracea is thin. In addition there are suture lines and foramina which assist the spread of infection. The other mechanism by which infection spreads is hematogenous. Retrograde thrombophlebitis of valveless veins can cause the infection to spread rapidly. Cellulitis if untreated can result in a preseptal abscess which can cause blindness and/or intracranial complications.

The patient is toxic presenting with high-grade fever, purulent nasal discharge, blocked nose and periorbital erythema and tenderness. Epistaxis may also be present. The affected eye will be proptosed and tender. A nasal swab will help identify the causative organism. A CT scan must be done and should be done in the axial and coronal planes. If the infection is thought to have spread intracranially then an MRI will also be needed.

Appropriate antibiotics given at the optimal dose for the appropriate period of time is essential. If cellulitis is present then a conservative line of treatment may be adopted. If an abscess has formed then it would need to be drained immediately. In this situation the sinus needs to be drained and the orbit decompressed as well. The principles of treatment under these circumstances are the following:
• Control and eradication of the infection with the appropriate antibiotic given in high doses for a sustained period of time until the infection has resolved successfully and completely.
• Prevention of the infection from spreading elsewhere especially intracranially.
• Adequate drainage of the sinus.
• Decompression of the orbit and drainage of the abscess.
Intracranial complications can also occur. Cavernous sinusitis is a dreaded complication. This is usually accompanied by high-grade fever, severe toxicity, impaired extraocular movements, decrease in visual acuity and signs and symptoms of meningitis. This needs to be identified quickly and treated aggressively with high doses of antibiotics and anticoagulants. When

cavernous sinusitis is recognized quickly and treated immediately the outcome is favorable. When the disease is well advanced morbidity and mortality are high.

A brain abscess in the frontal lobe can present differently as compared to a brain abscess in the posterior fossa. The patient usually has high-grade fever, signs and symptoms of meningitis and may have changes in behavior. CT scanning or MRI helps in identifying and localizing the abscess. Treatment lies in aggressive high-dose antibiotics and drainage of the abscess.

REFERENCES

1. Meltzer EO, Hamilos DL et al. Rhinosinusitis: Establishing definitions for clinical research and patient care. *Otolaryngol Head Neck Surg Suppl* 2004; 131(6):1–62.
2. Lanza DC, Kennedy DW. Adult rhinosinusitis defined. *Otolaryngol Head Neck Surg* 1997; 117(3):S1–7.
3. Gwaltney JM, Wiesinger BA, Patrie JT. Acute community acquired bacterial sinusitis: The value of antimicrobial treatment and the natural history. *Clin Infect Dis* 2004; 38: 227–233.
4. Blackwell DL, Collins JG, Coates. Summary health statistics for US adults. National Health Interview. *Vital Health Stat* 2002; 10:205.
5. Hughes R, Jones NS. The role of endoscopy in outpatient management. *Clin Otolaryngol* 1998; 23:224–226.
6. Jones NS. CT of the paranasal sinuses: A review of the correlation with clinical, surgical and histopathological findings. *Clin Otolaryngol* 2002; 27:11–17.
7. Kennedy DW. Prognostic factors, outcomes and staging in ethmoid sinus surgery. *Laryngoscope* 1992; 102:1–18.
8. Stankiewicz J, Chow J. Nasal endoscopy and the definition and diagnosis of chronic rhinosinusitis. *Otolaryngol Head Neck Surg* 2002; 126(6):623–627.
9. Flinn J, Chapman ME, Wightman AJ, Maran AG. A prospective analysis of incidental paranasal sinus abnormalities on CT head scans. *Clin Otolaryngol* 1994; 19(4): 287–289.
10. Asraf N, Bhattacharya N. Determination of the 'incidental' Lund score for the staging of chronic sinusitis *Otolaryngol Head Neck Surg* 2001; 125(5):483–486.
11. Bhattacharya T, Piccirilo Wippold FJ. Relationship between patient-based descriptions of sinusitis and paranasal sinus computed tomographic findings. *Arch Otolaryngol Head Neck Surg* 1997; 123:1189–1192.
12. Cassiano R. Correlation of clinical examination with computerized tomography in paranasal sinus disease. *Am J Rhinol* 1997; 11:193–196.
13. Norlander T, Westrin KM, Stierna P. The inflammatory response of the sinus and nasal mucosa during sinusitis: Implications for research and therapy. *Acta Otolaryngol Suppl* 1994; 515:38–44.
14. Perloff JR, Gannon FH, Bolger WE et al. Bone involvement in sinusitis: An apparent pathway for the spread of disease *Laryngoscope* 2000; 110:2095–2099.
15. Bolger WE, Leonard D, Dick EJ et al. Gram-negative sinusitis: A bacteriologic and histologic study in rabbits. *Am J Rhinol* 1997; 11:15–25.
16. Kennedy DW, Senior BA, Gannon FH et al. Histology and histomorphometry of ethmoid bone in chronic sinusitis. *Laryngoscope* 1998; 108:502–507.
17. Catalano PJ, Setliff RC, Catalano LA. Minimally invasive sinus surgery in the geriatric patient: Operative techniques. *Otolaryngol Head Neck Surg* 2001; 12(2):85–90.
18. Chiu AG. Osteitis in chronic rhinosinusitis. *Otolaryngol Clin North Am* 2005; 38:1237–1242.
19. Seiberling KA, Grammer L, Kern RC. Chronic rhinosinusitis and superantigens. *Otolaryngol Clin North Am* 2005; 38: 1215–1236.
20. Brook I. The role of bacteria in chronic rhinosinusitis. *Otolaryngol Clin North Am* 2005; 38:1171–1192.
21. Cervin A, Wallwork B. Antiinflammatory effects of macrolides antibiotics in the treatment of chronic rhinosinusitis. *Otolaryngol Clin North Am* 2005; 38:1339–1350.
22. Lund VJ. Maxial medical therapy for chronic rhinosinusitis. *Otolaryngol Clin North Am* 2005; 38:1301–1310.
23. Bhattacharya N. Symptom and disease severity differences between nasal septal deviation and chronic rhinosinusitis. *Otolaryngol Head Neck Surg* 2005; 133:173–177.
24. Yasan H, Dogru H, Baykal B et al. What isa the relationship between chronic sinus disease and isolated nasal septum deviation? *Otolaryngol Head Neck Surg* 2005; 133:190–193.

Evidence-based Management of Pediatric Chronic Rhinosinusitis

CHAPTER 12

Anthony E Magit

Creating evidence-based guidelines for the management of pediatric chronic rhinosinusitis (CRS) is a difficult, if not an impossible task, because of the paucity of literature investigating this disease. This opinion is supported in a paper by Chan, et al. Despite this situation, a rational approach to pediatric CRS can be created based upon available studies and clinical experience.

EPIDEMIOLOGY OF PEDIATRIC SINUSITIS

It is difficult to accurately assess the prevalence of sinusitis in the pediatric population because of the relatively non-specific signs and symptoms of sinusitis. Authors suggest that bacterial sinusitis complicates approximately 5 to 10% of viral upper respiratory infections in children. The average child has between six and eight viral upper respiratory infections per year with each episode lasting between five and ten days. The number and duration of upper respiratory infections leads to difficulty in distinguishing between recurrent viral infections and protracted bacterial sinusitis.

The economic impact of pediatric sinusitis on health care is significant. The estimated cost of medical therapy for pediatric sinusitis in the United States of America was estimated to have been 1.8 billion dollars in 1996. Chronic rhinosinusitis also influences the quality of life for pediatric patients. Validated scales are available to study the impact of CRS on pediatric patients. The SN-5 survey is validated and suitable for assessing outcomes for treatments for CRS in pediatric patients.

Various medical conditions predispose individuals to recurrent or chronic sinus infections. Environmental allergies leading to respiratory mucosal inflammation and stasis of upper respiratory secretions are a likely risk factor for sinusitis; although, the actual prevalence of recurrent or chronic sinusitis amongst allergic children

is unknown. One study reported that 80% of children with rhinosinusitis have a family history of environmental allergies, as compared to a prevalence of environmental allergies of 15 to 20% in the general population.

DIAGNOSIS OF PEDIATRIC SINUSITIS

Physical Examination

The physical examination is directed at assessing signs of active infection within the nose and sinuses. Additionally, the physical examination can provide information about factors contributing to sinusitis. As discussed previously, the signs and symptoms of sinusitis are non-specific, anterior rhinoscopy can be accomplished with an otoscope, allowing for an evaluation of the status of the nasal mucosa, presence of secretions or obstructing lesions. The characteristics of the secretions do not necessarily distinguish between viral rhinitis, allergic rhinitis or bacterial rhinosinusitis. Anterior rhinoscopy is easily performed and the necessary equipment is readily available.

Nasal endoscopy with a rigid or flexible telescope requires more elaborate equipment than anterior rhinoscopy and is less well tolerated by children. Office nasal endoscopy provides information about the nature of the nasal mucosa, including polypoid changes of the middle turbinates that may be associated with allergic disease. Additionally, the presence of nasal polyps may be associated with systemic conditions such as cystic fibrosis or conditions limited to the nose and paranasal sinuses such as allergic fungal sinusitis.

Radiographic Imaging

Standard radiographic imaging of the sinuses has a minor role in the evaluation of patients with suspected chronic rhinosinusitis. Plain radiographs are difficult to interpret as the appearance of the sinus mucosa and degree of aeration is non-specific and does not distinguish between inflammation secondary to bacterial, viral or allergic disease.

Computerized axial tomography (CAT) scans are the preferred method of paranasal sinus imaging and have been shown to correlate with the clinical diagnosis of chronic rhinosinusitis. CAT scans provide detailed anatomic information in addition to data regarding the degree of mucosal thickening and aeration of the sinuses. Despite the marked superiority of CAT scans compared to plain radiographs, findings from CAT scans are not sufficient to make the diagnosis of CRS in the absence of clinical correlation.

Medical Therapy

Oral antibiotics constitute the major antimicrobial therapy for chronic sinusitis. Although no scientific literature has determined the preferred length of treatment with oral antibiotics to treat pediatric CRS, short-term (7–10 days) use of oral antibiotics for chronic sinusitis has shown no benefit and common clinical practice suggests that longer periods (21 days to 6 weeks) are required to manage CRS in children.

Interest has been given to using intravenous antibiotics for pediatric chronic sinusitis. A review of three uncontrolled studies of outpatient intravenous antimicrobial therapy demonstrated efficacy for CRS. Short-term improvement ranged from 29 to 89% with a relapse rates as high as 89%. Complications ranged from 14 to 26%. These complications included problems directly related to the access catheters as well as reactions to the medications.

A retrospective review of intravenous antibiotics evaluated 70 patients who did not improve after 3 to 4 weeks of oral antibiotics. Patients then had a maxillary sinus aspiration with some patients having an adenoidectomy based on unreported clinical criteria. Patients then received 1 to 4 weeks of intravenous antibiotics. Outcomes assessed were: Clinical response, complications from the intravenous therapy, need for endoscopic sinus surgery and recurrent sinusitis. Follow-up for this study ranged from 6 to 62 months with a mean follow-up of 25 months. Sixty-two (89%) had complete clinical resolution, eight (11%) failed therapy and required endoscopic sinus surgery. No difference was noted in outcomes if patients had an adenoidectomy. All recurrent episodes of sinusitis responded to oral antibiotics.

Complications included six (9%) patients with thrombophlebitis from the intravenous therapy and three (4%) patients had antibiotic related complications.

Nasal saline irrigation is a potentially safe, inexpensive and beneficial tool for treating CRS. The body of literature reporting the use of saline for pediatric CRS patients is limited. One study compared hypertonic (3.5%) to normal saline (0.9%) irrigations in 30 patients ranging in age from 3 to 16 years. Treatment lasted for four weeks on outcomes were based on clinical symptoms and radiology results. The hypertonic saline group improved significantly for all clinical scores and the normal saline group improved only for postnasal drip. There was no difference between the groups one month after the study.

Adjuvant medical therapies include: Topical nasal steroids, antihistamines, decongestants and mucolytics. Topical nasal steroids are commonly used empirically with oral antibiotics although no studies support this type of use for patients without environmental allergies or non-allergic rhinitis. Antihistamines have not been proven to assist with the management of CRS; however, underlying allergic disease may improve. Mucolytics have theoretical benefits for treating the thickened secretions associated with CRS. The inability to recommend specific adjuvant therapies for CRS is supported by the American Academy of Pediatrics' clinical guideline for managing sinusitis. This guideline makes no recommendations regarding adjuvant therapy because of a lack of scientific evidence either for or against the efficacy of adjuvant therapy.

Gastroesophageal reflux (GER) has recently become identified as a contributor to diseases of the upper respiratory tract. For many patients, otitis media, sinusitis or laryngitis are considered to be extra-esophageal manifestations of gastroesophageal reflux. A study of the prevalence of GER in patients with chronic sinusitis used 24-hour pH monitoring of reflux and questionnaires as outcome tools. Sixty-three percent of 30 patients evaluated had esophageal reflux, six (32%) of 19 patients had nasopharyngeal reflux and 15 (79%) of 19 patients treated for GER showed improvement for their CRS.

A retrospective review of GER treatment for patients considered surgical candidates for CRS showed benefits for GER treatment. Thirty pediatric patients considered good candidates for endoscopic sinus surgery were treated for GER. Twenty-five (89%) of 28 patients improved with medical therapy and surgery was avoided. Two patients were not included in the analysis because of needing surgery for surgical conditions other than CRS.

Surgical Therapy

Adenoidectomy has been the primary surgical intervention for chronic nasal obstruction in children. The role of adenoidectomy has extended to the management of otitis media with studies demonstrating the benefits of adenoidectomy as an adjunct to medical and surgical management of chronic otitis media. The two major theories as to the underlying benefit of adenoidectomy for treating chronic sinusitis revolve around the adenoid being obstructive and acting as a reservoir for bacteria. From a mechanical standpoint, obstructing adenoid tissue may interfere with normal nasal drainage and lead to a stasis of secretions. As a bacterial reservoir, adenoid tissue serves as a repository of bacteria that occupy the paranasal sinuses during episodes of acute or chronic sinusitis.

Rosenfeld published a pilot study of adenoidectomy for the treatment chronic sinusitis. He concluded that a subgroup of children thought to be candidates for endoscopic sinus surgery can improve with adenoidectomy. A large-scale, prospective study of adenoidectomy for this group of patients has not been undertaken. The relationships between adenoid size, adenoid microbiology and results from maxillary sinus aspirates were evaluated in 30 children with clinical and radiographic evidence of sinusitis. Adenoid size was assessed with office flexible endoscopy and endoscopy during surgery. There was no statistical relationship between cultures obtained from the adenoid tissue and maxillary sinus aspirate. Additionally, there was no correlation between the size of the adenoid and culture results from the maxillary sinus.

In a non-randomized study, the efficacy of adenoidectomy with or without concurrent endoscopic sinus surgery for treatment of CRS has been reviewed. Ramadan presented a prospective, non-randomized study of 202 children treated surgically for CRS. Three groups were compared: Endoscopic sinus surgery with adenoidectomy (Group 1), endoscopic sinus surgery (Group 2) and adenoidectomy (Group 3). The study spanned 10 years and assessed clinical outcomes at 12 months. Group 1 had 87% improvement, Group 2, 75% improvement and Group 3, 52% improvement. Three independent predictors of clinical success emerged from this study: Asthma, passive smoke exposure and age of the patient.

ENDOSCOPIC SINUS SURGERY

Absolute clinical indications for endoscopic sinus surgery for pediatric patients with chronic rhinosinusitis do not exist. Sinus surgery is usually contemplated once the patient has received 'maximal medical therapy' and underlying medical conditions have been evaluated and treated. Due to the multifactorial nature of the causative factors for CRS, 'maximal medical' therapy varies between physicians and the extent of the evaluation for concurrent medical conditions is driven by the patient's history, family history and clinical presentation.

Experience with endoscopic sinus surgery in children has proliferated with advances in instrumentation and education amongst sinus surgeons. Prospective, randomized trials of pediatric endoscopic sinus surgery have not been completed. The studies available for evaluation tend to be either retrospective or non-randomized. Despite the limitations of available literature, guarded conclusions can be made with regard to clinical outcomes, surgical techniques and safety related to performing endoscopic sinus surgery in children.

A meta-analysis of pediatric endoscopic sinus surgery included 8 published articles consisting of 832 patients and unpublished data from 50 patients. Overall 'positive' outcomes for published, unpublished and combined data were: 88.4, 92, and 88.75%, respectively with an average combined follow-up of 0.6%. The major complications rate for the combined data was 0.6%.

Jiang, et al reported on 104 patients younger than 16 years of age who had FESS between April 1988 and March 1998. Postoperative improvement in this population was 84% with operative complications occurring in 5 (4.1%) of patients.

Lieu et al 10 attempted to correlate treatment success with the stage of sinus disease. Three hundred and eight patients with 2-year follow-up were evaluated using a questionnaire. Overall, 55% of patients were 'much improved'. Endoscopic surgery did not demonstrate benefit above medical therapy for patients with stage 1 (no predictive factors) or stage 4 (moderate to severe day cough). Endoscopic sinus surgery did have 79% overall improvement compared to 54% improvement for medical therapy for stage 2 (night cough, halitosis, no stage 3 or 4 symptoms) sinus disease. Surgery was associated with 68% overall improvement as compared to 42% overall improvement for medical therapy for stage 3 (headache, 2 or more co-morbid conditions, medications other than for sinusitis, and no day cough).

The impact of patient age on success related to endoscopic sinus surgery was investigated by Ramadan. Ninety-nine children underwent endoscopic sinus surgery between January 1994 and June 1999 with the primary outcome being a parent questionnaire at least one year after surgery. Failure was considered to be no improvement in symptoms or the need for revision surgery. For the entire cohort of patients, overall success was 82% with 89% of patients older than six years having 'successful' outcomes and 73% of patients younger than 6 years of age having 'successful' outcomes. Eleven (9%) of the entire study population required revision surgery.

Surgical Considerations

The type of endoscopic sinus surgery performed in children differs from that performed in adults. This discussion addresses sinus surgery in patients without underlying systemic disease, such as cystic fibrosis or ciliary dysfunction. Functional endoscopic sinus surgery in children is designed to achieve improved aeration of the paranasal sinuses without extensive mucosal resection. Chang evaluated the efficacy of a limited approach of FESS in pediatric patients with chronic rhinosinusitis refractory to medical therapy. Surgeons used drainage rather than an extirpation procedure. A retrospective review of records and parental questionnaire served as the outcome measures. One hundred and one patients had surgery between January 1995 and September 2002. Improvement of specific symptoms included: Nasal obstruction, 91%; purulent rhinorrhea, 90%: postnasal drip, 90%; headache, 97%; hyposmia, 89% and chronic cough, 96%. Eighty-seven parents (86%) were satisfied with the surgery.

A "second-look" endoscopic procedure was initially considered an integral aspect of pediatric FESS. Adult patients having FESS typically have several endoscopic debridements performed in the office setting following the operative endoscopic procedure. These procedures are directed at removing granulation tissue, crusts and thick secretion from the nose and sinus cavities. Surgeons performing pediatric FESS understood the difficulty in performing endoscopic debridements in the office setting and choose to return patients to the operating room 1 to 4 weeks after the initial surgical procedure to for a debridement procedure.

The efficacy of performing 'second-look' procedures was assessed in 100 children undergoing FESS, 50 having a 'second-look' procedure and 50 without a 'second-look' procedure. Children were excluded if they had any underlying systemic disease. There were no differences in clinical outcomes with regard to nasal obstruction, nasal discharge or cough when comparing the patients who did or did not have a 'second look' procedure.

Facial Growth

A long-term consideration in performing FESS in pediatric patients is the impact on facial growth. Surgical procedures involving the paranasal sinuses have the theoretic possibility of adversely affecting growth centers and subsequently altering development of the midface. Facial growth was evaluated in 67 patients with mean age at presentation of 3.1 years and 13.2 years at follow-up. Forty-six patients had FESS and 21 served as surgical controls. Anthropomorphic measures were used as the primary outcome measure and no statistical difference were found between the two groups.

Evaluating the Evidence

The information presented regarding the diagnosis and treatment of pediatric chronic sinusitis does not provide sufficient information to create an 'evidence-based' management scheme for pediatric CRS. Several factors contribute to the difficulty in obtaining high quality data in the form of prospective, randomized clinical trials investigating pediatric CRS. The multifactorial nature of CRS and the overlap in clinical presentations with other clinical situations (i.e. recurrent uncomplicated viral upper respiratory infections) makes identifying a cohort of similar subjects extremely difficult. Ensuring that all subjects enrolled in a study have the same environmental, medical and allergic risk factors would be expensive and time consuming. Nonetheless, enough information exists to create a clinically useful and reasonable approach to managing pediatric CRS. Recommendations are guided by clinical studies where possible.

Recommendations

Medical History and Physical Examination

The medical history and physical examination should address the possibility of underlying diseases and environmental conditions contributing to CRS. Possible contributing factors include environmental allergies, immunodeficiency, gastroesophageal reflux, cystic fibrosis, passive smoke exposure and participation in large daycare settings for pre-school age children. The basic physical examination should include anterior rhinoscopy to assess the status of the nasal mucosa in addition to the presence of secretions and polypoid tissue. Flexible nasopharyngoscopy is not a routine part of the initial physical examination in the evaluation of suspected CRS in all children; however, it will provide more information than anterior rhinoscopy regarding intranasal structures, the size and appearance of adenoid tissue and laryngeal findings suggestive of gastro-esophageal reflux. These recommendations are based upon the numerous factors associated with CRS and not prospective clinical studies.

Radiographic Imaging

Radiographic imaging plays a secondary role in diagnosing CRS in children. Plain radiographs can be difficult to interpret for young children and provide limited information regarding specific anatomy. CAT scans provide more information than plain radiographs; however, the findings must be interpreted in the context of the clinical presentation. CAT scans are usually performed once a thorough evaluation has been completed, the patient has received extensive medical therapy, and endoscopic sinus surgery is being contemplated. In the evaluation of chronic sinus disease, the CAT scan is preferably obtained after the patient has received prolonged medical therapy and in the spring or summer to lessen the likelihood of a concurrent viral upper respiratory infection being responsible for findings of mucosal thickening or sinus opacification.

Medical Therapy

Hypertonic nasal saline irrigations can be beneficial in the management of CRS. This treatment is inexpensive, readily available and has minimal risk. Empiric use of topical nasal steroids is appropriate for co-existent allergic disease and is commonly used in conjunction with prolonged oral antibiotics as part of 'maximal medical therapy' for CRS. The empiric use of antihistamines and decongestants for CRS is anecdotal but may provide symptomatic improvement without impacting upon the underlying sinus disease.

Antimicrobials are the mainstay for the treatment of CRS. Short courses of one week or less of oral antibiotics do not seem effective for chronic disease. The choice of antibiotic is based upon adequate coverage of suspected aerobic bacteria. The role of anaerobic bacteria and fungal infections for CRS in pediatric patients is not clear. Intravenous antibiotics may have a role in the treatment of CRS; however, published studies are not prospective and complications occur with the intravenous administration of the medications.

Treatment for gastroesophageal reflux in selected patients has been shown to reduce or eliminate signs and symptoms of CRS in selected patients. The empiric use of therapies intended to treat GERD may be appropriate for patients with clinical evidence of GERD, a family history of GERD or as a reasonable medical treatment prior to surgery for patient failing 'maximal medical therapy' with antibiotics and topical steroids.

Surgical Therapy

Adenoidectomy can alleviate nasal obstruction in appropriately selected patients and should be considered as a primary surgical intervention for patients with chronic nasal obstruction and clinical evidence of adenoid hypertrophy. The procedure is performed routinely with minimal morbidity and has been shown to provide benefit in patients with CRS. The value of maxillary sinus aspiration at the time of adenoidectomy to direct antimicrobial therapy may be supported in some situations based upon retrospective studies. The utility of adenoidectomy for managing CRS in patients without evidence of obstructive adenoid tissue is less clear.

Endosopic sinus surgery has been shown to be a safe procedure in children with a relatively low complication rate with no clinically relevant impact on facial growth. Prospective studies comparing pediatric endoscopic sinus surgery to specific medical therapies do not exist. For patients without underlying systemic disease contributing to CRS (i.e. cystic fibrosis, ciliary dysfunction), endoscopic sinus surgery has a role in management after a thorough medical evaluation and 'adequate' medical therapy. In contrast to surgery in adults with CRS, pediatric patients are usually managed with a more limited endoscopic procedure. As 'second-look' endoscopic procedure for debridement does not appear to have clinical benefit.

SUMMARY

Pediatric chronic rhinosinusitis is a difficult disease to manage because of diagnostic challenges and the vast array of treatment options. The overlap in signs and symptoms between CRS, allergic diseases and recurrent uncomplicated upper respiratory viral infections clouds clinical decision making and creates a challenge for designing and performing clinical research studies of CRS. Medical therapy should be instituted after a thorough history and medical evaluation. Surgery for CRS can be done safely; however, the goals and expected outcome of surgery should be clearly defined.

BIBLIOGRAPHY

1. American Academy of Pediatrics Subcommittee on Management of Sinusitis and Committee on Quality Improvement. Clinical practice guideline: Management of sinusitis. *Pediatrics* 2001; 108(3):798–808.

2. Bhattacharyya N, Jones DT, Hill M, Shapiro NL. The diagnostic accuracy of computed tomography in pediatric chronic rhinosinusitis. *Arch Otolaryngol Head Neck Surg* 2004; 130(9):1029–1032.

3. Bothwell MR, Parsons DS, Talbot A, Barbero GJ, Wilder B. Outcome of reflux therapy on pediatric chronic sinusitis. *Otolaryngol Head Neck Surg* 1999; 121(3):255–262.

4. Bothwell MR, Piccirillo JF, Lusk RP, Ridenour BD. Long-term outcome of facial growth after functional endoscopic sinus surgery. *Otolaryngol Head Neck Surg* 2002; 126(6):628–634.

5. Chan KH, Winslow CP, Levin MJ, Abzug MJ, Shira JE, Liu AH, et al. Clinical practice guidelines for the management of chronic sinusitis in children. *Otol Head Neck Surg* 1999; 120: 328–34.

6. Chang PH. Functional endoscopic sinus surgery in children using a limited approach. *Arch Otolaryngol Head Neck Surg* 2004; 130(9):1033–1036.

7. Don DM, Yellon RF, Casselbrant ML, Bluestone CD. Efficacy of a stepwise protocol that includes intravenous antibiotic therapy for the management of chronic sinusitis in children and adolescents. *Arch Otol Head Neck Surg* 2001; 127(9): 1099–1101.

8. Goldsmith AJ, Rosenfeld RM. Treatment of Pediatric Sinusitis. *Pediatric Clinics of North America* 2003; 50(2):413–26.

9. Hebert RL, Bent JP. Meta-analysis of outcomes of pediatric functional endoscopic sinus surgery. *Laryngoscope* 1998; 108(6):796–799.

10. Jiang RS, Hsu CY. Functional endoscopic sinus surgery in children and adults. *Ann Otol Rhinol Laryngol* 2000; 109: 1113–1116.

11. Kay DJ. Quality of life for children with persistent sinonasal symptoms. *Otolaryngol Head Neck Surg* 2003; 128(1):17–26.

12. Lieu JE, Piccirillo JF, Lusk RP. Prognostic staging system and therapeutic effectiveness for recurrent or chronic sinusitis in children. *Otolaryngol Head Neck* 2003; 129:222–232.

13. Mitchell RB, Pereira KD, Younis RT, Lazar RH. Pediatric functional endoscopic sinus surgery: Is a second look necessary? *Laryngoscope* 1997; 107(9):1267–1269.

14. Phipps CD, Wood WE, Gibson WS, Cochran WJ. Gastro-esophageal reflux contributing to chronic sinus disease in children: A prospective analysis. *Arch Otolaryngol Head Neck Surg* 2000; 126(7):831–836.

15. Ramadan HH. Relation of age to outcome after endoscopic sinus surgery in children. *Arch Otolaryngol Head Neck Surg* 2003; 12(92):175–177.

16. Ramadan HH. Surgical management of chronic sinusitis in children. *Laryngoscope* 2004; 114(12):2103–2109.

17. Ray NF, Baraniuk JN, Thamer M, Rinehart CS, Gergen PJ, Kaliner M, et al. Health care expenditures for sinusitis in 1996: Contributions of asthma, rhinitis, and other airway disorders. *J Allergy Clin Immunol* 1999; 103:408–414.

18. Rosenfeld RM. Pilot study of outcomes in pediatric sinusitis. *Arch Otol Head Neck Surg* 1995; 121:729–736.

19. Shapiro GG, Rachelevsky GS. Introduction and definition of sinusitis. *J Allergy Clin Immunol* 1992; 90:417-418.

20. Shoseyov D, Bibi H, Shai P, Shoseyov N, Shazberg G, Hurvitz H. Treatment with hypertonic saline versus normal saline nasal wash of pediatric chronic sinusitis. *J Allergy Clin Immunol* 1998; 101(5):602–605.

21. Tanner SB. Intravenous antibiotics for chronic rhinosinusitis: Are they effective? *Curr Opinion Otolaryngol Head Neck Surg* 2004; 12(1):3–8.

22. Tuncer V. Chronic rhinosinusitis and adenoid hypertrophy in children. *Am J Otolaryngol* 2004; 25(1):5–10.

23. Wald ER. Sinusitis. *Pediatr Ann* 1998; 27:811–818.

Nasal Polyposis: Current Concepts in Pathophysiology and Management

Nadim B Bikhazi

Nasal polyposis (NP) is a multifactorial disease which results in edematous masses that obstruct the nasal cavities and paranasal sinuses. It is clearly understood that NP results in dramatic impairment of quality-of-life issues often contributing to other common diseases such as sleep apnea and asthma.[1] An allergic cause of polyp development was initially purported in the Yonge's landmark article in 1907,[2] but better understanding of the pathophysiology has proven this to be a simplistic association. We now understand that the development of polyps involves a complex interaction between a variety of immunologic cells including eosinophils, neutrophils, and lymphocytes. The inflammatory cascade is more directly implicated than the allergic process, involving complex interactions between mucosal epithelium, matrix, and the cells themselves.

The delineation of the pathophysiology of NP has resulted in more directed and successful treatment towards the various causes of polyps. No longer is simple 'polypectomy' an accepted treatment approach due to the high rate of recidivism. Controversies in management still exist in the role fungi play in the process, the exact role and timing of surgical intervention, and specific disease processes such as cystic fibrosis and aspirin-sensitive patients.

EPIDEMIOLOGY

The exact prevalence of nasal polyps is not clearly known. The incidence is often noted to be 1–4% of the population[3] with higher rates among patients with asthma, cystic fibrosis, and allergic fungal disease (Table 13.1). Most of these reported rates are from review of patient records and questionnaires. More recent Danish studies by Larsen and Tos using endoscopy as the diagnostic modality have found an incidence of 0.627/thousand/year.[6] Anatomic studies have found higher rates in up to 40% of specimens examined. This may indicate that many polyps may be asymptomatic or difficult to identify on routine examination. There appears to be increased incidence with rising age and male gender. Polyps are rarely seen in children less than 10 years of age unless there is an accompanying diagnosis of cystic fibrosis. Patients with asthma have higher rates of nasal polyps and when present, polyps are associated with more severe and earlier onset asthma.[7]

CLASSIFICATION

The five groups of polyps have been delineated by Stammberger.[8] These have been separated based on differing histological characteristics and clinical presentation. They include:
- Antrochoanal polyps
- Isolated large polyps
- Polyps with chronic rhinosinusitis (non-eosinophil dominated)

Table 13.1: Prevalence of nasal polyposis in various disease states*	
Aspirin sensitivity	36–95%
Asthma	5–13%
IgE mediated	5%
Non-IgE mediated	13%
Chronic sinusitis	2%
Cystic fibrosis	7–56%
Allergic fungal sinusitis	66–100%
Primary ciliary dyskinesia	40%

*Adapted from Mygind et al. Nasal polyposis, eosinophil dominated inflammation, and allergy. Thorax 2000; 55 (Suppl 2): S79-S83.[4,5] Adapted and reproduced with permission from the BMJ Publishing Group.

- Polyps with chronic rhinosinusitis (eosinophil dominated)
- Polyps with specific diseases (i.e. cystic fibrosis).

Although they share a common pathological structure, these various disease states vary greatly in location, treatment and rates of recidivism.

PATHOPHYSIOLOGY

Allergic Inflammation

The development of a polyp results from chronic inflammation specifically in histological stromal edema with a variable cellular infiltrate. Initially, due to higher IgE levels and eosinophils/mast cells in polyp tissue, an allergic IgE-mediated response was postulated. However, several studies have shown no higher incidence of polyps in atopic individuals. This accounts for the lack of efficacy of most antihistamines in patients with nasal polyps.[9] Interestingly, several specific types of allergic reactions directed towards infectious organisms have been related to polyp development. Elevated IgE levels towards *Staphylococcus* and *Streptococcus* superantigens have been discovered in nasal polyp patients.[10] Although the exact mechanism is not known, the superantigens may either elicit a direct IgE response or instead bind directly to major histocompatibility (MHC) II sites resulting in T helper driven cytokine release. This suggests chronic colonization by *S. aureus* may promote a local allergic

cycle stimulating polyp development, again underscoring the multifactorial nature of NP. Additionally, fungi have been implicated in the development of a localized allergic response in the nasal mucosa. A high proportion of NP patients (40%) have shown skin reactivity to *C. albicans*[11] but it is unclear whether this is a cause of, or result of the NP development.

Greater emphasis has currently been placed recently on the active role of leukotrienes promoting NP development. Particularly, the proinflammatory effects of cysteinyl leukotrienes (cysLTs) are becoming more appreciated. Activation of mast cells, eosinophils, monocytes and macrophages results in arachidonic acid being released from cellular membranes which increases cysLT formation via the 5-lipoxygenase pathway (Fig. 13.1). The pro-inflammatory nature of cysLTs and their association with NP has been described.[12] This has particular import for aspirin-sensitive NP patients (discussed below).

Non-allergic Inflammation

The eosinophil plays a central role in the pathophysiology of polyp development. Conversely, in non-eosinophil dominated diseases (cystic fibrosis and primary ciliary dyskinesia), the neutrophil occupies center position. The pathophysiology of polyps in aspirin-sensitive patients will be discussed as a separate category.

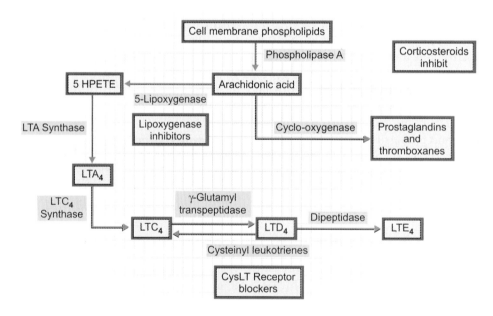

Fig. 13.1: Leukotriene synthesis pathway [Reprinted from *Oto Head Neck Surg*, Vol 129, Haberal and Corey, *The role of leukotrienes in nasal allergy*, 2003, pages 274–279 with permission from American Academy of Otolaryngology—Head and Neck Surgery Foundation Inc.

Eosinophils are potent initiator cells in inflammation releasing cytotoxic granule proteins, major basic protein (MBP) and eosinophil cationic protein. The presence of these mediators affects adhesion molecules, vascular permeability and other inflammatory cells. This accounts for the efficacy of steroids in downregulating the inflammatory process resulting in a diminution of polyp size.[13] There has been a strong association of MBP deposition in extracellular tissue and damage to the sinus mucosa.[14] It is thought that this persistent damage allows extravasation of the lamina propria. Elevated levels of albumin have also been found in polyps implicating plasma exudation as a driving force towards forming the polyp structure.[15] Eosinophils are attracted to the area by neutrophil-produced granulocyte colony stimulating factor (GCSF) and T helper cell-produced cytokines IL-4 and IL-5. IL-5 is found at high levels in NP tissue and at higher levels in asthma patients with polyps than in non-asthma polyp patients.[16] IL-5 therefore plays a key role in the pathophysiology of eosinophil-dominated polyps. Eosinophils also produce IL-5 (resulting in autocrine stimulation) thus lending evidence to the self-perpetuating process of polyp development.

HISTOLOGY

The surface of the nasal polyps is often covered by the same mucosa that lines the respiratory tract, pseudostratified columnar epithelium (Figs 13.2 and 13.3). Often, zones of transitional and squamous epithelium are seen. The subepithelium reveals a composition of eosinophils in 80–90% of all polyp patients and neutrophils in 10–20% (Fig. 13.4). An admixture of other cells including mast cells, lymphocytes and plasma cells can be seen. The histological picture of polyps in non-eosinophil polyps includes many more neutrophils and lymphocytes than eosinophils.

The polyp surface epithelium does not usually reveal epithelial defects even though this is postulated to occur during the polyp development. Tissue hydration is a *sine qua non* of polyps occurring secondary to lamina propria extravasation as has already been mentioned. The large quantities of extracellular fluid in polyps has promoted theories of dysregulation of Na-Cl transport caused by histamine release.[17] Polyps have no innervation and do not reveal any production of mucus but can have cystic degeneration.[18] It is this denervation and subsequent decreased secretion that leads to irreversible tissue edema. The vascularity of polyps appears to be much less than that of the surrounding nasal mucosa.

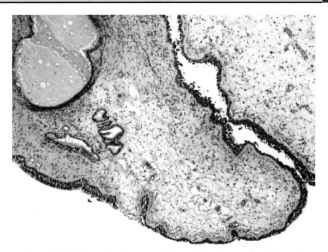

Fig. 13.2: Nasal polyp revealing ciliated pseudostratified respiratory epithelium. Original magnification x40

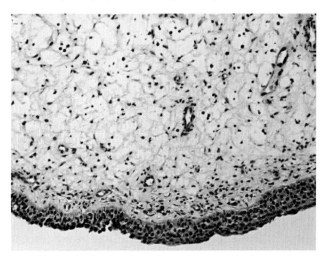

Fig. 13.3: Nasal polyp with respiratory epithelium and edematous stroma. Original magnification x100

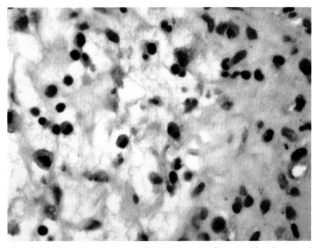

Fig. 13.4: Nasal polyp revealing plasma cells upon background of edematous stroma. Original magnification x400

ANATOMICAL OCCURRENCE

As opposed to antrochoanal polyps which are based off the maxillary sinus mucosa, most eosinophil-dominated polyps are pedicled off of the ostiomeatal area (Fig. 13.5). Stammberger has defined the most common areas of polyp origin in 200 consecutive patients (Table 13.2). He has speculated that narrow mucosal contact areas around ostial openings account for these sites of origin. Stasis of mucus occurs in these 'narrow clefts' and edema sets in eventually resulting in polyp development. Larsen and Tos have further defined that 75% of all polyps found on autopsy study were related to ostia, clefts, and recesses.[20] These 'catch areas' therefore are the sites of antigen deposition and subsequent reaction of the nasal lining to them.

DIAGNOSIS

Clinical Presentation and Evaluation

The diagnosis of NP is now easily ascertained due to advances in endoscopic and radiographic techniques. Most commonly symptoms of nasal obstruction, headache, sinus pressure, rhinitis, and hyposmia are noted by patients. Bilateral presentation is noted in 80–90% of patients and is associated with higher prevalence of asthma and aspirin sensitivity.[21] Infrequently, NP patients will present with other diseases such as asthma without any upper airway complaints. Many patients with NP experience difficulties with daily activities. These appear to be age-related as adolescents have more difficulty concentrating, adults have more emotional problems and children have difficulty performing practical problems due to NP.[1]

Table 13.2: Origination of polyps in 200 consecutive patients*	
80%	Uncinate-middle turbinate-infundibulum
65%	Anterior face of bulla-hiatus-infundibulum
48%	Frontal recess
42%	Turbinate sinus (between bulla and middle turbinates)
30%	Inside bulla
28%	Supra-/retrobulbar recess
27%	Posterior ethmoid/superior meatus
15%	Middle turbinate

*Stammberger H. *FESS*. Philadelphia: BC Decker 1991:204[19]

Diagnosis of NP is chiefly based on direct visualization. Because a majority of polyps are based high in the ethmoid cavity, evaluation by anterior rhinoscopy may miss smaller polyps. Nasal endoscopy provides excellent visualization of the aforementioned areas of polyp development. In patients who have undergone prior surgical extirpation, angled scopes (30° and 45°) can be used to view the maxillary sinus interior and nasofrontal recesses. Sometimes, severe congestion precludes clear endoscopic visualization and a combination of 0.25% neosynephrine and 2% lidocaine solution can be used to decongest the inferior and middle turbinates prior to visualization. Additionally, recurrent polyps can be addressed in the office in this manner after removing localized areas of recidivism with topical anesthesia.

Radiographic Appearance

The computerized tomography (CT) scan is considered gold standard to evaluate uncomplicated polyps. Radiographic appearance of NP is varied, extending from small isolated opacification in the ostiomeatal complex to pan-sinus opacification on CT scanning (Fig. 13.6).

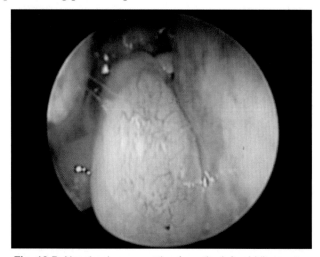

Fig. 13.5: Nasal polyp emanating from the left middle meatus

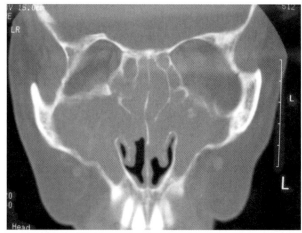

Fig. 13.6: CT scan revealing nasal polyposis resulting in pan-sinus opacification

Unilateral polyps should raise the possibility of an antrochoanal polyp or inverting papilloma and should always be biopsied to exclude a neoplastic process (Fig. 13.7). Often, bone erosion can be seen with benign nasal polyps thus mimicking a neoplastic disease. At other times, surrounding osteitis can occur raising the question of a primary osteogenic disease even though this is simply secondary to the reactive process surrounding the polyps (Fig. 13.8). Polyps associated with fungi often have calcifications within the affected sinus. Any appearance of intracranial pathology that is suspected to be NP should be further evaluated with magnetic resonance imaging (MRI) to exclude the possibility of an encephalocele (Fig. 13.9).

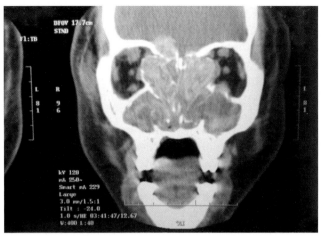

Fig. 13.9: Severe nasal polyposis causing cerebritis. Bowing of the lamina paparycea into both orbital cavites

MEDICAL MANAGEMENT

Although multiple etiologies exist, the end result of NP is an edematous structure that demonstrates a high density of inflammatory cells. Medical management of nasal polyps is directed towards minimizing inflammation while surgical control is focused on removing the mechanical obstruction within the sinus and nasal cavities.[22] Medical management is most effective when directed towards the early edematous initiation of NP and tends to fail when more extensive polyps are present. Even with surgery, NP remains a mucosal disease that often requires ongoing medical maintenance. Much like asthma, NP is a chronic disease that is active in 85% of patients 20 years after surgery.[23] Advances in medical management over the last several decades have relied on better understanding of the pathophysiology of polyp development. There continues to be controversy as to the exact role of medical and surgical approaches, but a combination of both these is often required to adequately manage polyps. When the exact cause of polyps is known, as in the case of aspirin-sensitive patients, treatment must be directed towards the disease process to prevent recurrence.

Because there is a higher association of asthma among NP patients, medical treatment of the polyps often improves associated bronchial hyper-responsiveness. When viewed another way, the presence of asthma is a negative predictor of successful medical and surgical outcomes.[24, 25] This is even more striking among aspirin-sensitive patients.

Systemic Corticosteroids

Corticosteroids are the mainstay of medical management of NP, being the only class of medication shown to have

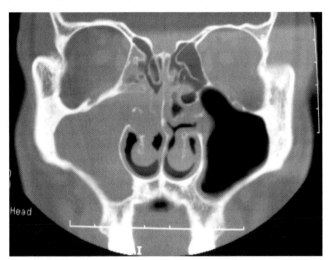

Fig. 13.7: Unilateral nasal polyposis causing effacement of the uncinate process. These findings can also be seen in inverting papilloma or other neoplastic processes

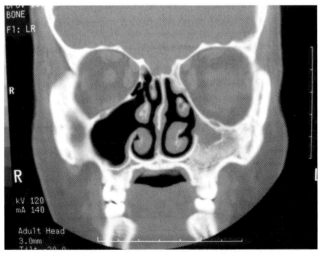

Fig. 13.8: Chronic osteitis secondary to nasal polypoid tissue in the left maxillary sinus

proven efficacy in reducing the signs and symptoms. Systemic steroids are often used as 'medical polypectomy' reducing inflammation in both eosinophil and non-eosinophil dominated polyps. Their effect has been less well-documented than intranasal steroids but several studies have detailed their symptomatic improvement in nasal polyposis especially for regaining the sense of the smell.[26–29] Often a systemic burst is used to shrink large obstructive polyps in order to provide more area to apply topical steroid therapy. Infrequently, systemic steroids may prevent the need of surgical extirpation. A recent study using this protocol in 152 patients reported 68.5% success after 1 year follow-up with 31.5% ultimately requiring surgical remedy.[30] Preoperative steroids are also used to minimize polyp size and blood loss and postoperative steroid pulses can be used for recurrent disease.

A typical steroid taper would be prednisone at 60 mg per day tapering of 10 mg every several days over 3 weeks. High-risk patients include patients who are smokers, obese, diabetic, have glaucoma, hypertension, or psychiatric disorders.[31] These patients need to be apprised of the risks of systemic steroid use. If problems do arise such as elevated blood sugar, the steroid dose can be tapered quickly over 2 to 3 days without side effects.

Intranasal Steroids

Intranasal steroids have been used extensively as first-line management of nasal polyposis with very few adverse effects. Topical steroids can be delivered either by drops or sprays. Usually, patients with small polyps and limited CT involvement are good candidates for topical therapy alone. Intranasal steroids have repeatedly been shown to reduce nasal congestion, drainage and polyp recurrence.[26,27,32,33] The effect of steroids appears to be non-specific in improving symptoms in both eosinophilic and non-eosinophilic dominant polyps. While there have not been any studies confirming reductions in mucoperiosteal thickening on CT scan, intranasal steroids can provide excellent mainstay therapy to help control polyp development and minimize their recurrence.[34,35]

After therapy is initiated, it is recommended that the patient be re-examined in 6–8 weeks to evaluate efficacy. Typically, the steroids are applied via nasal spray with only a small amount of medication reaching the middle meatus.[36] Generally, it is believed that clinical improvement may take several weeks, but a recent study has noted significant clinical changes within three days of treatment.[37] Nasal bleeding is the most common adverse sequelae which usually can be minimized by directing the medication away from the septum. Topical steroid therapy in children with polyps has also been shown to be safe with no overall effect on attainable height when using clinically indicated doses.[38,39] Most recently, nasal nebulizers have been used to control refractory rhinosinusitis with antibiotics, but no clinical studies have documented nebulized nasal steroid benefit as of yet.[40,41]

Antibiotic Therapy

Most of the data regarding antibiotic therapy is based on the efficacy of macrolides. The effectiveness of this group of antibiotics seems to be related to their anti-inflammatory properties rather than their antimicrobial characteristics.[42] Macrolides appear to decrease neutrophil and eosinophil degranulation as well as reduce fibroblast activity *in vitro*.[43] Most of the clinical studies of successful macrolide therapy in nasal polyposis emanate from Japan, but these are uncontrolled studies. Ichimura has noted that roxithromycin 150 mg per day for 8 weeks resulted in a diminution of polyps in 52% of the patients with smaller polyps more likely to diminish in size.[44] When cetirizine was added to the treatment group, the success rate increased to 68% although this was not a significant difference. Some authors have advocated using macrolides in patients where corticosteroids appear to fail,[45] but the exact role of macrolides in the paradigm of polyp management has not been defined. Randomization of CT staging and consistent definitions of clinical success need to occur before the utility of macrolide therapy can be stated in NP.

Antifungal Therapy

Controversy exists regarding the exact role fungi play in the development of nasal polyps. Some feel that due to the high prevalence of fungi noted in some studies,[46] polyps may occur secondary to chronic inflammation against fungal antigens. It is also unclear what the prevalence of this entity is as fungal exposure differs not only between countries but even within areas of the United States. One disease directly related to fungal exposure is allergic fungal rhinosinusitis where antifungal immunotherapy appears to effectively reduce mucosal edema and prevent recurrence in allergic fungal patients.[47] Another study using Amphotericin B nasal irrigations among general polyp patients noted 39% of patients experienced endoscopic disappearance of polyps after 4 weeks of irrigations, but again no control group was used.[48] Further controlled studies are needed to separate out factors of corticosteroid use and pre-treatment stage differences among patients before successes can be proven.

Leukotriene Modifiers

It is clear that zileuton, zafirlukast, and montelukast play an important role in the management of asthma but limited data exists to prove their value in nasal polyposis. Ulualp studied 18 previously operated sinus patients with aspirin-sensitive polyposis and found 9 of 15 who completed the study experienced clinical improvement confirmed by endoscopic findings.[49] A second study by Parnes and Chuma[50] confirmed the benefit of zileuton and zafirlukast among general polyp patients with 72% clinical improvement. While these initial results appear promising, controlled and randomized studies are needed before anti-leukotrienes become widely used.

Intranasal Capsaicin

Capsaicin, the pungent agent in hot pepper, has been used intranasally in general polyp patients with some success in ameliorating symptoms. Its mechanism appears to block neurogenic inflammation in the nose after topical application resulting in a depletion of neurokinins.[51] This has been used both prior to and after sinus surgery with improvement in nasal symptoms.[52] It appears that capsaicin provides a low-cost alternative to corticosteroids that may be used in developing countries.

Antihistamines

Although antihistamines may provide relief of allergic symptoms in patients with nasal polyposis, polyp regression is not seen. One study using cetirizine noted a reduction in concomitant nasal symptoms of sneezing and rhinorrhea in 45 patients over 3 months.[53] These medications are less efficacious on the symptom of nasal congestion. This is surprising given the large amount of mast cell degeneration found within polyps. Antihistamines are not currently indicated in the primary management of polyp patients unless there is an underlying allergic diathesis.

Intranasal Lysine-acetylsalicylic Acid (LAS)

More than a third of nasal polyp patients have association with aspirin sensitivity. LAS appears to have an anti-

proliferative effect on fibroblasts from nasal polyps *in vitro*.[54] A controlled study revealed that postoperative treatment with LAS in both aspirin-tolerant and aspirin-sensitive patients diminished recurrence rates of polyps.[55] The mechanism of LAS appears thus to be anti-inflammatory rather than through desensitization as both groups benefited equally.

Intranasal Furosemide

Since polyps absorb plasma and water into the lamina propria, intranasal furosemide has been theorized to reduce polyp size. Furosemide minimizes postoperative relapse in general nasal polyps when compared to intranasal mometasone.[56] Limited data exists to warrant widespread use at this point however.

SURGICAL MANAGEMENT

The exact role and extent of surgery in NP is not yet clear. It is known that NP is a chronic mucosal disease and that surgery is used only to control the disease process once it is refractory to medical therapy. The exact timing of this intervention is debatable. A position statement has noted that surgery should not be considered prior to 1 month of medical treatment as many patients will not require surgical therapy.[57] This appears reasonable given the often dramatic response that can be seen with a combination of systemic and topical steroids.

Surgery

The literature regarding the extent of surgery to be performed for NP is controversial. 'Polypectomy' by itself does not achieve aeration of diseased sinuses effectively and has largely been abandoned for more complete marsupialization. While recent attention in endoscopic sinus surgery has been focused on mucosa sparing techniques, extensive NP requires extensive exenteration. The severity of disease on CT scan should govern the extent of surgery. Many with limited disease in the ostiomeatal complex require only limited surgery while others with diffuse polypoid mucosa and large polyps will require a more radical removal of affected air cells. The introduction of microdebriders has also facilitated sinus surgery by preserving normal anatomy resulting in less blood loss during cases.

It is clear that endoscopic sinus surgery has improved our ability to obtain safe and thorough cleanout of sinus cavities with excellent outcomes even among extensive NP. In a retrospective follow-up in 170 chronic polypoid sinusitis patients undergoing ESS, Weber has noted 92% of patients obtained successful outcomes even up to 10 years after sinus surgery. Recurrent polyps were found in 25% of patients.[58] Surgery not only controls the severity of polyp obstruction but the resulting enlargement of orifices facilitates topical application of antibiotics and steroids. Many patients may experience radiographic mucoperiosteal thickening, but increased sinus patency allows application of nebulized medical therapy. In many other studies however, patients with NP experience high recidivism, especially among aspirin-sensitive patients.[21,59] Endoscopic surgical outcomes in NP patients have consistently shown improvement in quality of life issues postoperatively[60] but there is less symptom improvement when compared to non-polyp chronic sinus patients.[61] NP patients also experience higher rates of revision surgery resulting from the chronic nature of the disease. Although surgery does not appear to improve olfaction any more than medical treatment alone,[29] there may be a subset of patients who through improved aeration may be able to apply antibiotics to previously unreachable areas. Postoperative systemic steroid bursts may be required to control polypoid mucosa along the roof of the ethmoid/cribiform areas. The role of postoperative steroid lavages has not been studied well enough, but may provide periodic symptomatic relief. Clearly, surgery cannot be evaluated by itself but rather as one of many therapeutic modalities necessary to control NP due to the chronic mucosal inflammation, which occurs. Comparative studies of medical versus surgical therapy are often unrealistic as factors confound both groups and both treatment regimens often rely on one another.

SPECIAL CONSIDERATIONS

Aspirin-sensitive Patients

In 1922, the term 'aspirin triad' describing patients with aspirin sensitivity, nasal polyposis and asthma was described by Widal et al[62] and later popularized by Samter and Beers.[63] Since then a much more detailed understanding of the pathophysiology as detailed earlier has led to desensitization of these patients to control their asthma and polyp disease.

Polyps in aspirin-sensitive patients are generally viewed as more recalcitrant to both medical and surgical therapy. The abnormal regulation of cyclo-oxygenase pathways is critical to the high rate of polyp recurrence among these patients. It appears that aspirin-sensitive patients experience depressed formation of PGE_2

compared to controls which causes enhanced 5-lipoxygenase activity.[64] Reduction in PGE_2 eliminates its modulating effect on mast cells and the 5-lipo-oxygenase pathway. The overproduction of cysLTs results in bronchoconstriction and mucosal inflammation in aspirin-sensitive patients causing airway edema and secretions. PGE_2, which also has an anti-inflammatory effect on the activation and chemotaxis of eosinophils, is significantly decreased in aspirin-sensitive patients as compared to polyps in aspirin-tolerant patients.[65] The management of aspirin-sensitive patients therefore must include aspirin desensitization to disrupt the inflammatory cascade resulting in marked improvement of chronic sinus symptoms among these patients.

Donald Stevenson's group at The Scripps Clinic in La Jolla has developed protocols of inducing aspirin tolerance in these patients through desensitization. Once aspirin tolerance is induced in these patients, aspirin challenge still results in elevated leukotrienes but the response appears mitigated when compared to their original reactivity.[64] If aspirin is discontinued, aspirin sensitivity re-establishes within 48 to 96 hours therefore lifelong therapy is required. It is recommended that aspirin-sensitive patients have sinus surgery first followed by desensitization within several weeks as this decreases the bulk of tissue required to respond.

The protocol involves progressively increasing oral aspirin doses in a monitored setting until 450–600 mg of aspirin is tolerated.[66] Once this is done, daily aspirin is administered with doses ranging up to 650 mg bid. Nasal responsiveness appears better than bronchial, and polyp recurrence in these patients has been shown to be delayed an average of 6 years. These patients also experience a significant reduction in the need for both systemic and topical steroids and there is a concomitant decrease in sinus infections per year.

Currently aspirin desensitization is recommended for:
• Asthmatics unresponsive to medical therapy or requiring high systemic corticosteroid doses.
• Severe polyp patients who have required repeated sinus surgery.

Other investigators have also corroborated the beneficial results in chronic hyperplastic rhinosinusitis. Gosepath et al noted that an even lower dose of aspirin at 100 mg may work as well as higher doses.[67] Typical side effects during aspirin desensitization include bronchospasm and nasal-ocular symptoms both of which are readily controllable.[68] The asthma should be fully controlled prior to initiating desensitization as the most critical day is the first day where bronchospasm may occur.[66] Desensitization thus can be considered a critical component of mucosal disease control among these patients with minimal demerits.

Aspirin-sensitive patients deserve special attention with regard to surgical outcomes. Mc Fadden et al were one of the first to compare 'conservative' (simple ethmoidectomy) versus 'radical' (Caldwell Luc/trans-sphenoethmoidectomy) surgery in aspirin triad patients.[69] He noted that none of the 9 patients undergoing the more radical procedure had recurrence while 6 of 16 patients undergoing conservative therapy required revision. This retrospective study however did not control for disease severity. Other studies attest beneficial surgical outcomes among aspirin-sensitive patients.[70,71] When extirpative surgery is combined with desensitisation protocols, patients can experience prolonged disease-free sinus and asthma intervals. Long-term outcomes have shown that over 80% of patients will show improvement in nasal symptom score and asthma severity.[66] Usually, surgery required in aspirin-sensitive polyposis is more extensive in nature than in general polyp patients and postoperative systemic steroids may be needed to maintain patient's improvement prior to desensitization (Fig. 13.10).

Allergic Fungal Sinusitis

Since Millar's initial description, allergic fungal sinusitis (AFS) is recognized as a well-defined entity.[72] Diagnostic criteria has been proposed by Bent and Kuhn[73] to include:
- Nasal polyposis
- Atopy by skin or serological testing

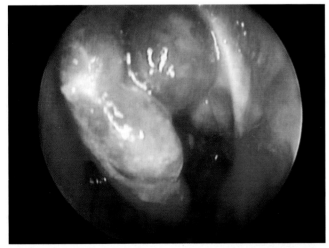

Fig. 13.10: Aspirin-sensitive patient within 3 months after endoscopic sinus surgery revealing recidivism with polyps occluding the ostiomeatal complex

- Characteristic CT scan features
- Histologic allergic mucin
- Non-invasive fungal hyphae.

Because fungus can be detected in high percentages of chronic sinus patients in the absence of allergic response,[74] the diagnosis of AFS should only be made in the presence of all criteria. Again the eosinophil occupies centerstage in the inflammatory response but most studies also implicate an IgE type I hypersensitivity response.[75] The presence of fungus in the nose does not necessarily lead to the diagnosis of AFS as many fungi can be saprophytic colonizers without eliciting an exaggerated inflammatory response. Treatment in these cases is not only directed at the polyps but must remove inflammation-producing fungal debris. Additionally, allergen specific immunotherapy, topical and systemic steroids, antihistamines, and anti-leukotrienes may all need to be used to prevent recurrence. The role of following serum IgE titres as a marker of recurrence has not been clearly established. Since fungi are frequently present in the sinuses and are difficult to eradicate in AFS, it is no surprise that this disease has high rates of recurrence.

Cystic Fibrosis

NP in children is an unusual occurrence and should raise the suspicion of the diagnosis of cystic fibrosis (CF). When polyps are noted in non-CF patients, over three-fourths of patients have associated asthma symptoms. Asthma symptoms may often be improved after surgical intervention. Surgery also significantly improves symptoms of nasal obstruction, rhinorrhea, and halitosis. Unlike non-CF patients, NP in CF tends to have high rates of recurrent symptoms despite aggressive surgical intervention.[76] Stammberger has noted that the term 'recurrence' is not entirely accurate as the widespread inflammatory process never really stops. These patients cannot only achieve excellent control of NP but also improvement in quality of life.[77] Maintenance therapy with saline rinses and nebulized antibiotics are often needed to decrease the viscosity of secretions. Higher rates of lower respiratory tract colonization with *Pseudomonas* have been associated with the presence of nasal polyps in CF patients but this has not necessarily lead to increased morbidity.[78, 79] Management of this organism, due its resistance profile and the lack of effective oral antibiotics, often relies on nebulized aminoglycosides for symptomatic improvement. Overall, CF remains a challenging chronic disease but substantial improvement in quality of life can be obtained by surgery and frequent sinus hygiene.

Antrochoanal Polyp

These polyps are solitary, unilateral polyps not associated with an allergic predisposition. They begin as a mucus retention cyst within the maxillary sinus expanding the natural ostium overtime frequently extending down the nasopharynx. Histologically, these polyps have a cystic intramaxillary portion and a solid extramaxillary portion.[80] Treatment is exclusively surgical as these polyps have few inflammatory cells and therefore do not respond well to corticosteroids. They tend to recur if not removed completely including their underlying mucosa; therefore, Caldwell-Luc approaches may be needed in anterior-based polyps to prevent recurrence.

ACKNOWLEDGMENTS

I would like to thank Andrew Murr, MD for his assistance with clinical photographs and Christopher Hall, MD for his assistance with microscopic photography.

REFERENCES

1. Radenne F, Lamblin C, Vandezande L, Tillie-Leblond I, Darras J, Tonnel A, et al. The quality of life in nasal polyposis. *J All Clin Immunol* 1999; 103:79–84.
2. Yonge ES. The determining cause of nasal polyps. 1907; *Br Med J* 2:964–969.
3. Bateman N, Fahy C, Woolford T. Nasal polyps: Still more questions than answers. *J Laryngol* 2003; 117:1–9.
4. Settipane G. Nasal polyps: Epidemiology, pathology, immunology and treatment. *Am J Rhinol* 1987; 1:119–126.
5. Mygind N, Dahl R, Bachert C. Nasal polyposis, eosinophil dominated inflammation, and allergy. *Thorax* 2000; 55 (Suppl 2): S79–S83.
6. Larsen P, Tos M. The estimated incidence of symptomatic nasal polyps. *Acta Otolaryngol* 2002; 122:179–182.
7. Slavin R. Sinusitis in adults and its relation to allergic rhinitis, asthma and nasal polyps. *J All Clin Immunol* 1988; 82:950–956.
8. Stammberger H. Examination and endoscopy of the nose and paranasal sinuses. In *Nasal polyposis: an inflammatory disease and its treatment,* N Mygind, T Lindholt. Copenhagen (Eds): Munksgaard, 1997; 120–136.
9. Settipane G, Chaffe F. Nasal polyps in asthma and rhinitis: A review of 6037 patients. *J All Clin Immunol* 1976; 59:17–21.
10. Tripathi A, Conley D, Grammer L, Ditto A, Lowery M, Seiberling K et al. Immunoglobulin E to Staphylococcal and Streptococcal toxins in patients with chronic sinusitis/nasal polyposis. *Laryngoscope* 2004; 114:1822–1826.
11. Asero R, Botazzi G. Hypersensitivity to molds in patients with nasal polyposis: A clinical study. *J Allergy Clin Immunol* 2000; 105:186–188.
12. Steinke J, Bradley D, Arango P, Crouse C, Frierson H, Kountakis S et al. Cysteinyl leukotriene expression in chronic hyperplastic sinusitis–nasal polyposis: Importance to eosinophilia and asthma. *J Allergy Clin Immunol* 2003; 111: 342–349.
13. Shin S, Lee S, Jeong H, Kita H. The effect of nasal polyp epithelial cells on eosionophil activation. *Laryngoscope* 2003; 113:1374–1377.
14. Harlin S, Ansel D, Lane S, Myers J, Kephart G, Gleich G. A clinical and pathologic study of chronic sinusitis: The role of the eosionophil. *J Allergy Clin Immunol* 1988; 1:867–875.
15. Rudack C, Prehm P, Stoll W, Maune S. Extracellular matrix components in nasal polyposis. *Acta Otolaryngol* 2003; 123: 643–647.
16. Bachert C. Comparison between polyp tissue, diseased sinus mucosa and normal tissue. In *Nasal polyposis: An inflammatory disease and its treatment,* Mygind N, Lildholdt T Copenhagen (Eds) Munksgaard, 1997; 78–87.
17. Drake-Lee A, McLauhlin P. Clinical symptoms, free histamine and IgE in nasal polyps. *Int Arch Allergy Appl Immunol* 1982; 69:268–271.
18. Mygind N. Advances in the medical treatment of nasal polyps. *Allergy* 1999; 54:12–16.
19. Stammberger H. *FESS.* Philadelphia: BC Decker, 1991; 204.
20. Larsen P, Tos M. Origin of nasal polyps: An endoscopic autopsy study. *Laryngoscope* 2004; 114:710–719.
21. Stammberger H. Surgical treatment of nasal polyps: Past, present and future. *Allergy* 1999; 54:S7–S11.
22. Bikhazi N. Contemporary management of nasal polyps. *Otolaryngol Clin North Am* 2004; 37:327–337.
23. Vento S, Ertama L, Hytönen M, Wolff C, Malmberg C. Nasal polyposis: Clinical course during 20 years. *Ann Allergy Asthma Immunol* 2000; 85:209–214.
24. Bonfils P, Avan P. Non-specific bronchial hyperresponsiveness is a risk factor for steroid insensitivity in nasal polyposis. *Acta Otolaryngol* 2004; 124:290–296.
25. Dinis P, Gomes A. Sinusitis and asthma: How do they interrelate in sinus surgery? *Am J Rhinol* 1997; 11:421–428.
26. Mygind N, Lildholt T. Medical management. In *Nasal polyps: Epidemiology, pathogenesis, and treatment,* Settipane G, Lund V, Bernstein J, Tos M. Rhode Island (Eds) Oceanside Publications, 1997; 147–155.
27. Lildholt T, Dahl R, Mygind N. Effect of corticosteroids. Evidence from controlled trials. In *Nasal polyposis: An inflammatory disease and its treatment,* Mygind N, Lildholdt T. Copenhagen (Eds) Munksgaard, 1997; 160–169.
28. Van Camp P, Clement P. Results of oral steroid treatment in nasal polyposis. *Rhinology* 1994; 32(1):5–9.
29. Heden Blomqvist E, Lundblad L, Anggard A, Haraldsson P, Stjarne P. A randomized controlled study evaluating medical treatment versus surgical treatment in addition to medical treatment of nasal polyposis. *J Allergy Clin Immunol* 2001; 107(2):224–228.
30. Nores JM, Avan P, Bonfils P. Medical management of nasal polyposis: A study in a series of 152 consecutive patients. *Rhinology* 2003; 41(2):97–102.
31. Holmstrom M, Holmberg K, Lundblad L, Norlander T, Stierna P. Current perspectives on the treatment of nasal polyposis: A Swedish opinion report. *Acta Otolaryngol* 2002; 122(7):736–744.
32. Bernstein JM. Nasal polyps: Finding the cause, determining treatment. *J Respir Dis* 1997; 18:847–856.

33. Bonfils P, Nores JM, Halimi P, Avan P. Corticosteroid treatment in nasal polyposis with a three-year follow-up period. *Laryngoscope* 2003; 113(4):683–687.

34. Virolainen E, Puhakka H. The effect of intranasal beclomethasone dipropionate on the recurrence of nasal polyps after ethmoidectomy. *Rhinology* 1980; 18(1):9–18.

35. Karlsson G, Rundcrantz H. A randomized trial of intranasal beclomethasone dipropionate after polypectomy. *Rhinology* 1982; 20(3):144–148.

36. Weber R, Keerl R, Radziwill R, Schick B, Jaspersen D, Dshambazov K et al. Videoendoscopic analysis of nasal steroid distribution. *Rhinology* 1999; 37(2):69–73.

37. Johansson L, Holmberg K, Melen I, Stierna P, Bende M. Sensitivity of a new grading system for studying nasal polyps with the potential to detect early changes in polyp size after treatment with a topical corticosteroid (budesonide). *Acta Otolaryngol* 2002; 122(1):49–53.

38. Agertoft L, Pedersen S. Short-term lower leg growth rate in children with rhinitis treated with intranasal mometasone furoate and budesonide. *J Allergy Clin Immunol* 1999; 104(5):948–952.

39. Schenkel E, Skoner D, Bronsky E, Miller S, Pearlman D, Rooklin A et al. Absence of growth retardation in children with perennial allergic rhinitis after one year of treatment with mometasone furoate aqueous nasal spray. *Pediatrics* 2000; 105(2):E22.

40. Desrosiers M, Salas-Prato M. Treatment of chronic rhinosinusitis refractory to other treatments with topical antibiotic therapy delivered by means of a large-particle nebulizer: Results of a controlled trial. *Otolaryngol Head Neck Surg* 2001; 125(3):265–269.

41. Vaughan W, Carvalho G. Use of nebulized antibiotics for acute infections in chronic sinusitis. *Otolaryngol Head Neck Surg* 2002; 127(6):558–568.

42. Iino Y, Sasaki Y, Kojima C, Miyazawa T. Effect of macrolides on the expression of HLA-DR and costimulatory molecules on antigen-presenting cells in nasal polyps. *Ann Otol Rhinol Laryngol* 2001; 110:457–463.

43. Nonaka M, Pawankar R, Saji F, Yagi T. Effect of roxithromycin on IL-8 synthesis and proliferation of nasal polyp fibroblasts. *Acta Otolaryngol Suppl* 1998; 539:71–75.

44. Ichimura K, Shimazaki Y, Ishibashi T, Higo R. Effect of new macrolide roxithromycin upon nasal polyps associated with chronic sinusitis. *Auris Nasus Larynx* 1996; 23:48–56.

45. Cervin A. The anti-inflammatory effect of erythromycin and its derivatives, with special reference to nasal polyposis and chronic sinusitis. *Acta Otolaryngol* 2001; 121(1):83–92.

46. Ricchetti A, Landis BN, Maffioli A, Giger R, Zeng C, Lacroix JS. Effect of anti-fungal nasal lavage with amphotericin B on nasal polyposis. *J Laryngol Otol* 2002; 116(4):261–263.

47. Mabry R, Mabry C. Allergic fungal sinusitis: The role of immunotherapy. *Otolaryngol Clin North Am* 2000; 33:433–440.

48. Ponikau J, Sherris D, Kern E, Homburger H, Frigas E, Gaffey T et al. The diagnosis and incidence of allergic fungal sinusitis. *Mayo Clin Proc* 1999; 74(9):877–884.

49. Ulualp S, Sterman B, Toohill R. Antileukotriene therapy for the relief of sinus symptoms in aspirin triad disease. *Ear Nose Throat J* 1999; 78(8):604–606, 608, 613, passim.

50. Parnes S, Chuma A. Acute effects of antileukotrienes on sinonasal polyposis and sinusitis. *Ear Nose Throat J* 2000; 79(1):18–20, 24–25.

51. Lacroix J, Buvelot J, Polla B, Lundberg J. Improvement of symptoms of non-allergic chronic rhinitis by local treatment with capsaicin. *Clin Exp Allergy* 1991; 21(5):595–600.

52. Zheng C, Wang Z, Lacroix J. Effect of intranasal treatment with capsaicin on polyp recurrence after polypectomy and ethmoidectomy *Lin Chuang Er Bi Yan Hou Ke Za Zhi* 2000; 14(8):344–346.

53. Haye R, Aanesen J, Burtin B, Donnelly F, Duby C. The effect of cetirizine on symptoms and signs of nasal polyposis. *J Laryngol Otol* 1998; 112(11):1042–1046.

54. Bruzzese N, Sica G, Iacopino F, Paludetti G, Schiavino D, Nucera E et al. Growth inhibition of fibroblasts from nasal polyps and normal skin by lysine acetylsalicylate. *Allergy* 1998; 53(4):431–434.

55. Nucera E, Schiavino D, Milani A, Del Ninno M, Misuraca C, Buonomo A et al. Effects of lysine–acetylsalicylate (LAS) treatment in nasal polyposis: Two controlled long-term prospective follow-up studies. *Thorax* 2000; 55 (Suppl 2): S75–S78.

56. Passali D, Bernstein JM, Passali FM, Damiani V, Passali GC, Bellussi L. Treatment of recurrent chronic hyperplastic sinusitis with nasal polyposis. *Arch Otolaryngol Head Neck Surg* 2003; 129(6):656–659.

57. Lildholdt T. Position statement on nasal polyps. *Rhinology* 1994; 32:126.

58. Weber R, Draf W, Keerl R, Schick B, Saha A. Endonasal microendoscopic pansinus operation in chronic sinusitis. II. Results and complications. *Am J Otolaryngol* 1997; (4):247–253.

59. Senior BA, Kennedy DW, Tanabodee J, Kroger H, Hassab M, Lanza DC. Long-term impact of functional endoscopic sinus surgery on asthma. *Otolaryngol Head Neck Surg* 1999; 121(1): 66–68.

60. Dufour X, Bedier A, Ferrie J, Gohler C, Klossek J. Diffuse nasal polyposis and endoscopic sinus surgery: Long-term results, a 65-case study. *Laryngoscope* 2004; 114:1982–1987.

61. Deal T, Kountakis S. Significance of nasal polyps in chronic rhinosinusitis: Symptoms and surgical outcomes. *Laryngoscope* 2004; 114:1932–1935.

62. Widal M, Abrami P, Lenmoyez J. Anaphylaxie et idiosyncrasie. *Presse Med* 1922; 30:189–192.

63. Samter M, Beers R. Intolerance to aspirin. Clinical studies and consideration of its pathogenesis. *Ann Intern Med* 1968; 68: 975–983.

64. Szczeklik A, Stevenson D. Aspirin-induced asthma in pathogenesis and management. *J Allergy Clin Immunol* 1999; 104: 5–13.

65. Mullol J, Fernandez-Morata J, Roca-Ferrer J, Pujols L, Xaubet A, Benitez P. Cyclooxygenase 1 and cyclooxygenase 2 expression is abnormally regulated in human nasal polyps. *J All Clin Immunol* 2002; 109:824–830.

66. Stevenson D, Hankammer M, Mathison D, Christiansen S, Simon R. Aspirin desensitization treatment of aspirin-sensitive patients with rhinosinusitis–asthma: long-term outcomes. *J Allergy Clin Immunol* 1996; 98:751–758.

67. Gosepath J, Schaefer D, Amedee RG, Mann W. Individual monitoring of aspirin desensitization. *Arch Otolaryngol Head Neck Surg* 2001; 127(3):316–321.

68. Mardiney M, Borish L. Aspirin desensitization for chronic hyperplastic sinusitis, nasal polyposis, and asthma triad. *Arch Otolaryngol Head Neck Surg* 2001; 127:1287.

69. McFadden E, Kany RJ, Fink J, Toohill R. Surgery for sinusitis and aspirin triad. *Laryngoscope* 1990; 100:1043–1046.

70. Nakamura H, Kawasaki M, Higuchi Y, Takahashi S. Effects of sinus surgery on asthma in aspirin triad patients. *Acta Otolaryngol* 1999; 119(5):592–598.

71. Uri N, Cohen-Kerem R, Barzilai G, Greenberg E, Doweck I, Weiler-Ravell D. Functional endoscopic sinus surgery in the treatment of massive polyposis in asthmatic patients. *J Laryngol Otol* 2002; 116:185–189.

72. Millar J, Johnston A, Lamb D. Allergic aspergillosis of the maxillary sinuses. *Thorax* 1981; 36:710.

73. Bent J III, Kuhn F. Diagnosis of allergic fungal sinusitis *Otolaryngol Head Neck Surg* 1994; 111:580–588.

74. Ponikau J, Sherris D, Kern E, Homburger H, Frigas E, Gaffey T et al. The diagnosis and incidence of allergic fungal sinusitis. *Mayo Clin Proc* 1999; 74:877–884.

75. Stewart A, Hunsaker D. Fungus-specific IgG and IgE in allergic fungal rhinosinusitis. *Otolaryngol Head Neck Surg* 2002; 127:324–332.

76. Triglia J, Nicollas R. Nasal and sinus polyposis in children. *Laryngoscope* 1997; 107:963–966.

77. Nishioka G, Barbero G, König O, Parsons D, Cook P, Davis W et al. Symptom outcome after functional endoscopic sinus surgery in patients with cystic fibrosis: A prospective study. *Otolaryngol Head Neck Surg* 1995; 113:440–445.

78. Henriksson G, Westrin KM, Karpati F, Wikstrom AC, Stierna P, Hjelte L. Nasal polyps in cystic fibrosis: Clinical endoscopic study with nasal lavage fluid analysis. *Chest* 2002; 121:40–47.

79. Kingdom T, Lee K, FitzSimmons S, Cropp G. Clinical characteristics and genotype analysis of patients with cystic fibrosis and nasal polyposis requiring surgery. *Arch Otolaryngol Head Neck Surg* 1996; 122:1209–1213.

80. Maldonado M, Martinez A, Alobid I, Mullol J. The antrochoanal polyp. *Rhinology* 2004; 42:178–182.

CHAPTER 14

Transsphenoidal Approaches to the Sella Turcica

Jeffrey G Neal, David J Osguthorpe, Rodney J Schlosser

Surgical access to the sella turcica is applied most commonly for pituitary adenomas. It can be accomplished by several different approaches that have evolved with innovations in surgical techniques and advances in instrumentation. Historically, Schloffer performed the first successful removal of a pituitary tumor in 1907 using an extracranial transsphenoidal approach.[1] In 1909, Hirsh pioneered the modified endonasal approach to the sella using the Killian submucosal resection of the septum and preserving intact intranasal mucosal flaps.[2] Halstead modified the technique by placing an incision in the gingivolabial sulcus.[3] In 1910, Harvey Cushing combined the submucosal resection of Hirsh with the sublabial incision of Halstead and thereby eliminated external incisions.[4] Cushing was credited with standardizing the sublabial transsphenoidal approach, which he used in 247 cases of pituitary tumors over a 20-year period. However by 1929 Cushing had reverted back to using the intracranial approach initially described by Frazier in 1912, as he had perceived a higher rate of recurrence and the occasional discovery of other kinds of lesions around the sella turcica such as meningiomas or craniopharyngiomas.

In the 1960s, Hardy reintroduced the sublabial transsphenoidal approach.[5] He advanced the technique by combining the use of binocular operating microscopes for a microsurgical dissection, and intraoperative radiofluoroscopy for orientation. The direct magnified view of the operation allowed complete tumor removal in the majority of the cases and overcame some of the previous major criticisms. The sublabial transsphenoidal approach has since remained the standard approach to pituitary tumors because it is perceived to be the most convenient and practical for neurosurgeons.

Over the last decade, due to postoperative complications of the sublabial approach including upper lip and incisor paresthesias, a complete transnasal approach has been developed. In this approach, a hemitransfixion or Killian incision is made in the nostril and the entire procedure is performed through one nostril, which with concomitant septal translocation usually allows the insertion of the regular transsphenoidal retractor. Although the transnasal approach signifies a major improvement in technique, it may occasionally be associated with postoperative complications including septal perforation and scarring. In addition, this approach requires that the nose be packed for several days because of the extensive submucosal septal dissection.[6-9]

In 1985, Kennedy first introduced the endoscopic transsphenoidal approach to remove pituitary lesions.[10] Advances in endoscopic sinus surgery and improvements in endoscopic instrumentation over the past two decades have allowed the implementation of endoscopy into the approach to the sella. While endoscopic procedures were first performed using the traditional sublabial and transseptal dissection routes, surgeons are now able to use a completely endoscopic approach that allows them to bypass the transseptal dissection.[11-17] Using this technique, both the endoscope and endoscopic instruments can be passed through one or both nostrils. The endoscopic approach has several advantages over the more traditional approaches in that it minimizes mucosa trauma, and does not require sellar reconstruction, sphenoid obliteration or usually postoperative nasal packings if there is no intraoperative CSF leak. All three approaches are described in this chapter.

SURGICAL APPROACHES

Sublabial Transsphenoidal Approach

Oxymetazoline or 5% cocaine soaked cottonoid pledgets are initially used to pack the nostrils, using a nasal speculum, bayonet forceps, and a headlight. The pledgets are allowed to remain in contact with the nasal mucosa for 5–10 minutes, and the nose and face are prepared with an aqueous antiseptic solution (SUR-CLEANS™). Using a 26-guage needle and making a conscious effort to dissect the nasal mucoperichondrium away from the cartilaginous septum, approximately 2–4 ml of 1% lidocaine with 1:100,000 epinephrine is injected submucoperichondrially along the side of nasal septum and floor of the nose on which the flap elevation is planned. Approximately 6 ml is then infiltrated along the upper gingivolabial sulcus to facilitate the subsequent elevation of soft tissues off the maxilla and to diminish bleeding.

The patient is then positioned in a supine or a semi-sitting position, with the head on a horseshoe headrest (as in all transfacial approaches to the sella, the oropharynx can be packed with moist sponges to help prevent aspiration of blood). A fluoroscopy unit is then positioned so that the horizontal beam is centered on the sella turcica. A foot pedal controlled by the surgeon is used to switch the fluoroscopy unit on and off during the operation.

Traditionally, the surgical procedure begins by making a left-sided (if the surgeon is right-handed and is standing on the right-side of the patient and the septum is relatively straight) hemitransfixion incision along the caudal aspect of the cartilaginous septum. Using sharp dissection the cartilaginous septum is exposed. Retracting the columella laterally to the patient's left, a muco-perichondrial flap is elevated off the left side of the bony-cartilaginous septum and a submucoperiosteal tunnel is created just under the left maxillary crest, across which the two mucosal flaps are then connected (Fig. 14.1). This is performed using a combination of sharp and blunt dissecting techniques. The premaxilla region is then undermined in a subperiosteal plane.

Attention is turned to making an incision in the buccogingival junction while retracting the upper lip. The incision is made from one canine tooth to the other. To expose the pyriform aperture and the anterior nasal spine, mucosa is elevated off the anterior 2 cm of each side of the floor of the nose, and the septal cartilage is separated from the anterior nasal spine, maxillary crest, vomer and perpendicular plate of the ethmoid with a Cottle knife and elevator, or similar Freer instruments. The freed cartilaginous septum can then be swung easily toward the right nasal side wall (Fig. 14.2). It remains attached to the nasal dorsum and to its overlying mucoperi-chondrium on the right. A right posterior mucosal tunnel is then developed along the right side of the bony septum,

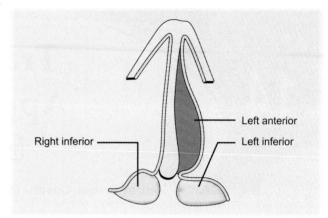

Fig. 14.1: Mucoperichondrial flaps are elevated from the left side of the septum back to bony-cartilaginous junction, forming the anterior tunnel. Elevating mucosa from the floor of the nose and then medially up to the level of the anterior tunnel forms the inferior tunnel. The left anterior and left inferior tunnels may be joined permitting wide exposure and the ability to mobilize the cartilaginous septum

so that the mucosa has now been elevated from both sides of the bony septum. The transsphenoidal retractor can then be inserted though the sublabial tunnel into the surgically formed intranasal tunnel. To prevent tears in the nasal mucosa the retractor is opened gently. Out fracture of the nasal turbinates occurs as the retractor is opened (Fig. 14.3). The vomer and perpendicular plate of the ethmoid are visualized once the retractor is in place, and much is removed with a Takahashi or similar instrument as submucosal dissection proceeds up to the face of the sphenoid sinus in the midline (20°–30° from the nasal floor, and usually 6–8 cm posterior to the anterior nasal spine), then sweeping mucosa laterally

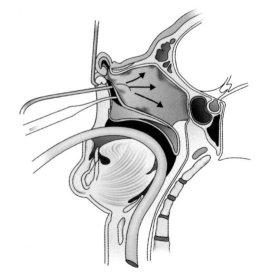

Fig. 14.2: Elevation of the mucoperichondrium from the nasal septum in the sublabial approach

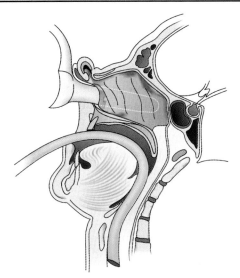

Fig. 14.3: A transsphenoidal retractor is inserted and then opened slowly to expose the anterior wall of the sphenoid sinus on both sides

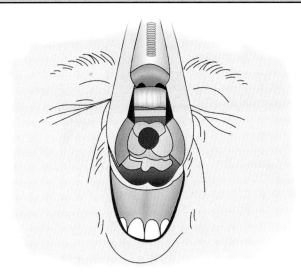

Fig. 14.5: Anterior view demonstrating direct midline path to the sella via the sublabial approach

from the central two-thirds of that sinus wall. At this point the transsphenoidal retractor is repositioned to just anterior to the face of the sphenoid. Any remaining bony septum and the anterior central face of the sphenoid are removed using cutting forceps, and small osteotomes as needed.

Fluoroscopy may be used to determine the relationship of the transsphenoidal retractor to bony landmarks and to aid in determining the pathway of surgical approach to the pituitary tumor. The operating microscope is then placed into the optimal position and the anterior face of the sella, and then the pituitary tumor, are resected under microscopic visualization by the neurosurgery service (Figs 14.4 and 14.5).

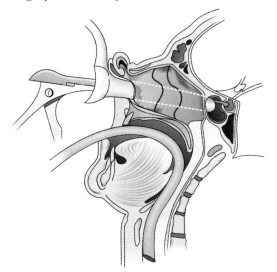

Fig. 14.4: The sella floor is removed using a small Kerrison rongeur

After the tumor has been removed by the neurosurgery service, the sella may be packed with homograft fat or muscle taken from the left lower quadrant of the abdomen if there is any evidence of a cerebrospinal fluid (CSF) leak. Using cup forceps a piece of fat is placed within the sella and secured by a piece of nasal bone or cartilage in the epidural position. A fascia lata graft may also be used to reconstruct the roof of the sella if a CSF leak occurs, and even the sphenoid sinus can be packed with muscle or fat. However, in the absence of a CSF leak the sphenoid sinus is left free of packing or foreign material.

The transsphenoidal retractor is then removed and the nasal cavity suctioned clean. Closure of the hemitransfixion incision is performed using interrupted 5-0 chromic sutures. The cartilaginous septum is repositioned on the anterior maxillary spine using a 3-0 chromic suture on a Keith needle. Bilateral nasal packs are placed in the nasal cavity. Finally, the gingivolabial incision is closed with loose, interrupted 3-0 chromic sutures. A nasal drip pad is then placed beneath the nostrils. The nasal packs are usually removed on the second postoperative day. Prophylactic antibiotics are continued until the packs are removed. Patients can generally be discharged on the third day after surgery in uncomplicated cases without CSF leak.

Transnasal Transsphenoidal Approach

The transnasal transsphenoidal approach to pituitary tumors proceeds in the same fashion as the sublabial approach except that no incision is made along the

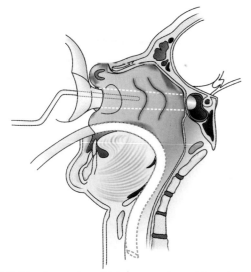

Fig. 14.6: The transsphenoidal retractor is positioned completely in the nose in the transnasal approach. This approach does not require a sublabial incision

gingivolabial sulcus (Fig. 14.6). As performed in the sublabial approach, oxymetazoline or 5% cocaine soaked cottonoid pledgets are packed in the nostrils using a nasal speculum, bayonet forceps, and a headlight. The pledgets are allowed to remain in contact with the nasal mucosa for 5–10 minutes and the nose and face are prepared with an aqueous antiseptic solution (SUR-CLEANS™). Using a 26-guage needle and making a conscious effort to dissect the nasal mucoperichondrium away from the cartilaginous septum, approximately 2–4 ml of 1% lidocaine with 1:100,000 epinephrine is injected submuco-perichondrially along the nasal septum and floor of the nose on which the flap elevation is planned.

The surgical procedure begins with a hemitransfixion incision along the caudal aspect of the cartilaginous septum. Using sharp dissection the cartilaginous septum is exposed. Retracting the columella laterally to the patient's right (if the surgeon is right-handed), a muco-perichondrial flap is elevated off the left side of the bony-cartilaginous septum and a submucoperiosteal tunnel is created just under the left maxillary crest, across which the two mucosal flaps are then connected. This is performed using a combination of sharp and blunt dissecting techniques. Using a Cottle elevator, the bony-cartilaginous junction is identified and separated in a vertical manner. Mucoperiosteal flaps are then created bilaterally from the perpendicular plane of the ethmoid bone. The dissection proceeds posteriorly until the sphenoid rostrum is visualized. The cartilaginous portion of the nasal septum is dislocated off the nasal spine and reflected to the patient's right. It remains attached to the

nasal dorsum and its overlying mucoperichondrium on the right. The transsphenoidal retractor can then be inserted into the surgically formed intranasal tunnel. The vomer and perpendicular plate of the ethmoid is visualized once the retractor is in place, and much is removed with a Takahashi or similar instrument as submucosal dissection proceeds up to the face of the sphenoid sinus in midline, and then mucosa on the central two-thirds of that anterior sinus wall is mobilized laterally. Any remaining bony septum and the anterior central face of the sphenoid are removed using cutting forceps, and small osteotomes as needed. The trans-sphenoidal retractor is then repositioned to insure optimal visualization for the neurosurgical resection of the pituitary tumor by either endoscopic or microscopic visualization.

An alternative transnasal approach if performed by gently outfracturing the inferior and middle turbinates using a Sayre instrument. This allows exposure of the superior turbinate and the posterosuperior septum. The mucosa of the posterior cartilaginous and bony septum can then be infiltrated with 1% lidocaine with 1:100,000 epinephrine. A 1.5 cm vertical line on the posterior septum 1 cm anterior to the face of the sphenoid is then cauterized using a suction monopolar cautery. The mucosa over the anterior central portion of the right side of the sphenoid can then be elevated using a combination of a sickle knife and Cottle elevators. The posterior perpendicular plate of the ethmoid and the mucosa from the anterior face of the central portion of the sphenoid can then be elevated using a transsphenoidal retractor. Again, cutting forceps and small osteotomes can then be used to remove the inferior half of the anterior sphenoid face to the intersinus septum. A small transsphenoidal retractor is then repositioned for optimal visualization for pituitary tumor removal.

As performed in the sublabial approach, if there is any evidence of a CSF leak, the sella is packed with homograft fat or muscle taken from the left lower quadrant of the abdomen. Using cup forceps a piece of fat is placed within the sella and secured by a piece of nasal bone or cartilage in the subdural position. A fascia lata graft may also be used to reconstruct the roof of the sella if a CSF leak occurs, and the sphenoid sinus may be packed with muscle or fat if necessary. In the absence of a CSF leak, the sphenoid sinus is left free of packing or foreign material.

Small nasal packs are then placed in the nasal cavity of both sides just inside the anterior face of the sphenoid along the nasal roof and medial to the middle turbinate.

A nasal drip pad is then placed beneath the nostrils. The packs are removed the day after surgery.

Endoscopic Transsphenoidal Approach

As performed in the sublabial approach and the transnasal approaches oxymetazoline or neosynephrine soaked cottonoid pledgets are initially used to pack and decongest the nasal cavities bilaterally. Greater palatine and sphenopalatine blocks are then performed by injecting 1% lidocaine with 1:100,000 epinephrine into the greater palatine foramen and the area of the sphenopalatine artery using a 26-gauge needle. The cottonoid pledgets are removed and under endoscopic visualization the middle turbinate is gently lateralized and the inferior one-third of the superior turbinate is resected (Figs 14.7 and 14.8). A large sphenoidotomy is then performed using Kerrison punches and mushroom punches. Then approximately 6–8 mm anterior to the face of the sphenoid a posterior nasal septectomy is performed. Through-cutting forceps are then used to resect the posterior nasal septum and the intersinus septum. If desired, a small transsphenoidal retractor can be inserted into the nasal cavity, once wide enough exposure is obtained by performing sphenoidotomies and the septectomy. The neurosurgeon may then position the microscope for excision of the pituitary tumor or they may hold the endoscope in one hand and resect the tumor using pituitary forceps and curettes (Fig. 14.9).

An alternative approach is for an assistant to hold the endoscope at the desired location or the endoscope can be securely fixed on a gooseneck holder in the position that provides optimal visualization, freeing the

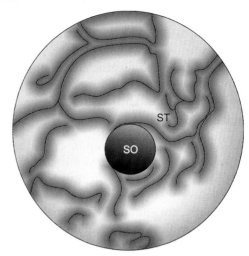

Fig. 14.8: Endoscopic view of the sphenoid ostia (SO), superior turbinate (ST) after the inferior one-third of the superior turbinate is resected and a large sphenoidotomy is then performed

neurosurgeon to resect the pituitary tumor bimanually. This approach can eliminate the need for the transsphenoidal retractor and both nostrils can be used to pass endoscopes and instruments, thus providing the ability for a three- or even four-handed technique.

Using angled endoscopes, the sella can then be inspected for CSF leaks and residual tumor. If a CSF leak occurs, a variety of materials may be used as grafts. Abdominal fat, fascia, muscle, or alloplastic materials such as cadaveric dermis, collagen substrate or fascia, have all been used successfully. We recommend that these repairs be performed at the level of the sella, and we avoid obliterating the entire sphenoid sinus due to the potential risk of mucocele formation. Fat, Gel Foam™

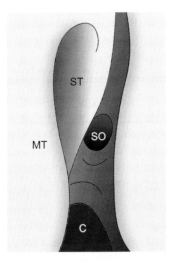

Fig. 14.7: Endoscopic view of the sphenoid ostia (SO), superior turbinate (ST), middle turbinate (MT), and choana (C)

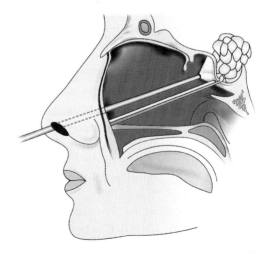

Fig. 14.9: The endoscopic approach through wide sphenoidotomies demonstrating removal of the face of the sella using a rongeur

or Surgicel™ may be used for temporary packing of the sinus, but the sphenoidotomies are intentionally left patent at the conclusion of the case. In the absence of a CSF leak, the sella is not reconstructed and nasal packing is generally not necessary with this approach.

Image-guided Surgery

As technology evolves, radiographic confirmation of surgical location may be performed with image-guided surgery (IGS), rather than fluoroscopy. These commercially available systems provide three-dimensional information to the surgeon and additional feedback as to the location of calibrated surgical instruments during the surgical procedures. It is important to note that intracranial anatomy shifts after entering the sella and removing tumor. Thus, image-guided surgery based on preoperative images is unreliable, except for bony landmarks before such are surgically disrupted. At our institution we typically do not use radiographic confirmation or IGS except in cases with extremely unusual anatomy.

Complications

Numerous complications may occur with the traditional sublabial approach including numbness of the maxillary dentition, loss of nasal tip projection, septal perforations or deviations and other nasal deformities.[12,13] In their review of 114 cases, Kennedy et al reported that sinusitis was the most common complication (15%) of the sublabial transsphenoidal approach.[18] CSF leaks occurred in 9.6% of cases. Septal perforations occurred in 7% and paresthesia of the upper lip in 5.3% of cases. Other less frequently encountered complications in their study included anosmia, meningitis, temporary diplopia, and temporal lobe epilepsy. Two operative mortalities were noted in their series. In a review of 267 cases by Eisele et al., 38% of the cases had either major or minor complications.[19] Major complications were noted in 6.7% of procedures and included 13 CSF leaks, 1 operative mortality, 2 visual losses, 1 epistaxis and sublabial hemorrhage. The most common minor complications included temporary numbness of the upper lip and/or incisor teeth (21.7%), septal peforations (7.1%), and intranasal synechiae (3.1%).

While fewer complications are encountered with the transnasal approach, they are similar to sublabial approach except that the transnasal approach avoids the sublabial incision and the subsequent upper lip and incisor paresthesias.[13] Since the transnasal approach also incorporates the use of a nasal speculum and mucosal dissections, septal perforations and intranasal synechiae continue to be common complications.

Several studies have shown the advantages of the endoscopic approach including quicker recovery, fewer cosmetic, dental and nasal complications when compared to the sublabial approach.[16,20–22] In their review of 180 cases of endoscopic transnasal pituitary surgery, Nasseri et al reported that their complication rate was equivalent to the rate reported for the transnasal approach.[21] Only 6 delayed CSF leaks (4.4%) and 12 intraoperative CSF (6.6%) were reported. One patient developed community-acquired pneumococcal meningitis and had a cerebrovascular accident complicated by hydrocephalus requiring a ventriculoperitoneal shunt. Minor complications included alar abrasions in 4 patients; epistaxis requiring packing in 2 patients; headache in 3 patients; and new onset of nasal congestion and rhinosinusitis in 2 patients.

CONCLUSION

The sublabial approach is the historic standard to which all other transnasal sellar approaches must be compared. Recent studies at our institution and others have demonstrated that strictly transnasal and endoscopic approaches as described in this chapter demonstrate a decreasing trend in all complications.[16,20–22] This trend was evident in fewer CSF leaks, fewer lumbar drains, shorter hospitalizations, and less nasal packing. Our recurrence rates were similar across all 3 groups (0–10%), but there has been relatively short-term follow-up regarding adenoma recurrence with the transnasal or endoscopic approaches,[22] so we anticipate some resistance in the general neurosurgical community until comparable adenoma eradication rates can be documented, and neurosurgical trainees gain experience with handling an endoscope.

Endoscopy does decrease the need for nasal packing, allows for shorter operative times, and hospital stays.[22–26] The adjunctive use of the IGS may increase patient safety during the management of tumors with unusual anatomy and is now allowing some surgeons to push the envelope in the approach for repair or resection of parasellar pathology such as lesions of the cavernous sinus, optic chiasm, and petrous apex.[27]

REFERENCES

1. Sonnenburg RE, White D, Ewend MG, Senior B. Sellar reconstruction: Is it necessary? *Am J Rhinol* 2003; 17:343–346.
2. Hirsch O. Symptoms and treatment of pituitary tumors. *Arch Otolaryngol* 1952; 55:268–306.

3. Halstead AE. Remarks on the operative treatment of tumors of the hypophysis. *Surg Gynecol Obstet* 1910; 10:494–502.

4. Henderson WR. The pituitary adenomata: A follow-up study of the surgical results in 338 cases (Dr. Cushing's series). *Br J Surg* 1939; 26:811–921.

5. Hardy J. Transsphenoidal hypophysectomy. *J Neurosurg* 1971; 33:582–594.

6. Griffith H, Veerapen R. A direct transnasal approach to the sphenoid sinus. *J Neurosurg* 1987; 66:140–142.

7. Cooke R. Experience with direct transnasal transphenoidal approach to the pituitary the pituitary fossa. *Br J Neurosurg* 1994; 8:193–196.

8. Jankowski R, Auque J, Simon C, et al. Endoscopic pituitary tumor surgery. *Laryngoscope* 1992; 102:198–202.

9. Yaniv E, Rappaport ZH. Endoscopic transseptal trans-sphenoidal surgery for pituitary tumors. *Neurosurg* 1997; 40:944–946.

10. Kenndy DW. Functional endoscopic sinus surgery technique. *Arch Otolaryngol* 1985;111:643–649.

11. Jarrahy R, Berci G, Shahinian HK. Assessment of the efficacy of endoscopy in pituitary adenoma resection. *Arch Otolaryngol Head Neck Surg* 2000; 126:1487–1490.

12. Jho HD, Carrau RL, Ko Y et al. Endoscopic pituitary surgery: An early experience. *Surg Neurol* 1997; 47:213–223.

13. Sheehan MT, Atkinson JL, Kasperbauer JL, Erickson BJ, Nippoldt TB. Preliminary comparison of the endoscopic transnasal vs the sublabial transseptal approach for clinically nonfunctioning pituitary macroadenomas. *Mayo Clin Proc* 1999; 74:661–670.

14. Badie B, Nguyen P, Preston JK. Endoscopic-guided direct endonasal approach for pituitary surgery. *Surg Neurol* 2000; 53: 168–173.

15. Jho HD, Carrau RL. Endoscopy assisted transsphenoidal surgery for pituitary adenoma. *Acta Neurochir (Wien)* 1996; 138:1416–1425.

16. Jho HD, Alfieri A. Endoscopic endonasal pituitary surgery: Evolution of surgical technique and equipment in 150 operations. *Minim Invasive Neurosurg* 2001; 44:1–12.

17. Moreland DB, Diaz-Ordaz E, Czajka GA. Endoscopic endonasal hemisphenoidotomy for resection of pituitary lesions confined to the sella: Report of 3 cases and technical note. *Minim Invasive Neurosurg* 2000; 43:57–61.

18. Kennedy DW, Cohn ES, Papel ID, Holliday MJ. Trans-sphenoidal approach to the sella: The Johns Hopkins experience. *Laryngoscope* 1984; 94:1066–1074.

19. Eisele DW, Flint PW, Janas JD, Kelly WA, Weymuller EA, Cummings CW. The sublabial transseptal transsphenoidal approach to the sellar and parasellar lesions. *Laryngoscope* 1988; 98:1301–1308.

20. Jho HD, Carrau RL. Endoscopic endonasal transsphenoidal surgery: Experience with 50 patients. *J Neurosurg* 1997; 87: 44–51.

21. Nasseri SS, Kasperbauer JL, Strome SE, McCaffrey TV, Atkinson JL, Meyer FB. Endoscopic transnasal pituitary surgery: Report on 180 cases. *Am J Rhinol* 2001; 15:281–287.

22. Adams CT, Burke CW. Current modes of treatment of pituitary tumours. *Br J Neurosurg* 1993; 7:123–128.

23. Neal JG, Patel SJ, Kulbersh JS, Osguthorpe JD, Schlosser RJ. Comparison of techniques for transsphenoidal pituitary surgery. *Am J Radiol* (Submitted).

24. Heilman CB, Shucart WA, Rebeiz EE. Endoscopic sphe-noidotomy approach to the sella. *Neurosurg* 1997; 41:602–607.

25. Rodziewicz GS, Kelley RT, Kellman RM, Smith MV. Trans-nasal endoscopic surgery of the pituitary gland: Technical note. *Neurosurg* 1996; 39:189–192.

26. Spencer WR, Das K, Nwagu C, Wenk E, Schaefer SD, Moscatello A, Couldwell WT. Approaches to the sellar and parasellar region: Anatomic comparison of the microscope versus endoscope. *Laryngoscope* 1999; 109:791–794.

27. Sethi DS, Pillay PK. Endoscopic management of lesions of the sella turcica. *J Laryngol Otol* 1995; 109:956–962.

Cerebrospinal Fluid Leak

Robert E Sonnenburg Jr, Brent A Sr

The leakage of cerebrospinal fluid (CSF) into the nose has been a topic of interest to physicians for centuries. In the second century AD Galen proposed that cerebrospinal fluid periodically purged by way of the pituitary and ethmoid regions into the nose. The idea that a free communication existed between the nose and brain continued until the seventeenth century.[1] Anterior skull base CSF fistulas were originally described in the literature by Willis in 1682 and later demonstrated at autopsy by Miller in 1826.[2] St. Clair Thompson reported the first series of cases in 1899 describing 20 patients.[3] More than 200 years after the initial description in the literature, Dandy reported the first surgical repair of a CSF fistula using a frontal craniotomy approach in 1926.[4] In an attempt to avoid the morbidity of a craniotomy, Dohlman described an extracranial approach using a naso-orbital incision in 1948.[5] Overtime less invasive approaches were developed. Hirsch, a pioneer in transnasal transseptal pituitary surgery wrote about repairing sphenoid sinus CSF fistulas transnasally in 1952.[6] Vrabec and Hallberg reported on an intranasal approach to cribriform plate CSF fistulas that included a submucous resection of the nasal septum and advancement flap from nearby turbinate in 1964.[7] The era of endoscopic management was ushered in with Wigand's 1981 description of endoscopic closure of a CSF fistula.[8] Since that time several authors have reported series on the endoscopic management of these lesions. Given the high success and low complication rates of endoscopic repair, otolaryngologists are increasingly being called upon to manage these complex cases.

The purpose of this chapter is to provide a broad overview of the management of anterior skull base CSF fistulas. Normal CSF physiology and composition will be discussed followed by the etiology and pathophysiology of CSF fistulas. Endoscopic, laboratory, and radiographic diagnostic tools for establishing the presence and location are reviewed. Finally, treatment plans are reviewed with attention to etiology, technique, graft materials, prophylactic antibiotics, lumbar drain usage, location, and outcomes.

NORMAL PHYSIOLOGY

Contugno first described cerebrospinal fluid in relation to the anatomy of the CSF system approximately 250 years ago. Subsequently, CSF production, flow, and resorption have been extensively studied. Most CSF is produced by the choroid plexuses that are located within the lateral, third, and fourth ventricles. A smaller contribution of CSF production is thought to arise from capillary ultrafiltrate and the metabolism of water. CSF flows from the lateral ventricles into the third ventricle via the foramen of Monro. The third ventricle then communicates with the fourth ventricle through the sylvian aqueduct. CSF leaves the fourth ventricle through the laterally positioned foraminas of Luschka and the midline foramen of Magendie to enter the subarachnoid space. Generally, the normal rate of CSF production is 0.3–0.4 ml/min with a total volume of approximately 140 ml. Using 0.35 ml/min as an estimate, 500 ml of CSF is produced daily. CSF resorption occurs at the arachnoid villi, which are invaginations of arachnoid membrane covered with venous sinus epithelium. The pressure gradient between the subarachnoid space and venous sinuses, typically on the order of 20–30 mm H_2O drives CSF resorption.[9]

CSF composition has been well characterized. The divergence of electrolyte composition from that of plasma indicates an active process is responsible for the formation of CSF. The amount and types of protein found in CSF differ from that of plasma. As we will discuss later, this can be useful in identifying CSF fistulas. Generally, very few cells exist in the CSF. Normal numbers of white blood cells would be < 4 cells/mm^3. The ratio of white blood cells to red blood cells is 1–2:1000.[10]

Normal intracranial pressures (ICP) typically range from 5 to 15 cm of H_2O. Multiple factors can influence the pressures including patient position, activity level, sleep, respiratory phase, time of day, and cardiac cycle. Pathologic alterations in ICPs may occur secondary to a mass lesion such as tumor growth, or change in one of the components of the intracranial compartment, such as decreased resorption of CSF. Pressure measurements are commonly obtained at the time of lumbar puncture. More sophisticated ICP monitoring devices are commercially available that allow continuous monitoring of ICP and ventricular pressure waves. Generally, increased ICP is defined as a sustained pressure over 20–30 cm of H_2O. Increased ICP puts patients at increased risk for the development of CSF fistulas. Patients with increased ICP are also more likely to have repair failure and recurrence after successful repair. Early symptoms of increased ICP can include headache, visual disturbances, and balance problems. Progression can lead to Cushing's triad of hypertension, bradycardia, and irregular respiratory rate. As pressure continues to increase herniation occurs leading to compression of the respiratory centers in the medulla oblongata and death.

PATHOPHYSIOLOGY

Hydrocephalus associated with increased ICP can be classified as non-communicating or communicating. Non-communicating hydrocephalus results when a pathologic process impinges on the outflow of CSF preventing it from reaching the arachnoid villi in the subarachnoid space for resorption. Communicating hydrocephalus results from a pathologic process that interferes with CSF resorption at the arachnoid villi. ICP can be increased without the presence of hydrocephalus as occurs in idiopathic intracranial hypertension, also commonly known as benign intracranial hypertension. These patients tend to be middle-aged, obese women with symptoms of visual disturbances, pulsatile tinnitus, vertigo, and headache. New evidence suggests that patients previously diagnosed with 'spontaneous' CSF leaks may in fact have BIH or a variant of BIH as the underlying cause. This will be discussed in further detail in the etiology section. The presence of hydrocephalus or increased intracranial pressure is an important consideration in planning the treatment of CSF fistulas, especially regarding the use of CSF diversion.

The main concern for patients with anterior cranial fossa CSF fistula is the risk of life-threatening meningitis. This risk has been calculated to be 10% annually and up to 40% with long-term follow-up.[11] In fact not uncommonly patients with subclinical CSF fistulas are referred for evaluation due to recurring episodes of meningitis. The high risk of developing meningitis has lead some to question whether or not traumatic CSF leaks should be repaired early to reduce this risk even though about 70% will heal spontaneously with bed rest or lumbar drainage. Another concern for these patients is the risk of developing pneumocephalus. Though this is less common it is a real concern for patients with concomitant obstructive sleep apnea on a nasal continuous positive airway pressure machine. There is a case report in the literature of a patient with obstructive sleep apnea developing pneumocephalus after transsphenoidal removal of a pituitary adenoma.[12] It also poses problems with mask ventilation if the patient were to undergo an operative procedure for an unrelated reason.

The etiology of a CSF leak is important for understanding the underlying pathophysiology, deciding upon when operative intervention is indicated, choosing the technique for repair, and deciding whether or not use CSF diversion. Classically, Ommaya characterized CSF leaks as traumatic or nontraumatic cases.[13] Traumatic cases include those secondary to accidental trauma and surgical trauma. Nontraumatic cases are further subdivided based on whether there is an elevated or normal intracranial pressure. Elevated intracranial pressure cases can be divided into those caused by tumors whether via direct or indirect effect, and those caused by hydrocephalus whether it is communicating or non-communicating. Normal pressure cases classically were divided into congenital, and spontaneous cases.[13]

Accidental trauma account for the majority of CSF leaks in most described series in the literature. This group accounts for 60–70% of cases; 1–3% of all head trauma patients and 20–30% of those with skull fractures will develop a CSF leak.[14] Most patients (66%), will show signs of CSF leakage within the first 48 hours. By 3 months 95% of patients will have presented.[15] There is a report in the literature of a traumatic CSF leak presenting 34 years after the presumed inciting event.[16] The reasons for delayed appearance of CSF leak include: delayed increase in ICP, lysis of blood clot in area, resolution of soft tissue edema, maturation and contraction of wound edges, or loss of vascularity and necrosis of soft tissue around the wound.[17] Patients with fine cracks in the skull base and dural tears often have a favorable prognosis.

Most commonly the cribriform plate and ethmoid roof will be the site of the CSF leak due to the thinness of bone and tight adherence of the dura in these locations. The olfactory neurons that penetrate the cribriform plate are surrounded by dura and subarachnoid space as they enter the nasal cavity. These may be the site of the CSF leak. Most of these cases will resolve with conservative treatment such as elevation of the head of bed, laxatives, and bedrest. Other cases will resolve with CSF diversion via a lumbar drain. The risk of meningitis with this can be as high as 40%. Antibiotic prophylaxis has not been reported to be beneficial in preventing meningitis in these patients.[18,19]

Surgical trauma is the second most common etiology of CSF leak. Most series will have 20–30% of cases attributable to surgical trauma though in more recent series in the literature a greater percentage are due to surgical trauma. This may indicate either referral bias or that an increased number of endoscopic sinus surgeries and skull base procedures are being performed. Surgical procedures associated with risk of CSF leak include open or endoscopic sinus surgery, transsphenoidal pituitary surgery, open or endoscopic resection of other anterior skull base tumors, and transcranial approaches to the optic chiasm, or cavernous carotid for aneurysm clipping. The risk of CSF leak has been reported to be < 1% during endoscopic sinus surgery.[20] A predilection for CSF leak has been noted for the right side as compared to the left. This is thought to be due to the tendency of a right handed surgeon to drift to a more medial direction, towards the thin lateral lamella of the cribriform plate. The most common sites of injury include the lateral lamella of the cribriform plate and the posterior ethmoid roof.

Tumors can cause CSF leaks via direct erosion through the skull base with large defects surrounded by diseased tissue, or by causing hydrocephalus either communicating or non-communicating. Both benign and malignant neoplasms may cause these fistulas. The origin may be intracranial, sinonasal, or metastatic. In most series these are responsible for less than 5% of cases. The mechanism of CSF leakage is important in planning treatment as cases with hydrocephalus will usually require CSF diversion for repair to be successful.

Congenital encephaloceles can be a source of CSF fistulas. They are the cause in < 5% of cases in most series. They can be classified as occipital, sincipital, or basal. Occipital encephaloceles are the most common, accounting for 75% of congenital encephaloceles. Sincipital encephaloceles which comprise about 15% of congenital encephaloceles can be further divided into nasofrontal, nasoethmoidal, and naso orbital types.

Finally, basal encephaloceles, the least common, can be further divided into transethmoidal, sphenoethmoidal, transsphenoidal, and sphenomaxillary types.[21] Encephaloceles may present externally on the glabella, external nose, or be completely intranasal. During embryological development encephaloceles that pass through the foramen cecum into the fontinculus nasofrontalis or prenasal space account for the glabellar and external nose presentations respectively. Typically, encephaloceles are compressible, pulsatile masses that increases in size with straining or crying (Furstenberg's sign). Differential diagnosis would include a nasal dermoid or glioma. Encephaloceles can also be acquired and associated with the other causes of CSF fistulas, particularly spontaneous cases. The presence of an encephalocele is an important consideration in preoperative surgical planning as it may influence technique chosen for repair and decision for postoperative CSF diversion. Additionally, the presence of an encephalocele is associated with an increased risk of complications.[22]

Traditionally, spontaneous CSF fistulas were thought to arise in patients with normal intracranial pressure. Several potential explanations exist to explain this phenomenon. It has been suggested that atrophy of the olfactory fili or pituitary lead to a a CSF filled space that can become an encephalocele CSF fistula.[23] Another alternative is that a previously unrecognized congenital defect in the skull base existed. Finally, it has been proposed that a focal osteomyelitis at the skull base led to a defect with resultant encephalocele and CSF fistula. Recently, the traditional dogma that spontaneous CSF fistula occur in patients with normal intracranial pressure has been challenged. In a series by Schlosser 10 patients developed symptoms such as headache, pulsatile tinnitus, and vertigo after successful repair of CSF fistula. In addition to symptoms, these patients shared clinical characteristics similar to patients with benign intracranial hypertension such as female preponderance, increased body mass index, and high incidence of empty sella syndrome. These findings suggest that increased intracranial pressures play a significant role in spontaneous CSF fistula (contrary to traditional belief).[28]

DIAGNOSIS (FIGS 15.1 TO 15.4)

The major presenting symptom of patients with a CSF leak will be clear, watery rhinorrhea. This is usually unilateral, but may be bilateral. The rest of the history will depend on the cause of the CSF leak. More than 50% of trauma patients will develop rhinorrhea within the first 48 hours; however, it can be delayed as edema

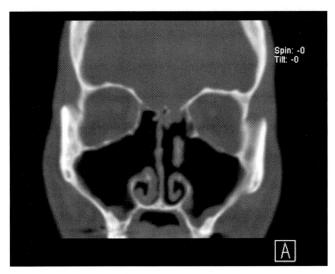

Fig. 15.1: Surgical trauma resulting in left cribriform plate cerebrospinal fluid fistula

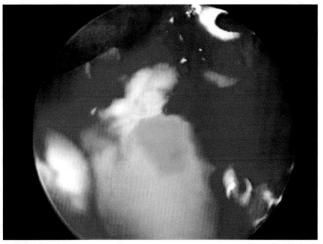

Fig. 15.3: Endoscopic identification in sphenoid sinus of 0.1 ml of 10% fluorescein diluted in 9.9 ml of cerebrospinal fluid and injected intrathecally

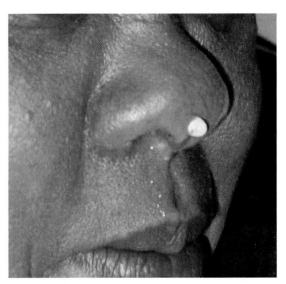

Fig. 15.2: Unilateral cerebrospinal fluid rhinorrhea

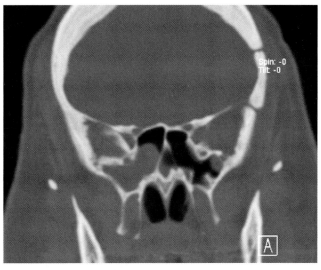

Fig. 15.4: Persistent spontaneous CSF fistula in lateral recess of left sphenoid sinus despite attempted repair via a temporal craniotomy

resolves and allows the CSF to flow out. These patients may have hyposmia or anosmia and headache. Iatrogenic CSF rhinorrhea patients may have undergone endoscopic sinus surgery, transsphenoidal pituitary tumor resection, or removal of a less common skull base tumor such as esthesioneuroblastoma. Patients with hydrocephalus as an underlying factor may complain of the common symptoms of increased ICP. Visual problems, vertigo, pulsatile tinnitus, and headache may indicate an underlying idiopathic intracranial hypertension. An intranasal mass that enlarges with Valsalva maneuver (Furstenberg's sign) may indicate a congenital encephalocele associated with the CSF leak. These patients can also present with recurrent episodes of meningitis.

Patients should receive a complete head and neck examination. Having the patient sit forward with their head down may reproduce the rhinorrhea. Nasal endoscopy is performed with careful attention to the cribriform plate, middle meatus, sphenoethmoidal recess, and eustachian tube. A Valsalva maneuver may increase the CSF flow and make it more detectable. The presence of an encephalocele may also be determined during initial nasal endoscopy. The use of intrathecal sodium fluorescein either preoperatively, or intraoperatively can be done for identification and localization of CSF fistulas. At the time of lumbar puncture 0.2 ml of 5% fluorescein is mixed in 9.9 ml of sterile saline and injected. The characteristic yellow-green color can be very helpful in detecting CSF leakage. Visual detection can be further improved with the use of a blue light filter. Prior to use of sodium fluorescein a detailed discussion is held with the patient regarding its use. Tinnitus, nausea, headache, seizures, and death have been reported to the Food and Drug Administration in connection with the use of intrathecal sodium fluorescein. In the United States the product label explicitly states 'Not recommended for intrathecal use'. Despite this several large studies have detailed hundreds of intrathecal sodium fluorescein administrations with very few complications.[24] The complication rate appears to be dose dependent with few side effects when less than 25 mg of drug is used. Several radiographic studies may detect the presence and location of the CSF fistula.[25,26]

Plain skull radiographs may demonstrate a fracture, pneumocephalus, or an air-fluid level in the sinus, but, generally have little value for the diagnosis and localization of CSF leak. High-resolution CT scanning is extremely useful for delineation of the skull base anatomy and identification of bony defects. The degree of sinus pneumatization can be an important factor particularly in spontaneous CSF fistulas. Shetty found 91% of patients with spontaneous CSF fistulas had significant pneumatization of the lateral recess of the sphenoid sinus compared to 23% of controls.[27] The diagnostic yield of CT can be improved with the injection of contrast agent into the intrathecal space. Water soluble contrast agents like metrizamide and iohexol have been used for this purpose. In addition to identification of the presence of a CSF leak these studies may indicate the location of the leak. Disadvantages include the need for an invasive procedure with injection of material into the intrathecal space, poor soft tissue definition to evaluate for the presence of a concomitant encephalocele, and possible false-negative result in patient with an intermittent or slow leak. Radionuclide cisternography can help identify a CSF leak. In this technique radioactive isotopes are introduced into the CSF via lumbar puncture. This can be done at the same time as injection of intrathecal contrast (iodine 131, radioactive serum albumin (RISA), ytterbium (Yb) 169 diethylenetriamine (DTPA), indium 111 DTPA, technetium (Tc99m) serum albumin, and Tc99m pertechnetate). Typically, cottonoid nasal pledgets

are placed in the nasal cavity in the middle meatus, sphenoethmoidal recess, and at the eustachian tube. After several hours the pledgets are removed and counts obtained from each of them. This technique may be particularly useful in detecting a slow or intermittent CSF leak. Disadvantages to the technique included exposure of the patient to radioactive material, inability to identify the exact location of the leak, and absorption of the isotope into the circulatory system with contamination of extracranial tissue. The inability of MRI to demonstrate bony anatomy at the skull base is a major limitation in its use for evaluation of CSF leak. It does, however, have several advantages: it is the modality of choice for identifying the presence of a co-existing encephalocele, and best identifies empty sella syndrome (ESS) that is associated with spontaneous CSF leaks. ESS occurs when dura herniates through the diaphragma sellae into the sella turcica and fills it with CSF. The CSF compresses the pituitary gland giving the sella turcica a characteristic 'empty' radiographic appearance.[28] About 90% of patients with spontaneous CSF fistulas were noted to have a partially or completely empty sella in one study.[27] MRI cisternography relies on the bright T2 signal of CSF, thereby obviating the need for lumbar puncture and injection of material into the subarachnoid space. This can be especially important in patients with increased intracranial pressure in whom lumbar puncture would be contraindicated. It may be better than CT cisternography at detecting dural lesions less than 2 mm in size and multiple lesions. MRI identification of CSF fistulas is maximized when sequences use heavy T2 weighting, high spatial resolution, suppress flow phenomena that promote signal attenuation or extinction, and use a short examination time as the prone or head down position is uncomfortable for patients.[29] The use of intrathecal gadopentetate dimeglumine enhanced MRI cisternography has also been reported and may enhance CSF leak detection compared to traditional MRI cisternography.[30]

There are reports in the literature on the use of SPECT and PET scanning to identify CSF leaks but these are less commonly used.[31,32] The differential composition of proteins in CSF compared to other body fluids can be useful for establishing the presence of a fistula.

Transferrin is an iron-binding glycoprotein found in several polymorphic forms in the serum and other body fluids. Beta-2 transferrin is a desialated isoform of transferrin that occurs only in the cerebrospinal fluid, perilymph, aqueous humor, and vitreous humor. Thus its detection can be very useful in determining whether the clear rhinorrhea is CSF or another fluid. In certain instances desialated isoforms of transferrin can be found in the serum including patients with a rare allelic variant of transferrin, severe liver disease, or those who chronically abuse alcohol.[33]

Originally described for detection of CSF leakage in 1979, testing for the presence of beta-2 transferrin is noninvasive, sensitive and specific.[34] Sensitivity and specificity of beta-2 transferrin has been reported in the literature to be 97 and 99% respectively.[35] In most clinical practice it has replaced methods of fluid analysis such as glucose concentration, protein concentration, and prealbumin index that have been used in the past. The fluid is analyzed by first using isoelectric focusing on agarose or polyacrylamide gels. Then either immunoblotting or immunofixation with antitransferrin and silver staining are used to identify beta-2 transferrin from other isoforms.[36] Disadvantages of this method were a lengthy time for the completion of the testing and need for 2–5 ml of fluid for analysis, however, a recent report in the literature describes an automated immunofixation electrophoresis system that can give accurate results in approximately 150 minutes with as little as 2–5 µl of fluid.[33]

Beta trace protein analysis has been offered as an alternative to beta-2 transferrin testing. Beta trace protein's presence in CSF was first described in 1961.[37] It has subsequently been discovered to be prostaglandin-D synthase, an enzyme responsible for catalyzation of prostaglandin H_2 to prostaglandin D_2.[38] It is the second most abundant protein in CSF after albumin. It is mainly produced in the meninges and choroid plexus. It can also be identified in perilymph, serum, urine, amniotic fluid, seminal plasma, breast cyst fluid, milk of lactating women, breast tumor extracts, placental extracts, fetal brain, and fetal heart tissues.[39] The high concentration of beta trace protein in CSF compared to other fluids makes it clinically useful in diagnosing CSF leakage. Concentrations of beta trace protein are known to be altered in patients with bacterial meningitis or renal insufficiency.[40,41] In one study of 187 patients evaluated for suspected CSF leakage, 30 patients were found to have a highly suspicious beta-trace protein test defined as a concentration greater than 1.31 mg/l. All 30 patients had CSF leak confirmed with surgical exploration. Beta-2 transferrin testing was positive in 28 of these patients and negative in 2 patients.[42] In another study evaluating 53 patients with suspected CSF leak beta trace protein and beta-2 transferrin testing correlated in all but 3 patients. These authors also note advantages of beta-trace protein testing compared to beta-2 transferrin testing to be that testing is fully automated, it takes less time (approximately 15 minutes), and is less expensive.[39] Once the diagnosis of CSF fistula has been established a treatment plan can be formulated.

Treatment (Figs 15.5 to 15.10)

The etiology of the CSF fistula is extremely important in determining when to operate. As mentioned earlier the

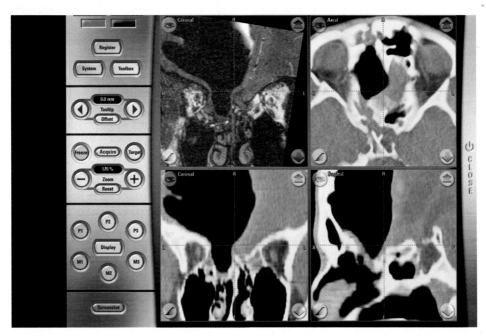

Fig. 15.5: Tension pneumocephalus resulting from skull base fracture after motor vehicle collision

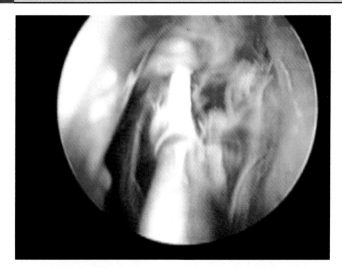

Fig. 15.6: Denudation of mucosa surrounding defect and cauterization

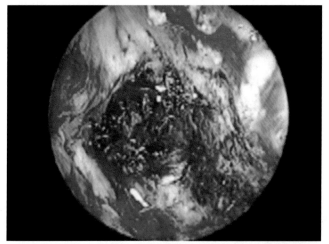

Fig. 15.7: Defect bed after removal of mucosa and cauterization

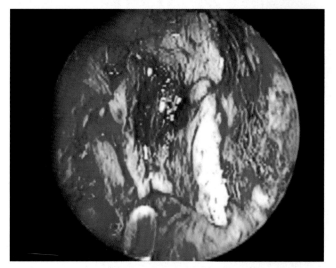

Fig. 15.8: Mucosal overlay graft. Epithelial surface has been marked to facilitate correct placement

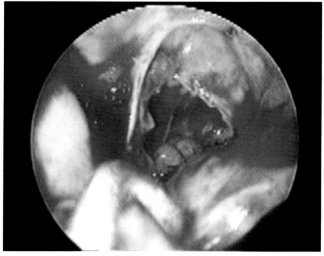

Fig. 15.9: Fat used to obliterate the lateral-most recess of the sphenoid sinus

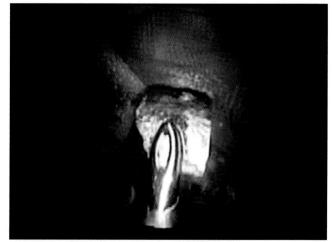

Fig. 15.10: Temporalis fascia graft

majority of patients with a CSF fistula due to accidental trauma will respond to conservative management such as elevating the head of bed, avoiding nose blowing and straining, and using stool softeners. Additional closures will occur with CSF diversion via lumbar drainage. One proposed treatment algorithm for these patients is conservative management for 3 days. Patients who fail conservative management go on to lumbar drainage for 4 days. Patients who fail this treatment proceed to surgical repair.

Accidental trauma patients can present with a heterogenous group of injuries. Patients in a motor vehicle collision (Fig. 15.5) with a fine skull base fracture and CSF leak will generally do well. Other patients with more severe injuries may go directly to surgical repair such as those who present with a delayed CSF leak, have penetrating missile trauma to the skull base, and/or have large fragments of skull base missing. Patients with increased intracranial pressures too may respond to medical interventions such as the use of acetazolamide, mannitol, and steroids. For patients who have failed conservative and medical management surgical intervention is indicated.

The following factors should be taken into consideration when planning surgical repair: etiology, technique, graft material, use of prophylactic antibiotics, need for CSF diversion, and location of the fistula. Understanding the cause and underlying pathophysiology of the CSF fistula is essential for successful surgical treatment. Classification of the lesion as occuring from accidental trauma, surgical trauma, erosive, congenital, or spontaneous is only the initial decision. Further consideration of factors such as likelihood for closure with conservative treatment, extent and location of the skull base defect, presence of increased intracranial pressure, previous or current symptoms consistent with meningitis, previous repair attempts, and coexisting medical conditions should be accounted for. A complete understanding of the unique characteristics of each patient will allow for designing an individualized treatment plan that has the highest likelihood of success.

Four techniques are described for the endoscopic repair of CSF fistulas: overlay, underlay, bath plug, and obliteration. Hegazy reported in his meta-analysis the use of overlay technique in 79% of cases, and use of underlay technique in 12% of cases.[43] With the overlay technique, after identification of the leakage site the surrounding mucosa is denuded from the skull base defect. The graft material, usually a free graft, is placed over the defect and the cleared bone edges. The graft is supported with intranasal packing material. A second more technically challenging technique is the underlay technique. With this technique after identification of the leakage site, dura is carefully elevated intracranially around the skull base defect. Then a graft material such as bone, cartilage, or other supporting graft is placed intracranially. An additional piece of graft material is then placed over this site. The graft is supported with intranasal packing material. This technique is often used in instances where there is a large skull base defect. Another technique that has been reported is the bath plug technique. In this technique after identification of the fistula and preparation of the site, a piece of appropriately sized abdominal fat is fashioned. A vicryl suture is placed through the length of the fat plug. The fat plug is gently placed intracranially, then traction on the suture seals it

into the bony defect. The vicryl suture is then placed through a free mucosal graft that is placed in an overlay fashion on the fat plug. Finally, intranasal packing is placed. The final technique is sinus obliteration. This is most commonly used for fistula in the sphenoid sinus, particularly in the lateral recess of the sphenoid. In this technique mucoperisoteum is stripped from the sinus. The sinus is then obliterated with fat or muscle. The anterior face of the sphenoid can be reconstructed with bone, cartilage or a bioabsorbable plate. This will assist in holding the obliterative material in place. A variation of this technique that has been reported to have good success is to obliterate the sinus with hydroxyapatite.[44]

Multiple materials exist for use as graft in repair. These materials can be simply be categorized as pedicled or free grafts, and self or non-self materials. Pedicled grafts are from adjacent turbinate or septum. These may or may not include cartilage or bone. The free grafts can come from a variety of sites. Locally mucoperichondrium or mucoperiosteum from adjacent turbinate or septum are favored. The use of fascia lata, and temporoparietal fascia have also been described. Abdominal fat and muscle plugs are often used for obliteration. A wide variety of non-self materials are commercially available to use alone or with other graft material. These include: Alloderm, Medpor, Gelfoam, Tisseal, Fibrin glue, Floseal, and hydroxapatite.

While prophylactic antibiotics have not been shown to be effective in reducing the risk of meningitis after traumatic CSF fistula, most authors use prophylactic antibiotics in the perioperative period. There are no randomized clinical trials investigating their use at the present time. We routinely continue prophylactic antibiotics while patients have intranasal packing in place.

The use of CSF diversion via a lumbar drain is debatable in the literature: 67% of members of the American Rhinologic Society (ARS) who responded to a survey about repairing CSF fistulas and encephaloceles used lumbar drains for an average of 4 days.[22] In a meta-analysis of 14 series on the endoscopic management of CSF leaks, 48% of the total 204 repairs with that information available used a lumbar drain.[43] Since then four more series using lumbar drain have been published . In one of those articles that dealt only with patients who had a spontaneous etiology of their CSF leak, lumbar drainage was used in all cases for 5–8 days.[45] Another series notes their use in 46.2% of their patients for a mean duration of 3.4 days.[46] The other two series did not specifically comment on lumbar drain usage but stated they were more likely to be used for spontaneous etiologies, revisions, and repair failures.[11,47] Casiano and Jassir report the largest series in the literature[33] where lumbar drainage was never used.[48] These included some patient with small skull base defects who were treated as outpatients. While CSF diversion intuitively makes sense in reducing the pressure head against the repair, it also has potential complications. Lumbar drainage has been reported to cause headache in 59% of patients undergoing the procedure. In this same study 16% (5/32) patients developed culture proven meningitis, 6% (2/32) had radicular pain, 2 patients had suspected vocal cord dysfunction attributed to traction on the vagal nerve rootlets, 1 patient had posterior lateral infarction of the left occipital lobe thought to be due to kinking of the left posterior cerebral artery across the tentorium cerebelli, and 1 patient had L5 nerve root inflammation, all thought to be due to the lumbar drainage of CSF.[49] Clearly, lumbar drainage should be used cautiously with skilled nursing staff facile with care of the lumbar drain available. It is most likely to be useful in cases where the etiology of the CSF leak is associated with increased ICP, or is of longstanding duration.

Usually, the location of the lesion has been identified preoperatively by nasal endoscopy and radiographic studies. Occasionally, the exact location is not identified until the time of the operation with surgical exploration and the use of intrathecal fluorescein. The exact location has important ramifications for choosing an approach. CSF fistulas involving the frontal sinus are most often approached using an osteoplastic flap with or without obliteration approach. In certain cases of extensive trauma we use a frontal craniotomy and cranialization as a joint procedure with the neurosurgical service. A coronal, pretrichial, or midbrow incision is used based on the patient's hairline, and previous surgical scars. The bone cuts are made with the assistance of transillumination, six foot Caldwell plain films, or stereotactic CT guidance based upon the experience and preference of the surgeon. We routinely used stereotactic CT guidance for this purpose and have shown that its use is more accurate than transillumination or six foot Caldwell films.[50] Once the fistula is repaired a decision is made regarding obliteration. Important considerations in this decision are the status of the frontal sinus outflow tract, the condition of remaining frontal sinus mucosa, the presence of supraorbital ethmoid and frontal sinus cells, and perhaps most important, the reliability of the patient. In most cases we do not obliterate; instead adequate frontal sinus outflow drainage is established in an effort to re-establish

healthy sinus function and physiology. The patient is followed with serial endoscopic and radiographic examinations. A well planned algorithm for this approach in patients sustaining frontal sinus fractures has been described in the literature.[51]

CSF fistulas that involve the ethmoid roof can be approached via a craniotomy, external ethmoidectomy, or endoscopic approach. As mentioned earlier there is a somewhat higher incidence of these lesions after endoscopic sinus surgery on the right side for right handed surgeons. The lateral lamella of the cribriform plate is a common site due to the thinness of bone, the tight adherence of the dura, and the entry point of the anterior ethmoidal artery making a natural area of dehiscence in this area. Another common area for injury is the posterior ethmoid roof when the surgeon fails to lower the angle of approach with the endoscope as he penetrates the basal lamella of the middle turbinate and approaches the face of the sphenoid. In the frontal craniotomy approach a coronal incision is made. If the side of the CSF fistula is known the bone flap is removed from that side. Mannitol may be given, or CSF removed via a lumbar drain to reduce the size of the brain and minimize retraction on the frontal lobes. The ipsilateral olfactory tract is divided behind the olfactory bulb. If during exploration no fistula site is found the coronal incision allows for bifrontal craniotomy and exploration of the other side. Once the fistula site is identified it can be repaired using a pedicled dural, pedicled falx cerebri flap, or free pericranial flap.[52] External extracranial approaches use a naso-orbital incision similar to that originally described by Dohlman. A complete external ethmoidectomy is performed to expose the ethmoid roof. The frontoethmoidal suture line is used as a landmark of the position of the cribriform plate. The anterior ethmoidal artery is ligated. Once the defect is identified usually a pedicled flap of middle turbinate or septum is used for closure. McCabe reported the use of a flap from middle turbinate with mucosa and bone rotated laterally against the ethmoid roof and secured with intranasal packing.[53] Montgomery has described a mucoperiosteal septal flap that is posteriorly based and rotated 90° to cover the defect.[54] In most cases an endoscopic approach is used for ethmoid CSF fistula. A complete endoscopic sphenoethmoidectomy is performed exposing the anterior skull base. The fistula is identified and an intraoperative decision made on which repair technique to employ: Overlay, underlay, or bath plug. The graft material is chosen and a decision is made regarding the use of a free graft or pedicled graft. In most cases we use an overlay technique with a free graft. An effort is made to preserve the middle turbinate in all cases if not previously resected. This both maintains anatomic landmarks for orientation and helps prevent frontal sinus outflow stenosis due to turbinate remnant lateralization. After repair absorbable nasal packing is placed over the repair site. This is reinforced with nonabsorbable packing.

Lesions involving the sphenoid roof or posterior wall can be approached via a craniotomy, transseptal, or endoscopic approach. The craniotomy approach is identical to that used for ethmoid roof leaks with the exception that in some cases the tuberculum sellae will be removed, the mucosa of the posterior wall of the sphenoid sinus pushed away and the sphenoid filled with muscle or fat. A sublabial or transnasal trans-septal approach can also be employed. The approach is identical to that used for a transseptal transsphenoidal approach to pituitary tumor removal. After sublabial or transnasal incision and septum removal, a Hardy speculum is placed. The rostrum and intersinus septum are removed and the sphenoid sinus mucosa stripped. A free graft can be placed against the defect, then the sinus is packed with muscle or fat. The anterior wall of the sphenoid sinus can be reconstructed with septal bone or cartilage. Endoscopically, the technique is quite similar to that used for the ethmoid. The more challenging problem in sphenoid lesions is the CSF fistula in a lateral recess of a well pneumatized sphenoid. The acute angle, distance from the front of the nose, and presence of vital structures such as the carotid artery and optic nerve make these lesions much more interesting. Using 70° endoscopes and specialized instruments we often repair these lesions in the same fashion as the ethmoid roof lesions. In some instances, however, we use one of two additional techniques: Sphenoid obliteration or the transpterygoid approach. For sphenoid obliteration all mucoperiosteum is removed from the sinus. The entire sinus, or if an intersinus septum is intact the affected side is obliterated with abdominal fat. The rostrum of the sphenoid may be repaired using cartilage, bone, or a bioabsorbable plate.[55] Another alternative is the use of the transpterygoid approach as described by Bolger. In this technique a wide maxillary antrostomy is performed exposing the posterior wall of the maxillary sinus. The wide sphenoidotomy is also performed. A flap of mucosa is raised off the posterior maxillary sinus wall, then the underlying bone is removed. A hemaclip is used to ligate the sphenopalatine artery. An effort is made to identify and preserve the pterygopalatine ganglion, vidian nerve, and infraorbital nerve as dissection continues throught the pterygopalatine fossa. The anterior aspect of the ptery-

goid process is identified and removed using a drill thus entering the lateral recess of the sphenoid sinus.[56]

Traditional craniotomy approaches to CSF fistula repair have been reported to be successful in 60–80% of cases after the first attempt.[57,58] In a series of 53 patients 27% developed recurrences after the initial repair. Of these 10% continued despite multiple attempts at closure.[52] Extracranial open approaches have a success rate of 86–100% after initial repair and 97–100% after subsequent attempts.[1,59] In addition to avoiding the morbidity of open procedures, endoscopic repair of CSF fistulas and encephaloceles has an success rate of approximately 90% on the first attempt and 96% by the second attempt. Success rates are slightly lower for patients with increased intracranial pressure and lesions of the far lateral recess of a well pneumatized sphenoid sinus; complication rates for endoscopic techniques is quite low. For endoscopic repair of CSF fistulas the overall complication rate is 2.5%. The most common of these would be meningitis at 1.1% with all other complications occurring less than 1% of the time. Endoscopic repair of encephaloceles has a higher complication rate of 8.6%. The most common complicaton of this category would be seizures, 3.1%, followed by meningitis, 2.3%. The higher incidence of complications is attributed to greater manipulation of brain tissue in these repairs.

REFERENCES

1. Calcaterra TC. Extracranial repair of cerebrospinal rhinorrhea. *Ann Otol Rhinol Laryngol* 1980;89(2 Pt 1):108-116.
2. Gross CW. The diagnosis and treatment of cerebrospinal fluid rhinorrhea. *Trauma* 1975;45:11–14.
3. Thompson SC. *Cerebrospinal fluid: Its Spontaneous Escape from the Nose with Observations of its Composition and Function in Human Subjects*. London: Cassell and Co Ltd, 1899.
4. Dandy WD. Pneumocephalus (intracranial pneumocele or aerocele). *Arch Surg* 1926;12:949–982.
5. Dohlman G. Spontaneous cerebrospinal fluid rhinorrhea. *Acta Otolaryngol Suppl* (Stockholm) 1948;67:20–23.
6. Hirsch O. Successful closure of cerebrospinal fluid rhinorrhea by endonasal surgery. *Arch Otolaryngol* 1952;56:1–13.
7. Vrabec DP, Hallberg OE. Cerebrospinal fluid rhinorrhea. *Arch Otolaryngol* 1964;80:218–229.
8. Wigand WE. Transnasal ethmoidectomy under endoscopic control. *Rhinology* 1981;19:7–15.
9. Tindall GT et al (Eds). *The Practice of Neurosurgery*. Baltimore: Williams and Wilkins, 1996.
10. Greenberg MS. *Handbook of Neurosurgery*, 2nd edn. Florida: Greenberg Graphics Inc., 1991.
11. McMains KC, Gross CW, Kountakis SE. Endoscopic management of cerebrospinal fluid rhinorrhea. *Laryngoscope* 2004;114:1833–1837.
12. Shields CB, Valdes-Rodriguez AG. Tension pneumocephalus after transsphendoidal hypophysectomy: Case report. *Neurosurgery* 1982;11(5):687–689.

13. Ommaya AK. Spinal fluid fistula. *Clin Neurosurg* 1976; 23: 363–392.

14. Dagi FT, George ED. Management of cerebrospinal fluid leaks. In *Operative Neurosurgical Techniques*: Indications, methods, and results, Schmidek HH, Sweet WH (Eds). Florida: Grune and Stratton, 1988;49–69.

15. Zlab MK, Moore GF, Daly DT et al. Cerebrospinal fluid rhinorrhea: A review of the literature. *Ear Nose Throat J* 1992; 72:314–317.

16. Russell T, Cummins BH. Cerebrospinal fluid rhinorrhea 34 years after trauma: A case report and review of the literature. *Neurosurgery* 1984;15:705–706.

17. Applebaum EL, Chow JM. Cerebrospinal fluid leaks. In *Otolaryngology–Head and Neck Surgery*, Cummings CW (Eds) et al, 2nd edition. St Louis: Mosby-Year Book, 1993.

18. Klastersky J, Sadeghi M, Brihaye J. Antimicrobial prophylaxis in patients with rhinorrhea or otorrhea: A double blind study. *Surg Neurol* 1976;6:111.

19. MacGee EE, Cauthen JC, Brackett CE. Meningitis following acute traumatic cerebrospinal fluid fistula. *J Neurosurg* 1970;33:312.

20. Stankiewicz JA. Cerebrospinal fluid fistula and endoscopic sinus surgery. *Laryngoscope* 1991;101:250–256.

21. Sessions RB, Picken C. Congenital anomalies of the nose. In *Head and Neck Surgery–Otolaryngology*, BJy et al (Eds), 3rd edn. Philadelphia: Lippincott Williams and Wilkins, 2001.

22. Senior BA, Jafri K, Benninger M. Safety and efficacy of endoscopic repair of CSF leaks and encephaloceles: A Survey of the Members of the American Rhinologic Society. *Am J Rhinol* 2001;15(1):21–25.

23. Schlosser RJ, Wilensky EM, Grady MS, Bolger WE. Elevated intracranial pressures in spontaneous cerebrospinal fluid leaks. *Am J Rhinol* 2003;17(4): 191–195.

24. Keerl R, Weber RK, Draf W, Wienke A, Schaefer SD. Use of sodium fluorescein solution for detection of cerebrospinal fluid fistulas: An analysis of 420 administrations and reported complications in Europe and the United States. *Laryngoscope* 2004;114:266–272.

25. Stammberger H, Greisdorfer K, Wolf G, Luxenberger W. Surgical occlusion of cerebrospinal fistulas of the anterior skull base using intrathecal fluorescein. *Laryngorhinootologie* 1997; 76:595–607.

26. Moseley J, Carton C, Stern E. Spectrum of complications in the use of intrathecal fluorescein. *J Neurosurg* 1978;48:765–767.

27. Shetty PG, Shroff MM, Fatterpekar GM et al. A retrospective analysis of spontaneous sphenoid sinus fistula: MR and CT findings. *Am J Neuroradiol* 2000;21:337–342.

28. Schlosser RJ, Bolger WE. Significance of empty sella in cerebrospinal fluid leaks. *Otolaryngol Head Neck Surg* 2003; 128(1):32–38.

29. Eberhardt KEW, Hollenbach HP, Deimling M, Tomandl BF, Huk WJ. MR cisternography: A new method for the diagnosis of CSF fistulas. *Eur Radiol* 1997; 7:1485–1491.

30. Aydin K, Guven K, Sencer S, Jinkins JR, Minareci O. MRI cisternography with gadolinium-containing contrast medium: Its role, advantages and limitations in the investigation of rhinorrhoea. *Neuroradiology* 2004; 46:75–80.

31. Servadei G, Moscatelli G, Giuliani G, Cremonini AM, Piazza G, Agostini M, Riva P. Cisternography in combination with single photon emission tomography for the detection of the leakage site in patients with cerebrospinal fluid rhinorrhea: Preliminary report. *Acta Neurochirurgica* 1998;140:1183–1189.

32. Bergstrand G, Bergstrom M, Eriksson L, Edner G, Widen L. Positron emission tomography with 68Ga-EDTA in the diagnosis and localization of CSF fistulas. *J Comput Assist Tomogr* 1982;6(2):320–324.

33. Papadea C, Schlosser RJ. Rapid method for beta-2 transferrin in cerebrospinal fluid leakage using an automated immuno-fixation electrophoresis system. *Clin Chem* 2005;51(2):1–7.

34. Meurmann OH, Irjala K, Suonpaa J, Laurent B. A new method for the identification of cerebrospinal fluid leakage. *Acta Otolaryngol* 1979;87:366–369.

35. Warnecke A, Averbeck T, Wurster U, Harmening M, Lenarz T, Stover T. Diagnostic relevance of B2-transferrin for the detection of cerebrospinal fluid fistulas. *Arch Otolaryngol Head Neck Surg* 2004;130:1178–1184.

36. Roelandse FW, van der Zwart N, Didden JH, van Loon J, Souverijin JH. Detection of cerebrospinal fluid leakage by isoelectric focusing on polyacrylamide gel, direct immuno-fixation of transferrins and silver staining. *Clin Chem* 1998; 44:351–353.

37. Clausen J. Proteins in normal cerebrospinal fluid not found in serum. *Proc Soc Exp Biol Med* 1961;107:170–172.

38. Hoffmann A, Conradt HS, Gross G et al. Purification and chemical characterization of beta-trace protein from human cerebrospinal fluid: Its identification as prostaglandin D synthase. *J Neurochem* 1993;61:451–456.

39. Meco C, Oberascher G, Arrer E, Moser G, Albegger K. Beta-trace protein test: New guidelines for the reliable diagnosis of cerebrospinal fluid fistula. *Otolaryngol Head Neck Surg* 2003; 129:508–517.

40. Tumani H, Reiber H, Nau R, et al. Beta-trace protein concentration in cerebrospinal fluid is decreased in bacterial meningitis. *Neurosci Lett* 1998;242:5–8.

41. Melegos DN, Grass L, Pierratos A et al. Highly elevated levels of prostaglandin D synthase in serum of patients with renal failure. *Urology* 1999;53:32–37.

42. Arrer E, Meco C, Oberascher G, Piotrowski W, Albegger K, Patsch W. Beta-trace protein as a marker for cerebrospinal fluid rhinorrhea. *Clin Chem* 2002; 48:939–941.

43. Hegazy HM, Carrau RL, Snyderman CH, Kassam A, Zweig J. Transnasal endoscopic repair of cerebrospinal fluid rhinorrhea: A meta-analysis. *Laryngoscope* 200;110:1166–1172.

44. Costantino PD, Hiltzik DH, Chandranath S, Friedman CD, Kveton JF, Snyderman CF, Gnoy AR. Sphenoethmoid cerebrospinal fluid leak repair with hydroxyapatite cement. *Arch Otolaryngol Head Neck Surg* 2001;127:588–593.

45. Lopatin AS, Kapitanov DN, Potapov AA. Endonasal endoscopic repair of spontaneous cerebrospinal fluid leaks. *Arch Otolaryngol Head Neck Surg* 2003;129:859–863.

46. Lee T, Huang C, Chuang C, Huang S. Transnasal endoscopic repair of cerebrospinal fluid rhinorrhea and skull base defect: Ten-year experience. *Laryngoscope* 2004;114:1475–1481.

47. Lindstrom DR, Toohill RJ, Loerhl TA, Smith TL. Management of cerebrospinal fluid rhinorrhea: The Medical College of Wisconsin experience. *Laryngoscope* 2004;114:969–974

48. Casiano RR, Jassir D. Endoscopic cerebrospinal fluid rhinorrhea repair: Is a lumbar drain necessary? *Otolaryngol Head Neck Surg* 1999;121:745–750.

49. Roland PS, Marple BF, Meyerhoff WL, Mickey B. Complications of lumbar spinal fluid drainage. *Otolaryngol Head Neck Surg* 1992;107:564–569.

50. Melroy CT, Dubin MG, Hardy SM, Senior BS. Analysis of methods to assess frontal sinus extent in osteoplastic flap surgery: Transillumination vs. six foot Caldwell vs. image guidance. *Am J Rhinol* – accepted for publication.

51. Smith TL, Han JK, Loerhl TA, Rhee JS. Endoscopic management of the frontal recess in frontal sinus fractures: a shift in the paradigm? *Laryngoscope* 2002;112(5):784–790.

52. Ray BS, Bergland RM. Cerebrospinal fluid fistula: Clinical aspects, techniques of localization and methods of closure. *J Neurosurg* 1969;30:399–405.

53. McCabe BF. The osteomucoperiosteal flap in repair of cerebrospinal fluid rhinorrhea. *Laryngoscope* 1976;86:537–539.

54. Montgomery WW. Cerebrospinal rhinorrhea. *Otolaryngol Clin North Am* 1973;6:757–771.

55. Mehendale NH, Marple BF, Nussenbaum B. Management of sphenoid sinus cerebrospinal fluid rhinorrhea: Making use of an extended approach to the sphenoid sinus. *Otolaryngol Head Neck Surg* 2002;126:147–153.

56. Bolger WE, Osenbach R. Endoscopic transpterygoid approach to the lateral sphenoid recess. *Ear Nose Throat J* 1999;78: 36–46.

57. Park JI, Strelzow VV, Friedman WH. Current management of cerebrospinal fluid rhinorrhea. *Laryngoscope* 1983;93: 1294–1300.

58. Aarabi B, Leibrock LG. Neurosurgical approaches to cerebrospinal fluid rhinorrhea. *Ear Nose Throat J* 1992;71:300–305.

59. McCormack B, Cooper PR, Persky M et al. Extracranial repair of cerebrospinal fluid fistulas: technique and results in 37 patients. *Neurosurgery* 1990;27:412–417.

Optic Nerve Decompression

Kevin C McMains, Stilianos E Kountakis

Early descriptions of traumatic blindness appear in the writings of Hippocrates and Galen.[1,2] Battle first distinguished between direct penetrating injuries to the optic nerve and those which do not penetrate the optic nerve, but involve it indirectly.[3] In their text, Walsh and Hoyt defined indirect injury as 'traumatic loss of vision which occurs without external or initial ophthalmoscopic evidence of injury to the eye or its nerve'.[4] Between 0.7 and 5% of head trauma involves the afferent and efferent visual pathways.[5,6] The optic nerve is injured in 0.5 to 1.5% of cases of closed head injury.[7] The optic canal is fractured in 6–92% of cases of traumatic blindness.[8,9] The most common injury resulting in TON has been variably reported as a blow to the ipsilateral brow or forehead, a MVA, a bicycle accident, or a fall.[2,9,10] In American women, up to one-third of orbital trauma is the result of sexual assault and domestic violence.[11] Though widely recognized and investigated, the precise pathophysiology of and optimal treatment modalities for traumatic optic neuropathy (TON) continue to be the source of some debate. A thorough understanding of the relevant anatomy, suspected mechanisms of injury, available diagnostic testing modalities, and treatment strategies is important to inform and tailor individual patient care.

ANATOMY/MECHANISMS OF INJURY

The optic nerve is not a true cranial nerve, but is a fiber tract of brain white matter. Afferent fibers course posteriorly from the retina to the bony optic canal located at the postero-superior aspect of the bony orbit which passes through the lesser wing of the sphenoid. The optic canal contains the optic nerve, ophthalmic artery, post-ganglionic sympathetic fibers, and meningeal extensions (Fig. 16.1). From the bony canal, optic nerves course posteriorly to the optic chiasm, interdigitating there

before passing posteriorly to the lateral geniculate nuclei and subsequently to the primary visual cortex. While the intraorbital segment of the optic nerve is permitted limited motion, the optic nerve is tethered within the optic canal where the optic nerve dura fuse with the periorbita.[12] This places the intracanalicular nerve at risk

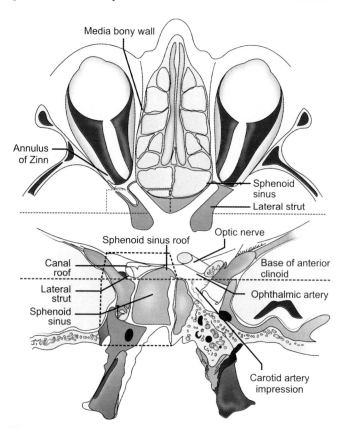

Fig. 16.1: Axial and coronal views of surrounding anatomy in a transethmoid/transorbital approach. (Reprinted from *Ophthalmology Plastic Reconstructive Surgery*, 12(3):163–170, Goldberg and Steinsapir. 'Extracranial optic canal decompression: Indications and technique.' © 1996, Lippincott Williams and Wilkins)

for both primary and secondary ischemic injury shearing and swelling within the fixed cross-sectional area of the bony canal.[6] The optic canal bone is thickest at the optic ring.[13] While the ophthalmic artery generally courses laterally to the optic nerve within the optic canal, in 16% of cases it travels medial to the nerve.[14] While 4% of optic nerves are dehiscent within the sphenoid sinus,[15] the optic nerve may be present within a posterior ethmoid Onodi cell in up to 25% of cases.[16]

Hager and colleagues described and illustrated mechanisms of indirect optic nerve.[17] Kline's group described mechanisms of injury to the optic nerve.[5] These include:

- Laceration
- Bone deformation
- Vascular insufficiency
- Concussion
- Contusion
- Hemorrhage

While laceration of the nerve or bony impingement may not fit neatly within the definition of indirect TON, these conditions may be seen in conjunction with indirect causes. In a postmortem study of patients with traumatic head injuries, 44% were found to have shearing with ischemic necrosis and 36% were found to have interstitial hemorrhage.[18] In two-thirds of those with interstitial hemorrhage, this injury occurred within the optic canal.

More recently, the role of excitatory amino acids and their involvement in free radical production has been explored. Glutamate is an excitatory neurotransmitter that exists in high concentration within neurons. It is released in response to damage sustained by these cells. Glutamate activates NMDA receptors which allow increased levels of calcium to enter cells, ultimately inducing nitric oxide synthase and producing free radicals.[19] In addition, cation influx activates phospholipase C which degrades cell membranes and releases fatty acids and arachidonic acids.[20,21] The end result of these pathways is secondary neuronal damage.

DIAGNOSIS

TON is a clinical diagnosis and, as such, a thorough history and physical examination remain the cornerstones of diagnosis. In addition to the most complete medical history possible under the circumstances of presentation, specific history should include the mechanism of injury, including direction and relative force of the trauma. Supporting history of visual compromise, especially of progressive nature, suggests the possibility of TON.

Patients with a lucid interval of unaffected sight before deterioration have a better prognosis than those with no light perception (NLP) from the time of injury.[22] Physical examination should include complete primary and secondary surveys, though it may be limited by the overall condition of the patient. The most commonly associated optic abnormality is subconjunctival hemorrhage.[23] Thorough ophthalmologic exam should be performed at the earliest instance possible.

Patients with TON can present with any level of visual acuity ranging from no light perception to normal vision, though some degree of visual impairment is standard. The prognostic importance of visual acuity following injury has been demonstrated by several authors.[2,10,24] In patients with isolated TON, the integrity of the globe is maintained. Intraorbital optic nerve trauma is suggested by an abnormal funduscopic exam; however, in the acute phase of posterior segment injury, the optic nerve head appears normal.[12] The most common findings include afferent papillary defect (APD) with normal retina and disc.[25] The swinging flashlight test is a good tool for APD; however, analgesic opioids can inhibit this test.[26] Visual evoked potentials (VEP) is the recommended study tool in comatose patient,[27] though swinging flashlight test can be as accurate in the acute trauma setting.[22] Visual field loss can be present in patients with TON. Hughes notes that, in 75% of patients with visual loss, the loss was limited to the lower visual fields. The mechanism suggested for this distinction was greater adherence of the pia and arachnoid in the upper canal.[2,10] Despite normal funduscopic exam at initial presentation, later in the course optic atrophy may be noted.[22]

Contrasted CT scanning is critical in assessment of the integrity of the optic canal and identification of points of bony impingement. Guyon et al noted the most common fracture site in patients with TON was the inferomedial sphenoid sinus.[28] This group also demonstrated two previously undiagnosed carotid-cavernous fistulas and recommend cerebral angiography in cases of demonstrated canal fracture. Seiff et al note that failure to demonstrate canal fracture does not rule out TON.[29] Further delineation of the intracanalicular subarachnoid space can be provided by an intrathecal metrizimide study of the region.[30]

TREATMENT

In patients with TON who receive no therapy, 20–38% will experience spontaneous recovery of vision.[2,31-33] High-dose steroids in treatment of TON were first used by Anderson et al to evaluate whether surgical decompression could be avoided.[34] Corticosteroids (CS) were initially used reduce edema and vasospasm with the thought that these effects would limit ischemic nerve cell death. The CS regimen used in this study was initial dose of dexamethasone 0.75 mg/kg body weight, followed by 0.33 mg/kg every 6 hours for 24 hours. Subsequently, the dose was decreased by 1 mg/kg/day for up to 48 additional hours and the taper extended for 5–7 days in patients showing improvement. In their study, 3 of 6 patients improved within the first 6 hours following administration of CS.

The multicenter National Acute Spinal Cord Injury Studies (NASCIS I, II, III) demonstrated benefit to patients with spinal cord injuries receiving high-dose CS within the first 8 hours following injury.[35-37] Methlyprednisone is thought to be a better choice than dexamethasone in trauma patients because it does not interact with anticonvulsant medications often used in this setting.[38] Neuroprotection provided by glucocorticoids results from inhibition of free radicals rather than as a direct result of GC receptor activity.[35] The dosing regimen used in the NASCIS study involved bolus delivery of 30 mg/kg body weight of methylprednisone followed by 5.4 mg/kg/h infusion for the subsequent 23 hours. Because of the biphasic antioxidant effect of CS, doses of 60 mg/kg result in loss of effect and doses of 90 mg/kg result in increased lipid peroxidation.[39] In models of injured spinal cords, methylprednisone delivered at high levels has been shown to improve blood flow, decrease breakdown of microfilaments, and decrease lipid per oxidation of cell membranes, thereby decreasing arachidonic acid byproducts and eliminating local vasospasm.[40-42]

The results of the NASCIS trials have been used as justification for high-dose CS for treatment of TON; however, important differences exist between these structures. The spinal cord consists of both grey and white matter whereas the optic nerve consists exclusively of white matter. These tissue types differ in their response to trauma.[43] Clinical data remain inconclusive about the role of CS. Seiff retrospectively analyzed uncontrolled historical cohort data from 36 patients treated expectantly or with dexamethasone 1 mg/kg/day. Although initiation of steroid treatment was delayed for up to 48 hours and there was no statistical difference in the percentage of patients with improved eyesight, patients treated with CS has more rapid return of sight.[33]

Corticosteroids are not a risk-free treatment. CS has a significant risk profile including GI bleeding, psychomotor agitation, glycemic dysregulation, decreased immune capacity, and cardiac arrhythmia. Additionally, research suggests that glucocorticoids are neurotoxic with concentrated effect on the hippocampal CA1 cells.[44,45] In a rat model, Steinsapir and colleagues demonstrated methylprednisone caused a dose-dependent reduction in optic nerve myelin sheaths following crush injury.[46] They hypothesize that methylprednisone interferes with mechanisms to limit secondary neuronal injury. Additionally, further analysis of the NASCIS data demonstrated a harmful effect of high dose CS is begun later than 8 hours following injury.[47] In a recent review, Steinsapir and colleagues state that the evidence supporting use of CS in TON is 'weak at best' and that withholding corticosteroids in these patients is 'no longer unethical'.[48]

In the face of uncertain evidence of CS benefit and in attempts to broaden the range of available treatments, other medical therapies are currently being studied. The lazaroids, 21-aminosteroids that possess free-radical scavenging capabilities, may have equal or superior neuroprotective effects without the risks attendant with high-dose CS.[37,49] MK-801, a non-competitive NMDA receptor antagonist, has shown promise in animal models with respect to visual performance and mixed results with respect to ganglion cell survival.[50,51]

Some authors recommend surgical intervention alone or in conjunction with CS for certain presentations of TON. Walsh established early criteria for surgical decompression of the optic canal via transcranial approach. These criteria were:

1. In the unconscious patient, surgery is never performed as a selective procedure.
2. In a patient with visual loss, non-reactive pupil, and immediate visual loss from time of injury, surgery is contraindicated.
3. If visual loss or loss of pupillary response occur after injury, surgery can be considered.
4. If it is unclear whether a lucid interval existed, observation for 4–6 days to allow for recovery can be appropriate.[6]

Lubben and colleagues used the following criteria for surgical exploration using a fronto-ethmoid approach:

a. Post-traumatic visual loss or decrease in acuity (< 20/100 to 20/60).
b. Increasing restriction of visual field.
c. APD in unconscious patients.[52]

Surgical decisions made using these indications were further supported by optic disc swelling resulting from damage to the optic nerve and CT evidence of bony fragment impinging on the nerve within the optic canal.

Kountakis et al recommended that surgical decompression be performed for:

- Progressive vision loss
- Documented canal fracture
- No improvement following administration of high-dose corticosteroids.[53]

In later work, Kountakis' group noted that patients who presented with visual acuity of 20/200 or better improved with CS therapy alone while patients presenting with visual acuity of 20/400 or worse required surgical decompression as well.[24]

Several studies have been published evaluating the benefits of decompression. Though outliers like Fukado exist who reported improvement in 100% of patients,[54] these results have not been reproduced elsewhere. Other reports demonstrate measurable benefit in 31–82% of cases undergoing surgical intervention with or without CS therapy.[24,55–62] In a retrospective comparison of optic nerve decompressions in 13 comatose patients with TON and 52 conscious patients, Lubben and colleagues found rates of visual recovery of 61.5 and 57.7% respectively, which was not statistically significant.[52]

Although most studies used surgical decompression for patients not improving on CS therapy, Giraud et al demonstrated visual improvement in 8 of 11 patients receiving decompression alone.[63] Caution advised in repair of LeFort III fractures in patients with concomitant orbital apex or optic canal fractures given possibility of secondary optic nerve damage and resultant blindness following repair.[64] Li and colleagues recommend delay of midfacial fracture repair for 10–14 days in a patient with concomitant TON.[57] They additionally state that severe nasal or naso-orbital-ethmoid fracture are poor candidates for decompression by external ethmoidectomy approach used by their group. Kountakis et al included conchal pneumatization as a contraindication for surgery.[24] In the study by Lubben et al, the time interval before surgical intervention did not correlate with outcome.[52] In contrast, Rajiniganth et al showed benefit of combined therapy undertaken before 7 days and go as far as to encourage weighing the risk/benefit ratio of undertaking therapy beyond 7 days.[23]

In their work on TON, Steinsapir and Goldberg concluded that the benefit of intervention of any kind had not clearly been established.[65] The International Optic Nerve Trauma Study (IONTS) aimed to provide conclusive data regarding the best pathway for TON management. Unfortunately, IONTS was discontinued secondary to insufficient enrollment. From data collected on the 127 enrolled patients, no clear benefit was shown from either CS therapy or optic nerve decompression.[66] However, in a meta-analysis of smaller studies, Cook et al concluded that some intervention, whether CS or decompression alone or in conjunction, resulted in better outcomes than no intervention.[55]

Given that surgery carries risk of loss of vision, CSF leak, carotid injury, cavernous sinus injury, and death, surgical decompression should not be undertaken lightly.[67] Because of the variable presentations and time courses of patient treatment and because of differing treatment approaches, results from these studies are difficult to compare and conclusions more difficult still to draw. Significant questions remain regarding what constitutes the best treatment in cases of TON.

SURGICAL APPROACHES

In 1916, Pringle reported the first optic nerve decompression for treatment of an optic nerve sheath hematoma using an orbital approach.[68] Dandy described the frontotemporal craniotomy approach to the optic nerve for patients requiring this approach for treatment of other lesions.[69] This procedure became the most common surgery for TON for several decades. In 1951, Takahashi described the first endonasal approach.[70] Niho et al, described a transethmoidal approach to the optic canal in cases of TON (Fig. 16.2).[71] This approach involved complete extirpation of the mucosal lining of the antrum, ethmoid, sphenoid, and frontal sinus as well as the medial orbital wall. This technique, referred to as Grade I surgery, provided access to the medial canal wall, an area which is difficult to reach via frontal craniotomy. These procedures were performed under local anesthesia. If vision did not subjectively improve following Grade I surgery, Grade II surgery was undertaken: This consisted of a transfrontal approach to the optic canal roof. This approach provided access to this region with less morbidity than via frontal craniotomy.[72]

Goldberg and Steinsapir used a transethmoid/transorbital approach similar to Niho's Grade I surgery in patients with pathology limited to the optic canal (see Fig. 16.1).[73] Kennerdell's group further expanded the range of available options for extracranial access, describing a trans-antralethmoidal approach.[74] This technique involved a Caldwell-Luc, elevation of an inferiorly based mucosal flap, ethmoidectomy with mucosa-stripping followed by microscopic removal of the posterior lamina papyracea, removal of the anterior sphenoid and dissection of the canal.

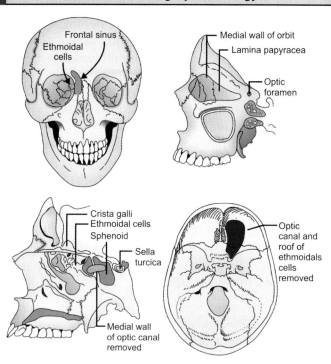

Fig. 16.2: Transethmoidal approach to the optic canal. (Reprinted from *American Journal of Ophthalmology*, Vol 51, Niho et al. Decompression of the optic canal by the transethmoidal route, Pages 659–665, © 1961, with permission from Elsevier)

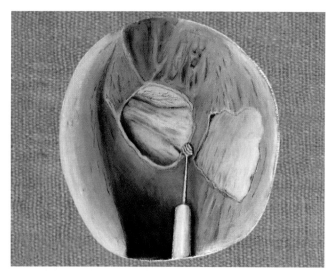

Fig. 16.3: Endoscopic dissection of medial orbital wall and medial optic canal (bone over Annulus of Zinn intact)

Sofferman introduced the microscopic sublabial sphenoethmoid approach to combat limited visibility afforded by other techniques and increase the operative angle of incidence with respect the canal.[75] This technique

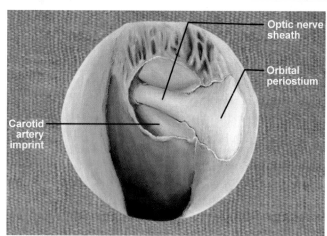

Fig. 16.4: Endoscopic dissection of medial orbital wall and medial optic canal (bone over Annulus of Zinn removed). (Reprinted from *American Journal of Otolaryngology*, V16(6):422–427, Kountakis et al: 'Optic neuritis secondary to sphenoethmoiditis: Surgical treatment' © 1995 Elsevier Inc.)

also uses a Caldwell-Luc antrotomy but relies on wider resection of bone and preservation of a posterior septal mucosal flap for reconstruction. The canal is dissected infero-medially, though a buttress of bone is preserved between the OC and the internal carotid artery.[76] In its original conception, this procedure was intended for treatment of depressed OC fractures.[75]

Call used the transorbital-sphenoid decompression, dividing and reflecting the medial canthal tendon, retracting the periorbita laterally, and proceeding under microscopic vision in a manner similar to Niho's Grade I surgery.[77] Resulting defects were reconstructed with silicone to prevent enophthalmos.

In the context of patients with multiple facial fractures, Knox's group applied the lateral facial approach to TON.[78] This approach involves reflecting the temporalis muscle, retracting the zygomatic arch, removing the greater wing of the sphenoid, identifying and preserving the superior orbital fissure, and transecting the lesser wing en route to unroofing the optic canal. In accord with Sofferman who stated that the benefit of sheath incision unclear,[22] the optic nerve sheath was left intact in this procedure. This procedure is specifically aimed at treating patients with lateral OC fractures. As fiberoptic technology has improved, completely endoscopic optic nerve decompression has been accomplished to good effect (Figs 16.3 and 16.4).[79] Completely endoscopic techniques hold promise for accomplishing optic nerve decompression with improved visualization and comparatively low morbidity.

CONCLUSION

Traumatic optic neuropathy involves complex processes occurring within intricate anatomy with dramatic consequences on the way a patient will interact with his or her surroundings. Though high-dose corticosteroids have been widely used, mixed results have been reported. Some basic science research now suggests that steroids may actually have a negative effect on survival of damaged neurons. The role of optic nerve decompression surgery is no less clear. Though several series have reported benefit, these studies have not been controlled. Additionally, slow enrollment into the International Optic Nerve Trauma Study resulted in data insufficient to resolve this question. Further difficulty is introduced into comparisons between or among interventions based on variables such as time between injury and initiation of treatment, degree of visual impairment at presentation, effects of patient's age, and surgical approach used. Ultimately, decisions about care of the specific patient would take all factors into account and treatment plans would weigh risks and benefits, knowns and unknowns to best treat the specific patient with TON.

REFERENCES

1. Chadwick J, Mann WN. *The Medical Works of Hippocrates*. Oxford: Blackwell, 1950.
2. Hughes B. Indirect injury of the optic nerves and chiasma. *Bull Johns Hopkins Hosp* 1962; 3:98–126.
3. Battle WH. Some points relating to injuries to the head. *Lancet* 1890; 2:57.
4. Walsh FB, Hoyt WF. *Clinical Neuro-ophthalmology*, 3rd edn. Baltimore: Williams and Wilkins, 1969;2375–2386.
5. Kline LB, Morawetz RB, Swaid SN. Indirect injury of the optic nerve. *Neurosurgery* 1984;14(6):756–764.
6. Walsh FB. Pathological-clinical correlations: I. Indirect trauma to the optic nerves and chiasm. II. Certain cerebral involvements associated with defective blood supply. *Invest Ophthalmol* 1966;433–449.
7. Obenchain TG, Killeffer FA, Stern WE. Indirect injury of the optic nerves and chiasm with closed head injruy. Report of three cases. *Bull Los Angeles Neurol Soc* 1973;38(1):13–20.
8. Osguthorpe JD, Sofferman RA. Optic nerve decompression. *Otolaryngol Clin North Am* 1988;21(1):155–169.
9. Noble MJ and McFadzean R. Indirect injury to the optic nerves and optic chiasm. *Neuroophthalmology* 1987;7:341–348.
10. Davidson M. The indirect traumatic optic atrophies. *Am J Ophthalmol* 1938;21:7–21.
11. Hartzell KN, Botek AA, Goldberg SH. Orbital fractures in women due to sexual assault and domestic violence. *Ophthalmology* 1996;103(6):953–957.
12. Pomeranz HD, Rizzo JF, Lessell S. Treatment of traumatic optic neuropathy. *Int Ophthalmol Clin* 1999;39(1):185–194.
13. Maniscalco JE, Habal MB. Microanatomy of the optic canal. *J Neurosurg* 1978;48(3):402–406.
14. Lang J. *Clinical Anatomy of the Nose, Nasal Cavity, and Paranasal Sinuses*. Stuttgart: Thieme Verlag, 1989;85–98:125–128.
15. Fujii K, Chambers SM, Rhoton AL Jr. Neurovascular relationships of the sphenoid sinus. A microsurgical study. *J Neurosurg* 1979;50(1):31–39.
16. Maniscalco JE, Habal MB. Microanatomy of the optic canal. *J Neurosurg* 1978;48(3):402–406.
17. Hager G, Gerhardt H-J, Maruniak M. Indications and results of operative exposure of traumatically damaged optic nerves (author's transl). *Klin Monatsbl Augenheilkd* 1975;167(4):515–526.
18. Crompton MR. Visual lesions in closed head injury. *Brain* 1970;93(4):785–792.
19. Farkas RH, Grosskreutz CL. Apoptosis, neuroprotection, and retinal ganglion cell death: An overview. *Int Ophthalmol Clin* 2001;41(1):111–130.
20. Schoepp D, Bockaert J, Sladeczek F. Pharmacological and functional characteristics of metabotropic excitatory amino acid receptors. *Trends Pharmacol Sci* 1990;11(12):508–515.
21. Sugiyama H, Ito I, Hirono C. A new type of glutamate receptor linked to inositol phospholipid metabolism. *Nature* 1987;325(6104):531–533.
22. Sofferman RA. Harris P. Mosher Award thesis. The recovery potential of the optic nerve. *Laryngoscope* 1995;105(7 Pt 3 Suppl 72):1–38.
23. Rajiniganth MG, Gupta AK, Gupta A, Bapuraj JR. Traumatic optic neuropathy: Visual outcome following combined therapy protocol. *Arch Otolaryngol Head Neck Surg* 2003;129(11):1203–1206.
24. Kountakis SE, Maillard AA, El-Harazi SM, Longhini L, Urso RG. Endoscopic optic nerve decompression for traumatic blindness. *Otolaryngol Head Neck Surg* 2000;123(1 Pt 1):34–37.
25. Levin LA, Beck RW, Joseph MP, Seiff S, Kraker R. The treatment of traumatic optic neuropathy: The International Optic Nerve Trauma Study. *Ophthalmology* 1999;106(7):1268–1277.
26. Lagreze WA. Neuro-ophthalmology of trauma. *Curr Opin Ophthalmol* 1998;9(6):33–9.
27. Gellrich NC, Zerfowski M, Eufinger H, Reinert S, Eysel UT. [Interdisciplinary diagnosis and therapy of traumatic optic nerve damage.] *Mund Kiefer Gesichtschir* 1998;2 Suppl 1:S107–112.
28. Guyon JJ, Brant–Zawadzki M, Seiff SR. CT demonstration of optic canal fractures. *Am J Roentgenol* 1984;143(5):1031–1034.
29. Seiff SR, Berger MS, Guyon J, Pitts LH. Computed tomographic evaluation of the optic canal in sudden traumatic blindness. *Am J Ophthalmol* 1984;98(6):751–755.
30. Jinkins JR. The optic neurogram: evaluation of CSF 'block' caused by compressive lesions at the optic canal. *Am J Neuroradiol* 1987;8(1):135–139.
31. Lessell S. Indirect optic nerve trauma. *Arch Ophthalmol* 1989;107(3):382–386.
32. Wolin MJ, Lavin PJ. Spontaneous visual recovery from traumatic optic neuropathy after blunt head injury. *Am J Ophthalmol* 1990;109(4):430–435.
33. Seiff SR. High dose corticosteroids for treatment of vision loss due to indirect injury to the optic nerve. *Ophthalmic Surg* 1990;21(6):389–395.
34. Anderson RL, Panje WR, Gross CE. Optic nerve blindness following blunt forehead trauma. *Ophthalmology* 1982; 89(5):445–455.

35. Bracken MB, Collins WF, Freeman DF, Shepard MJ, Wagner FW, Silten RM, Hellenbrand KG, Ransohoff J, Hunt WE, Perot PL Jr et al. Efficacy of methylprednisolone in acute spinal cord injury. *JAMA* 1984;251(1):45–52.

36. Bracken MB, Shepard MJ, Collins WF, Holford TR, Young W, Baskin DS, Eisenberg HM, Flamm E, Leo-Summers L, Maroon J, et al. A randomized, controlled trial of methylprednisolone or naloxone in the treatment of acute spinal-cord injury. Results of the Second National Acute Spinal Cord Injury Study. *N Engl J Med* 1990;322(20):1405–1411.

37. Bracken MB, Shepard MJ, Holford TR, Leo-Summers L, Aldrich EF, Fazl M, et al. Administration of methylprednisolone for 24 or 48 hours or tirilazad mesylate for 48 hours in the treatment of acute spinal cord injury. Results of the third national acute spinal cord injury randomized controlled trial. National acute spinal cord injury study. *JAMA* 1997;277(20):1597–1604.

38. Miller JD, Sakalas R, Ward JD, Young HF, Adams WE, Vries JK, Becker DP. Methylprednisolone treatment in patients with brain tumors. *Neurosurgery* 1977;1(2):114–117.

39. Hall ED. The neuroprotective pharmacology of methylprednisolone. *J Neurosurg* 1992;76(1):13–22.

40. Braughler JM, Hall ED, Means ED, Waters TR, Anderson DK. Evaluation of an intensive methylprednisolone sodium succinate dosing regimen in experimental spinal cord injury. *J Neurosurg* 1987;67(1):102–105.

41. Young W, Flamm ES. Effect of high-dose corticosteroid therapy on blood flow, evoked potentials, and extracellular calcium in experimental spinal injury. *J Neurosurg* 1982;57(5):667–673.

42. Young W. Bloodflow, metabolic and neurophysiologic mechanisms in spinal cord injury. In: *Central Nervous System Trauma Status Report*, Becker D, Povlishock JT (Eds). Rockville: National Institutes of Health, 1985;6373.

43. Stys PK. Anoxic and ischemic injury of myelinated axons in CNS white matter: From mechanistic concepts to therapeutics. *J Cereb Blood Flow Metab* 1998;18(1):2–25.

44. Sapolsky RM, Pulsinelli WA. Glucocorticoids potentiate ischemic injury to neurons: Therapeutic implications. *Science* 1985;229(4720):1397–1400.

45. Sapolsky RM. The physiological relevance of glucocorticoid endangerment of the hippocampus. *Ann NY Acad Sci* 1994;746:294–304; discussion 304–307.

46. Steinsapir KD, Goldberg RA, Sinha S, Hovda DA. Methylprednisolone exacerbates axonal loss following optic nerve trauma in rats. *Restor Neurol Neurosci* 2000;17(4):157–163.

47. Bracken MB, Holford TR. Effects of timing of methylprednisolone or naloxone administration on recovery of segmental and long-tract neurological function in NASCIS 2. *J Neurosurg* 1993;79(4):500–507.

48. Steinsapir KD, Seiff SR, Goldberg RA. Traumatic optic neuropathy: Where do we stand? *Ophthal Plast Reconstr Surg* 2002;18(3):232–234.

49. Hall ED, Braughler JM, McCall JM. Role of oxygen radicals in stroke: effects of the 21-aminosteroids (lazaroids). A novel class of antioxidants. *Prog Clin Biol Res* 1990;361:351–362.

50. Schmitt U, Sabel BA. MK–801 reduces retinal ganglion cell survival but improves visual performance after controlled optic nerve crush. *J Neurotrauma* 1996;13(12):791–800.

51. Yoles E, Muller S, Schwartz M. NMDA-receptor antagonist protects neurons from secondary degeneration after partial optic nerve crush. *J Neurotrauma* 1997;14(9):665–675.

52. Lubben B, Stoll W, Grenzebach U. Optic nerve decompression in the comatose and conscious patients after trauma. *Laryngoscope* 2001;111(2):320–328.

53. Kountakis SE, Maillard AA, Stiernberg CM. Optic neuritis secondary to sphenoethmoiditis: Surgical treatment. *Am J Otolaryngol* 1995;16(6):422–427.

54. Fukado Y. Results in 400 cases of surgical decompression of the optic nerve. *Mod Probl Ophthalmol* 1975;14:474–481.

55. Cook MW, Levin LA, Joseph MP, Pinczower EF. Traumatic optic neuropathy. A meta-analysis. *Arch Otolaryngol Head Neck Surg* 1996;122(4):389–392.

56. Levin LA, Joseph MP, Rizzo JF 3rd, Lessell S. Optic canal decompression in indirect optic nerve trauma. *Ophthalmology* 1994;101(3):566–569.

57. Li KK, Teknos TN, Lai A, Lauretano A, Terrell J, Joseph MP. Extracranial optic nerve decompression: A 10-year review of 92 patients. *J Craniofac Surg* 1999;10(5):454–459.

58. Maurer J, Hinni M, Mann W, Pfeiffer N. Optic nerve decompression in trauma and tumor patients. *Eur Arch Otorhinolaryngol* 1999;256(7):341–345.

59. Luxenberger W, Stammberger H, Jebeles JA, Walch C. Endoscopic optic nerve decompression: The Graz experience. *Laryngoscope* 1998;108(6):873–882.

60. Schroder M, Kolenda H, Loibnegger E, Muhlendyck H. Optic nerve damage following craniocerebral trauma. A critical analysis of trans-ethmoid decompression of the optic nerve. *Laryngorhinootologie* 1989;68(10):534–538.

61. Schmidbauer JM, Muller E, Hoh H, Robinson E. Early trans-sphenoid decompression in indirect traumatic optic neuropathy. *Head Neck Oncol* 1998;46(2):152–156.

62. Joseph MP, Lessell S, Rizzo J, Momose KJ. Extracranial optic nerve decompression for traumatic optic neuropathy. *Arch Ophthalmol* 1990;108(8):1091–1093.

63. Giraud BC, Bouzas EA, Lamas G, Soudant J. Visual improvement after transethmoid-sphenoid decompression in optic nerve injuries. *J Clin Neuroophthalmol* 1992;12(3):142–148.

64. Weymuller EA Jr. Blindness and LeFort III fractures. *Ann Otol Rhinol Laryngol* 1984;93(1 Pt 1):2–5.

65. Steinsapir KD, Goldberg RA. Traumatic optic neuropathy. *Surv Ophthalmol* 1994;38(6):487–518.

66. Levin LA, Beck RW, Joseph MP, Seiff S, Kraker R. The treatment of traumatic optic neuropathy: The International Optic Nerve Trauma Study. *Ophthalmology* 1999;106(7):1268–1277.

67. Soudant J, Lamas G, Girard B, Fougeront B, Guenon P. Post-traumatic decompression of the optic nerve. Ophthalmologic and x-ray computed tomographic evaluation. Results in a series of 23 cases. *Ann Otolaryngol Chir Cervicofac* 1990;107(5):299–303; discussion 303–304.

68. Pringle JH. Monocular blindness following diffuse violence to the skull: Its causation and treatment. *Br J Surg* 1916-17;4:373–385.

69. Dandy WE. Prechiasmal intracranial tumors of the optic nerves. *Am J Ophthalmol* 1922;12:169–188.

70. Takahashi R. Exposure of the optic canal. *Operation* 1951;5:300–302.

71. Niho S, Yasuda K, Sato T et al. Decompression of the optic canal by the transethmoidal route. *Am J Ophthalmol* 1961; 51:659–665.

72. Niho S, Niho M, Niho K. Decompression of the optic canal by the transethmoidal route and decompression of the superior orbital fissure. *Can J Ophthalmol* 1970;5(1):22–40.

73. Goldberg RA, Steinsapir KD. Extracranial optic canal decompression: indications and technique. *Ophthal Plast Reconstr Surg* 1996;12(3):163–170.

74. Kennerdell JS, Amsbaugh GA, Myers EN. Transantral-ethmoidal decompression of optic canal fracture. *Arch Ophthalmol* 1976;94(6):1040–1043.

75. Sofferman RA. An extracranial microsurgical approach to the optic nerve. *J Microsurg* 1979;1:195–202.

76. Sofferman RA. Sphenoethmoid approach to the optic nerve. *Laryngoscope* 1981;91(2):184–196.

77. Call NB. Decompression of the optic nerve in the optic canal. A transorbital approach. *Ophthal Plast Reconstr Surg* 1986; 2(3):133–137.

78. Knox BE, Gates GA, Berry SM. Optic nerve decompression via the lateral facial approach. *Laryngoscope* 1990; 100(5): 458–462.

79. Kountakis SE, Maillard AA, Urso R, Stiernberg CM. Endoscopic approach to traumatic visual loss. *Otolaryngol Head Neck Surg* 1997;116(6 Pt 1):652–655.

Midfacial Degloving Approach to the Nose, Sinuses, and Skull Base

Gady Har-El, Daniel M Zeitler

The procedure of midfacial degloving was first mentioned in the French literature in 1927. However, it was only in the mid 1970s when more detailed and systematic descriptions of the procedure began to appear in the plastic and otolaryngologic literature.[1–7] The procedure combines the principles of extensive sublabial sinus surgery with the surgical principles and maneuvers of cosmetic nasal procedures. The result is an open, wide exposure of the external and internal nose, all sinuses, orbits, nasopharynx, and anterior skull base. The midfacial degloving approach (MFD) does not require any external facial incisions.[2–17] We have used the MFD approach extensively for tumor management, most commonly performing wide medial maxillectomy for a variety of lesions, mainly inverted papilloma. Having gained experience with the MFD approach, we extended the histologic and the anatomic indications for this procedure. Currently, we use the MFD approach to manage different benign and malignant neoplasms, odontogenic lesions, vascular lesions, massive midfacial trauma, and penetrating trauma.[14–17] Anatomic regions that may be approached by MFD include the anterior skull base, frontal sinuses, sphenoid sinuses, clivus and pterygopalatine space.[14–17]

SURGICAL TECHNIQUE

The technique we currently use includes a few modifications of the techniques described in the literature. After induction of general anesthesia with an orotracheal tube in place, temporary tarsorrhaphy is performed. We use a fine 6-0 nylon suture which is passed through the conjunctival aspect of the edge of the eyelids. Placing the suture through the skin side of the eyelashes may cause inversion of the eyelashes with potential corneal trauma. Before tightening the sutures, eye ointment is placed on the cornea.

Extensive infiltration with a vasoconstrictive solution is advised. It will reduce bleeding and facilitate dissection and exposure. We use 30–40 ml of 1:200,000 epinephrine. We begin with a standard rhinoplasty infiltration through the intracartilaginous space on both sides. Through that space, we infiltrate the nasal bones, the midline, the glabella, the nasomaxillary grooves, and both medial canthal regions. Transcutaneous infiltration of the frontal bone as well as both medial orbital walls is also performed. This is followed by extensive sublabial infiltration as well as transoral greater palatine foramen injection on the involved side.

The procedure is begun with a complete transfixion incision which is connected at the dome with bilateral intercartilaginous incisions. This will allow complete separation of the nasal septum and the upper lateral cartilages from the lower lateral cartilages and the medial crurae (the columella). Through the intracartilaginous space, elevation of the soft tissue of the nasal dorsum is performed. In contrast to standard rhinoplasty, undermining is extensive and complete from the anterior wall of the maxillary sinus on one side to the anterior wall on the contralateral side. Undermining and elevation is also continued superiorly to the glabella and the frontal bone (Fig. 17.1). Then, the intercartilaginous incision is extended laterally and caudally, through the anterior aspect of the nasal floor, and connected to the caudal aspect of the transfixion incision. This will result in complete bilateral circumvestibular incision (Fig. 17.2).

The sublabial incision is usually made between the first molars, about 4 mm above the teeth (Fig. 17.3). However, the incision may be extended to the third molar on the involved side if lateral exposure is required or if ligation of the internal maxillary artery posterolateral to the maxillary tuberosity is planned. Using periosteal elevators, the soft tissues are elevated off the anterior

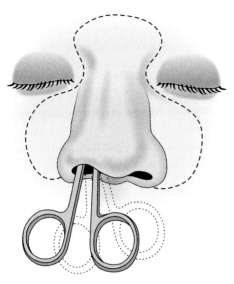

Fig. 17.1: Extensive elevation and undermining of the midfacial skin of the nose, maxilla, glabella and frontal bone

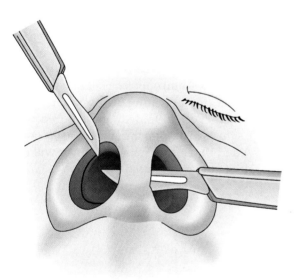

Fig. 17.2: Bilateral complete circumvestibular incisions

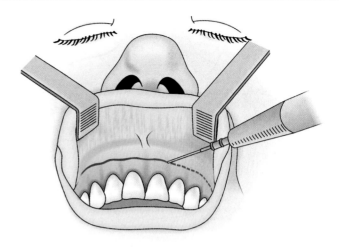

Fig. 17.3: Sublabial incision

maxillary wall on both sides. Elevation continues superiorly to the level of the orbital rim while identifying, protecting and preserving both infraorbital nerves. In the pyriform aperture region, the sublabial incision is connected with the intranasal incision. As elevation continues, the entire midfacial skin, including the lower lateral and medial crural cartilages, is separated from the maxilla and the nasal pyramid.

Complete elevation is performed from one zygomatic buttress to the contralateral one. In the midline, elevation

is continued superiorly at the glabella and both medial canthal regions. Dissection continues onto the frontal bone. Two Penrose rubber drains are placed through the nostrils and around the upper lip and are used to retract the midfacial flap superiorly. One of these drains should be released every 20–30 minutes to allow perfusion of the central lip.

The 'degloving' part of the procedure is now completed (Fig. 17.4). Additional surgical steps depend on the exact type and location of the lesion and the exposure desired. For example, if the procedure is performed for repair of midfacial and periorbital trauma, such as in the case of bilateral LeFort fractures, reduction and plating may be performed at this stage with good exposure of the alveolar ridge, maxillary bones, and the inferior, lateral and medial orbital rims, as well as the nasal and frontal bones. The medial aspect of the superior orbital rim can also be accessed through this exposure.

One of the most common procedures we performed through MFD is medial maxillectomy with ethmoidectomy. The procedure may be done for wide resection of a tumor, such as inverted papilloma, or for wide exposure of deeper structures. The procedure of medial maxillectomy is begun with removing the anterior wall of the maxillary sinus while preserving and protecting the infraorbital neurovascular bundle (Fig. 17.5). Anterior maxillary bone removal continues superomedially toward the ethmoid complex and superolaterally toward the zygomatic buttress.

There are different modifications for medial maxillectomy. The 'classic' one includes a complete en bloc resection of the lateral nasal wall, including the bone

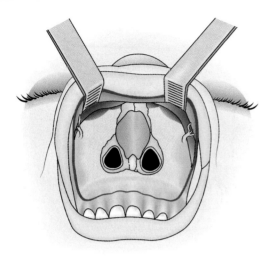

Fig. 17.4: The 'degloving' part is completed, exposing the nasal pyramid, pyriform apertures, infraorbital rims, orbits and glabella. Both infraorbital nerves are identified and protected throughout the procedure

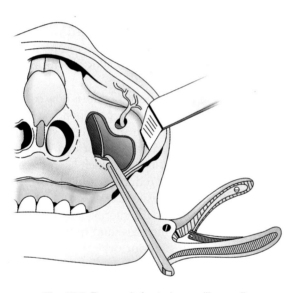

Fig. 17.5: Removal of anterior maxillary wall

at the lateral and superolateral aspects of the pyriform aperture, the medial 25–35% of the orbital floor and orbital rim, together with the lamina papyracea and the lacrimal fossa. A modification of this approach includes preservation of the inferior and medial orbital rim, as well as a rim of bone around the pyriform aperture.[10] The resection part of the procedure is performed deep to this preserved 'frame' of bone. With a third modification, a similar bony frame is removed and replaced at the end of the procedure using microplates to fix it to the alveolar ridge, orbital rim, and glabella.[8] Although the second and

third techniques were developed to achieve better cosmetic results, it is our opinion that these complicated and time-consuming maneuvers are not necessary as the final cosmetic result depends mainly on the preservation of the nasomaxillary angle by preservation of the nasal bone, alveolar bone, and 65–75% of the orbital rim. These structures are well preserved during the 'classic' medial maxillectomy.

Before starting the resection itself, the nasolacrimal sac/duct system (NLS) needs to be addressed. Different techniques of management of the NLS were described in the literature. They range from a simple transection at the orbital floor level without any reconstruction or stenting, to drilling the entire bone of the nasolacrimal canal and preservation of the entire length of the nasolacrimal duct with a cuff of nasal mucosa around its inferior meatal orifice. Some surgeons stent the NLS after any type of maxillectomy. We prefer to transect the duct at a level of about 10–15 mm distal to the periorbita. This is accomplished by first removing the anterior wall of the bony canal using a mastoid drill for 10–15 mm from the orbital rim (Fig. 17.6). The NLS is then elevated off its bony canal and transected distally with a No. 11 blade or a myringotomy knife. The NLS is then removed from the bony canal. Two, 3–4 mm opposing cuts are then made in the distal duct, thus creating two semicircular flaps which are then everted, folded, and sutured with 5-0 absorbable sutures to the proximal duct or to the periorbita (Figs 17.7A and B). This eversion maneuver will prevent stenosis. No stenting is required.

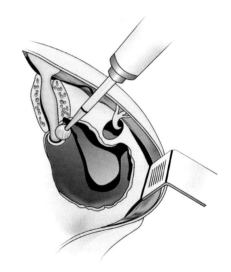

Fig. 17.6: The anterior wall of the nasolacrimal bony canal is removed with a mastoid drill

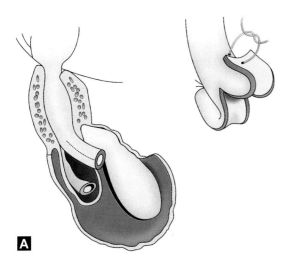
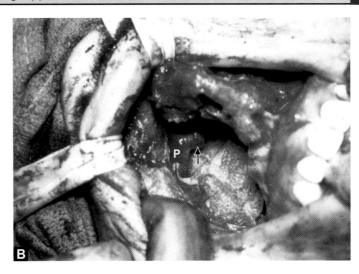

Figs 17.7A and B: (A) The NLS is transected distally and elevated off the bony cancel. Inset: Two distal semicircular flaps are everted, folded and sutured proximally. (B) Marsupialization of NLS (arrow) is completed. P: periorbita

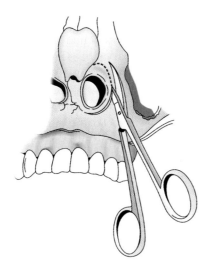
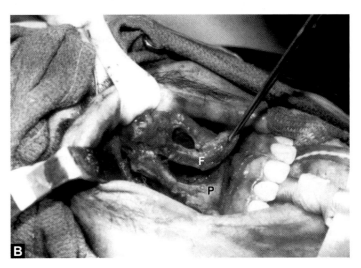

Figs 17.8A and B: (A) A bipedicled vestibular skin flap is created (Reprinted with permission from the American Journal of Rhinology[14]). (B) Bipedicled vestibular flap (F). P: Edge of bony pyriform aperture (Reprinted with permission from the American Journal of Rhinology[14])

The bone cuts for medial maxillectomy with ethmoidectomy are now performed. The procedure is done the same way it is done via lateral rhinotomy. Although we usually remove the entire anterior wall of the maxilla and the lateral wall of the nose including the edge of the pyriform aperture, we recommend leaving a 10–12 mm wide strip of inner nasal vestibular skin, caudal to the pyriform aperture edge. This bipedicled vestibular skin flap is created by making an incision at the pyriform aperture bony edge into the nose. It extends from the cranial aspect of the pyriform aperture at the junction with the upper lateral cartilage, along the pyriform aperture, to the floor of the nose (Figs 17.8A and B). At the end of the procedure, the edge of this bipedicled flap will be sutured to the cut edge of the circumvestibular incision.[9] In our experience, this is an excellent maneuver for prevention of postoperative nasal valve stenosis.[14–17] The following bony cuts are made for medial maxillectomy (Fig. 17.9): A cut along the nasal bone from the pyriform aperture to the glabella, a few millimeters anterior to the nasomaxillary groove; a horizontal cut just below the glabella directed posteriorly toward the frontoethmoid suture line; anterior-to-posterior cut along the frontoethmoid suture line or below and parallel to it. The posterior limit of this cut

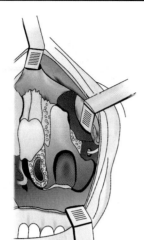

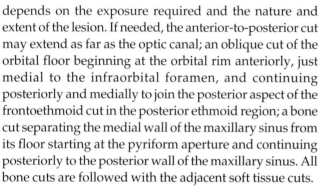

Fig. 17.9: Bone cuts for medical maxillectomy

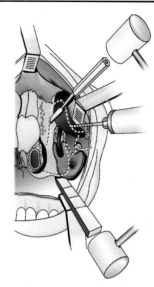

Fig. 17.10: Medial maxillectomy with ethmoidectomy is completed

depends on the exposure required and the nature and extent of the lesion. If needed, the anterior-to-posterior cut may extend as far as the optic canal; an oblique cut of the orbital floor beginning at the orbital rim anteriorly, just medial to the infraorbital foramen, and continuing posteriorly and medially to join the posterior aspect of the frontoethmoid cut in the posterior ethmoid region; a bone cut separating the medial wall of the maxillary sinus from its floor starting at the pyriform aperture and continuing posteriorly to the posterior wall of the maxillary sinus. All bone cuts are followed with the adjacent soft tissue cuts.

At this point, the specimen is almost free. It is still attached at the posterior aspect of the lateral nasal wall and the ascending process of the palatine bone. The posterior cut is now made with curved osteotomes and heavy curved scissors. The specimen is removed quickly and the bleeding sphenopalatine artery (within or as it exits from the sphenopalatine foramen) is clamped and ligated. If needed, the ascending process of the palatine bone is removed using an osteotome. This will require proximal control of the internal maxillary artery in the pterygopalatine space.

The classic medial maxillectomy with ethmoidectomy is now complete (Fig. 17.10). If additional exposure of other compartments is required, it may be now achieved through the wide exposure provided. The orbital contents are now widely exposed. The optic canal may be drilled out, and the optic nerve will be exposed throughout its length. Removal of the anterior wall of the sphenoid sinus will provide wide exposure to the cavernous carotid artery and the pituitary gland. The nasopharynx and the clivus may also be approached. The posterior aspect of the nasal cavity

and nasal septum as well as the nasopharyngeal aspect of the soft palate are also seen (Figs 17.11A to C). The pterygo-palatine fossa may be approached by removing the posterior wall of the maxillary sinus (Figs 17.12A and B). The posterior wall of the sinus may also be removed en bloc with the pterygoid plate to expose the skull base at the central aspect of the middle cranial fossa (foramen lacerum) and the medial aspect of the infratemporal fossa (foramen ovale). The roof of the ethmoid sinuses is well exposed, and if the middle turbinate is removed, the cribriform plate may be approached. This provides exposure of the anterior cranial base.

Some authors believe that the MFD does not provide a good approach to the frontal sinus.[4–6] Our experience is different.[14,15] The frontal outflow tract is easily identified anterior to the anterior ethmoid cells and the anterior ethmoid artery. Additional retraction of the midfacial flap on the ipsilateral side may be achieved by some release of the Penrose rubber drain on the contralateral side. More retraction may be achieved by transecting the medial canthal ligament and separating it from the medial orbital wall. With the use of Kerrison rongeurs, or a mastoid drill, the floor of the frontal sinus is removed from the frontal ostium, which is located at the posterior aspect of the sinus floor, in a posterior-to-anterior direction. With the same instruments, the anterior wall of the frontal sinus may be completely removed. This may also be extended super-olaterally above the orbit.

At the end of the procedure, the surgical cavity is packed with ½" iodoform gauze soaked with non-petrolatum based antibiotic ointment. The gauze is passed cranial to the bipedicled vestibular flap and brought out through

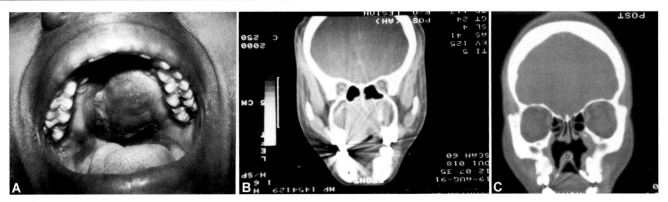

Figs 17.11A to C: Bilateral inverted papilloma with hard palate erosion. (A) Intraoral view. (B) Coronal CT scan. (C) CT scan 6 months after bilateral medial maxillectomy as well as septectomy and palatectomy via the MFD approach O:palatal obturator in place (Reprinted with permission from the American Journal of Rhinology[14])

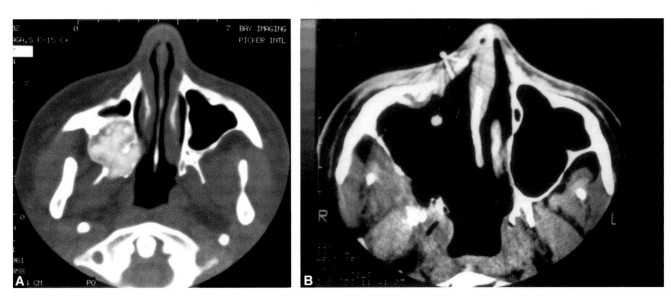

Figs 17.12A and B: Tumor of pterygopalatine fossa. (A) Preoperative axial CT scan (Reprinted with permission from the American Journal of Rhinology[14]). (B) Axial CT scan 3 months after posterior and medial maxillectomy with ethmoidectomy, sphenoidectomy and pterygopalatine dissection via the MFD approach

the nostril. All intranasal incisions are now meticulously closed with 4-0 absorbable sutures, carefully restoring the preoperative projection and rotation of the nose. The sublabial incision is closed with 3-0 absorbable sutures. A dorsal nasal splint, aluminum or thermoplastic, may be applied to reduce postoperative nasal edema. The packing is removed in 1–3 days and aggressive nasal irrigation is begun.

We have also been using the MFD approach to treat large juvenile angiofibroma.[16] The procedure includes medial maxillectomy followed by removal of the posterior maxillary sinus wall and the ascending process of the palatine bone. This provides excellent exposure to the pterygopalatine space and the infratemporal fossa (Figs 17.13A to E). The procedure is usually done 48 hours after embolization.

The MFD approach can be also used for anterior craniofacial resection for benign or malignant tumors of the anterior skull base.[17,18] The MFD approach can be either combined with a conventional frontal craniotomy or with the subcranial approach through the posterior wall of the frontal sinus and the anterior ethmoid complex.[17,18] With

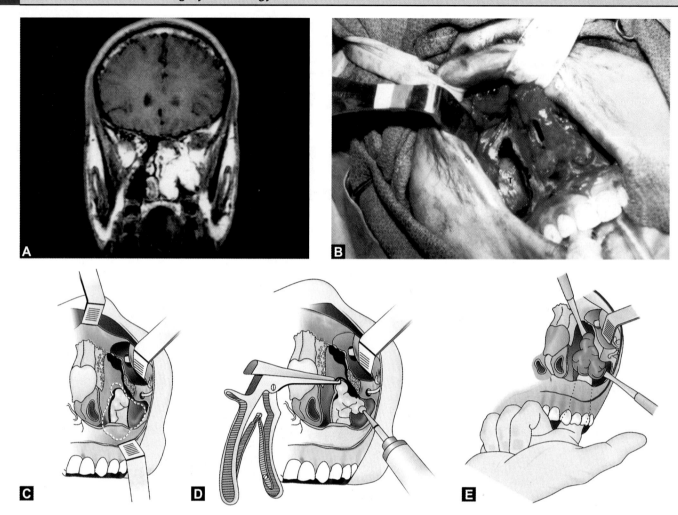

Figs 17.13A to E: Juvenile angiofibroma. (A) Preoperative coronal MR. Tumor in pterygopalatine space and nasopharynx with extensions to the sphenoid sinus and infratemporal fossa. (Reprinted with permission from Elsevier[16]). (B) MFD procedure is completed. The tumor (T) is seen bulging through the posterior wall of the maxillary sinus. (C) Tumor extensions to the pterygopalatine fossa, sphenoid sinus and oropharynx. (D) Bone removal to expose all tumor extensions. (E) Transmaxillary removal of tumor with transoral digital assistance

either approach, excellent exposure of the anterior skull base is provided while avoiding external facial incisions.

COMPLICATIONS

Only complications that are specifically related to the MFD approach are discussed. Temporary infraorbital anesthesia or hypesthesia is quite common, affecting 50–60% of the patients. It may be bilateral. However, almost all patients will completely recover midfacial sensation in 2–4 months. In our experience, the rate of permanent infraorbital anesthesia is less than 1%. Rarely, changes in the appearance of the nose will occur. Permanent epiphora occurs in less than 0.5%. In our experience, nasal valve stenosis occurred only before we began using the bipedicled skin flap. Today, with the routine use of this flap, symptomatic nasal valve stenosis occurs in 0.5% of our patients. In none of our patients were there any limitations on the exposure and or respectability of the lesion because the MFD approach was used.

REFERENCES

1. Carson PR, Bonanno PC, Converse JM. The midfacial degloving procedure. *Plast Reconstruct Surg* 1974;53:102–103.
2. Conley JJ, Price JC. Sublabial approach to the nasal and nasopharyngeal cavities. *Am J Surg* 1979;138:615–618.
3. Price JC. The midfacial degloving approach to the central skull Base. *ENT J* 1986;65:46–53.
4. Price JC. The midfacial degloving approach. In: *The Principles and Practice of Rhinology*, Goldman JL (Ed.) New York: Churchill Livingstone, 1987;615–638.

5. Price JC, Holliday MJ, Johns ME, Kennedy DW, Richtsmeier WJ, Mattox DE. The versatile midfacial degloving approach. *Laryngoscope* 1988;98:291–295.

6. Price JC, Koch WM. The midfacial degloving approach to the paranasal sinuses and skull base. In: *Surgery of the Paranasal Sinuses*. Blitzer A, Lawson W, Friedman WH. 2nd edn. Philadelphia: WB Saunders, 1991;309–315.

7. Maniglia AJ. Indications and techniques of midfacial degloving. *Arch Otolaryngol Head Neck Surg* 1986;112:750–752.

8. Draf W. Juvenile angiofibroma. In: *Surgery of Cranial Base Tumors*, Sekhar LN, Janecka IP (Eds). New York: Raven Press, 1993; 485–496.

9. Sachs ME, Conley JJ, Rabuzzi, DD, et al. Degloving approach for total excision of inverted papilloma. *Laryngoscope* 1984; 94:1595–1598.

10. Anand VK, Conley JJ. Sublabial surgical approach to the nasal cavity and paranasal sinuses. *Laryngoscope* 1983; 93:1483–1484.

11. Allen GW, Siegel GJ. The sublabial approach for extensive nasal and sinus resection. *Laryngoscope* 1981;91:1635–1640.

12. Howard DJ, Lund VJ. Surgical options in the management of nose and sinus neoplasia. Ch 20. In: *Tumors of the Upper Jaw*. Harrison DFN, Lund VJ (Eds). Edinburgh: Churchill Livingstone, 1993;329–335.

13. Nuss DW, Janecka IP. Surgery of the anterior and middle cranial base. In: *Otolaryngology*—Head and Neck Surgery, Cummings CW, (Eds) et al St. Louis: Mosby-Year Book, 1993;3300–3337.

14. Har-El G, Lucente FE. Midfacial degloving approach to the nose, sinuses and skull base. *Am J Rhinol* 1996;10:17–22.

15. Har-El G. Medical maxillectomy via midfacial degloving approach. *Oper Tech Otolaryngol Head Neck Surg* 1999;10: 82–86.

16. Har-El G. Management of juvenile angiofibroma via midfacial degloving with medial maxillectomy. *Oper Tech Otolaryngol Head Neck Surg* 1999;10:107–108.

17. Har-El G. Anterior craniofacial resection without facial skin incisions – A review. *Otolaryngol Head Neck Surg* 2004;130: 780–787.

18. Fliss DM, Zucker G, Amir A, Gatot A. The combined subcranial and midfacial degloving technique for tumor resection: Report of three cases. *J Oral Maxillofac Surg* 2000;58:106–110.

Robotics in Otolaryngology

Cherie-Ann O Nathan, Vinaya Chakradeo

While robots have been widely used in various industries for nearly 40 years, medical robots designed to support surgeons have existed for only a decade and a half. The pace of development of robotic assistance for surgery has been slow since safety is a primary consideration. Surgical robotics is a broad term that refers to the use of robotic technology in the operating room.

The term robot was first coined by the Czech author Kopek and is defined by the Robot Institute of USA as 'a programmable multifunction manipulator designed to move materials, parts, tools or specialized devices through variable programmed motions for performance of a variety of tasks'.

An increasing number of robot and robotic devices are in clinical use.[1] Current robotic technology had its genesis in the 1980s when researchers at the National Aeronautics and Space Administration (NASA) conceived the idea of a surgeon-controlled robotic hand piece.[2] The United States Department of Defense became interested in this technology because of its application in the battlefield, where a surgeon could operate on a wounded soldier from a remote location. This would protect the surgeon from danger while allowing life-saving measures to the soldier. That initial vision was put to use but not on the battlefield. Surgical robotic technology has seen its greatest growth and development in commercial systems, with its main application in minimally invasive surgical procedures.

ROBOTIC SURGERY

Robotic surgery implies the use of surgical robots for the performance of a surgical procedure. Surgical robots may be active, semiactive, and passive. An *active* robot can be programmed to perform an entire procedure without input

from the surgeon and can function independently during the performance of a task. No truly active robot has yet received Food and Drug Administration (FDA) approval. A *semiactive* robot requires input from the surgeon to carry out powered, directed activity. A *passive* robot does not have any powered movement but rather is completely controlled by the surgeon. These are more appropriately described as telemanipulators rather than robots.[3] Semiactive and passive robots currently function as an extension of minimally invasive surgery and are used to hold endoscopes and other instruments. FDA approval has been granted for semiactive and passive robots in minimally invasive cardiac and gastrointestinal surgery, general non-cardiac thoracoscopic surgical procedures—surgeries involving the lungs, esophagus, and the internal thoracic artery, and for radical prostatectomy.

Surgical Robotic Devices are best classified in terms of their current applications. The **Robodoc** (Integrated Surgical Systems, Sacramento, CA, USA) was the first clinically successful robotic device and is used in total hip replacement, to core out the femoral shaft to match the exact hip replacement prosthesis. It is the only commercially available true active robot and has been used in more than 5000 human total hip replacement procedures in Europe, but is not yet FDA approved.[3] The **Acrobot** (The Acrobot Company Ltd., London, UK), another active robot, has recently been developed for use in total knee replacement, and clinical trials to test its utility are in progress. The **Probot** is an active robot currently in development at the Imperial College of London and is designed to perform a transurethral resection of the prostate after registration with a transurethral ultrasound.[2,4]

Robotic surgery can also be classified as:

Telerobotic Surgery

This allows a surgeon to operate from a remote console with a virtual three-dimensional vision projection system, using robotically controlled instruments that reproduce surgical maneuvers.[5] This system provides depth perception, uses specially created articulating instruments that mimic the natural range of articulation of the human wrist, and maintains a stable camera platform. There were two telerobotic surgical systems that were commercially available. The da Vinci surgical system (Intuitive Surgical Co., Sunnyvale, CA, USA) and the Zeuss Robotic Surgical System (Computer Motion, Inc.) Recently, Computer Motion has been brought out by Intuitive as a result of which there has been support provided for the da Vinci surgical system. At our institution we have had experience with the Zeuss system, which uses the same principles as Da Vinci. These are also called telemanipulators or master/slave systems (Figs 18.1 to 18.3).

Both systems consist of a surgical workstation containing a three-dimensional imaging system at which the surgeon is seated. The Zeuss system evolved from Aesop and incorporates Aesop as the camera arm component of the Zeuss system. It consists of three arms: one arm holds the camera, and two arms hold the surgical instruments.

The da Vinci system was recently upgraded to include an additional operative arm, for a total of four arms. The learning curve for both systems is significant. The main difference between the two systems is in the workstation itself. Both these systems were designed to facilitate minimally invasive cardiac surgery, especially coronary artery bypass surgery. Both of them have been shown to be safe for closed chest coronary artery bypass grafting, and median sternotomy is avoided in most patients. These systems are also used in gastrointestinal surgery like laparoscopic cholecystectomy and laparoscopic Nissen fundoplication. The Zeuss system lagged behind due to limited FDA approval in gastrointestinal surgery in 2001. The da Vinci system is used to perform gastric bypass, colectomy, laparoscopic radical prostatectomy, and nephrectomy.

Telerobotic Video Assistance

The first robot for which FDA approval was granted was the automated endoscopic system for optimal positioning, or AESOP (Computer Motion, Inc., Goleta, CA, USA) in 1994. Initially, this was controlled by foot or hand controls, but newer versions are voice activated (Hermes

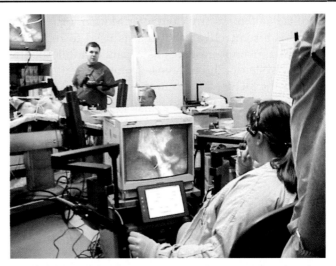

Fig. 18.1: The Zeuss system with robotic arms and workstation

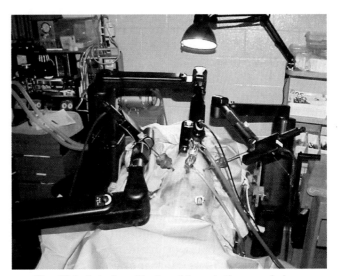

Fig. 18.2: Actual positioning of the robotic arms during a procedure

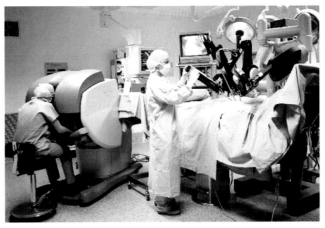

Fig. 18.3: Set-up for da Vinci system in the operating room

voice activation system; Computer Motion, Inc.). Thus, Aesop is a semiactive robot that is used to replace a surgical assistant or serves as a part of a telerobotic surgical system). Through voice commands, a surgeon controls the picture and position of the endoscope, thus allowing the surgeon to get a steadier operative image. The Endoassist (Armstrong Healthcare Ltd., High Wycombe, UK) is a newer modification of a robotic camera holder that moves in response to the surgeon's head movements and is currently being investigated.

Telepresence Robotic Surgery

It refers to the extension of telerobotic surgery to a remote site to allow a surgeon to receive a virtual image of the operative site and telecast their hand motions to a remote telerobot to perform a surgical procedure without ever physically encountering the patient. This technology was recently used to perform a laparoscopic cholecystectomy on a patient in Strasbourg, France, by a surgeon 3800 miles away in New York City.[6]

Telementoring

It is an extension of telepresence that allows dissemination of new techniques virtually anywhere by allowing a skilled surgeon to demonstrate or teach a technique to surgeons, in remote locations. In 2001, the FDA approved the Socrates Telecollaborative system (Computer Motion, Inc.) as the first robotic telemedicine device.[5] Socrates works in conjunction with Aesop, Hermes and Zeuss. The telementor is able to collaborate interactively with a surgeon in a remote operating room in real time, and can share the control of surgical robotic equipment (Aesop and Zeuss) in the operating room through voice activation.

Advantages and Disadvantages of a Robotic System

Robots are not going to replace surgeons, but they will provide assistance with increasing intelligence. They increase the accuracy and dexterity of the surgeon, reduce the tremor of the human hand and can amplify or reduce the movements and/or forces applied by the surgeon and improve ergonomics; they can help with hazardous removal from the environment, image- guided positioning and telecollaborative surgery.

Medical robots are built to be under human control rather than autonomous. Many levels of safeguard measures have been designed to prevent the robot moving outside its permitted safe area and to limit its

speed and force. Sensors are fitted to detect excessive contact pressure or undue proximity. Also an extensive level of self-checking is provided so that the robot monitors its own performance. Critical components are duplicated so that failure of one can be immediately detected. Another critical feature of success for medical robot is its user-friendliness. Thus, while validating a robot- assisted task, the key requirements considered are safety, accuracy, sterility, integration in the operating room, and measurable benefits (such as reduced operative time, reduced surgical trauma, and improved clinical outcomes).

Typical surgical tasks being robotized include instrument positioning and micropositioning, trajectory planning and precise needle insertion, free motion allowing the instrument to be arbitrarily positioned and oriented, motion in a constrained region, motion and force scaling, bone cutting, drilling, milling, shaping and soft tissue cutting and destruction.

Although robots have certain advantages, they are unable to match the human capability in large number of areas. The range and flexibility of the human hand greatly exceeds today's robotic manipulators. The mobility of the human body through one's legs and torso is another capability far beyond the reach of today's robotic technology. The sense of 'touch' received from our fingers (often called haptic feedback) comprises force feedback, as well as texture, viscosity, temperature and other characteristics that provide the surgeon with much information. The human visual processing that allows us to distinguish anatomy during a procedure greatly exceeds the capabilities of today's image processing computers. Finally, the human brain and the reasoning capability of a surgeon are far beyond the ability of today's computational algorithms and artificial intelligence technology.

ROBOTIC APPLICATION IN OTOLARYNGOLOGY

The number and the range of robotic applications in surgery are rapidly growing. Robots are used in neurosurgery, urology, orthopedics, general surgery and ophthalmology. But the use of robot in the field of otolaryngology is fairly recent. Only a few published studies that explore the use of robotics in surgical procedures. In 2002, we performed the first voice controlled robotic assist for endoscopic sinus surgery after perfecting the technique in cadavers.[7] In the same year, a robot was used for micropick fenestration of the stapes footplate, a difficult step in stapedotomy.[8] A quantitative improvement in performance during simulated ear surgery using robot assistance was shown. In 2003, the

Germans reported the first development of a functional robotic milling procedure for otoneurosurgery with forced-base control.[2] Their future plans include implementation of ultrasound based local navigation and performance of robotic mastoidectomy.

Endoscopic neck surgery has recently been described in both porcine and human cadaveric models as an alternative to conventional open surgical approaches for selective neck dissection and removal of submandibular and thyroid gland.[9-11] A telerobotic surgical system has been used successfully in a porcine model of endoscopic neck surgery and is the first report of the application of robotic surgery in the neck.[12] The da Vinci telerobotic system has also been used to assist in direct laryngoscopy and for excision of a vallecular cyst.[13]

We will now describe our experience with voice-controlled robotic assist (Aesop) for endoscopic sinus surgery (ESS).

The robotic arm automates the critical task of endoscope positioning, providing the surgeon with direct control over a smooth, precise and stable view of the surgical field. It mimics the human arm in form and function, with seven degrees of freedom, while never fatiguing or misinterpreting the surgeon's commands. The elimination of the need for manual stabilization of the scope permitted the use of both hands for the actual procedure. This resulted in the ability to use the suction at all times thus obtaining a clean operative field (Fig. 18.4). Another advantage was the ability of AESOP to store and return to a specific camera position. It also eliminates the fine tremor. This reduces eye fatigue, provides a steady field when passing instruments and can allow for positioning the scope closer to the target tissue with less collision. This eliminates the frequent need of cleaning the endoscope.

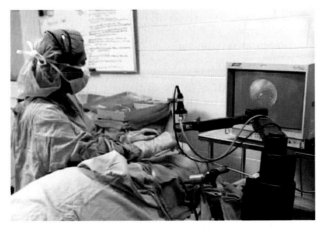

Fig. 18.4: Set-up of AESOP for functional endoscopic sinus surgery

More recently we have extended the above robotic application for the endoscopic approach to the pituitary.[14] The endoscopic endonasal approach to the sellar has gained popularity in recent times. However, the inherent difficulty with holding the endoscope thus having only one hand for the surgical procedure or the need for a second surgeon to hold the scope has hindered its widespread use by neurosurgeons. The voice-activated robotic scope holder is safe and has several advantages over the current scope holders. Its utility may result in reduced operative time and eliminates the need for a second surgeon to hold the scope. The above study was performed in cadavers and hence further studies need to be done to establish its effectiveness in a clinical setting.

Recently, the application of transoral robotic surgery (TORS) using da Vinci system has been described in animal, cadaver as well as on live human subjects. Weinstein et al[15] noted the benefits of TORS for laryngeal surgery in a canine model. Traditional microlaryngeal surgery is associated with certain disadvantages. Surgery is limited secondary to long working distance, two-dimensional visualization rather than three-dimensional and the need to maintain a straight line between the microscope and the surgical site. In transoral robotic laryngeal surgery, robotic arms were used to introduce one videoscope and two, 360°- rotating, 5 and 8 mm instruments in mongrel dogs. The surgeon performed the actual procedure from another suite. It provided excellent photography, controlled microdissection and increased manueuverability. Further studies need to be performed in human subjects.

O'Malley et al[16,17] have described use of TORS for base of tongue neoplasms. Over the past decade base of tongue tumors have been treated with primary radiation or chemoradiation secondary to significant morbidity from standard surgical approaches. The TORS avoids the need for mandibulotomy with lip split thus improving the functional and cosmetic outcome. The three-dimensional axes and 0° and 30° angles provided by the robotic arms enables the surgeon to perform en bloc resection with negative margins thus providing more benefits than laser microsurgery through a rigid laryngoscope. Robotic instrumentation offers hand tremor buffering and greater degree of movement, which improves the precision needed for oropharyngeal tumors. TORS might shift the paradigm of management of these tumors back to surgery avoiding the significant morbidity from chemoradiation.

CONCLUSION

Along with helping surgeons perform minimally invasive surgical tasks, robots have superhuman capabilities that make surgery easier. Robotic surgical systems can also improve depth perception, giving surgeons three-dimensional vision, compared with the two-dimensional vision they would normally get with endoscopic procedures. Robotics also offers motion scaling, which means that a surgeon's gross hand movements can be reduced to fine movements, allowing for accuracy in tight spaces. So far, there have not been indications that robotic surgery is any more risky than standard laparoscopic procedures. No patient injuries or deaths related to robotic system failures have been recorded. There is always a risk of technical difficulty when it comes to automated products. However there are fail-safe mechanisms that help protect against such problems. Studies of da Vinci indicate that surgery using the robotic device took about 50 minutes longer—nearly twice as long as with standard laparoscopic surgery. The increase in length of time is largely attributed to lack of experience with the new technology.

The FDA requires manufacturers to train surgeons before they can use robotic surgical systems on patients. Training involves having surgeons come to the company's headquarters and training at hospitals. The current robotic surgical systems are just the beginning of an exciting new era in surgical innovations. The products will likely evolve to correct their limitations. Often sight can compensate for touch, but force feedback remains an area that needs more attention.

The numerous benefits of robotic surgery namely accuracy, minimal invasiveness, novel surgical approaches and telepresence surgery deserve recognition and demand commitment for greater adoption on a global scale. The learning curve will be steep as it is with any newer and more advanced technology. Rigorous investment of time, effort and money to increase and perfect the uses of robotic surgery will reap immense rewards and blaze a new trial in the field of surgery.

REFERENCES

1. Gourin CG, Terris DJ. Surgical robotics in otolaryngology: Expanding the technology envelope. *Curr Opin Otolaryngol Head Neck Surg* 2004; 12(3):204–208.
2. Satava RM. Surgical robotics: the early chronicles: A personal historical perspective. *Surg Laparosc Endosc Percutan Tech* 2002; 12(1):6–16.
3. Federspil PA, Geisthoff UW, Henrich D, et al. Development of the first force-controlled robot for otoneurosurgery. *Laryngoscope* 2003; 113(3);465–471.
4. Guyton SW. Robotic surgery: The computer-enhanced control of surgical instruments. *Otolaryngol Clin North Am* 2002; 35(6):1303–1316.
5. Ballantyne GH. Robotic surgery, telerobotic surgery, telepresence, and telementoring. Review of early clinical results. *Surg Endosc* 2002; 16(10):1389–1402.
6. Marescaux J, Leroy J, Gagner M et al. Transatlantic robot-assisted telesurgery. *Nature* 2001; 413(6854):379–380.
7. Rothbaum DL, Roy J, Stoianovici D, Berkelman P, Hager GD, Taylor RH, Whitcomb LL, Francis HW, Niparko JK. Robot-assisted stapedotomy: Micropick fenestration of the stapes footplate. *Otolaryngol Head Neck Surg* 2002; 127(5):417–426.
8. Monfared A, Saenz Y, Terris DJ. Endoscopic resection of the submandibular gland in a porcine model. *Laryngoscope* 2002; 112(6):1089–1093.
9. Terris DJ, Monfared A, Thomas A, Kambham N, Saenz Y. Endoscopic selective neck dissection in a porcine model. *Arch Otolaryngol Head Neck Surg* 2003; 129(6):613–617.
10. Terris DJ, Haus BM, Gourin CG. Endoscopic neck surgery: Resection of the submandibular gland in a cadaver model. *Laryngoscope* 2004; 114(3):407–410.
11. Haus BM, Kambham N, Le D, Moll FM, Gourin C, Terris DJ. Surgical robotic applications in otolaryngology. *Laryngoscope* 2003; 113(7):1139–1144.
12. Nathan CO, Dixie L, Stucker F. Voice controlled robotic assist for endoscopic sinus surgery. *Otolaryngol Head Neck Surg* 2002; 127(2):57.
13. McLeod IK, Melder PC. Da Vinci robot-assisted excision of a vallecular cyst: A case report. *Ear Nose Throat J* 2005;84(3):170-172.
14. Nathan CO, Chakradeo V, Malhotra K et al. The voice-controlled Robotic Assist scope holder Aesop for the endoscopic approach to the sella. *Skull Base*. 2006;16(3):123–131.
15. Weinstein GS, O'malley BW Jr, Hockstein NG. Transoral robotic surgery: Supraglottic laryngectomy in a canine model. *Laryngoscope*. 2005; 115(7):1315-1319.
16. O'Malley BW Jr, Weinstein GS, Snyder W, Hockstein NG. Transoral robotic surgery (TORS) for base of tongue neoplasms. *Laryngoscope*. 2006; 116(8):1465-1472.
17. Hockstein NG, O'Malley BW Jr, Weinstein GS. Assessment of intraoperative safety in transoral robotic surgery. *Laryngoscope*. 2006; 116(2):165-168.

Image-guided Endoscopic Sinus Surgery

Todd T Kingdom, Richard R Orlandi

Image-guided surgery (IGS) of the paranasal sinuses has steadily grown as an important tool. In a relatively short period of time IGS has evolved from a novelty, with limited utility, into a technology with broad applications in the field of rhinology and minimally invasive skull-base surgery. As a result of this rapid advancement in technology many issues have surfaced which present challenges to the universal application of this technology. There remains a learning curve for the user to master, and decreased surgical complications and improved patient outcomes have yet to be clearly established. Moreover, the large capital investment required makes economic justification illusive and issues of 'standard of care' remain unresolved and acutely debated. Thus, despite the increasing availability of image guidance systems, the proper role of this new technology remains to be defined. Nonetheless, IGS of the sinuses and skull-base appears have become an important adjunctive tool and its future growth certain. The objective of this chapter is to review these issues as they pertain to the current and future use of IGS in the field of rhinology.

HISTORICAL PERSPECTIVE

The origin and evolution of IGS of the sinuses is rich and fascinating. Anon's Triologic Thesis published in 1998 provides an outstanding review for the interested reader.[1] A brief synopsis of the history of IGS follows.

The roots of IGS can be found in the field of stereotactic intracranial surgery. Work began in the early 1900s with the development of a stereotactic apparatus for neuro-surgical navigation. After the creation and refinement of stereotactic frames in the 1950s, stereotactic surgery was being performed throughout the world. The introduction of computed-tomography (CT) in the 1970s help facilitate a surge in the development of stereotactic techniques. Software development in the 1980s allowed for the marriage between CT data and stereotactic surgery which resulted in 3-dimensional surgical targeting. In the early 1990s the development of frameless stereotactic systems allowed probes and instruments to be tracked during procedures while CT or MRI images were displayed in relation to the target area. The first such systems, developed for neurosurgery, used mechanical arms to track pointers.

Interest in the use of image guidance systems in otolaryngology increased with the development of endoscopic sinus surgery and the development of frameless systems. The initial experiments using IGS in the field of rhinology were performed by a group of surgeons in Aachen, Germany in the late 1980s using a passive robot arm.[1] In 1993, the Aachen group published their experience using the technology in 212 rhinologic cases.[2] They concluded that IGS was useful for intra-operative orientation and they suggested a 2% reduction in complication rate could be expected. In 1994, Anon et al published the first report of computer-assisted endoscopic sinus surgery in the United States.[3] The Viewing Wand (ISG Technologies, Mississauga, Ontario, Canada) was used in 70 cases. The arm-based Viewing Wand had a sterilizable, detachable probe attached to a multijointed mechanical arm linked to an intraoperative computer with a high-resolution monitor. In 1995, Roth et al added to the US experience using the Viewing Wand in 12 cases.[4] Like Anon, they found accuracy to fall into the range of 2 mm and concluded the technology was generally useful. However, they did articulate several important deficiencies and outlined five goals that needed to be set in order for future systems to be adopted widely. Their stated goals were:

- Accuracy within 2–3 mm should be maintained.
- The requirement for a second CT should be eliminated.
- The computer should update for head movement.

- Suctions and dissection instruments should be tracked.
- The device must be easily operated by the surgeon in order to eliminate the technician.

By the late 1990s these goals had been reached through further advances in technology and clinical application. The refinement of optical-based and electromagnetic systems resulted in a growing surgical experience within rhinology. Several important publications then followed confirming accuracy, establishing utility, and outlining future development of these navigational systems.[5–8]

OVERVIEW OF CURRENT TECHNOLOGY

Simply stated, image guidance systems convert preoperative images, such as CT or MRI, into maps of the area of targeted surgery. The actual movements of the surgical instruments are tracked by the system and projected onto the preoperative image data set displayed on the system's monitor. This integration of data and computing technology provides precise surgical guidance to the surgeon.

System Components

An IGS system consists of a computer workstation, image-processing software, a display monitor, a localization system, and specialized instrumentation that can be tracked (Fig. 19.1).

Computer Workstation

The computer workstation and its operating software are the 'guts' of any navigational system. Current operating systems include UNIX-based and Windows-based systems. While the UNIX systems tend to be more powerful, Windows systems are perhaps more widely used in today's hospital environments. This fact combined with the lower costs associated with Windows-based platforms explains the increased use of this operating system in current system design.

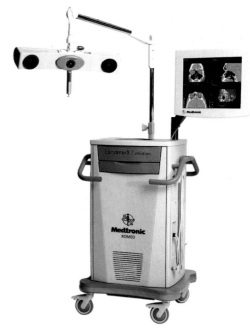

Fig. 19.1: The standard image-guided surgical system includes a computer workstation, display monitor, and tracking system. This tracking system is optical-based (LandmarX Evolution)

Display Monitor

IGS systems include a computer monitor to handle the output of the visual data. The data is typically displayed in multiplanar format with options of videoscopic feeds as well (Figs 19.2A to D).

Localization System

The localization unit uses preoperative CT or MRI data to provide the surgeon with a 'real-time' 3-D visual localization of the surgical instruments relative to the patient's anatomy during the image-guided procedure. Tracking systems can be optical, electromagnetic, or electromechanical. The majority of currently available systems for sinus surgery are optical-based with the exception of the InstaTrak system (GE Medical Systems, Lawrence, Massachusetts) which uses electromagnetic technology (Table 19.1).

Table 19.1: Summary of available image guidance systems in the United States (list is not exhaustive)

Digitizer	Product	Company	Registration method	Head-frame required in CT	Website
Optical	LandmarX	Medtronic	Anatomic fiducial Surface mapping	No	www.medtronic.com
	Vector Vision	BrainLab	Surfacing mapping	No	www.brainlab.com
	Stryker Navigation	Stryker Corporation	Anatomic fiducial Surface mapping	No	www.strykercorp.com
Electromagnetic	InstaTrak	GE Medical	Autoregistration	Yes	www.vitech.com

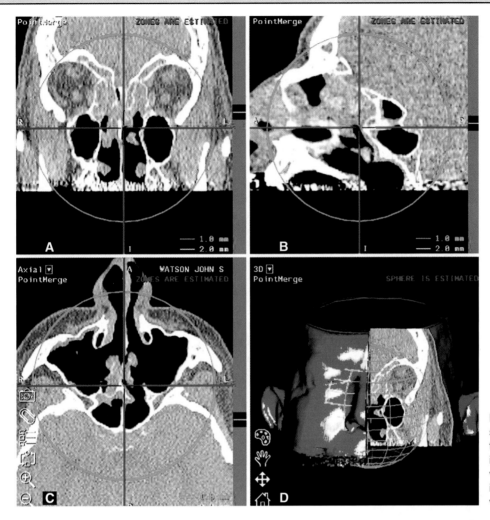

Figs 19.2A to D: Each image-guided system incorporates a display monitor to project the visual information. CT data is displayed in three planes with a fourth viewing quadrant available for various image manipulations or endoscopy video input

Optical tracking systems use infrared light for the tracking of surgical instruments. These systems include a camera with a view of the surgical field as well as optical sensors placed on the surgical instruments. In addition, optical sensors are placed on a reference frame or head-frame worn by the patient (Fig. 19.3). Active optical systems use a camera to track the position of the flashing infrared emitters (LEDs) attached to the instruments and head frame. This type of system requires either a cable connection to the instrument and head frame (LandmarX Evolution, Medtronic Xomed, Jacksonville, Florida) or the incorporation of batteries to power the LEDs (Stryker Navigation System, Stryker Corporation, Kalamazoo, Michigan). In passive optical tracking systems, the camera arrays track reflection of infrared light from reflective markers placed on the cordless instruments (LandmarX Evolution; Vector Vision, Brainlab, Germany). The key benefit of a passive system is the availability of cordless

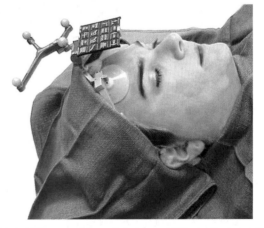

Fig. 19.3: With optical-based systems, LEDs (active) or reflective markers (passive) are placed on the reference frame which is worn by the patient during the surgical procedure. These reflective spheres are in a known geometric configuration and secured to the patient's head. The infrared light reflected by these points is then tracked, allowing the system to localize the patient's head throughout the procedure (LandmarX Evolution)

instrumentation. Regardless of the type of optical tacking system employed, line-of-sight must be maintained between the system components or navigation will be temporarily disrupted.

Electromagnetic tracking systems consist of a transmitter, located near the operative site, and a receiver, placed on the surgical instrument. This system uses radiofrequency electromagnetic sensors and relies on detection of variations within the electromagnetic field caused by instrument or patient movement. These systems are relatively inexpensive and do not require line-of-sight between the transmitter and the receiver. However, signal interference due to metallic objects in the operating field may be a disadvantage.

Electromechanical systems are in the form of a mechanical arm with multiple mechanical linkages and articulating joints between the instrument and a computer processor. Instrument tip location is computed by measuring angular rotations at these joints using special sensors. These systems are not widely used in sinus surgery because of their obtrusive design.

Surgical Instrumentation

A wide array of surgical instrumentation can be tracked by the majority of the currently available IGS systems. There are differences between the various vendors in instrumentation, but in most cases the differences are small and a vast degree of functionality is now available to the endoscopic surgeon. Options include straight and angled suction devices, forceps, straight and angled probes, and powered instrumentation such as microdebriders and drills (Figs 19.4A to C). Several systems have a universal tracking adapter device that can be attached to various rigid surgical instruments providing even greater flexibility in navigation.

Data Storage and Transfer

The radiologic data must be transferred from the radiology suite to the IGS system. Most systems support DICOM compatible data formats for data transfer via an Ethernet link. However, issues of incompatibility may arise depending on CT or MRI systems and software

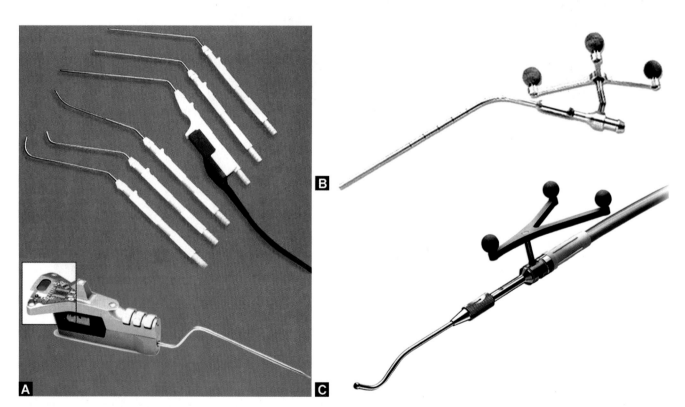

Figs 19.4A to C: A wide array of instruments are available with most systems for surgical navigation. (A) Several types of aspirators are available with the electromagnetic InstaTrak system. (B) Passive cordless IGS instruments are available with the LandmarX Evolution system. (C) Cordless, battery powered navigational pointers and suctions are available with the Stryker Navigational system

version used. A more common, and often more straight-forward option, is the use of portable media such as CD-ROM or optical disks.

THE REGISTRATION PROCESS

The registration process required to set-up IGS systems can be an intimidating and confusing element for many users. A comprehensive treatment of IGS registration is beyond the scope of this review, however, an overview with an emphasis on the clinically important highlights follows.

Registration is the process of matching preoperative image data (virtual) to the physical space occupied by the patient during surgery. The accurate correlation (matching) of these two data sets subsequently provides for localization of the surgical tools within the surgical volume of interest. A variety of registration strategies have been developed and are currently in use with today's systems. Perhaps the major limiting factor in accuracy of present navigational systems is the matching procedure that links the computer data to the anatomy of the patient on the operating table.[9] A key feature of this process is the method of selecting the registration points which will define the surgical volume for navigation. Generally, speaking two types of approaches are in use today. The use of 'intrinsic' markers includes anatomic points selected directly from the patient's anatomy (anatomic fiducial registration). 'Extrinsic' markers include skin-affixed fiducials, bone-anchored markers, and head-frame mounted reference points (autoregistration). A brief review of the various registration methods follows.[10]

Anatomic Fiducial Registration

Anatomic points are selected directly on the patient's head or face and may include the tragus, lateral canthus, nasion, and rhinion. The LandmarX Evolution (Point Merge) and Stryker systems use this registration strategy. The patient is not required to wear a special head-frame during the CT with this method.

Skin-affixed Fiducials

Radiopaque makers are attached to the patient's skin prior to the CT scan and must remain in place until registration is complete. This provides for an accurate and fast registration process but is impractical in the majority of elective sinus surgery cases.

Bone-anchored Fiducial Registration

Pins or screws can be inserted into the facial skeleton prior to the CT scan. Though very accurate, the invasive nature of this process makes it impractical for routine sinus procedures.

Autoregistration

Head-frame mounted fiducial makers may be used for registration. The InstaTrak uses this registration process. This requires a special head-frame that must be worn by the patient at the time of the CT and repositioned in the operating room at the time of surgery. These special head-frames provide a 'fixed' arrangement of registration markers relative to the patient's head (Fig. 19.5).

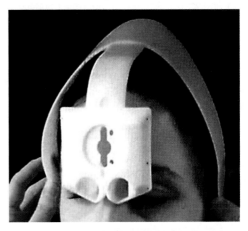

Fig. 19.5: Head-frame mounted fiducial markers may be used for autoregistration protocols with some systems. The device shown is the InstaTrak head-frame. This device must be worn by the patient at the time of the CT and re-positioned on the patient's head at the time of surgery in order to complete the autoregistration process

Surface Mapping Registration

A variation of anatomic fiducial registration, this process uses surface mapping strategies to define the contour of the patient's face. With this strategy multiple data points (50–400) are gathered in a relatively short period of time using a variety of available techniques. The LandmarX Evolution (Tracer) gathers multiple points rapidly by dragging the registration probe along the patient's face (Figs 19.6A and B). The Vector Vision (Z-Touch) unit uses a cordless laser registration probe to map the face and gather points (Figs 19.7A and B). The Stryker system offers an automated surface registration option (the Mask) using a battery powered disposable mask that is applied to the patient's face (Fig. 19.8). The Mask contains multiple active

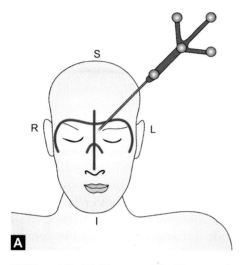

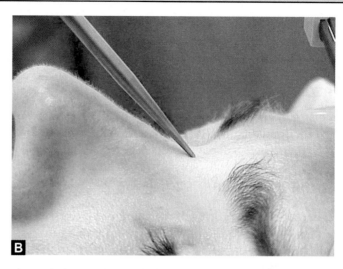

Figs 19.6A and B: (A) Diagram of the Tracer surface registration technique available with the LandmarX Evolution (Medtronic). The cordless probe is dragged along the patient's face rapidly collecting multiple anatomic points. (B) Demonstrating the use of the probe to gather points on the patient's face

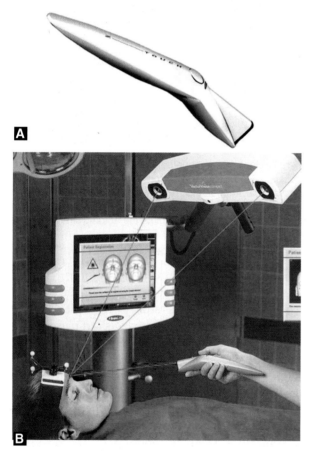

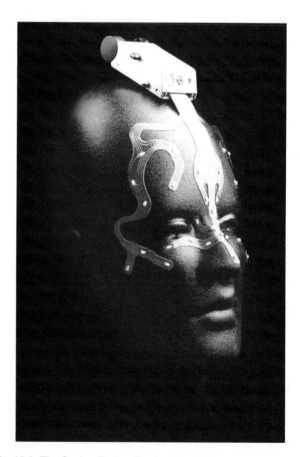

Figs 19.7A and B: Z-Touch (Vector Vision, BrainLab) is a cordless registration pointer used to gather anatomic points from the patient's face

Fig. 19.8: The Stryker Patient Registration Mask provides automatic registration using a battery powered disposable mask placed on the patient's face

LEDs that the system's infrared camera detects as part of the registration process. With all of these techniques the computer then matches the patient's facial contour to the preoperative image data set. These methods have proven efficient and accurate though they also add to the cost

The registration process is a major factor in the accuracy of IGS. Overall, these various registration methods have proven accurate and user-friendly to the surgeon and staff. However, a learning curve does exist and must be overcome before one is comfortable and proficient. This fact is not unique to any single system or method but a reality with all aspects of IGS.

ISSUES RELATED TO ACCURACY

Obviously, if the IGS systems are not accurate they are not useful. Perhaps the major limiting factor in the accuracy of IGS systems is the matching or registration strategy used. Other theoretical factors related to electromagnetic vs. optical tracking protocols or passive vs. active tracking methodologies may have an impact on navigational accuracy. Though still debated, most authors believe accuracy within 2 mm is sufficient for endoscopic paranasal sinus surgery.

Extensive clinical experience and multiple publications have confirmed the accuracy of the currently available systems. In 1997, Fried et al reviewed their experience using the InstaTrak system in 55 cases of endoscopic sinus surgery.[5] Registration accuracy was reported as 1.97 mm using anatomic fiducial registration and 2.28 mm using autoregistration (head-frame). A mean anatomic drift of 0.6 mm was estimated in the anterior-posterior plane during the procedures. In 2000, Metson et al reviewed their experience with the optical-based LandmarX system.[7] This review included 754 cases performed by 34 surgeons. The measured accuracy of anatomical localization at the start of surgery was reported to be 1.69 mm for this cohort. An earlier report by Metson et al found a mean anatomic drift of 0.89 mm in cases using both the InstaTrak and LandmarX systems.[8]

Based on the work by Claes et al the spatial distribution of the registration points chosen and their distance from the surgical site will influence the accuracy of navigation.[9] In general, the number of anatomic points used and their spread on the skull seem to be of significance.[7] Thus, the registration points should be nonlinear and should not lie in the same virtual plan. This concept suggests that matching strategies that use surfacing mapping or multiple widely distributed anatomic points will provide a more accurate registration than the head-frame mounted autoregistration protocols. Though a sound theoretical argument, this concept remains to be proven clinically. Other important factors that may impact on accuracy include head-frame displacement during surgery (anatomic drift), variations in the facial skeleton, skin laxity, head-frame positioning-repositioning (autoregistration), and CT image acqui-sition methodology (spiral vs. conventional).[9] Spiral CT techniques are faster, thus, reducing motion artifact. Sub-millimeter imaging is also possible, though not widely used currently, and may further help improve registration accuracy.[11, 27]

Despite the powerful technology built into these image guidance systems, there may be inaccuracies due to head-frame displacement, poor CT image acquisition, or unfavorable patient anatomy for registration: the surgeon must be aware of this. It is imperative at the beginning of the case, and throughout the procedure, that the surgeon verify accuracy 'visually'.[12] This means identifying intranasal landmarks and confirming that the endoscopic picture matches the multiplanar IGS view. This internal check takes priority over calculated accuracy figures generated by the system's operating system.

CURRENT USE AND CONCERNS

Although image-guided sinus surgery has the potential to improve safety and efficacy, the impact this technology has on current practice still remains ill-defined. It seems logical that complications would be reduced, management of disease become more 'complete', and patient outcomes improved. However, these assumptions currently are unproven and need further analysis. Adding to this area of controversy is the growing debate surrounding 'standard of care' and the role of IGS in elective sinus surgery. As a guide, the American Academy of Otolaryngology—Head and Neck Surgery has issued the following policy statement regarding the use of image guidance in surgery:

The American Academy of Otolaryngology—Head and Neck Surgery endorses the intraoperative use of computer-aided surgery in select cases to assist the surgeon in providing localization of anatomic structures.

These appropriate, specialty-specific, and surgically indicated procedural services should be reimbursed whether used by neurosurgeons or other qualified physicians regardless of the specialty.

Examples of indications in which use of computer aided surgery may be deemed appropriate include:

1. Revision sinus surgery.
2. Distorted sinus anatomy of development, post-operative, or traumatic origin.
3. Extensive sinonasal polyposis.
4. Pathology involving the frontal, posterior ethmoid and sphenoid sinuses.
5. Disease abutting the skull base, orbit, optic nerve or carotid artery.
6. CSF rhinorrhea or conditions where there is a skull-base defect.
7. Benign and malignant sinonasal neoplasms.

Source: http://www.entlink.net/practice/rules/image-guiding.cfm

While image guidance can be a powerful tool in endoscopic sinus surgery, it should be used with caution. Essentially, the major danger of this technology is over-reliance upon it. As previously noted, the accuracy of currently available systems is about 2 mm. While this is an impressive accomplishment of engineering, 2 mm is a large distance compared to the thickness of the lateral lamella of the cribriform plate or the thin bone covering the optic nerve. Image guidance must always be used as an anatomy-*confirming* device, not an anatomy-*seeking* device.

Many authors argue that image guidance makes endoscopic sinus surgery safer. It is probably more accurate to say that it can make the surgery safer. In his review of 34 surgeons performing 754 cases, Metson found that 'increased confidence during surgery' was cited as the major advantage of using an image guidance system.[7] When a surgeon well versed in sinus anatomy, in general, and in the individual patient's anatomy, in particular, uses this technology to confirm position within the sinuses then safety is probably enhanced. Conversely, when a surgeon who is not familiar with the anatomy relies on a tool with variable accuracy to tell him/her where to operate, safety may instead be compromised.

It has been stated that 'reliance upon anatomic landmarks and proper vigilance during dissection can never be replaced by a monitoring device.'[13] This statement was made in relation to facial nerve monitoring during otologic surgery, which in many ways is analogous to image guidance in sinus and skull-base surgery. The goals of facial nerve monitoring and image guidance nearly parallel one another (Table 19.2). Many experienced otologic surgeons use facial nerve monitoring in order to enhance the safety during mastoid and stapes procedures.[14] Nevertheless, it is also well accepted that while the monitoring device can be helpful, it is not infallible. The surgeon must primarily rely on knowledge and technique to safeguard the facial nerve, not the monitor. The same healthy mistrust is appropriate for image guidance in sinus surgery.

INDICATIONS FOR IMAGE-GUIDED SINUS SURGERY

Revision Sinus Surgery

Image guidance can confirm anatomical landmarks in the surgical field, especially with altered skull-base anatomy, either due to previous surgery, trauma, or anatomical variations. Aggressive resection of structures such as the middle turbinate can leave a smooth-walled ethmoid cavity where few if any landmarks exist. In these cases, persistent cells along the lamina papyracea, face of the sphenoid, or along the roof of the ethmoid sinus may be very difficult to identify. Image guidance can confirm identification of these cells and furthermore confirm opening of the ethmoid cells to their anatomic limits. Altered landmarks due to previous surgery remains one of the principal uses of image guidance.

Sphenoid and Posterior Ethmoid Surgery

Occasionally, it may be difficult to differentiate the sphenoid sinus from the posterior ethmoid cells. A number of anatomical descriptions have been presented to aid in the identification of the sphenoid sinus.[15,16]

Table 19.2: A comparison of the goals of facial nerve monitoring and image guidance	
Goals of facial nerve monitoring	*Goals of image guidance*
Early identification of the facial nerve	Early identification of the skull-base
Warning the surgeon of unexpected facial stimulation	Warning the surgeon of unexpected skull-base breach
Mapping course of facial nerve	Mapping course of skull-base
Reducing mechanical trauma to the facial nerve during tumor resection	Reducing mechanical trauma to the skull-base during tumor resection

Adapted from: Olds MJ, Rowan PT, Isaacson JE, Silverstein H. Facial nerve monitoring among graduates of the Ear Research Foundation. *Am J Otol* 1997;18(4):507–511.

Nevertheless, this area can present a challenge for a number of surgeons. Image guidance can confirm the position of the anterior face of the sphenoid sinus and, therefore, aid in the accomplishment of a sphenoidotomy.

Frontal Sinus Surgery

The intricate and variable anatomy of the frontal sinus drainage challenges even the most accomplished sinus surgeon. Due to the variability of the anatomy in this region, image guidance is often helpful even in the absence of previous surgery. In addition to these intraoperative advantages, the image guidance workstation can be used preoperatively to better understand each patient's individual anatomy. The surgeon can identify points of interest and then compare their relationships in all three anatomical planes. By scrolling through each plane, obliquely oriented pathways, like the frontal drainage, can be followed and thus better understood. This preoperative planning capability afforded by these IGS systems is one of the most important benefits of using this technology.

Extended Endoscopic Applications

The role of endoscopic techniques in nasal, sinus, and skull-base surgery continues to expand. As more areas at the borders and outside the borders of the sinuses are explored, image guidance can again assist in confirming this less familiar anatomy. Optic nerve decompression, pterygopalatine tumor resection, and lateral sphenoid encephalocele resection are examples where image guidance can be useful, if not nearly essential.

BALANCING COSTS AND BENEFITS

There are many substantial benefits that can result from the use of image guidance in endoscopic sinus and skull base surgery. By quickly and accurately confirming the surgeon's appreciation of the anatomy, this technology may shorten surgery time, allow for more thorough dissection within the sinuses, and potentially decrease complications due to inadvertent dissection beyond the confines of the surgical field. In addition to the confirmation of anatomy, the tri-planar display can greatly enhance the surgeon's understanding of the anatomy of the sinuses, particularly in the frontal recess. This advantage is true not just for residents and medical students but for experienced surgeons as well.

The many potential benefits of image guidance must be balanced by its real and potential drawbacks. The systems currently marketed are major capital expenditures and the degree to which third party payers will reimburse for this technology is not yet clear. There is a distinct 'learning curve' with the use of these devices, although they have become more 'user friendly.' Nevertheless, user inexperience may affect accuracy and may also lead to long set-up times. While this has been a major point of detractors of this technology, with very limited user experience the additional time for set-up rarely extends beyond 15 minutes for most systems.[7,12,17–19] It is likely that this additional time is easily offset by the time saved during the procedure that results from the rapid confirmation of anatomy. Gibbons et al reviewed their experience before and after the availability of image guidance at the University of Alabama.[20] In their retrospective analysis, they found the times of surgery for these two groups were in fact not different. They did, however, find a small (2.6%) increase in charges for patients who underwent image guidance. These charges were for a disposable headset and localization instruments as well as a hospital shared-resource fee. The study was performed prior to extension of CPT 61795 to include extracranial applications so that additional professional charges were not included in the analysis. Economic factors may vary considerably, as not all systems require disposable equipment, hospital fees vary, and professional charges may be charged. The reimbursement of these variable charges by third party payers brings another considerable level of variability so that the true economic impact of image guidance is difficult to assess.

It needs to be stressed that there is little objective data to truly assess not only the costs but also the benefits of image guidance. While there are many *potential* benefits, no data exist to confirm that there is a decrease in complications or improved patient outcome. Numerous studies have examined the risk of major complication (bleeding requiring transfusion, intracranial penetration, or visual injury) in endoscopic sinus surgery.[21–26] Taken as an aggregate, they show the risk of such a complication ranges from 0.1–0.25%. While obviously fortunate for the patient, this low-risk limits the researcher's likelihood of demonstrating an intervention's ability to change the complication rate. For example, we can assume that a 50% reduction in the complication rate would be clearly meaningful. Taking the higher complication rate (0.25%) and using widely accepted statistical cut-off values ($\alpha = 0.05$, $\beta = 0.20$), such a study would require about 32,000 patients in order to have sufficient power to show such a difference. In the absence of such a study, experts may offer opinions or clinical vignettes supporting the safety of image guidance but should not definitively draw any conclusions.

The limitations on objective data make balancing costs and benefits difficult. Nevertheless, the inability to measure a phenomenon does not disprove its existence. It is certainly the opinion of many experts that image guidance has great potential to enhance the safety and outcomes of endoscopic sinus surgery.[17,21] The authors share this belief as well. Metson's recent review of the first 1000 cases performed with image-guided technology by a group of 42 surgeons emphasizes many important points when one considers the implementation of this technology (Table 19.3).[28] Depending on the level of complexity in a particular practice, image guidance likely brings a significant benefit that is simply difficult to measure.

Table 19.3: Image-guided sinus surgery: Lessons learned from the first 1000 cases
1. Surgeons should start with relatively easy cases first when first learning to use an image-guidance system
2. Image-guidance systems are relatively accurate and reliable
3. The use of an image-guidance system is associated with increased operative time and expense
4. Image-guidance systems enhance surgeon confidence
5. Image-guidance systems are not meant for every surgeon
6. Image-guidance systems are not meant for every patient
7. The image-guidance system should not be used to make millimeter decisions about how to proceed during surgery
8. When information from the image-guidance system conflicts with your own judgment, trust your judgment
9. The effect of image-guidance on clinical outcome from sinus surgery is unknown
10. Technology is no substitute for technique

Source: Metson R. Image-guided sinus surgery: lesions learned from the first 1000 cases. *Otolaryngol Head Neck Surg* 2003;128: 8–13.

STANDARD OF CARE

'Is image guidance the standard of care?' This is a commonly asked and debated question. It has significant implications in that image guidance is an expensive technology that is available to many but certainly not all sinus surgeons. Moreover, its commonplace use may actually increase the risks of sinus surgery in inexperienced hands, as discussed above. The issue of standard of care therefore has medical as well as legal implications.

Each physician has a duty to comply with the standard of care:

A physician is required to exercise the same degree of learning, care, skill, and treatment ordinarily possessed and used by other qualified physicians in good standing practicing in the same medical field. The law does not require that the physician exercise the highest degree of care. It requires the physician to exercise the degree of care that other qualified physicians would ordinarily exercise under the same circumstance. (Model Utah Jury Instructions 6.1).

'Standard of care' is a legal term and therefore varies from jurisdiction to jurisdiction. Nevertheless, the example above demonstrates that the standard of care is a minimum acceptable level of quality of care and that providing care below this standard presents unacceptably high-risks to the patient. It is the level of care generally accepted by the medical community such that surgeons who cannot achieve this level of quality care should be excluded from providing care. Where there is no consensus among the medical community regarding a procedure or piece of equipment, the physician may or may not elect to utilize the procedure or equipment but there is no standard.

Examined in this light, it is clear that at this time image guidance is currently not the standard of care for routine sinus surgery. 'Will it become the standard in the future?' follows closely on the answer to the first question. Technology evolves rapidly and as it does so it may decrease in cost and become more universally available. As the technology becomes 'ordinarily possessed and used by other qualified physicians,' it will then become the standard. While this may and probably will occur in the not too distant future, it is not the case now for routine endoscopic sinus surgery.

The issue is not as clear for advanced techniques where the level of surgical skill, and probably technology, is usually higher. A good example of such a situation is endoscopic optic nerve decompression. In a sphenoid sinus which is not particularly well pneumatized, the impression of the optic nerve on the lateral wall can be difficult to see. In these cases its position may be difficult to differentiate from the internal carotid artery. Failure to differentiate between the two can lead to catastrophic consequences. Image guidance can be very helpful in this situation. Were an injury to occur in such a case and image guidance was not employed by the surgeon, the case may be less legally defensible. This would particularly be the case if the technology was available to the surgeon and not used or if it was available by referral to another surgeon in the community. This example demonstrates where image guidance is becoming the standard of care in advanced sinus procedures.

NEW APPLICATIONS AND FUTURE CONSIDERATIONS

Image-guided sinus surgery has firmly established its role as a valuable technology in the management of paranasal sinus disease. However, many questions regarding the optimal application and positioning of this powerful tool in today's clinical practice remain. With growing computing capabilities we can expect smaller, faster, easier to use, and more economical IGS options. Several smaller and more affordable IGS platforms are now available to meet some of these growing demands (iNAV from Medtronic, the Kolibri from BrainLab). This in turn may lead to a more widespread use of IGS as experience grows and these questions are answered. New uses for IGS are also being researched for cardiovascular, oncology, general surgery, ophthalmic, and dental applications. Tracking technology is evolving and soon it may be possible to track objects such as catheters or flexible endoscopes.

Evolution in the imaging technology has also begun to shape future development in this area. Fusion of CT and MRI images has proven promising in the operative approaches to soft tissue tumors and lesions in close proximity to major vessels. Termed CT-MRI fusion this technology is still in the early stages of application in paranasal sinus surgery.[29] Ultimately, the future will probably see a greater emphasis on the use of intra-operative real-time imaging to improve accuracy where structural changes may have taken place. Currently, MRI is the predominant intraoperative imaging modality available. Its application to endoscopic sinus surgery is severely limited due to costs and poor definition of bony anatomy.[30] However, the use of these intraoperative imaging technologies in endoscopic sinus surgery remains an exciting area for research and development. The era of computer-aided medicine has arrived and now includes robotics and surgical simulators. Exactly how these newer concepts will fit into the field of otolaryngology is unclear at this time, but we can expect a steady growth in our understanding and use of these technologies.

SUMMARY

Image-guided surgery has been established as an important adjunctive tool for rhinologic surgery. The technology has evolved since the middle of the last century and continues to do so at a rapidly increasing rate. A number of systems exist, each with its relative benefits and drawbacks. Image guidance can assist the endoscopic sinus surgeon by confirming position within challenging anatomical fields. Many issues remain, however, before the widespread application of this technology can be justified. Many advantages exist, yet significant limitations are also evident. Nonetheless, the role of image guidance in routine and advanced paranasal sinus surgery is certain to grow. Discussion and debate of the issues regarding the use of image guidance are likely to grow with it.

ACKNOWLEDGMENT

The authors wish to thank Bryon J Benevento, JD for his invaluable input regarding standard of care.

Financial Disclosures

Todd T Kingdom and Richard R Orlandi are consultants for Medtronic.

REFERENCES

1. Anon JB. Computer-aided endoscopic sinus surgery. *Laryngoscope* 1998; 108:949–961.
2. Mosges R, Klimek L. Computer-assisted surgery of the paranasal sinuses. *J Otolaryngol* 1994; 104:901–905.
3. Anon JB, Lipman SP, Oppenheim D, Halt RA. Computer-assisted endoscopic sinus surgery. *Laryngoscope* 1994;104: 901–905.
4. Roth M, Lanza DC, Zinreich J, Yousem D, Scanlan KA, Kennedy DW. Advantages and disadvantages of three-dimensional computed tomography intraoperative localization for functional endoscopic sinus surgery. *Laryngoscope* 1995; 105:1279–1286.
5. Fried MP, Kleefield J, Gopal H, Reardon E, Ho BT, Kuhn FA. Image-guided endoscopic surgery: Results of accuracy and performance in a multicenter clinical study using an electromagnetic tracking system. *Laryngoscope* 1997;107: 594–601.
6. Metson R, Gliklich RE, Cosenza M. A comparison of image guidance systems for sinus surgery. *Laryngoscope* 1998; 108:1164–1170.
7. Metson RB, Cosenza MJ, Cunningham MJ, Randolph GW. Physician experience with an optical based image guided system for sinus surgery. *Laryngoscope* 2000; 110:972–976.
8. Metson R, Cosenza M, Gliklich RE, Montgomery WW. The role of image-guidance systems for head and neck surgery. *Arch Otolaryngol Head Neck Surg* 1999; 125:1100–1104.
9. Claes J, Koekelkoren E, Wuyts FL, Claes GME, Van den Hauwe L, de Heying V. Accuracy of computer navigation in ear, nose, throat surgery: The influence of matching strategy. *Arch Otolaryngol Head Neck Surg* 2000; 126:1462–1466.

10. Citardi MJ. Computer-aided frontal sinus surgery. *Otolaryngol Clin North Am* 2001; 34(1):111–122.

11. Kalender WA, Polacin A, Suss C. A comparison of conventional and spiral CT: An experimental study on the detection of spherical lesions. *J Comp Assist Tomogr* 1994; 18:167–176.

12. Koele W, Stammberger H, Lackner A, Reittner P. Image guided surgery of paranasal sinuses and anterior skull base: Five years experience with the InstaTrak system. *Rhinology* 2002; 40:1–9.

13. Pensak ML, Willging JP, Keith RW. Intraoperative facial nerve monitoring in chronic ear surgery: A resident training experience. *Am J Otol* 1994; 15(1):108–110.

14. Olds MJ, Rowan PT, Isaacson JE, Silverstein H. Facial nerve monitoring among graduates of the Ear Research Foundation. *Am J Otol* 1997; 18(4):507–511.

15. Bolger WE, Keyes AS, Lanza DC. Use of the superior meatus and superior turbinate I the endoscopic approach to the sphenoid sinus. *Otolaryngol Head Neck Surg* 1999;120(3): 308–313.

16. Orlandi RR, Lanza DC, Bolger WE, Clerico DM, Kennedy DW. The forgotten turbinate: The role of the superior turbinate in endoscopic sinus surgery. *Am J Rhinol* 1999;13(4):251–259.

17. Fried MP, Moharir VM, Shin J, Taylor-Becker M, Morrison P. Comparison of endoscopic sinus surgery with and without image guidance. *Am J Rhinol* 2002;16:193–197.

18. Caversaccio M, Nolte LP, Hausler R. Present state and future perspectives of computer aided surgery in the field of ENT and skull base. *Acta Oto-Rhino-Laryngolica Belg* 2002;56:51–59.

19. Reardon EJ. Navigational risks associated with sinus surgery and the clinical effects of implementing a navigational system for sinus surgery. *Laryngoscope* 2002;112:1–19.

20. Gibbons MD, Gunn CG, Niwas S, Sillers MJ. Cost analysis of computer-aided endoscopic sinus surgery. *Am J Rhinol* 2001; 15(2):71–75.

21. Keerl R, Stankiewicz J, Weber R, Hosemann W, Draf W. Surgical experience and complications during endonasal sinus surgery. *Laryngoscope* 1999;109(4):546–550.

22. Nguyen QA, Cua DJ, Ng M, Rice DH. Safety of endoscopic sinus surgery in a residency training program. *Ear Nose Throat J* 1999;78(12):898–904.

23. Gross RD, Sheridan MF, Burgess LP. Endoscopic sinus surgery complications in residency. *Laryngoscope* 1997; 107(8): 1080–1085.

24. Marks SC. Learning curve in endoscopic sinus surgery. *Otolaryngol Head Neck Surg* 1999;120(2):215–218.

25. Ramadan HH, Allen GC. Complications of endoscopic sinus surgery in a residency training program. *Laryngoscope* 1995; 105(4):376–379.

26. Kinsella JB, Calhoun KH, Bradfield JJ, Hokanson JA, Bailey BJ. Complications of endoscopic sinus surgery in a residency training program. *Laryngoscope* 1995;105(10):1029–1032.

27. Chiu A, Vaughan WC. Revision endoscopic frontal sinus surgery with surgical navigation. *Otolaryngol Head Neck Surg* 2004;130:312–318.

28. Metson R. Image-guided sinus surgery: Lessons learned from the first 1000 cases. *Otolaryngol Head Neck Surg* 2003;128:8–13.

29. Cohen NA, Kennedy DW. Endoscopic sinus surgery: Where we are and where we're going. *Curr Opin Otolaryngol Head Neck Surg* 2005;13:32–38.

30. Fried MP et al. Endoscopic sinus surgery with magnetic resosance imaging guidance: Initial experience. *Otolaryngol Head Neck Surg* 1998;119:374–380.

Powered Instrumentation in Endoscopic Sinus Surgery

Jonathan M Owens, Todd T Kingdom

The use of powered debriding instrumentation in otolaryngology dates to the 1960s, when the House-Urban dissector was introduced for use in vestibular schwannoma surgery. This instrument featured a rotating inner blade housed in a stationary sheath, effecting a guillotine-like cutting mechanism; debrided material was suctioned down the hollow blade.[1,2] Similar equipment was incorporated into arthroscopic and temporomandibular joint surgery in the succeeding decades. Each of these applications of powered dissectors involved a fluid-filled field and involved the cutting of soft tissue and rarely any bone.

The introduction of powered instrumentation to rhinology is credited to Setliff and Parsons, who described the use of the Hummer (Stryker Corporation, Kalamazoo, Michigan) device for polypectomy in 1994.[1] Setliff and Parsons noted the utility of the device which allowed for precise tissue dissection while providing continuous suction, thus avoiding the 'grab and tear' technique. The Hummer device originated as an arthoscopic shaver and lacked irrigation. Plugging of the unlubricated blade by the dry tissues of the nasal and sinus cavities was clearly a drawback of this device. The suction line in this handpiece required two 90° turns, as the motor was in-line with the blade. This design reduced the efficiency of the suction the device was able to deliver. Straight and curved blades were available for this instrument; however, the radius of curved blades was approximately 6–7 cm, prohibitively long for many rhinologic applications.

Medtronic (Jacksonville, Florida) introduced its first rhinologic powered debrider, the Wizard, in 1994. This instrument has been followed by several other iterations, including the Straightshot, Straightshot Magnum, Straightshot II, Straightshot II Magnum, and, most recently, the Straightshot M4 (Figs 20.1A and B).

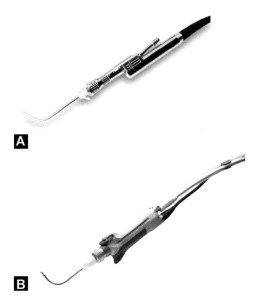

Figs 20.1A and B: Straighshot II. (A) and Straightshot M4. (B) microdebrider handpiece designs marketed by Medtronic-Xomed (Jacksonville, FL). The newer model M4 features a more ergonomically designed handpiece as well as a rotatable blade tip. (*Courtesy*: Medtronic-Xomed)

Innovations introduced in these handpieces have included gravity and pump irrigation, straight-through suction, short radius curved blades, and rotating blade heads. A variety of cutting blades and drill burs are available for this system, with varying angles and diameters to meet most rhinologic applications.

The Diego microdebrider was introduced by Gyrus ENT (Memphis, Tennessee) in 2002. This device incorporates a pistol-grip style ergonomic handpiece as well as a revolving nosecone which allows the entire blade to be turned with the fingertips (Fig. 20.2). The handpiece was designed to be a low-profile, light device and houses the motor in the pistol-grip. The suction and

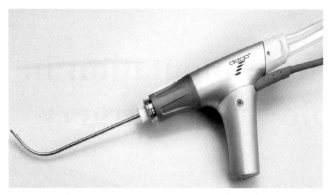

Fig. 20.2: Diego microdebrider handpiece marketed by Gyrus ENT (Memphis, Tennessee) which features an ergonomic design, rotatable blade and nosecone, and true in-line suction (*Courtesy:* Gyrus ENT)

irrigation tubing connects as a single housing to the back end of device, removing the irrigation component from the blade and allowing more rapid blade exchange. The device also has a wide assortment of blades and burs, with application not only in rhinology but also in laryngology and adenoidectomy.

ENGINEERING AND DESIGN CONSIDERATIONS

The basic components of contemporary microdebrider systems include a power source, a handpiece, interchangeable blades, an irrigation system, and a suction source. The microdebrider handpiece has evolved significantly since the Hummer was introduced. Initial products incorporated the motor directly in-line with the blade, necessitating the suction line to curve around the periphery. This created significant issues with efficiency of suction and clogging, as the suction line was forced to turn 90° twice. Later handpiece designs featured more eccentric motor placement, allowing a direct suction path and consequently less clogging. This placement of the motor also allowed the creation of more ergonomic handpieces, with current models being configured in a pistol-grip arrangement while prior versions were linear or resembled bayonet forceps.

The basic design of microdebrider blades incorporates a static, blunt outer sheath with a lateral fenestration and a mobile inner blade which possesses cutting edges which oppose the fenestration (Figs 20.3A and B). The smooth surface and blunt tip of the outer sheath prevents damage to surrounding tissue, allowing meticulous dissection of only the tissue which is suctioned into the fenestration and cutting blade. This design feature eliminates avulsion of adjacent tissue, which can be common when using more traditional instrumentation.

The edges of the sheath fenestration may be serrated, which facilitate soft tissue cutting, or smooth. Several factors guide design of debrider blades. The size difference between the inner and outer components must be sufficiently small (0.05 mm) to allow close approximation of the cutting edge and the fenestration for efficient cutting. The shape of the fenestration is also critical in determining the efficiency of the blade. A square configuration of the fenestration coupled with a straight cutting blade produces a guillotine cutting motion. This is less efficient than the scissors cutting motion afforded by an angled fenestration, allowing cutting along the entire stroke of the cutting blade[3] (Figs 20.3A and B).

The addition of irrigation systems to powered dissection devices is unique to sinus equipment versus

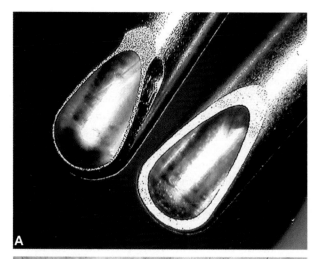

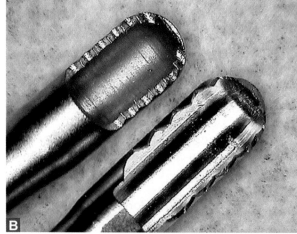

Figs 20.3A and B: Microdebrider blade design. (A) Smooth-edged fenestration window with angled (scissor-type) configuration. (B) Serrated fenestration window which allows greater cutting ability

arthroscopic equipment. The application of the arthroscopic technology requires a fluid-filled space in contrast to the air-filled cavities of the paranasal sinuses. Thus, it quickly became evident that lubrication of the oscillating blade was a requirement for optimal use in the sinuses. The first irrigation systems introduced were simple gravity-fed lines introduced through a separate irrigation port on the blade sheath. Subsequent versions featured powered infusion pumps which deliver a metered flow of irrigation fluid to the handpiece when power is applied. The flow rate is adjustable to suit the preference of the surgeon (Fig. 20.4). While anecdotal evidence strongly suggests these innovations have decreased device clogging, no data to support this notion have been published.

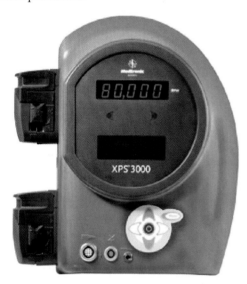

Fig. 20.4: Medtronic-Xomed XPS 3000 power unit which coordinates blade speed and direction as well as irrigation pump functions. Surgeon-controlled foot pedal plugs directly into the face of this unit (*Courtesy*: Medtronic-Xomed)

Suction is an integral component of the microdebrider system, serving to remove cut tissue and bone as well as irrigating fluid and blood from the operative field. A malfunctioning or clogged suction apparatus cripples the entire microdebrider system. Several iterations of suction design have been incorporated in handpiece design, with varying degrees of successful function. As noted previously, early devices such as the Hummer included a sideport, with the suction tubing connecting to the handpiece perpendicular to the long axis of the cutting blade. Experience dictated that the circuitous route of debris suctioned away from the field led to significant clogging and subsequent lost operative time to clean the

device. More recent designs have incorporated linear suction paths, such that suctioned debris travel in a straight line to the suction tubing, thereby reducing the opportunity for clogging. Another important design modification addressing the plugging issue was the optimization of blade speed. If the blade oscillation speed is too slow, too much tissue will be pulled into the blade and cut in each motion and plugging is more likely to occur. Conversely, too rapid a blade speed does not allow tissue to be suctioned into the cutting mechanism. Thus, a balance must be reached between efficiency of tissue removal and the ability to remove excised fragments from the blade.

APPLICATION OF POWERED INSTRUMENTATION

It is clear that the evolution and subsequent application of powered instrumentation in endoscopic sinus surgery (ESS) has been widely accepted. This tool has expanded the rhinologist's ability to efficiently manage many conditions encountered in the sinuses. Though powerful, the application of powered instrumentation in rhinologic surgery must be measured as significant complications and poor outcomes are possible. This technology is not a replacement for sound endoscopic surgical training and mastery of the more traditional techniques. An overview of the current applications and uses of powered instrumentation in ESS is as follows.

Polypectomy

Polypectomy was the initial rhinologic application of the microdebrider described by Setliff and Parsons, and continues to be an important use for this equipment.[1,4] This instrumentation offers the advantages of pinpoint dissection of polypoid tissue, relatively low blood loss, removal of tissue from the field via suction, and less trauma to surrounding tissue than with avulsive techniques. Furthermore, polypoid tissue in areas poorly accessible to standard instrumentation such as the floor of the maxillary sinus may be accessed with curved blades currently available. It is safe to say that the nasal polypectomy is perhaps the most common routine application of powered instrumentation in rhinologic surgery.

Maxillary Antrostomy and Sphenoethmoidectomy

As the use of microdebriders for polyposis became common, the scope of applications of the technology expanded to encompass other aspects of ESS. The meticulous soft-tissue dissection afforded by the instruments was soon found to be useful in maxillary antrostomy, ethmoidectomy, frontal recess dissection, and sphenoidotomy.[5] As with polyposis, the continuous removal of tissue and blood from the field by the microdebrider allows the surgeon to operate without removing the instrument from the nose. In addition, various blade design modifications enhanced to surgeon's control during tissue removal.

Removal of the uncinate is typically the first step in maxillary sinus surgery and multiple techniques have been described.[6] Use of a microdebrider for removal of the uncinate has been described and proven to be an efficient technique. Angled blade have been developed for this purpose and include 12° and 40° designs. In conjunction with angled endoscopes, the ostium may be debrided of polypoid tissue or widened as appropriate with curved cutting blades. Newer blade designs (90° and 120°) allow for access to the inferior and lateral reaches of the antrum in select cases (Figs 20.5A and B).

Similarly, an ethmoidectomy and sphenoidotomy can be performed using powered instrumentation. Dissection of diseased tissue without stripping adjacent normal

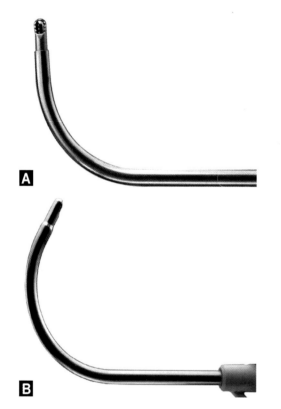

Figs 20.5A and B: Advances in curved blade design have allowed development of 90°. (A) and 120°. (B) blades which facilitate removal of tissue in the maxillary sinus (*Courtesy*: Medtronic-Xomed)

mucosa is a major advantage of this technique for each of these applications. In most, but not all, situations this technology is sufficient to remove the thin partitions of the ethmoid labyrinth as well thus adding further efficiency. One concern, however, is that tactile feedback afforded by standard instrumentation while dissecting in these areas may be lessened when using powered instrumentation. Complications (discussed later) are often devastating with powered instrumentation is involved. Furthermore, the ease of dissection afforded by powered instruments mandates that the surgeon be cognizant of the functional aspects of the endoscopic procedure and avoid unnecessarily excessive tissue removal.

Inferior Turbinate Reduction

Another rhinologic application of powered instrumentation is submucous resection of inferior turbinates. Inferior turbinate hypertrophy is a commonly encountered clinical phenomenon which is often treated surgically when medical treatments fail. Numerous procedures have been advocated for treatment of hypertrophic inferior turbinates, including turbinectomy, submucous turbinectomy, partial resection of the inferior turbinates, inferior turbinoplasty, cryotherapy, electrosurgery, CO_2 laser turbinoplasty, and radiofrequency ablation.[7] Each surgical technique has merits and shortcomings, particularly bleeding and atrophic rhinitis. Experience has dictated that preservation of turbinate mucosa may limit these complications.

The development of specific inferior turbinate microdebrider blades facilitated the application of the technology to submucous resection of inferior turbinates. This technique was first described by Friedman et al, who reported their experience in 120 patients. Friedman's technique involved injection of the inferior turbinates and sphenopalatine ganglion with lidocaine with epinephrine.[8] With operative endoscopy, a vertical incision is made in the anterior aspect of the inferior turbinate and a sharp elevator used to create a submucosal pocket. The microdebrider blade is then inserted into this pocket with the cutting blade facing laterally, away from the mucosal flap. The submucosal erectile tissue and turbinate bone are then debrided with the device. Hwang recommends that the cutting blade face the mucosal surface to maximize resection of soft tissue.[7] He also emphasizes more aggressive dissection anteriorly, where the anterior aspect of the inferior turbinate and lateral nasal wall at the insertion of the bony turbinate contribute significantly to the nasal valve (Figs 6A and B).

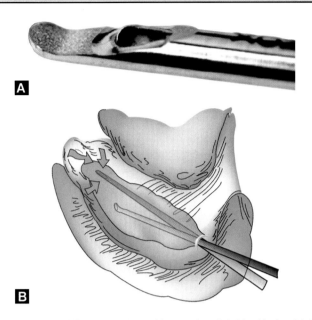

Figs 20.6A and B: (A) Inferior turbinate microdebrider blade which features a broad leading edge which protects overlying mucosa from the cutting blade. (B) Illustration of the inferior turbinate submucosal dissection technique in which the microdebrider blade is inserted into the anterior portion of the turbinate and several passes of the blade are performed between the turbinate bone and overlying mucosa

Friedman et al reported a decrease in size in each turbinate treated in this manner. Two patients (1.6%) experienced bleeding requiring a return to the operating room. Mucosal tears were noted in 55% of patients; none experienced mucosal loss. Postoperatively, no patients noted crusting or dryness, while 5% experienced synechia to the nasal septum.[8] While not providing data, Hwang noted that crusting may temporarily occur when flap tears complicate dissection.[7]

The advantages of submucous resection of inferior turbinate include perservation of mucosa, controlled volume reduction under direct visualization, and meticulous dissection of specific areas of hypertrophy. Disadvantages cited by authors include the risks of bleeding, mucosal tear, and adverse scarring. This is the technique preferred by the senior author (Kingdom).

Frontal Sinus Surgery

The surgical management of chronic frontal sinusitis remains one of the most difficult challenges facing rhinologists. Advances in surgical instrumentation and imaging technology have permitted successful endoscopic management of complicated frontal sinus disease. The extent of surgical treatment necessary for manage-

ment of the frontal sinus depends on the extent and pathophysiology of the disease process. Weber et al recently reviewed current techniques available to approach the frontal sinus endoscopically and emphasized the importance of a stepwise algorithm.[9] While conservative approaches such as complete ethmoidectomy (Draf I) or limited frontal recess dissection (Draf IIa) will suffice in most cases, situations may arise that require more aggressive removal of osteitic bone or extensive scar formation. Improved designs in non-powered instrumentation such as curettes, angled forceps, and angled biting punches are available for endoscopic frontal sinusotomy. These instruments, however, may have limitations in the efficiency of tissue removal, mucosal trauma, and precision when extended procedures are indicated (Draf IIb and III).

The introduction of powered instrumentation to frontal sinus surgery has augmented the surgeon's ability to efficiently and atraumatically operate in this region. In conjunction with angled endoscopes, a variety of microdebrider blades are available with a range of angles and widths to accommodate controlled and delicate dissection of the frontal recess and frontal sinus outflow tract (Fig. 20.7).[10] When using powered instrumentation for frontal sinusotomy, the operator needs to proceed very cautiously. Excessive removal of mucosa, penetration of the skull base, and orbital injury are still possible and typically more catastrophic with powered instrumentation. Visualization must be excellent and the surgeon's skill sound in order to safely utilize these techniques in frontal sinus surgery.

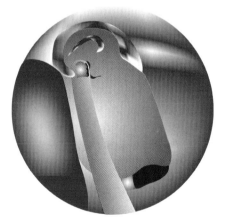

Fig. 20.7: Meticulous dissection in the left frontal recess using curved microdebrider blades. Powered endonasal instruments allow such careful dissection while maintaining a clean, dry operative field. (Reprinted with permission from American Journal of Rhinology, Vol 14, Friedman et al, 'Frontal sinus surgery: Endoscopic technique and preliminary results', Copyright 2000, Pages 393–493, with permission of the American Rhinologic Society)

Continued refinement in surgical instrumentation has allowed for refinements in extended endoscopic frontal sinusotomy approaches. These techniques include the Draf IIb frontal sinusotomy, the Draf III transseptal frontal sinusotomy and the endoscopic modified Lothrop procedure (EMLP). The EMLP has been established as a viable alternative to external fronto-ethmoidectomy or osteoplastic flap with fat obliteration techniques for recalcitrant frontal sinus disease or to gain extended access for neoplasm.[11–14] Consistent with the extensive disease typically present, these extended techniques often require removal of thickened and osteitic bone which may not be feasible with traditional instrumentation. The initial descriptions of EMLP included use of straight or minimally curved burs and noted significant limitations with these designs. Recently, Chandra et al reported their experience using a 70° diamond bur (Medtronic-Xomed) in the management of complicated frontal sinus disease (Figs 20.8A and B).[15] They used this bur design in Draf IIb (4 patients) and Draf III (6 patients) procedures. They reported that the 70° angle appeared optimal for access to the frontal recess and floor of the frontal sinus while minimizing trauma to surrounding bone and mucosa. Additional advantages noted by the authors included the diamond design to resist skipping and simultaneous suction and irrigation at the tip. Precise and efficient removal of bone is a prerequisite for successful extended frontal sinus procedures. The new available bur designs provide this function and have become an important instrument option in select cases.

Orbital Surgery

Powered endoscopic dacrocystorhinostomy (DCR) has been recently advocated as a viable alternative to more traditional external techniques.[16] Historically, Endonasal DCR techniques have been plagued by lower success rates when compared to the external DCR approach championed by our ophthalmology colleagues.[17] Poor intranasal visualization combined with inadequate understanding of the intranasal surgical anatomy is the main reason for these discrepancies in outcomes and acceptance. Intranasal visualization is no longer a limiting factor with widely available high-resolution videoscopic equipment of varying sizes and designs. It is generally accepted that the size of the ostium created during DCR surgery is an important factor impacting on the success of the procedure.[18] Therefore, a thorough understanding of the endoscopic surgical anatomy of the lacrimal system and the ability to efficiently expose the lacrimal sac are two elements critical to the success of an endoscopic DCR.

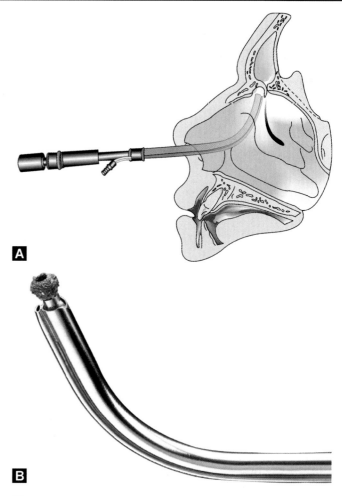

Figs 20.8A and B: (A) Dissection of the floor of the frontal sinus with a 70-degree bur. (B) 70-degree burr with integrated suction and irrigation function. (Figure reprinted with permission from The Laryngoscope, Vol 114, Chandra, et al. 'Use of the 70-degree diamond bur in the management of complicated frontal sinus disease,' Copyright 2004, Pages 188–192, with permission of the Triological Society)

In 2000, Wormald et al published their important work describing the intranasal location of the lacrimal sac.[19] They found that the location of the sac was consistently higher relative to the middle turbinate insertion than previously reported. Thus, it became evident that removal of the frontal process of the maxilla must be extended more superiorly in order to completely expose the sac. The frontal process of the maxilla is extremely hard bone in most patients. Thus, its removal is often difficult with traditional endoscopic instrumentation. As early as 1996, the use of cutting powered burs for endoscopic DCR had been reported.[20] In 2002, Wormald presented his experience with 47 powered endoscopic DCRs using a 15° coarse diamond bur

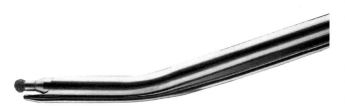

Fig. 20.9: The 20° DCR bur which includes irrigation and suction components in addition to diamond bur. The unique angulation of this blade is useful for endoscopic dacryocystorhinostomy (*Courtesy*: Medtronic-Xomed)

attached to a microdebrider (Medtronic-Xomed).[16] Wormald reported a 95% success rate and emphasized the importance of total lacrimal sac exposure which he felt is most efficiently accomplished via the use of powered instrumentation. Additional validation of the powered endoscopic DCR technique as outlined by Wormald can be found in a recent publication comparing this technique to traditional external DCR approaches.[17] Currently available diamond burs for endoscopic DCR include the 15° 4 mm diameter and 20° 2.5 mm diameter, both are typically run at 12,000 rpm (Medtronic-Xomed) (Fig. 20.9). Based on data presented in the recent literature and the senior author's personal experience, powered instrumentation provides an excellent option for endoscopic removal of bone during DCR with outcomes at least equivalent to traditional techniques.

Endoscopic optic nerve decompression (EOND) is a surgical technique in which the use of powered instrumentation has also been advocated. The indications, patient selection and treatment outcomes for surgical decompression remain controversial and are beyond the scope of this chapter. However, EOND has been established as the preferred technique when surgical decompression is indicated.[21–24] Luxenberger et al in 1998 published the Graz Experience with EOND and introduced an irrigating diamond drill (Karl Storz, Tuttlingen, Germany) for thinning the bony optic canal.[24] To the best of our knowledge, additional burs specific to EOND have not been developed. However, the currently available high-speed burs with their simultaneous suction and irrigation, different sized diamond heads, and varying shaft angles proved ample alternatives to the rhinologic surgeon. The senior author (Kingdom) has found the 15° diamond DCR bur (Medtronic-Xomed) to be useful for this procedure.

Endoscopic Surgery of the Skull Base

With the rapid and continued refinements in instrumentation, imaging and minimally invasive endonasal endoscopic surgical techniques, it is not surprising that endoscopic surgery of the skull base has become an area of major focus for rhinologists, neurosurgeons, and skull base surgeons. Transnasal and trans-sinus routes to the skull base universally require the surgeon to traverse thick bone for access to the area of interest. Therefore, efficient bone removal is mandatory and the application of powered instrumentation ideal. The design of instrumentation specific to endoscopic skull base surgery is in its infancy but new options should be available soon. Technical challenges include longer shafts with smaller cutting surfaces, unique shaft or tip angles, and the development of malleable or flexible instrumentation. Endonasal endoscopic approaches to the pterygo-maxillary fossa[25] lateral recess of the sphenoid sinus,[26] clivus,[27,28] infratemporal fossa,[29] anterior cranial fossa[30] cavernous sinus,[31] and the posterior cranial fossa via a transclival[32] route are examples of described techniques often requiring powered instrumentation using high-speed burs for bone removal. The future of minimally invasive endoscopic skull base surgery is exciting. The continued application and development of powered instrumentation will certainly play an important role in the future.

Endoscopic Removal of Neoplasms

The endoscopic resection of nasal cavity and paranasal sinus neoplasms in select patients has gained in popularity as technology has evolved and as experience has grown.[33–39] Reported experience is greatest with the endoscopic management of inverted papillomas (IP). The use of powered instrumentation in endoscopic tumor removal appears to include three general applications:

1. Debulking of tumor in order to precisely define attachments,[40]
2. Removal of bone to gain extended access,[15] and
3. Removal of bone corresponding to location of tumor attachment.[34]

The use of the microdebrider to rapidly debulk IP has been reported as a reasonable adjunctive technique as long as several important tenets are followed. First, care must be taken not to directly remove tumor adjacent to nasal or sinus mucosal surfaces.[40] The origin of the neoplasm and its site of attachment must be removed adequately in order to minimize recurrence rates. Secondly, all specimen dissected with the microdebrider must be collected and sent for pathologic analysis.[41] Suction traps are available to collect the specimen after it passes through the microdebrider and prior study has demonstrated that the passage of histologic material through the microdebrider does not adversely affect the pathologist's ability to make an accurate diagnosis.[42]

USE OF POWERED INSTRUMENTATION WITH IMAGE-GUIDED SURGERY

Image-guided endoscopic sinus and skull base surgery is another powerful technology that has been successfully applied to the field of rhinology. Most available image-guided systems have a variety of instrument options for intraoperative navigation, including the ability to track the tip of a microdebrider.[43] Options for tracking powered instrumentation include directly mounted optical arrays or a universal adapter that can be placed on most instruments for subsequent tracking (Figs 20.10A and B). A word of caution, however: when considering using image-guided surgical navigation during powered

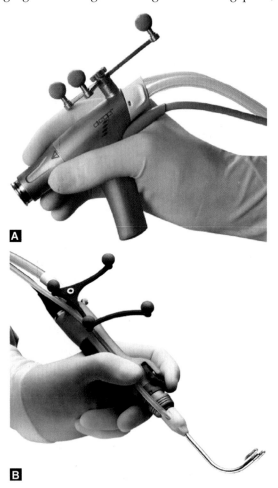

A

B

Figs 20.10A and B: IGS arrays may be attached to both the Diego. (A) and the Straightshot. (B) Microdebrider handpieces to allow navigation of the blade when using surgical navigation systems (*Courtesy*: Gyrus ENT and Medtronic-Xomed)

dissection in the paranasal sinuses, the potential for disastrous complications must always be kept in mind. Complications associated with powered instrumentation will be discussed later in this chapter. Over-reliance on image-guided technology in place of a sound understanding of the surgical anatomy is also a serious potential pitfall for the rhinologic surgeon. Thus, the combination of powered dissection and concurrent image-guided navigation should only be performed with great care and an even greater appreciation of the limitations which accompany both technologies.

COMPLICATIONS

Few reports of complications specific to powered instrumentation exist in the literature. Given the widespread use of this technology and the reported rates of major complications in endoscopic sinus surgery, it is likely many complications are unreported. Generally, speaking, 'minor' complications which would prove to be trivial using conventional instrumentation have the potential of turning into 'major' complications when powered instrumentation is used.

Orbital Injury

Orbital injury is a major complication of endoscopic sinus surgery which occurs infrequently with traditional as well as powered instrumentation. The injury may be direct or indirect. Direct orbital injury with powered instrumentation involves the debridement of periorbita, orbital fat, rectus muscle, or optic nerve with the surgical device. Indirect injury occurs via orbital hemorrhage, which may be arterial or venous. Arterial hemorrhages occur following laceration of the anterior or posterior ethmoid artery while venous hemorrhages result from venous disruption following breach of the lamina papyracea.[44] These injuries were described in endoscopic sinus surgery prior to the advent of powered instrumentation.

The proximity of orbital contents including the medial rectus muscle to the lamina papyracea and periorbita place them directly in harm's way. In cases with significant amount of nasal polyposis within the anterior and posterior ethmoid cavities in particular, delineation of polypoid mucosa from periorbita may be difficult. The bone of the lamina papyracea may be very thin or absent in places, juxtaposing these structures. Furthermore, the loss of tactile feedback with powered instrumentation may predispose to orbital injury.

Two case series have been published of orbital injuries during endoscopic sinus surgery with powered instrumentation. Graham and Nerad reported two cases of medial rectus injury and a third case with ethmoid artery laceration and subsequent orbital hematoma as well as medial rectus injury.[45] Bhatti et al reported a case with breach of the lamina papyracea which resulted in global ophthalmoplegia as well as a case of medial rectus injury.[46] Both authors noted that the severity of orbital trauma was significantly increased with the microdebrider versus standard endoscopic instrumentation due to the ability of the powered instrumentation to suck orbital contents (which might otherwise remain in place) into the cutting blades. Furthermore, with the high rate of oscillation of the blade, considerable damage to orbital structures may occur prior to the surgeon becoming aware of encountering orbital contents. The extent of medial rectus injury in the cases reported precluded strabismus surgery to provide meaningful recovery of function.[45] Graham and Nerad recommended great care be taken to keep the mouth of the microdebrider blade at 90° to the lamina papyracea when operating along the medial orbital wall and dissecting only superiorly or inferiorly to avoid entering the orbit (Figs 20.11A to D).

CSF Leaks

Intracranial penetration has also been documented prior to the use of powered instrumentation in endoscopic sinus surgery, with published rates of incidence from 0–3%.[47] Reports attributing this complication to the use of microdebriders are also scarce. To the surgeon unfamiliar with the anatomy of the skull base, dissection in this area may be difficult for many reasons. The skull base bone along the ethmoid fovea may be attenuated or absent prior to surgery. Furthermore, considerable variation exists in the configuration of the bony skull base in this area.[48] As with the orbit, the soft tissue structures of dura and brain matter which lie immediately superior to the skull base are readily dissected by powered instrumentation. The extent of intracranial injury following breach of skull base is compounded by the suction capability of the microdebrider to pull intracranial structures into the cutting blade.

Church et al reported three cases of large skull base defects (< 2 cm) created by the use of powered instrumentation.[49] In each case, brain tissue was noted in the pathology report from the original procedure. Berenholz, et al reported a case of skull base breach with subarachnoid hemorrhage following powered endoscopic sinus surgery.[50] Three of these patients immediately reported severe headaches following the procedure

(Fig. 20.12). In order to prevent such occurrences, Church, et al recommended judicious use of the microdebrider along the skull base and suggested that cutting instruments and curettes may be safer. The lack of tactile feedback afforded by the microdebrider in dissecting this area was noted by both authors.

Tissue Effects and Outcomes

Theoretically the use of powered instrumentation in ESS provides efficient atraumatic tissue removal leading to more rapid mucosal recovery and improved outcomes. Though believed to be true by the majority of surgeons favoring this technology, scientific evidence is lacking. Hackman and Ferguson recently published an excellent overview of the tissue effects of powered instrumentation in the nose and paranasal sinuses.[51]

Krouse and Christmas were the first to compare postoperative healing following endoscopic sinus surgery performed with powered instrumentation versus traditional endoscopic techniques.[52] In a retrospective, non-blinded fashion they evaluated 250 patients undergoing ESS with a microdebrider and 225 patients undergoing ESS with traditional endoscopic techniques. They reported more rapid mucosal healing with less crusting, less bleeding, decreased synechia formation, and a lower ostial occlusion rate in the microdebrider group as compared to the traditional group. Bernstein et al in 1998 published their experience with powered instrumentation in 40 patients undergoing ESS.[53] This was a retrospective review without a control or comparator group. They reported improved mucosal healing and a low synechiae formation rate however standardized objective outcome measures were not used and there was not a control group for comparison. Selivanova et al recently compared conventional sinus surgery with the use of powered instrumentation with respect to mucosal healing, tissue trauma, and efficacy.[54] The authors evaluated 24 patients undergoing ESS using a microdebrider on one side and traditional techniques of the other side. Outcome measures included nasal endoscopy, saccharin testing time, presence of complications, and clinical symptoms. Based on this criteria both groups demonstrated the same degree of improvement at 13 months follow-up. The authors attributed the lack of difference between the patient groups to the meticulous mucosal sparing techniques employed regardless of the instruments used. Operative time requirements were not discussed in this paper, however.

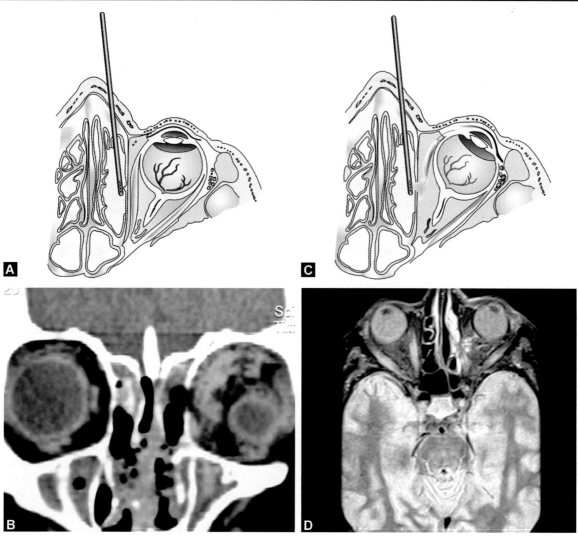

Figs 20.11A to D: (A) Use of powered microdebrider along the lamina papyracea. The suctioning function of the device will remove soft tissue along this bony partition. (B) If the bone of the lamina is breached, the orbital contents are easily drawn into the cutting window of the blade and may be readily injured. (C) Coronal CT which demonstrates a bony defect of the left lamina with orbital hematoma. (D) Axial T1 MRI with contrast which reveals left orbital injury with medial rectus injury. (Figures 20.11A and B reprinted from Otolaryngology–Head and Neck Surgery, Vol 125, Bhatti MT, Giannoni CM, Eaynor E, Monshizadeh R, Levine LM, 'Ocular motility complications after endoscopic sinus surgery with powered cutting instruments', pages 501-509, Copyright 2001, with permission from the American Academy of Otolaryngology – Head and Neck Surgery Foundation, Inc.)

The ability of microdebriders to remove tissue with minimal injury to surrounding tissue has been described as a major advantage of this technology versus standard techniques. Clinical experience suggests that mucosal recovery, intraoperative efficiency, and outcomes are improved when powered instrumentation is used in ESS. Limited clinical studies support this observation as well. However, scientific evidence to confirm this is still lacking and further study is required.

FUTURE DIRECTIONS

Powered instrumentation has become standard in ESS. The technology has evolved rapidly from arthroscopic instrumentation to the current sophisticated portfolio of rhinologic instruments now available. Research and development in this area remains a significant focus for many medical equipment manufacturers. As new applications are defined and refined blade designs to adapt. New applications may include the ability to

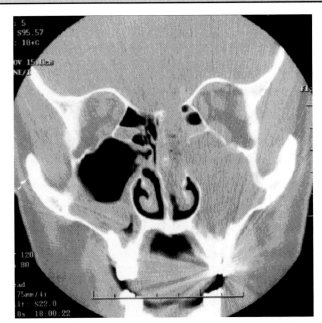

Fig. 20.12: Injury to the left ethmoid skull base following endoscopic sinus surgery with powered instrumentation (Reprinted from Otolaryngology–Head and Neck Surgery, Vol 129, Church et al, 'Endoscopic repair of large skull base defects after powered sinus surgery', Pages 204-209, Copyright 2003, with permission from the American Academy of Otolaryngology – Head and Neck Surgery Foundation, Inc.)

provide hemostasis while performing powered dissection, flexible instrumentation, and smaller and more efficient blade/bur designs. Continued redesign and modification of existing products is also likely to allow powered instruments to dissect more cleanly, suction more efficiently, and continue to offer the rhinologic surgeon greater flexibility in their use.

Financial Disclosures

Todd T Kingdom is a consultant for Medtronic.

REFERENCES

1. Setliff RC, Parsons DS. The "hummer": New instrumentation for functional endoscopic sinus surgery. *Am J Rhinol* 1994; 8:275–278.
2. Gross CW, Becker DG. Power instrumentation in endoscopic sinus surgery. *Oper Tech Otolaryngol Head Neck Surg* 1997; 7:236–241.
3. Becker DG. Technical considerations in powered instrumentation. *Otolaryngol Clin North Am* 1997; 30:421–434.
4. Krous JH, Christman DA. Powered nasal polypectomy in the office setting. *ENT J* 1996; 75:608–610.
5. Christmas DA, Krouse JH. Powered instrumentation in functional endoscopic sinus surgery I: Surgical technique. *ENT J* 1996; 75:33–40.
6. Kennedy DW. Functional endoscopic sinus surgery: Anesthesia, technique, and postoperative management. In *Diseases of the Sinuses*, Kennedy DW, Bolger WE, Zinreich SJ (Eds). Hamilton: BC Decker, 2001; 211–221.
7. Lee KC, Hwang PH, Kingdom TT. Surgical management of inferior turbinate hypertrophy in the office: Three mucosal sparing techniques. *Oper Tech Otolaryngol Head Neck Surg* 2001; 12:107–111.
8. Friedman M, Tanyeri H, Lim J, Landsberg R, Caldarelli D. A safe, alternative technique for inferior turbinate reduction. *Laryngoscope* 1999; 109:1834–1837.
9. Weber R, Draf W, Kratzsch B, Hoseman W, Schafer SS. Modern concepts of frontal sinus surgery. *Laryngoscope* 2001; 111:137–146.
10. Friedman M, Bliznikas D, Vidyasagar R, Landberg R. Frontal sinus surgery 2004: Update of clinical anatomy and surgical techniques. *Oper Tech Otolaryngol Head Neck Surg* 2004; 15(1):23–31.
11. Becker DG, Moore D, Lindsey WH, Gross WE, Gross CW. Modified transnasal endoscopic Lothrop procedure: Further considerations. *Laryngoscope* 1995; 105:1161–1166.
12. Scott NA, Wormald P, Close D, Gallagher R, Anthony Adrian, Maddern GJ. Endoscopic modified Lothrop procedure for the treatment of chronic frontal sinusitis: A systematic review. *Otolaryngol Head Neck Surg* 2003; 129:427–438.
13. Samaha M, Cosenza MJ, Metson R. Endoscopic frontal sinus drillout in 100 patients. *Arch Otolaryngol Head Neck Surg* 2003; 129:854–858.
14. Gross CW, Zachman GC, Becker DG, et al. Follow-up of the University of Virginia experience with the modified Lothrop procedure. *Am J Rhinol* 1997; 11:49–54.
15. Chandra RK, Schloser R, Kennedy DW. Use of the 70-degree diamond bur in the management of complicated frontal sinus disease. *Laryngoscope* 2004; 114:188–192.
16. Wormald PJ. Powered endoscopic dacrocystorhinostomy. *Laryngoscope* 2002; 112:69–72.
17. Tsirbas A, Davis G, Wormald PJ. Mechanical endonasal dacrocystorhinostomy versus external dacrocystorhinostomy. *Ophthal Plast Reconstr Surg* 2004; 20(1):50–56.
18. Welham RA, Wulc AE. Management of unsuccessful lacrimal surgery. *Br J Ophthalmol* 1987; 71:152–157.
19. Wormald PJ, Kew J, Hasselt AV. Intranasal anatomy of the nasolacrimal sac in endoscopic dacrocystorhinostomy. *Otolaryngol Head Neck Surg* 2000; 123:307–310.
20. Sprekelsen NM, Barberan MT. Endoscopic dacrocystorhinostomy: Surgical technique and results. *Laryngoscope* 1996; 106:187–189.
21. Rajiniganth MG, Gupta AK, Gupta A, Bapuraj JR. Traumatic optic neuropathy: Visual outcome following combined therapy protocol. *Arch Otolaryngol Head Neck Surg* 2003; 129(11):1203–1206.
22. Jiang RS. Hsu CY. Shen BH. Endoscopic optic nerve decompression for the treatment of traumatic optic neuropathy. *Rhinology.* 2001; 39(2):71–74.
23. Kountakis SE, Maillard AA, El-Harazi SM, Longhini L, Urso RG. Endoscopic optic nerve decompression for traumatic blindness. *Otolaryngol Head Neck Surg* 2000; 123:34–37.
24. Luxenberger W, Stammberger H, Jebeles JA, Walch C. Endoscopic optic nerve decompression: The Graz experience. *Laryngoscope.* 108(6):873–882.

25. Lane AP, Bolger WE. Endoscopic transmaxillary biopsy of pterygopalatine space masses: A preliminary report. *Am J Rhinol* 2002; 16(2):109–112.

26. Al–Nashar IS. Carrau RL, Herrera A, Snyderman CH. Endoscopic transnasal transpterygopalatine fossa approach to the lateral recess of the sphenoid sinus. *Laryngoscope* 2004; 114(3):528–532.

27. Puxeddu R, Lui MWM, Chandrasekar K, Nicolai P, Sekhar LN. Endoscopic-assisted transcolumellar approach to the clivus: An anatomical study. *Laryngoscope* 2002; 112:1072–1078.

28. Kingdom TT, Delgaudio JM. Endoscopic approach to lesions of the sphenoid sinus, orbital apex, and clivus. *Am J Otolaryngol* 2003; 24:317–322.

29. Roger G, Tran Ba, Huy P, Froehlich P, Van Den Abbeele T, Klossek JM, Serrano E, Garabedian EN, Herman P. Exclusively endoscopic removal of juvenile nasopharyngeal angiofibroma: Trends and limits. *Arch Otolaryngol Head Neck Surg* 2002; 128:928–935.

30. Jho HD, Ha HG. Endoscopic endonasal skull base surgery: The midline anterior fossa skull base. *Minim Invasive Neurosurg* 2004; 47:1–8.

31. Alfieri A, Jho HD. Endoscopic endonasal approaches to the cavernous sinus: Surgical approaches. *Neurosurgery* 2001; 49:354–360.

32. Jho HD, Ha HG. Endoscopic endonasal skull base surgery: The clivus and posterior fossa. *Minim Invasive Neurosurg* 2004; 47:16–23.

33. Roh HJ, Batra PS, Citardi MJ, Lee J, Bolger WE, Lanza DC. Endoscopic resection of sinonasal malignancies: A preliminary report. *Am J Rhinol* 2004; 18:239–246.

34. Wolfe SG, Schlosser RJ, Bolger WE, Lanza DC, Kennedy DW. Endoscopic and endoscope-assisted resections of inverted sinonasal papillomas. *Otolaryngol Head Neck Surg* 2004; 131:174–179.

35. Tomenzoli D, Castelnuovo P, Pagella F, et al. Different endoscopic surgical strategies in the management of inverted papilloma of the sinonasal tract: Experience with 47 patients. *Laryngoscope* 2004; 114:193–200.

36. Pasquini E, Sciarretta V, Frank G, Cantaroni C, et al. Endoscopic treatment of benign tumors of the nose and paranasal sinuses. *Otolaryngol Head Neck Surg* 2004; 131:180–186.

37. Mann WJ, Jecker P, Amedee RG. Juvenile angiofibromas: Changing surgical concept over the last 20 years. *Laryngoscope* 2004; 114:291–293.

38. Stammberger H, Walch W, Papaefthyiou G. Possibilities and limitations of endoscopic management of nasal and paranasal sinus malignancies. *Acta Oto-Rhino-Laryngologica Belg* 1999; 53:199–205.

39. Walch C, Stammberger H, Anderhuber W, Unger F, Kole W, Feichtinger K. The minimally invasive approach to olfactory neuroblastoma: Combined endoscopic and sterotactic treatment. *Laryngoscope* 2000; 110:635–640.

40. Wormald PJ, Ooi E, van Hasselt CA, Nair S. Endoscopic removal of sinonasal inverted papilloma including endoscopic medial maxillectomy. *Laryngoscope* 2003; 113:867–873.

41. Kennedy DW. Commentary–Routine histopathology in uncomplicated sinus surgery: Is it necessary? *Otolaryngol Head Neck Surgery* 2005; 132:413.

42. Zweig JL, Schaitkin BM, Fan CY, Barnes EL. Histopathology of tissue samples removed using the microdebrider technique: Implications for endoscopic sinus surgery. *Am J Rhinol* 2000; 14:27–32.

43. Kingdom TT, Orlandi RR. Image-guided surgery of the sinuses: Current technology and applications. *Otolaryngol Clin N Am* 2004; 37:381–400.

44. Stankiewicz JA, Chow JM. The two faces of orbital hematoma in intranasal (endoscopic) sinus surgery. *Otolaryngol Head Neck Surg* 1999; 120:841–847.

45. Graham SM, Nerad JA. Orbital complications in endoscopic sinus surgery using powered instrumentation. *Laryngoscope* 2003; 113:874–878.

46. Bhatti MT, Giannoni CM, Eaynor E, Monshizadeh R, Levine LM. Ocular motility complications after endoscopic sinus surgery with powered cutting instruments. *Otolaryngol Head Neck Surg* 2001; 125: 501–509.

47. May M, Levine HL, Mester SJ, Schaitkin B: Complications of endoscopic sinus surgery: Analysis of 2108 patients—Incidence and prevention. *Laryngoscope* 1994; 104:1080–1083.

48. Keros P. On the practical value of differences in the level of the lamina cribrosa of the ethmoid. *Z Laryngol Rhinol Otol* 1962; 41:809–813.

49. Church CA, Chiu AG, Vaughan WC. Endoscopic repair of large skull base defects after powered sinus surgery. *Otolaryngol Head Neck Surg* 2003; 129:204–209.

50. Berenholz L, Kessler A, Sarfaty S, Segal S. Subarachnoid hemorrhage: A complication of endoscopic sinus surgery using powered instrumentation. *Otolaryngol Head Neck Surg* 1999; 121: 665–667.

51. Hackman TG, Ferguson BJ. Powered instrumentation and tissue effects in the nose and paranasal sinuses. *Curr Opin Otolaryngol Head Neck Surg* 2005; 13:22–26.

52. Krouse JH, Christmas DA. Powered instrumentation in functional endoscopic sinus surgery. II: A comparative study. *ENT J* 1996; 75: 42–44.

53. Bernstein JM, Lebowitz RA, Jacobs JB. Initial report on postoperative healing after endoscopic sinus surgery with the microdebrider. *Otolarygnol Head Neck Surg* 1998; 118:800–803.

54. Selivanova O, Kuehnemund M, Mann WJ, Amedee RG. Comparison of conventional instruments and mechanical debriders for surgery of patients with chronic sinusitis. *Am J Rhinol* 2003; 17:197–202.

Minimally Invasive Sinus Surgery

Peter J Catalano

Since its introduction in the mid-1980s, functional endoscopic sinus surgery (FESS) has become the standard surgical intervention for patients with chronic sinusitis refractory to medical therapy. Unlike prior sinus procedures such as the Caldwell-Luc, FESS represented a targeted intervention, aimed at restoring normal sinus mucosal physiology. FESS was the first surgical model for sinus intervention to address the underlying pathophysiologic mechanisms of sinusitis as first described by Messerklinger in 1978.[1]

Through his endoscopic examination of the nose, Messerklinger made a number of instrumental discoveries to the development of FESS. In his book entitled *Endoscopy of the Nose*, he described a pattern of shifting light reflexes seen on the mucosal surface of the sinuses representing mucociliary movement that we now recognize as mucociliary transport or clearance. Using endoscopy in conjunction with time-lapse photography, he examined the direction of mucus movement and found that clearance was directed from the larger sinuses to their respective ostia. He also noted that contact between mucosal surfaces leads to disruption of mucociliary movement thereby causing retention of secretions with subsequent obstruction of the subordinate maxillary, frontal and anterior ethmoid sinuses. Furthermore, he recognized that contact is most likely to occur in the narrow transition spaces (i.e. ethmoidal infundibulum, hiatus semilunaris superior, and retroaggar space/ nasofrontal recess). While contact may be due to a number of causes, such as inflammation from environmental irritants, allergic rhinitis, viral infection, or ciliary dysfunction (i.e. Kartagener's disease), these factors are most influential to the disruption of sinus physiology and development of sinusitis when they directly affect the aforementioned transition spaces. The theory that transition spaces represent the primary physiologic/

anatomic bottleneck for the development of sinusitis is further supported by the high frequency with which both CT and clinical exam findings demonstrate inflammation limited to the maxillary, frontal and anterior ethmoid sinuses (the posterior ethmoid and sphenoid sinuses do not drain into transition spaces).

Another critical realization in the development of FESS was that mucosal damage and mucociliary dysfunction is a reversible process. Prior to this, many believed that mucosal damage found in chronic sinusitis was irreversible and therefore, procedures such as the Caldwell-Luc involved stripping of sinus mucosa. In his clinical experience with more than 2500 patients, Stammberger showed that once the transition spaces are cleared off disease, the larger sinuses usually heal without being touched even if mucosal damage seemed 'almost irreversible'.[2] Recent studies examining mucociliary clearance have shown that patients with chronic sinusitis have impaired mucociliary movement and that FESS is capable of correcting mucociliary dysfunction in these patients thus demonstrating the reversibility of disease.[3-6] Moreover, others have shown that mechanical damage to nasal mucosal epithelium results in loss of cilia and decreased mucociliary transport.[7-8] In order to create optimal conditions for reversal of disease to occur, surgical intervention should avoid destruction of cilia in order to maintain mucociliary clearance and normal sinus physiology.

Following the discoveries of mucociliary clearance, reversible mucosal damage in chronic sinusitis, and the role of transition spaces as a nidus for sinusitis, FESS was a logical advancement. The technique, based on conservatism, served as a targeted intervention addressing the narrowed transition spaces and re-establishing drainage through birth ostia while avoiding direct manipulation of the larger sinuses themselves. Kennedy demonstrated the favorable long-term results of FESS with 98.4% of 72 patients reporting improvement compared to before surgery over an average 7.8 year follow-up period.[9] Although there was a steep initial learning curve, many studies have since highlighted the relative paucity of complications associated with the procedure. In a study of 250 patients undergoing FESS, Levine reported that 8.3% of patients developed minor complications while only 0.7% developed major complications.[10] In comparison, a study of 670 patients undergoing the Caldwell-Luc procedure, the previous gold standard intervention for chronic maxillary sinusitis, reported a 19% rate of major complications as result of the operation.[11] Finally, since FESS is based on a minimally invasive approach compared to conventional surgeries, there was less overall postoperative discomfort and shorter hospital stays.

While FESS initially established itself as a less invasive, more targeted, and more effective technique than its predecessors, *conventional FESS* has evolved beyond this description. Originally, proponents emphasized that FESS provides a conservative and effective surgical intervention, rarely requiring a middle meatal antrostomy or stripping of diseased nasal mucosa. Overtime, however, there has been a departure from these conservative principles with a tendency towards more aggressive intervention. As a result, surgeons have excessive freedoms in the nose and the procedures are not standardized. If a patient were to report a history of parotidectomy, one would know exactly what was done. To the contrary, if the patient reported a history of FESS, one could only speculate as to what interventions were actually performed. Since there is no longer a systematic reproducible surgical model called FESS, the surgical intervention and decision-making varies widely depending on the surgeon. Routine resection of middle turbinates, creation of large maxillary antrostomies, aggressive removal of all ethmoid bone, and manipulation of normally functioning sinus ostia are just some examples of how the original FESS procedure has morphed over time. One would hope and expect that procedures and treatment philosophies would and should be modified over time. However, we should also expect that there be reasonable scientific proof in support of such change.

Although endoscopy offered a window for more precise visualization of nasal pathology, advances in other sinus instrumentation lagged. The original instruments used in FESS offered minimal precision, were associated with shear damage to normal mucosal tissue, and caused inadvertent stripping of mucus membranes. Technological breakthroughs, coupled with a surgical model based on Messerklinger's principles, led to the next major advance in rhinology—MIST.

THEORETICAL CONCERNS

The minimally invasive sinus technique (MIST) is a targeted endoscopic intervention, introduced in 1994, with virtually identical goals to those originally reported for FESS; however, there are distinct differences. Unlike FESS, MIST strictly upholds Messerklinger's functional concepts so that the surgeon performs a very minimal initial intervention. Although sinus ostia are rarely enlarged, MIST is much more than *not* performing a middle meatal antrostomy. The procedure, described below, is the only stepwise intranasal intervention with a defined beginning and end for all patients regardless of disease severity, thereby standardizing the procedure for surgeons and patients alike. By starting at the most medial aspect of the lateral nasal wall and moving laterally, the surgeon is able to preserve the delicate tissue of the lamina papyracea and critical ciliary function of the sinus ostia. Furthermore, the procedure still allows for extension into the less involved posterior ethmoid and/or sphenoid cavities while maintaining an anatomic based progression. This elegant, reproducible method avoids unnecessary disruption of normal mucosa while restoring mucociliary clearance through the primary birth ostia.

Although not specific to MIST, endoscopically guided powered instrumentation was first introduced with this procedure and is now routinely used. In comparison to the early handheld instruments used in FESS, powered instruments provide true cutting blades for improved precision and preservation of non-diseased mucosa which is key to the restoration of normal mucociliary function. In one study, a powered microdebrider termed the *HUMMER*, was shown by Setliff et al to be associated with accelerated healing and reduced synechiae formation.[12] Real-time continuous suctioning at the tip of the instrument obviates the need for frequent instrument removal for cleaning, thereby reducing mucosal trauma and decreasing operating time. Continuous real-time suction also improves intraoperative visibility with the potential for reduced operative morbidity. Finally, because the minimally invasive technique markedly reduces nasal trauma, eliminates exposed sinus bone, and decreases blood loss, the healing burden placed on the nose is minimal and the need for uncomfortable nasal packing eliminated.

MIST clearly offers a number of advantages over traditional methods used in FESS. While proponents of

MIST recognize FESS as an effective surgical option for patients with chronic sinusitis, they question the need for departure from Messerklinger's functional concepts. MIST is a true embodiment of these principles and improves upon FESS by providing an anatomically based reproducible approach to sinus surgery, invokes powered instrumentation with real-time suctioning, preservation of mucosa and turbinate tissue, leaves the primary birth ostia undisturbed in most patients, and decreases operative morbidity.

Turbinate tissue is critical to proper nasal and sinus physiology. Routine resection of the middle turbinate often leads to edema and/or stenosis of the nasofrontal duct, and can produce compensatory glandular hypertrophy of the remaining nasal tissue. Powered shaving (i.e. thinning) of the lateral aspect of the middle turbinate and powered resection of the lateral wall of concha bullosa can each improve middle meatal airflow without incurring the risks associated with turbinate resection.

Creation of a middle meatal antrostomy (MMA) is occasionally required. Absolute indications include the biopsy of an antral mass, presence of one or more accessory ostia leading to maxillary recirculation, resection of a maxillary sinus fungal ball or inverted papilloma, and to allow for the application of topical medications or repeated antral lavage in select cases. The problem with creation of an MMA is not whether it works, but whether it is necessary. There is no study to date that demonstrates the routine need for, nor the proper size of, an MMA. However, Silva et al recently reported that for every surgical candidate with CRS, they performed an MMA on one maxillary sinus but not the other.[13] The results show **no difference** in the control of maxillary sinus symptoms or disease between the two sides. Thus, the potential risks of increased middle meatal scarring, interruption of mucociliary clearance and proper ostial function, development of maxillary recirculation by not including the natural ostia in the MMA, and the likely need for revision maxillary surgery preclude the routine creation of an MMA.

Aggressive ethmoid surgery, with routine removal of all ethmoid partitions, is another component of conventional FESS with yet unproven benefit. This topic will be discussed later in this chapter.

THE MIST PROTOCOL

Preoperative Protocols

In the holding area, patients receive a series of nasal sprays with the aim of causing vasoconstriction and thus greater operative visibility with decreased bleeding. Two

sprays of oxymetazoline (0.05%) solution are administered in each nostril. Three doses are delivered at five-minute intervals. Following these three doses of oxymetazoline, a cocaine/epinephrine solution is delivered via an atomizer containing 8 ml cocaine (10%) and 0.16 ml of 1:100,000 epinephrine (diluted 1:50,000). Two sprays of this solution are administered every 5 minutes for the 15 minutes prior to surgery for a total of three doses. Of note, the oxymetazoline sprays must be taken before and not concurrently with the cocaine/epinephrine solution as the former plays a role in limiting the systemic absorption of the cocaine solution.

Intraoperative Protocols

Anesthesia is achieved with general anesthesia, preferentially via a laryngeal mask technique (LMA). Three injections of lidocaine 1% with epinephrine 1:100,000 are given. The first is injected into the anterior and lateral attachment of the middle turbinate to the lateral nasal wall. The subsequent two injections are placed directly into the body of the middle turbinate. If the surgeon plans to operate on the contralateral nasal cavity as well, then pre-injection should be avoided because more bleeding may result from a rebound effect of the injections.

After the injections, a 0° endoscope is introduced and the middle turbinate gently medialized with a freer elevator. Surgery then progresses anatomically in a stepwise manner, beginning with identification of the uncinate process at the hiatus semilunaris. The transition space located behind the uncinate and associated with this landmark is the ethmoidal infundibulum. A pediatric back-biter is used, via a retrograde approach described by Parsons,[14] to incise the uncinate process from the hiatus semilunaris toward the nasolacrimal duct (posterior to anterior). This provides an added measure of safety by starting the uncinectomy at the farthest point from the lamina papyracea. The uncinotomy should be inspected to ensure that all three layers of the uncinate have been transected and the lamina papyracea has not been violated. Powered instruments can then be used to extend the uncinate resection superiorly to uncover the aggar nasi cells, as well as anterior and inferior to uncover the primary maxillary sinus ostium. These steps serve to open the transition space of the maxillary sinus, aggar nasi cells (anterior ethmoid), and frontal recess.

The next landmark is the posteromedial wall of the aggar nasi cell. The retro-aggar space or naso-frontal recess (transition space for the frontal sinus) lies just behind the posteromedial wall of the aggar nasi cell. On occasion, the posterior wall of the aggar dome must be removed in order to further enlarge this transition space. This area is best viewed with a 30° or 45° telescope. A frontal seeker and giraffe forceps can be used to safely remove the aggar dome when indicated. Extreme polyposis and/or tissue edema may obscure the frontal recess during this initial procedure. It is prudent to allow the potential benefit from complete uncinectomy, application of topical medications, and subsequent improvement of the patient's nasal/sinus physiology to reverse the mucosal swelling in this area. If symptoms relevant to this frontal region persist three months after surgery, the frontal recess can be re-addressed with a greater chance of success and reduced morbidity (i.e. synechia formation).

The next anatomic landmark is the face of the ethmoidal bulla. The associated transition space is the hiatus semilunaris superior (HHS), a space between the lateral edge of the middle turbinate and medial edge of the ethmoid bulla (this is the transition space for the remainder of the anterior ethmoid sinus). Powered instrumentation is used to remove the **medial** wall of the bulla (beginning at the HHS and working laterally) thereby exposing the anterior ethmoid sinus ostium and enlarging the transition space of the anterior ethmoid sinus. Projections of the anterior ethmoid sinus through the basal lamella, termed the retro-bulla space, are now visualized. Dissection with the micro-debrider is begun inferior and medial to minimize risk to both the lamina papyracea (laterally) and a potentially low cribriform plate (superior and medial).

The middle turbinate is repositioned and the medial corridor, that space between the middle turbinate and the septum, is inspected. Natural contact synechia in this area are lysed with a freer and the superior meatus and spheno-ethmoidal recess are inspected.

If no disease is noted in the medial corridor, the standard MIST procedure is now complete. For all patients who receive an anterior and/or posterior ethmoidectomy, or the mucosa of the lateral edge of the middle turbinate is violated, a 1 cm wide and 2 cm long piece of Merogel is rolled in the shape of the number '9', and placed into the middle meatus to prevent synechia.[15] Additionally, and for the same reason, a 1.5 cm square piece of moistened gel film is placed in the medial corridor. No other nasal packing is placed. The nasopharynx, oropharynx, and hypopharynx are suctioned free of blood and debris that might have accumulated. The patient can then be safely extubated.

If a posterior ethmoidectomy is required, then the microdebrider is used to pierce the inferomedial quadrant of the basal lamella. This is the safest entry point into the posterior ethmoid cells and can be done without the need for surgical navigation technology. From this position, the basal lamella is removed both laterally and superiorly under direct visualization. In severely diseased sinuses, surgical navigation is recommended. All ethmoid partitions are not removed, exposing bare bone is avoided, and reversal of diseased mucosa is expected. Once this portion is completed, the medial corridor is entered and the superior meatus inspected. Obstructing polypoid disease is often found in this location and is easily removed with the microdebrider. This provides dual ventilation/drainage for this region. The spheno-ethmoidal recess is examined next and polypoid obstruction of the sphenoid sinus addressed with the microdebrider. Entry into the sphenoid sinus is rarely necessary (i.e. total obstruction/mucocele) and, in those cases, may require the aid of surgical navigation technology.

Postoperative Protocols

All patients are prescribed an oral antibiotic for the first 5 days after surgery. Nasal saline irrigations are begun within 24 hours of surgery and maintained for a minimum of 4 weeks. Middle meatal debridement is rarely required postoperatively.

Most patients are able to return to work or school in 24–48 hours following the procedure. There are no diet or activity limitations for most patients. Pain is usually minimal and well controlled with acetaminophen.

OUTCOME STUDIES INVOLVING MIST

Since its introduction in the literature in 1996, MIST has grown in popularity worldwide.[12,14] However, it was not until January 2002, that a formal outcome study was published comparing MIST to FESS.[15] This study used the chronic sinusitis survey (CSS) as the quality of life outcome instrument to assess improvement following MIST. The CSS was chosen because it has been proven a reliable, sensitive and easily administered test to evaluate patient disability from chronic sinusitis. The CSS has also been used in previous outcome reports on FESS, allowing a direct comparison of the two techniques. To summarize: outcome from MIST as measured by the CSS medication, CSS symptom, and CSS total subscales either equaled or surpassed those after FESS; compared to FESS, many more patients after MIST were improved to a level that was better than the normative symptom data for healthy individual in the general population; the follow-up period for the MIST study was twice as long (23 months compared to 12 months) as the FESS study, yet still demonstrated improvement; and the surgical revision rate following MIST was 5.9% compared to an average of 10% following FESS. Furthermore, the results seen following MIST were consistent across the spectrum of disease severity (using CT grades I through IV), disproving the opinion that the procedure was only effective for minimal disease.

These findings strongly support the recommendation that MIST be considered the initial surgical intervention for the treatment of chronic sinusitis. It strongly suggests that an excellent quality of life for chronic sinus sufferers could be achieved with minimal surgical manipulation of the nose and sinuses, it validates Messerklinger's transition space theory and the reversibility of diseased nasal membranes, and it contradicts the rationale for the routine creation of a middle meatal antrostomy.

Another, less formal outcome study on MIST titled *Minimally Invasive Sinus Surgery in the Geriatric Patient*, was published in 2001.[16] The study used a geriatric population (age 65–93) of 100 patients undergoing MIST for chronic sinusitis, to assess whether, due to their age, they had a greater potential for intra- or postoperative complications. Quality of life outcome following surgery was also assessed subjectively 6 months after surgery by the study patients: 84% of patients reported feeling significantly better, 10% somewhat better, and 6% unchanged. In comparison, another study of 119 patients with chronic sinusitis reported that 80.2% of patients experienced relief after FESS.[10] Interestingly, 8 of 10 patients who reported feeling 'somewhat better' after MIST, and 2 of 6 patients who experienced no improvement, had previously undergone aggressive FESS elsewhere. This supports the opinion that aggressive FESS may have 'irreversible adverse effects on nasal and sinus function'.

The study also assessed whether there was any exacerbation of preexisting medical conditions, or an increase in surgical morbidity after MIST. The 100 patients presented a spectrum of preexisting medical conditions including hypertension, coronary disease, gastrointestinal disorders, diabetes, bronchitis and asthma, thyroid disorders, gout, stroke, renal disease, prostate disease, dysrhythmias, and others. Early medical complications (within 72 hours of surgery) following MIST included 12 patients with headache, 6 with postoperative sinusitis, 4 had nausea and vomiting, 3 had fatigue, and 1 each with ataxia, hyposmia, syncope, incontinence and hypoxia. The ataxia and syncope were self-limited and appropriate evaluation obtained. The nausea, vomiting, incontinence and hypoxia all occurred in the recovery area following surgery and were self-limited. In addition to verifying the efficacy of MIST for the treatment of chronic sinusitis, the results highlight the fact that minimal medical/surgical morbidity is experienced by geriatric patients following MIST, making the procedure equally safe for the oldest and potentially most frail portion of the population.

A more recent article evaluated the efficacy of various middle meatal stents used during the MIST technique.[17] In this study of 100 patients, a rolled gel-film stent was placed into the right middle meatus, while a rolled Merogel stent was used on the left. Laterality of the stents was kept constant throughout the study. Perioperative morbidity associated with stent use was also assessed. Follow-up was a minimum of 3 months following surgery. Retention time for the gel-film stent was 5 days, whereas it was closer to 8 days for Merogel (a statistically significant difference). Four patients developed visible middle meatal synechia on the right (gel film) side, none were seen on the left. The perioperative morbidity associated with the use of stents was negligible and not side specific. Merogel appeared to be an excellent middle meatal spacer during sinus surgery. Compared to the literature, where the rates of middle meatal synechia vary from 27 to 4%, the overall synechia rate in this study was only 2% (0% for the Merogel side).

The findings of this study are significant because it introduces several new concepts and confirms others:

1. Middle meatal stents are beneficial following sinus surgery and can minimize synechia.
2. A biodegradable stent is well tolerated post-operatively and eliminates the need for middle meatal debridement.
3. Merogel (avian derived hyaluronic acid) may be a better material than gelfilm because of its longer retention time and/or enhanced biocompatibility.
4. Due to a combination of minimally invasive mucosal sparing surgery, and biocompatible, biodegradable middle meatal stents, synechia following MIST are rare.
5. Because MIST does not manipulate the primary maxillary sinus ostium, the latter remains in the oblique or horizontal plane making it less likely to be obstructed by a lateralized middle turbinate. Whereas the final position of an MMA is in the para-sagittal plane, making it much more vulnerable to obstruction by a lateralized middle turbinate.

The results of these peer-reviewed articles validate MIST as an effective surgical treatment option for chronic sinusitis.

THE FESS DEPARTURE FROM FUNCTIONAL PRINCIPLES

A rationale has been provided for the aggressive ethmoidectomy seen in contemporary FESS, however, the basis for it remains unproven. It has been shown in both animal and human studies that osteitis of ethmoid and maxillary sinus bone can occur in the face of chronic sinusitis.[18,19] It is proposed that the osteitic bone serves as a nidus for recurrent infection or mucosal inflammation and, therefore, may be responsible for persistent/recurrent disease following medical/surgical intervention. Thus, it is proposed, that aggressive removal of all ethmoid sinus partitions will theoretically minimize the risk of recurrence.

However, osteitis is a histopathologic diagnosis which cannot be made in the operating room. How will the surgeon know which bone is osteitic; what if it involves the lamina or fovea? Furthermore, what remains unproven is whether the osteitis is reversible surgically or medically, and if so, how much medicine and/or surgery is required to do so? Until we know the answers to these pivotal questions, surgical conservatism is warranted.

Recent studies have shown that SPECT bone scanning of the paranasal sinuses in patients with chronic sinusitis may be helpful in identifying foci of osteitis preoperatively.[20] These foci were correlated with histopathology of osteitis in 94% of cases examined. Longitutinal studies to determine the potential for reversing osteitic bone changes after MIST are underway. Yet another study recently compared pre-treatment bone scans to CT scans in the same patients being treated for CRS. Although there was overall good correlation between patients with abnormal CT scans and those with positive bone scans, there was poor correlation between the individual sinuses themselves. For example, a patient with mucosal disease by CT in the right maxillary sinus could have a positive bone scan in the left ethmoid sinus. Both scans were abnormal in a given patient, but the location of 'disease' frequently varied. Thus, there is much to be learned about osteitis and its role in etiology of sinusitis.

REFERENCES

1. Messerklinger W. *Endoscopy of the nose.* Baltimore: Urban and Schwarzenberg, 1978.
2. Stammberger H. Endoscopic endonasal surgery – Concepts in treatment of recurring rhinosinusitis. Part II. Surgical technique. *Otolaryngol Head Neck Surg* 1986; 94(2):147-156.
3. Katsuhisa I, Takeshi O, Masayuki F, Yukio K, Akira S, Tomonori T, Shin M. Restoration of the mucociliary clearance of the maxillary sinus after endoscopic sinus surgery. *J Allergy Clin Immunol* 1997; 99(1,pt1):48-52.
4. Asai K, Haruna S, Otori N, Yanagi K, Fukami M, Moriyama H. Saccharin test of maxillary sinus mucociliary function after endoscopic sinus surgery. *Laryngoscope* 2000; 110(1):117–122.
5. Elwany S, Hisham M, Gamaee R. The effect of endoscopic sinus surgery on mucociliary clearance in patients with chronic sinusitis. *Eur Arch Otorhinolaryngol* 1998; 255:511–514.
6. Min YG, Yun YS, Song BH, Cho YS, Lee KS. Recovery of nasal physiology after functional endoscopic sinus surgery: Olfaction and mucociliary transport. *J Oto–Rhino–Laryngol Rel Specialt* 1995; 57(5):264–268.
7. Yang TQ, Majima Y, Guo Y, Harada T, Shimizu T, Takeuchi K. Mucociliary transport function and damage of ciliated epithelium. *Am J Rhinol* 2002; 16(4):215–219.
8. Melgarejo-Moreno PJ, Hellin-Meseguer D, Alpay F. Disturbances in mucociliary clearance after maxillary sinus surgery. Experimental study. *Acta Otorrinolaringologica Espanola* 1997; 48(2):105–108.
9. Senior BA, Kennedy DW, Tanabodee J, Kroger H, Hassab M, Lanza D. Long-term results of functional endoscopic sinus surgery. *Laryngoscope* 1998; 108:151–157.
10. Levine HL. Functional endoscopic sinus surgery: Evaluation, surgery, and follow-up of 250 patients. *Laryngoscope* 1990; 100:79–84.
11. Penttilä MA, Rautiainen MEP, Pukander JS, Karma PH. Endoscopic versus Caldwell–Luc approach in chronic maxillary sinusitis: Comparison of symptoms at one-year follow-up. *Rhinology* 1994; 32:161–165.
12. Setliff III RC, Parsons DS. The 'Hummer': New instrumentation for functional endoscopic sinus surgery. *Am J Rhinol* 1994; 8(6):275–278.
13. Silva A, Albu, Tomescu (Romania). *Oto Head Neck Surg* 2004; 31(4):542–547.
14. Setliff RC. Minimally invasive sinus surgery: Rationale and technique. *Otolaryngol Clin North Am* 1996; 29:115–129.
15. Catalano PJ, Roffman E. Outcome of patients with chronic sinusitis after the minimally invasive sinus technique. *Am J Rhinol* 2003; 17(1):17–22.
16. Catalano PJ, Setliff III RC, Catalano LA. Minimally invasive sinus surgery in the geriatric patient. *Oper Tech Otolaryngol Head Neck Surg* 2001; 12(2):85–90.
17. Catalano PJ, Roffman E. Evaluation of middle meatal stenting after the minimally invasive sinus technique (MIST). *Oto Head Neck Surg* 2003; 128(6):875–881.
18. Kennedy DW, Senior BA, Gannon FH, Montone KT, Hwang P, Lanza DC. Histology and histomorphometry of ethmoid bone in chronic sinusitis. *Am J Rhinol* 1998; 108 (4 Pt 1):502–507.
19. Giacchi RJ, Lebowitz RA, Yee HT, Light JP, Jacobs JB. Histopathologic evaluation of the ethmoid bone in chronic sinusitis. *Am J Rhinol* 2001; 15(3):193–197.
20. Catalano PJ, Dolan R, Romanow JH, Payne SC, Silverman M. Correlation of Bone SPECT Scintigraphy with histopathology of the ethmoid bulla: Preliminary investigation. *Ann Otol Laryngol Rhinol* 2007; 116(12):875–879.

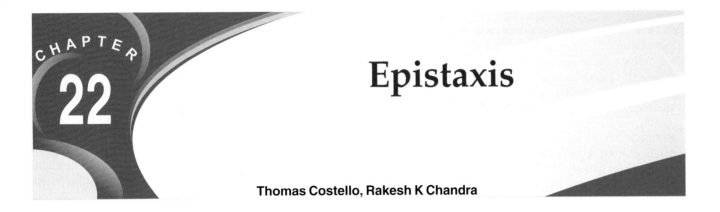

Thomas Costello, Rakesh K Chandra

Epistaxis arises from a perturbation in the normal hemostatic mechanisms of the nose. This is usually a self-limiting process; the majority of the cases are evaluated and managed as outpatients. However, a subset of patients may have persistent recurrences, dangerous hemorrhage, or life-threatening sequels including anemia and hypotensive shock. Furthermore, recurrent epistaxis may be a sign of occult neoplasm or underlying systemic disease associated with coagulopathy. Complete evaluation and effective treatment begins with an understanding of the vascular anatomy of the nose, identification of anatomic abnormalities of the sinonasal tract, and careful evaluation of the patient's general medical condition. The objective of this chapter is to present a comprehensive approach to understanding, evaluating, and managing epistaxis.

EPIDEMIOLOGY

It is difficult to obtain an exact incidence of epistaxis given its variable presentation and often self-limiting nature. Up to 60% of people will have an episode of epistaxis over their lifetime with approximately 6% requiring medical attention. There is a male predominance, and it occurs more frequently in colder, drier months. Age may also play a role with clustering seen in the young (2nd decade) and older (6th to 8th decades) age groups.[1,2]

Another theory focuses on sustained hypertension as a causative factor, and some experts suggest that epistaxis may be the presenting symptom of hypertension.[3] It has also been observed that vasculature in the nasal cavity shows changes similar to that of the cerebral system in patients with longstanding hypertension, and epistaxis may thus represent the nasal correlate of end organ damage secondary to hypertensive disease (Table 22.1).[4]

ETIOLOGY

There are various causes of epistaxis, ranging from the trivial and mundane to life-threatening disorders. It is useful to separate the etiologic factors into local and systemic causes.

Local Causes

Among the various local causes (Table 22.2), trauma is one of the most common causes. Certainly external trauma with or without nasal bone fracture can cause intranasal lacerations. Habitual nose rubbing or picking can lead to superficial mucosal interruption which may progress to ulceration. This is more common in children but may also be seen in adults. Surgery, or other instrumentation, in the nose can also leave disrupted mucosa that can be a site of hemorrhage. Less commonly, an arterial vessel may be

	Odd ratio	95% confidence interval	P
History of hypertension—crude	2.7	1.4 to 5.2	0.002
Adjusted for age and gender	2.6	1.3 to 5.0	> 0.001
Adjusted for age, gender, rhinitis, diffuse bleeding, and malignant diseases	2.8	1.4 to 5.6	> 0.001

Table 22.1: Association between active epistaxis at ED presentation and history of hypertension adjusted by multivariate logistic regression modeling[13]

Table 22.2: Local causes of epistaxis

Traumatic
- External trauma with or without fracture
- Surgery or other instrumentation of the nose
- Digital trauma (more common in children)
- Chemical inhalants (e.g. Afrin, nasal steroids, cocaine, snuff, etc.)

Anatomic
- Septal deviation or spur
- Septal perforation

Inflammation
- Rhinosinusitis (infectious or noninfectious)
- Granulomatous diseases

Tumors
- Angiofibroma
- Hemangioma
- Aneurysms
- Malignant or benign epithelial lesions

damaged leading to a more severe form of epistaxis. Both external trauma and intranasal surgery have the rare, but devastating complication of cartico-cavernous fistula. This may occur in a delayed fashion and is characterized by massive epistaxis followed by pulsating exophthalmos, ophthalmoplegia, and headache.[5]

Topical nasal sprays can also cause mucosal irritation leading to epistaxis. These include nasal corticosteroids, particularly the aerosol formulations, as well as over-the-counter vasoconstrictors. Cocaine can cause tissue necrosis and ultimately epistaxis. Any factor which results in dry nasal mucosa can predispose to bleeding. This includes changes in weather, medical conditions, or systemic medications.

Any anatomic abnormality associated with exposure of one area of the mucosa to excess or turbulent airflow may, over time, result in excessive dryness, crusting, and bleeding. In a study examining the sites of hemorrhage in epistaxis patients, bleeding areas occurred frequently in front of septal spurs and only in the posterior nasal cavity if the nasal airway was wide and patent, presumably to allow drying air to flow by.[6] Epistaxis may also be the most common presenting symptom of a patient with a septal perforation.[7] Again, the underlying pathophysiology is thought to be the drying effect of air on the edge of the perforation causing crusting and bleeding.

Local inflammation must also be considered in unexplained epistaxis or in the presence of a septal perforation or ulcer of unclear etiology.[7] Sinonasal inflammatory disease is often due to any combination of allergic rhinitis, nonallergic rhinitis, acute bacterial

sinusitis, and chronic sinusitis. Other diseases that must be included in the differential diagnosis include sarcoidosis and Wegener's granulomatosis.[7,8] Tuberculosis and syphilis are still prevalent worldwide and increasing in some areas of North America and may cause epistaxis from nasal manifestation of the disease.[9]

Systemic Causes

There are many systemic causes of epistaxis (Table 22.3). Most of these causes are related to an interruption in the normal clotting mechanism. For example, there are increasing numbers of indications to begin patients on anti-coagulation therapy. Each patient responds differently to the same level of anti-coagulation therapy. Low dose anti-platelet therapy with aspirin may be just as likely to induce epistaxis as high-intensity anti-coagulation therapy with warfarin. Often, the indications for initiating anti-coagulation can be so compelling that the otolaryngologist, in conjunction with the medical specialist, may be reluctant to stop the offending agent despite recurrent or severe epistaxis. In this situation an escalating approach to epistaxis control is warranted which may include invasive procedures in an attempt to allow the patient to continue anti-coagulation therapy.

Both inherited and acquired disorders of the clotting pathways are also a possible source for recurrent epistaxis. Frequent unprecipitated epistaxis, particularly, but not exclusively, in younger patients should raise the suspicion of an inherited clotting disorder. These include von Willebrand's disease, the most common inherited coagulopathy, and hemophilia types A and B.[10,11] Von Willebrand's disease is an inherited disorder resulting in

Table 22.3: Systemic causes of epistaxis

Coagulation defects
- Inherited
- Iatrogenic
- Hematologic malignancies
- Hepatic dysfunction
- Malnutrition and vitamin deficiency
- Alcohol abuse
- Renal failure

Cardiovascular disorders
- Atherosclerosis
- Collagen disorders
- Hereditary hemorrhagic telangiectasias (Osler-Weber-Rendu)
- Hypertension (possible link)
- Venous congestion (e.g. from heart failure)

either a quantitative or qualitative deficiency of von Willebrand factor. This circulating protein plays two roles in the clotting pathway. It serves as a link between platelets and an injured vessel wall, as well as in a secondary capacity as a carrier for factor VIII. It is a heterogeneous defect in the gene located in chromosome 12, with the most common variation (type I, 70% of those with von Willebrand's disease and 1% of the general population) is inherited in an autosomal dominant fashion.[11] Hemophilia A (factor VIII) and hemophilia B (factor IX) are both X-linked recessive traits.[11]

Diseases of the liver or the kidney are examples of acquired coagulopathies. Alcohol, even in small amounts, can significantly prolong bleeding times and lead to epistaxis.[12] Any hematologic dyscrasia or malignancy can adversely impact the coagulation cascade, thereby promoting the tendency for epistaxis.

An association between hypertension and epistaxis remains controversial. Herkner and colleagues investigated the link between blood pressure and epistaxis in patients seen at a non-trauma emergency department. Blood pressure was found to be significantly higher in patients with active epistaxis than in those with other emergency conditions.[3] In another study conducted by the same group of investigators, they noted that patients presenting with active epistaxis, were nearly three times more likely to have a history of hypertension than patients without epistaxis, even after controlling for confounding variables (see Table 22.1).[13] Other investigators have also reported that 17% of patients with hypertensive crises present with active epistaxis.[14] However, many other studies failed to established any relationships between hypertension and epistaxis.[15] This is exemplified by a study conducted by Neto, who examined a cohort of hypertensive patients and were unable to demonstrate an association between blood pressure and incidence of epistaxis.[15]

The exact mechanistic link between hypertension and epistaxis, should one truly exist, has not been clearly elucidated. Theories include hypertension as result of sympathetic arousal from hemorrhage in a region rich in autonomic innervation. This theory is supported by a subset of patients who presented with active epistaxis and hypertension in the emergency department but who did not have sustained elevated blood pressures upon follow-up. This scenario is similar to the well known phenomenon of 'white coat hypertension'.[3]

Of special note is the inherited disease hereditary hemorrhagic telangiectasia (HHT), also known as Osler-Weber-Rendu syndrome. HHT is inherited in an autosomal

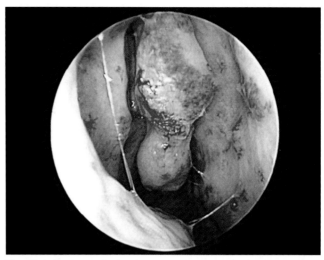

Fig. 22.1: Endoscopic view into right nasal cavity revealing multiple foci of HHT involving the mucosa of the nasal septum and middle turbinate. (*Courtesy:* Dr James Palmer, Assistant Professor, Division of Rhinology, Department of Otorhinolaryngology, University of Pennsylvania)

dominant fashion and causes telangiectasias along any mucocutaneous surface of the body (Fig. 22.1). These friable vessels are more prone to vessel wall rupture and hemorrhage (Fig. 22.2). Recent epidemiologic studies have suggested that HHT may be more common than was once believed, with an estimated incidence of 1 in 5000 to 8000 individuals.[16,17] Although the disease-causing genes have been isolated on chromosomes 9 and 12, the diagnosis remains a clinical one secondary to genetic and locus heterogeneity.[17] Classically, the triad of epistaxis,

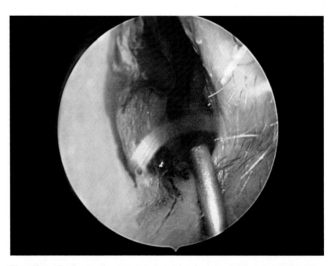

Fig. 22.2: Endoscopic view into left nasal cavity demonstrating active hemorrhage from an HHT lesion. (*Courtesy:* Dr James Palmer, Division of Rhinology, Department of Otorhinolaryngology, University of Pennsylvania)

telangiectasias and family history was considered pathognomonic for HHT. With greater understanding of the potentially lethal involvement of the pulmonary and cerebral vascular systems, more stringent criteria have been suggested (Table 22.4). Over 90% of patients will have epistaxis. If the patient has infrequent epistaxis, episodic control may be sufficient. However, with more frequent, or life-threatening bleeding episodes, more aggressive treatment may be necessary. Epistaxis in patients with HHT can be difficult to manage because the chronicity and the recurrence of epistaxis episodes can be life-threatening. The use of hormonal therapy and/or pro-thrombotic agent to induce a hypercoagulable state is the main medical treatment option.[16,18] Various surgical approaches can also be used to specifically attempt control of the epistaxis. Various wavelength lasers have been used including KTP, argon, neodymium-YAG, and pulsed dye laser. Septodermoplasty with skin grafting to the nasal septum is also a potential therapeutic modality.[19]

Recurrent epistaxis may also be a sign of a sino-nasal neoplasm.[20,21] Exhaustive coverage of this topic is beyond the scope of this chapter, but consideration will be given to angiofibromas since this is of particular interest to the topic of epistaxis.

Juvenile nasopharyngeal angiofibroma (JNA) is an entity unique to young males. It is a rare tumor comprising only about 0.05 to 0.5% of head and neck neoplasms.[22–24] The exact etiology and histologic origin of angiofibromas are uncertain, but anatomically they arise in the lateral nasal wall, specifically from the junction of the pterygopalatine fossa and the foramen of the sphenopalatine artery into the nasal cavity (Figs 22.3 and 22.4). Its predilection for adolescent males with an average age of onset of 15 years, suggests a hormonal connection.[24] The predilection toward males is so strong that the diagnosis must be questioned in a female, or genetic testing should

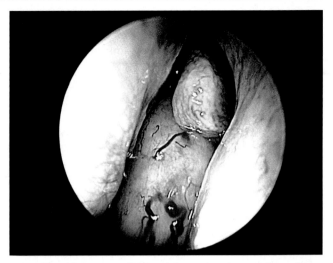

Fig. 22.3: Endoscopic view into left nasal cavity revealing a JNA. Note the vascularity apparent on the tumor surface

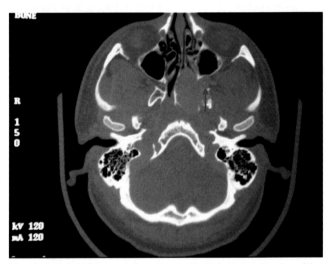

Fig. 22.4: Axial CT image of a patient with JNA. Note widening of the sphenopalatine foramen (arrow), consistent with the characteristic tendency of this neoplasm to extend along the sphenopalatine artery into the pterygopalatine space

be considered to look for XX–XY mosaicism. However, the link of this disease to estrogen, progesterone or androgen receptors have not been demonstrated or observed in any studies.[24–27] Other theories include an abnormal connective tissue response to an ectopic nidus of vascular tissue or an aberrant and unrestrained growth of the embryonic occipital plate (including the basilar process, body of the sphenoid, medial pterygoid process, foramen lacerum and vicinity, and the pterygopalatine fossa).[25]

The clinical presentation of JNA classically includes a male patient with nasal airway obstruction, often unilateral, with recurrent epistaxis.[27] On physical examination it appears as a red-purple nodular mass in the

---

Table 22.4: The Curacao criteria for the diagnosis of HHT

Diagnosis
- Definite, if 3 criteria are present
- Possible or suspected, if 2 criteria are present
- Unlikely, if fewer than 2 criteria are present

Criteria
- Epistaxis—spontaneous, recurrent nose bleeds
- Telangiectasias—multiple at characteristic sites such as lips, oral cavity, fingers, or nose
- Visceral lesions—GI telengectasia ± bleeding, pulmonary AVM, hepatic AVM, cerebral AVM or spinal AVM
- Family history—a first-degree relative with HHT by these criteria

nasopharynx which displaces the soft palate as it grows. If untreated, it can continue to grow to involve the soft tissues of the face, the orbit, and extend intracranially. Intracranial involvement has been reported in 10–36% of cases, with the pituitary region, anterior, and middle cranial fossae being the most commonly involved sites.[22–27] Some proposed routes of spread include direct extension through the floor of the middle fossa from the infratemporal fossa, extension through the superior and inferior orbital fissures, erosion through the sphenoid sinus into the cavernous sinus, and erosion through the ethmoid skull base and cribriform into the anterior fossa.[22] Microscopically, a highly vascular tumor is seen with a dense fibrous stroma background. There are two main classification systems, but the Fisch's classification has become the standard classification system (Tables 22.5 and 22.6). CT and MRI imaging are very helpful in ascertaining the extent of the disease and in preoperative planning.

Surgery is the mainstay of treatment with the underlying paradigm being complete removal of all disease. Historically, this may require surgical approaches such as midfacial degloving, lateral rhinotomy, craniofacial resection, or transpalatal. With the advent of endoscopic surgery, selected tumors can be managed without incisions.[24,27] Scholtz et al, propose a surgical approach based on tumor location (Table 22.7). The use of preoperative arteriogram aids in identifying the vascular supply and in assisting with resection through embolization within the preceding 12 to 48 hours.[24] Nonetheless, intraoperative blood loss often exceeds 1000 ml or more.[22,23] Radiation therapy may be considered for extensive lesions involving the orbit or intracranial structures.[22,27,28]

Table 22.5: Fisch's classification for juvenile nasopharyngeal angiofibromas[57]

Class I : Tumors limited to the nasopharynx and nasal cavity with no bone destruction

Class II: Tumors invading the pterygopalatine fossa and the maxillary, ethmoidal, and sphenoidal sinuses with bone destruction

Class III: Tumors invading the infratemporal fossa, orbit, and parasellar region remaining lateral to the cavernous sinus

Class IV: Tumors with massive invasion of the cavernous sinus, optic chiasma, or pituitary fossa

Table 22.6: Chandler's classification for juvenile nasopharyngeal angiofibromas[57]

Stage I: Tumor confined to the nasopharynx

Stage II: Tumor extending into the nasal cavity and/or the sphenoid sinus

Stage III: Tumor extending into one or more of the following: antrum, ethmoid sinus, pterygomaxillary and infratemporal fossae, orbit and/or cheek

Stage IV: Tumor extending into cranial cavity

MANAGEMENT

Before attempting to manage a patient with epistaxis, one must have a clear understanding of the vascular supply of the nose. The external carotid artery (ECA) and internal carotid artery (ICA) both contribute to the blood supply of the nose. Both the nasal septum (Fig. 22.5) and the lateral nasal wall (Fig. 22.6) receive contributions from both

Table 22.7: Different surgical approaches corresponding to tumor location					
Tumor location	*Transnasal/Endoscopic*	*Transpalatal*	*Lateral rhinotomy*	*Midfacial degloving*	*Infratemporal*
Sphenopalatine foramen	X	X	X	X	X
Nasal cavity	X	X	X	X	
Nasopharynx	X	X	X	X	X
Pterygopalatine fossa	X		X	X	X
Sphenoid fossa	X	X	X	X	X
Ethmoids	X		X	X	
Maxillary sinus			X	X	
Orbit			X	X	X
Medial infratemporal fossa			X	X	X
Lateral infratemporal fossa				X	X
Middle cranial fossa				X	X
Medial cavernous sinus			X	X	
Lateral cavernous sinus				X	X

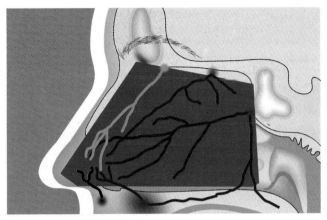

Fig. 22.5: Nasal septum demonstrating anastomoses of the anterior ethmoid (green), posterior ethmoid (blue), sphenopalatine (red), greater palatine (lavendar), and superior labial (black) arteries in Little's area. The greater palatine re-enters the nasal cavity via the nasopalatine foramen. The superior labial is a branch of the facial artery

vascular arcades. The major conduits from the ECA are the internal maxillary artery (via the sphenopalatine and greater palatine branches) and the facial artery (external maxillary artery). In contrast, the anterior and posterior ethmoid arteries are terminal branches of the ICA via the ophthalmic artery.

Most anterior epistaxis arises from Kiesselbach's plexus (Little's area) where branches from the spheno-palatine, greater palatine, and facial arteries anastamose.[29] Posterior epistaxis arises from the sphenopalatine branch and from the ethmoidal perforators.

The vast majority of epistaxis is self-limiting and often patients do not present to a physician for treatment. Those

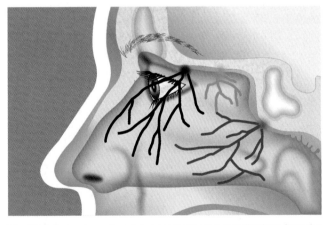

Fig. 22.6: Lateral nasal wall demonstrating the contributions from the anterior ethmoid (black), posterior ethmoid (green), sphenopalatine (red)

that present for medical management are still most likely to be anterior in nature with the bleeding site visible and accessible to local treatment.[6] The first effective measure, which is often forgotten, is simply to pinch the nasal tip. This affords tamponade of Little's area. Acute epistaxis with voluminous blood loss is approached with a slightly different protocol than either chronic or recurrent epistaxis.

Chronic or Recurrent Epistaxis

With chronic or recurrent epistaxis, control of hemorrhage is usually not as important as discovering the reason for the recurrent and chronic bleeding. Coagulopathies and various sinonasal tumors must be considered. A complete discussion of these entities is beyond the scope of this chapter. However, a few points need to be emphasized. First, a comprehensive laboratory evaluation for coagulopathy is not indicated in isolated acute epistaxis. Laboratory evaluation with possible hematologic consultation should be considered if the patient has chronic or recurrent episodes of bleeding, or if the patient has a personal or family history suggesting an underlying disorder, such as easy bruising or heavy menses. It should be remembered that the most common 'coagulopathy' is secondary to oral anti-coagulants or antiplatelet medications. Thus, a complete medication history should be obtained for each patient. Patients with recurrent, but limited episodes of epistaxis secondary to medications are often best treated with nasal saline spray, humidity, and counseling.

Nonetheless, the otolaryngologist must retain a high index of suspicion of a neoplasm, and this can be further investigated by nasal endoscopy and/or imaging. If the otolaryngologist is unable to appreciate the site of the bleeding with anterior rhinoscopy, diagnostic endoscopy should be undertaken. If a complete examination is confounded by bleeding in the acute setting, a careful endoscopy should be conducted during a follow-up visit. Diagnostic imaging (i.e. CT scan) can provide complementary data but does not circumvent the role of endoscopic examination.

Acute Epistaxis

During an acute epistaxis episode, as circumstances permit, a focused but thorough history should be obtained. Assessment must be made of duration and severity of bleeding, frequency of epistaxis episodes, any known predisposing medical conditions, current medications (including non-prescription medication and dietary supplements), allergies, and any history of trauma. If a significant amount of blood loss is suspected, the patient should be treated in a monitored setting with intravenous access. Control of bleeding should commence simultaneously with laboratory evaluation, but only after the overall hemodynamic stability of the patient has been assessed. Blood products, if indicated, should be requested as early as possible to allow adequate time for preparation.

A thorough examination of the nasal cavity is critical for effective treatment of epistaxis. It is often difficult thoroughly examine the patient secondary to briskness of bleeding and the anxiety level of the patient, which can often exacerbate hypertension. The patient should be examined with a headlight or a mirror, wall suction with a Frazier tip, suction, and a nasal speculum. All clots in the nasal cavity should be evacuated to allow inspection of the nasal mucosa. If the site of bleeding is not readily visible, endoscopes can be used to facilitate examination of the posterior nasal cavity.

A stepwise approach from the least to the most invasive interventions is often appropriate for the patient with non-exsanguinating epistaxis. Contrary to a widely held belief, ice packs probably do not have any beneficial effect on epistaxis.[30] There are a number of topical vasoconstrictors available which can be useful during physical examination and may also be therapeutic for mild hemorrhage (Table 22.8). These agents can be sprayed into the nose or placed on cottonoids and laid on the nasal mucosa under direct visualization or with the use of rigid endoscopes. Reflex vasoconstriction is of historical interest. William Buchan, in 1769, stated *"If the genitals be immersed for some time in cold water, it will generally stop a bleeding nose; I have seldom known this to fail."*[31]

Every effort should be made to find a discrete source of bleeding. Once found, it can be cauterized at the bedside or in the operating room. For a slow hemorrhage, silver nitrate can be used. This has been used for generations and is a clinically proven effective way to control epistaxis. Silver nitrate acts as a strong oxidizer causing a wave of free radical release which will oxidize tissue, kill bacteria, and coagulate vessels.[32] The histological effects of silver

nitrate on tissue were demonstrated by Hanif and colleagues, who also reported that five seconds would be the optimal duration of application.[32] Complications of silver nitrate include septal perforation, particularly if apposing sides of the septum are cauterized, transient pain, and chemical burns to the skin. If the bleeding is brisk, electrocautery may be required.

Packing

When a specific site of hemorrhage is not identifiable, packing of the nose may be required. In general these types of hemorrhage can be considered anterior or posterior. These are not specific anatomic divisions and, historically, have been attributed to the nasal septum if anterior and branches of the sphenopalatine artery if posterior (Fig. 22.7). The vast majority of epistaxis is anterior, involving the nasal septum.[33] The clinical distinction between anterior and posterior bleeding often depends on physical examination and patient's symptomatology—whether the patient has more blood coming from the nares or draining into the pharynx. There are several methods and products available for packing the nose, all of which use the basic principle of tamponade to control bleeding.

A number of different materials have been used for anterior packing. Ribbon gauze of different weaves with or without impregnated additives such as bismuth and iodoform have been used. This is inserted with a bayonet forceps and headlight into the nasal cavity, with the goal of filling the space between the septum and the lateral nasal wall. While this procedure is very effective, it is time consuming, prolongs patient discomfort, carries the risk

Table 22.8: Commonly used topical vasoconstrictors
• Oxymetazoline
• Neosynephrine
• Phenylephrine
• Cocaine
• Epinephrine

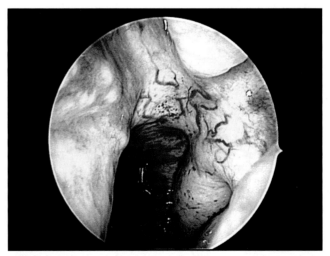

Fig. 22.7: Endoscopic view into the posterior nasal cavity revealing dilated mucosal vasculature. These branches of the sphenopalatine artery can be responsible for posterior epistaxis

of aspiration of part of the ribbon gauze, and must be inserted by an individual with at least rudimentary knowledge of nasal anatomy who is familiar with the instrumentation.[34,35]

Alternatively, preformed nasal packs have been developed that may been inserted even by inexperienced practitioners quickly and effectively. There are prefabricated devices too for controlling epistaxis: The prototype of these is the hydroxylated polyvinyl acetal nasal pack (Fig. 22.8). This nasal pack is a compressed material that triples in size when hydrated with either blood or saline. Instead of passive expansion with hydration, there are also other nasal packs which need to be inflated to provide adequate tamponading effect. They are available in a variety of sizes targeting either anterior or posterior sources of bleeding; they have been demonstrated to be effective, easily placed even by inexperienced practitioners, and fairly well-tolerated by patients.[35] Typically, with packs such as these, they are left in place for 3 to 5 days in order to allow adequate repair of the bleeding vessel and to allow the unavoidable mucosal abrasions to heal. Removal can be facilitated by moistening the pack with saline or a topical vasoconstrictor such as oxymetazoline.

An alternative strategy is to use a resorbable hemostatic material which does not need to be removed. This may be preferable in patients with underlying coagulation disorders, which the mere act of removing a nasal pack would be traumatic enough to restart bleeding. Examples of resorbable hemostatic materials include Gelfoam, oxidized cellulose, microfibrillar collagen, or newer proprietary agents such as Floseal® (microfibrillar collagen and thrombin, Baxter Pharmaceuticals). The effects of these agents on the nasal mucosa have not been well-studied, but most clinicians agree that they are not inert.[36]

Although complications from anterior nasal packing are rare, they do occasionally occur. While most are minor, serious adverse events during and subsequent to anterior nasal packing rarely occur and these are summarized in Table 22.9.

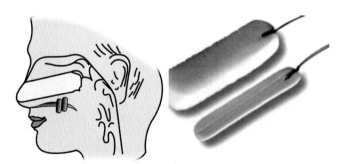

Fig. 22.8: Hydroxylated polyvinyl acetal packing prehydrated, after hydration, and *in situ* when inserted properly

Table 22.9: Complications of nasal packing[34]

Cardiovascular collapse
- Hypovolemia, shock, syncope
- Nasal-vagal reflex
  - Bradycardia
  - Reduction of cardiac output
  - Hypotension
  - Apnea
- Reaction to topical agents
  - Technical problems
- Continued bleeding
- Dislodgement of packing
- Laceration of nose or soft palate
- Septal injury
  - Hypoxia or hypoxemia
- Disorientation
- Myocardial infarction or cerebrovascular accident
  - Iatrogenic obstructive sleep apnea
  - Infection
- Local or topical
- Bacteremia
- Toxic shock syndrome

Adapted from Fairbanks 1986

The nasal cardiopulmonary reflex has been well-documented. It is most likely mediated through the afferent trigeminal nerve and uses the vagus nerve as its efferent conduit.[37,38] This reflex is highly developed in aquatic mammals and birds that experience peripheral vasoconstriction and decreased cardiac output but with preserved cerebral blood flow mediated through baroreceptors in the nose.[39] In some individuals, the presence of even trivial noxious stimulation such as insertion of anesthesia probes or even strong noxious odors may stimulate this response, even to the point of cardiac arrest.[37,38] However, the use of topical anesthesia in the nose may attenuate this reflex.

Toxic shock syndrome (TSS) was first described in a population of young menstruating women associated with retained superabsorbent tampons containing synthetic materials such as polyester. TSS has also been reported in cases of nasal packing.[34,40,41] TSS is a systemic disease caused by the *Staphylococcal* exotoxin TSST-1. The major diagnostic criteria are fever greater than 38.9°C, a characteristic desquamating rash, hypotension, and shock (Table 22.10).[40] Symptoms may begin shortly after packing or may be delayed by several hours to a day. Once suspected, observation at the intensive care unit, administration of parenteral antibiotics, and removal of all packing materials should be considered. Jacobson and colleagues estimated that the incidence of TSS following nasal operations to be 16.5 per 100,000.[41] Rapid

Table 22.10: Diagnostic criteria for TSS
• Fever >38.9°C
• Exanthem with erythoderma
• Subsequent desquamation
• Hypotension or shock

development of multisystem organ failure has been reported. It is generally believed that coating the packing material with antibiotic ointment will help reduce the incidence of TSS. However, the benefits of this approach and routine administration of systemic anti-staphylo-coccal antibiotics has never been proven or studied. Breda and colleagues studied the ability of *Staphylococcus aureus* to use either nasal tampon or gauze packing strip as a matrix for bacterial proliferation following nasal surgery. Gauze packing strip was found to support a higher growth rate of *Staphylococcus* than nasal tampon and that the only toxic shock toxin forming bacteria in vitro were in isolates from the gauze packing strip. Further, neither coating of the gauze with antibiotic ointment nor administering systemic antibiotics completely prevented the *in vitro* growth.[40]

If anterior packing fails to control the hemorrhage, reinforcing it with more packing or packing the contra-lateral nasal cavity sometimes aids tamponade. However, if physical examination reveals a posterior source of bleeding, anterior packing alone will not be successful, and more advanced maneuvers including anterior-posterior packing, arterial ligation, and/or embolization may be required.

While preparing for a more definitive method of control, the use of transoral local anesthetic injection of the sphenopalatine artery via the greater palatine foramen can be a useful adjunct to temporize posterior epistaxis. In this procedure, a 3 cc syringe containing 2.5 cc of 1% lidocaine with 1:100,0000 epinephrine is mounted onto a 25-gauge needle, which is acutely bent 2.5 cm from the tip. The needle is passed into the greater palatine foramen, which can be localized in a depression just medial to the second molar (Figs 22.9A and B). The local anesthetic is instilled slowly, and frequent aspiration is necessary to prevent intra-vascular injection. Although rare, both temporary and permanent blindness are theoretical complications of this maneuver. This procedure may allow additional, more definitive procedures to be performed while slowing the rate of acute blood loss.

Classically, anterior-posterior packing is with a gauze ball placed through the mouth with a suture attached to it.

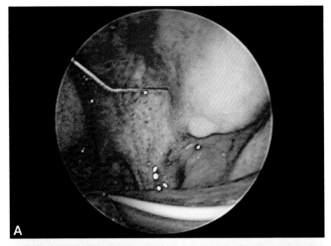
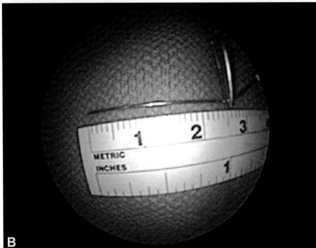

Figs 22.9A and B: Transoral injection of the sphenopalatine artery. The greater palatine foramen can be cannulated in a palpable depression just medial to the second molar (note that this particular patient is edentulous). The needle is acutely bent 2.5 cm from the tip to insure that the needle is not passed overly superiorly into the orbital apex

The suture is drawn through the nose via a flexible catheter which is passed transnasally, brought out through the mouth and attached to the suture prior to placement. A more expedient method involves passing a Foley urinary catheter through the nose, inflating the balloon, and then impacting it into the nasopharynx. It is held tightly in place with a clamp just outside the nose, but carefully padded to protect against the disfiguring possibility of alar and columellar pressure necrosis. There are also preformed balloon devices currently manufactured to accomplish the same goal (Fig. 22.10). The anterior nose must be packed as well. Often the posterior pack is not resting over the hemorrhaging vessel, and it is only by combining anterior and posterior packing that adequate

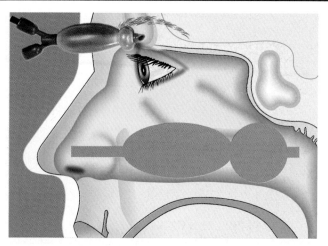

Fig. 22.10: Commercially available combined anterior-posterior balloon pack, with diagrammatic representation of device placement *in situ*

pressure builds up in the nasal cavity to tamponade the bleeding. It is not uncommon to have bloody tears or hemotympanum as a result of bloody reflux upwards in the associated ducts. A common mistake is to place a posterior pack and then place a 10 cm tampon as an anterior pack. This length of nasal tampon will protrude into the nasopharynx and an adequate seal by the posterior pack, undermining the desired tamponade effect.

Anteroposterior packs are associated with a higher morbidity rate than anterior packs alone. In one study, the overall rate of complications approached 70% with nearly 20% being classified as life-threatening.[42] Cardiac complications (most commonly bradycardia) alone were observed in almost 8% of patients in a study by Wang and Vogel.[42] This incidence is even greater in patients with comorbidities. Patients in whom anterior and posterior packs are placed should thus be monitored in an intensive care unit or other monitored location for the development of cardiac complications from their pack.

The efficacy of anterior-posterior nasal packing has also been called into question. Although previous studies have reported its usefulness, recent studies have reported failure rates to range from 25 to 50%.[42–44] With the medical morbidity of anterior-posterior packing, its dubious success rate, and the degree of discomfort experienced by the patient, there has been interest in examining alternative treatment for posterior epistaxis. In general anteroposterior packing should be viewed as a temporizing measure until definitive control of epistaxis can be obtained.

Invasive Procedures

Surgery has been a traditional treatment for epistaxis. Historically, it was reserved for packing failures and

consisted of carotid artery ligation. The first artery to be ligated was the common carotid artery, but was abandoned secondary to the high rate of morbidity. Since the blood supply to the nasal cavity is mostly from the external carotid system, the external carotid artery was the next candidate for ligation. External carotid artery ligation, both ipsilateral and bilateral has been shown to be a safe, effective and a quick way of controlling intractable epistaxis.[31,45] In some cases, anterior ethmoid artery ligation must be performed concurrently to provide total hemostasis. Selective arterial ligation is also an option, which is more appealing because the hemorrhage will be controlled closer to the source. However, it does have the drawback of being technically difficult and sometimes requiring special instruments.

Many approaches to the branches of the external carotid system have been described and shown to be effective. One approach is clipping the internal maxillary artery through a sublabial transantral approach (Figs 22.11 and 22.12). This approach is effective, but is made difficult by the tortuosity of the vessels at this point. Complications of this procedure include re-bleeding (9.5–10%), oralantral fistula, dental problems, and anesthesia in the distribution of the infraorbital nerve or the superior alveolar nerve.[46,47]

According to a retrospective review of 100 patients with epistaxis by Metson and colleagues, the most common cause of failure of the surgical intervention to control bleeding was failure of the surgeon to identify the internal maxillary artery or its terminal branches in the pterygopalatine fossa.[46] Nasal endoscopic surgery has allowed for identification and control of an even more distal site,

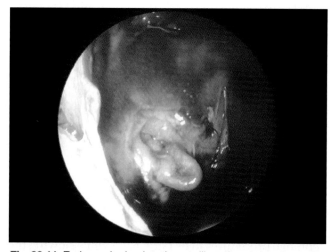

Fig. 22.11: Endoscopic view into the maxillary sinus in a cadaver. The mucosa has been incised, and the posterior wall of the sinus opened. A branch of the internal maxillary artery has been delivered from the surrounding fatty tissue in the pterygopalatine space

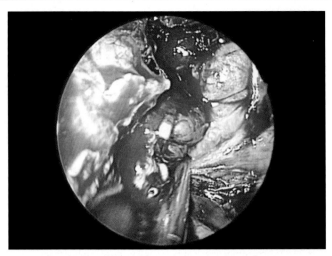

Fig. 22.12: Endoscopic view of the internal maxillary artery *in vivo* status postclipping

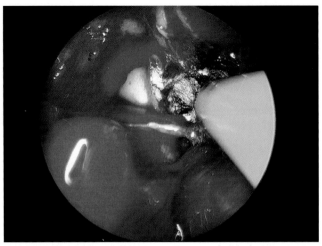

Fig. 22.14: Endoscopic view of the right sphenopalatine as it exists its foramen. The vessel has been controlled with a suction electrocautery. The landmarks and orientation of this image are an *in vivo* correlate of the image shown in Fig. 22.13

the sphenopalatine artery as it enters the nasal cavity. It is approached by developing a vertical mucosal flap on the palatine bone at the posterior attachment of the middle turbinate. The sphenopalatine artery enters the nasal cavity through a foramen just posterior and inferior to the attachment of the orbital process of the palatine bone with the sphenoid body, seen as a bony crest (the *Crista ethmoidalis*) in the nose (Figs 22.13 and 22.14).[48] The artery may either be cauterized or clipped at this point. If the bleeding is not controlled by addressing the external carotid branches, the anterior ethmoid artery should also be controlled.[47–49] This is most often done through an external incision, but may also be approached with the assistance of endoscope.[50,51] It is critical to keep the

relationship of the ethmoidal arteries in mind while operating in this area. The anterior ethmoidal artery is 24 mm deep to the lacrimal crest, 12 mm deep to this is the posterior ethmoidal artery and 6 mm deep to that is the optic canal (Fig. 22.15).[52]

Selective arterial endovascular occlusion is another alternative method in managing intractable epistaxis. Several studies have shown that this method is safe and effective.[53,54] However, its usefulness is limited to branches of the external carotid system only, as embolization off the

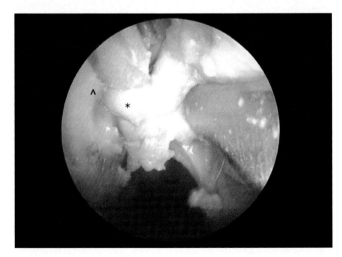

Fig. 22.13: Endoscopic view of the right sphenopalatine artery as its exits its foramen as seen in a cadaveric dissection. The crista ethmoidalis (arrowhead) and artery (asterisks) are identified

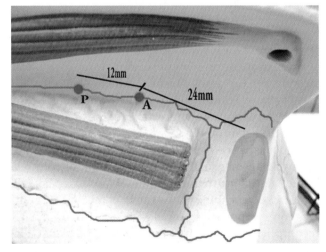

Fig. 22.15: Medial orbital wall demonstrating the relationship of the anterior ethmoid artery (A) and posterior ethmoid artery (P). The former is approximately 24 mm posterior to the lacrimal crest, and the latter is approximately 12 mm posterior to that. The optic nerve (not shown) is just 6 mm posterior to the posterior ethmoid foramen. The foramina for these arteries lie along the frontoethmoid suture line

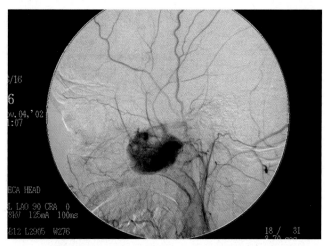

Fig. 22.16: Angiographic image demonstrating the intense vascularity of a JNA

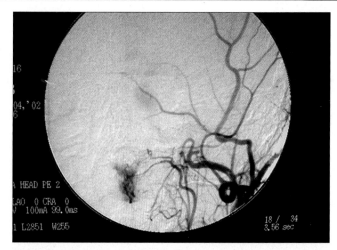

Fig. 22.17: Angiogram after internal maxillary artery embolization (same case as that shown in Fig. 22.16) revealing a marked decrease in tumor vascularity. The primary feeding vessel was the sphenopalatine artery, but other internal maxillary branches and collaterals were also implicated

Circle of Willis is not feasible. A variety of occlusive agents may be used with this method, including coils or thrombogenic particles. The endovascular approach can be complicated by groin hematomas, trigeminal nerve hypersensitivity, facial nerve paralysis, myocardial infarction, hemiplegia, or cheek necrosis.[55] The most common minor complication was facial parasthesias and jaw pain which occurred in 3–19% of the cases. The risk of cerebrovascular accident with embolization is approximately 1%.[54,55]

Studies which have compared the efficacy, safety, and cost of arterial ligation and endovascular embolization, have failed to demonstrate one modality to be superior to the other.[42,54–56] One important note is that failure of one modality does not preclude an attempt with the other. However, following endovascular occlusion of a major artery, such as the internal maxillary, any further episodes of epistaxis in the distribution of that vessel are typically secondary to the development of collateral blood vessels distal to the site of embolization. This complicates further attempts at endovascular occlusion of the main vessel to control the hemorrhage.

Endovascular embolization is an important component in the management of JNA, where this typically precedes surgical resection to reduce operative blood loss (Figs 22.16 and 22.17). Depending on the extent of the tumor and the surgeon's experience, excision of the tumor may be accomplished with any combination of transfacial, transpalatal, and endoscopic approaches (Fig. 22.18).

SUMMARY

Epistaxis is caused by multiple factors. It is largely a self-limiting disease of trivial consequence; occasionally, it may

be severe and life-threatening. Furthermore, underlying etiologies such as malignancy, JNA, and hematologic diseases must at least be considered in the differential diagnoses, and ruled out with further evaluation as indicated.

There are many modalities available for treating even the most severe epistaxis, and it should be emphasized that angiographic embolization has potential risks, is not always *immediately* available, and may not be feasible in all centers. Thus, angiographic embolization has not

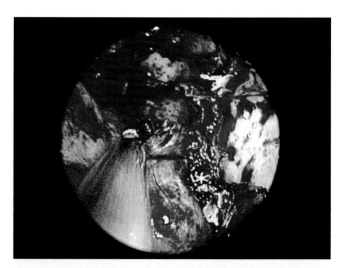

Fig. 22.18: Endoscopic resection of a JNA. The suction is displacing the tumor mass inferiorly and medially. The sphenopalatine artery has been cauterized (asterisk), and the tumor has been freed from its posterosuperior attachments

supplanted the surgeon's role in the definitive management of this disease, and all otolaryngologists must be well-versed in the various procedures to manage epistaxis.

REFERENCES

1. Danielides V, Kontogiannis N, Bartzokas A, Lolis CJ, Skevas A. The influence of meteorological factors on the frequency of epistaxis. *Clin Otolaryngol* 2002;27(2):84–88.
2. Okafor BC. Epistaxis: A clinical study of 540 cases. *Ear Nose Throat J* 1984;63(3):153–159.
3. Herkner H, Laggner AN, Mullner M et al. Hypertension in patients presenting with epistaxis. *Ann Emerg Med* 2000; 35(2):126–130.
4. Shaheen OH. Arterial epistaxis. *J Laryngol Otol* 1975;89(1): 17–34.
5. Pothula VB, Reddy KT, Nixon TE. Carotico-cavernous fistula following septorhinoplasty. *J Laryngol Otol* 1999;113(9): 844–846.
6. Padgham N. Epistaxis: Anatomical and clinical correlates. *J Laryngol Otol* 1990;104(4):308–311.
7. Diamantopoulos II, Jones NS. The investigation of nasal septal perforations and ulcers. *J Laryngol Otol* 2001;115(7):541–544.
8. Baum ED, Bondousquie AC, Shiyong Li, Mirza N. Sarcoidosis with nasal obstruction and septal perforation. *Ear Nose Throat J* 1998;77(11):896–898.
9. Batra K, Chaudhary N, Motwani G, Raj AK. An unusual case of primary nasal tuberculosis with epistaxis and epilepsy. *Ear Nose Throat J* 2002;81(12):842–844.
10. Hambleton J. Advances in the treatment of von Willebrand disease. *Sem Hematol* 2001;38(4 Suppl 9):7–10.
11. Lee JW. Von Willebrand disease, hemophilia A and B, and other factor deficiencies. *Int Anesthesiol Clin* 2004;42(3):59–76.
12. McGarry GW, Gatehouse S, Vernham G. Idiopathic epistaxis, haemostasis and alcohol. *Clin Otolaryngol Allied Sci* 1995;20(2):174–177.
13. Herkner H, Havel C, Mullner M, Active epistaxis at ED presentation is associated with arterial hypertension. *Am J Emerg Med* 2002;20(2):92–95.
14. Zampaglione B, Pascale C, Marchision M, Cavallo-Perin P. Hypertensive urgencies and emergencies: Prevalence and clinical presentation. *Hypertension* 1996;27(1):144–147.
15. Neto JFL, Fuchs FD, Facco SR et al. Is epistaxis evidence of end-organ damage in patients with hypertension? *Laryngoscope* 1999;109(7 Pt 1):1111–1115.
16. Begbie ME, Wallace GM, Shovlin CL. Hereditary haemorrhagic telangiectasia (Osler-Weber-Rendu syndrome): A view from the 21st century. *Postgrad Med J* 2003;79(927):18–24.
17. Shovlin CL, Guttinachen AE, Buscarini E et al. Diagnostic criteria for hereditary hemorrhagic telangiectasia (Rendu-Osler-Weber syndrome). *Am J Med Genet* 2000;91(1):66–67.
18. Jameson JJ, Cave DR. Hormonal and antihormonal therapy for epistaxis in hereditary hemorrhagic telangiectasia. *Laryngoscope* 2004;114(4):705–709.
19. Shah RK, Dhingra JK, Shapshay SM. Hereditary hemorrhagic telangiectasia: A review of 76 cases. *Laryngoscope* 2002; 112(5):767–773.
20. Osguthorpe JD. Sinus neoplasia. *Arch Otolaryngol Head Neck Surg* 1994;120(1):19–25.
21. Resto VA, Deschler DG. Sinonasal malignancies. *Otolaryngol Clin North Am* 2004;37(2):473–487.
22. Lee JT et al. The role of radiation in the treatment of advanced juvenile angiofibroma. *Laryngoscope* 2002;112(7 Pt 1): 1213–1220.
23. Liu L, Wang R, Huang D et al. Analysis of intra-operative bleeding and recurrence of juvenile nasopharyngeal angio-fibromas. *Clin Otolaryngol Allied Sci* 2002;27(6):536–540.
24. Mann WJ, Jecker P, Amedee RG. Juvenile angiofibromas: Changing surgical concept over the last 20 years. *Laryngoscope* 2004;114(2):291–293.
25. Chandler JR, Goulding R, Moskowitz L et al. Nasopharyngeal angiofibromas: Staging and management. *Ann Otol Rhinol Laryngol* 1984;93(4 Pt 1):322–329.
26. Howard DJ, Lloyd G, Lund V. Recurrence and its avoidance in juvenile angiofibroma *Laryngoscope* 2001;111(9):1509–1511.
27. Scholtz AW, Appenroth E, Kamen-Jolly K et al. Juvenile nasopharyngeal angiofibroma: Management and therapy *Laryngoscope* 2001;111(4 Pt 1):681–687.
28. Beriwal S, Eidelman A, Micaily B. Three-dimensional conformal radiotherapy for treatment of extensive juvenile angiofibroma: Report on two cases. *Orl J Oto-Rhino-Laryngol Rel Specialt* 2003;65(4):238–241.
29. Koh E, Frazzini VI, Kagetsu NJ. Epistaxis: Vascular anatomy, origins, and endovascular treatment. *Am J Roentgenol* 2000; 174(3):845–851.
30. Teymoortash A, Sesterhenn A, Kress R et al. Efficacy of ice packs in the management of epistaxis [see comment]. *Clin Otolaryngol Allied Sci* 2003;28(6):545–547.
31. Malcomson K. The surgical management of massive epistaxis. *J Laryngol Otol* 1963;77(3):299–314.
32. Hanif J, Tasca RA, Frosh A et al. Silver nitrate: Histological effects of cautery on epithelial surfaces with varying contact times. *Clin Otolaryngol Allied Sci* 2003;28(4):368–370.
33. Viducich RA, Blanda MP, Gerson LW. Posterior epistaxis: Clinical features and acute complications. *Ann Emerg Med* 1995;25(5):592–596.
34. Fairbanks DN. Complications of nasal packing. *Otolaryngol Head Neck Surg* 1986;94(3):412–415.
35. Pringle MB, Beasley P, Brightwell AP. The use of Merocel nasal packs in the treatment of epistaxis. *J Laryngol Otol* 1996; 110(6):543–546.
36. Chandra RK, Conley DB, Kern RC. The effect of FloSeal on mucosal healing after endoscopic sinus surgery: A comparison with thrombin-soaked gelatin foam. *Am J Rhinol* 2003;17(1): 51–55.
37. Bailey PL. Sinus arrest induced by trivial nasal stimulation during alfentanil–nitrous oxide anaesthesia. *Br J Anaesthesia* 1990;65(5):718–720.
38. Patow CA, Kaliner M. Nasal and cardiopulmonary reflexes. *Ear Nose Throat J* 1984;63(2):22.
39. Angell JE, Daly M de B. Nasal reflexes. *Proc Royal Soc Med* 1969;62(12):1287–1293.
40. Breda SD, Jacobs JB, Leibowitz AS, Tierno PM. Toxic shock syndrome in nasal surgery: A physiochemical and microbiologic evaluation of Merocel and NuGauze nasal packing. *Laryngoscope* 1987;97(12):1388–1391.
41. Jacobson JA, Kasworm EM. Toxic shock syndrome after nasal surgery: Case reports and analysis of risk factors. *Arch Otolaryngol Head Neck Surg* 1986;112(3):329–332.
42. Wang L, Vogel DH. Posterior epistaxis: Comparison of treatment. *Otolaryngol Head Neck Surg* 1981;89(6):1001–1006.

43. Klotz DA, Winkle MR, Kichmon J, Hengerer AS. Surgical management of posterior epistaxis: A changing paradigm *Laryngoscope* 2002;112(9):1577–1582.

44. Cannon CR. Effective treatment protocol for posterior epistaxis: A 10-year experience *Otolaryngol Head Neck Surg* 1993; 109(4):722–725.

45. Hunter K, Gibson R. Arterial ligation for severe epistaxis. *J Laryngol Otol* 1969;83(11):1099–1103.

46. Metson R, Lane R. Internal maxillary artery ligation for epistaxis: An analysis of failures. *Laryngoscope* 1988;98(7): 760–764.

47. Spafford P, Durham JS. Epistaxis: Efficacy of arterial ligation and long-term outcome. *J Otolaryngol* 1992;21(4):252–256.

48. Srinivasan V, Sherman IW, O'Sullivan G. Surgical management of intractable epistaxis: Audit of results. *J Laryngol Otol* 2000;114(9):697–700.

49. Singh B. Combined internal maxillary and anterior ethmoidal arterial occlusion: The treatment of choice in intractable epistaxis. *J Laryngol Otol* 1992;106(6):507–510.

50. Douglas SA, Gupta D. Endoscopic-assisted external approach anterior ethmoidal artery ligation for the management of epistaxis. *J Laryngol Otol* 2003;117(2):132–133.

51. Woolford, TJ and NS Jones. Endoscopic ligation of anterior ethmoidal artery in treatment of epistaxis. *J Laryngol Otol* 2000;114(11):858–860.

52. Lander MI, Terry O. The posterior ethmoid artery in severe epistaxis. *Otolaryngol Head Neck Surg* 1992;106(1):101–103.

53. Elahi MM, Parnes LS, Fox AJ et al. Therapeutic embolization in the treatment of intractable epistaxis. *Arch Otolaryngol Head Neck Surg* 1995;121(1):65–69.

54. Elden L, Montanera W, Terbrugge K et al. Angiographic embolization for the treatment of epistaxis: A review of 108 cases. *Otolaryngol Head Neck Surg* 1994;111(1):44–50.

55. Cullen MM, Tami TA. Comparison of internal maxillary artery ligation versus embolization for refractory posterior epistaxis. *Otolaryngol Head Neck Surg* 1998;118(5):636–642.

56. Strong EB, Bell DA, Johnson LP, Jacobs JM. Intractable epistaxis: Transantral ligation vs embolization: Efficacy review and cost analysis. *Otolaryngol Head Neck Surg* 1995;113(6):674–678.

57. Fisch U, Fagan P, Valavanis A. The infratemporal fossa approach for the lateral skull base. *Otolaryngol Clin North Am* 1984;17(3):513–552.

CHAPTER 23

Disorders of the Nasal Septum

Thomas Costello, Rakesh K Chandra

The nasal septum is a highly conserved structure across all mammals. Despite this, its function has not been fully elucidated. It probably has some function in reducing total nasal resistance by forming a parallel circuit (two nasal valves and two nasal cavities) rather than a circuit in series. Many disorders, both local and systemic, may manifest as a nasal septal disorder. Symptoms include epistaxis, nasal airway obstruction, facial pressure or pain, sinusitis or are asymptomatic. The nasal septum has both bony and cartilaginous components which are covered by a type of respiratory mucosa which is different from that of the remaining respiratory tract. In order to diagnose and manage nasal septal disorders, a broad understanding of many local and systemic problems is required. It should be noted that simple epistaxis is most often a disorder of the nasal septum. The topic of epistaxis is covered comprehensively elsewhere within this text. In the present chapter, we attempt to classify disorders of the nasal septum in the following categories: Deviation, perforation, infection, inflammatory, neoplastic, and reactive. It should be clarified, however, that this scheme is intended only as a framework, since the clinical presentations of these unique disorders could lead them to be classified under multiple headings.

SEPTAL DEVIATION

Perhaps the most common nasal septal disorder is deviation of the septum, often brought to medical attention by unilateral nasal obstruction. Deviation may be classified as congenital or acquired, though the distinction is somewhat cloudy. One theory of congenital septal deviation is that pressure is exerted on the nose and maxilla during the birth process. This theory is weakened by the presence of septal deviations in children delivered by cesarean section.[1] Other theories speculate that a deviated

nasal septum is an inevitable result of the evolution of the human skull. This theory was supported by the observation published in 1978 by Gray that septal deviation is very rare in lower mammals but was about 37% in apes and baboons.[2] Acquired septal deformity is almost universally caused by trauma (Fig. 23.1), however chronic pressure from mass effect (e.g. inflammatory polyp or neoplasm) may gradually displace the septum (Fig. 23.2).

Deviation of the nasal septum may be asymptomatic, for which no therapy is necessary. However, it may be a cause of nasal airway obstruction. This may be from direct blockage of the nasal airway, compromise of the cross-sectional area with exacerbation by mucosal inflammation such as from allergy, or contralateral obstruction from a hypertrophied turbinate. There is also some evidence that mucosal clearance is decreased on the concave side of septal deformity.[3] Since the cause of nasal airway obstruction may be partially due to a mucosal process, treating with a

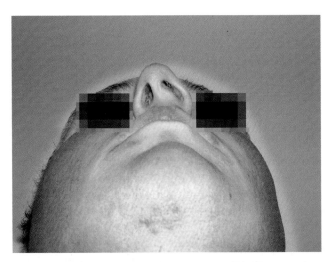

Fig. 23.1: Traumatic deviation of the nasal pyramid with concomitant deflection of the septum as seen in basal view

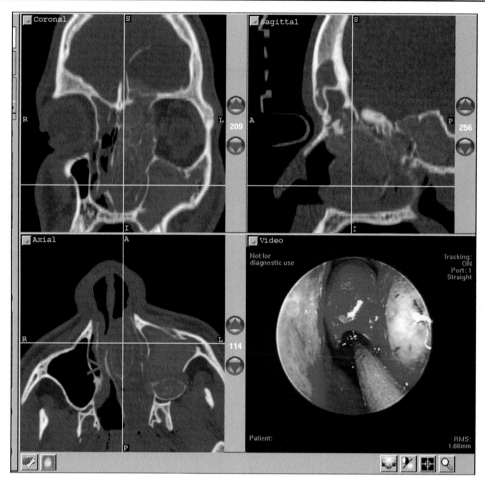

Fig. 23.2: Triplanar CT reconstruction as used for stereotactic image-guided surgical navigation. In the coronal image (upper left panel), note that the more severe inflammatory disease (allergic fungal sinusitis) on the left side has resulted in septal displacement to the right. The septum contacts the right lateral nasal wall (arrowhead shown on axial image in lower left panel), resulting in bilateral nasal obstruction

nasal steroid is advisable. If medical management does not relieve the symptom, a septoplasty procedure can be considered. There are many different approaches to correcting the deformed nasal septum,[4] and a full discussion is beyond the scope of this chapter. In brief, after elevating a subperichondrial flap on the nasal septal cartilage, the deformed areas are either removed or weakened enough to allow repositioning to the midline. The main tenets are to remove as little of the bony and cartilaginous septum as possible to create a widely patent airway. It is mandatory to leave enough suprastructure along the dorsum and the columella to prevent postoperative saddle nose deformity. Often septal correction is augmented with reduction of the inferior turbinates to increase the cross-sectional area of the nasal

airway. It should be noted that surgery for a nasal septal deviation should be avoided on a prepubescent child, as the septum is a facial growth center, and septoplasty in these patients may stunt final nasal height. The exact minimum age for elective septoplasty (or rhinoplasty) is somewhat controversial, but age 15 is a good rule of thumb, at least when the primary goal of the procedure is aesthetic.

One particular disorder that may be associated with septal deviation is the contact point headache. A full discussion of headache and facial pain syndromes is beyond the scope of this chapter, and the exact influence of sinonasal pathology in the development of these conditions is unclear. Some hypothesize that pain can be elicited by contact between the nasal septum and one or more turbinates. Typically, a septal spur is observed in the region of contact. These findings are certainly present in many asymptomatic patients. Thus, it remains questionable why some patients would manifest headache or facial pain as a result of this anatomy. Diagnosis of a contact point headache can be supported by a diagnostic application of vasoconstrictive agent to the region of contact followed by injection of the contact points with 1% lidocaine (Figs 23.3A and B). The patient is observed in the office for 15 minutes. If the pain is aborted, the diagnosis of contact point headache may be considered. Parsons and colleagues demonstrated 85% success rate with a combination of septoplasty, turbinoplasty, and endoscopic sinus surgery in *carefully selected* patients.[5] Prior to considering surgery, a trial of topical nasal steroids (at least one month) should be attempted. Overall, given the debatable nature of the disorder, we reserve septal and turbinate surgery for those who also report nasal obstruction and only perform endoscopic sinus surgery in patients who manifest chronic sinusitis that has failed medical management. The patient must be counseled that the role of septal deviation in headaches is controversial and that the effect of surgery on the headache itself is somewhat unpredictable.

SEPTAL PERFORATION

Nasal septal perforations are another anatomic abnormality of the septum which may be symptomatic or asymptomatic. If symptomatic, the patient most commonly complains of whistling during inspiration, crusting or bleeding (Table 23.1).[6,7] The presence of a through-and-through defect in the nasal septum is never normal and should prompt an investigation into the cause. Despite a

Table 23.1: Symptoms of nasal septal perforation
• Whistling
• Crusting
• Bleeding
• Pain
• Rhinorrhea
• Nasal obstruction
• Voice changes
• Headache
• Dry nose or mouth

thorough work-up, in approximately half the patients the cause remains unclear.[6] There could be many causes of a septal perforation and the presumptive idiopathic cause must be a diagnosis of exclusion (Table 23.2).

Iatrogenic

Previous surgery is one of the most common causes of septal perforation. It can occur from any nasal procedure which either directly or indirectly traumatizes the septum. The most common procedure is septoplasty (Fig. 23.4). Bateman, et al conducted a literature review the results of which estimate a 2–8% perforation rate from submucous resection and a 1.6–5.4% rate from septoplasty.[8] This most often results from the creation of opposing mucoperichondrial lacerations on each side of the septum.

Traumatic

Traumatic injuries involving the nasal septum can leave a septal perforation after healing. This is particularly true in cases where a septal hematoma develops following nasal or facial trauma. Any collection of blood between

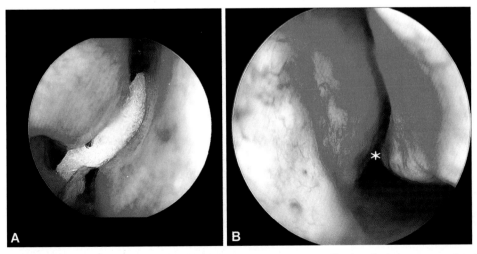

Figs 23.3A and B: The nasal cavity is decongested with a cottonoid soaked in phenylephrine or oxymetazoline.
(A) After decongestion. (B) The contact point (asterisk) can be injected with 1% lidocaine

Table 23.2: Causes of a nasal septal perforation (Adapted from Kridel 1999)[7]

Trauma
- External
- Fracture
- Septal hematoma
- Piercing injuries
- Self-inflicted
- Nose picking
- Foreign bodies
- Iatrogenic
- Nasal surgery
- Septoplasty
- Sinus surgery
- Turbinate surgery
- Rhinoplasty
- Septal cauterization
- Septal packing
- Septal splinting
- Cryosurgery
- Trans-sphenoidal hypophysectomy
- Postoperative suctioning
- Nasotracheal intubation

Drugs: Legal and otherwise
- Vasoconstrictive nasal sprays
- Steroid nasal sprays
- Cocaine
- Smoking

Chemical irritants
- Chromic, sulfuric, and hydrochloric acids
- Chlorines and bromines
- Agricultural aerosolized dust
- Rice and grain elevator dust
- Chemical and industrial dusts
- Lime
- Cement
- Glass
- Salt
- Dust
- EMSP, heavy metal
- Cyanide, arsenicals

Neoplastic causes
- Adenocarcinoma
- Squamous cell carcinoma
- Metastatic carcinoma
- Midline destructive granuloma

Inflammatory causes
- Vasculitides
- Collagen vascular diseases
- Sarcoidosis
- Wegener's granulomatosis

Contd...

Contd...

Infections
- Tuberculosis
- Syphilis
- Rhinoscleroma
- Lepromatous leprosy
- Rhinosporidiosis
- Multiple fungal species
- *Mucor*
- Typhoid
- Diphtheria

cartilaginous component of the septum and the overlying mucoperichondrium deprives the underlying cartilage from its blood supply, which is exclusively provided by the perichondrial layer. As a result, cartilaginous necrosis can occur, which in the long-term may lead to septal perforation and/or severe cosmetic deformity, particularly a saddle nose. In the acute post-traumatic setting, the otolaryngologist must be vigilant to make the diagnosis. Management requires prompt endonasal incision and drainage of the hematoma. The mucoperichondrium can then be bolstered to the underlying cartilaginous framework by a short period (3–4 days) of nasal tampon packing. To prevent toxic shock syndrome, it is also prudent to cover the patient with antistaphylococcal antibiotics while packing is in place, although it should be noted that antibiotics have not been proven to eliminate bacterial proliferation.[9]

In cases of delayed diagnosis, bacterial translocation (most commonly *Staphylococcus aureus*) into the milieu of hematoma and necrotic cartilage will result in abscess development. Additional suppurative complications including cavernous sinus thrombosis, meningitis and brain abscess are then likely.[10] Septal hematoma is most common in males, and in children, and often occurs after minor external nasal trauma. Self-inflicted trauma such as nose piercing or obsessive nose picking have also been known to result in septal perforation.[7]

Drug-induced

Chronic use of vasoconstrictive agents in the nose can lead to septal perforation. The classic example of this is cocaine abuse,[7,12–14] however, it can occur with over-the-counter sprays such as oxymetazoline, neosynephrine and others or secondarily from smoking nicotine containing products.[7] Chronic vasoconstriction leads to ischemic necrosis.[15] There have also been reported perforations from the intranasal abuse of narcotics.[16] Silver nitrate should

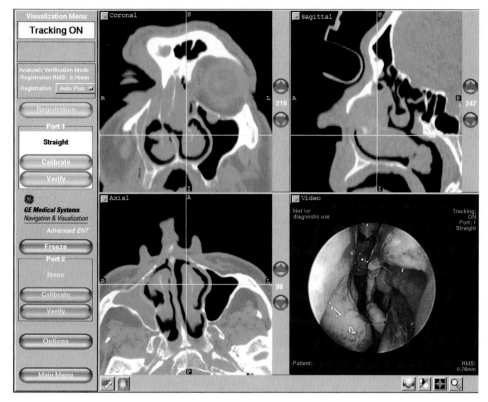

Fig. 23.4: Triplanar CT reconstruction as used for stereotactic image-guided surgical navigation in a patient who had septoplasty in the remote past. The coronal image (upper left panel) suggests a septal defect. This is clearly apparent in the endoscopic view into the right nasal cavity (lower left panel). Polyps from the left nasal cavity are visible through the perforation

be included in this discussion as well. Aggressive use of chemical (or thermal) cautery can also cause a septal perforation, particularly when apposing places on the septum are cauterized.[17]

Management of Septal Perforations

The first step in the management of a septal perforation is to rule out an underlying inflammatory or infectious cause and to rule out cocaine abuse. One should not hesitate to obtain a toxicology screen even in the most unlikely cases. Once all treatable or life-threatening disorders are ruled out and the perforation is symptomatic, the patient may desire therapeutic intervention. If the patient does have an underlying non-traumatic (or noniatrogenic) cause, the condition should be quiescent for 6 months to one year before septal reconstruction is contemplated. Often these patients require formal rhinoplasty to address saddle deformity.

Conservative measures to provide symptomatic relief include nasal saline sprays and lavage, which help with crusting and epistaxis. However, if the sensation of turbulent airflow or whistling is the main complaint, surgical intervention may be indicated. The goals of surgery are both to address symptoms and to attempt to regain nasal function. Many authors have reported good success rates (> 90%) using septal flaps with a connective tissue autograft interposed between the two muco-perichondrial flaps.[7,18,19] The key predictor of success is not the absolute size of the perforation, but the proportion of septum remaining. For example, a smaller perforation in a child may be more difficult to repair than a larger one in an adult. Also, the location influences the technical difficulty of the repair, with those perforations extending all the way to the floor being more difficult to access. Both closed (endonasal) and open techniques have been described.[7,18,19] Many different materials have been used to serve as the connective tissue graft between the septal flaps. These include temporalis fascia, pericranium, acellular dermis, and synthetics such as bioglass.[7,20] Unfortunately, most septal perforations large enough to be symptomatic are also less likely to be closed successfully, making a septal button an attractive option.

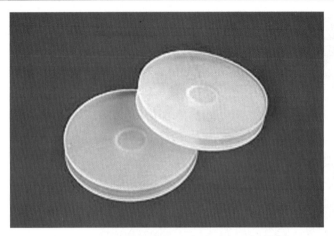

Fig. 23.5: Septal button. This silastic material is trimmed to the appropriate size and can be secured across the margins of the perforation

Alternatives to septal mucosal flaps include a pedicled flap from the inferior turbinate,[21] silicone septal buttons (Fig. 23.5), or surgically enlarging the perforation. The latter two techniques are concerned with alleviating symptomatology rather than repairing the perforation. Septal buttons must be fashioned to the particular dimensions of the pathology. They have a fair rate of success with 59% reporting improvement in crusting and 77% in epistaxis in a series by Price et al.[22]

INFECTIONS

There are many infectious processes which can lead to septal peforations. Some of these presentations overlap with those of non-infectious granulomatous processes, and many of these conditions represent nasal manifestations of diseases that are typically systemic in nature.

The nasal septum may become involved by fulminant invasive fungal sinusitis (Figs 23.6 and 23.7). This process is seen in diabetic and immunocompromised patients and involves invasion of fungal elements through tissue planes with subsequent angioinvasion, infarction, and ischemic necrosis. The offending organisms typically include *Aspergillus flavus or fumigatus* (septated hyphal forms) or members of the Zygomyctes class/Mucorales order, particularly *Rhizopus oryzae* (non-septated hyphae). Classically, it was thought that Aspergillus was associated with the immunocompromised state and that mucormycosis is associated with diabetes, but certainly either group of organisms may be implicated in either condition, and *Aspergillus* is more common overall. Early in the course of the disease, symptoms and endoscopic examination may mimic chronic sinusitis, but the

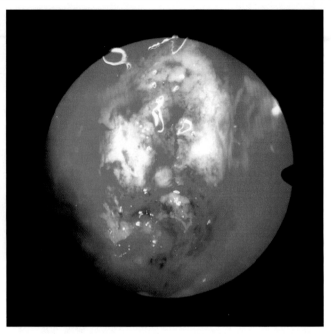

Fig. 23.6: Endoscopic view into the right nasal cavity in a patient with diabetes who was treated with high-dose prednisone for autoimmune disease. The nasal septum demonstrates significant mucosal ulceration with blackened punctate areas involving the surrounding mucosa and the exposed cartilage

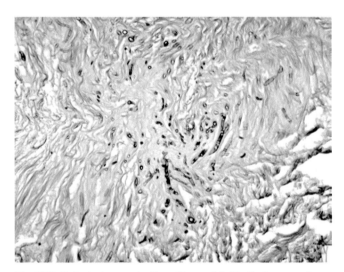

Fig. 23.7: Pathologic examination of tissue debrided in the case shown in Fig. 23.4 revealed this area to be consistent with invasive *Aspergillus* (Grocott silver stain)

condition rapidly progresses to severe pain, facial anesthesia, cranial neuropathy, proptosis, chemosis, and/ or change in visual acuity. Treatment requires aggressive debridement, intravenous antifungal therapy, and possible hyperbaric oxygen. Management of the underlying condition is essential. The prognosis is nonetheless dismal given the fulminant nature of the process and the severity of the predisposing condition.

Syphilis, the sexually transmitted disease caused by infection with *Treponema pallidum*, is nearly ubiquitous in all medical differentials. Interestingly, the disease is named after a cursed shepherd in the 1546 poem by Fracastorius entitled *Syphilis sive morbus Gallicus* (syphilis, or the French disease). Of course, the French called it the Italian disease or the Spanish disease! A full discussion of the manifestations of syphilis even when limited to just the head and neck region is beyond the scope of this section. In the nose, syphilis appears different depending on which stage in which it is discovered. Primary syphilis in the nose is rare. When it does occur a chancre is seen at the mucocutaneous border of the nasal vestibule or septum. It is difficult to diagnose because it may appear neoplastic, erosive, scabbed or have a change in skin pigmentation.[23] The usual history is that these lesions tend to ulcerate and form a minimally painful sore with disproportionate lymphadenopathy in the adjacent nodal basins. Secondary, syphilis is often confused with acute rhinitis; however, careful examination may reveal discrete mucous patches, erythema, or a solitary plaque on the external nose.[23,24] It may or may not be associated with syphilitic pharyngitis or laryngitis. Septal perforation is a consequence of tertiary syphilis and may result in enough cartilage destruction to cause a saddle nose deformity. The diagnosis is made with a screening RPR or VDRL serology and an FTA-ABS specific fluorescent treponemal antibody test for confirmation or in patients that have a high clinical risk. The treatment is with penicillin or other antibiotics.

Tuberculosis, caused by *Mycobacterium tuberculosis* is also able to affect the nose either primarily (rare) or as an extension from a primary pulmonary infection. While cervical lymphadenopathy is the most common head and neck manifestation, it is followed by nasal obstruction as the second most frequently encountered presenting complaint.[25–27] The diagnosis may be difficult because the organism is not easily cultured and the characteristic caseating granulomas may not be found in a nasal biopsy specimen.[27–29] The diagnosis may become simplified with the advent of newer technology including polymerase chain reaction. The treatment is prolonged anti-tuberculous chemotherapy using a multi-drug regimen that is effective in the specific geographic locale that the patient is being treated.

Leprosy is uncommon in North America but affects a large number of people worldwide. In some countries, it may be the most common cause of chronic nasal symptoms.[30] It is an ancient disease with written records in India dated to 600 BC. The Chinese also referred to it as early as 190 BC. It was most likely brought to the West by soldiers in Alexander the Great's army following an Indian campaign. The disease is caused by infection with the acid-fast bacillus *Mycobacterium leprae* which has a natural reservoir in the footpads of mice and the nine-banded armadillo.[30] It selectively invades peripheral nerves and causes irreversible cutaneous anesthesia and paralysis of muscles. The estimated incubation period is 3 to 10 years. Nasal symptoms including obstruction, bleeding, crusting and hyposmia are present in up to 94% of people with septal perforation being a relatively late manifestation.[30] Treatment is with anti-leprosy antibiotics such as dapsone, kanamycin, rifampin or minocycline.

Physical findings consistent with rhinoscleroma have been found in Mayan head masks dated between 300 and 600 AD.[31] The disease is caused by an infection with *Klebsiella rhinoscleromatis* and can affect the entire respiratory tract. The first phase is known as the catarrhal atrophic stage and is characterized by a foul smelling purulent nasal discharge which may persist for months. This is also known as *ozaena*. The second or granulomatous stage (sometimes referred to as the florid phase) is when most cases are diagnosed and is associated with nasal deformity. This eventually subsides into the sclerotic phase where there is growth of granulomas and possible bony destruction.[31] Particularly, in the granulomatouos phase, multinucleated macrophages with numerous vacuoles containing viable or non-viable bacteria can be seen and are referred to as *Mikulicz* cells. Russell bodies, which are eosinophilic structures within the cytoplasm of plasma cells, are also seen. Giemsa, Warthin–Starry, or periodic acid-Schiff stains demonstrate the gram-negative rods in the macrophages and are useful for diagnosis.[31,32] There is no definitive cure for rhinoscleroma but treatment with antibiotics and ablation may alter the evolution of the disease.

Rhinosporidiosis is a nasal infection which occurs most commonly in India, Sri Lanka and South-East Asia but has been know to occur in North America as well.[33] It is caused by a fungus, *Rhinosporidium seeberi*, which is easily seen on routine light microscopy.[34] The walls of the fungal spores are birefringent under crossed polarized filters and a host granulomatous response with mostly histiocytes and some neutrophils and lymphocytes can be seen.[35] It seems to be transmitted with very low efficiency in nasal secretions. The natural reservoir seems to be contaminated water, but the host, postulated to be everything from fish to cattle, remains undetermined.[34] Surgical excision is the treatment of choice for localized lesions. Dapsone may also be considered for recurrent or disseminated infections.[33] It is considered to be unresponsive to systemic anti-mycotics.[35]

INFLAMMATORY DISEASES

This diverse group of illnesses may be caused by infections with many of the above mentioned pathogens or may be due to a different cause altogether. This group includes Wegener's granulomatosis, sarcoidosis and angiocentric T-cell lymphomas. Giant cell reparative granulomas have also been reported to occur in the nasal cavity.[36]

WEGENER'S GRANULOMATOSIS

Wegener's granulomatosis is the prototype disease in this broad category. It is a systemic disease characterized by necrotizing granulomatous inflammation of the upper and lower respiratory tract, vasculitis of small and medium sized blood vessels and focal or proliferative glomerulonephritis.[37] The incidence ranges from one to ten cases per million people.[37,38] The cause is unknown but is believed to be immune-mediated. Though systemic in nature, rhinologic complaints are the most common presenting symptoms and the otolaryngologist is often the diagnosing physician.[38,39] Prior to the introduction of cytotoxic pharmacotherapy the prognosis was dismal with a mean survival of 5 months and 90% dead within two years. With the advent of cyclophosphamide in combination with corticosteroids the 5-year survival is now approximately 72%.[38] While Wegener's granulomatosis may affect multiple head and neck sites including the middle and inner ears, the larynx, especially the subglottic region, the mouth and eye, rhinologic manifestations are the most common.[37] The nasal examination often reveals crusting, erythematous mucosa, and granulation tissue. Vasculitic involvement of Kiesselbach's plexus may result in tissue necrosis that does not develop into a septal perforation until disease remission periods. So, the presence of a perforation does not necessarily correlate with active disease.[37] A high index of suspicion must be maintained in order to make the diagnosis. Cytoplasmic antineutrophil antibodies (c-ANCA) are a specific serum marker. However, c-ANCA may also be elevated in cocaine abuse,[15] leprosy, invasive amebiasis and infectious endocarditis.[37] Additionally a biopsy can be useful but lacks sensitivity (paranasal sinus tissue is the highest yield in these cases).[37] In patients with high suspicion of Wegener's and in whom the c-ANCA and biopsy are both negative, repeated serology with c-ANCA may reveal the diagnosis over time.[40] The treatment

of Wegener's is primarily medical and needs to be approached in coordination with other specialties.

Sarcoidosis

Sarcoidosis is another granulomatous disease which may involve the nasal septum. This is a poorly understood disease characterized by systemic non-caseating granulomas in the absence of other identifiable cause. The incidence is widely variable between geographic locations and between racial groups. The highest incidence is in Sweden and has been reported to be 67 per 100,000 people, however, autopsy studies suggest it may be much higher.[41] The incidence is higher in African-Americans than Caucasians in North America and in West Indian populations than Caucasians in London.[41,42] Otolaryngologic involvement is present in 10–15% of cases.[41,43] The most common otolaryngic manifestation is cervical lymphadenopathy.[41–43] Nasal complaints are rare with only 1% of patients having nasal complaints in the absence of other symptoms.[44] The disorder can manifest as nasal obstruction, rhinosinusitis, nasal polyposis, or septal perforation (Fig. 23.8).[41–45] Diagnosis is that of exclusion and consists of characteristic radiologic findings in the chest, serology especially elevated angiotensin converting enzyme (ACE) levels, and biopsy demonstrating non-caseating granulomas. It must be remembered that none of these tests are pathognomonic and tuberculosis, Wegener's, syphilis, leprosy, and Gaucher's disease must be excluded.[41,43] Stains of nasal biopsies for acid-fast bacilli are mandatory, and fine needle aspirate of any head and neck lymphadenopathy may also be of diagnostic value.[46] The natural history of sarcoidosis is often marked with spontaneous remission and therefore continuous therapy is not always indicated. Corticosteroids are the mainstay for exacerbations. Central nervous system or ocular involvement constitute medical emergencies and need to be addressed. Topical corticosteroids for nasal symptoms are beneficial.[43]

Angiocentric T-cell Lymphoma

Angiocentric T-cell lymphoma deserves to be included here rather than the section on neoplasms because it can be confused for a more benign granulomatous disease upon examination (Figs 23.9 and 23.10). This aggressive disease was among those which had previously been placed in a group of diseases collectively referred to as lethal midline granulomas syndrome.[47–49] It can be confused with any of the disorders previously discussed. A rare site for lymphoma, it shows a predilection for people of Asian,

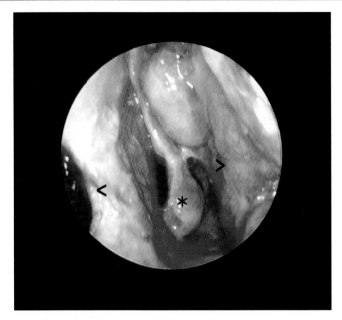

Fig. 23.8: View into left nasal cavity revealing nodular appearing mucosa (right arrowhead) and chronic (mature) septal perforation (left arrowhead) in a patient with sarcoidosis. A mucosal biopsy would reveal subepithelial deposits of non-caseating granulomatous inflammation. The patient also has a nasal polyp (asterisk) pedicled to the middle turbinate. The inferior turbinate is atrophic

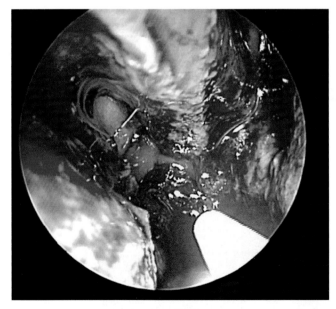

Fig. 23.9: Large septal perforation with bleeding edges and an obvious destructive quality. Biopsy from the margin of this perforation revealed angiocentric T-cell lymphoma. Other pathologies (i.e. cocaine abuse, Wegener's granulomatosis) may have a similar endoscopic appearance, making biopsy essential

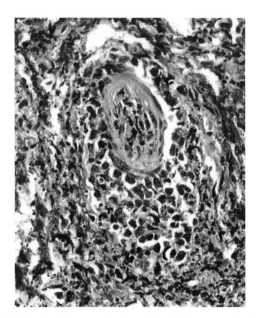

Fig. 23.10: Pathologic examination of the patient shown in Fig. 23.6 revealing a monomorphic lymphocyte population with an giocentric pattern. Flow cytometry was performed to confirm the diagnosis

Mexican, and South American descent.[47,49,50] A biopsy is diagnostic with the help of immunohistochemistry and flow cytometry. Histology shows pleomorphic tumor cells variably associated with angiocentric infiltration or angiodestructive growth as well as zonal coagulative necrosis.[50]

There is growing evidence that the clonal cell may not be T-cells but rather NK (natural killer) cells or a common progenitor.[49–51] EBV antigens are present in nearly all nasal T-cell lymphomas and may be of use in diagnosis and prognosis with higher EBV involvement signifying a more aggressive disease.[49] Treatment options, in general, are unsatisfactory with neither chemotherapy nor radiation therapy alone or in combination greatly increasing survival rates. For patients with local regional disease at presentation 5-year survival rates are about 40% and in those with systemic disease it drops to 7–25%.[47,49–51] New strategies including using cisplatinum as a radiation sensitizer or high-dose chemotherapy are being explored.

SEPTAL NEOPLASMS

Many tumors can affect the nasal septum. Any neoplasm with a predilection for the upper respiratory tract can involve all or part of the septum. These include squamous cell carcinoma, minor salivary gland neoplasms and olfactory neuroblastomas. In a 25-year review of cases from the Armed Forces Institute of Pathology, Thompson found 17% of 115 melanomas of the sinonasal tract involved the nasal septum alone.[52] In general, however, these are exceedingly rare and comprise about 0.5% of all sinonasal neoplasms. Other rare tumors include chordomas,[53] chondromas,[54] glomus tumors,[55] paragangliomas (Figs 23.11 and 23.12), and chondrosarcomas.[56,57]

Papillomas of the nasal septum deserve special mention. The mucosa of the nasal cavity originates from the neuroectoderm which also gives rise to the olfactory placode. Also called the Schneiderian membrane, it is bounded posteriorly by the choanae and is in contrast to the remainder of the respiratory tract which is of endodermal origin.[58,59] Secondary to the unique nature of the mucosa, there are neoplastic processes that occur in this area that do not occur elsewhere. The World Health Organization divides sinonasal papilloma into three distinct histologies: Exophytic (fungiform), inverted, and cylindrical (oncocytic schneiderian papilloma – OSP).

Inverted papillomas have a predilection for the lateral nasal wall and are characterized by squamous cell architecture with classic papilloma-like features extending into the underlying stroma. Mucinous cysts or cells can be identified either grossly or by special stains.[59] Hyams found

46% recurrence rate and a 13% malignancy rate in this type of papilloma.[59] Other studies have supported these findings with respect to malignant degeneration; however the recurrence rate has decreased with development surgical approaches.[60–64] It frequently appears polypoid and bulky. Historically, the treatment was surgical excision using a medial maxillectomy through a lateral rhinotomy approach.[59,60,63,64] Recent studies show that endoscopic approaches may yield equally good results.[62,65] The important concept is to ensure complete removal of affected tissue and close surveillance for recurrence and malignant transformation. Cylindrical cell papilloma or OSP (also called columnar cell papilloma) is a rare sinonasal neoplasm which also has a predilection for the lateral nasal wall. It is characterized by proliferating multilayered columnar cells with scant or absent overlying squamous mucosa.[59] It has a ragged or beefy appearance.[59] Because of its rarity it is difficult to quantify its malignant potential. In the Hyams series (n = 10), one malignancy was observed.[59] Exophytic or fungiform papilloma has the highest tendency to occur on the nasal septum (Fig. 23.13). It is similar to papilloma found elsewhere on the body. In contrast to the inverting and cylindrical forms, the exophytic form does not have any malignant potential and complete excision is the treatment of choice.[58–60]

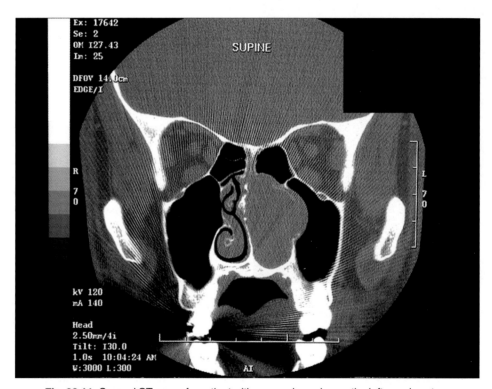

Fig. 23.11: Coronal CT scan of a patient with a mass-based upon the left nasal septum

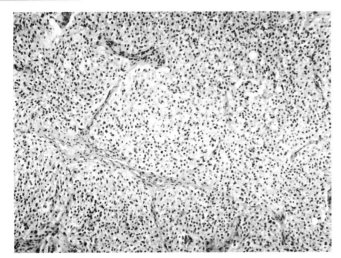

Fig. 23.12: Pathology from the patient in Fig. 23.6 revealed a paraganglioma. This lesion demonstrates the characteristic zellballen, or nests of eosinophilic tumor cells separated by vascular channels

endoscopic sinus surgery. The finding of a 'septal turbinate' may be observed in patients who have had resection or partial resection of the middle turbinate. The mucosa of the adjacent septum undergoes focal compensatory hypertrophy in an attempt to fill the void (Fig. 23.15). The resulting region may have similar dimensions as the resected portion of middle turbinate. No specific treatment is necessary, as the focus of hypertrophy rarely causes symptomatic nasal obstruction. This variant, however, must be recognized during endoscopic sinus surgery, as it may incorrectly lead the surgeon to dissect medially in the nasal cavity towards the cribriform area.

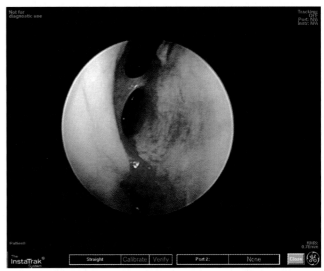

Fig. 23.14: Adhesions between the nasal septum and lateral nasal wall in a patient who has had prior endoscopic sinus surgery

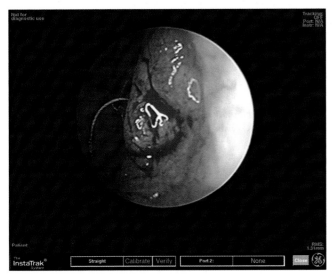

Fig. 23.13: Simple papillomatous mass of the right nasal septum. This lesion, unlike an inverting papilloma, has no malignant potential

REACTIVE SEPTAL LESIONS

It should be noted that inflammatory nasal polyposis infrequently originates with attachment to the nasal septum, and neoplastic change must be considered in the evaluation of masses of the septum. The septal mucosa, however, should be considered a dynamic tissue which is susceptible to the development of reactive pathology including adhesions, the so-called 'septal turbinate,' and pyogenic granuloma.

Adhesions to the lateral nasal wall (Fig. 23.14) may appear after nasal intubation or surgery, underscoring the importance of avoiding trauma to the septal mucosa during

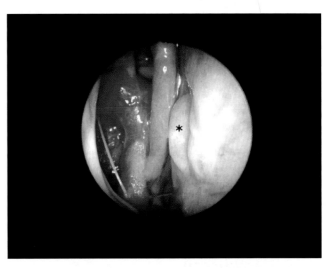

Fig. 23.15: Endoscopic view into right nasal cavity demonstrating the so-called 'septal turbinate' (asterisk)

Pyogenic granuloma is a reactive lesion that develops secondary to mucosal trauma and hormonal factors (pregnancy, oral contraceptive, estrogen replacement), although the exact pathophysiology is unknown. The overall incidence of these lesions in pregnancy is 2–5%. Mucosal lesions more commonly involve the oral cavity rather than the nasal mucosa, but when originating in the nasal cavity, the anterior septum is the most common site, presumably secondary to nose picking. The most common presentation is unilateral epistaxis followed by nasal obstruction. A reddish to purple mass is observed on physical examination of the anterior septum. Pathology reveals numerous vascular channels and chronic inflammation, leading some to term the lesion a lobular capillary hemangioma. It is notable that the lesion does not exhibit either acute bacterial infection or granulomas, making the term 'pyogenic granuloma' a misnomer. Growth may be rapid, and for lesions that do not involute after pregnancy, surgical resection with or without the KTP laser is indicated.[66]

SUMMARY

The septal mucosa is a dynamic, reactive tissue that may become involved in numerous infectious, inflammatory states, and systemic processes beyond the mundane deviations and perforations that are often encountered by the otolaryngologist. The otolaryngologist must be very familiar with the multitude of local and systemic entities that can manifest with nasal septal lesions, particularly as many of these disease entities can be life-threatening and require prompt medical or surgical intervention.

REFERENCES

1. Roblin DG, Eccles R. What, if any, is the value of septal surgery? *Clin Otolaryngol Allied Sci* 2002;27(2):77–80.
2. Gray LP. Deviated nasal septum: Incidence and etiology. *Ann Otol Rhinol Laryngol* 1978;87(3 Pt 3 Suppl 50):3–20.
3. Jang YJ, Myong NH, Park KH et al. Mucociliary transport and histologic characteristics of the mucosa of deviated nasal septum. *Arch Otolaryngol Head Neck Surg* 2002;128(4):421–424.
4. Marshall AH, Johnston MN, Jones NS. Principles of septal correction. *J Laryngol Otol* 2004;118(2):129–134.
5. Parsons DS, Batra PS. Functional endoscopic sinus surgical outcomes for contact point headaches. *Laryngoscope* 1998;108(5):696–702.
6. Diamantopoulos II, Jones NS. The investigation of nasal septal perforations and ulcers. *J Laryngol Otol* 2001;115(7):541–544.
7. Kridel RW. Septal perforation repair. *Otolaryngol Clin North Am* 1999;32(4):695–724.
8. Bateman ND, Woolford TJ. Informed consent for septal surgery: The evidence base. *J Laryngol Otol* 2003;117(3):186–189.
9. Breda SD, Jacobs JB, Leibowitz AS, Tierno PM. Toxic shock syndrome in nasal surgery: A physiochemical and microbiologic evaluation of Merocel and NuGauze nasal packing. *Laryngoscope* 1987;97(12):1388–1391.
10. Canty PA, Berkowitz RG. Hematoma and abscess of the nasal septum in children. *Arch Otolaryngol Head Neck Surg* 1996; 122(12):1373–1376.
11. Chukuezi AB. Nasal septal haematoma in Nigeria. *J Laryngol Otol* 1992;106(5):396–398.
12. Daggett RB, Haghighi P, Terkeltaub RA. Nasal cocaine abuse causing an aggressive midline intranasal and pharyngeal destructive process mimicking midline reticulosis and limited Wegener's granulomatosis. *J Rheumatol* 1990;17(6):838–840.
13. Smith JC, Kacker A, Anand VK. Midline nasal and hard palate destruction in cocaine abusers and cocaine's role in rhinologic practice. *Ear Nose Throat J* 2002;81(3):172–177.
14. Talbott JF, Gorti GK, Koch RJ. Midfacial osteomyelitis in a chronic cocaine abuser: A case report. *Ear Nose Throat J* 2001;80(10):738–740.
15. Seyer BA, Grist W, Muller S. Aggressive destructive midfacial lesion from cocaine abuse. *Oral Surg Oral Med Oral Pathol Oral Radiol Endodont* 2002;94(4):465–470.
16. Yewell J, Haydon R, Archer S, Manaligol JM. Complications of intranasal prescription narcotic abuse. *Ann Otol Rhinol Laryngol* 2002;111(2):174–177.
17. Hanif J, Tasca RA, Frosh A et al. Silver nitrate: Histological effects of cautery on epithelial surfaces with varying contact times. *Clin Otolaryngol Allied Sci* 2003;28(4):368–370.
18. Fairbanks DN. Closure of nasal septal perforations. *Arch Otolaryngol* 1980;106(8):509–513.
19. Newton JR, White PS, Lee MS. Nasal septal perforation repair using open septoplasty and unilateral bipedicled flaps. *J Laryngol Otol* 2003;117(1):52–55.
20. Stoor P, Grenman R. Bioactive glass and turbinate flaps in the repair of nasal septal perforations. *Ann Otol Rhinol Laryngol* 2004;113(8):655–661.
21. Friedman M, Ibrahim H, Ramakrishnan V. Inferior turbinate flap for repair of nasal septal perforation. *Laryngoscope* 2003l;113(8):1425–1428.
22. Price DL, Sherris DA, Kern EB. Computed tomography for constructing custom nasal septal buttons. *Arch Otolaryngol Head Neck Surg* 2003;129(11):1236–1239.
23. McNulty JS, Fassett RL. Syphilis: An otolaryngologic perspective. *Laryngoscope* 1981;91(6):889–905.
24. Sturm HM. Secondary syphilis appearing as a solitary plaque of the nose. *Int J Dermatol* 1976;15(9):678–679.
25. Al-Serhani AM. Mycobacterial infection of the head and neck: Presentation and diagnosis. *Laryngoscope* 2001;111(11 Pt 1):2012–2016.
26. Messervy M. Primary tuberculoma of the nose with presenting symptoms and lesions resembling a malignant granuloma. *J Laryngol Otol* 1971;85(2):177–184.
27. Nayar RC, Al Kaabi J, Ghorpade K. Primary nasal tuberculosis: A case report. *Ear Nose Throat J* 2004;83(3):188–191.
28. Batra K, Chaudhary N, Matwani G, Raj AK. An unusual case of primary nasal tuberculosis with epistaxis and epilepsy. *Ear Nose Throat J* 2002;81(12):842–844.
29. Choi YC, Park YS, Jeon EJ, Song SH. The disappeared disease: Tuberculosis of the nasal septum. *Rhinology* 2000;38(2):90–92.

30. Lalwani AK, Tami TA, Gelber RH. Lepromatous leprosy: Nasal manifestations and treatment with minocycline. *Ann Otol Rhinol Laryngol* 1992;101(3):261–264.

31. Hart CA, Rao V. Rhinoscleroma. *J Med Microbiol* 2000;49(5): 395–396.

32. Thompson LD. Rhinoscleroma. *Ear Nose Throat J* 2002; 81(8):506.

33. Gaines JJ Jr, Clay JR, Chander FW, Powell ME et al. Rhinosporidiosis: Three domestic cases. *Southern Med J* 1996;89(1):65–67.

34. Batsakis JG, El-Naggar AK. Rhinoscleroma and rhinosporidiosis. *Ann Otol Rhinol Laryngol* 1992;101(10):879–882.

35. Mears T, Amerasinghe C. Rhinosporidiosis. *J Laryngol Otol* 1992;106(5):468.

36. Morris JM, Lane JI, Witte RJ, Thompson DM. Giant cell reparative granuloma of the nasal cavity. *Am J Neuroradiol* 2004;25(7):1263–1265.

37. Gubbels SP, Barkhuizen A, Hwang PH. Head and neck manifestations of Wegener's granulomatosis. *Otolaryngol Clin North Am* 2003;36(4):685–705.

38. Takwoingi YM, Dempster JH. Wegener's granulomatosis: An analysis of 33 patients seen over a 10-year period. *Clin Otolaryngol Allied Sci* 2003;28(3):187–194.

39. Nagai H, Takahaslu H, Yao K et al. Clinical review of Wegener's granulomatosis. *Acta Oto–Laryngologica Supplement* 2002;547:50–53.

40. Jones NS. Nasal manifestations of rheumatic diseases. *Ann Rheumat Dis* 1999;58(10):589–590.

41. Fergie N, Jones NS, Havlat MF. The nasal manifestations of sarcoidosis: A review and report of eight cases. *J Laryngol Otol* 1999;113(10):893–898.

42. Baum ED, Boudousquie AC, Shiyong Li, Mirza N et al. Sarcoidosis with nasal obstruction and septal perforation. *Ear Nose Throat J* 1998;77(11):896–898.

43. Dash GI, Kimmelman CP. Head and neck manifestations of sarcoidosis. *Laryngoscope* 1988;98(1):50–53.

44. Braun JJ, Gentine A, Pauli G. Sinonasal sarcoidosis: Review and report of fifteen cases. *Laryngoscope* 2004;114(11): 1960–1963.

45. Shah UK, White JA, Gooey JE, Hybels RL et al. Otolaryngologic manifestations of sarcoidosis: Presentation and diagnosis. *Laryngoscope* 1997;107(1):67–75.

46. Frable MA, Frable WJ. Fine-needle aspiration biopsy: Efficacy in the diagnosis of head and neck sarcoidosis. *Laryngoscope* 1984;94(10):1281–1283.

47. Chen HL, Cheng PW, Tsai CC. Pathology quiz case: Nasal T/NK-cell lymphoma. *Arch Otolaryngol Head Neck Surg* 2003;129(10):1135–1136.

48. Pickens JP, Modica L. Current concepts of the lethal midline granuloma syndrome [see comment]. *Otolaryngol Head Neck Surg* 1989;100(6):623–630.

49. Yih WY, Stewart JCB, Kratochwil FM, Zieper MB. Angiocentric T-cell lymphoma presenting as midface destructive lesion: Case report and literature review. *Oral Surg Oral Med Oral Pathol Oral Radiol Endodont* 2002;94(3):353–360.

50. Li CC, Tien HF, Tang JL et al. Treatment outcome and pattern of failure in 77 patients with sinonasal natural killer/T-cell or T-cell lymphoma. *Cancer* 2004;100(2):366–375.

51. Cheung MM, Chan JK, Lan WH et al. Early stage nasal NK/T-cell lymphoma: Clinical outcome, prognostic factors, and the effect of treatment modality. *Int J Radiation Oncol Biol Physics* 2002;54(1):182–190.

52. Thompson LD, Wieneke JA, Miettinen M. Sinonasal tract and nasopharyngeal melanomas: A clinicopathologic study of 115 cases with a proposed staging system. *Am J Surg Pathol* 2003;27(5):594–611.

53. Scartozzi R, Couch M, Sciubba J. Chondroid chordoma of the nasal septum. *Arch Otolaryngol Head Neck Surg* 2003; 129(2):244–246.

54. Unlu HH, Unlu Z, Ayhan S, Egrilmez M. Osteochondroma of the posterior nasal septum managed by endoscopic transnasal transseptal approach. *J Laryngol Otol* 2002;116(11):955–957.

55. Li XQ, Hisaolia M, Morio T et al. Intranasal pericytic tumors (glomus tumor and sinonasal hemangiopericytoma-like tumor): Report of two cases with review of the literature. *Pathol Intl* 2003;53(5):303–308.

56. Blotta P, Carinci F, Pelucchis S et al. Chondrosarcoma of the nasal septum. *Ann Otol Rhinol Laryngol* 2001;110(2):202–204.

57. Matthews B, Whang C, Smith S. Endoscopic resection of a nasal septal chondrosarcoma: First report of a case. *Ear Nose Throat J* 2002;81(5):327–329.

58. Batsakis JG. Pathology consultation: Nasal (Schneiderian) papillomas. *Ann Otol Rhinol Laryngol* 1981;90(2 Pt 1): 190–191.

59. Hyams VJ. Papillomas of the nasal cavity and paranasal sinuses: A clinicopathological study of 315 cases. *Ann Otol Rhinol Laryngol* 1971;80(2):192–206.

60. Buchwald C, Franzmann MB, Tos M. Sinonasal papillomas: A report of 82 cases in Copenhagen County, including a longitudinal epidemiological and clinical study. *Laryngoscope* 1995;105(1):72–79.

61. Kaufman MR, Brandwein MS, Lawson W. Sinonasal papillomas: Clinicopathologic review of 40 patients with inverted and oncocytic schneiderian papillomas. *Laryngoscope* 2002;112(8 Pt 1):1372–1377.

62. Kraft M, Simmen D, Kautmann D, Holzmann D. Long-term results of endonasal sinus surgery in sinonasal papillomas. *Laryngoscope* 2003;113(9):1541–1547.

63. Lawson W, Ho BT, Shaari CM, Biller HF. Inverted papilloma: A report of 112 cases. *Laryngoscope* 1995;105(3 Pt 1):282–288.

64. Outzen KE, Grontved A, Jorgensen K, Clausen PP. Inverted papilloma of the nose and paranasal sinuses: A study of 67 patients. *Clin Otolaryngol Allied Sci* 1991;16(3):309–312.

65. Kraft M, Simmen D, Casas R, Pfaltz M. Significance of human papillomavirus in sinonasal papillomas. *J Laryngol Otol* 2001;115(9):709–714.

66. Jones JE, Nguyen A, Tabaee A. Pyogenic granuloma (pregnancy tumor) of the nasal cavity: A case report. *J Reprod Med* 2000;45(9):749–753.

Nasal Allergy: Diagnosis, Evaluation and Management

Rebecca E Fraioli, Suman Golla

Allergic rhinitis has been reported to affect 20–40% of the people in the USA; the incidence continues to rise.[1] An estimate of the worldwide prevalence of allergic rhinitis comes from the International Study of Asthma and Allergies in Childhood (ISAAC). This study used a written questionnaire translated from English to the subject's local language to assess symptoms of allergy and asthma: Children in the age group 6–7 years from 38 countries and those in the age group 13–14 years from 56 countries. The prevalence of rhinoconjunctivitis was shown to vary from 0.8–4.9% in 6–7-year-old, and from 1.4–39.7% in 13–14-year-old.[2]

The burden of allergic rhinitis to society is substantial. On an economic level, there are both direct and indirect costs associated with allergic rhinitis. Direct costs (cost of doctor visits and medical treatment) in the USA alone have been estimated at USD 1.1–3.4 billion (1990 and 1993 estimates, respectively).[1] Indirect costs are those due to lost work days and lost productivity. For the US in 1990, these have been estimated at USD 800 million.[1] Finally, the incidence of rhinosinusitis, asthma, and otitis media with effusion (OME) appear to be more prevalent in patients with allergic rhinitis. If the cost of treating these disorders is taken into account, the direct cost of allergic rhinitis has been estimated to grow from USD 1.9 billion to over USD 4 billion (1996 USD).[3]

The combined direct and indirect costs represent the total economic burden to society, but the true impact of allergic rhinitis cannot be measured by economics alone. The effect of allergic rhinitis on quality of life (QOL) has been assessed by survey. Rhinitis has been reported to reduce sleep, emotional well-being, and concentration levels, and to increase headache and malaise.[1,4] Studies of learning, memory, and decision-making show a decrease in these skills during the allergy season. In addition, body image may be affected. Adolescents (15 to 19 years) have a high agreement with the statements that they are 'feeling tired' or 'feeling unattractive' due to allergic rhinitis.[1]

PATHOPHYSIOLOGY OF ALLERGIC RHINITIS

Allergy is a result of a hypersensitivity of the immune response to a particular antigen.[5] Activation of the immune system by exposure to triggering allergen causes release of inflammatory mediators and the subsequent inflammation and tissue destruction that are responsible for the symptoms of allergy. Hypersensitivity reactions are generally classified into four types as initially described by Gel and Coombs.[6] Allergic rhinitis and, indeed, most allergy treated by otolaryngologists, is caused by Type I IgE-mediated hypersensitivity.

Type I: Immediate Hypersensitivity

Type I hypersensitivity reactions are mediated by specific IgE antibodies to allergen. IgE antibody exists bound to mast cells. Binding of antigen to its specific IgE causes cross-linking of IgE molecules and the subsequent degranulation of the mast cells with release of preformed inflammatory mediators and newly formed mediators.

The mediators stored in mast cells, including histamine, proteases, leukotrienes, prostaglandins, and cytokines, are responsible for the almost immediate allergic response upon exposure to allergen, which occurs within seconds to minutes.[7,8] Upon mast cell degranulation, chemical mediators cause edema, vasodilation, and stimulation of nerve endings. The result of the combined action of these mediators is the swelling, itching, congestion, and bronchospasm that are the classic signs and symptoms of an allergic reaction.[6] The release of these preformed mediators and the resulting symptoms together make up the 'early phase' of the type I hypersensitivity response.

The 'late phase' of the type I hypersensitivity response, although also initiated at the time of mast cell degranulation, occurs several hours following the early response. This phase affects approximately 50% of allergy sufferers. The chemical mediators released from mast cells, in addition to their direct local effects, also cause lysis of the cell wall and release of newly formed chemical inhibitors, including the leukotrienes and prostaglandins.[6] These newly formed mediators in turn recruit inflammatory cells to the site of the mast cell degranulation. Eosinophils and neutrophils, in particular, are recruited, and they release toxic substances which add to the inflammation and tissue damage.

Type II: Antibody-mediated Cytotoxicity

These reactions are caused by IgG and IgM antibody targeted against a patient's own cells. Once antibody binds to the targeted cells, natural killer cells or complements mediate cytotoxicity or cell lysis, respectively. Examples of type II hypersensitivity reactions are myasthenia gravis, pemphigus vulgaris, and hemolytic disease of the newborn.[6]

Type III: Immune Complex-mediated

Type III hypersensitivity reactions occur when a large number of antibody-antigen complexes accumulate in tissues. The immune complexes activate complement, which in turn recruits neutrophils and begins the cascade of inflammation and tissue destruction.

Type IV: Cell-mediated Hypersensitivity

Type IV hypersensitivity reactions are also known as delayed hypersensitivity reactions, as the reaction takes over 12 hours to appear.[6] These reactions are mediated by T-cells that have previously been sensitized to antigen. After the initial sensitization, exposure of a T-cell to antigen causes the T-cell to secrete cytokines, which then trigger the inflammatory cascade. An example of type IV hypersensitivity is tuberculin sensitivity, which serves as the basis for the tuberculin skin test.

RHINOSINUSITIS AND ALLERGY

Diagnosis

As in other areas of medicine, a thorough history and physical examination is crucial to understanding the patient's symptoms and complaints. The differential diagnosis, as well as initial diagnostic testing is based on the history. Often the treatment paradigm is also based on the patient's history, initial interview, and office examination.

History

The importance of a good patient history in the diagnosis of nasal allergy cannot be overstated. First, the patient's symptoms should be described in his or her own words. Next, the duration, location, timing, context, quality, and severity of the symptoms should be determined, as well as aggravating or alleviating factors.[9] A good history alone may be enough to strongly suggest or strongly exclude allergy as a cause of a patient's symptoms. For example, a chief complaint of nasal obstruction may be due to myriad causes, including septal deviation, tumor, or rhinosinusitis in addition to nasal allergy. However, a history of sneezing followed by nasal congestion which worsens with exposure to air conditioning strongly suggests an allergic cause.

Less intuitive, but equally important to a good allergy history is a thorough review of systems. The review of systems entails determining from the patient whether certain specific symptoms are present or absent. It may help refine, rule out, or suggest an alternative diagnosis.[9] It is also important to remember that allergy is a systemic disorder, and as such, strange or seemingly unconnected symptoms may in fact be related to the patient's nasal symptoms through the common denominator of allergy. Symptoms such as sneezing and pruritus of the nose, eyes, and palate are strongly suggestive of allergy. Other, less obvious symptoms such as fatigue, abdominal pain, and headache are also commonly caused by allergy.[9] Fever, although often a sign of infection, does not rule out allergy, as an acute allergic attack may cause a fever.[9]

Past medical history, current medications, family history, and social history are also important in making the diagnosis of allergy. Chronic dermatological or gastrointestinal conditions may in fact be due to allergy to foods or inhalants.[9] Allergy is a systemic inflammatory disorder, and just as the mucous membranes of the upper airway may react to the local tissue inflammation, so may the skin or the mucous membranes of the gastrointestinal tract as the food passes through. Medications may have side effects that mimic allergy. For example, angiotensisn converting enzyme (ACE) inhibitors can cause cough. In addition, other medications can affect the immune system or the inflammatory response and thereby modify a patient's response to an allergen. Beta-blockers, for example, lower the threshold for mediator release from mast cells because stimulation of beta-receptors inhibits the degranulation of mast cells.[9] Knowing a patient's past surgical history is obviously critical, as changes in the nasal mucosa and turbinates from allergy may have necessitated the surgery. Family history is important because allergic disease is heritable. Thirty-five percent of the offspring of a single allergic parent will have some form of allergy; this number increases to 65% if both parents have allergy. Social history is important because a patient may be allergic to a substance in the home or work environment. Patients with food allergy frequently experience an exacerbation of symptoms within an hour of eating or in the late afternoon.[9]

Physical Examination

Certain findings on physical examination are indicative of allergy.[4] When found in conjunction with a history suggestive of allergy, one may assume allergy to be the cause of the patient's symptoms and move straight to initial treatment. This may then obviate the need for allergy testing. A meticulous physical examination may therefore prevent the need for further testing and save the patient from formal allergy testing.

Many facial stigmata, which may be apparent to the physician prior to the physical examination, are classic signs of allergy. *Adenoid facies* is the term used to describe the characteristic pattern of facial development that occurs when chronic nasal obstruction is present. This consists of flattened malar eminences, a low nasal bridge, and a shortened mandible. Protrusion of the front teeth is also frequently present, as well as a moderately open mouth at rest.[10, 11] Eye findings characteristic of allergy include dark circles under the eyes, known as 'allergic shiners,' and horizontal creases in the lower eyelid skin, known as 'Dennie's lines'. Both of these findings are caused by venous congestion in the lower eyelid skin resulting from chronic nasal congestion. Venous drainage from the orbit occurs through the marginal and angular veins to the sphenopalatine veins and the pterygoid plexus.

Venous stasis in the lower eyelid is directly responsible for the initial discoloration of the lower eyelid skin. Eventually, hemosiderin deposits make the discoloration permanent. Eyelid creasing results from spasm of the Müller muscle caused by the low oxygen tension that result from venous stasis. Other characteristic eye findings in allergy include conjunctival edema and erythema, which are a result of sensitivity of the conjunctiva to histamine and other mediator release in response to airborne allergens.[10]

Nasal findings suggestive of allergy include external signs such as a horizontal supra-tip crease, which results from a gesture known as the 'allergic salute.' This gesture involves using the palm of the hand to push the nasal tip upward, which serves the dual purpose of temporarily opening the nasal airway and alleviating the nasal itch. This is also used by children as a maneuver to tackle rhinorrhea. Frequent saluting for 2 years or more is sufficient to make this crease permanent. Other external signs include erythema of the philtrum due to chronic nasal drip and irritation, as well as crusting or frank nasal discharge. Anterior rhinoscopy performed with a headlight and a nasal speculum is also an essential component of the physical examination. Characteristic findings in the patient with nasal allergy include pale, edematous turbinate mucosa, enlarged turbinates, and abundant clear nasal secretions. These findings are distinct from the nasal findings in other disorders. Rhinitis medicamentosa, the rebound rhinitis caused by overuse of topical decongestants such as over-the-counter nasal sprays or cocaine, causes the nasal mucosa to appear atrophic, dry, erythematous, and friable.[11] Posterior rhinoscopy must be performed using either flexible or rigid telescopes. Findings in the posterior nasal cavity that are consistent with, but not diagnostic for, nasal allergy include cobblestoning of the mucosa or nasal polyposis. One may also see clear mucosal streaking between the turbinates and septum on nasal endoscopy. Nasal polyps may arise from causes other than allergy; for example, they are found as a part of Samter's triad, which includes aspirin sensitivity and asthma in addition to nasal polyposis. Nasal polyps caused by allergy are expected to be bilateral, as the hypersensitivity is systemic. Therefore, unilateral nasal polyposis requires a high level of suspicion for a neoplastic process (mainly in adults) or a foreign body reaction (especially in children). Nasal polyps in children are uncommon, and should raise suspicion of cystic fibrosis.[12,13]

Although the facial appearance (eyes and nose) manifest allergic signs the most, the remainder of the physical examination is also important. Oral cavity manifestations include dry chapped lips, a high-arched palate caused by long-term mouth breathing, as well as foul breath and dental caries caused by pH changes. Oropharyngeal findings of allergies include enlarged or cryptic tonsils from the recurrent infections and cobblestoning of the oropharyngeal mucosa due to hypertrophy of small patches of submucosal lymphoid tissue.[11] Laryngeal findings in allergy may include thick mucus overlying the vocal folds, mild edema of the vocal folds, and erythema of the arytenoids. Neck examination may reveal lymphadenopathy of the jugulodigastric chain resulting from frequent infections in the allergic patient. Hypertrophy of the neck musculature may be present, caused by the frequent swallowing to clear nasal secretions.[11] Otologic examination includes examination of the pinna for contact dermatitis or eczema, which are common in allergic patients. The tympanic membrane may be retracted or thickened due to recurrent episodes of acute otitis media or chronic eustachian tube dysfunction.

TREATMENT OF ALLERGIC RHINITIS

The first-line treatments for allergic rhinitis include nasal steroids and non-sedating antihistamines. These medications have few side effects, are relatively inexpensive, and are also efficacious.[14-17] Because the potential benefits of treatment exceed potential harm, the threshold to treat should be low.[18] In a patient with signs and symptoms strongly suggestive of allergy, a negative allergy test does not lower the probability of allergy enough to preclude a trial of treatment.[18] Therefore, empiric treatment is warranted if negative results of testing would not change the treatment algorithm.

Allergen Avoidance

Allergen avoidance is often recommended as one of the first-line treatments for allergic rhinitis. Avoiding allergen exposure may be one of the most effective and cost-effective management strategies. Simple strategies such as limiting pollen exposure by closing windows, using an air conditioner, or incorporating a high-efficiency particulate arresting (HEPA) filter. Dust mites, another common allergen, may be avoided by using allergen-impermeable covers on bedding and pillows, washing bedding in water of at least 150°F temperature, or replacing bedding frequently. More thorough elimination of environmental allergens, however, may require removing carpets, curtains, and even pets from the home. The bedroom should be an area which is the 'allergy free' focus as this is the region where most working people spend the majority of their time. Occasionally initial avoidance techniques may be best used after allergy testing has definitively identified the allergen to be avoided.[5,18] One must be aware of the impact and practicality of recommended changes. For example, if the person recommending the change, whether it be the allergy support staff or the physician find it difficult to implement the suggestion into their own lives, the recommendation should be reconsidered.

Pharmacotherapy

The choice of first-line pharmacotherapy should be based on both the nature and the severity of an individual patient's symptoms. The available medications include oral and topical antihistamines, oral or topical corticosteroids or decongestants, topical nasal cromolyn, topical anticholinergics, and antileukotrienes.

Antihistamines

Oral antihistamines have been a mainstay of allergic treatment since their discovery in the 1930s.[5] Antihistamines reversibly bind to H1 histamine receptors and block histamine action.[19] Because histamine is largely responsible for the early allergic response, antihistamines are most effective at blocking the sneezing, itching, and rhinorrhea that characterize this response.[4,8] Antihistamines are only minimally effective at controlling nasal congestion. The side effect of sedation that characterized the first-generation antihistamines has been virtually eliminated in the second-generation antihistamines, as these newer medications do not cross the blood-brain barrier.[19] Antihistamines are available in oral and topical forms, and are useful as first-line treatment for mild or intermittent allergic rhinitis. In more severe or chronic allergic rhinitis, where nasal congestion is a prominent complaint, other treatment options in combination with or in lieu of antihistamines are more appropriate.

Corticosteroids

Topical corticosteroids are the most effective first-line agents approved to treat allergic rhinitis.[8] Although they are used primarily to treat nasal congestion, some reports indicate that they may also control eye symptoms in addition to treating sneezing, rhinorrhea, and nasal itch.[18] Topical corticosteroids are useful as a first-line treatment for severe allergic rhinitis or allergic rhinitis refractory to initial treatment. Unlike antihistamines, corticosteroids do not prevent the allergic event, but attenuate the effects of the allergic response by decreasing the release of pro-inflammatory cytokines and decreasing capillary permeability, and inhibiting the recruitment of eosinophils and other inflammatory cells.[5,19,20] Corticosteroids therefore act by inhibiting both the early and late phases of the allergic response.[19] Side effect profiles of intranasal corticosteroids are mild, and despite concern of systemic effects and growth-inhibition in children, recent studies demonstrate no significant systemic effects from topical corticosteroids.[16,21] Minor side effects such as nasal irritation, burning, epistaxis, sore throat and foul taste may be minimized with thorough instructions on proper use of these topical sprays.

Mast Cell Stabilizers

Cromolyn sodium is a mast cell stabilizer that has the capability of preventing the allergic response if used prior to allergen exposure. Cromolyn is safe and has long been available without prescription in the US; in addition, if used frequently it is effective at controlling symptoms of sneezing, pruritis, and rhinorrhea. The major disadvantage of intranasal cromolyn is that it must be used many times a day during allergy season to achieve maximum benefit. Side effects are typically not a problem.[5] Cromolyn may be a good first-line agent for a patient with mild allergy and an identifiable trigger such as dusting or mowing.[5]

Anticholinergics

The main role of intranasal ipratropium is for controlling rhinorrhea. Many of the other agents described above are also effective at controlling this symptom, therefore, the main role of this medication is as an adjunctive medication for refractory rhinorrhea.[5]

Decongestants

Nasal congestion can be a prominent and troublesome symptom of allergic rhinitis. In addition, nasal congestion predisposes to the development of related symptoms such as sinusitis and serous otitis media. Although chronic nasal congestion is best-treated with intranasal corticosteroids or immunotherapy, nasal congestion in the setting of acute sinusitis is best-treated aggressively with an oral or topical decongestant. Oral decongestants may also be useful on a daily basis during a period of intense allergen exposure, and for this purpose the patient may prefer the convenience of combined oral antihistamine/ decongestant combinations. Topical nasal decongestants (oxymetazaline/neo-synephrine) are also available and are very effective; however, use of topical decongestants for 5 days or more can cause rebound rhinitis (rhinitis medicamentosa). Oral decongestants need to be used cautiously secondary to their system side effects. This is especially true in patients with hypertension, benign prostatic hypertrophy and cardiovascular disease.

Allergy Testing

Allergy testing is indicated when a patient's symptoms are not controlled by routine medical therapies. Allergy tests are used to determine the specific antigens that trigger the allergic response in the patient. This in turn allows treatment or allergen-avoidance to be antigen-specific.[22] Allergy tests can be divided into two broad categories: *in vivo* and *in vitro* tests. *In vitro* testing measures the level of IgE to a particular antigen present in a patient's serum. Elevated IgE levels demonstrate that a patient has been previously sensitized to the allergen in question. *In vivo* testing consists of direct inoculation of antigen onto the patient in a controlled fashion to allow direct and objective measurement of the patient's reaction to the allergen. The two testing methods have been shown to have similar diagnostic efficacy. *In vivo* testing has been demonstrated to be lower in cost, but the patient must be able to tolerate the testing process.[22] In addition, skin carries with it a risk of serious allergic reactions, although this risk is small.[23]

In Vivo Testing

Skin testing for allergens has been performed for over a century. Several testing methods have been used. Patch testing consists of applying an allergen to intact skin and measuring the skin response. Because antigens as large as 30,000 daltons can penetrate intact skin, most allergens can generate a skin reaction from patch testing. Patch testing measures the late phase of Type I hypersensitivity reactions as well as Type IV delayed hypersensitivity reactions. Although patch testing is still useful when a suspected antigen is a solid (such as a fabric or metal), the reproducibility of allergy testing is lower for patch testing than for the other methods of skin testing, and it may be difficult to differentiate skin irritation from a true allergic response.[24]

Scratch testing consists of making a superficial (2 mm deep) cut through the epidermis and placing a drop of concentrated antigen onto the cut surface. The wheal and flare of the surrounding skin are measured 10–20 minutes later, and the response is determined based on their size. Scratch testing has a low sensitivity and specificity, and is not a recommended method of allergen testing.[23] Skin prick testing, similar to scratch testing, uses a small amount of concentrated antigen and has a low risk of systemic reaction. However, skin prick testing is more sensitive and more reproducible than scratch testing, and is also a rapid test that allows the testing of many antigens in a short period of time.[23,24] There are many methods of skin prick testing, but the general method involves placing a drop of concentrated antigen on the skin and placing a solid needle through the drop into a controlled distance through the epidermis. Although the needle may pass to the dermal-epidermal junction, skin prick testing does not include passing the needle into the dermis.[23]

Intradermal or IDT testing requires introduction of antigen into the dermis. Because the dermis is more vascular than the epidermis, the potential for systemic allergic reaction is higher with intradermal than with scratch or skin prick testing. However, the sensitivity and reproducibility of intradermal testing is also higher than with these other methods.[23] The intradermal test, unlike the more superficial tests, does not use concentrated antigen but instead uses a precise volume of dilute antigen injected superficially into the dermis. In order to determine the safe concentration of antigen to be used, intradermal testing should be preceded by screening prick tests or should start with a highly dilute antigen concentration.[23,25]

Skin endpoint titration or progressive intradermal testing is a modification of intradermal testing that involves the sequential injection of a constant volume of progressively less dilute allergen until a positive skin reaction occurs. Once a positive response has been obtained, one additional intradermal test using the next stronger dilution or more concentrated allergen is injected to confirm that the resulting skin wheal is larger than the initial wheal. If the second wheal is larger, this demonstrates that the allergen dilution being tested is on the ascending portion of the dose-response curve, where wheal size is directly related to the dose of antigen injected.[24] The main advantage to skin endpoint titration is that it allows the determination of a starting dose for immunotherapy that carries with it a low-risk of systemic allergic reaction. It is also safer and more reliable than intradermal skin testing performed with a single antigen dilution.[24] The dilution of the allergen in this type of testing varies among general allergists and the otolaryngic allergist.

In Vitro Testing

In vitro testing does not directly measure the patient's response to an allergen challenge; rather, it measures the quantity of preformed IgE antibody to a specific allergen present in the patient's serum. As the early type I hypersensitivity reaction is directly dependent on the level of preformed IgE antibody to a specific allergen present in the patient's serum at the time of antigen challenge, elevated allergen-specific IgE in the serum is a sign that the patient has been sensitized to the allergen previously. The simplest form of *in vitro* testing is a measurement of the total IgE antibody level in a patient's serum. Total IgE is a nonspecific test that nonetheless has utility in certain situations. A normal total IgE screen does not rule out an elevated IgE to a specific antigen, and therefore a normal

result warrants further testing. However, measurement of total IgE may prove useful if elevated, as this may prompt more thorough allergen testing if the initial allergy screen is negative.[26]

The classic *in vitro* test for allergen-specific IgE is the radioallergosorbent test (RAST). Although this test has largely been replaced with the similar but non-radioactive enzyme-labeled immunoassay (ELISA), the concept of RAST testing is important to understand. In RAST testing, the allergen is linked to a solid support and then incubated with the patient's serum. If the serum contains allergen-specific IgE, this IgE will bind to the allergen on the solid support. Washing then removes antibody that is not bound specifically to the allergen. Next, the solid support and its attached allergen-antibody complexes are incubated with a radiolabeled anti-IgE antibody that binds to the allergen-antibody complexes but not to free allergen. The amount of radioisotope bound to the solid support at the end of the experiment is a reflection of the amount of allergen-specific IgE present in the serum at the time of the test.[26]

There are certain situations in which *in vitro* allergy testing is preferred over *in vivo* testing. These include testing for young children who cannot tolerate skin testing, patients with severe anaphylactic reactions in whom *in vivo* testing may be risky, and patients with dermatological conditions that make skin testing difficult. Overall, both methods have comparable efficacy and the clinical situation should dictate the type of testing used.[26] IDT is more sensitive, while RAST testing may be more specific.

Immunotherapy

In additional to environmental controls and medical management, immunotherapy or immune modulation exists as a treatment option. Immunotherapy is the most specific treatment for allergic rhinitis. It is indicated for patients who require constant pharmacotherapy (for at least two to three consecutive seasons) or in whom pharmacotherapy either cannot be tolerated or is not effective.[8] Immunotherapy has been proven to be effective inpatients whose symptoms from both hay fever and perennial dust mites were not controlled by antihistamines and intranasal corticosteroids. Immunotherapy decreased both symptoms and medication use in these patients.[27,28] Disadvantages to immunotherapy include the requirement for an identifiable allergy on allergy testing, as well as a long-term commitment. Patients need to commit at least one year for effect and up to five years for completion. In about 80% of patients, treatment may be discontinued after three to five years without a return of symptoms.[29] Many patients have allergies to multiple allergens, making immunotherapy impractical. In addition, immunotherapy has low efficacy for several antigens, including molds. Relative contraindications to immunotherapy include an uncontrolled asthmatic patient, beta adrenergic blocker treatment, therapy initiation and escalation during pregnancy, and patients with immune dysregulation.[30]

FOOD ALLERGY

The previous section focused on airborne or inhalant allergens. Food or ingested allergens have also been shown to contribute to the allergic response. There are numerous clinical manifestations of food allergy. Unlike inhalant allergens, reactions related to food allergens can present outside of the upper airway tract. One or numerous organ systems may be involved. For example, a patient may present with headache, dermatologic or asthma type reactions. One needs to differentiate complaints that are related to food sensitivity or gastrointestinal reactions, rather than true food allergies.

In general, there are two types of food allergies; 'fixed' and 'cyclic'. The presentations of 'fixed' food allergies are quite clear. These are the immediate reactions seen after the ingestion of a substance which leads to an IgE mediated response. The prevalence of fixed food allergies is estimated to constitute 5–20% of all food hypersensitivities.[31] The presentation of fixed allergies varies; however, they are consistent and regular with the ingestion of the offending food. The reactions are immediate, rapid, dose-independent and often severe. The typical reaction is to either nuts, or seafood. Concerning manifestations include airway edema and hyperreactivity. The treatment is complete and life-long avoidance.

Unlike fixed reactions, cyclic reactions can be immediate or delayed. They are dose and frequency related. Immunologic reactions involving complement, immune complexes, and other nontype 1 hypersensitivity reactions have been implicated. These complexes, which are associated with IgG mediated type III hypersensitivity reactions, may affect numerous areas within the body. This explains the multiplicity of the clinical manifestations. Cyclic food allergies account for approximately 60–80% of food sensitivity.[7]

The initial work-up for a suspected cyclic food allergen includes patient documentation in the form of a food diary. After a two-week journal of ingested foods, the clinician can perform an objective assessment of the frequency and quantity of ingested foods. Thorough knowledge of food additives and food families must be ensured prior to the analysis of the diary. In addition, associated symptoms should also be entered into the food diary.

Cross-reactivity can occur between inhalants and foods, as well as among food families themselves. This phenomenon occurs because of common antigen epitopes shared between the offending food and the inhalant or other food to which the patient is allergic. There are excellent references which list these common food cross-reactions.[32] In addition, there are common inhalant-food cross reactions. A few examples include birch pollen to apples; dust mites to shrimp; grasses and ragweed to melons; mugwort with carrots, and latex with avocado.[7]

After the food diary is analyzed with these reactions in mind, the principal ingested foods can be identified. At another scheduled time, an oral antigen challenge may be performed. The challenge involves the elimination of a particular suspected food for a period of 4 to 5 days. The food is then introduced in large amounts, preferably early in the morning. If an allergy to that food is present, the patient will present with exaggerated symptoms. This is explained by the large deposition of immune complexes after the elimination period where there is an excess of free antibody circulating. After the offending food is introduced, the excess antigen-antibody binding leads to complex deposition.[7] Later, in terms of treatment, avoidance is advocated for 3 to 5 months. During this time of omission, or avoidance, the decreased antigen levels led to decrease antibody levels. Eventually, ingestion of the food in controlled amounts does not produce symptoms. This is considered to be the tolerance phase.[7] If the particular food continues to be ingested in moderate amounts, symptoms should remain tolerable; if however, it is consumed frequently or in large amounts, symptoms may recur.

In vitro or RAST based, IgE testing may also be performed for a history of previous severe reactions, or for patients with brittle diseases such as asthma. For those with a history of less severe reactions, or no known serious reactions, skin prick or patch testing may be cautiously performed.[7]

ALLERGIC FUNGAL SINUSITIS

Allergic rhinitis may predispose the paranasal lining to inflammation. This inflammatory process is thought to play a primary role in both acute and chronic sinusitis. One related entity which has attracted much attention is allergic fungal sinusitis (AFS). The exact incidence of this disease process is unknown, however, it is thought to affect 7–10% of chronic sinusitis cases.[33]

This disease process should be separated from other paranasal fungal infections such as invasive fungal sinusitis, noninvasive fungal balls (mycetoma or aspergilloma), and chronic fungal growth (saprophytic growth), and eosinophilic mucin sinusitis. While the first of the previously-mentioned entities primarily afflicts immunocompromised hosts, the other processes affect immune competent patients. Allergic fungal sinusitis is an inflammatory condition, and therefore is extramucosal and noninvasive.

The patients with allergic fungal sinusitis may present with a range of symptoms from mild nasal obstruction to orbital complications with extensive disease. Often these patients have polyposis which manifests primarily as nasal obstruction. Radiologic evaluations reveal heterogeneous areas of signal intensity on computed tomography scans with occasional remodeling or expansion of the involved paranasal sinus. On magnetic resonance imaging, there is a decrease in signal intensity in both the T1 and T2 weighted images secondary to the high protein concentrations within the allergic mucin.[34]

The combination of the above radiologic findings with intraoperative retrieval of thick, tenacious material may convince one of the diagnosis of allergic fungal sinusitis. These findings, however, only partially fulfill the diagnostic criteria. Many authors have proposed inclusive criteria, however, one commonly cited reference is that delineated by Bent and Kuhn. Initially they outlined five common characteristics in these patients to include: Type 1 hypersensitivity (by history, skin test, or serology), nasal polyposis, characterisitic radiographic findings, and eosinophilic mucus demonstrating fungus without tissue invasion.[35] More recently, there have been the previously mentioned five major criteria, in addition to six minor or associated characteristics related to AFS. These minor criteria include asthma, unilateral predominance, radiographic bone erosion, fungal culture, Charcot Leyden crystals, and serum eosinophilia.[36] The authors conjecture that it may take a patient several years to develop each of the inclusive criteria.

Essential to the treatment for allergic fungal sinusitis is the exenteration or complete removal of the allergic mucin. Surgery in these patients should re-establish and occasionally enlarge physiologic drainage pathways between the affected sinus cavities and the nasal cavity. Prior to the surgery, intravenous steroid use may decrease inflammation encountered intraoperatively[37] especially in the cases of massive polyposis. Medical approaches afterwards have included the use of steroids, antifungals, and immunotherapy. There is some evidence that the use of steroids in the postoperative period may decrease recurrence of this process.[38] Others, too, have included postoperative steroids for at least a period of 6 months in their treatment.[36] Immunotherapy has traditionally been recommended as optimum postoperative treatment. In a recent review, however, patients who had been not received immunotherapy fared the same as those who had immunotherapy as part of their postperative treatment plan.[39] The authors' conclusions were encouraging in that patients did well regardless of the initial treatment modality.

ANAPHYLAXIS

Anaphylaxis accounts for approximately 500 deaths in the USA every year, and approximately 3% of anaphylaxis is fatal.[25] In otolaryngologic allergy, only 0.005% of immunotherapy injections caused major systemic reactions, and all patients responded to treatment. Nevertheless, health care professionals involved in *in vivo* allergy testing or allergen immunotherapy should be educated on the prevention and treatment of anaphylaxis. Skin endpoint titration allergy testing helps to determine a safe starting point for immunotherapy, and so may decrease the risk of anaphylaxis as it makes the injection of too high a dose of allergen less likely. Other situations can also affect the patient's ability to tolerate allergen without anaphylaxis. Immunotherapy injections given too frequently or dosing increased too rapidly may predispose to anaphylaxis. Injection of an allergen during its peak environmental season may significantly increase the allergen burden and lead to anaphylaxis.[25]

True anaphylaxis must be rapidly identified and treated. Anaphylaxis must be differentiated from other patient conditions such as a severe local reaction to injection or a vasovagal event.[25] Symptoms of a vasovagal event include paleness and clamminess of the skin, sweating, slow pulse, and normal blood pressure in a resting position. Symptoms of anaphylaxis are quite different, consisting of flushed, warm, dry skin, rapid pulse, and low blood pressure. Bronchospasm, pruritis, urticaria, and angioedema may also be seen.[25] Thorough knowledge of the treatment of anaphylaxis is essential in any allergy practice. Provisions for the establishment of the airway, cardiac monitoring, epinephrine, oxygen, intravenous supplies should be readily available. Other medications such as albuterol and ipratropium inhalers, dopamine, phentolamine, nitroglycerin, lidocaine, atropine, and others may ultimately also be necessary, but the extent of medications and supplies stocked in the office should be determined based on the proximity of the office to the nearest emergency care center.[25]

SUMMARY

Allergy is a worldwide problem. Allergic symptoms, combined with comorbities such as sinusitis and otitis continue to account for extensive health care costs. Recognition and proper diagnosis based on history, physical examination, and (if necessary) allergy testing is essential. The *in vitro* and *in vivo* techniques available for allergy testing need to be patient specific. Medical treatment strategies are usually safe and effective for this problem, including immunotherapy in select cases. Other related disease processes exist, such as food allergy, and allergic fungal sinusitis. Treatment approaches also exist for these entities. Finally, all health care providers testing and treating for allergic disease need to be equipped with the knowledge and materials to respond to an allergy emergency.

REFERENCES

1. Fineman SM. The burden of allergic rhinitis: Beyond dollars and cents. *Ann Allergy Asthma Immunol* 2002; 88(4 Suppl 1): 2–7.
2. Sly RM. Changing prevalence of allergic rhinitis and asthma. *Ann Allergy Asthma Immunol* 1999;82(3):233–48; quiz 248-252.
3. Ray NF, Baraniuk JN, Thamer M et al. Direct expenditures for the treatment of allergic rhinoconjunctivitis in 1996, including the contributions of related airway illnesses. *J Allergy Clin Immunol* 1999;103(3 Pt 1):401–407.
4. Hadley JA. Overview of otolaryngic allergy management. An eclectic and cost-effective approach. *Otolaryngol Clin North Am* 1998;31(1):69–82.
5. Marple BF. Allergy and the contemporary rhinologist. *Otolaryngol Clin North Am* 2003;36(5):941–955.
6. Hadley JA. Immunology of allergic upper respiratory disorders. In: *Allergy and immunology: An otolaryngic approach*, Krouse JH, Chadwick SJ, Gordon BR et al (Eds). Philadelphia: Lippincott, Williams and Wilkins 2002;19–34.
7. Trevino RJ, Gordon BR, Veling MC. Food allergy and hypersensitivity. In: *Allergy and Immunology: An Otolaryngic Approach*, Krouse JH, Chadwick SJ, Gordon BR (Eds) et al. Philadelphia: Lippincott, Williams and Wilkins, 2002;50–80.
8. Borish L. Allergic rhinitis: Systemic inflammation and implications for management. *J Allergy Clin Immunol* 2003; 112(6):1021–1031.
9. Boyd EL. Patient history. In *Allergy and Immunology: An Otolaryngic Approach*, Krouse JH, Chadwick SJ, Gordon BR (Eds) et al. Philadelphia: Lippincott, Williams and Wilkins, 2002;81–86.
10. King HC, Mabry RL, Mabry CS. *Allergy in ENT Practice: A Basic Guide*. New York: Thieme, 1998;452.
11. Miller JJ, Osguthorpe JD. Physical examination of the allergic patient. In: *Allergy and Immunology: An Otolaryngic Approach*, Krouse JH, Chadwick SJ, Gordon BR et al (Eds). Philadelphia: Lippincott, Williams and Wilkins, 2002;87–98.
12. Schramm VL Jr, Effron MZ. Nasal polyps in children. *Laryngoscope* 1980;90(9):1488–1495.
13. Triglia JM, Nicollas R. Nasal and sinus polyposis in children. *Laryngoscope* 1997;107(7): 963–966.
14. Dykewicz MS. Rhinitis and sinusitis. *J Allergy Clin Immunol* 2003;111(2 Suppl): S520–S529.
15. van Cauwenberge P, Bachert C, Passalacqua G et al. Consensus statement on the treatment of allergic rhinitis. European Academy of Allergology and Clinical Immunology. *Allergy* 2000;55(2):116–134.
16. Stanaland BE. Once-daily budesonide aqueous nasal spray for allergic rhinitis: A review. *Clin Ther* 2004;26(4): 473–492.
17. Nathan RA. Pharmacotherapy for allergic rhinitis: A critical review of leukotriene receptor antagonists compared with other treatments. *Ann Allergy Asthma Immunol* 2003;90(2):182–90; quiz 190–1:232.
18. Gendo K, Larson EB. Evidence-based diagnostic strategies for evaluating suspected allergic rhinitis. *Ann Intern Med* 2004;140(4):278–289.
19. Berger WE. Overview of allergic rhinitis. *Ann Allergy Asthma Immunol* 2003;90(6 Suppl 3):7–12.
20. Salib RJ, Drake-Lee A, Howarth PH. Allergic rhinitis: Past, present and the future. *Clin Otolaryngol Allied Sci* 2003; 28(4):291–303.
21. Wilson AM, Sims EJ, McFarlane LC et al. Effects of intranasal corticosteroids on adrenal, bone, and blood markers of systemic activity in allergic rhinitis. *J Allergy Clin Immunol* 1998;102 (4 Pt 1):598–604.
22. Krouse JH, Stachler RJ, Shah A. Current *in vivo* and *in vitro* screens for inhalant allergy. *Otolaryngol Clin North Am* 2003;36(5): 855–868.
23. Fornadley J. Skin testing in the diagnosis of inhalant allergy. In: *Allergy and immunology: An Otolaryngic Approach*, Krouse JH, Chadwick SJ, Gordon BR et al (Eds). Philadelphia: Lippincott, Williams and Wilkins, 2002;114–23.
24. Gordon BR. Allergy skin tests for inhalants and foods. Comparison of methods in common use. *Otolaryngol Clin North Am* 1998;31(1):35–53.
25. Gordon BR. Anaphylaxis: Prevention and treatment. In: *Allergy and Immunology: An Otolaryngic Approach*, Krouse JH, Chadwick SJ, Gordon BR et al (Eds). Philadelphia: Lippincott, Williams and Wilkins, 2002;99–113.
26. Emanuel I. *In vitro* testing for allergies. In: *Allergy and Immunology: An Otolaryngic Approach*, Krouse JH, Chadwick SJ, Gordon BR et al (Eds). Philadelphia: Lippincott, Williams and Wilkins, 2002;124–132.
27. Varney VA, Gaga M, Frew AJ et al. Usefulness of immunotherapy inpatients with severe summer hay fever uncontrolled by antiallergic drugs. *Br Med J* 1991;302(6771):265–269.
28. Varney VA, Tabbah K, Mavroleon G et al. Usefulness of specific immunotherapy inpatients with severe perennial allergic rhinitis induced by house dust mite: A double-blind, randomized, placebo-controlled trial. *Clin Exp Allergy* 2003;33(8):1076-1082.
29. King HC, Mabry RL, Mabry CS. Vial preparation and immunotherapy. In: *Allergy in ENT Practice: A Basic Guide*, New York: Thieme, 1998;205–267.

30. Haydon RC, Gordon BR. Aeroallergen immunotherapy. In: *Allergy and Immunology: An Otolaryngic Approach*, Krouse JH, Chadwick SJ, Gordon BR et al (Eds). Philadelphia: Lippincott, Williams and Wilkins, 2002;151–184.

31. Mabry RL. Food allergy. In: *Allergy in ENT Practice: A Basic Guide*, King HC, Mabry RL, Mabry CS (Eds). New York: Thieme, 1998;319–349.

32. Mabry RL. Appendix 5. In: *Allergy in ENT Practice: A Basic Guide*, King HC, Mabry RL, Mabry CS (Eds). New York: Thieme, 1998;439–441.

33. Corey JP. Allergic fungal sinusitis. *Otolaryngol Clin North Am* 1992;25(1):225–230.

34. Marple BF, Mabry RL. Allergic fungal sinusitis. In: *Allergy and Immunology: An Otolaryngic Approach*, Krouse JH, Chadwick SJ, Gordon BR et al (Eds). Philadelphia: Lippincott, Williams and Wilkins, 2002;232–248.

35. Bent JP 3rd, Kuhn FA. Diagnosis of allergic fungal sinusitis. *Otolaryngol Head Neck Surg* 1994;111(5):580–588.

36. Kuhn FA, Swain R Jr. Allergic fungal sinusitis: Diagnosis and treatment. *Curr Opin Otolaryngol Head Neck Surg* 2003; 11(1): 1–5.

37. Marple BF, Mabry RL. Comprehensive management of allergic fungal sinusitis. *Am J Rhinol* 1998;12(4):263–268.

38. Schubert MS, Goetz DW. Evaluation and treatment of allergic fungal sinusitis: II. Treatment and follow-up. *J Allergy Clin Immunol* 1998;102(3):395–402.

39. Marple B, Newcomer M, Schwade N, Mabry R. Natural history of allergic fungal rhinosinusitis: A 4- to 10-year follow-up. *Otolaryngol Head Neck Surg* 2002;127(5):361–366.

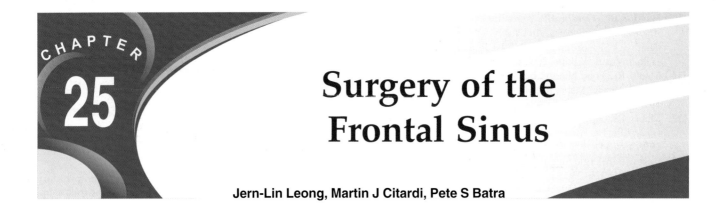

Surgery of the Frontal Sinus

Jern-Lin Leong, Martin J Citardi, Pete S Batra

Since the late nineteenth century, the surgical management of frontal sinus disease has been fraught with controversy. Overtime, many schools of thought have developed on the optimal management of frontal sinus disease. In its historical evolution, the type of surgical approaches has swayed repeatedly between external and intranasal.

The first published record of surgery on the frontal sinus was by Wells in 1870.[1] He cured a patient with a frontal pyocele through both external and intranasal drainage. In the late 1880s, anterior wall trephination was first performed by Ogston and later by Luc.[2] However, this Ogston-Luc technique fell into disrepute due to the high rate of nasofrontal stenosis.[3]

During the early twentieth century, several intranasal approaches were attempted for management of frontal sinus disease.[4-6] Using a combination of mallet, chisel and burr, Halle enlarged the frontal sinus outflow tract intranasally by removing the frontal process of the maxilla and frontal sinus floor.[7] Schaeffer performed a 'direct' intranasal puncture technique to re-establish the frontal sinus drainage.[8] These procedures were abandoned due to unacceptable high failure and mortality rates, primarily because of inadequate visualization.[9-12]

A more aggressive approach, the ablation of the anterior wall, was also explored as an alternative to the intranasal approaches during this period. These procedures involved stripping of the frontal sinus mucosa in its entirety and removal of varying extent of anterior frontal sinus wall.[9] The main drawback was the resulting unsightly cosmetic deformity.[9,13-17] In 1903, Killian proposed preserving a portion of the supraorbital rim which ameliorated the cosmetic defect.[9,18] These procedures again were discontinued due to serious complications like supraorbital rim necrosis, restenosis and even death.

In order to avoid cosmetic disfigurement of anterior table ablation, external frontoethmoidectomy approaches (via the medial orbital wall) followed, in an attempt to restore the frontonasal function. In 1914, Lothrop described a combined intranasal ethmoidectomy and external Lynch-type approach to create a common nasofrontal communication, by resecting the floor, intersinus septum of the frontal sinus and the superior nasal septum.[15] In 1921, Lynch and Howarth also reported their success in addressing the frontoethmoid complex via the external approach.[19,20] However, high failure rate due to medial collapse of orbital soft tissue, resulting in narrowing, scarring and late restenosis, lead to these procedures falling out of favor.[19]

From 1920 to 1960, various modified external frontoethmoidectomy approaches were attempted to prevent restenosis by preserving mucosa and providing buttresses, and/or by placement of stents, grafts and flaps. Temporary stents were made of rubber, tantalum foil or acrylic, while long dwelling stents consisted of gold or Dacron.[21-24] Various mucoperiosteal flaps were also devised to line the surgically enlarged frontal recess. The flaps were either based medially or laterally within the nasal cavity.[25] In addition, the use of mucosal free grafts[26] and split-thickness skin grafts[27] also yielded disappointing results.[28] The long-term results of all these procedures however, remained poor, with reported failure rates as high as 30%.[29]

During the 1960s, osteoplastic procedures with frontal sinus obliteration became the standard approach for treatment of frontal sinus disease.[10,30] This procedure was widely popularized by Montgomery in the US.[31] However, in a series of 250 consecutive osteoplastic procedures, an overall operative complication rate of 19% and an intraoperative cerebrospinal fluid (CSF) leak rate of 2.8% were reported.[32]

The advent of operating microscopes and nasal endoscopes resulted in renewed interest in intranasal management of frontal sinus disease.[33–36] In 1991, Draf described a medial endoscopic drainage approach to the frontal sinus combining microscopic and endoscopic techniques.[37] While re-establishing the intranasal frontonasal tract, the lateral bony walls were preserved, thus preventing medial collapse of the orbital soft tissues. In 1995, Gross et al described an extended endoscopic approach to create a similar common frontal opening.[38] As more experience was accumulated, the endoscopic intranasal approaches rapidly became a viable alternative to the conventional approach.[39]

ANATOMY

Knowledge of the frontal sinus and its drainage pathway is paramount for understanding the concepts and techniques of contemporary frontal sinus surgery. The frontal sinuses are generally paired, asymmetric structures found within the squamosal portion of the frontal bones. The adult size averages 28 mm in height, 24 mm in width, and 20 mm in depth.[40] The posterior table is the thinner of the two tables and lies in direct contact with the dura.

The Frontal Recess

The anatomy of the frontal sinus outflow tract, otherwise known as the frontal recess, is complex. This concept was initially described by Killian in 1903.[18] The term nasofrontal duct has also been used by authors; however, this is an anatomic misnomer, since the frontal outflow tract is not a rigid, tubular structure. The frontal recess is a potential space that is pneumatized by various cells, and, thus, the use of the term nasofrontal duct is discouraged. This was also recognized by Mosher through his cadaveric works.[41] The boundaries of this recess are as follows:
- *Anterior:* Agger nasi region.
- *Posterior:* Skull-base.
- *Medial:* Middle turbinate
- *Lateral:* Lamina papyracea

The drainage pathway, as described by Kuhn, has an hourglass configuration with the frontal internal ostium as the narrowest portion, between the frontal sinus infundibulum superiorly and frontal recess inferiorly. The frontal ostium is usually found in the medial floor of the sinus. The posterior boundary of the frontal recess consists of the skull-base. An important structure, the anterior ethmoidal artery resides here and forms the posterior boundary of the frontal recess along the skull base (Fig. 25.1). The path of the anterior ethmoid artery is important to recognize when performing frontal sinus

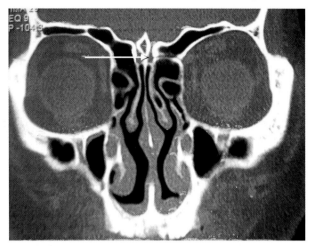

Fig. 25.1: Coronal sinus CT shows left anterior ethmoidal artery crossing the ethmoidal roof (arrow)

surgery. The skull-base at the site of entry of the artery, or the ethmoid sulcus, has been measured to be only 0.05 mm thick, which represents a ten-fold reduction in the thickness of the skull base.[42] This is the most common site for iatrogenic cerebrospinal fluid leaks during functional endoscopic sinus surgery (FESS).

The exact configuration of the frontal recess can be quite variable. It is dependent on the three-dimensional pneumatization pattern of the anterior ethmoidal cells into the frontal recess. These cells include:
- Agger nasi cell
- Frontal cells
- Supraorbital ethmoid cell
- Suprabullar cell
- Frontal bullar cell
- Intersinus septal cell

The agger nasi area (nasal mound) is found just anterior and superior to the insertion of the middle turbinate into the lateral nasal wall.[43] The rate of pneumatization of the agger nasi region has been documented as high as 98.5%.[44] The agger nasi cell is the most anterior and constant frontal recess cell, located at the anterior boundary of the frontal recess (Fig. 25.2). Extensive pneumatization of the agger nasi cell can narrow the frontal recess and may predispose the patient to frontal sinusitis.

A variety of frontal cells can pneumatize anteriorly into the frontal recess in conjunction with the agger nasi cell. They have been classified into type I to IV by Bent and Kuhn.[45] They are defined as follows:
- *Type I frontal cell (FC1):* A single cell pneumatizing above the agger nasi cell (Fig. 25.2).

- *Type II frontal cells (FC2):* Tier of two or more cells pneumatizing above the agger nasi cell and extending into the frontal sinus.
- *Type III frontal cell (FC3):* A single large cell pneumatizing above the agger nasi cell and extending into the frontal sinus (Fig. 25.3).
- *Type IV frontal cell (FC4):* An isolated cell within the frontal sinus that arises from a narrow stalk or pneumatization tract from the anterior frontal recess (Fig. 25.4).

The prevalence of FC1, FC2, FC3 and FC4 has been quoted as 37%, 19%, 8%, and rare.[46]

Laterally, presence of a supraorbital ethmoid cell can determine the frontal recess caliber as well[47] (Fig. 25.5). This cell has recently been found to occur as often as 62% of the time,[46] much higher than the previously quoted 6[48] to 15%.[49] This was thought to be due to the cells being previously wrongly identified as part of a septated frontal sinus.[46] This cell may pneumatize extensively and is commonly mistaken for the frontal sinus. In general, the ostium leading to the supraorbital ethmoidal cell lies posterolateral to the internal ostium of the frontal sinus. In some individuals, more than one supraorbital ethmoid cell may be present on one side. Missed supraorbital cells are a frequent source of iatrogenic frontal sinus disease.

Frontal bullar and suprabullar cells reside superior to the ethmoidal bulla. Their pneumatization pattern can cause significant compromise from the posterior portion of the frontal recess. Their definitions have been recently refined by Lee et al.[46] Frontal bullar cell pneumatizes along the skull-base in the posterior frontal recess, and extends into the frontal sinus. The suprabullar cell, on the other hand, has the same configuration except that it does not pneumatize into the frontal sinus.

Intersinus septal cell, as the name suggests, pneumatizes the frontal intersinus septum and may result in substantial narrowing of the recess medially.[50] Extensive pneumatization of this cell may be associated with a pneumatized crista galli. The opening for the interfrontal sinus cell is in the medial frontal recess. In fact, this pattern of pneumatization may be used to surgically widen a narrow frontal recess.[51]

Physiology

The normal mucociliary transport of the frontal sinus is important, as this serves as the basis for functional endoscopic frontal sinus techniques. The pattern of mucous transport in the frontal sinus is superiorly along the intersinus septum, laterally along the roof and then

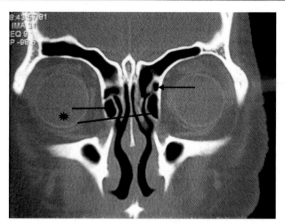

Fig. 25.2: Coronal sinus CT depicts bilateral agger nasi cells (asterisk) and a type I frontal cell (arrow)

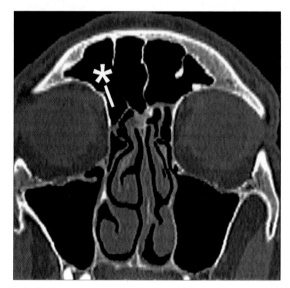

Fig. 25.3: Coronal sinus CT depicts a right type III frontal cell (asterisk) (From Lee W, Kuhn F, Citardi M. 3D computed tomographic analysis of frontal recess anatomy in patients without frontal sinusitis. Otolaryngol Head Neck Surg 2004;131(3):164–73; with permission)

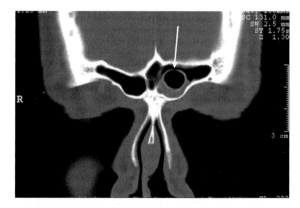

Fig. 25.4: Coronal CT sinus shows a type IV frontal cell (arrow)

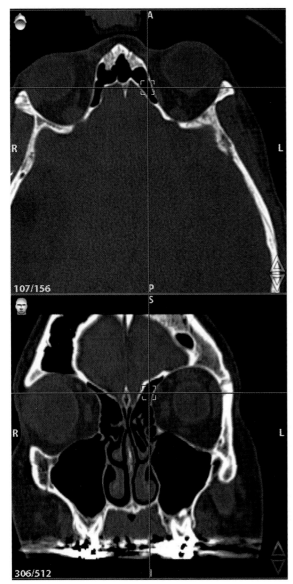

Fig. 25.5: The supraorbital ethmoid cell (indicated by the cross hairs in these orthogonal axial and coronal CT images) pneumatizes over the orbit (coronal image, bottom) and enters the frontal recess posterior and lateral to the true frontal sinus (axial image, top). (From Lee W, Kuhn F, Citardi M. 3D computed tomographic analysis of frontal recess anatomy in patients without frontal sinusitis. Otolaryngol Head Neck Surg 2004; 131(3):164–73; with permission)

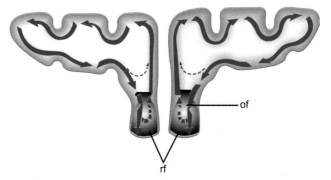

Fig. 25.6: Schematic drawing of frontal sinus circulation (of = frontal sinus ostium and rf = frontal recess), (From Stammberger H. Functional endoscopic sinus surgery. In Secretion transportation. 1st edition. Philadelphia: BC Decker Inc, 1999; p 31)

ADVANCES IN ENDOSCOPIC SINUS SURGERY

Functional Endoscopic Sinus Surgery (FESS) Paradigm

The surgical management of chronic frontal sinusitis commences after the disease is deemed refractory to maximal medical therapy. Over the last quarter of a century, the advent of rigid telescopes and improved imaging techniques (CT scans) has revolutionized the management of chronic sinus disease, and more specifically chronic frontal sinus disease. The 'traditional' open approaches were all limited by the absence of proper imaging and visualization of the frontal recess. The paradigm has shifted from 'ablative' to 'preservative' approaches with the wide acceptance of the concept of FESS (i.e. mucosal preservation and re-establishment of sinus ventilation and drainage).[34,52–55] With improved understanding of the pathophysiology of rhinosinusitis and the recent technological advances, a new algorithm for management of chronic frontal sinusitis is proposed.

The proposed stepwise approach is as follows:
- Endoscopic frontal sinusotomy.
- Endoscopic frontal sinusotomy with endoscopic frontal trephination (above and below approach).
- Frontal sinus rescue procedure.
- Modified endoscopic Lothrop procedure (including transseptal endoscopic frontal sinusotomy)
- Endoscopic frontal sinusotomy with osteoplastic flap (osteoplastic procedure without obliteration).
- Osteoplastic flap with frontal sinus obliteration.

Some of the important considerations in formulating this approach include:
- Frontal sinus surgeries performed in tertiary centers 86.6% are standard endoscopic sinus surgery.[55]

medially along the floor of the sinus (Fig. 25.6). The mucus then exits laterally out of the frontal ostium. However, a substantial portion of the mucus does not exit the sinus and recirculates along the medial frontal recess for another cycle. The frontal sinus is the only sinus with active transportation of mucus in an inward direction. Thus, debris or pathogens present in the frontal recess may be actively swept into the sinus.[52,53]

- Osteoplastic flap can be performed without obliteration.
- Frontal sinus drillout procedures are performed infrequently.
- Frontal sinus obliteration is the absolute last resort.

Based on the above approach, the philosophy essentially translates to the graduated approach of performing minimal or no surgery to advanced surgical techniques, depending on the severity of the disease state.

Image-guided FESS Paradigm

Computer-aided surgery (CAS) is increasingly being used in endoscopic sinus surgery over the last 15 years.[56] The indications include a variety of complex rhinologic procedures including endoscopic frontal sinusotomy.[57] CAS helps to simplify the complex frontal sinus anatomy by aiding the surgeon in understanding the anatomy in a three-dimensional manner. This then translates into a better safety profile, decreasing the morbidity and increasing the efficacy of the surgery. Image-guided surgery (IGS), which is a part of CAS, refers to the use of surgical navigation and localization technology for execution of FESS. To incorporate CAS into FESS, a new paradigm has been termed, namely, image-guided FESS (IG-FESS).[56]

Principles of IG-FESS include:

- Precise anatomic dissection and mucosal preservation remains important.[33]
- Preoperative CT review on computer work-station aids in formulation of a precise surgical plan.
- Surgical navigation allows direct correlation between preoperative imaging data and surgical plan to the operative field.
- Intraoperative tracking of surgical instruments allows for integration of the surgical navigation system in the implementation of the surgical plan.

Frontal Instrumentation

The advances in surgical instrumentation have been critical to the implementation of the endoscopic frontal sinus surgery paradigm. A wide array of surgical instruments is now available the surgeon's for the management of frontal sinus disease. In particular, the refinement has revolved around the development of angled instruments, micro-through-cutting forceps, and angled rigid endoscopes.

The following instruments may help facilitate frontal recess dissection for the endoscopic surgeon including:

- Angled endoscopes (30°, 45° and 70°).
- Frontal recess suctions (45° and 90°).

- Curettes (suction and nonsuction, 45° and 90°).
- Frontal seekers.
- Giraffe forceps (through- and non-throughcutting, front-to-back and side-to-side biting orientation).
- Frontal sinus (Hosemann) punch.
- Heuweisser through-cutting forceps.

Microdebriders and drills may serve as important adjuncts to the endoscopic techniques in selective cases.

Endoscopic Frontal Sinusotomy

The majority of frontal sinus disease can be managed by standard endoscopic techniques using the IG-FESS paradigm outlined earlier. This also represents the first step in the graduated approach.

Indications
- Chronic frontal sinusitis refractory to maximal medical therapy (both primary and revision cases).
- Frontal sinus mucoceles.[58]
- Frontal recess inverting papillomas.[59]

Contraindications
- Frontal sinus tumors.
- Frontal sinus inverting papilloma.
- Broad-based osteomas.
- Frontal recess stenosis.
- Laterally-based mucoceles.

Advantages
- Less morbidity compared to open procedures.
- Can be performed as an outpatient procedure.
- Shorter convalescent time.
- No facial scars.

Disadvantages
- Difficult technique as entire procedure is performed with angled endoscopes and curved frontal recess instruments.
- Risk of skull-base injury and consequent CSF leak.

Surgical Techniques
There are several prerequisites to performing a successful endoscopic frontal sinusotomy. These include intimate knowledge of frontal sinus anatomy, availability of frontal instrumentation, and commitment to meticulous postoperative care. CAS technology is also desirable, albeit not absolutely necessary.

Principles of the endoscopic technique include:
- Understanding of the three-dimensional anatomy of the frontal recess by the surgeon. This can be achieved through an endoscopic examination, review of preoperative CT scan and IGS technology (if available).

- The entire procedure is performed under visualization with 30° and 70° telescopes.
- Frontal recess curettes are used to fracture each frontal recess cell, advancing in a medial to lateral direction and from a posterior to anterior direction.
- The instruments should never be advanced from anterior to posterior or lateral to medial direction, as this may result in inadvertent penetration of the skull-base.
- All bone fragments must be removed with giraffe forceps as they can serve as a nidus for infection or incite scar tissue formation in the postoperative period.
- Mucosal preservation is of utmost importance in the frontal recess.
- The internal ostium of the frontal sinus should be directly visualized at the completion of the procedure. Simple cannulation of the frontal sinus is insufficient (Fig. 25.7).
- Powered instrumentation should be used with extreme care.
- Rasp-type instruments should not be used as they may cause circumferential tissue damage and result in iatrogenic stenosis.

Close postoperative follow-up is essential to ensure optimal outcome from the surgical procedure. The patient should be seen weekly to biweekly with meticulous removal of all fibrin clot and debris under endoscopic visualization. The patient is placed on a daily regimen of nasal saline irrigations. Culture-directed antibiotics and systemic steroids, if clinically indicated, are continued in the postoperative period until complete healing of the frontal recess is ensured[60] (Fig. 25.8).

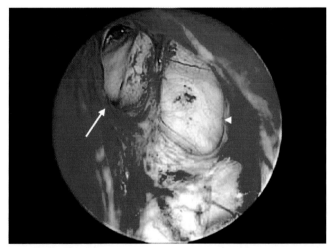

Fig. 25.7: Immediate postoperative endoscopic view of the left frontal internal ostium (arrow). An adjacent supraorbital ethmoid cell has also been dissected (arrowhead)

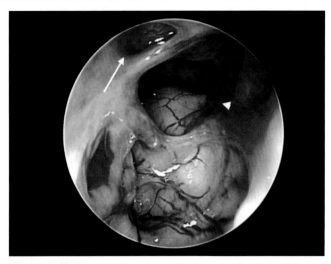

Fig. 25.8: Postoperative endoscopic view of a healed left frontal ostium (arrowhead). A remnant agger nasi cell cap is also noted anteriorly (arrow)

Outcomes

The surgical outcomes of endoscopic frontal sinusotomy have been very encouraging. The results have also been reported to be better than the external approaches by some centers.[11] Success rates are reported at over 90% for symptomatic relief, with 2 to 11% rate of persistent frontal sinusitis symptoms. Approximately, 1–5% of the patients eventually required revision surgery.[11,39,61,62]

Endoscopic Frontal Trephination and Endoscopic Frontal Sinusotomy (the 'above and below' approach)

This approach was first described by Wigand in 1978.[58] It offers an extension to the pure endoscopic technique, obviating the need for more invasive approaches with their associated morbidity.

Indications

- Certain patterns of frontal recess pneumatization that are beyond the reach of standard endoscopic frontal recess instrumentation.
- Alteration of frontal sinus/recess anatomy that proves inaccessible with standard endonasal endoscopic approach due to the extensive inflammatory disease, previous surgery or neoplasm. The additional 'porthole' allows visualization and instrumentation with the endoscopic approach.

Contraindications

- Acute frontal sinusitis with suppurative complications (relative contraindication).
- Extensive new bone formation within frontal sinus/recess.
- Previous frontal sinus obliteration.

Advantages

- Allows preservation of natural frontal sinus outflow tract.
- Small external facial wound/scar.
- Allows postoperative surveillance by intranasal endoscopy and radiographic means.

Disadvantages

Difficult technique as entire procedure is performed with angled endoscopes and curved frontal recess instruments.

Surgical Technique [55,59]

The classic frontal sinus trephination is performed for drainage of acute frontal sinusitis, through the floor of the frontal sinus below the medial brow. However, variations of the placement of the site of trephination may be performed (Fig. 25.9). Trephination of the anterior table allows visualization of the frontal sinus in all four directions (Fig. 25.10). The maximum diameter of this trephine is about 4 mm to avoid cosmetic deformity and at the same time, allow standard frontal recess instruments to pass through. The trephination of the anterior table is not to be used for acute frontal sinusitis due the possibility of causing frontal bone osteomyelitis.

Placement of the trephine in the frontal sinus floor allows the size to be as large as 10 mm without concern for frontal deformity. The main advantage of this larger opening is that it allows the simultaneous admission of a nasal telescope and additional surgical instrumentation to endoscopically address the pathology. Care must be taken to ensure that the trephine is through the frontal sinus floor and not the frontal recess cells.

Trephination is performed in a mucosa-sparing manner. Using a diamond drill and concurrent irrigation, the frontal bone is first 'blue-lined'. Then, frontal sinus mucosa is incised with a scalpel knife. Further enlargement of the trephine may be achieved by using the Kerrison rongeur. This mucosal preservation is critical for success of this approach.

Frontal stents may be used to ensure potency in the postoperative period. As in the frontal sinusotomy approach, meticulous postoperative care is essential. Culture-directed antibiotics and steroids may be prescribed through the early healing phase.

Outcomes

The management of frontal mucoceles by this approach has been reported by Bent et al.[59] They noted that all 11 patients were cured or improved by this approach at a mean follow-up of 19 months. Benoit and Duncavage also

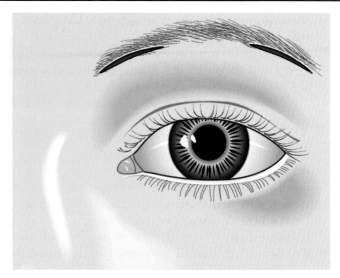

Fig. 25.9: Frontal view demonstrating medial and lateral trephine incisions

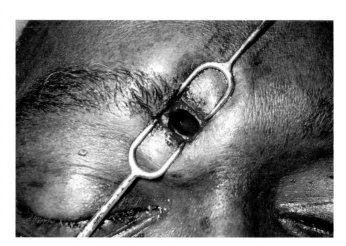

Fig. 25.10: Frontal view demonstrating right frontal sinus floor trephine

reported good results with this approach with stent placement.[63] Overall frontal recess patency was 79% with subjective improvement in 78% of patients. In a series of 22 patients with varied complex frontal sinus disease, Batra et al noted an overall patency rate of 86% with a mean follow-up of 16.2 months.[64]

Frontal Sinus Rescue (Revision Endoscopic Frontal Sinusotomy with Mucoperiosteal Flap Advancement)

Frontal sinus rescue (FSR) was first introduced by Kuhn in 1997 for management of frontal recess stenosis after middle turbinate resection. It is essentially a modification of the standard endoscopic frontal sinusotomy technique with mucoperiosteal flap advancement.[65,66] The mucoperiosteal flap is used for repositioning an iatrogenically stenosed frontal recess or ostium and aims to restore normal function to a diseased frontal sinus.

Indications
- Recurrent or persistent frontal sinusitis due to a scarred frontal recess or ostium, most likely secondary to middle turbinate resection with lateralization and stenosis of the frontal recess (Fig. 25.11).
- Frontal sinusitis associated with intracranial complication (definitive management after initial treatment failure).
- Frontal recess tumors, e.g. osteoma.
- Frontal sinus fractures.

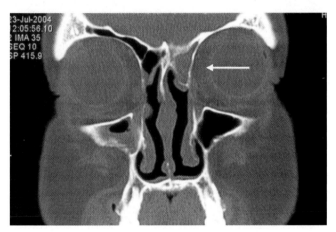

Fig. 25.11: Coronal sinus CT demonstrates a lateralized left middle turbinate remnant (arrow) causing iatrogenic frontal sinusitis

Contraindications
- Patients with an intact middle turbinate.
- Acute frontal sinusitis.
- Frontal osteomyelitis with inadequate medical treatment.

Advantages
- Mucociliary clearance restored since lateral frontal recess mucosa is preserved.
- Compensation of both bony and soft tissue stenosis due to middle turbinate resection.
- Mucoperiosteal flap minimize granulation tissue formation and stenosis.

Disadvantages
- Mucoperiosteal flap is extremely delicate and may tear easily.
- Difficult technique as entire procedure is performed with angled endoscopes and curved frontal recess instruments.

- Risk of skull-base injury and consequent CSF leak as cribriform plate is just posterior to the site of manipulation.
- Revision FSR might be indicated in some cases.

Surgical Technique
Today most procedures are done with intraoperative surgical navigation. Instrumentation with angled endoscopes is vital for the successful execution of this procedure. A parasagittal incision is first made with a sickle knife along the anterior edge of the middle turbinate remnant. A portion of the middle turbinate remnant is removed with through-biting forceps. The mucosa on both medial and lateral aspects of the bony remnant is then elevated atraumatically. The medial mucosa and a small area of adjacent nasal roof mucosa are then removed. The bony remnant of the middle turbinate is then removed with through-biting giraffe forceps. The preserved lateral mucosa then forms the mucoperiosteal flap. This flap is then laid medially over the denuded area of the former bony middle turbinate.[65,66]

Outcomes
The preliminary results of FSR have been encouraging. In a preliminary report, success rate of 87.5% was attained in 12 patients on 16 sides with an average follow-up of 8.5 months.[65] Subsequently, Kuhn et al reported a 91% success rate in maintaining frontal recess patency and complete resolution of symptoms in 24 patients (32 sides) with a mean follow-up of 9.6 months.[66]

Endoscopic Modified Lothrop Procedure (The Frontal Sinus Drill-out)

The Lothrop procedure was originally devised to create a large common drainage pathway from the frontal sinus to the nasal cavity via an external ethmoidectomy approach.[15] This essentially involved the removal of the frontal floor and intersinus septum as well as part of the nasal septum. However, this technique had a high failure rate due to the prolapse of orbital contents into the frontal recess. The endoscopic modified Lothrop procedure (EMLP) was later introduced to achieve the same surgical goals via the endonasal approach.[38,67] This avoided the external incision and prevented orbital content prolapse by preserving the lamina papyracea.[68,69]

Indications
- Chronic frontal sinusitis after failed endoscopic sinus surgery, especially in the setting of 'neo-osteogenesis' or middle turbinate resection.
- Frontal sinus mucocele formation.
- Inverted papilloma.

- Sinonasal malignancy.
- Fibro-osseous lesions.
- Trauma.

Relative Contraindications
- Large frontal recess comprising multiple partitions, e.g. frontal cells, supraorbital ethmoidal cells.
- Narrow AP dimensions (< 1.2 cm) may not allow for successful completion of the procedure and may place the patient at higher risk of CSF leak.

Advantages
- Low reported morbidity.
- Good cosmesis.
- Able to evaluate patient endoscopically for recurrent disease postoperatively.

Disadvantages
- Technically difficult even in experienced hands.[67]
- Require specialized instrumentation.

Surgical Technique
The surgery is performed under general anesthesia. The adjacent paranasal sinus disease, which is often present due to previous surgeries, should be addressed first. This prevents bleeding from the 'drill-out' from being an issue when dealing with the adjacent disease.

A superiorly based 1.5–2 cm iatrogenic septal perforation is first created just across from the leading edge of the middle turbinate/agger nasi region below the skull-base. This helps to provide adequate exposure and an enlarged frontal sinus outflow tract for ventilation. This maneuver also facilitates postoperative endoscopic inspection and debridement. The initial septal incisions are made with an ophthalmic crescent knife. Then, using a through-cutting forceps or micro-debrider, the perforation is completed. Throughout the procedure, it is important to keep bony and cartilaginous exposure to a minimum.

The surgery is begun by first identifying the frontal sinus floor. This is done either by intraoperative surgical navigation, or using surgical landmarks to help gauge the relative position of the sinus. This is an essential step as it defines the posterior limit of the drill-out, which helps to minimize potential intracranial injury. The midline position of the frontal sinus floor is typically located posterosuperior to the most anterosuperior aspects of the septal bony-cartilaginous junction. This location is also approximately adjacent to the most anterior remnant or root of the middle turbinate and agger nasi (ascending process of the maxilla). This site is also noted to be more anterior than the position of the naturally occurring frontal recess area.

The bony frontal sinus floor is then removed with an angled suction-irrigation drill using the lamina papyracea as the two lateral boundaries. The direction of drilling is directed laterally and anteriorly to minimize possible injury to the anterior ethmoidal artery and intracranial penetration. Alternatively, straight drills may be used with concurrent irrigation. If the sinus floor thickness allows it, curetting may be sufficient to enter the frontal sinus. The lower portion of the intersinus septum is also removed to create a common cavity (Fig. 25.12). Mucosal preservation technique is to be observed to prevent delayed stenosis. Again, meticulous postoperative care is essential. However, some contracture of this neo-ostium is to be expected from this procedure.

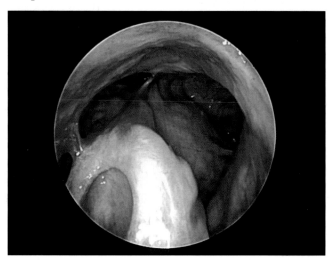

Fig. 25.12: A postoperative endoscopic view of the 'drill-out' frontal neo-ostium

A novel technique, endoscopic trans-septal frontal sinusotomy (TSFS) has been recently described.[70] It builds upon the concepts of the endoscopic modified Lothrop procedure and uses the unique relationship of the nasal septum to the midline floor of the frontal sinus (Figs 25.13A and B). The advantages that this technique offers are the preservation of intersinus septum and that it can be performed in cases where severity of the stenosis prohibits cannulation of the frontal recess as a primary landmark.

Outcomes
Long-term outcomes reported by Schlosser et al on 44 patients over a mean follow-up period of 40 months were favorable.[71] The overall success rate was 82% with failures occurring at a mean of 12 months after the initial Lothrop procedure. Batra et al reported on drill-out procedures on 25 patients with a wide variety of indications.[72] Endoscopic patency of the neo-ostium was

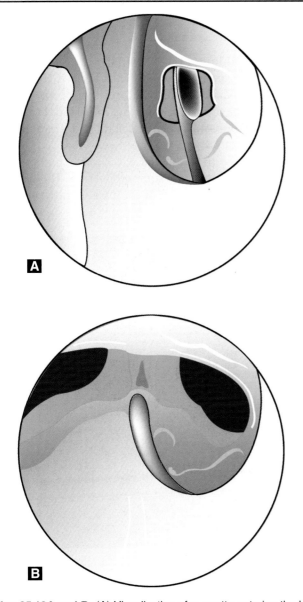

Figs 25.13A and B: (A) Visualization of a curette entering the left frontal sinus floor via a septal perforation. (B) C-shaped 'neo-ostium' created via endoscopic modified Lothrop procedure

achieved in 92% of cases at an average follow-up of 16.3 months. In a comparative review of EMLP versus osteoplastic flap procedure (OFP), it was found that EMLP caused fewer adverse postoperative outcomes but is more likely to produce perioperative cerebrospinal fluid leak. EMLP was also found to be superior to OFP with lower morbidity, shorter operative time, and lower perioperative blood loss. However, due to the relatively short follow-up period in the majority of the studies, the long-term efficacy of EMLP could not be determined.[73]

Frontal Osteoplastic Flap without Obliteration (OFWO)

The preservation of frontal sinus function with osteoplastic flap surgery has emerged in recent years due to the paradigm shift in the concepts of FESS. Proponents of the obliteration procedure state that it has a high success rate and that it prevents late mucocele or pyocele formation. However, this argument may be flawed, as it has been observed to take an average of seven years for mucoceles to present clinically after the obliteration procedure.[74] Moreover, with frequent endoscopic surveillance of the frontal recess with the endoscopic techniques, early failure due to stenosis can easily be detected before mucocele formation.

Indications
- Frontal sinus disease refractory to previous surgical attempts.
- Frontal diseases manifested by altered physiology (e.g. primary ciliary dyskinesia and cystic fibrosis).
- Frontal bone osteomyelitis with bone necrosis.
- Fractures of the frontal sinus with posterior table involvement.
- Fractures of the frontal recess.
- Frontal sinus disease with orbital or intracranial extension.
- Cases where complete removal of sinus mucosa is difficult or dangerous, e.g. comminuted fracture, mucocele with densely adherent mucosa to dura mater or periorbita.
- Previous frontal sinus obliteration with complication, e.g. fat necrosis, mucocele.

Surgical Technique
The approach is essentially similar to that of the 'obliterative' procedure with regard to the skin incision and raising of the flap. However, the main difference is that the mucosa of the frontal sinus is preserved. A standard intranasal endoscopic frontal sinusotomy is then performed to ensure patency of the frontal recess and frontal sinus function. This step is important to ensure that both the frontal sinus and recess are visible endoscopically for subsequent surveillance. As part of postoperative monitoring, serial nasal endoscopy and CT scans are also essential.

More recently, a technique for the 'unobliteration' of a previously obliterated frontal sinus has been introduced.[75] After frontal sinus obliteration, many patients complain of persistent headaches, which might be indicative of mucocele formation or fat necrosis. The osteoplastic frontal sinusotomy then provides maximum exposure to inspect and address the intrasinus pathology. Mucocele is opened and the diseased sinus contents are removed. Islands of mucosa that are still present in the cavity are carefully preserved to help remucosalization of the sinus cavity. In most instances, a stent composed of a thin silastic sheeting is placed both in the frontal sinus and in the frontal recess. Although the stent is mostly in the frontal sinus, it may be easily removed under endoscopic visualization in the office. The frontal sinus is then left to recover its mucociliary clearance.

Frontal Osteoplastic Flap with Obliteration (OFO)

This procedure was once the gold standard for the surgical treatment of frontal sinus pathology as it has a fairly high success rate.[31,32] The philosophy of the procedure is to completely obliterate the frontal sinus so that it will no longer serve as an air space.[76] However, with the wide acceptance of FESS concepts and the advancement of endoscopic surgical techniques (frontal sinusotomy and modified Lothrop procedure), the frequency of use of the 'osteoplastic flap' surgery has dwindled.

Indications

- Frontal sinus disease refractory to previous surgical attempts.
- Frontal diseases manifested by altered physiology (e.g. primary ciliary dyskinesia and cystic fibrosis).
- Frontal bone osteomyelitis with bone necrosis.
- Fractures of the frontal sinus with posterior table involvement.
- Fractures of the frontal recess.
- Frontal sinus disease with orbital or intracranial extension.

Contraindications

- Frontal sinus mucocele with erosion of the posterior table or orbital roof.
- Frontal sinus allergic fungal sinusitis.
- Frontal sinus neoplasms.

Advantage

Technically easier compared to endoscopic modified Lothrop surgery.

Disadvantages

- Poor cosmesis.
- Forehead anesthesia.
- Bone flap necrosis.
- Neuralgia.
- Orbital fat exposure.
- Unintentional fracture of frontal sinus anterior wall.
- Incorrect placement of anterior bony cuts.

- Dural lacerations.
- Late mucocele formation.

Surgical Technique

Access to the anterior frontal sinus table is first made through the skin incision. This can either be via a brow, forehead, or bicoronal incision (Fig. 25.14). The boundary of the frontal sinus must then be determined. Traditionally, a sterilized standard 6-foot Caldwell view radiograph template of the frontal sinus was used.[77] It should be placed accurately over the supraorbital rims. This can also be achieved with the aid of an intraoperative image-guidance system.[78]

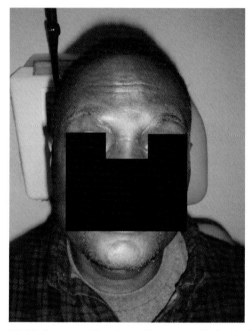

Fig. 25.14: Postoperative view of brow or 'gull wing' incision for an osteoplastic flap procedure

The incision over the periosteum should be made with a 1 cm cuff beyond the planned osteotomy site. This would help ensure the blood supply for the flap, which is derived inferiorly from the periosteum. Using a saw or drill, the inferiorly based bone flap with its periosteum is raised. It is also important to bevel the incision to facilitate alignment during closure. Once the flap is raised, and the sinus entirely exposed, the intrasinus work is done (Fig. 25.15). All diseased bony septations and mucosa within the frontal sinus, frontal recess, and posterior aspect of the flap are removed. This is done with an otologic drill, using both cutting and diamond burrs. In all cases, the sinus cavity may be obliterated by various means to prevent late mucocele or pyocele formation. By placing no material,

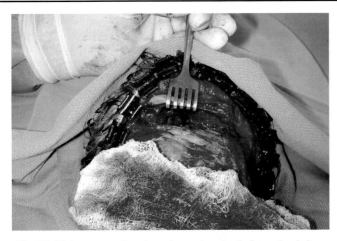

Fig. 25.15: Intraoperative view of an osteoplastic flap raised via a bicoronal incision, exposing the frontal sinuses

spontaneous osteoneogenesis occurs, resulting in self-obliteration of the sinus.[79,80] Most commonly fat autograft is used, but other autologous materials, such as bone, muscle, hydroxyapatite, and polymethacrylate have also been used.[81–84] The flap is then replaced and secured with either suture or microplates.

Outcomes

The success rates of OFO are variable, with complication rates varying from 18 to 65%. In consecutive series of 250 patients, Hardy et al reported a 93% overall cure rate and 6% revision surgery rate. Operative complications in 19% and intraoperative CSF leak rate of 2.8% was also noted.[32] On the other hand, Weber et al described a total complication rate of 65.8%.[85] Moreover, this procedure precludes endoscopic and radiographic surveillance postoperatively; thus these patients cannot be adequately assessed if they develop frontal symptoms (a relatively common occurrence).

CONCLUSION

Surgery of the frontal sinus is technically difficult and continues to challenge even the most experienced endoscopic surgeons. A clear understanding of the anatomy and physiology is a prerequisite to a successful outcome in any surgical procedure, but this is especially true in the frontal sinus. By tracing its controversial history, we are able to understand some of the issues faced by surgeons of the past, and will help us to manage patients with frontal sinus disease.

With the technical advances in imaging, instrumentation and increasingly, intraoperative surgical navigation systems, there has been a paradigm shift in the graduated approach to the frontal sinus from 'ablative' to 'preservative' procedures. However, this does not mean that we abandon the external or 'ablative' approaches, since they are indicated in specific situations.

REFERENCES

1. Wells R. Abscess of the frontal sinus. *Lancet* 1870; 1:694.
2. Ogston A. Trephining the frontal sinus for catarrhal diseases. *Men Chron Manchester* 1884; i:235.
3. Coakley CG. Frontal sinusitis: Diagnosis, treatment, and results. *Trans Am Laryngol Rhinol Otol Soc* 1905; 11:101.
4. Goode RH. An intranasal method for opening the frontal sinus establishing the largest possible drainage. *Laryngoscope* 1908. 18:266.
5. Ingals EF. New operation and instruments for draining the frontal sinus. *Ann Otol Rhinol Laryngol* 1905; 14:512–20.
6. Van Alyea OE. Frontal sinus drainage. *Ann Otol Rhinol Laryngol* 1946; 55:267.
7. Halle M. External and internal operation for suppuration of the accessory nasal sinuses. *Laryngoscope* 1907; 17:115.
8. Schaeffer JP. Cited by Sier: Rouillons. *Arch Int Laryngol* 1911; 709.
9. Donald PJ. Surgical management of frontal sinus infections. In *The sinuses* PJ Donald et al (Ed). New York: Raven Press, 1995; 201.
10. Becker D, Moore D, Lindsey W, Gross W, Gross C. Modified transnasal endoscopic Lothrop procedure: Further considerations. *Laryngoscope* 1995; 105(11):1161–1166.
11. Schaefer S, Close L. Endoscopic management of frontal sinus disease. *Laryngoscope* 1990; 100(2 Pt 1):155–160.
12. Pratt JA. The present status of the intranasal ethmoid operation. *Arch Otolaryngol* 1925; 1:42–50.
13. Williams H, Holman C. The causes and avoidance of failure in surgery for chronic suppuration of the frontoethmo-sphenoid complex of sinuses: With a previously unreported anomaly which produces chronicity and recurrence, and the description of a surgical technique usually producing a cure of the disease. *Laryngoscope* 1962; 72:1179–1227.
14. Hosemann W, Gode U, Wigand M. Indications, technique and results of endonasal endoscopic ethmoidectomy. *Acta Otorhinolaryngol Belg* 1993; 47(1):73–83.
15. Lothrop HA. Frontal sinus suppuration. *Ann Surg* 1914; 59:937–957.
16. Lyman EH. The place of the obliterative operation in frontal sinus surgery. *Laryngoscope* 1950;60:407–441.
17. Riedel-Schenke H. Cited by Gosdale RH. The radical obliterative frontal sinus operation: A consideration of technical factors in difficult cases. *Ann Otol Rhinol Laryngol* 1955; 64:470–485.
18. Killian G. Die killianische radical operation chronischer stirnhohleneiterungen: Weiteres kasui stisches material und zasammenfassung. *Arch Laryngol Rhinol* 1903.
19. Lynch RC. The technique of a radical frontal sinus operation which has given me the best results. *Laryngoscope* 1921; 31(1):1–5.
20. Howarth WG. Operations on the frontal sinus. *J Laryngol* 1921; 36:417–421.
21. Harris HE. The use of tantalum tubes in frontal sinus surgery. *Cleve Clin Q* 1948; 15:129–133.

22. Erich JB, New JB. An acrylic obturator employed in the repair of an obstructed frontonasal duct. *Trans Am Acad Ophthalmol Otolarygol* 1947; 51:628–640.

23. Anthony DH. Use of Ingala gold tube in frontal sinus operations. *South Med J* 1940; 33:949–955.

24. Barton RT. Dacron prosthesis in frontal sinus surgery. *Laryngoscope* 1972; 82(10):1799–1805.

25. Sewall E. The operative technique of nasal sinus disease. *Ann Otol Rhinol Laryngol* 1935; 44:307–316.

26. Mihoefer W. External operation on the frontal sinnus: Critical review. *Arch Otolaryngol* 1928; 7:133.

27. Negus VE. The surgical treatment of chronic frontal sinusitis. 1947; *Br Med J* 1:135.

28. McNaught R. A refinement of the external frontoethmosphenoid operation: A new nasofrontal pedicle flap. *Arch Otolaryngol* 1936; 23:544–549.

29. Goodale RL. Some causes for failure in frontal sinus surgery. *Ann Otol Rhinol Laryngol* 1942; 51:648–652.

30. May M, Schaitkin B. Complications of endoscopic sinus surgery. *Oper Tech Otolaryngol Head Neck Surg* 1995.

31. Goodale R, Montgomery W. Experiences with the osteoplastic anterior wall approach to the frontal sinus. Case histories and recommendations. *Arch Otolaryngol* 1958; 68(3):271–283.

32. Hardy J, Montgomery W. Osteoplastic frontal sinusotomy: An analysis of 250 operations. *Ann Otol Rhinol Laryngol* 1976; 85(4 Pt 1):523–532.

33. Kennedy DW. Functional endoscopic sinus surgery technique. *Arch Otolaryngol* 1985; 111(10):643–649.

34. Stammberger H. Endoscopic endonasal surgery—Concepts in treatment of recurring rhinosinusitis. Part II. Surgical technique. *Otolaryngol Head Neck Surg* 1986; 94(2):147–156.

35. Wigand ME. Transnasal ethmoidectomy under endoscopical control. *Rhinology* 1981; 19(1):7–15.

36. May M. Frontal sinus surgery: Endonasal endoscopic osteoplasty rather than external osteoplasty. *Oper Tech Otolaryngol Head Neck Surg* 1991; 2:247–256.

37. Draf W. Endonasal micro-endoscopic frontal sinus surgery: The Fulda concept. *Oper Tech Otolaryngol Head Neck Surg* 1991; 2:234–240.

38. Gross W, Gross C, Becker D, Moore D, Phillips D. Modified transnasal endoscopic Lothrop procedure as an alternative to frontal sinus obliteration. *Otolaryngol Head Neck Surg* 1995; 113(4):427–434.

39. Hosemann W, Kuhnel T, Held P, Wagner W, Felderhoff A. Endonasal frontal sinusotomy in surgical management of chronic sinusitis: A critical evaluation. *Am J Rhinol* 1997; 11(1):1–9.

40. Schaeffer J. *The Nose, Paranasal Sinuses, Nasolacrimal Passage-ways, and Olfactory Organ in Man.* New York: McGraw-Hill. 1920.

41. Mosher H. The applied anatomy and intranasal surgery of the ethmoid labyrinth. *Trans Am Laryngol Assoc* 1912; 34:25–39.

42. Kainz J, Stammberger H. The roof of the ethmoid: A place of least resistance in the skull-base. *Am J Rhinol* 1989; 4:191–199.

43. Van Alyea OE. Ethmoid labyrinth: Anatomic study with consideration of the clinical significance of its structural characteristics. 1939; *Arch Otolaryngol* 29:881–902.

44. Bolger W, Butzin C, Parsons D. Paranasal sinus bony anatomic variations and mucosal abnormalities: CT analysis for endoscopic sinus surgery. *Laryngoscope* 1991; 101(1 Pt 1): 56–64.

45. Bent JP, Cuilty-Siller C, Kuhn FA. The frontal cell as a cause of frontal sinus obstruction. *Am J Rhinol* 1994; 8:185–91.

46. Lee W, Kuhn F, Citardi M. 3D computed tomographic analysis of frontal recess anatomy in patients without frontal sinusitis. *Otolaryngol Head Neck Surg* 2004;131(3):164–173.

47. Owen RG Jr, Kuhn FA. Supraorbital ethmoid cell. *Otolaryngol Head Neck Surg* 1997; 116(2):254–261.

48. Van Alyea OE. Frontal cells: An anatomic study of these cells with consideration of their clinical significance. *Arch Otol* 1941; 34:11–23.

49. Owen RG Jr, Kuhn FA. Supraorbital ethmoid cell. *Otolaryngol Head Neck Surg* 1997. 116(2):254–261.

50. Merritt R, Bent JP, Kuhn FA. The intersinus septal cell. *Am J Rhinol* 1996; 299–302.

51. Chiu A, Vaughan W. Using the frontal intersinus septal cell to widen the narrow frontal recess. *Laryngoscope* 2004; 114(7):1315–1317.

52. Stammberger H. *Functional endoscopic sinus surgery: Secretion transportation,* 1st (ed) Philadelphia: BC Decker, 1991; 30–31.

53. Messerklinger W. On the drainage of the normal frontal sinus of man. *Acta Otolaryngol* 1967; 63(2):176–181.

54. Kennedy DW, Zinreich SJ, Rosenbaum AE, Johns ME. Functional endoscopic sinus surgery. Theory and diagnostic evaluation. *Arch Otolaryngol* 1985; 111(9):576–582.

55. Batra PS, Lanza DC. *Endoscopic transseptal frontal sinusotomy: The frontal sinus,* 1st ed. Heidelberg: Springer, 2005; 251–259.

56. Olson G, Citardi MJ. Image-guided functional endoscopic sinus surgery. *Otolaryngol Head Neck Surg* 2000; 123(3):188–194.

57. Citardi MJ. Computer-aided frontal sinus surgery. *Otolaryngol Clin North Am* 2001; 34(1):111–122.

58. Wigand M, Steiner W, Jaumann M. Endonasal sinus surgery with endoscopical control: From radical operation to rehabilitation of the mucosa. *Endoscopy* 1978; 10(4):255–260.

59. Bent J 3rd, Spears R, Kuhn F, Stewart S. Combined endoscopic intranasal and external frontal sinusotomy. *Am J Rhinol* 1997; 11(5):349–354.

60. Kuhn FA, Citardi MJ. Advances in postoperative care following functional endoscopic sinus surgery. *Otolaryngol Clin North Am* 1997; 30(3):479–490.

61. Jacobs J, Lebowitz R, Lagmay V, Damiano A. Conservative approach to inflammatory nasofrontal duct disease. *Ann Otol Rhinol Laryngol* 1998; 107(8):658–661.

62. Kennedy D. Prognostic factors, outcomes and staging in ethmoid sinus surgery. *Laryngoscope* 1992; 102(12 Pt 2 Suppl 57):1–18.

63. Benoit C, Duncavage J. Combined external and endoscopic frontal sinusotomy with stent placement: A retrospective review. *Laryngoscope* 2001; 111(7):1246–1249.

64. Batra PS, Citardi MJ, Lanza DC. Combined endoscopic trephination and endoscopic frontal sinusotomy for management of complex frontal sinus pathology. *Am J Rhinol.* 2005; 15(1):48–55.

65. Citardi M, Javer A, Kuhn F. Revision endoscopic frontal sinusotomy with mucoperiosteal flap advancement: The frontal sinus rescue procedure. *Otolaryngol Clin North Am* 2001; 34(1):123–132.

66. Kuhn F, Javer A, Nagpal K, Citardi M. The frontal sinus rescue procedure: Early experience and three-year follow-up. *Am J Rhinol* 2000; 14(4):211–216.

67. Close L, Lee N, Leach J, Manning S. Endoscopic resection of the intranasal frontal sinus floor. *Ann Otol Rhinol Laryngol* 1994; 103(12):952–958.

68. Gross C, Zachmann G, Becker D, Vickery C, Moore D Jr, Lindsey W, Gross W. Follow-up of University of Virginia experience with the modified Lothrop procedure. *Am J Rhinol* 1997; 11(1):49–54.

69. Casiano R, Livingston J. Endoscopic Lothrop procedure: The University of Miami experience. *Am J Rhinol* 1998. 12(5): 335–339.

70. Lanza D, McLaughlin R Jr Hwang. The five year experience with endoscopic transseptal frontal sinusotomy. *Otolaryngol Clin North Am* 2001; 34(1):139–152.

71. Schlosser R, Zachmann G, Harrison S, Gross C. The endoscopic modified Lothrop: Long-term follow-up on 44 patients. *Am J Rhinol* 2002; 16(2):103–108.

72. Batra PS. Lanza DC. Surgical outcomes of drillout procedures for management of complicated frontal sinus pathology. Presented at the American Rhinologic Society, COSM 2005, Boca Raton Resort & Spa, Boca Raton, Florida. May 2005.

73. Scott NA, Wormald P, Close D, Gallagher R, Anthony A, Maddern GJ. Endoscopic modified Lothrop procedure for the treatment of chronic frontal sinusitis: A systematic review. *Otolaryngol Head Neck Surg* 2003; Oct. 129(4):427–438.

74. Bordley J, Bosley W. Mucoceles of the frontal sinus: Causes and treatment. *Ann Otol Rhinol Laryngol* 1973; 82(5):696–702.

75. Javer A, Sillers M, Kuhn F. The frontal sinus unobliteration procedure. *Otolaryngol Clin North Am* 2001; 34(1):193–210.

76. Montgomery WW. *Surgery of the Upper Respiratory System,* 3rd ed. Baltimore: Williams & Wilkins, 1996; 233.

77. Tato JM, Sibbald DW, Bergaglio DE. Surgical treatment of the frontal sinus by the external route. *Laryngoscope* 1954; 64:504.

78. Carrau R, Snyderman C, Curtin H, Weissman J. Computer-assisted frontal sinusotomy. *Otolaryngol Head Neck Surg* 1994; 111(6):727–732.

79. Bergara AR. Itoiz AO. Present state of the surgical treatment of chronic frontal sinusitis. *Arch Otolaryngol* 1955.;61(6):616–628.

80. Mickel T, Rohrich R, Robinson J Jr. Frontal sinus obliteration: A comparison of fat, muscle, bone, and spontaneous osteoneogenesis in the cat model. *Plast Reconstr Surg* 1995; 95(3): 586–592.

81. Janeke J. Frontal sinus obliteration with an allograft. *S Afr Med J* 1982; 61(8):272–273.

82. Owens M, Klotch D. Use of bone for obliteration of the nasofrontal duct with the osteoplastic flap: A cat model. *Laryngoscope* 1993; 103(8):883–889.

83. Rohrich R, Mickel T. Frontal sinus obliteration: In search of the ideal autogenous material. *Plast Reconstr Surg* 1995; 95(3): 580–585.

84. Anderson TD, Kennedy DW. Surgical intervention for sinusitis in adults. *Curr Allergy Asthma Rep* 2001; 1(3):282–288.

85. Weber R, Draf W, Kahle G, Kind M. Obliteration of the frontal sinus: State of the art and reflections on new materials. *Rhinology* 1999; 37(1):1–15.

Granulomatous Diseases of the Nose and Paranasal Sinuses

Steven B Cannady, Martin J Citardi, Pete S Batra

A wide spectrum of infectious, inflammatory and neoplastic diseases can produce granulomatous inflammation in the nose and paranasal sinuses. In fact, sinonasal symptoms may be the initial manifestation of a serious systemic disease process. The initial presentation of sinonasal granulomatous disease is quite variable. On occasion, these diseases may even involve adjacent vital structures, such as the brain or the orbit. In most instances, patients will initially present with non-specific sinonasal complaints. An inordinate delay in diagnosis may result in serious adverse sequelae. A high index of suspicion, coupled with a comprehensive laboratory work-up, and on occasion, biopsy for histopathologic confirmation, will help arrive at the proper diagnosis.

DEFINITION

The hallmark of the diseases discussed herein is the presence of granulomatous inflammation. In particular, the disease processes are characterized by 'a distinctive pattern of chronic inflammatory reaction characterized by focal accumulations of activated macrophages, which often develop an epithelial-like (epithelioid) appearance. Granulomas are characterized by lesions consisting of a focus of chronic inflammation that includes macrophages transformed into epithelium—like cells, with a collar of mononuclear leukocytes.'[1] Variation to the granulomatous architecture may exist depending on the inciting event.[1] A granulomatous inflammation may develop as a response to a foreign body or as an immune-mediated reaction; in both cases, an insoluble material incites the immune response seen in granulomas.

CATEGORIES

The three major categories of granulomatous disease include the inflammatory, infectious, and neoplastic

varieties.[2] This classification scheme describes granulomatous disease as it relates to its pathogenesis. The first group is inflammatory and includes diseases like Wegener's granulomatosis (WG), Churg–Strauss syndrome (CSS), sarcoidosis, and cholesterol granuloma (CG). The neoplastic group includes various T-cell lymphomas and was previously termed midline lethal granuloma. The third group of diseases is the largest and includes a wide range of infectious etiologies (Table 26.1).[2]

Table 26.1: Sinonasal granulomatous diseases (Adapted from Lund[2])

Inflammatory		
Rheumatologic		Wegener's granulomatosis
		Churg–Strauss syndrome
		Sarcoidosis
Other		Cholesterol granuloma
Neoplastic		
Lymphomas		T-cell lymphoma
		B-cell lymphoma
Infectious		
Bacterial	Tuberculosis	*Mycobacterium tuberculosis*
	Leprosy	*Mycobacterium leprae*
	Rhinoscleroma	*Klebsiella rhinoscleromatis*
	Syphilis	*Treponema pallidum*
	Actinomycosis	*Actinomyces israeli*
Fungal	Aspergillus	*Aspergillus fumigatus, flavus, niger*
	Zygomycosis	*Conidibolus coronatus, Rhizopus oryzae*
	Rhinosporidiosis	*Rhinosporidiosis seeberi*
	Blastomycosis	*Blastomyces dermatitidis*
	Histoplasmosis	*Histoplasma capsulatum*
	Sporotrichosis	*Sporotrichum schenkii*
	Coccidiomycosis	*Coccidiodes imitis*
Protozoa	Leishmaniasis	*Leishmania spp.*

INFLAMMATORY DISEASES

Wegener's Granulomatosis

Although Friedrich Wegener was credited with discovering the disease that bears his name in 1936,[3] the first case was reported by Klinger as a variant of polyarteritis nodosa in 1931.[4] The actual prevalence of WG remains elusive, as the data reported is dependent on the inclusion criteria, the population surveyed, and the method of diagnosis. Further confounding the diagnosis is the occurrence of a systemic form and the more limited form of WG first recognized by Carrington in 1966.[5] Diagnosis of WG has been made more readily with the addition of the antineutrophil cytoplasmic antibody test (ANCA) in 1985.[6]

Definition

The definition of WG was refined by the international consensus committee convened in Chapel Hill, NC in 1994.[7] This consensus defined WG as a 'granulomatous inflammation involving the respiratory tract, and necrotizing vasculitis affecting small- to medium-sized vessels (e.g. capillaries, venules, and arteries) with necrotizing glomerulonephritis commonly.'[8] Diagnosis is based on both clinical and laboratory data as outlined by the American College of Rheumatology.[8] Four selected criteria are described in the 1990 WG definition update: Abnormal urinary sediment, abnormal chest radiograph, oral or nasal pathology, and granulomatous inflammation on biopsy. The presence of two findings confirms WG with 88.2% sensitivity and 92% specificity.[8]

Laboratory data, including cytoplasmic antineutrophil cytoplasmic antibodies (cANCA) and erythrocyte sediment rate (ESR) have been used to aid clinicians in the diagnosis of WG. Overall, the use of combined ANCA testing in the diagnosis of vasculitis demonstrated 82% sensitivity and 99% specificity for the use of both cANCA and perinuclear antineutrophil cytoplasmic antibodies (pANCA) testing.[9]

Both cANCA and pANCA are autoantibodies directed against neutrophil granules or monocyte lysozymes in patients with primary vasculitides. The former has been associated with the antigen proteinase-3 (PR3) within the secretory vesicles and azurophil granules of neutrophil cytoplasm in WG. The latter has been linked to the antigen myeloperoxidase (MPO) within the azurophil granules. Testing for both now frequently involves immunofluorescent staining against cANCA and pANCA as well as molecular testing for PR3 and MPO.[13]

Epidemiology

The best estimate for the prevalence of WG is at least 3 per 100,000 in the US population.[10] Men and women contract the disease in equal numbers and the mean age at time of diagnosis is 40–55 years, although the disease can occasionally be diagnosed in children or older patients.[10] The majority of those afflicted with this disease are Caucasians (30–97%), followed by African-Americans (2–8%).[10]

Prognosis

The disease and its treatment are associated with a significant degree of morbidity. In patients diagnosed with WG early in their working years (< 40 years), 27% are on full disability three years after diagnosis. In addition, half of the patients in this study were hospitalized at least once in the previous 12 months, and most patients reported the need for frequent physician office visits necessitating over 14 days off work in the same time period.[11]

Etiology

A complete review of all current hypotheses of WG etiology is beyond the scope of this chapter. The most important of these are highlighted below.

First among these, 'superantigens' derived from microbes have been associated with WG. Superantigens are known to activate T-cell populations that express B-chain variable segments of the T-cell receptor. They can directly stimulate the B-cells to produce autoantibody (i.e. c-ANCA) in a T-cell dependent, or independent fashion.[13] In fact, 60-70% of patients with WG have been shown to be chronic nasal carriers of *Staphylococcus aureus*, and this carrier-state is associated with an eight-fold increased rate of recurrence.[12,13] This led to attempts to treat WG with anti-staphylococcal based antibiotics, such as trimethoprim/sulfamethoxazole. This strategy was met with some success in preventing relapses of WG (82% relapse free versus 60% in placebo).[14] Though successful in the upper airway, this does not carry over to prevention of relapses in other organ system.

Circulating autoantibodies probably play an important role in the pathogenesis of WG. These antibodies are directed towards neutrophil granules and monocyte lysosomes.[13] The two main ANCA antigens are PR3 and MPO; there is a strong association of WG with PR3-ANCA (c-ANCA). ANCA levels have even been shown to correlate with disease activity scores.[15] However, the mechanisms of ANCA production and the inciting events are not fully understood. It is postulated that ANCA may prevent programmed neutrophil death, a normal mechanism of controlling inflammation via a complex interaction of antibody with natural inactivators of PR3 or other ANCA antigens.[13] Irrespective of the exact method of interaction, rising c-ANCA titer may indicate pending relapse.[16]

General Clinical Evaluation

The American College of Rheumatology criteria for diagnosis of WG remain the gold standard.[8] Laboratory work-up including urinalysis (casts and red cells), complete blood count (CBC), complete metabolic panel (CMP), and serum markers of WG, including ESR, c-ANCA, and p-ANCA are effective as initial screening tests in detecting kidney disease. The rheumatologic tests for c-ANCA and p-ANCA can be useful to help bolster the diagnosis of WG and determine disease activity.[15] The c-ANCA is positive in patients with active and localized disease in 95 and 60%, respectively.[16]

Radiologic evaluation includes an initial chest X-ray to assess for the presence of cavitation or fibrosis of the lungs. Further imaging is directed based upon the disease course and can include CT of the paranasal sinuses, brain/head, orbits, abdomen (kidney), and chest (lung) and/or MRI of the same structures.

Tissue biopsy can be useful, but often pathology offers only nonspecific findings. A recent review of 51 biopsy specimens revealed 'typical' diagnostic specimens in only 24% of single biopsies. Furthermore, among patients with multiple biopsies, typical findings resulting in diagnosis was achieved in only 42% of cases.[17] The

histologic features of pyogenic granulation tissue (a polypoid form of capillary hemangioma[1]), granulomas of epithelioid-cell type, and vasculitis confirm WG on biopsy from any involved site (Figs 26.1A and B).[2]

Systemic Manifestations

The triad of upper airway, lung, and kidney involvement is classic pattern of WG. The brain, eyes, skin, and central nervous system (CNS) may also be affected. On the other hand, in limited WG one organ system is affected and other sites are spared typical involvement.

WG of the lung is present in as many as 94% of patients with systemic disease and can manifest as alveolar, bronchial, or pleural tissue damage.[18] Frequent symptoms include wheezing, dyspnea and hemoptysis. Necrotizing glomerulonephritis, the most serious kidney complication of WG, is the hallmark of renal involvement. Estimates of renal involvement range from 10 to 85%, depending on the level of disease activity and the duration of the disease process.

It is important to highlight the concept of limited WG, which is defined as disease that 'includes manifestations of WG that pose no immediate threat to either the patient's life or the function of a vital organ.[11,19] In a report of the Wegener's Granulomatosis Etanercept Trial (WGET) Research Group in 2003, 52 patients with limited WG were reviewed.[20] Specific inclusion criteria were patients with diagnosis of WG based on the American College of Rheumatology criteria and the absence of several key exclusionary criteria:

1. The patient must not have red blood cell casts in the urine.

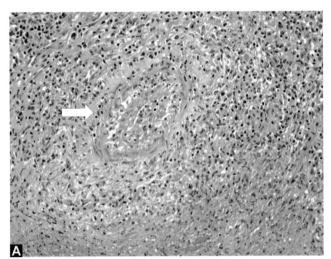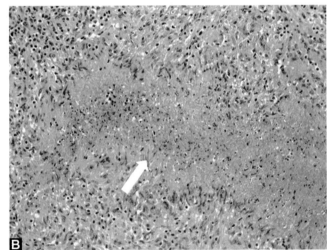

Figs 26.1A and B: Representative histology from a sinonasal mucosal biopsy of WG. Dense inflammatory infiltrate in tissues and vasculitis (black arrow) Granuloma formation with central necrosis (white arrow) (*Courtesy*: Dr Richard Prayson, Department of Anatomic Pathology, The Cleveland Clinic Foundation)

2. If hematuria is present the creatinine must be ≤ 1.4 mg/dl, with no evidence of rise in creatinine > 25% above baseline.
3. Limited pulmonary involvement so that room air PO_2 is > 70 mm Hg or room air O_2 saturation > 92% by pulse oximetry.
4. No disease within any other critical organ that if not treated immediately with maximal therapy threatens the function of that organ or the patient's life.[20]

Patients with limited disease generally presented at an earlier age (10 years younger on average at diagnosis), tended to have longer disease duration, greater frequency of exacerbation, and higher rate of destructive upper airway disease at presentation. They were less likely to have c-ANCA or p-ANCA positivity at diagnosis. A significantly greater incidence of bloody nasal discharge/nasal crusting/ulcer (67.3% versus 56.3%), and sinus involvement (59.6% versus 41.4%) led to an overall greater incidence of ear, nose, and throat manifestations in the limited WG versus severe group.[20]

Head and Neck Manifestations

Head and neck manifestations of WG are exhibited in 72–99% of patients at some point in their disease course.[21,22] The importance of the head and neck sites is highlighted by their integral role in the modified Birmingham Vasculitis Activity Score (BVAS) Survey that includes sections detailing 'mucous membrane, and ear, nose, and throat manifestations.'[21] Rasmussen reviewed the results with the BVAS and frequency of symptoms in the first 124 WG patients enrolled in the European Vasculitis Study Group (EUVAS) (Table 26.2).[23] The most commonly occurring head and neck manifestations of WG rhinologic, otologic, oral, orbital, and laryngeal. Salivary gland and cutaneous manifestations are less frequent.[24]

Table 26.2: BVAS head and neck symptom categories and frequency of occurrence in the first 124 patients enrolled by the EUVAS with WG[27]	
BVAS for WG	*Frequency of involvement in EUVAS*
Bloody nasal discharge	50%
Nasal crusting	56%
Paranasal sinus involvement	33%
Salivary gland enlargement	Not specified
Subglottic inflammation	19%
Conductive hearing loss	30%
Sensorineural hearing loss	Not specified

Otologic manifestations of WG occur in 19–38% of cases.[25] These can be limited to the external, middle, or inner ear, but most commonly involve the middle ear[26] usually, with chronic serous otitis media secondary to eustachian tube dysfunction, granulation tissue resulting in chronic suppurative otitis media, or scarring in the middle ear. Chronic infection can be associated with intracranial complications and conductive hearing loss.[24]

Oral manifestations of WG are multiple, and rarely encountered, with ulceration being the most common. The occurrence of strawberry gingival hyperplasia is considered by some authors to be pathognomonic for WG.[27]

The most ominous manifestation of WG in the larynx is that of subglottic stenosis (SGS). SGS due to WG occurs more frequently in patients diagnosed at a younger age and those with the systemic form.[28] Studies suggest that 40–50% of patients presenting with SGS in WG will ultimately require tracheotomy.[28,29] In contrast, dilation coupled with injection of long-acting glucocorticoids into the stenotic segment of the subglottis can produce significantly improved results.[30,31]

Nasal and Sinus Manifestations

Sinonasal sites are the most frequently affected in the head and neck region, afflicting up to 85% of patients.[24,28] Patients may suffer from foul smelling rhinorrhea secondary to chronic *S. aureus* colonization, epistaxis, nasal crusting, and smell disturbances.[26] Long-term sequelae include septal perforation, saddle-nose deformity, chronic rhinosinusitis (CRS), and mucocele formation from scarring and outflow obstruction, most commonly in the frontal and sphenoid sinuses.[24] As one may expect, frontal and sphenoid mucoceles are more common than maxillary and ethmoid mucoceles. In general, sinonasal manifestations can be separated into active vasculitis symptoms and chronic sequelae of inflammation.

Clinical Evaluation of Sinonasal WG

Office evaluation by an otolaryngologist has become part of the standard comprehensive assessment of WG patients. Since some WG patients may have limited upper airway disease, otolaryngologists may facilitate the initial diagnosis. Routine office evaluation for sinonasal involvement encompasses both a thorough clinical history (including standardized survey instruments) and physical examination. Nasal endoscopy may be used to evaluate the integrity of the sinonasal mucosa and assess

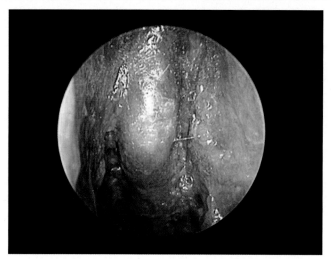

Fig. 26.2: Endoscopic view of left nasal cavity in Wegener's granulomatosis. Note evidence of scarring between the middle turbinate and the septum and the lateral nasal wall. Diffuse crusting is present

for potential sequelae of WG. The acute and chronic manifestations of WG can be readily seen on endoscopy. Areas of vasculitis with crusting and scarring are often noted (Fig. 26.2). Flexible fiberoptic laryngoscopy is essential in the evaluation of laryngotracheal manifestations of WG.

Endoscopic cultures can be useful in the treatment of CRS by helping guide antibiotic therapy, especially in the scenario of an acute bacterial exacerbation of the baseline CRS of WG. Given the potential role of *S. aureus* in the disease process, its presence on cultures may also have prognostic significance.[12,13]

Imaging modalities are often used in the evaluation of sinonasal disease. Benoudiba et al recently reviewed the CT characteristics of nine patients in an attempt to describe 'typical' CT findings in WG. They noted four specific CT findings that should warrant further investigation with c-ANCA testing: Nodular appearing mucosa, punctate bony destruction of the septum and 'internasosinusal wall' sparing the ethmoid labyrinth, periantral soft tissue infiltration in association with bone demineralization or orbital extension, and midline bone destruction.[32] Lloyd et al reviewed their experience with 28 patients from 1990 to 2001. They demonstrated that 85.7% of patients exhibited mucosal thickening, 75% bony destruction, 50% new bone formation, and 30% orbital involvement on imaging. They concluded that in an undiagnosed patient without history of sinus surgery, the combination of bony destruction and bone formation when accompanied by MR finding of fat signaling in sclerotic bone was virtually diagnostic for WG.[33]

Sinonasal biopsy is frequently requested for by other physicians when the diagnosis of WG cannot be confirmed but the clinical suspicion of WG is high. Maguchi et al reviewed 51 biopsy specimens from c-ANCA seropositive WG patients. Twenty-nine of these biopsies were from the nose or paranasal sinuses. Despite relatively low distribution of 'typical' findings of WG, paranasal sinus and nasal sites resulted in a slightly increased rate of diagnosis (50% and 25% respectively, compared with 24% overall).[17] In a histopathologic study specific to the head and neck, Devaney et al found that the three hallmark findings of WG were present in just 16% of all biopsy specimens.[34] This stresses the importance of other diagnostic testing to aid in the overall workup of WG.

Acute Vasculitic Sinonasal WG

Symptoms and Management

The acute vasculitic symptoms of WG can be attributed to the result of granulomatous inflammation and vasculitis in the upper airway. Nasal obstruction, epistaxis, crusting, and CRS are directly attributable to inflammation of the sinonasal lining. In actuality, all of the 'acute vasculitic' symptoms can also be encountered in the chronic stage, even when the disease is not active. Chronic crusting and epistaxis is caused by both chronic inflammation and dryness, and on occasion by granuloma formation. CRS may result from functional occlusion of the sinus ostia by mucosal inflammation and scarring in WG patients. Taken together, these symptoms lead to acute and chronically inflamed mucosa with subsequent scarring that results in non-functional sinonasal lining.

Treatment of acute vasculitic sinonasal disease requires the combination of systemic and local treatments (Table 26.3). The management strategy is based on careful consideration of multiple factors including the age, length of diagnosis, limited versus systemic disease, and clinical manifestations of each individual patient. The mainstay of systemic treatment involves the use of corticosteroids and immunosuppressive agents. Corticosteroids are given in an initial pulsed regimen either intravenously or orally dependent on disease severity for the first several months, followed by a tapering regimen (Table 26.4). Systemic steroids are also prescribed for maintenance therapy intended to prevent relapses and to treat symptom exacerbations.

The cytotoxic medications frequently employed in addition to steroids include cyclophosphamide,

Table 26.3: Summary of systemic and local sinonasal treatments for acute vasculitic disease

Type of treatment	Symptom	Treatment
Systemic		*Corticosteroids*
		Immunosuppressives: Cyclophosphamide, methotrexate, azathioprine, cyclosporin, chlorambucil, others
		Antibiotics: sulfamethoxazole/trimethoprim
Local sinonasal	Nasal obstruction	Nasal steroids
	Nasal crusting	Sinonasal irrigations
	Epistaxis	Irrigations, nasal cream
	Chronic rhinosinusitis	Culture-specific antibiotics, plus above
	Acute rhinosinusitis	
	S. aureus colonization	Sulfamethoxazole/trimethoprim, mupirocin irrigations

Table 26.4: Selected induction and maintenance doses for Wegener's granulomatosis

Medication	Induction dose	Maintenance
Corticosteroids	1. Methylprednisolone 500–1000 mg IV qd for 3 days 2. Prednisone 1 mg/kg/d for first few months	1. Prednisone – tapered and adjusted for symptom control
Immunosuppressives	1. Cyclophosphamide (CTX) 500–750 mg/m^2/month IV for 6–12 months, then every other month for 6–12 months 2. Methotrexate 20–25 mg/week	1. CTX 2 mg/kg/day 2. Methotrexate 20–25 mg/week 3. Azathioprine 2–2.5 mg/kg/day 4. Trimethoprim/sulfamethoxazole

methotrexate (MTX), and azathioprine. The induction phase of treatment can involve the use of cyclophosphamide for the first 6 to 12 months every month, followed by every other month for an additional 6 to 12 months.[24] MTX has been used in patients with limited disease for induction.[35] MTX and azathioprine can also be used for maintenance therapy, and trimethoprim/sulfamethoxazole can decrease incidence of upper airway exacerbations.[24]

Investigational treatment modalities include selective immunomodulatory agents such as Etanercept, an antibody to tumor necrosis factor-alpha. However, the WGET Research Group demonstrated that it was not an effective medication for maintenance of remission and, thus, does not recommend its use currently.[36]

Before the 1970s, more than 82% of patients with active WG died within one year. These outcomes have been greatly impacted by the recognition that the disease is at least in part immunogenic. Thus, long-term survival has been achieved with various regimens of immunosuppression with use of these agents.[37]

Medical treatment of sinonasal disease requires a regimen of systemic medications and topical irrigations. Topical nasal steroids may help with nasal obstruction and assist in controlling chronic inflammation. Topical saline irrigations and alkaline douches are important in helping optimize nasal health. Antibiotic irrigations, containing mupirocin ointment and saline, can assist in minimizing crusting and improve the moisture of the nasal lining. This will also help decrease the frequency of epistaxis and may also potentially reduce *S. aureus* colonization. Infectious exacerbations are managed with culture-specific antibiotics. Many WG patients benefit from the use of trimethoprim/sulfamethoxazole. This has been effective in decreasing frequency of sinonasal relapse, as well as in prevention of *Pneumocystis carinii* pneumonia, a potentially fatal complication of cytotoxic and glucocorticoid immunosuppression.[14]

Long-term Sequelae and their Treatment

Long-term sinonasal sequelae of WG include nasal septal erosion, saddle-nose deformity, facial/nasal pain, smell disturbances, nasolacrimal duct obstruction, and orbital complications such as orbital apex syndrome. In addition, all of the acute vasculitic symptoms can become chronic as the mucosa progressively scars and loses function.

Nasal septal erosion and saddle-nose deformity are a consequence of the progressive vasculitis of Kiesselbach's plexus causing necrosis and loss of the cartilaginous support of the nose. Given the adverse aesthetic consequences of this complication, patients may seek advice regarding repair. WG provides poorly vascularized tissue and inadequate bony and cartilaginous structures to support the repair. Most attempts at repair during the active phase of the disease process are fraught with failure. Disease remission is a requisite prior to any attempt at repair.[38] Congdon et al reported on a series of 13 patients undergoing augmentation rhinoplasty with 92% satisfaction rate. Nasal reconstruction with calvarial bone via an extranasal approach that spares violations of the nasal mucosal lining may provide an optimal technique for correction of saddle nose deformity due to WG.

Epiphora may result from progressive nasolacrimal duct obstruction. Aggressive treatment of sinonasal disease may be sufficient, although dacrocystorhino-stomy (DCR) may also be required for definitive relief. Open DCR has been found to produce symptomatic relief without negative effects in 13/14 surgeries on 11 patients as reported by Kwan and Rose in 2000.[39] Alternatively, endoscopic DCR can also produce acceptable results.[40] Procedures should be preferably performed in the periods of remission to increase the success rate of the procedure and to decrease the need for postoperative immuno-suppression.

Granulomatous orbital masses can occasionally present to the otolaryngologist. The symptoms are generally dependent upon the location of granuloma. Limited inflammatory masses can result in subtle proptosis, pain, or ocular muscle paresis. On the other hand, lesions in the orbital apex can be vision-threatening (Fig. 26.3). Surgical intervention to decompress the orbit, in conjunction with aggressive anti-inflammatory medical therapy, is crucial in this setting to preserve vision.

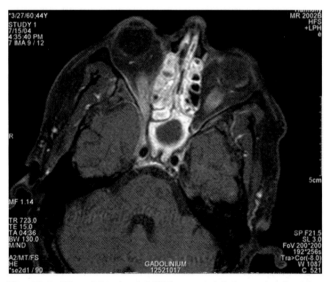

Fig. 26.3: T1-weighted axial MRI postgadolinium administration demonstrating high signal intensity in the right orbital apex with adjacent sphenoid mucocele formation

CRS in the setting of WG refractory to medical management may require surgical intervention. Given the risk of subsequent scarring in the nose and paranasal sinuses, all conservative efforts should be exhausted prior to proceeding with surgery. Functional endoscopic sinus surgery (FESS) principles should be maintained including mucosal sparing techniques and preservation of retained structures. Meticulous postoperative care with at least weekly postoperative debridement, irrigations, and culture-directed antibiotics are essential. In cases of limited sinus disease, or mucocele formation, only the site of pathology should be addressed to prevent scarring in other areas.

Sarcoidosis

Sarcoidosis is a systemic granulomatous disease afflicting primarily young to middle-aged adults. Major organ systems affected include the lungs, liver, spleen, muscles, bones, kidneys and central nervous system.[41] However, the disease can also have noticeable involvement of head and neck sites at any stage of the disease course.[42] Commonly affected sites include the salivary glands, larynx, nose and sinuses, orbit, ear, and the lymph nodes. Since sarcoidosis may initially present with head and neck complaints, the otolaryngologist must be prepared to facilitate the diagnosis both clinically and by histologic tissue confirmation.

Epidemiology

Sarcoidosis most frequently affects adults in the age range between 20 and 40, with a predominance among women. Approximately, 6 per 100,000 people are affected in the US, with a higher prevalence among African, Americans and Hispanics.[41] Overall, people of Scandinavian or Northern European descent are most at risk for develop-ment of the disease. Most fatalities associated with sarcoidosis are related to progressive pulmonary disease that results in death in 1–5% of patients.[41]

Etiology

The classic histopathologic finding on biopsy is non-caseating epithelioid granuloma but definitive diagnosis requires further exclusion of diseases that demonstrate similar pathologic findings.[41] A definitive etiology has not been identified in sarcoidosis, however several clues to its origin have been identified. Clusters of patients living close proximity have been identified in the United Kingdom, Sweden, Greece, Spain, and Japan.[43-45] Other studies have suggested that patients sharing common environments, such as aircraft servicemen or fire fighters, are more likely to be affected by the disease.[46,47] These studies have suggested that a causative agent may be contracted by susceptible individuals. Multiple studies have led to the identification of two potentially inciting agents: mycobacteria and propionibacterium. Although no definitive evidence exists to implicate these bacteria, several studies have demonstrated their presence in patients with sarcoidosis.[48,49]

Furthermore, some studies have shown a genetic predisposition to development of sarcoidosis. Several specific gene alleles have been identified as conferring susceptibility to disease presentation: HLA DR 11, 12, 14, and 17.[50] Regardless of the cause, sarcoidosis is a multifactorial disease process that presents in genetically predisposed individuals exposed to an unidentified trigger leading to over-exuberant inflammatory response and multisystem granuloma formation.

General Clinical Evaluation

The clinical presentation of sarcoidosis is quite variable and may mimic other clinical entities. The intent of the clinical evaluation of a patient with suspected sarcoidosis is to exclude other conditions that may present with granulomatous inflammation. Exclusion of tuberculosis, fungal infection, malignancy, vasculitis, or other granulomatous diseases is essential and has been included in a recent expert panel's approach to the diagnosis of sarcoidosis.[51]

The Joint Statement of the American Thoracic Society, the European Respiratory Society, and the World Association of Sarcoidosis and other Granulomatous Disorders recommended initial evaluation guidelines in 1999. These included a thorough history and physical examination, chest X-ray, pulmonary function tests, peripheral blood counts, serum chemistries, urinalysis, ophthalmologic exam and tuberculin skin test.[51] Other studies that may help arrive at the diagnosis include ACE level, protein electrophoresis, and electrocardiogram.

Biopsy demonstrating granulomatous features can help facilitate diagnosis. However, biopsy can be often unfruitful with random lip biopsy giving 40–50% yield rate in patients with mediastinal adenopathy. Salivary gland biopsy is diagnostic 58% of the time, while conjunctival biopsy yields positive results in just 38% of specimens from patients with proven sarcoidosis.[42]

Classic clinical features including bilateral hilar adenopathy on chest X-ray, erythema nodosa, uveitis, or maculopapular skin lesions in conjunction with biopsy evidence of granuloma formation can be sufficient for diagnosis.[62] Even in the face of a negative biopsy, other findings suggestive of sarcoidosis include elevated ACE level, bronchoalveolar lavage lymphocytosis, panda sign on gallium scan (scan activity in the lacrimal or salivary glands when they are involved), or lupus pernio (purple plaques on the nose, cheeks, and ear lobes).

Radiologic work-up for sarcoidosis involves CT and/or MR imaging of involved sites to assist in the assessment of pulmonary and extrapulmonary sites. Positron emission tomography (PET) scanning can also show disease activity on whole-body scanning.

Systemic Manifestations

Up to 50% of patients diagnosed with sarcoidosis will be asymptomatic and are diagnosed via routine chest X-ray.[41] Other patients will present with constitutional symptoms such as fever, chronic fatigue, weight loss, or fatigue. The lungs are involved in 90% of patients with sarcoidosis.[41] The typical pulmonary pattern is interstitial disease, and symptoms may include cough, dyspnea, and chest pain. A variable pattern ranging from progressive loss of function to no progression of disease exists. Remission can ensue in 5–90% of patients depending upon the clinical stage of disease.[51]

Other organ system may be involved in sarcoidosis. The sites in order of frequency include mediastinal lymph nodes (95–98%), liver (50–80%), spleen (40–80%), eyes (20–50%), musculoskeletal (25–39%), peripheral lymph nodes (30%), hematologic (4–40%), skin (25%), neurologic (10%), cardiac (5%), endocrine with hypercalcemia (2–10%), parotid glands (< 6%), gastrointestinal (< 1%), and kidneys (rare).[51]

Treatment

Treatment of sarcoidosis may in fact involve expectant management for the asymptomatic patient. For patients with chronic disease (not resolving after 2–5 years), long-term therapy may be necessary.[52] Active sarcoidosis of the heart, lungs, and central nervous system, as well as hypercalcemia due to sarcoidosis, are specific indications for active treatment. Other systemic constitutional symptoms that disturb daily function may also be considered relative indications for treatment.

The mainstay of treatment for sarcoidosis remains corticosteroids. The regimen may include prednisone 20–40 mg daily initially followed by 5–10 mg QOD maintenance dose to achieve remission. The exact duration of the steroid treatment depends on the clinical response and disease activity. Long-term complications of systemic steroids must always be factored into the decision-making process. Non-steroidal regimens include antimalarial (chloroquine or hydroxychloroquine) and cytotoxic agents (MTX, azathioprine, cyclophosphamide, cyclosporine, and infliximab).

Head and Neck Manifestations

In a large series reported by the Mayo Clinic in 1982, 9% of patients with sarcoidosis manifested head and neck involvement.[53] As reviewed by Lund, involvement of other otolaryngologic related organ systems in those patients with nasal sarcoidosis include lung (66%), skin (56%), peripheral lymph node (30%), lupus pernio (26%), eye (22%), larynx (19%), lacrimal gland (15%), conjunctiva (11%), and uveitis (11%).[2]

Nasal and Sinus Manifestations

Sinonasal involvement in sarcoidosis is infrequent. Most large studies report the incidence of upper airway involvement to be in the range of 1–5%.[2] The largest series published by McCaffrey and McDonald in 1983, suggested a rate of less than 1% (23 patients identified out of 2319 reviewed).[54] However, this study was retrospective and may have failed to detect such frequently occurring symptoms as stuffiness and obstruction (88%), crusting (63%), bloody discharge (37%), purulent sinusitis (30%), facial pain (22%), mucus discharge (15%) or anosmia (4%) if not specifically posed to patients.[2] A recent prospective study of 159 consecutive patients identified sinonasal disease in over 60% of patients with careful history.[55] When upper airway disease is identified, the nose and paranasal sinuses are frequently involved. In fact, the rate of involvement of the nose approaches 100% in those afflicted with upper airway disease.[54,56]

Although the presentation of sinonasal sarcoidosis is variable, the 'most common presentation [is] a chronic, often crusty, rarely destructive inflammatory rhinosinusitis with nodules on the septum and/or turbinates.'[57] Extensive disease can involve adjacent structures, including the brain, orbit and adjacent cranial nerves.

Clinical Evaluation

Specific work-up should include a thorough history and physical examination with attention directed towards frequent sites of head or neck involvement. Nasal endoscopy frequently demonstrates dry and crusty

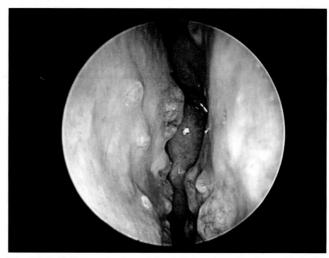

Fig. 26.4: Endoscopic view of the left nasal cavity of a patient with sinonasal sarcoidosis. Note the pale to yellow submucosal deposits present on the nasal mucosa

mucosa with pale, yellowish submucosal nodules (Fig. 26.4). DeShazo et al have suggested that the diagnosis of nasal sarcoidosis be considered when histopathology confirms noncaseating granuloma with negative stains for acid-fast bacilli, serologic tests are negative for WG or syphilis, and no other disease process associated with nasal and sinus granulomas is present (Fig. 26.5).[58]

CT imaging may reveal mucoperiosteal thickening with occasional granulomatous masses. Rarely, extensive bony remodeling with new-bone formation may be noted (Fig. 26.6).[58] Occasional orbital involvement is identified

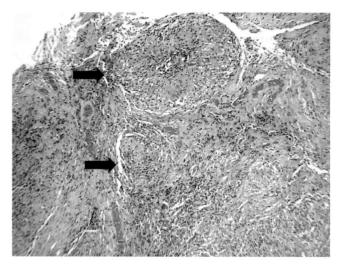

Fig. 26.5: Representative histology from sinonasal biopsy in sarcoidosis. Note evidence of non-caseating granuloma formation (black arrows) and marked inflammation (*Courtesy:* Dr Richard Prayson, Department of Anatomic Pathology, The Cleveland Clinic Foundation)

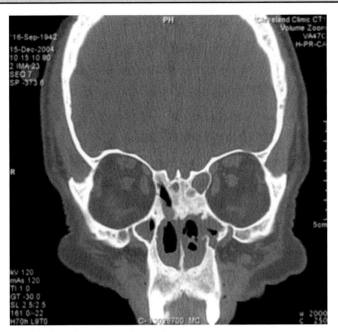

Fig. 26.6: Coronal CT scan of a patient with sinonasal sarcoidosis. Note extensive bony remodeling and mucoperiosteal thickening in the ethmoid and maxillary sinuses

and may include orbital mass formation with exophthalmus, thickening of the extraocular muscles, or cuffing of the globe.[59]

Management

In confirmed cases of sinonasal sarcoidosis, a logical approach that addresses the primary symptoms should ensue. Systemic treatment with corticosteroids or immunosuppressants yields poor long-term satisfaction with respect to nasal complaints.[57] Therefore, the emphasis should be on control of sinonasal symptoms with local therapy. As in WG, antibiotic nasal irrigations and topical nasal steroids are frequently used for general maintenance and reducing inflammation within the nose.

Other medical treatment has included local nasal corticosteroid injection. Krespi reported good results with this modality in selected patients with sinonasal sarcoidosis. However, other studies have reported less success with injected steroids.[57]

Although surgery should be avoided, surgical treatment may sometimes be necessary in patients with recalcitrant symptoms despite local and systemic medical treatments. Sinonasal obstruction by sarcoid deposits, mucocele formation, or extension into contiguous structures such as the eye are indications for surgery. A relative indication is refractory rhinosinusitis. Two series recently reported success with FESS for sinonasal

sarcoidosis. Marks and Goodman performed nasal surgery on six patients; short-term symptom improvement was noted in all patients, though recurrence of symptoms ensued in most patients on long-term follow-up.[60] Kay and Har-El reported success with FESS in symptom relief where specific obstructive pathology was identified preoperatively. They considered ESS to be a viable option in these specific patients to relieve anatomic blockage.[61] As with WG, meticulous postoperative care is essential to the healing process.

Churg-Strauss Syndrome

Definition

Churg-Strauss syndrome (CSS) has been defined by the Chapel Hill Consensus Committee (CHCC) as an 'eosinophil-rich and granulomatous inflammation involving the respiratory tract, necrotizing vasculitis affecting small to medium sized vessels, associated with asthma.'[7] According to the American College of Rheumatology, the diagnosis of CSS rests upon meeting four of five specific criteria: Eosinophilia (>10% on CBC); mononeuropathy or polyneuropathy; pulmonary infiltrates (non-fixed, i.e. migratory or transitory); paranasal sinus abnormalities (pain, tenderness, or radiographic opacification); and extravascular eosinophils (biopsy including artery, arteriole or venule showing accumulation of extravascular eosinophils).[62]

Head and Neck Manifestations

The percentage of patients exhibiting ear, nose, or throat manifestations can be 44% at presentation and 55% throughout the disease course.[62] Sinonasal symptoms include polyps, crusting, rhinitis, epistaxis, and septal perforation. The disease can mimic WG symptoms, but can usually be differentiated by other systemic manifestations such as asthma. CSS rarely exhibits the severity of symptoms associated with WG or midline bony destruction classic to WG.[63]

General Clinical Evaluation

Clinical evaluation for CSS is similar to WG and consists of laboratory testing including c-ANCA and p-ANCA, ESR, C-reactive protein (CRP), CBC, CMP, and urinalysis. ANCA testing allows for the exclusion of other vasculitides, such as WG. Diagnosis is also in part based on history (neuropathy, sinusitis), radiographic findings (pulmonary infiltrate on chest X-ray), and biopsy data.[64] Histology demonstrates necrotizing giant-cell vasculitis, interstitial granulomas, and eosinophilic inflammation.[2]

Sinonasal CSS Evaluation

Sinonasal evaluation should consist of endoscopy and CT of the sinuses in CSS patients. Endoscopy generally shows less severe findings than WG, but still demonstrates mucosal hypertrophy, crusting, and possibly chronic rhinosinusitis. Sinonasal CT often demonstrates mucosal thickening and radiographic evidence of rhinosinusitis.

Treatment

The systemic treatment for CSS generally involves use of oral steroids. Local sinonasal treatment consists of optimizing nasal hygiene with saline irrigations, nasal steroids for mucosal hypertrophy, and selective management of chronic sequelae as with WG. When present, sinonasal polyposis can be surgically treated using the mucosal sparing techniques of FESS. The 5 years survival of CSS was reported to be 68.1% in one recent series.[62]

Cholesterol Granuloma

This is characterized by the presence of granulation tissue, hemosiderin, histiocytes, and fusiform clefts (sites where cholesterol was present prior to processing), all of which may be present extracellularly, or within multinucleated giant cells.[65] It is theorized that the combination of hemorrhage and impaired ventilation and drainage of a mucosa-lined space of the paranasal sinuses or middle ear and mastoid leads to granuloma formation.[51] Most frequently associated with chronic ear disease, CG has been reported rarely to involve the maxillary and frontal sinus.[65,66] The expansile growth and subsequent impingement of adjacent structures by the CG can result in headache, diplopia, visual changes, ptosis, proptosis, and nasal obstruction. The differential diagnosis for CG includes other expansile, benign lesions of the sinuses (such as dermoid cyst, epidermoid cyst, bone cyst, ossifying fibroma, polyposis, or less frequently, metastases). The CT scan reveals a circumscribed homogenous mass with expansion rather than invasive characteristics. MRI is characterized by high-signal intensity on all imaging protocols.[2,65,66]

Treatment involves complete surgical resection of the granuloma to prevent recurrence when possible but marsupialization may be sufficient. Endoscopic techniques are frequently effective in successful management of the lesions. Rarely, accessory open approaches such as the Caldwell-Luc or the osteoplastic flap may be necessary to achieve successful removal of the granuloma in the maxillary and frontal sinuses, respectively.[51,52]

NEOPLASTIC DISEASES

Sinonasal T-cell Lymphoma (Midline Lethal Granuloma)

History and Definition

First described by McBride in 1897, this clinical entity has recently been more clearly defined clinico-pathologically to include T-cell and B-cell non-Hodgkin's lymphomas.[67] Nomenclature has been confusing in the past as the clinical entity is known by many other names: Stewart syndrome, lethal midline granuloma, idiopathic midline granuloma, non-healing midline granuloma, malignant midline granuloma, and idiopathic midline destructive disease.[68] In the 1970s and 80s, as specific disease processes such as WG, polymorphic reticulosis (lymphomatoid granulomatosis), and extranodal non-Hodgkin's lymphoma became recognized, this lead to the use of the term 'midline destructive granuloma'.[68,69]

Polymorphic reticulosis was defined by Eichel as a process that lies pathologically between atypical lymphoid proliferation and frank malignant lymphoma.[70] On the other hand, the rapidly progressive granuloma initially reported by McBride, is probably caused by T-cell lymphoma with extensive angiolymphatic invasion and destruction.[67,68,71]

Epidemiology

Extranodal lymphoma represents less than 0.05% of lymphoma cases in the USA. However, there is a significantly higher degree of involvement in parts of Asia. In China, it is the second most common extranodal non-Hodgkin's lymphoma.[72-74] Average age at onset is 45 years worldwide, and a slight male predominance exists in Asian and western studies.[74] An association with Epstein-Barr virus has been noted and may contribute to the regional differences in prevalence.[67,72] In Asia, T-cell lymphoma predominates, but B-cell variants seem to occur more frequently in western populations.[67]

Clinical Presentation

Clinically, the disease can range from indolent symptoms like nasal obstruction and drainage to rapid midline facial destruction in its most severe form resulting in sinonasal and palatal necrosis. Systemic symptoms are common and include constitutional symptoms indicative of lymphoma.[68,69,74]

Clinical Evaluation

The most important aspect of diagnosis is to exclude possibility of this disease early in its course. Clinical evaluation includes general medical history and review of systems, comprehensive head and neck exam, nasal endoscopy, and CT and/or MRI of paranasal sinuses and orbits. Both CT and MRI characteristics are nonspecific and are more useful as adjunctive measures to define the extent of the disease process.[75] Grossly, lesions appear grey to yellow and friable, and arise in the midline of the nose or palate.[72] When biopsy is obtained, histology frequently demonstrates neutrophil, macrophage, eosinophil and atypical lymphocyte infiltration.[67,72] However, biopsy can be unreliable and immunohistochemical analysis can be helpful in identifying the specific cell lineage. Studies suggestive of T-cell pathology include monoclonal lymphocytic proliferation as evidenced by CD2, CD5, CD7, CD43, CD45 and CD45RO staining.[68,72] B-cell pathology is identified by the presence of the CD19, CD20, CD22, and CD10 antigens.[72]

Treatment

Radiation therapy offers the best chance for long-term survival with maintenance of maxillofacial structures. In a study of 29 patients, the 1-year survival of patients treated with radiation therapy and chemotherapy was 70% and 15%, respectively.[76] The main predictor of survival appears to be early recognition and treatment with radiation prior to dissemination of the lymphoma systemically.[77] Additional studies are required to investigate the possibility of a combined chemotherapy and radiation approach to improve survival.

INFECTIOUS DISEASES

A wide spectrum of bacterial, fungal, and parasitic organisms can infect the nose and paranasal sinuses and produce granuloma. Most of these diseases are rare, but treatable. Prompt diagnosis and treatment are thus important. These infectious causes of granulomatous inflammation are summarized in Table 26.1.

Mycobacteria

Mycobacterium species, causing tuberculosis (TB) and leprosy, can result in granulomatous inflammation. Sinonasal TB (caused by *Mycobacterium tuberculosis*) can manifest in the presence or absence of pulmonary tuberculosis.[78] The rise of HIV has lead to an increase in the percentage of tuberculosis cases arising in extrapulmonary, including sinonasal, sites.[78] However, scattered reports of sinonasal tuberculosis emphasize its rarity, with one recent study reporting a 6.7% incidence of sinonasal extrapulmonary TB.[79] Symptoms include nasal congestion, fever, facial pain, and sinusitis. Diagnosis is made on the basis of culture and staining for acid-fast bacilli or PCR for the tuberculous species. The extent of pulmonary and systemic involvement is assessed by history and physical examination, chest X-ray, and purified protein derivative (PPD) testing.[79] When clinically apparent, upper airway TB should be treated with three- or four-drug antituberculosis therapy, including regimens of rifampin, isoniazid, pyrazinamide, and on occasion ethambutol, for 9 to 18 months.[79]

Similarly, leprosy (caused by *Mycobacterium leprae*) can present with nasal symptoms with tuberculoid skin or mucosal nodules, ulcerations, and nasal collapse. Leprosy is treated with dapsone.

Rhinoscleroma

Rhinoscleroma is caused by *Klebsiella rhinoscleromatis*. The prevalence of this infection is greatest in Eastern Europe and Central America. It is generally a three-stage disease: rhinitic, florid or granulomatous, and cicatricial stages. In the initial stage patients complain of rhinorrhea and nasal crusting. Granulomatous nodules define the second stage. In the final stage, fibrosis can result in stenosis of the nasal vestibule, larynx, or distal airways. Diagnosis can be made on clinical grounds by the stage and pathologically by biopsy demonstrating pseudo-epitheliomatous hyperplasia (a benign proliferation of the superficial epithelium into irregular squamous strands extending down into the deeper epithelial layers), Russell bodies (deposits of gamma globulin seen as small spherical hyaline bodies in cancerous and simple inflammatory growth and in degenerating plasma cells), and Mikulicz cells (large, round or oval vacuolated phagocyte with small pyknotic nucleus). Treatment consists of prolonged therapy with streptomycin or tetracycline. Local therapy in the nose can consist of nasal irrigation to prevent crusting and reduce rhinorrhea. Surgical intervention for stenosis may be required on occasion.[80]

Syphilis

Syphilitic infection of the nose and sinuses is caused by *Treponema pallidum*. The nose and sinuses can be affected either in the early or late stage of syphilis. If infection afflicts the nose or sinuses in primary stage, chancre formation can occur. In late stage involvement, or tertiary syphilis, gummas form at various sites in the body. Both chancre and gumma formation represent granulomatous inflammation and can occur in the sinonasal mucosa. Diagnosis is achieved on dark-field microscopy or immunofluorescence staining to confirm the presence of spirochetes. Alternatively, fluorescent treponemal antibody absorption test (FTA-ABS) may be used. Early recognition and treatment with penicillin is still effective for treatment of the disease process; saline irrigations may be required for nasal and sinus disease.[1,2,80]

Actinomycosis

Actinomycosis, most commonly caused by *Actinomyces israeli,* usually results from dental manipulation and causes mass formation in the nasal or sinus mucosa. The classic finding is that of a painless mass at the angle of the mandible, but actinomycosis should be considered with any painless mass of the head or neck. Extension from the maxillary bone to the maxillary or ethmoid sinuses can occur. Temporary improvement is usually observed with empiric antibiotic therapy. The potential for unrestricted extension to contiguous structures, including the carotid artery, cranium, cervical spine, trachea, or thorax, can occur. On biopsy, the granulomatous mass will demonstrate sulfur granules. Actinomycosis can be treated with surgical debridement and penicillin, erythromycin, tetracycline, doxycycline, or clindamycin.[1,2,80]

Rhinosporidosis

Rhinosporidiosis is caused by the organism *Rhinosporidium seeberi*. This infection is usually seen in Asian and African countries. Contraction is usually via submersion into infected water. The infection results in a nasal lesion that is initially flat but grows to become polypoid and can fill the entire nasal cavity. Diagnosis can be made by history and physical examination. Effective treatment requires surgical excision of the polypoid lesion.[81]

Fungi

Blastomycosis

Blastomycosis is caused by *Blastomyces dermatitidis.* Nasal disease can occur, but more commonly the triad of pulmonary, cutaneous, and constitutional symptoms

prevails. Diagnosis is via culture for the organism or with serologic testing demonstrating sandwich enzyme immunoassay positive or 120-kd antigen radioimmunoassay. Pathology shows pseudoepitheliomatous hyperplasia and single bifringent broad-based buds. Treatment is with amphotericin B, ketoconazole, itraconazole or fluconazole.

Histoplasmosis

Histoplasmosis is endemic to Missouri, Mississippi, and Ohio River valleys in the US, but has been reported in over 30 countries. Dust that harbors *Histoplasma capsulatum* is inhaled from the soil. Nasal involvement can consist of nodules, ulcers, or masses of organisms surrounded by macrophages (Fig. 26.7A). Diagnosis is confirmed by biopsy, which demonstrates evidence of epithelioid granulomas. The organism can be identified with periodic acid-Schiff, Gridley, or Grocott-Gomori methenamine-silver nitrate stain (Fig. 26.7B). Treatment consists of amphotericin B for a 2–3 months (1 to 10 mg per day progressing to 1 mg/kg for a total of 2 g over the treatment period).[80,81]

Invasive Granulomatous Fungal Sinusitis

Primary paranasal aspergillus granuloma (PPAG) is a type of granulomatous fungal sinusitis that has primarily been diagnosed in the Sudan and India. This chronic infection, caused by *Aspergillus flavus*, is contracted by

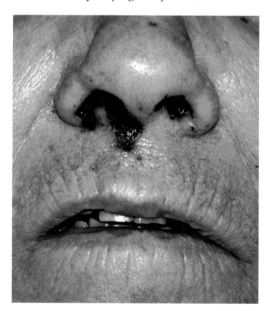

Fig. 26.7A: Representative ulcer formation in nasal histoplasmosis

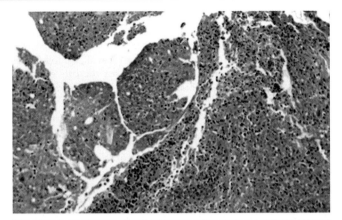

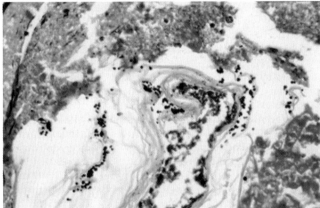

Fig. 26.7B: Routine hematoxylin and eosin stain demonstrates inflammation and granuloma formation in histoplasmosis (top). Grocott-Gomori methenamine-silver nitrate stain identifies causative organisms (bottom). (Reprint permission from Otolaryngology Head and Neck Surgery. Nasal Histoplasmosis: Report of a Case. In press)

susceptible individuals when exposed to contaminated food products. Currens et al also implicated type I (IgE) and type III (IgG) responses to *A. flavus* in the etiology of PPAG in a patient who presented with this disease.[82]

PPAG is slowly progressive but can extend beyond the confines of the paranasal sinuses. Symptoms can include nonspecific sinonasal complaints or even orbital symptoms such as orbital apex syndrome or proptosis.[82] The diagnosis of PPAG is suggested by nasal endoscopy that demonstrates grey-white tissue replacing the mucosa which is firm and irregular on its surface. Confirmation of diagnosis is achieved with surgical removal of affected areas and histopathologic evaluation of the tissue. Pathology demonstrates 'pseudotubercles, consisting of granulomatous reaction with giant cells, histiocytes, lymphocytes, plasma cells, and newly formed capillaries[82] (Fig. 26.8).

Treatment of PPAG involved surgical removal and antifungal therapy, although recurrences are common.

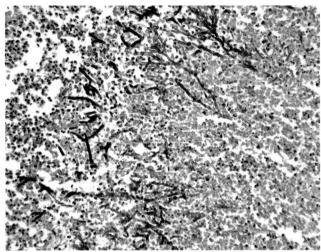

Fig. 26.8: Representative histologic appearance of chronic Aspergillus granulomatous sinusitis. Note presence of A. fumigatus in the sinonasal tissues. (*Courtesy:* Dr Richard Prayson, Department of Anatomic Pathology, The Cleveland Clinic Foundation)

Chronic disease often leads to outflow obstruction of the paranasal sinuses and can cause CRS over time.

Parasites

Leishmaniasis

Leishmaniasis can result in mucosal involvement of the head and neck. Epidemic outbreaks of infection have occurred in India, Bangladesh, and Sudan. Infection probabaly arises from exposure to the sandflies of the genus *Lutzomyia* in the Americas and *Phlebotomus* elsewhere. Transmission of the protozoa, *Leismania braziliensis* (others more rarely), is responsible for the clinical syndromes resulting in mucosal involvement. Symptoms often include nasal congestion, obstruction, rhinitis, and epistaxis, progressing to nasal collapse due to cartilage destruction in the later stages. Pathologic specimens are characterized by intense inflammation surrounding the organisms. Diagnosis can be made by culture, skin testing, ELISA, or antibody testing. Treatment is with pentavalent-antimony containing agents including stibogluconate sodium (Pentostam) and meglumine antimonate (Glucantime), amphotericin B, pentamidine, topical paromomycin, or INF-gamma depending on presentation site and host status.[83]

CONCLUSION

The presentation of sinonasal granulomatous disease can be quite variable. The disease processes may present insidiously with non-specific sinonasal symptoms or the presentation can be quite drastic, and potentially lethal, as in midline lethal granuloma. Many of these patients will initially present to the otolaryngologist with head and neck complaints, and, thus, a high index of suspicion is required on part of the clinician to initiate the appropriate work-up to arrive at the proper diagnosis. Clinical evaluation should include thorough clinical history, physical examination, endoscopy assessing the status of the nose and the larynx, laboratory testing, and possibly biopsy and radiologic imaging, as clinically indicated. An enhanced understanding of many of these disease processes has lead to advances in treatment and improvement in prognosis of this patient population.

REFERENCES

1. Acute and chronic inflammation. In Robbins and Cotran, *Pathologic Basis of Disease,* Kumar V, Abbas A, Fausto N (Eds) 7th (edn) Philadelphia: Elsevier Saunders, 2005; 47–86.
2. Lund V. Granulomatous diseases and tumors of the nose and paranasal sinuses. In *Diseases of the Sinuses: Diagnosis and management,* Kennedy DW, Zinreich J, Bolger WE (Eds), 1st edn. Ontario: BC Decker, 2001; 85–106.
3. Wegener F. Uber generalisierte, septische gefaberkrankugen. *Verh Dtsch Ges Pathol* 1936; 29:202–210.
4. Klinger H. Grenzformen deer pariarteritis Nodosa. *Frankfurt Z Pathol* 1931; 42:455–480.
5. Carrington CB, Liebow A. Limited forms of angiitis and granulomatosis of Wegener's type. *Am J Med* 1966; 41: 497–527.
6. Van der Woude FJ, Rasmussen N, Lobarto S, et al. auto-antibodies against neutrophils and monocytes: Tools for diagnosis and marker of disease activity in Wegener's granulomatosis. *Lancet* 1985; 1:425–429.
7. Jernette JC, Falk RJ, Andrassey K et al. Nomenclature of systemic vasculitides. Proposal of an international consensus conference. *Arthritis Rheum* 1994; 37:187–192.
8. Leawitt RY, Fauci AS, Bloch DA et al. The American College of Rheumatology 1990 criteria for the classification of Wegener's granulomatosis. *Arthritis Rheum* 1990; 33: 1101–1107.
9. Choi HK, Liu S, Merkel PA et al. Diagnostic value of ANCA testing for idiopathic systemic vasculitis syndromes. A meta-analysis with focus on anti-myeloperoxidase, p-ANCA and combined testing systems. *Arthritis Rheum* 1999; 42:S175.
10. Cotch MF, Hoffman GA, Yeng DE, et al. The epidemiology of Wegener's granulomatosis. *Arthritis Rheum* 1996; 39:87–92.
11. Reinhold-Keller E, Herlyn K, Wagner-Bastmeyer R. Effect of Wegener's granulomatosis on work disability, need for medical care, and quality of life in patients younger than 40 years at diagnosis. *Arthritis Rheum* 2002; 47:320–325.
12. Stageman CA, Tarvaert JW, Sluiter WG et al. Association of chronic nasal carriage of *Staphylococcus aureus* and higher relapse rates in Wegener granulomatosis. *Ann Intern Med* 1994; 120:12.
13. Reumaux D, Duthilleul P, Roos D. Pathogenesis of diseases associated with antineutrophil cytoplasm autoantibodies. *Human Immun* 2004; 65:1–12.
14. Stageman CA, Tervaert JW, de Jong PE et al. Trimethoprim-sulfamethoxazole (co-trimoxazole) for the prevention of relapses of Wegener's granulomatosis. Dutch Co-trimoxazole Wegener Study Group. *N Eng J Med* 1996; 335:16.
15. Cohen Tervaert JW, van der Woude FJ, Fauci AS et al. Association between active Wegener's granulomatosis and anticytoplasmic antibodies. *Arch Intern Med* 1989; 149:2461.
16. Cohen Tervaert JW et al. Prevention of relapses of Wegener's granulomatosis by treatment based on antineutrophil cytoplasmic antibody titre. *Lancet* 1990; 336:709–711.
17. Maguchi S, Fukuda S, Takizawa M. Histological findings in biopsies from patients with cytoplasmic-antineutrophil cytoplasmic antibody (cANCA)-positive Wegener's granulomatosis. *Auris Nasus Larynx* 2001; 28:S53–S58.
18. Yucel EA, Keles N, Ozturk AS. Wegener's granulomatosis presenting in the sinus and orbit. *Otolaryngol Head Neck Surg* 2002; 127:349–351.
19. Hoffmann GS, Kerr G, Leavitt R et al. Wegener's granulomatosis: An analysis of 158 patients. *Ann Intern Med* 1992; 116:488–498.
20. Wegener's Granulomatosis Etanercept Trial Research Group (WGET). Limited versus severe Wegener's granulomatosis: Baseline data on patients in the Wegener's granulomatosis etanercept trial. *Arthritis Rheum* 2003; 48:2299–2309.
21. Rasmussen N. Management of ear, nose, and throat manifestations of Wegener's granulomatosis: An otorhinolaryngologist's perspective. *Curr Opin Rheum* 2001; 12:3–11.
22. McDonald TJ, DeRemee RA. Head and neck involvement in Wegener's granulomatosis. In *ANCA-associated vasculitides: Immunological and clinical aspects,* Gross WL (Ed). New York: Plenum Press, 1993; 309–313.
23. Stone JH, Hoffmann GS, Merkel PA et al. A disease–specific activity index for Wegener's granulomatosis. *Arthritis Rheum* 2001; 44:912–920.
24. Gubbels SP, Barkhuizen A, Hwang PH. Head and neck manifestations of Wegener's granulomatosis. *Otol Clin N Am* 2003; 36:685–705.
25. McCafferey TV, McDonald TJ, Facer GW. Otologic manifestations of Wegener's granulomatosis. *Otolaryngol Head Neck Surg* 1980; 88:586–593.
26. Takagi D, Nakamaru Y, Maguchi S. Otologic manifestations of Wegener's granulomatosis. *Laryngoscope* 2002. 112: 1684–1690.
27. Knight JM, Hayduk MJ, Summerlin DJ et al. Strawberry gingival hyperplasia: A pathognomomic mucocutaneous finding in Wegener's granulomatosis. *Arch Dermatol* 2000; 136:171–173.
28. Lebovics RS, Hoffmann GS, Leavitt RY et al. The management of subglottic stenosis in patients with Wegener's granulomatosis. *Laryngoscope* 1992; 102:1341–1345.
29. Gluth MB, Shinners PA, Kasperbauer JL. Subglottic stenosis associated with Wegener's granulomatosis. *Laryngoscope* 2003; 113:1304–1307.
30. Langford CA, Sneller MC, Hallahan CW. Clinical features and therapeutic management of subglottic stenosis in patients with Wegener's granulomatosis. *Arthritis Rheum* 1996; 39:1754–1760.

31. Hoffman GS, Thomas-Golbanov CK, Chan J et al. Treatment of subglottic stenosis, due to Wegener's granulomatosis, with intralesional corticosteroids and dilation. *J Rheumatol* 2003; 30:1017–1021.

32. Benoudiba F, Marsot-Dupuch K, Hadj Rabia M. Sinonasal Wegener's granulomatosis: CT characteristics. *Neuroradiology* 2003; 45:95–99.

33. Lloyd G, Lund VJ, Beale T. Rhinologic changes in Wegener's granulomatosis. *J Laryngol Otol* 2002; 116:565–569.

34. Devaney KO, Travis WD, Hoffmann G et al. Interpretation of head and neck biopsies in Wegener's granulomatosis. A pathologic study of 126 biopsies in 70 patients. *Am J Surg Pathol* 1990; 14:555–564.

35. Sneller MC, Hoffmann GS, Talar-Williams C et al. An analysis of forty-two Wegener's granulomatosis patients treated with methotrexate and prednisone. *Arthritis Rheum* 1995; 38: 698–713.

36. Stone JH, Hoffman GS, Holbrook JT, (WGET). Etanercept plus standard therapy for Wegener's granulomatosis. *N Engl J Med* 2005; 352:351–361.

37. Langford CA. Wegener's granulomatosis: Current and upcoming therapies. *Arthritis Res Ther* 2003; 5:180–191.

38. Congdon D, Sherris DA, Specks U et al. Long-term follow-up of repair of external nasal deformities in patients with Wegener's granulomatosis. *Laryngoscope* 2002; 112:731–737.

39. Kwan ASL, Rose GE. Lacrimal drainage surgery in Wegener's granulomatosis. *Br J Ophthalmol* 2000; 84:329–331.

40. Wong RJ, Gliklich RE, Rubin PA et al. Bilateral nasolacrimal duct obstruction managed with endoscopic techniques. *Arch Otolaryngol Head Neck Surg* 1998; 124:703–706.

41. Wu JJ, Schiff KR. Sarcoidosis. *Fam Physician* 2004; 70:312–322.

42. Shah UK, White JA, Gooey JE et al. Otolaryngologic manifestations of sarcoidosis: Presentation and diagnosis. *Laryngoscope* 1997; 107:67–75.

43. Hills SE, Parkes SA, Baker SB. Epidemiology of sarcoidosis in the Isle of Man-2: Evidence for space-time clustering. *Thorax* 1987; 42:427–430.

44. Panayeas S, Theodorakopoulos P, Bouras A et al. Seasonal occurrence of sarcoidosis in Greece. *Lancet* 1991; 338:510–511.

45. Hosoda Y, Hiraga Y, Odaka M et al. A cooperative study of sarcoidosis in Asia and Africa: Analytic epidemiology. *Ann NY Acad Sci* 1976; 278:355–367.

46. Sarcoidosis among US Navy enlisted men, 1965–1993. *MMWR Morb Mort Wkly Rep* 1997; 46:539–543.

47. Kern DG, Neill MA, Wrenn DS et al. Investigation of the unique time–space cluster of sarcoidosis in firefighters. *Am Rev Respir Dis* 1993; 148:974–980.

48. Baughman RP, Lower EE, du Bois RM. Sarcoidosis. *Lancet* 2003; 361:1111–1118.

49. Ishige I, Usui Y, Takemura T et al. Quantitative PCR of Mycobacterial and Proprionibacterial DNA in lymph nodes of Japanese patients with sarcoidosis. *Lancet* 1999; 354: 120–133.

50. Foley PJ, McGrath DS, Petrek M et al. HLA-DRB1 position 11 residues are a common protective marker for sarcoidosis. *Am J Respir Cell Mol Biol* 2001; 25:272–277.

51. Hunninghake GW, Costabel U, Ando ME et al. ATS/ERS/WASOG statement on sarcoidosis. American Thoracic Society/European Respiratory Society/World Association of Sarcoidosis and other Granulomatous Disorders. *Sarcoidosis Vasc Diffuse Lung Dis* 1999; 16:149–173.

52. Johns CJ, Michele TM. The clinical management of sarcoidosis: A 50-year experience at the Johns Hopkins Hospital. *Q J Med* 1983; 78:65–111.

53. Neel HB, McDonald TJ. Laryngeal sarcoidosis, report of 13 patients. *Ann Otol Rhinol Laryngol* 1982; 91:359–362.

54. McCaffrey TV, McDonald TJ. Sarcoidosis of the nose and paranasal sinuses. *Laryngoscope* 1983; 93:1281–1284.

55. Zeitlin JF, Tami TA, Baughman R et al. Nasal and sinus manifestations of sarcoidosis. *Am J Rhinol* 2000; 14:157–161.

56. Wilson R, Lund V, Sweatman M et al. Upper respiratory tract involvement in sarcoidosis and its management. *Eur Respir J* 1988; 1:269–272.

57. Braun JJ, Gentine A, Pauli G. Sinonasal sarcoidosis: Review and report of fifteen cases. *Laryngoscope* 2004; 114:1960–1963.

58. De Shazo RD, O'Brien MM, Justice WK et al. Diagnostic criteria for sarcoidosis of the sinuses. *J All Clin Immunol* 1999; 103:789–795.

59. Damrose EJ, Huang RY, Abemayor E. Endoscopic diagnosis of sarcoidosis in a patient presenting with bilateral exopthalmos and pansinusitis. *Am J Rhinol* 2000; 14:241–244.

60. Marks SC, Goodman RS. Surgical management of nasal and sinus sarcoidosis. *Otolaryngol Head Neck Surg* 1998; 118: 856–858.

61. Kay DJ, Har-El G. The role of endoscopic sinus surgery in chronic sinonasal sarcoidosis. *Am J Rhinol* 2001; 15:249–254.

62. Lane SE, Watts RA, Shepstone L et al. Primary systemic vasculitis: Clinical features and mortality. *Q J Med* 2005; 98: 97–111.

63. Metaxaris G, Prokopakis EP, Karatzanis AD. Otolaryngologic manifestations of small vessel vasculitis. *Auris Nasus Larynx* 2002; 29:353–356.

64. Gross WL, Trabandt A, Reinhold-Keller E. Diagnosis and evaluation of vasculitis. *Rheumatology* 2000; 29:245–252.

65. Shykhon ME, Trotter MI, Morgan DW et al. Cholesterol granuloma of the frontal sinus. *J Laryngol Otol* 2002; 116: 1041–1043.

66. Aferzon M, Millman B, O'Donnel TR et al. Cholesterol granuloma of the frontal bone. *Otol Head Neck Surg* 2002; 127:578–581.

67. Westreich RW, Lawson W. Midline necrotizing nasal lesions: Analysis of 18 cases emphasizing radiological and serological findings with algorithms for diagnosis and management. *Am J Rhinol* 2004; 18:209–219.

68. Borges A, Fink J, Villablanca P et al. Midline destructive lesions of the sinonasal tract: Simplified terminology based on histopathologic criteria. *Am J Neuroradiol* 2000; 21:331–336.

69. Cleary KR, Batsakis JG. Sinonasal lymphomas. *Ann Otol Rhinol Laryngol* 1994; 103:911–914.

70. Eichel BS, Mabery TE. The enigma of the midline granuloma. *Laryngoscope* 78:1367–1386.

71. Friedman I. McBride and the midfacial granuloma syndrome. *J Laryngol Otol* 1982; 96:1–23.

72. Hartig G, Montone K, Wasik M et al. Nasal T-cell lymphoma and the lethal midline granuloma syndrome. *Otol Head Neck Surg* 1996; 114.

73. Yamanaka N, Harabuchi Y, Sambe S et al. Non-Hodgkins' lymphoma of Waldeyer's ring and nasal cavity. *Cancer* 1985; 56:768–776.

74. Ho FCS, Choy D, Loke SL et al. Polymorphic reticulosis and conventional lymphomas of the nose and upper aerodigestive tract: A clinicopathologic study of 70 cases and immuno-phenotypic studies in 16 cases. *Hum Pathol* 1990; 21:1041–1050.

75. Marsot-Dupuch, Cabane J, Raveau V et al. Lethal midline granuloma: Impact of imaging studies on the investigation and management of destructive midfacial disease in 13 patients. *Neuroradiology* 1992; 34:155–161.

76. Sobrevilla-Calvo P, Meneses A, Alfaro P et al. Radiotherapy compared to chemotherapy as initial treatment of angiocentric centrofacial lymphoma (polymorphic reticulosis). *Acta Oncol* 1993; 32:69–72.

77. Itami J, Itami M, Mikata A et al. Non-Hodgkin's lymphoma confined to the nasal cavity: Its relationship to polymorphic reticulosis and the results of radiation therapy. *Int J Radiat Oncol Biol Phys* 1991; 20:197–802.

78. Beltran S, Douadi Y, Lescure FX et al. A case of tuberculous sinusitis without concomitant pulmonary disease. *Eur J Clin Microbiol Infect Dis* 2003; 22:49–50.

79. Al-Serhani AM. Mycobacterial infection of the head and neck: Presentation and diagnosis. *Laryngoscope* 2001; 111:2012–2016.

80. Shah A. Granulomatous diseases of the head and neck. Updated 20 September 2006. http.//www.emedicinc.com/ent/topic768.htm.

81. McDonald TJ. Manifestations of systemic diseases of the nose. In *Otolaryngology: Head and neck surgery*, ed C Cummings, 3rd edn. St. Louis: Mosby-Year Book, Inc., 1998; 844–851.

82. Currens J, Hutcheson P, Slavin RG. Primary paranasal aspergillus granuloma: Case report and review of the literature. *Am J Rhinol* 2002; 16:165–168.

83. Pearson RD, De Queiroz Sousa A, Jeronimo SMB. *Leishmania* species: Visceral (kala-azar), cutaneous, and mucosal leishmaniasis. In *Principles and Practice of Infectious Diseases*, 5th edn, GL Mandell (Ed) et al. Philadelphia: Churchill Livingstone, 2000; 2831–2841.

CHAPTER 27

Imaging of the Paranasal Sinuses

Venna A Nagar, Meher A Ursekar, Bhavin G Jankharia

The structure of the paranasal air sinuses is complex and poses unique challenges to effective and meaningful imaging. CT and MRI have eclipsed the role of plain radiography in sinus evaluation.

ANATOMY OF THE NASAL CAVITY AND PARANASAL SINUSES

The Nose and Nasal Fossae

The external nose has an overall pyramidal shape.[1] At the apex of the pyramid is the cribriform plate of the ethmoid bone. At the base are the hard and soft palates and the sides are formed by the lateral nasal walls. It is divided down in the midline by the septum. The osteocartilaginous nasal septum is formed by the perpendicular plate of the ethmoid bone posteriorly and the septal cartilage anteriorly. The vomer contributes to the posteroinferior margin of the septum. The flexible articulation of the septal cartilage with adjacent bones permits septal deviation without fracture or dislocation.

The lateral nasal wall of the nose is an undulating surface with three distinct projections: The superior, middle, and inferior turbinates. The air space beneath and lateral to each turbinate is called the meatus. Thus, there are three distinct meatus running from anterior to posterior: The superior, middle, and inferior meatus (Fig. 27.1). The inferior meatus is the largest of the three nasal meatus. It receives the nasolacrimal duct in its anterior aspect. Small channels from the posterior ethmoidal air cells drain into the superior meatus. All other major drainage is into the middle meatus. Therefore, historically, more attention has been paid to the anterior osteomeatal unit, which is the volume around the middle meatus and its relationship to the surrounding anatomy.

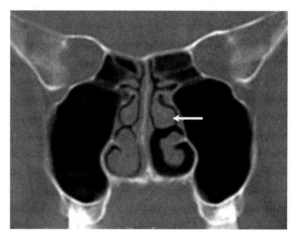

Fig. 27.1: Coronal CT (bone window) image showing the superior, middle and inferior meatus

The Paranasal Sinuses

All the paranasal sinuses originate as evaginations from the nasal fossae.[2] They are lined by pseudostratified columnar ciliated epithelium that contains both mucinous and serous glands.

Frontal Sinus

The paired, normally asymmetric frontal sinuses are located in the frontal bone. The inferior wall of the frontal sinus is also the anterior portion of the orbital roof. The posterior wall abuts the anterior cranial fossa. The frontal sinus most frequently (85% of cases) drains via the nasofrontal duct into the frontoethmoidal recess (Fig. 27.2). The nasofrontal duct is strictly speaking not a duct, rather an internal channel between the sinus and the frontoethmoidal recess.

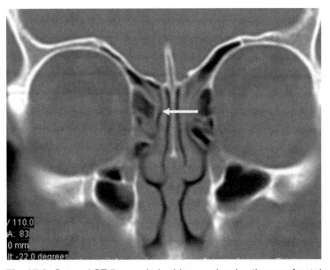

Fig. 27.2: Coronal CT (bone window) image showing the nasofrontal duct draining into the frontoethmoidal recess (arrow)

Ethmoidal Sinus

The ethmoid bone consists of four parts: The horizontal lamina above called the cribriform plate; a perpendicular plate; and two lateral masses, called the ethmoid labyrinths. The roof of the ethmoid labyrinth is called the fovea ethmoidalis. It is also the floor of the anterior cranial fossa (Fig. 27.3). The posterior labyrinth contains the posterior ethmoid air cells. They are intimately related to the orbit, especially the optic canal. The most anterior extramural ethmoid air cells are the agger nasi cells (Fig. 27.4). The ground lamella or the basal lamella from which the middle turbinate (concha) springs, runs upwards to the roof of the labyrinth. It divides the labyrinth into two compartments. All the cells in front of the basal lamella are called the anterior cells. They are relatively small and the biggest of these is known as the ethmoid bulla (bulla ethmoidalis) (Fig. 27.5). All cells posterior to the basal lamella are called the posterior cells. The lateral wall of the labyrinth constitutes medial orbital wall as a thin membranous bone called the lamina papyracea (Fig. 27.6). The ethmoidal uncinate process is a superior extension of the lateral nasal wall that lies posterior and inferior to the agger nasi cells. Secretions from the frontal sinus, anterior ethmoidal cells, and the maxillary antrum drain into the unciform groove and make their way down to the ethmoidal infundibulum at the semilunar hiatus. The semilunar hiatus is a curvilinear opening of the lateral nasal wall delimited by the ethmoidal uncinate process inferiorly, inferomedial orbit cranially, and the ethmoidal bulla superiorly (Fig. 27.7).

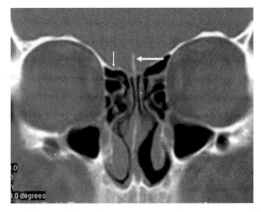

Fig. 27.3: Parts of the ethmoid bone as seen on coronal CT (bone window) image: Crista galli forming the perpendicular plate (thick arrow), ethmoid labyrinths and the cribriform plate. Fovea ethmoidalis (thin arrow) forms the roof of ethmoid labyrinths

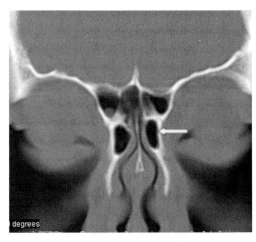

Fig. 27.4: Coronal CT (bone window) image shows the anterior most paired ethmoid air cells also known as the agger nasi cells (arrow)

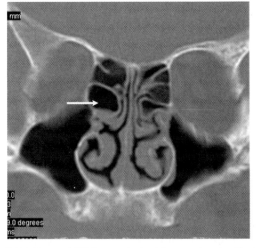

Fig. 27.5: Coronal CT (bone window) image showing the largest ethmoidal air cell (arrow) also called bulla ethmoidalis

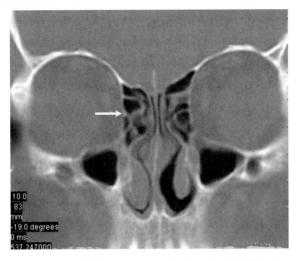

Fig. 27.6: Coronal CT demonstrates the lateral wall of the ethmoid sinuses formed by lamina papyracea (arrow), which also forms the medial wall of the orbits

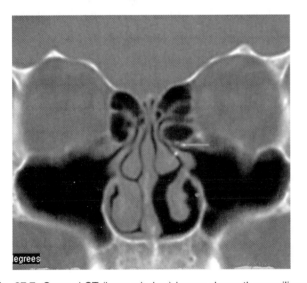

Fig. 27.7: Coronal CT (bone window) image shows the curvilinear opening of the lateral nasal wall, i.e. the hiatus semilunaris (solid long arrow). Note that the uncinate process (small arrow) forms the inferior limit of this opening

Maxillary Antrum

The antra are pyramidal air cavities within the maxillary bodies and are the largest paranasal sinuses. The sinus roof is the orbital floor and the floor is the alveolar process of the maxilla. The medial wall is a portion of the lateral nasal wall of the nose and the posterior wall abuts the retromaxillary fat pad and pterygopalatine fossa. Maxillary sinus drainage is into the inferior recess of the semilunar hiatus.

Sphenoid Sinus

This is the most posterior of paranasal air sinuses. The intersphenoidal septum is midline and typically aligned with the nasal septum. The roof (planum sphenoidale) of the sphenoid sinus underlies the anterior cranial fossa, sella turcica, optic chiasm, and juxtasellar space. The lateral wall is closely opposed to the orbital apex, the optic canal, and the cavernous sinus. Behind the sphenoidal sinus lie the clivus and the prepontine cistern, and below it lie the roof of the nasopharynx and posterior wall of the nasal fossa (Fig. 27.8). Drainage of the sphenoid sinus is into the superior meatus via the sphenoethmoidal recess or the posterior osteomeatal unit.

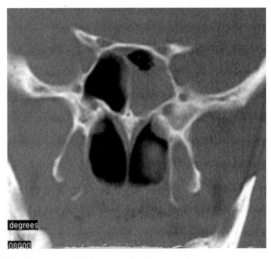

Fig. 27.8: Coronal CT (bone window) image shows the posterior wall of the nasal fossa seen lying below the body of the sphenoid sinus. Note the opacification of the left sphenoid sinus

Normal Mucociliary Clearance and the Osteomeatal Channels

The mucosa of the paranasal sinuses is made up of a ciliated cuboidal epithelium, and a mucus blanket is secreted on its surface. The cilia are in constant motion and act in concert to propel the mucus in a specific direction.[3] In the maxillary sinus the mucus flow is directed centripetally towards the primary ostium and then transported through the infundibulum to the hiatus semilunaris, from where it is passes into the middle meatus. In the frontal sinus the mucus travels down the frontoethmoidal recess into the middle meatus. The posterior ethmoid and sphenoid sinuses clear their mucus into the sphenoethmoidal recess. There are two main osteomeatal channels. The anterior osteomeatal unit (OMU) includes the frontal sinus ostium, frontoethmoidal recess, maxillary sinus ostium, infundibulum, and the middle meatus. The posterior OMU consists of the sphenoid sinus ostium, sphenoethmoidal recess, and the superior meatus. The important components of the anterior osteomeatal unit include the infundibulum, uncinate process, ethmoid bulla, hiatus semilunaris, and the middle meatus (Fig. 27.9). Since the development of functional endoscopic sinus surgery (FESS), the osteomeatal unit has become the center of interest. The osteomeatal unit is best visualized with coronal CT.

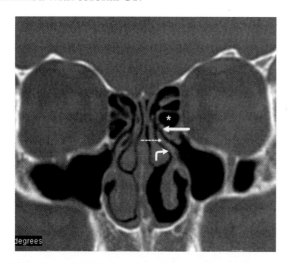

Fig. 27.9: Coronal CT (bone window) image displays the parts of anterior osteomeatal unit: Uncinate process (thin arrow), ethmoid bulla (asterisk), hiatus semilunaris (thick arrow), and the middle meatus (curved arrow)

PARANASAL SINUS DEVELOPMENT

Developmentally, the paranasal sinuses represent nasal 'diverticula'. All the paranasal sinuses may be opaque in an infant younger than 1 year of age. The maxillary sinus is the first aerated sinus to be visualized on plain radiographs or CT scans. Lateral growth of the maxillary sinuses beneath the orbits continues until 15 years of age. Hypoplasia of the maxillary sinuses occurs with an incidence of 9%. Small maxillary and ethmoid sinuses may be present at birth. The ethmoid sinus pneumatization extends from medial to lateral and from anterior to posterior. Aeration of the sphenoid sinuses generally is apparent by age 3 years. Growth proceeds from anterior to posterior underneath the sella and continues into early adulthood. The frontal sinuses are the last paranasal sinuses to be aerated. They are not visible on plain radiographs until age 6 years.

Anatomic Variations

Even though the nasal anatomy varies significantly from patient to patient, certain specific anatomic variations are observed. The real importance in identifying these variations is in presurgical mapping.

Concha Bullosa

A concha bullosa refers to an aerated middle turbinate and may be unilateral or bilateral. It may enlarge the middle turbinate so that it obstructs the middle meatus or the infundibulum (Fig. 27.10). It may also get infected and show an air-fluid level or be completely opacified.

Nasal Septum Deviation

Asymmetric bowing of the septum may compress the middle turbinate laterally and narrow the middle meatus. Bony spurs are often associated with a deviated septum (Fig. 27.11).

Paradoxical Middle Turbinate

The middle turbinate usually curves medially towards the nasal septum. A lateral convexity of the middle turbinate near the middle meatus may obstruct the anterior osteomeatal unit (Fig. 27.12).

Variations in the Uncinate Process

There are several variations of the free edge of the uncinate process. Its superior edge may deviate medially to obstruct the middle meatus or there may be pneumatization of its tip (Fig. 27.13). Sometimes, the free edge of the uncinate adheres to the orbital floor or lamina papyracea. This is referred to as an atelectatic uncinate process. This variation is usually associated with a hypoplastic ipsilateral maxillary sinus due to closure of the infundibulum.

Haller Cells

These are infraorbital ethmoid air cells that extend along the medial roof of the maxillary sinus (Fig. 27.14). When large they may cause narrowing of the infundibulum.

Onodi Cells

These are lateral and posterior extensions of the ethmoid air cells. These cells may surround the optic nerve tracts and put the nerve at risk during surgery.

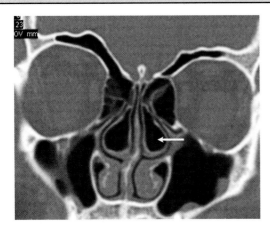

Fig. 27.10: Coronal CT (bone window) image shows pneumatization of the middle turbinates bilaterally, i.e. concha bullosa (arrow)

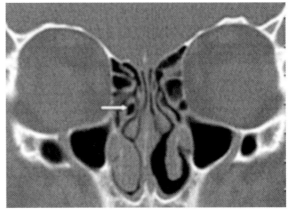

Fig. 27.13: Uncinate bulla. Coronal CT image at the level of the osteomeatal unit demonstrates pneumatization of the uncinate process at its tip

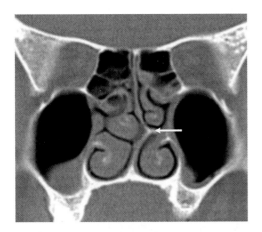

Fig. 27.11: Nasal septal deviation. Coronal CT image demonstrates the deviation of the nasal septum to the left with a nasal spur (arrow)

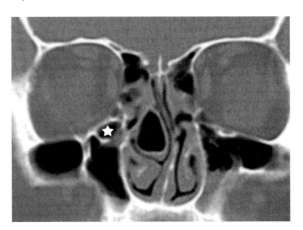

Fig. 27.14: Haller cell. Coronal CT (bone window) image demonstrates a large Haller (infraorbital ethmoid) cell (asterisk), which extends along the medial roof of the right maxillary sinus

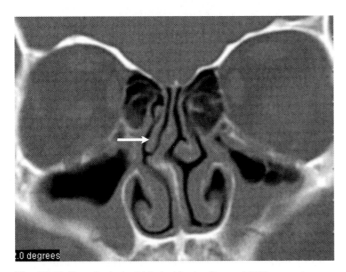

Fig. 27.12: Paradoxical middle turbinate. Coronal CT image shows a right-sided paradoxical middle turbinate (arrow) obstructing the osteomeatal unit on the same side

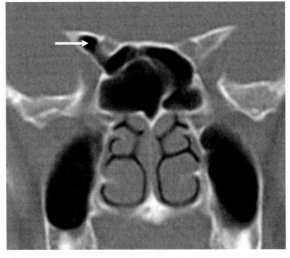

Fig. 27.15: Pneumatization of anterior clinoid process. Coronal CT image demonstrates pneumatization of the anterior clinoid process (arrow) on the right side. Note its close proximity to the optic nerve

Giant Ethmoid Bulla

The largest of the ethmoid air cells may enlarge and narrow the middle meatus and infundibulum.

Extensive Pneumatization of the Sphenoid Sinus

Pneumatization of the sphenoid sinus can extend into the anterior clinoids, clivus, and wings of the sphenoid (Fig. 27.15).

Medial Deviation or Dehiscence of the Lamina Papyracea

It is difficult to differentiate post-traumatic from congenital dehiscence. This finding places the intraorbital contents at risk especially if there is partial or total muscular prolapse.

Low-lying Fovea Ethmoidalis

It is often associated with a low position of the cribriform plate. There is higher incidence of intracranial penetration during FESS when this anatomic variation occurs.

IMAGING TECHNIQUES

Although CT and MRI have for the most part replaced routine plain film examination of the paranasal sinuses, these plain film studies are still often performed as the first roentgen examination. There are a number of radiographic views available for the evaluating the paranasal sinuses. However, only the Caldwell and Waters views are routinely obtained. If possible these views should be obtained in an erect position so as to allow clear identification of an air-fluid level. If the patient cannot tolerate erect position then a cross table lateral film should be obtained.

Coronal CT is necessary when any form of traditional or endoscopic surgery is anticipated. In weeks, before the CT examination, an attempt to treat reversible disease maximally should be made. Fifteen minutes before the study a vasoconstrictor spray should be applied in each nostril followed by vigorous nose blow. The study is usually performed with the patient in prone position with head hyper-extended. If the patient is unable to assume this position then supine coronal CT is performed. Axial images are also obtained. The technical details of the examination are beyond the scope of this chapter.

Under normal conditions, the sinonasal secretions form a complex solution that is in equilibrium with the interstitial fluids. By weight, the composition of these secretions is about 95% water and 5% macromolecular proteins. Thus, normal sinonasal secretions are predominantly water and on MR images have long T1 and T2 relaxation times. When normal sinonasal secretions are chronically obstructed, a number of predictable changes occur that progressively increase the protein concentration of the obstructed secretions. As a result of these alterations, the secretions change from a primarily serous composition into a loose mucus collection and finally into a desiccated, stone like mucus plug. These changes are predictable; what is not known is how long it takes for them to occur. In some patients, such changes are found to happen more rapidly in one sinus than in another, whereas in other patients all of the chronically obstructed secretions appear to undergo these changes at nearly the same rate (Fig. 27.16).

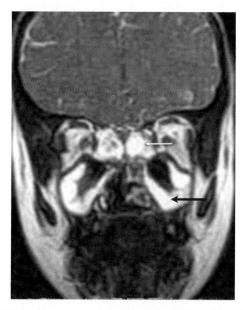

Fig. 27.16: MR appearance of sinusitis. Coronal T2-weighted image of the paranasal sinuses shows mucosal thickening of both the maxillary sinuses (thick black arrow), which appear hyperintense on T2-weighted images. Also note the hyperintense secretions in the ethmoid sinuses (thin black arrow)

As the protein content rises from 5% to about 25%, both the T1 and T2 relaxation times shorten. Since the protein content is about 25 to 30%, significant cross-linking occurs between protein molecules. These changes slow the macromolecular motion, which, in turn, allows dipole-dipole dephasing to become a more significant factor. As a result, the T2 relaxation time and signal intensity plummet. The T1-weighted signal intensity falls back to a low value between the protein content range of 25 and 40%. At protein content above 35 and 40%, virtually all of the free water has been eliminated from the secretions. These semisolid and solid protein mixtures have ultrashort T2 relaxation times. These are noted first as low signal intensities and then as signal voids on T1-weighted MR images and as signal voids on T2-weighted images.

In the case of the most concentrated secretions that give signal voids on both T1-weighted and T2-weighted MR images, distinction from an aerated sinus may be impossible with MR imaging. On CT scans, such secretions are dense, reflecting their high protein concentration, while air appears black. Thus, the radiologist can easily underestimate the presence of such chronic secretions and the severity of the sinus disease if MR imaging is the only imaging examination used.

Multiplanar CT with contrast or MRI is indicated in mainly two clinical settings. In patients suspected of having complications of sinusitis or surgery and radiologic staging of tumors of the sinuses where it is critical to evaluate fully the true deep-tissue extension of the tumor.[4]

Sinonasal Disease

Congenital Disease

Anterior cephalocele: Preoperative CT scanning is useful to assess congenital abnormalities, such as cephaloceles. These may be congenital, or may occur as a result of previous surgery or trauma. About 15% of all cephaloceles occur in the anterior cranial fossa. The anterior cephaloceles are classified depending on their craniofacial pathway. They are frontonasal cephalocele, nasoethmoidal and naso-orbital cephaloceles. When diagnosing an isolated soft tissue mass adjacent to the ethmoid or

sphenoid roof, the radiologist must consider cephalocele, especially if there is adjacent bone erosion. A child with suspected nasal polyp or nasopharyngeal mass should undergo CT or MRI before surgical intervention (Figs 27.17A and B).

Choanal atresia: This is a relatively rare anomaly of the upper airway, which can result in significant respiratory distress in the newborn. Congenital choanal atresia is a rare developmental anomaly characterized by failure of communication of the posterior nasal cavity with the nasopharynx. It may present as a component of the CHARGE association (coloboma; heart disease; atresia choanae; retarded growth and development; genital hypoplasia; and ear anomalies and/or deafness). It is often associated with other anomalies.[5] The oronasal membrane perforates during the seventh fetal week. If it fails to complete this process, some degree of choanal atresia will result. The lesion may be unilateral or bilateral, membranous or bony. CT plays a significant role in the diagnostic and therapeutic approach to congenital choanal atresia and should be the examination method of choice to evaluate neonates with nasal obstruction (Fig. 27.18).

Sinonasal Inflammatory Disease

Viral and Bacterial Rhinosinusitis: Sinusitis is rarely isolated to the paranasal sinuses and is nearly always accompanied or preceded by rhinitis. Sinusitis cannot be diagnosed on the basis of radiographic findings alone. It is important to remember that minor mucosal thickening is common in asymptomatic patients and its presence may

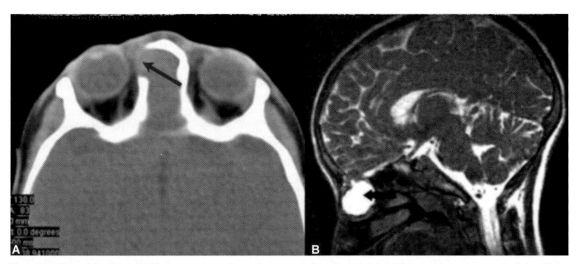

Figs 27.17A and B: CT and MR appearance of anterior encephalocele. (A) Axial CT image demonstrates a defect in the right half of the nasal bone with herniation of a soft tissue mass (thin black arrow). (B) Mid-sagittal T2-weighted MR image shows the outline of brain tissue, meninges, and cerebrospinal fluid (thick black arrow)

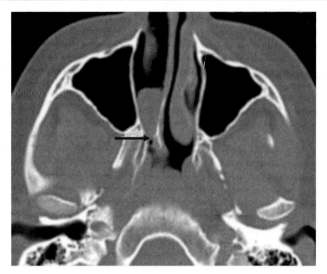

Fig. 27.18: Choanal atresia. Axial CT image demonstrates choanal atresia on the right side (arrow)

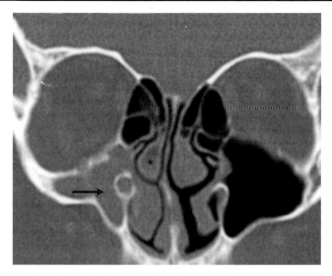

Fig. 27.19: Maxillary sinusitis. Coronal CT image showing opacification of the right maxillary sinus

be of no clinical significance. Sinusitis can be conventionally classified as acute or chronic, although recurrent acute and subacute patterns are recognized as well.[6] The most commonly implicated viruses for acute sinusitis are rhinovirus, parainfluenza and influenza viruses, adenoviruses, and repiratory syncytial virus.[7] The typical cold remains primarily a viral rhinitis with little significant sinusitis. However, if mucopurulent discharge develops, a secondary bacterial infection has occurred. In cases of non-complicated viral infections, imaging of the sinonasal cavities usually shows that they are normal or show minimal sinus mucosal thickening, but the mucosa in the nasal fossae is thickened and there is swelling of the turbinates. Obstruction of a sinus ostium leads to secondary bacterial infection. The most commonly implicated pathogens are *Streptococcus pneumoniae*, *Haemophilus influenzae*, and beta-hemolytic *Streptococcus*. Rarely *Staphylococcus aureus* and *Pseudomonas* infections occur.[8]

Multiple patterns of inflammatory sinonasal disease can be identified during coronal sinus CT. These include maxillary infundibular pattern, nasofrontal pattern, ostiomeatal pattern, sphenoethmoidal recess pattern, and sinonasal polyposis.

Maxillary infundibular pattern is a limited form of inflammatory disease involving a focal area of the osteomeatal unit. Only the maxillary infundibulum and the ipsilateral maxillary sinus are diseased in this pattern. The ipsilateral frontal and ethmoid sinuses are normal. Coronal sinus CT shows opacification of the maxillary infundibulum with secondary inflammatory changes within the maxillary sinus (Fig. 27.19).

In the nasofrontal duct pattern, inflammatory changes occur due to obstruction of the nasofrontal duct. This results in sinus disease limited to the frontal sinus. CT shows nasofrontal duct opacification with partial or complete opacification of the ipsilateral frontal sinus.

Osteomeatal pattern is the best understood pattern of inflammatory diseases seen on coronal sinus CT. Coronal sinus CT shows opacification of the middle meatal area of the lateral nasal wall, with associated chronic or acute inflammatory changes in the adjacent maxillary, anterior ethmoid and frontal sinuses (Fig. 27.20). This pattern requires more surgery than the infundibular or nasofrontal patterns, because multiple sinuses are involved.

Sphenoethmoidal recess pattern results from obstruction of the sphenoethmoidal recess, with secondary sinus inflammatory changes seen in the sphenoid sinus and ipsilateral posterior ethmoid sinus (Fig. 27.21).

Sinonasal Polyposis

Sinonasal polyposis is related to allergic sinusitis. In this inflammatory polyps fill the nasal vault and sinuses bilaterally. Coronal CT features included polypoid masses in the nasal cavity, partial or complete pansinus opacification, enlargement of infundibula, bony attenuation of the ethmoid trabeculae and nasal septum, opacified ethmoid sinuses with convex lateral walls and air-fluid levels. Recognition of sinonasal polyposis is important to the endoscopic surgeon since it can be the most troubling sinonasal inflammatory disease to manage due to its aggressive nature and tendency to recur despite appropriate treatment[9] (Fig. 27.22).

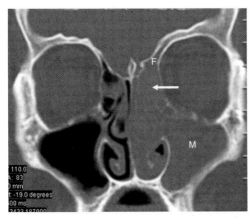

Fig. 27.20: Osteomeatal pattern of sinusitis. Coronal CT image demonstrates opacification of the left middle meatus with resultant opacification of the adjacent maxillary (M), anterior ethmoid (arrow) and frontal sinus (F)

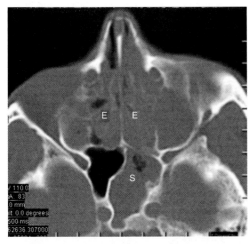

Fig. 27.21: Sphenoethmoidal recess pattern of sinusitis. Axial CT image shows opacification of bilateral posterior ethmoid sinuses (E) with opacification of the left sphenoid sinus (S)

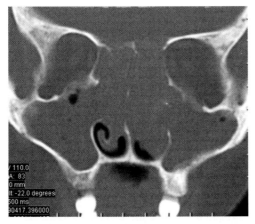

Fig. 27.22: Sinonasal polyposis. Coronal CT image shows opacification of all the paranasal sinuses with obliteration of the boundaries of the sinuses and enlargement of the infundibula

Imaging issues in sinusitis: The findings of sinusitis, regardless of the imaging modality, are quite nonspecific. Even an air/fluid level, the most definitive finding of acute bacterial sinusitis, may be due to other causes such as acute intrasinus hemorrhage from trauma or blood dyscrasia, crying and accumulation of tears, or redundant mucosa.[10] Mucoperiosteal thickening, another finding in sinusitis, has an even longer differential, including acute inflammation, resolving sinusitis, chronic sinusitis, viral rhinitis, or allergic rhinitis.[11]

Mucoperiosteal thickening, one of the most common incidental findings, is not synonymous with 'chronic sinusitis'. This diagnosis can only be suggested if serial sinus studies show that the mucoperiosteal disease, together with the symptoms, is chronic. Sclerosis and thickening of the sinus walls, and small volume sinuses are reliable signs of chronic sinusitis.

Fungal Sinusitis

A variety of fungal diseases involve the sinonasal cavities. These include aspergillosis, mucormycosis, candidiasis, histoplasmosis, cryptococcosis, coccidiodomycosis and rhinosporidiosis. There are four clinicopathologic classification of mycotic sinonasal disease:

* Acute invasive, fulminant disease
* Chronic invasive infection
* Noninvasive mycotic colonization (fungus ball)
* Allergic mycotic sinusitis.

These four types of infections are most commonly a result of *Aspergillus* infection.

Acute fulminant fungal sinusitis is a rapidly progessive disease that is most commonly seen in poorly controlled diabetics or immunosuppressed patients. CT scan of the paranasal sinuses reveals a soft-tissue density mass within the involved sinus with aggressive destruction of the sinus wall. Contiguous extension into the periantral soft tissues, orbital apex and intracranial extension can result. Vascular occlusion with an associated hemorrhagic infarct of the underlying brain parenchyma can also be seen.

Chronic invasive fungal sinusitis is characterized by an indolent course. Patients usually present with decreased vision and ocular immobility owing to the orbital apex syndrome. A non-contrast CT study reveals a hyperdense mass owing to tightly packed hyphae within the involved sinus with associated erosion of the sinus wall.[12] Contiguous extension into the region of the orbital apex produces the orbital apex syndrome.

Non-invasive mycotic colonization (commonly called a fungal ball) has been formally referred to as a mycetoma or aspergilloma. The disease usually occurs in a single sinus, most commonly the maxillary one. It may occur in association with a chronically diseased sinus to a polyp.[12] Non-contrast CT shows a well-defined mass of high attenuation within the involved sinus. A hypodense rim is seen adjacent to the sinus wall due to inflammatory mucosal thickening. Occasionally calcification may also be seen. MRI shows hypointense mass on T1 and T2 weighted sequences.

Allergic fungal sinusitis usually occurs in adolescent or young patients with histories of recurrent sinusitis. Nasal polyposis is frequently associated. Allergic fungal sinusitis usually involves multiple sinuses and expands them. High attenuation masses with sinus expansion and bone remodeling on an unenhanced CT raise suspicion of this entity.

Local Mucosal Complications of Sinusitis

Inflammatory polyp: This is the most common mucosal complication of chronic sinusitis. A polyp is composed of heaped up mucosa elevated by inflammation into polypoidal shape.[13] Polyps may occur in an isolated fashion when inflammatory or fill the entire sinonasal cavity as in sinonasal polyposis. A large polyp may fill the sinus cavity and then obstruct sinus drainage. An antral polyp may expand and prolapse through the sinus ostium, presenting as a nasal polyp. These are referred to as antrochoanal polyp. As the polyp continues to grow, it fills the ipsilateral nasal fossa and extends back into the nasopharynx (Fig. 27.23).

Mucus retention cyst: Inflammatory obstruction of the seromucinous glands of the sinus lining causes the mucus retention cyst. CT commonly demonstrated a low-density, smooth-walled mass in the dependant portion of the affected sinus. The maxillary sinus is most commonly affected (Fig. 27.24). Imaging studies cannot differentiate a small intrasinus polyp and the retention cyst clearly.

Mucocele: Mucoceles consist of mucoid secretions surrounded by cuboidal epithelium.[14] Unlike retention cysts mucocele completely fills the sinus and expands the sinus. There is bone remodeling from chronic expansion without reactive sclerosis. Mucoceles most commonly occur in frontal sinus, followed by ethmoid sinus. Symptoms may result from local mass effect. CT scans show the affected sinus to be expanded and filled with low attenuation mucoid material. Typically, there is no enhancement. The sinus wall is thin, remodeled, or dehiscent. On MR the signal intensity of the mucocele may

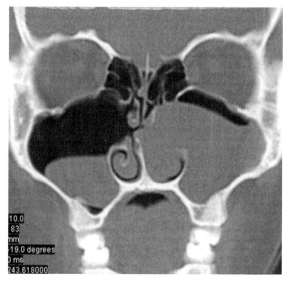

Fig. 27.23: Antrochoanal polyp. Coronal CT image shows low attenuation masses in both the maxillary sinuses. Note the expansion of the left infundibulum caused by herniation of the polyp into the left nasal cavity

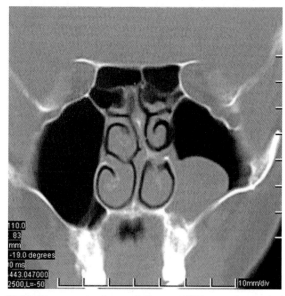

Fig. 27.24: Mucous retention cyst. Coronal CT image demonstrates a low density, well-defined mass in the dependant portion of the left maxillary sinus

vary depending on the age. With increase in protein content, there may be increase in T1 signal intensity. When desiccated, T2 signal intensity will decrease.

Regional Complications of Acute Sinusitis

These complications occur due to spread of infection through the emissary veins of the skull or due to extensive contiguous spread.

Orbital cellulitis and abscess: Ethmoid sinusitis can lead to subperiosteal abscess along the medial orbital wall. CT scan with contrast is performed when orbital involvement is suggested clinically (Fig. 27.25).

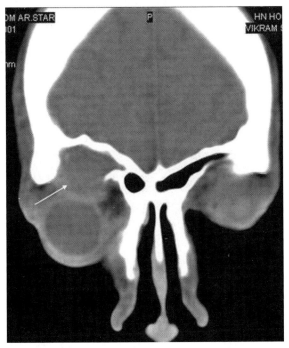

Fig. 27.25: Orbital cellulitis as a complication of sinusitis. Coronal CT image through the orbits shows downward displacement of the right globe caused by a subperiosteal abscess (arrow). Note the destruction of the inferior wall of the right frontal sinus

Intracranial complications: These include meningitis, subdural empyema, brain abscess and cavernous sinus thrombosis. Contrast enhanced MR is far superior to CT in identifying the presence of these diseases. In meningitis, MR would show meningeal enhancement. Brain abscess may be seen either in conjunction with subdural empyema or alone. Cavernous sinus thrombosis causes multiple cranial nerve neuropathy (cranial nerves III, IV, VI, V1, V2). CT and MR scans show enlarged cavernous sinus with non-enhancing areas within the sinus itself.

Noninfectious Destructive Sinonasal Disease

Wegener's granulomatosis is a necrotizing granulomatous vasculitis involving the upper and lower respiratory tracts and causes renal necrotizing glomerulonephritis. Wegener's granulomatosis is a systemic vasculitis that can affect any organ system, but primarily involves the upper and lower respiratory tracts and the kidneys. Chronic sinusitis is a well-known clinical feature of the disease. Specific bony findings include bony erosion and

destruction of the septum and turbinates; erosion of the ethmoid sinuses; neo-osteogenesis of the maxillary, frontal, and sphenoid sinuses; and complete bony obliteration of the maxillary, frontal, and sphenoid sinuses. Although these findings are suggestive of Wegener's granulomatosis, they are not pathognomonic. Bony changes on sinus CT scan may provide radiologic evidence of underlying Wegener's granulomatosis when clinical suspicion is high.[15]

Idiopathic midline granuloma is a more lympho-reticular disorder than a real granulomatous disease. It is now referred to as malignant midline reticulosis or polymorphic reticulosis. Idiopathic midline granuloma (IMG) is a rare, slowly progressive inflammatory process producing localized destruction of the nasal mucosa, septum, paranasal sinuses, and palate, often associated with erosion through central facial tissue and bone. The CT findings are not specific. Any large mass in the nose and nasal fossa with little associated bone destruction should, however, raise the differential diagnosis of polymorphic reticulosis.[16]

Midfacial necrosis due to the abuse of inhaled cocaine is included in the differential diagnosis of the midline destructive diseases such as Wegener's granulomatosis, polymorphic reticulosis, nasal lymphoma, infections and the idiopathic midline destructive disease. Cocaine-induced granuloma of the nasal septum is the primary component of this lesion.

Sarcoidosis of the sinuses should be considered in the differential diagnosis of sinusitis, especially in association with nasal polyposis, even when the sarcoidosis has not been otherwise diagnosed. Radiologic studies showed extensive and often complete opacification of the sinuses and nose similar to that seen in diffuse polyposis associated with chronic bacterial and fungal sinusitis.[17]

Tumors

Over half the patients with tumors of the sinonasal tract, benign or malignant, present initially with at least one of the following symptoms: Pain, nasal obstruction, epistaxis, and/or persistent nasal secretion. The first goal for the radiologist is to recognize the disease and to attempt to differentiate benign from malignant disease. Histological characterization of the disease process is usually not possible based on imaging. CT and MR imaging play complementary roles in defining the extent of the tumor. CT allows evaluation of the fine bony detail and infiltrative osseous involvement. MR imaging provides excellent delineation of tumor surrounding soft tissue, inflamed mucosa and retained secretions. About 95% of the tumors on MR appear hypo- to isointense on T1-weighted images, hyperintense on T2-weighted images and enhance with contrast administration.

A wide variety of benign and malignant tumors may affect the nasal cavity or paranasal sinuses. Primary tumors are derived from the lining of these structures, the nerves passing through, or the supporting elements i.e. the bone and cartilage of the sinuses and nose.[18]

Angiofibroma

The nasopharyngeal angiofibroma is a benign but locally aggressive tumor arising from the fibrovascular stroma on the posterolateral nasal wall adjacent to the sphenopalatine foramen. The common clinical presentation is of an adolescent male with a nasal mass and history of epistaxis. Extension into the pterygopalatine fossa occurs in 89% of the cases and results in widening of this fossa with resultant anterior bowing of the posterior ipsilateral antral wall. Other directions of tumor spread include: posteriorly into the nasopharynx, via the foramen rotundum into the middle cranial fossa and through the inferior orbital fissure into the orbits. The diagnosis by computed tomography (CT) is based upon the site of origin of the lesion in the pterygopalatine fossa. There are two constant features:

1. An enhancing mass in the posterior nasal cavity and pterygopalatine fossa.
2. Erosion of bone behind the sphenopalatine foramen with extension to the upper medial pterygoid plate.

Good bone imaging on CT is essential to show invasion of the cancellous bone of the sphenoid. This is the main predictor of recurrence: The deeper the extension, the larger the potential tumor remnant likely to be left following surgery. The characteristic features on MRI are due to the high vascularity of the tumor causing signal voids and strong postcontrast enhancement. MRI shows the preoperative soft tissue extent of angiofibroma optimally, but its more important application is to provide postoperative surveillance: To show any residual or recurrent tumor, record tumor growth or natural involution and monitor the effects of radiotherapy (Fig. 27.26).[19]

Papilloma

The mucosa of the nasal cavity and paranasal sinuses can give rise to three histologically distinct papillomas: Fungiform, inverted, and cylindric cell. Collectively they are also called Schneiderian papillomas.[18] Fungiform papillomas usually occur in males between the ages of

40 to 70 years. About 95% arise on the nasal septum and have a warty or verrucous appearance. They are quite unlikely to undergo malignant transformation.

The inverted papillomas also commonly occur in the same age group. Characteristically, they tend to arise from the lateral wall of the nose, 90% from the central portion of the middle meatus and extend into the sinuses. Secondary sinusitis and tumor extension into the sinuses and orbits can cause pain, purulent nasal discharge, proptosis, and diplopia. An associated squamous carcinoma has been reported in 2 to 56%. On CT, a lobulated mass is seen which tends to remodel bone rather than destroy bone (Fig. 27.27).

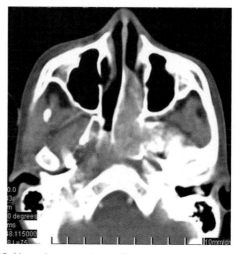

Fig. 27.26: Nasopharyngeal angiofibroma. Contrast-enhanced axial CT of the paranasal sinus shows an enhancing soft tissue mass that fills the left posterior nasal cavity and extends into the left pterygopalatine fossa

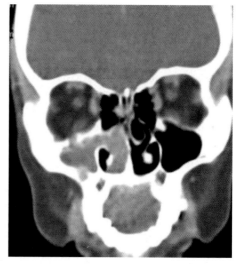

Fig. 27.27: Inverted Papilloma. Coronal CT image shows a soft tissue lesion arising from the right middle meatus, extending into the right maxillary sinus

The cylindrical cell papillomas arise in the maxillary sinus and are relatively rare.

Squamous Cell Carcinoma

Squamous cell carcinoma is the most common neoplasm of the nasal cavity and paranasal sinuses, and the maxillary sinus is the most common site of occurrence, either by primary or secondary involvement. The next common site of origin is the nasal cavity, followed by the ethmoids. Elderly males are affected, and the incidence is markedly increased in patients with exposure to wood, dust, nickel, snuff and chrome pigment. The American Joint Cancer Commission stages maxillary sinus tumors as follows:[20]

T1 stage: Tumor confined to the antral mucosa with no erosion or destruction of bone.

T2 stage: Tumor with erosion or destruction of the infrastructure including the hard palate or middle nasal meatus.

T3 stage: Tumor with invasion of any of the following: skin of the cheek, posterior wall of the maxillary sinus, floor or medial wall of the orbit, anterior ethmoid sinus.

T4 stage: Tumor involves orbital contents or any of the following: cribriform plate, posterior ethmoid or sphenoid sinuses, nasal pharynx, soft palate, pterygoid maxillary or temporal fossa, or base of skull.

The maxillary sinus can be divided into an inferior-anterior portion and a superior-posterior portion, the infrastructure and a suprastructure, respectively, by Ohngren's line, which is drawn from the medial canthus to the angle of the mandible. In general, tumors arising in the infrastructure of the sinus have a better prognosis than tumors arising in the suprastructure of the sinus.

Symptoms are often indolent, and because they are similar to benign sinusitis complaints, delay in diagnosis is common. Presenting symptoms include unilateral nasal obstruction, minor epistaxis, nasal discharge, and low-grade infection. Tooth pain, proptosis and diplopia, trismus, and headache imply extension to the palate, orbit, infratemporal fossa, or anterior skull base, respectively.

On CT, these tumors appear as sinonasal masses with bone infiltration and destruction. The mass is homogenous except for the areas of necrosis (Fig. 27.28). On T1-weighted images the mass is iso- to hypointense; on T2 the mass is slightly hyperintense. After contrast administration, on CT or MR, mild, heterogeneous enhancement is noted. Perineural involvement along the branches of the

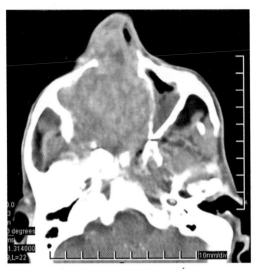

Fig. 27.28: Squamous cell carcinoma. Contrast-enhanced axial CT image shows a large destructive lesion of the right ethmoid sinus that has extended into the nasal cavity and the right maxillary sinus

trigeminal nerve may be evaluated with CT, which shows fine bony erosion, or MR, which can show the tumor extension directly. Nodal groups more commonly involved include submandibular, high internal jugular, and retropharyngeal. The incidence of nodal metastases increases with local recurrence.

Adenocarcinoma

Adenocarcinomas are the second most common malignancy involving the sinonasal tract. They typically occur in middle-aged or elderly and the most common site of origin is the ethmoid sinus. On CT, the lesion may either remodel bony margins or destroy bone with high-grade tumors. Commonly, tumors extend into the nasal cavity; less commonly there is extension intracranially through the cribriform plate.

Adenoid Cystic Carcinoma

The sinonasal tract is a common area of minor salivary gland involvement with adenoid cystic carcinoma. The hallmark of this tumor is perineural spread. The tumor is slow-growing but locally aggressive.

Mucoepidermoid Carcinoma

Mucoepidermoid carcinomas arise from the minor salivary glands. Most of these tumors involve the antrum and the nasal cavity. They are usually intermediate or high-grade lesions resembling adenocarcinomas.

Esthesioneuroblastoma

These arise from the neurosensory receptor cells in the olfactory epithelium of the high nasal vault. They have a bimodal age distribution occurring at 10–20 years and at 50–60 years. These tumors typically grow inferiorly into the nasal cavity and extend into the ethmoid sinuses. Common routes of spread are up through the cribriform plate into the anterior cranial fossa, and through the ethmoid sinus into the orbit. Enhanced CT or MR scans show a moderately enhancing mass centered in the cephalad nasal cavity with associated cribriform plate and sinus wall destruction. An uncommon finding for esthesioneuroblastoma is cysts seen along the intracranial margin of the mass (Fig. 27.29).

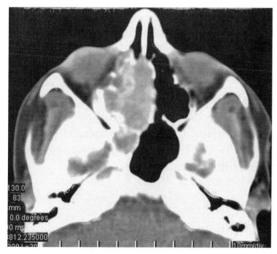

Fig. 27.29: Esthesioneuroblastoma. Axial contrast-enhanced CT scan shows a enhancing mass lesion destroying the medial wall of the right orbit

Malignant Melanoma

Sinonasal tract melanomas are rare. Melanomas are more common in the nasal cavity than in the sinuses. They tend to remodel bone, although bone erosion may also be present. As they are very vascular, they enhance on contrast CT and MR scans. Some melanomas have high signal intensity on T1WI primarily because of the presence of hemorrhage.

Rhabdomyosarcoma

This is one of the common soft tissue tumors in children under 15 years of age, with head and neck as principal locations. On imaging, these tumors are found within the maxillary sinus; they show a poorly defined homogenous mass, and there is destruction of the adjacent bone.

Lymphoma

The paranasal sinuses and nasal cavity are not common sites for lymphoma. The majority of sinonasal lymphomas are immunotyped as T-cell lymphoma.[21] The maxillary sinuses are most frequently involved. On CT and MRI, lymphomas in the sinonasal cavities tend to be bulky soft tissue masses that enhance to a moderate degree with evidence of bony remodeling and destruction.

Chondrosarcoma

Chondrosarcomas of the sinonasal cavities are rare. About 60% arise in the anterior maxillary alveolus: patients usually complain of nasal obstruction, loose teeth, poorly fitting dentures or an expansile painless mass. On CT these tumors have areas of nodular or plaque-like calcification. These tumors expand and destroy the bone.

Osteosarcoma

Osteosarcomas account for 0.5 to 1% of sinonasal tumors. They may arise de novo or be associated with radiation, Paget's disease, or fibrous dysplasia. They usually occur in adult men. The lesion appears as soft tissue masses with aggressive bone destruction. New bone formation with a sunburst pattern may be present.

Giant Cell Tumors

Giant cell lesions of the sinonasal tract are rare. They may be divided into giant cell reparative granulomas and giant cell tumors. The giant cell reparative granulomas most frequently involve the mandible or maxilla of young women, while the giant cell tumors present later in life. Radiologically, these lesions are indistinguishable, presenting as an expansile soft tissue mass with local bony invasion.

Fibro-osseous Lesions

Osteomas

Osteoma is a benign proliferation of bone that occurs almost exclusively in the skull and facial bones. Osteoma of the paranasal sinuses is a rare and benign entity that develops slowly. If they occur, locations within the frontal sinus and ethmoid cells are more frequent, whereas osteomas in the sphenoid or maxillary sinus are very rare. Osteomas are usually small and incidental findings on plain films. When multiple osteomas are seen, primarily in the skull and mandible, the diagnosis of Gardner syndrome should be considered. On CT, osteomas arise from the sinus walls (Fig. 27.30) or the intersinus septum. The degree of bone-matrix density seen within the lesion depends on the type of osteoma: Compact, cancellous, and fibrous. MRI shows these lesions to be of low to intermediate densities on all sequences.

Other rare fibro-osseous tumors involving the paranasal sinuses include osteochondromas, osteoid osteomas, and osteoblastomas.

Fibrous dysplasia and Paget's disease also involve the paranasal sinuses. The imaging appearance in Paget's disease depends on the phase of the disease. Fibrous dysplasia may be mono-ostotic or polyostotic. The radiological appearance varies, according to the degree of fibrous tissue present. Thus, the bone texture can range from a non-homogeneous mixture of bone and fibrous tissues to a predominantly fine bony, ground glass appearance (Fig. 27.31).

Ossifying fibroma is a dense cellular, well-circumscribed fibrous tumor that ossifies, starting at the periphery. In ossifying fibromas, the initial lesion is radiolucent, but it progressively becomes radiopaque, with sharp margins and dilated vascular channels.

It may be difficult on imaging and pathology to differentiate between fibrous dysplasia and ossifying fibromas (Fig. 27.32).[22]

Odontogenic Cysts

Odontogenic cysts arise from the various components of the dental apparatus.

Dentigerous cyst arises in an unerupted tooth, after the crown of the tooth has developed. Radiographically, it is a cyst into which the crown of the tooth projects. Small cysts are usually unilocular, while large ones may be multilocular. Maxillary dentigerous cysts extend into the maxillary antra or nasal cavities and cause expansion of the antral cavity (Fig. 27.33).

Periapical, radicular or dental cyst arises in erupted, infected tooth. Radiographically, the radicular cyst is a well-circumscribed radiolucency arising from the apex of the tooth and is bordered by a thin rim of cortical bone. Extension into the maxillary sinus can be observed if the cyst occurs in the maxilla (Fig. 27.34).

Odontogenic keratocysts are aggressively growing lesions and are associated with Marfan's syndrome and the basal cell nevus syndrome. They are more common in the mandible than the maxilla. CT shows a water density, sharply defined, cystic lesion. These cysts may be destructive and invade the adjacent bone.

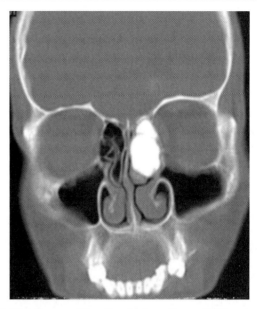

Fig. 27.30: Osteoma of the ethmoid sinus. Coronal CT image shows a bone density lobulated mass in the left ethmoid bone

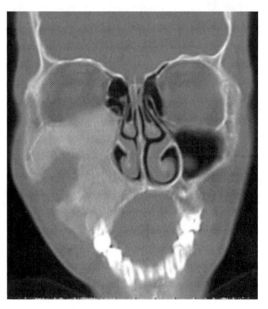

Fig. 27.31: Fibrous dysplasia. Coronal CT image shows expansion and ground glass appearance of the right maxilla

Odontogenic Tumors

Ameloblastoma is a slowly growing solid and cystic tumor. About 80% of these tumors are located in the mandible and 20% in the maxilla.[23] Radiographically, ameloblastoma may be a unilocular or multilocular radiolucent lesion. The CT findings of ameloblastoma consist of low attenuation cystic areas intermixed with isodense areas, reflecting the solid component of this lesion

(Fig. 27.35). The other odontogenic tumors to involve the paranasal sinuses are cementoma, odontoma, and fibromyxoma.

Metastases to the Paranasal Sinuses

The majority of metastases to the sinonasal tract are through hematologic spread to the bone. Renal, breast, lung, and prostate are among the most common primary sites. The most common site of involvement is the maxillary antrum.[24]

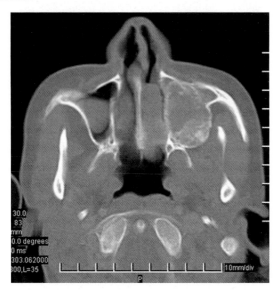

Fig. 27.32: Ossifying fibroma: Axial CT image shows a non-ossified mass with surrounding cortex in the left maxillary sinus

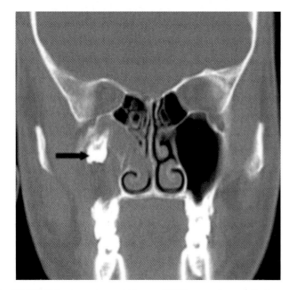

Fig. 27.33: Odontogenic cyst. Coronal CT image demonstrates an ill-defined cystic structure arising from the roof of the right alveolar arch. The lesion contains an unerupted tooth within (black arrow)

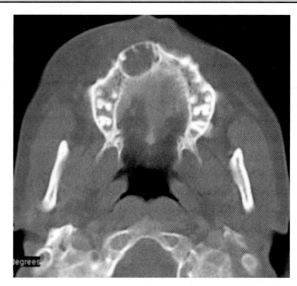

Fig. 27.34: Dental cyst. Axial CT image shows a well-defined corticated lucency arising from the apices of the incisor teeth

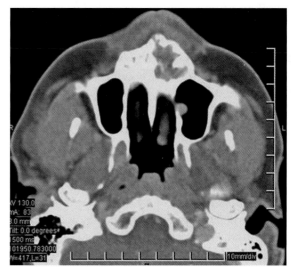

Fig. 27.35: Ameloblastoma. Axial CT image shows an ill-defined, lytic lesion arising from the alveolar arch. There is an isodense soft tissue seen within this lesion

ACKNOWLEDGMENT

We thank Dr Arpit M Nagar, DMRD, DNB, Department of Radiology, KEM Hospital, Mumbai for helping with editing of manuscript and the figures.

REFERENCES

1. Mafee MF. Endoscopic sinus surgery: Role of radiologist. *Am J Radiol* 1991; 157:1099–1104.
2. Lloyd GAS, Lund VJ, Phelps PD, Howard DJ. Magnetic resonance imaging in the evaluation of nose and paranasal sinus disease. *Br J Radiol* 1987; 60(718):957–968.

3. Shankar L, Evans K, Hawke M. *An atlas of imaging of the paranasal sinuses.* Toronto: Imago Publishing Ltd, 1994; 41–72.

4. Laine FJ, Kuta AJ. Imaging the sphenoid bone and basiocciput: Pathologic considerations. *Semin Ultrasound CT MR* 1993; 14(3):160–177.

5. Faust RA, Phillips CD. Assessment of congenital bony nasal obstruction by 3-dimensional CT volume rendering. *Int J Pediatr Otorhinolaryngol* 2001; 61(1):71–75.

6. Kalinger MA, Osguthorpe JD, Fireman P, Anon J, Georgitis J, Davis ML, *et al.* Sinusitis: Bench to bedside. Current findings, future directions. *Otolaryngol Head Neck Surg* 1997; 116(6 Pt 2):S1–S20.

7. Potsic WP, Wetmore RF. Pediatric rhinology. In *The Principles and Practice of Rhinology,* JL Goldman (Ed). New York: John Wiley & Sons Inc, 1987; 801–845.

8. Fried MP, Relly JH, Strome M. Pseudomonas rhinosinusitis. *Laryngoscope* 1984; 94:192–196.

9. Drutman J, Harnsberger HR, Babbel RW, Sonkens JW, Braby D. Sinonasal polyposis: Investigation by direct coronal CT. *Neuroradiology* 1994; 36(6):469–472.

10. Towbin R, Dunbar JS, Bove K. Antrochoanal polyps. *Am J Roentgenol* 1979; 132(1):27–31.

11. Gwaltney Jr JM, Phillips CD, Miller RD, Riker DK. Computed tomographic study of the common cold. *N Engl J Med* 1994; 330:25–30.

12. deShazo RD, Chapkin K, Swain RE. Fungal sinusitis. *N Engl J Med* 1997; 337(4):254–259.

13. Jacobs M, Som PM. The ethmoidal 'polypoidal mucocele'. *J Comput Assist Tomogr* 1982; 6(4):721–724.

14. Som PM, Shugar JM. CT classification of ethmoid mucoceles. *J Comput Assist Tomogr* 1980; 4(2):199–203.

15. Yang C, Talbot JM, Hwang PH. Bony abnormalities of the paranasal sinuses in patients with Wegener's granulomatosis. *Am J Rhinol* 2001; 15(2):121–125.

16. Teng MM, Chang CY, Guo WY, Li WY, Chang T. CT evaluation of polymorphic reticulosis. *Neuroradiology* 1990; 31(6):498–501.

17. deShazo RD, O'Brien MM, Justice WK, Pitcock J. Diagnostic criteria for sarcoidosis of the sinuses. *J Allergy Clin Immunol* 1999; 103(5 Pt 1):789–795.

18. Barnes L, Verbin RS, Gnepp DR. Disease of the nose, paranasal sinuses, and nasopharynx. *Surgical Pathology of the Head and Neck* Vol I. New York: Marcel Dekker Inc, 1985; 403–451.

19. Lloyd G, Howard D, Lund VJ, Savy L. Imaging for juvenile angiofibroma. *J Laryngol Otol* 2000; 114(9):727–730.

20. American Joint Committee on Cancer. Maxillary sinus. In *AJCC Cancer Staging Manual.* Philadelphia: Lippincott-Raven, 5th edn, 1997; 47–52.

21. Harnsberger HR, Bragg DG, Osborn AG, Smoker WR, Dillon WP, Davis RK et al. Non-Hodgkin's lymphoma of the head and neck: CT evaluation of nodal and extranodal sites. *Am J Neuroradiol* 1987; 149(4):785–791.

22. Barnes L. Verbin RS, Gnepp Dr. Diseases of the nose, paranasal sinuses and nasopharynx. In *Surgical Pathology of the Head and neck,* Vol.1, Barnes L (Ed). New York: Marcel Dekker Inc, 1985; 883–1044.

23. Mehlisch DR, Dahlin DC, Masson JK. Ameloblastoma: A clinicopathologic report. *J Oral Surg* 1972; 30(1):9–22.

24. Kubal WS. Sinonasal imaging: Malignant disease. *Semin Ultrasound CT MR.* 1999; 20(6):402–425.

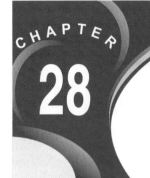

CHAPTER 28

The Subcranial Approach to the Anterior Skull Base

Ziv Gil, Dan M Fliss

The surgical treatments used for tumors involving the anterior skull base have evolved over the past 30 years. The rationale for craniofacial resection initially described by Smith et al,[1] Ketcham et al,[2] and Van Buren et al[3] has been well established by improved preoperative imaging assessment, technical advances in tumor resection and reconstruction, improved postoperative care, and the fruitful cooperation of multidisciplinary teams involving otolaryngologists, neurosurgeons, craniomaxillofacial surgeons, and plastic and reconstructive surgeons. Despite the technical reproducibility of the classic approaches, modifications are continually being designed to enhance access to this anatomical region and improve the functional and the cosmetic postoperative results.[4–14]

The concept of a broad subcranial approach to the entire anterior skull base from the ethmoidal labyrinth roof to the clivus and laterally to the orbital roofs was first introduced by Raveh in 1978, in cases of traumatic injuries of the anterior skull base as an alternative to the traditional transfacial-transcranial skull base approaches. It was later adapted for the surgical extirpation of tumors involving this anatomic region.[15–21] This technique has several major advantages. It affords broad exposure of the anterior skull base from below rather than through the transfrontal route, providing excellent access to the orbital, sphenoethmoidal, and clival regions, as well as to the nasal and paranasal cavities. This allows intradural and extradural tumor removal and precise repair of traumatic fractures with dural tears, cerebrospinal fluid (CSF) leakage, and brain tissue herniation. The procedure is performed with minimal frontal lobe manipulation, the avoidance of external facial incisions, and adequate drainage of the paranasal spaces.

Reconstruction of skull base and craniofacial defects are essential following tumor excision in order to:

- Form a watertight dural seal.
- Provide a barrier between the contaminated naso-sinusoidal space and the sterile subdural compartment.
- Prevent airflow into the intracranial space.
- Maintain a functional sinonasal system.
- Provide a good cosmetic outcome.

A variety of approaches have been developed to accomplish these goals. A split calvarial bone graft, hydroxyapatite paste or titanium mesh may be used for bony cranial reconstruction. Autologous flaps (pericranial flap, galeal flap), temporalis fascia or fascia lata grafts, free flaps (rectus abdominis flap, radial forearm flap, latissimus dorsi flap) and artificial substitutions are often used for reconstruction of the skull base. Unfortunately, these methods have significant disadvantages. Local flaps are often insufficient in size for reliable restoration of extensive anterior skull base defects.[22] The microvascular technique for free flap reconstruction requires a highly specialized team, is more costly and carries significant morbidity.[23] Synthetic substitutions of dura and bone can induce chronic inflammation, carry high-risk of infection and are inferior to biological sources in terms of strength and sealing quality.[24] Autografts, such as fascia lata and temporalis fascia, had been used in the past for skull base reconstruction, but they were usually covered with a vascularized flap (e.g. free muscular flaps, pericranial or galeal flaps), assuming that an overlying vascular tissue was essential in order to preserve long-term viability of the fascial graft.[25]

The purpose of this chapter is to review the medical and surgical management of patients operated for anterior skull base tumors via the subcranial approach. The postoperative results and quality of life of these patients, as well as the cytogenetics analysis of anterior skull base tumors is reviewed.

PREOPERATIVE EVALUATION AND ANESTHESIA

All patients scheduled for operation are evaluated preoperatively by a head and neck surgeon, a neurosurgeon and an anesthesiologist. Patients younger than 18 years are also examined by a pediatrician. If a free flap is planned, preoperative physical examination by a plastic surgeon is essential. Radiological evaluation of the patients includes axial and coronal CT and MRI of the head and neck. Neuroangiographic evaluations may also be performed in cases of highly vascular tumors such as juvenile angiofibroma or hemangiopericytoma invading the skull base or the cavernous sinus.

Patients who underwent prior skull base or craniofacial procedures for extirpation of tumors are also evaluated using a positron emission tomography-CT hybrid (PET-CT) using the Discovery LS PET/CT system (GE Medical) prior to the operative procedure. The PET part of PET-CT is performed twice, using a 2D and a 3D acquisition protocols for comparison purposes. We reported an upstaging of 20% of the patients (10 of 50) using this method. Electromyographic monitoring of the cranial nerves may be carried out in selected cases. Neuronavigation (BrainLab® Interface) was also used in selected cases.

Broad-spectrum antibiotics consisting of a combination of cefuroxime and metronidazole are instituted perioperatively. All the patients are operated under general anesthesia, in the supine position and without shaving the hair at the surgical site.[26] No tracheostomy is performed.[27] A lumbar spine catheter is inserted for 3–5 days for CSF drainage to facilitate frontal lobe retraction and to reduce the risk of postoperative CSF leak.

THE SURGICAL TECHNIQUE OF THE SUBCRANIAL APPROACH

After the induction of anesthesia, the patient's hair is shampooed vigorously with 4% w/v chlorhexidine (Septal Scrub®), parted with a sterile comb along the proposed incision line, and tied in clumps by rubber bands. The operative field is then scrubbed with surgical sponges containing chlorhexidine solution (0.05% w/v) and draped with sterile towels that were clipped in place with surgical staples.

The skin is incised above the hairline and a bicoronal flap is created in a supraperiosteal plane. A flap is elevated anteriorly beyond the supraorbital ridges and laterally superficial to the temporalis fascia. The pericranial flap is elevated up to the periorbits, and the supraorbital nerves and vessels are carefully separated from the supraorbital notch (Fig. 28.1). The lateral and medial walls of the orbits are then exposed, and the anterior ethmoidal arteries are clipped or ligated. The pericranium is elevated above the nasal bones, and the flap is rotated forward and held over the face throughout the rest of the procedure (Fig. 28.2). Titanium micro- or miniplates are applied to the frontal bones and removed before the performance of the osteotomies to ensure the exact repositioning of the bony segments at the end of the operation. An osteotomy of the anterior or the anterior and posterior frontal sinus walls, together with the nasal bony frame, part of the medial wall of the orbit, and a segment of the superoposterior nasal septum, is then performed.[28–30] For a type A osteotomy, the anterior frontal sinus wall as well as the nasal frame are osteotomized and removed in one block (Figs 28.3A and B). If a type B osteotomy is planned, burr holes are made and the posterior frontal sinus wall is resected after the dura has been detached from the frontal, orbital and ethmoidal roofs (Figs 28.4 and 28.5A and B). A part of the distal nasal bone is preserved in order to support the nasal valve. In cases of lateral invasion of a tumor, the osteotomy lines can be extended to include the lateral segments of the orbital roofs. After the frontonaso-orbital (NFO) bone segment is osteotomized, it is stored in saline until the reconstructive procedure. A bilateral ethmoidectomy and a sphenoidotomy are then performed: This approach enables the exposure and assessment of the tumor in its circumference. The tumor is extirpated at this stage and the dura or brain parenchyma are also resected when involved by tumor. Frozen sections are taken during surgery in order to ensure tumor-free margins. One or both sides of the cribriform plate and olfactory filaments are preserved whenever possible.

COMBINATIONS OF THE SUBCRANIAL APPROACH

In cases of massive involvement of the lower and lateral segments of the maxilla, the pterygomaxillary fossa, or the orbitofrontal segment, a maxillectomy and a craniotomy are performed using a combination of the subcranial approach with the transfacial approach, the facial translocation approach, the transorbital approach or the midfacial degloving approach (Figs 28.6A and B to 28.7A and B).[31]

The orbitozygomatic approach along with the subcranial approach is used if the tumor extends to the middle cranial fossa or for lesions involving the cavernous sinus.[32] While using this technique, the bicoronal flap is extended anterior to the tragus. The zygomatic process

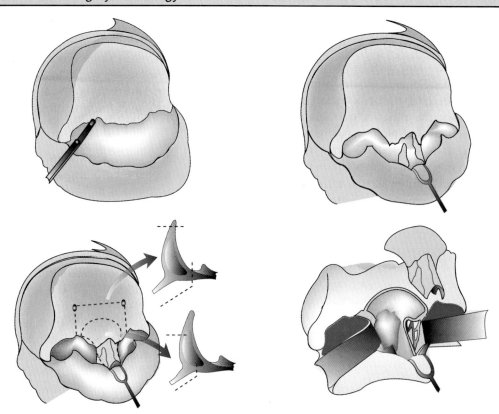

Fig. 28.1: The pericranial flap is elevated up to the periorbits, and the supraorbital nerves and vessels are carefully separated from the supraorbital notch. The superior and medial walls of the orbits are exposed, and the anterior ethmoidal arteries are clipped or ligated. The pericranium is elevated above the nasal bones, and the flap is rotated forward and held over the face throughout the rest of the procedure. The Nasofrontal-orbital (NFO) segment is osteotomized and stored in saline. (Adapted with permission from Fliss et al 2000, Operative Techniques in Otolaryngology Nasofrantal arbital Head and Neck Surgey)

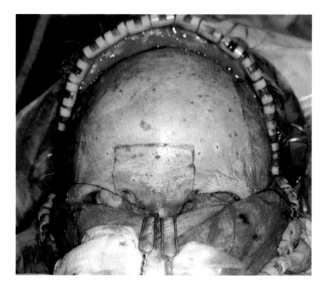

Fig. 28.2: Intraoperative picture of the surgical field following elevation of the pericranial flap and pericranium

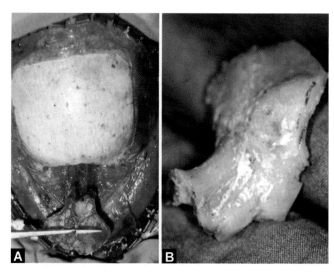

Figs 28.3A and B: Type A osteotomy; the anterior frontal sinus wall as well as the nasal frame are osteotomized and removed in one block. (A) the craniotomy. (B) The nasofronto-orbital segment

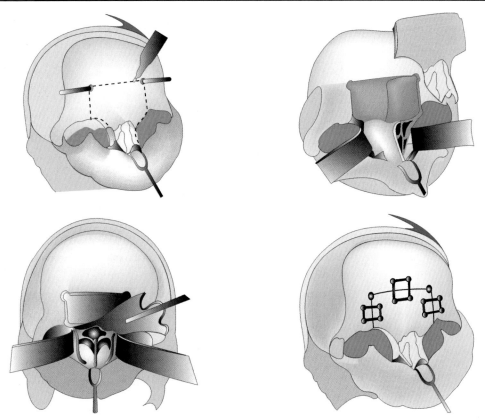

Fig. 28.4: Type B osteotomy. Burr holes are made and the posterior frontal sinus wall is resected after the dura has been detached from the frontal, orbital, and ethmoidal roofs. Adapted with permission from Fliss et al 2000, Operative Techniques in Otolaryngology Head and Neck Surgey

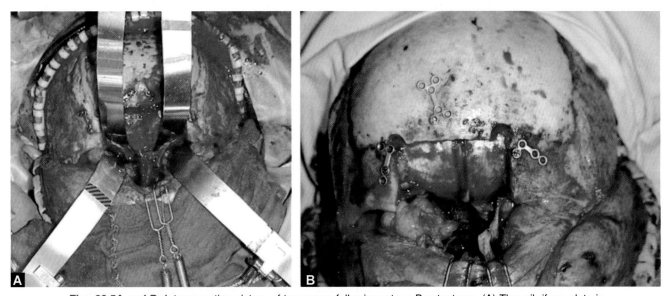

Figs 28.5A and B: Intraoperative picture of two cases following a type B osteotomy. (A) The cribriform plate is partially preserved. (B) Osteotomy of the NFO segment, and anterior skull base

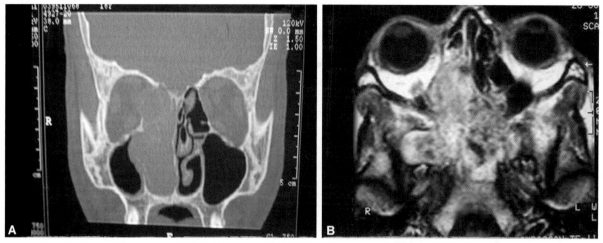

Figs 28.6A and B: A 17-year-old child with juvenile nasopharyngeal angiofibroma. (A) A coronal CT scan. (B) An axial T1 MRI with gadolinium

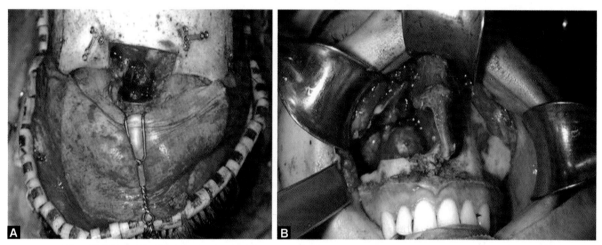

Figs 28.7A and B: (A) A partial maxillectomy was performed. (B) Along with the subcranial approach

along with the lateral orbital wall is osteotomized and removed and the temporalis muscle is displaced inferiorly. Care is taken not to injure the zygomatic branch of the facial nerve. This allows exposure of the pterional and infratemporal areas. A single bone flap craniotomy is then performed which allows access to the middle cranial fossa (Figs 28.8A and B). A two-piece craniotomy (i.e. a subcranial craniotomy followed by an osteotomy of the roof of the orbit, the zygomatic process of the frontal bone and part of the glabella across the midline) may be also performed.

RECONSTRUCTION FOLLOWING SUBCRANIAL SURGERY

Various surgical techniques for reconstruction of anterior skull base tumors have been established during the past 30 years.[33] Tumors that are located in this anatomical area may invade both soft and hard tissues of the skull base. In such cases, an en bloc tumor resection may create extensive skull base defects and produce a free conduit between the paranasal sinuses and the intracranial space. Following tumor extirpation, cranial base defects require reconstruction in order to provide a secure barrier between these two compartments. Reconstructive failure carries potential life-threatening complications (e.g. CSF leakage and meningitis) that may delay the initiation of adjuvant therapy.

Reconstruction of the anterior skull base is technically challenging and may be further complicated by several factors. First, there is a paucity of local tissue that is available for transfer into the defect. Second, previous radiation treatment significantly reduces tissue perfusion that delays normal wound healing. Finally, many of these patients have undergone multiple surgeries prior to the

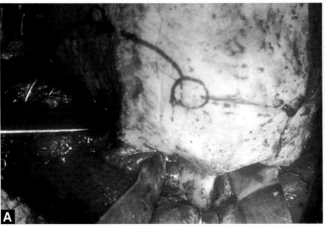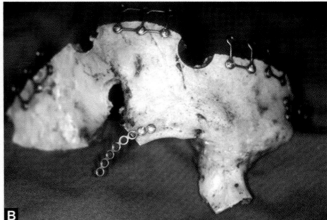

Figs 28.8A and B: The combined subcranial-orbitozygomatic approach. A subfrontal craniotomy is followed by an osteotomy of the roof of the orbit, the zygomatic process of the frontal bone part of the glabella across the midline and a pterional craniotomy. (A) Prior to the craniotomy. (B) The bone segment after the craniotomy

index operation, thus increasing its complexity and, secondary to scar tissue formation, decreasing tissue perfusion.

The reconstruction technique is designed according to the size of the cranial defect, based on radiological and intraoperative calculations. Primary closure of the dura is performed whenever possible. A graft of temporalis fascia is used if the defect is limited. In cases of extensive skull base defects, a second surgical team simultaneously harvests a large fascia lata sheath (20 × 10 cm).[34] The size of fascia used for reconstruction is tailored according to the dimension of the dural and skull base defects. The fascia is tucked under the edges of the dura and carefully sutured in place (Fig. 28.9). The dural repair is then covered with a second layer of fascia that is applied against the entire undersurface of the ethmoidal roof, the sella, and the sphenoidal area. Fibrin glue is used in order to provide additional protection against CSF leak. We initially had stented the subcranial area by means of polyethylene tubes externalized in the nasal lumen, with the tubes being left in place for a period of 6 months. However, in the last 40 operations in our series we cranialized the frontal area. A centripetal compression method is used to reduce the telecanthus. In this method, two threads are guided through the medial canthal ligament and driven underneath the frontonaso-orbital segment. The threads are tightened and fixed to the contralateral frontal plates in order to enable medial compression and alignment, thereby avoiding the telecanthus altogether. Vaseline gauze is applied to the reconstructed skull base to provide additional support against dural pulsation. After removing all the mucosa from its undersurface, the earlier

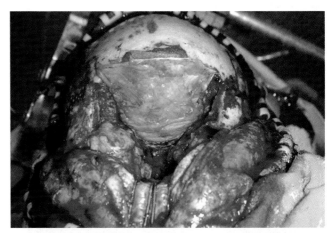

Fig. 28.9: The multilayered fascia lata for anterior skull base reconstruction. The first layer is tacked under the edges of the dura and carefully sutured in place. The dural repair is then covered with a second layer of fascia that is applied against the entire undersurface of the ethmoidal roof, the sella and the sphenoidal area. Fibrin glue is used in order to provide additional protection against CSF leak

osteotomized segment is repositioned in its original anatomical place and fixed with pre-bent titanium plates.

When the tumor involves the nasal bone or other fronto-orbital segments, a split calvarial bone graft or the posterior frontal sinus wall is used (Figs 28.10A and B). A bone graft can also be used for dorsal nasal support if the nasal septum has been resected. Reconstruction of the medial orbital walls is performed only in cases in which the total removal of this segment is necessary or if the periorbit is resected. In such cases, we use split calvarial bone grafts or 3-dimensional titanium mesh covered by pericranium (Figs 28.11A and B). Hydroxyapatite paste (Bonesource[©]) is used for small or medium defects of the calvarium following removal of the outer table.

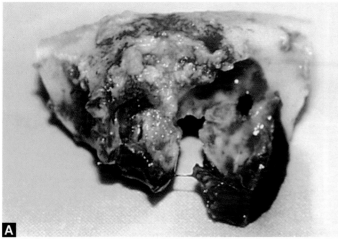
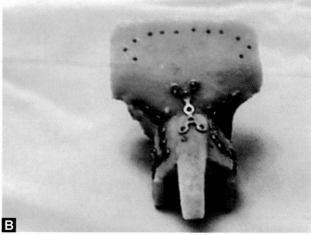

Figs 28.10A and B: When the tumor involves the nasal bone or other fronto-orbital segments, a split calvarial bone graft or posterior frontal sinus wall is used to reconstruct the excised bony segment. (A) The NFO segment infiltrated by the tumor. (B) The reconstructed segment from split calvarial bone graft

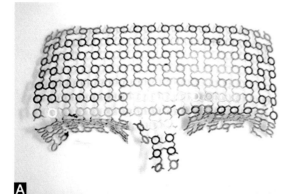

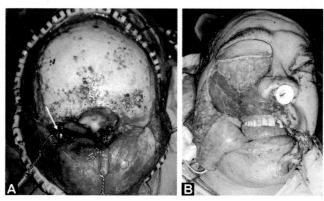

Figs 28.12A and B: In cases of eye globe exenteration, we use a temporalis muscle flap to cover the orbital socket: the anterior skull base is reconstructed using our standard method of double layer fascial graft. (A) This 42-year-old man had SCC of the ethmoid sinuses invading the anterior skull base and orbit (white arrow). (B) following reconstruction

In cases of eye globe exenteration, we use a temporalis muscle flap to cover the orbital socket. A composite rectus abdominus free flap is used to cover the orbital socket in cases of eye globe exenteration with radical maxillectomy, as well as in cases of a large anterior skull base tumor resection which also required radical maxillectomy (Figs 28.12A and B).

We did not use pericranial or galeal flaps or other regional flaps in order to reconstruct the skull base.

The pericranium is used only for patients undergoing extirpation of malignant tumors and for whom adjuvant radiation therapy is planned. This vascularized local flap is used in order to wrap the NFO segment for prevention of osteoradionecrosis (Figs 28.13A and B). This procedure begins with the removal of all the mucosa from the

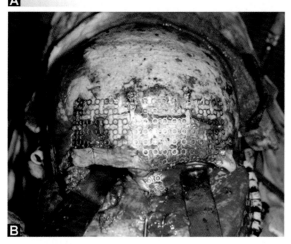

Figs 28.11A and B: If the orbital part of the NFO segment is excised, we use a 3-dimensional titanium mesh covered by pericranium. In this case the whole NFO segment was reconstructed by a titanium mesh. This 37-year-old man had recurrent SCC of the paranasal sinuses. In the second operation the NFO segment was partially damaged by the radiation. (A) 3D reconstruction of the NFO segment by titanium mesh. (B) The titanium mesh is attached to the skull using titanium screws

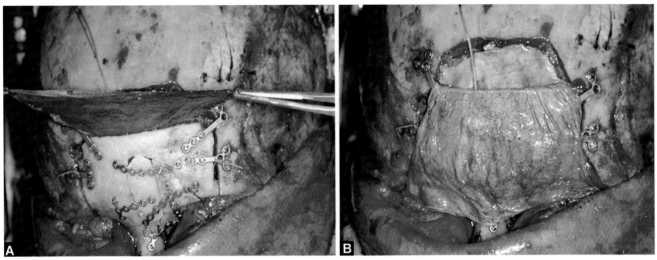

Figs 28.13A and B: (A) An intraoperative photograph showing the wrapping of the FNO segment with a pericranial flap, in a patient with SCC. (B) The entire bone flap is covered with a pericranial flap. This vascularized tissue is guided underneath the bony segment to cover the intranasal surface and then externalized over the entire frontal area. The patient was scheduled for radiation therapy following the operation

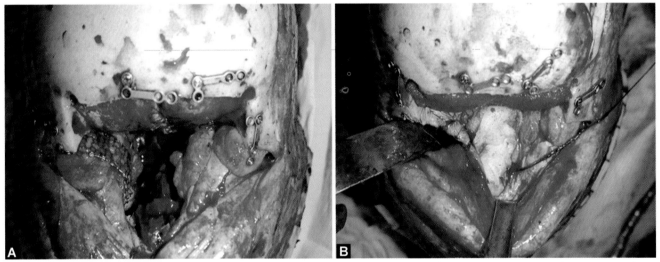

Figs 28.14A and B: A pericranial flap is also used in cases of medial orbital wall reconstruction, to cover the bone-graft segments or the titanium mesh. (A) Reconstruction of the orbit with a titanium mesh. (B) Wrapping of the titanium mesh

undersurface of the previously osteotomized bone segment. The frontal sinus bone is cranialized and the NFO segment is repositioned in its original anatomical position. Wrapping is accomplished by a double-sided covering of the bone segment with the pericranial flap. This vascularized tissue is guided underneath the bony segment to cover the intranasal surface and then it is externalized over the entire frontal area. The NFO segment and its overlying pericranial flap are fixed with the pre-bent titanium plates. A pericranial flap is also used in cases of medial orbital wall reconstruction to cover the bone-graft segments or the titanium mesh (Figs 28.14A and B).

In recent years, progress in various microvascular and surgical techniques has enabled the development and implementation of free tissue transfer. Free flaps may be used for massive skull base defects, with excellent surgical results and low complication rates.[35] The rectus abdominis is the most commonly used free flap in this anatomical area, followed by the radial forearm and latissimus dorsi flaps. Furthermore, free tissue transfer promises flexibility in flap content and design, and provides the opportunity to introduce a large quantity of well-vascularized tissue to the reconstructed area in a single-stage operation. Significant morbidity and mortality rates, however, were documented among elderly patients undergoing free flap reconstructions.[23] Free tissue transfer is a relatively complex surgical procedure, requiring especially high technical qualifications. Another drawback of this method is the bulk of the muscular free flap, which may mask local recurrence and make radiological follow-up more difficult.

In our series, we used a double layer fascial sheath as the standard procedure for anterior skull base reconstruction. In a previous report[1] we described a simple technique for harvesting large fascia lata sheaths which affords a low complication rate and low donor limb morbidity. The thin and low mass properties of the fascia lata enable the surgeon to cover large dural defects with a single fascial sheath. Furthermore, the flexibility of the fascia lata enables coating of extensive cranial defects, including parts of the orbit and paranasal sinuses. Large cranial base defects and prior surgery and radiotherapy (previously considered indications for free flap reconstruction[37]) were managed by fascia alone. Free flaps, autologous fat, or skin grafts were not necessary for achieving a reliable skull base reconstruction with excellent surgical outcome.

Several authors believe that bony reconstruction of the skull base is necessary to support the newly reconstructed skull base and to prevent herniation of the cranial content. However, our results showed that reconstruction with a double layer fascia does not require a rigid support of bone or of synthetic materials: Not one brain herniation occurred in our series.

The overall duration of the reconstructive procedure described herein is not longer than that of a pericranial flap,[8] and takes considerably less time than free tissue transfer procedures.[38] Routine postoperative radiological follow-up of patients after extirpation of malignant anterior skull base tumors is required in all cases. The relatively low bulk of the fascia lata assists in radiological follow-up in patients with an increased risk of local recurrence.

Vacuum drains are left in place and the incision is closed with inverted absorbable sutures and skin staples. After closing, the wound is covered with a thin film of antibiotic ointment. No dressing is used to cover the wound in order to permit easy access to the area of incision for examination and treatment.

POSTSURGICAL TREATMENT

After surgery, the patients are extubated and immediately transferred to the critical care unit for 24 hours.[33] The wound is kept clean by rinsing it with hydrogen peroxide 3 times a day during the first 10 days after the operation, and covered with antibiotic ointment after each cleansing. The drains are removed either 3 days after the operation or when the fluid was less than 20 ml in 24 hours. Broad-spectrum antibiotics (a combination of cefuroxime and metronidazole) are instituted preoperatively and continued for another 5–7 days. For pain control the patients are treated with tramadol 50–100 mg. Stool softeners are administered if there is a need to reduce the chance of Valsalva induced increase intracranial pressure. The lumbar drain is removed 3–5 days after the operation and the nasal packing is removed 7 days following the operation. The average stay in hospital is 10 ± 2 days. Routine CT is performed at the end of the procedure and 7 days following the operation.

Surgical Results

A retrospective evaluation of patients undergoing anterior skull base surgery was based on a review of the hospital charts and the outpatient clinical and radiological data of 189 consecutive cases operated between 1994 and 2005. All the resections and reconstructions were carried out by means of the subcranial approach to the anterior skull base. The patient age ranged from 2 to 81 years (mean 42 years): 102 patients were operated for extir-pation of anterior skull base tumors, 55 following craniobasal fractures, 15 due to cerebrospinal fluid leak, 7 to treat fungal and other infections (i.e. abscess and osteomyelitis) and 3 for reconstructive procedures following neurosurgical procedures (Fig. 28.15). There were no cases of recurrent CSF leak following anterior skull base reconstruction using the subcranial approach. In this chapter we report our experience with tumor resections of 44 malignant tumors (43%) and 58 had benign tumors (57%). Figures 28.16 and 28.17A and B show a typical case of a patient with juvenile

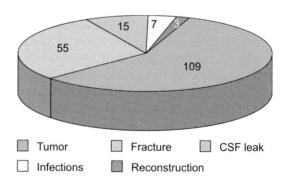

Fig. 28.15: We have used the subcranial approach in 189 cases. The graph shows the indications for using this approach

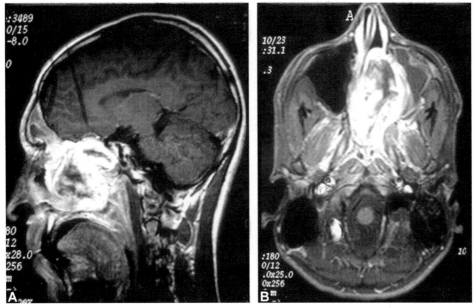

Figs 28.16A and B: A 17-year-old patient with juvenile angiofibroma invading. (A) Paranasal sinuses, anterior skull base, pterygopalatine fossa and cavernous sinus. (B) T1 MRI with gadolinium showing the extension of the tumor

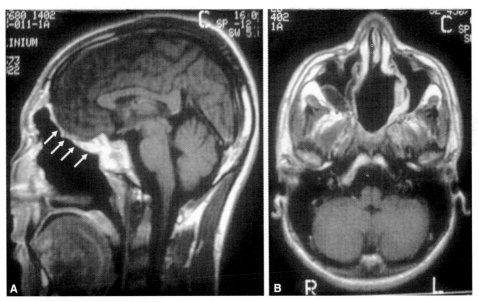

Figs 28.17A and B: A postoperative T1 MRI with gadolinium of the same patient as in Fig. 28.16 showing complete removal of the tumor. Arrows point at the anterior skull base reconstruction with two layers fascia lata

angiofibroma. Figures 28.18 to 28.20 show a case of a patient with malignant peripheral nerve sheath tumor.

There was no significant difference in age or sex between the two groups. The most common malignant tumor was squamous cell carcinoma and the most common benign pathology was meningioma. Table 28.1

provides a summary of the underlying tumors of the patients.

As many as 32 patients (31%) had undergone at least one previous operation and radiotherapy. The subcranial approach was used as a single procedure in 83 cases. It was combined with a midfacial degloving procedure in

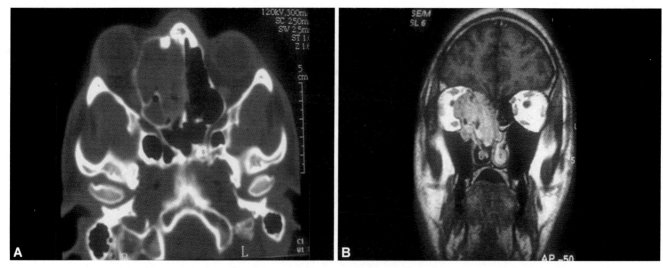

Figs 28.18A and B: A 21-year-old man with malignant peripheral nerve sheath tumor invading the right orbit. (A) An axial CT scan (B) T1 MRI with gadolinium

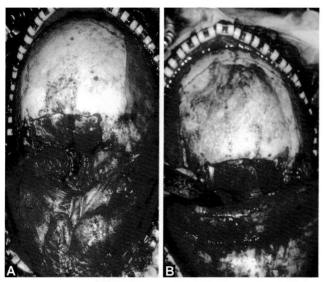

Figs 28.19A and B: Intraoperative picture of the patient in Fig. 28.18, following tumor extirpation. (A) The right orbital socket was reconstructed with a titanium mesh. (B) Following reconstruction of the skull base with fascia lata

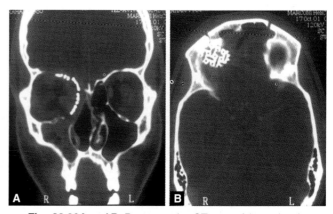

Figs 28.20A and B: Postoperative CT scan of the patient in Figs 28.18 and 28.19 showing complete removal of the tumor

11 cases, with transfacial/transorbital approaches in 7, with a pterional approach in another 6 and with transnasal endoscopic approach in 3 patients.

The mean hospital stay was 10 days. The overall complication rate among patients operated for extirpation of tumors was 30%. However, the incidence of CSF leak, intracranial infection and tension pneumocephalus was 3%. One patient who was operated upon for a pituitary adenoma and who suffered from meningitis and died 42 days after surgery. The overall postoperative complications associated with skull base and cranial reconstructions are listed in Table 28.1. Osteoradionecrosis with fistula was found in 5 patients, 4 of whom had undergone perioperative radiotherapy. Because of the risk for osteoradionecrosis of the frontonaso-orbital segment in patients who undergo perioperative radiation therapy, we developed a new method for skull base reconstruction. In these cases we used the pericranial flap for wrapping the NFO segment. There were no cases of bone flap necrosis in the patients who underwent this procedure. Two patients had wound dehiscence, which was associated with temporalis muscle transfer following

Table 28.1: Complications of skull base reconstruction procedures

Complication	N	(%)
Meningitis	2	2
CSF leak*	1	1
Tension pneumocephalus	1	1
Intracranial hematoma	2	2
Osteoradionecrosis and fistula	5	5
Wound infection	5	5
Mucocele	2	2
Telecanthus	5	5
Ptosis	2	2
Epiphora	5	7
Facial nerve paresis	1	1
Total	**31**	**29**

* Repaired following revision surgery.

orbital exenteration. They were successfully treated with local flaps several days after surgery. The oncological outcome in this series is shown in Table 28.2. All patients with malignant tumors were scheduled for radiation therapy (6000–7000 cGy).

We investigated the healing process of fascia lata grafts in 4 patients who had undergone a second surgery. Fragments of fascia lata that had previously been used for skull base reconstruction and had not been involved with the tumor were excised and submitted for histological examination. The fascia lata segment was fixed in 10% buffered formalin. Each specimen was embedded in paraffin and serially sliced (4 micrometers in thickness). The microsections were stained with hematoxylin and eosin. The degree of vascular proliferation and fibrotic reaction was evaluated by a senior pathologist. Microscopic examination revealed that the entire graft was composed of viable dense fibro-collagenous tissue. In large areas the bipolar, wavy nuclei of the fibroblasts were embedded in a collagenous stroma. The fibroblastic reaction was accompanied by proliferation of neovascular channels lined by plumped endothelial cells. The

Table 28.2: Histopathology of anterior skull base tumors

Pathology	No	A and W	AWD	DOD	DOC
Meningioma	16	15	1		
Mucocele	9	8			1
Osteoma	9	9			
Meningioencephalocele- encephalocele	9	9			
Inverted papilloma	6	5			1
A-V malformatiom	3	3			
Chordoma	3	2	1		
Neurofibromatosis I	2	2			
Angiofibroma	2	2			
Pituitary adenoma	1	1			
Hemangioma	1	1			
Epidermoid cyst	1	1			
Fibrous dysplasia	1	1			
Squamous cell carcinoma	12	10		1	1
Esthesioneuroblastoma	12	8	1	3	
Sarcoma	6	5	1		
Adenocarcinoma	3	1	2		
Malignant schwannoma	3	3			
Melanoma	3	2			1
Hemangiopericitoma	3	2			1
Plasmocytoma	2		2		
Adenoid cystic carcinoma	1	1			
Lymphoma	1	1			
Total (%)	**109**	**89 (80)**	**10 (10)**	**4 (4)**	**6 (6)**

A-V = arteriovenous malformation
A and W= alive and well; AWD= alive with disease; DOD = died of disease; DOC = died of other causes.

histological findings demonstrated an almost complete fibrous replacement of the fascia lata allograft.

USE OF THE SUBCRANIAL APPROACH IN THE PEDIATRIC PATIENT

There are several differences between cranial base tumors of adults and children. First, skull base tumors are relatively uncommon in children. Second, the types of tumors as well as the oncological management and prognosis of patients vary between adults and children. Third, anatomical differences, such as the size of the cranial fossa and paranasal sinuses or stage of tooth eruption, may also influence the choice of surgical approach.[39] A major concern of skull base procedures in children is the potential impact of osteotomies on the subsequent development of the face and paranasal sinuses. The feasibility of standard skull base procedures on the pediatric population and their potential effect on the long term esthetic results of these patients have not been established.

In a recent retrospective study we have reviewed the hospital charts and the outpatient clinical and radiological data of 67 consecutive pediatric surgeries for skull base tumors between May 1998 and May 2004. Eleven of these patients (14%) were operated via the subcranial approach to the anterior skull base (Fig. 28.21). These tumors include juvenile angiofibromas, sarcomas, squamous cell carcinomas and esthesioneuroblastoma.

From the study population, we have evaluated the maxillofacial growth of 11 children younger than 18 years on the day of surgery (mean 13.5 ± 4.5; range 6–18 years). X-ray films were analyzed in order to investigate the effect of the anterior subcranial approach on craniofacial development. Lateral cephalograms were taken

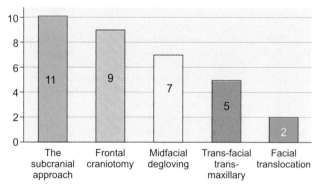

Fig. 28.21: The various approaches used for anterior skull base oncological extirpations of tumors in the pediatric population. Thirty-four children younger than 18 years were operated, among them 11 via the subcranial approach

post-operatively in order to assess facial growth. The results were matched against age-correlated standard Israeli population norms. Cephalometric studies included lateral cephalometric X-ray (time interval from surgery 1–7 years, mean 3.2 ± 2 years). Linear and angular measurements were made to the nearest 0.5 mm and 0.5°. A cephalometric analysis was performed on each cephalogram as described previously.[40] The data were compared to age-matched norms for the corresponding Israeli population. The errors were 0.1–0.8 mm for the linear measurements and 0.2°–0.9° for the angular measurements. The measurements performed were according to Riolo et al.[41] The reference planes used were:
1. SNA: Angle between sella turcica, nasion and A point (deepest point of maxillary alveolar ridge).
2. SNB: Angle between sella turcica, nasion and B point (deepest point of mandibular ridge).
3. The angle between the line connecting the Sella, Nasion and Occlusal plane (SN-OCC).

The average SNA showed non-significant deference from the norms (83.5° ± 4.8° and 82° for the study population and norms respectively), as well as the SNB (83.3° ± 5.4° and 80° respectively). The average SN-OCC in our group of children was also not significantly different from the norm (10.3° ± 4° and 14° respectively). These preliminary results show no significant difference between the study group and the normal values in the cranial base growth.

The most significant anatomical difference between children and adults is the size of the cranial base and maxillofacial complex. Another difference is the inconsistency of specific anatomical landmarks in children in comparison with the fully developed cranium of adults. For example, in children younger than 3 years, the mastoid tip may not be fully developed and so the facial nerve is more superficial and inferior than in adults. The mastoid air cells are also not fully pneumatized in very young children since the mastoid and middle fossa reach adult size after the age of 10.[42] The superior orbital fissure, which serves as a landmark for orbital and orbitozygomatic approaches, may also be absent in children younger than 8 years.[39] Another important anatomical discrepancy is the developmental stage of the paranasal sinuses: the frontal sinus starts to develop from the age of 6 years and reaches its full size at the end of puberty.[42] The surgeon must cautiously consider the variability in size of the frontal sinus if a frontal craniotomy is required. For example, a type A craniotomy of the subcranial approach involves osteotomy of the anterior frontal sinus wall alone. In such a case, we use intraoperative transnasal illumination of the frontal sinus in order to outline its borders before the osteotomies are carried out.

One of our key observations is that a child's brain is somewhat tighter than an adult's. For example, in a few cases neither ventriculostomy nor opening the basal cisterns was effective enough in reducing brain tightness during surgery. In contrast, similar measures carried out in an adult patient would have provided a marked improvement in brain relaxation. We could not find any data relating to the differences in brain elasticity in various age groups. We hypothesize, however, that the pediatric brain may be tighter because the sulci, fissures, and cisterns that comprise the subarachnoid space are generally smaller, leaving a relatively larger portion of the intracranial volume for the parenchyma. In addition, neurovascular elements in children are thinner and more fragile than in adults. Therefore, CSF drainage results in less brain relaxation than in adults. We suggest that using the subcranial or orbitozygomatic approaches can reduce brain retraction in the pediatric population, which might be even more significant than in adult neurosurgery.

A major issue in pediatric craniofacial surgery is the need to avoid disruption of the permanent dentition within the maxillary complex during maxillotomy, since permanent tooth eruption does not take place before the age of 10 years.[43] We also have avoided the use of the LeFort I down-fracture and transpalatal approaches for this reason. In order to avoid injury to the tooth buds, a dental panoramic X-ray or coronal CT scan is required for presurgical planning of the osteotomies. In our opinion, the midfacial degloving and transmaxillary approaches are suitable for wide exposure and extirpation of tumors originating in the paranasal sinuses and nasal cavity with preservation of normal tooth eruption.

The possibility of skull and craniofacial osteotomies having an impact on the growing head and face is of major importance. Our preliminary results of X-ray cephalometric analysis indicate that no significant deformation occurred in these patients. The youngest patient who underwent anterior skull base surgery was a 2-year-old child, and she has had normal craniofacial development throughout the 36 months following her operation.

POSTOPERATIVE CONTROL OF ACUTE PAIN FOLLOWING SUBCRANIAL EXTIRPATIONS

Pain was evaluated in 209 patients, 16 of them were scheduled for oncological subcranial surgery. In this group analgesics were administered only 'as needed' if the patient asked for them or if the nurses felt it to be necessary (PRN protocol). This treatment regimen consisted of an NSAID (diclofenac 75 mg intramuscularly or orally, or Rofecoxib 50 mg). Secondline treatment consisted of intramuscular meperidine 1 mg/kg (50 to 100 mg) repeated every 3 to 4 hours if required, but not exceeding a maximum of 150 mg as a single dose, or morphine via slow intravenous injection (4–10 mg, titrated according to effect).

On day one, 25% of the patients requested pain control medication. There was a 50% decline during the following 2.8 days, and fewer than 7% required pain control medication at one week following surgery. The most commonly prescribed drug was diclofenac.

A moderate degree of pain was recorded for the patients undergoing skull base surgery: pain varied from 3.5 ± 2.5 immediately following surgery to 1.3 ± 0.6 one week later (mean 2.65 ± 1) and its decline was slow ($t_{0.5} = 6$ days). There was a significant reduction in the level of pain one hour following drug application 'as needed' ($p < 0.001$) after all operations. Our data clearly showed that these patients reported the return of a substantial degree of pain as soon as the drug effect subsided several hours later.

In the second part of our study, we tailored a specific pain control protocol which included NSAIDs once daily and PRN tramadol 50–100 mg. These patients were treated with analgesics given at predetermined hours. Relative to the first group, there was a significant reduction in the level of pain for patients undergoing skull base surgeries ($p < 0.001$).

The overall results of the study show that a PRN protocol is not adequate for management of pain following surgery. Similar results were found for patients undergoing maxillofacial and major neck surgeries. Although we did find a reduction in the level of pain following drug administration, the patients reported a significant degree of pain during the intervals between drug administration as well as throughout the postoperative period. Based on these findings, we suggest treating these patients with scheduled NSAIDs, regardless of whether the patient complains of pain. Our results clearly showed a sharp reduction in the level of pain during the postoperative period among the patients who were medicated according to this protocol. Patients scheduled for skull base procedures also suffered a moderate degree of pain shortly after surgery: Unlike patients undergoing maxillofacial osteotomies, however, these patients reported a slow reduction in the level of pain. Patients undergoing skull base procedures most frequently required continuous drainage of CSF due to violation of the dura during surgery, and this mandates bed rest for five days until the drain is removed. These patients complained mainly of musculoskeletal and back pain due to lying in a supine position for a prolonged period of time. We therefore prescribed NSAIDs for these patients whether or not it was requested by the patient.

Patients after intracranial and skull base procedures are at risk for developing severe intracranial complications, such as meningitis, tension pneumocephalus and hemorrhage. Treatment of pain with a nonopiate analgesic allows close monitoring of the patient's neurological and mental conditions. We therefore preferred to administer tramadol PRN as an adjuvant pain control, since this drug is not very sedating.

NSAIDs have analgesic properties that are associated with opioid-sparing options and few side effects. Adequate postoperative analgesia may be provided by the routine administration of these drugs.[44] Furthermore, because these drugs do not induce respiratory depression or sedation, their administration may facilitate less intensive postoperative monitoring and allow close neurological follow-up following intracranial procedures. In addition, NSAIDs do not require sophisticated delivery mechanisms. If administered at regular intervals, regardless of whether or not the patient requested pain relievers, NSAIDs can decrease patient dependence on opioids with satisfactory results.

In summary, the PRN protocol was found to be inadequate for the management of pain following skull base surgeries. Our results suggest that patients undergoing skull base surgery should be treated with scheduled NSAIDs or tramadol for 5–7 days, whether or not they complain of pain.

CYTOGENETIC ANALYSIS OF SKULL BASE TUMORS

We have performed cytogenetics analysis on 100 tumors involving the anterior skull base; of these 18 were squamous cell and undifferentiated carcinomas.[45,46] G banding and spectral karyotyping (Figs 28.22 and 28.23) were used in order to find specific chromosomal aberrations. SCC of the nasal cavity and paranasal sinuses is a rare malignant neoplasm with an incidence of less than 1:200,000 per year. Nonkeratinizing (NK) squamous cell carcinoma (SCC) (also known as transitional cell carcinoma, intermediate cell carcinoma or schneiderian carcinoma) is considered a variant of SCC, whereas sinonasal undifferentiated carcinoma is a pathologically distinctive neoplasm which also lacks squamous differentiation. Both SNUC and NK SCC of the paranasal

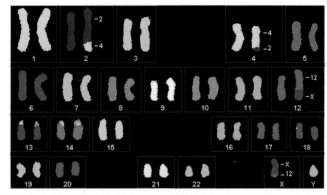

Fig. 28.22: A representative karyotype from the poorly differentiated non-keratinizing SCC. The karyotype of this tumor cell was: 46, XX, t(5; 11; 16) (q13; q13; q23), der (6)t(6; ?) (q23; ?), t(9; X) (q3; q23)

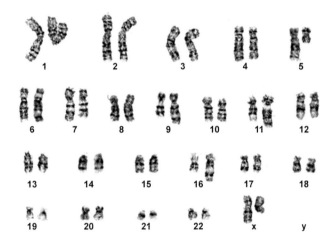

Fig. 28.23: Spectral karyotyping of a cell derived from a conventional chordoma: 46,XX,t(2;9),-3,t(3;19),t(5;15),+der(8)

sinuses are locally aggressive, and usually present as a large paranasal mass spreading into the anterior skull base, orbit, and dura. Complete surgical resection, followed by irradiation is the mainstay of treatment in these cases, and the 5-year survival prognosis for patients is 20–70%.[47,48]

The classification and different diagnosis of sinonasal carcinomas may be difficult. Due to their low frequency, the cytogenetic data on these tumors is limited, and the only previous study, which included 2 cases of adenocarcinoma and 3 of SCC reported various complex chromosomal abnormalities, with no specific karyotypic patterns.[49]

We have cytogenetically characterized the short-term cultures of NK SCC, and SNUC originating in the nasal cavity and paranasal sinuses. Most of these patients were operated via the subcranial approach.

Our study involves 18 patients who were operated in our institution in 2001-2004 for extirpation of sinonasal carcinomas. Of the 18 tumors 15 pathologically confirmed samples have successfully analyzed using conventional cytogenetic methods. Nine tumors originated in the maxillary sinus and 5 in the ethmoidal sinuses. One patient had undergone several excisions of SCC of the scalp. In his current operation the tumor invaded his ethmoid and sphenoid sinuses. All patients had received postoperative radiation therapy except one patient who had tumor recurrence and received 7700 cGy two years previous to her current operation. The oncological outcome of the patients is based on 10–42 months of clinical and radiological follow-up. Tumor staging was performed using the American Joint Committee on Cancer-Union Internationale Contre le Cancer (AJCC-UICC) 2002.

Cytogenetic Results

Fresh tumor samples were excised during surgery and submitted for pathological and cytogenetic analysis. Using G-banding technique 10–30 metaphase cells from primary cultures were studied in each specimen (230 metaphase overall). Seven of the 14 sinonasal carcinomas had an abnormal karyotype (50%).

Four of the nine NK SCC had chromosomal abnormalities. One tumor displayed two cytogenetically related clones and one subclone with 45–47 chromosomes. The principal chromosomal abnormality found in all cells of this case was inv(2)(p11;q13), which is frequently found in the Jewish population in Israel.[7] Another tumor had a near diploid complex karyotype with multiple structural abnormalities involving chromosomes: 1–3, 5–12, 14, 16–17, 19–22 and X. A third case showed a near diploid karyotype with loss of chromosome Y in 12 of the examined cells and a normal karyotype in 3 cells. The fourth tumor, which had suffered from NK-SCC originating in the maxillary sinus also had a complex karyotype involving 1p, 2p, 3q, 4p, 5p, 6q, 7p, 7q, 10p, 15q and 17p (data not shown). Among the cases with complex karyotype recurrent chromosomal abnormalities (ten tumor breakpoints per arm or more) were found in 1p, 1q, 2q, 6q, 7p, 8q, 12q and q13.

Of the 5 patients with SNUC, 3 had an abnormal karyotype. One of the 5 SNUC had a complex karyotype, with 2 translocations involving chromosomes 1, 6, 12 and 17 in three cells. Another patient had a karyotype showing t(5; 18)(q13; q23) in 1/20 cells. The third patient with SNUC originating in the maxillary sinus had a complex karyotype with 60–69 chromosomes.

All patients were followed on regular bases using both clinical and radiological examinations. Four of the patients enrolled in this study have died of disease and all displayed a complex karyotype. In the other hand, 2 of the 9 patients who are alive had a complex karyotype. Statistical analysis of the data suggested that abnormal karyotype may be associated with poor prognosis of patients with paranasal SCC (P = 0.01 Fisher Exact test).

Clinical Relevance

Cytogenetic information on sino-nasal SCC is scarce due to the low incidence of this tumor. Three reports with 5 cytogenetically abnormal karyotypes of paranasal SCC[49–51] and one of undifferentiated carcinoma have been described.[52] All of the previously reported tumors displayed a complex karyotype with unbalanced translocations and deletions. In our study we have found that 7 of the 14 analyzed sinonasal specimens displayed an abnormal karyotype. Most of the chromosomal abnormalities involved few clones with complex karyotypes.

This report is also the first to describe two abnormal karyotypes of sinonasal carcinoma: One with two novel translocations t(1; 6)(p22; p23) and t(12; 17)(q13; p13) and a second with loss of chromosome Y. The cytogenetic features of sinonasal NK SCC described herein resemble those previously reported by Jin et al,[49,50] while the karyotype of the SNUC is different from that previously described by Gollin and Janecka, which had a complex diploid karyotype.[52]

SCC of the upper aerodigestive tracts frequently harbors a highly complex karyotype as found in our study. Chromosomal aberrations involving similar breakpoints were previously described in SCC of the oral cavity, larynx, hypopharynx, and nasopharynx.[49,50,53]

Translocation (12; 17)(q13; p13) as found in case 1, was previously described in breast adenocarcinoma and acute monoblastic leukemia,[54,55] whereas t(1; 6)(p22; p23) was never described before. The karyotype described in case 9 (45,X) is also frequently found in SCC of the upper aerodigestive tracts.[49,53,56]

Recurrent chromosomal abnormalities involving 1p, 6q and 12q were found in 3 of our cases. Although not specific, such aberrations may be found in SCC of the oral cavity, larynx nasopharynx and hypopharynx.[57]

In our series, 7 of the 15 patients had a normal tumor karyotype. This may suggest that the tumor cells have not undergone cytogenetic changes and therefore the biological behavior of the tumor is relatively slow. Another explanation for a normal karyotype is that the analyses represent normal stromal cell proliferation in culture rather than tumor cell growth, and therefore represent the constitutional karyotype of the patient.

In addition to the cytogenetic data, we described the association between karyotype and prognosis. We have found that all of the 4 patients who died of disease, displayed a complex karyotype, whereas only 2 of the 9 patients who are free of tumor had a complex karyotype. These differences were statistically significant (p < 0.01).

Taking together, this finding suggests that abnormal karyotype may be associated with poor prognosis in patients with sinonasal SCC or SNUC.

In our series, 7 patients had a normal tumor karyotype. This may suggest that the tumor cells have not undergone cytogenetic changes and therefore the biological behavior of the tumor is relatively slow. Another explanation for a normal karyotype is that the analyses represent normal stromal cell proliferation in culture rather than tumor cell growth, and therefore represent the constitutional karyotype of the patient.

Previous studies have demonstrated the prognostic value of cytogenetic data in head and neck SCC.[58] To date, the extent of the cytogenetic data on sinonasal carcinomas is too limited to furnish precise association between karyotype and prognosis. Additional studies are required in order to determine whether cytogenetic data may serve as an adjunct to conventional pathology for the diagnosis and prognosis assessment of these rare and highly aggressive tumors.

QUALITY OF LIFE FOLLOWING SUBCRANIAL SURGERY FOR ANTERIOR SKULL BASE TUMORS

The importance of topics addressing quality of life (QoL) of patients with cancer is increasingly being acknowledged. QoL is assessed in an effort to improve treatment modalities, to promote restoration of the patient's daily function, and to accelerate his return to normal life. Estimation of the influence of surgical procedures on QoL can serve as a means by which the most appropriate surgical approach can be selected for a given patient. Detailed understanding of the different aspects of QoL may help surgeons improve assessment and management of patients, identify specific impediments as early as possible during follow-up, and direct specific medical interventions to patients with increased risk and poor outcome.[59] Furthermore, early access of patients to detailed information about their disease can yield better adjustment to an imminent medical condition.[60] A multidimensional evaluation of QoL involves retrieving information on the physical, emotional, social and economical aspects of the patient's lifestyle, as well as on specific symptoms associated with their disease. Valid interpretation of the data requires disease-specific instruments, which cover the morbidity associated with the site of cancer and its treatment.[61]

Subsequent reports have established the subcranial approach as a reliable treatment for anterior skull base tumors, but tumor control should not be the only goal of patient care. During the last decade, numerous studies have assessed QoL issues in patients with head and neck cancer,[62,63] however, the physical and psychological sequelae of anterior skull base surgery in general and of the subcranial approach in particular have not been systematically evaluated.

We assessed the influence of surgery for extirpation of anterior skull base tumors on patients' QoL and to investigate possible predictors of functional outcome after surgery. Since skull base surgery differs from other head and neck procedures, the psychological, social and physical well-being of this group of patients were assessed using a disease-specific multidimensional questionnaire.

Our study is based on a review of the hospital charts of 69 patients (76 consecutive cases) operated between 1994 and 2002 for extirpation of anterior skull base tumors at our institution. All operations were performed via the subcranial approach to the anterior skull base and carried out by the same interdisciplinary team.

Inclusion criteria dictated that at least three months had to have passed since surgery. Of the 69 potential study candidates, 13 died of various causes, 5 do not reside in Israel, 5 were lost to follow-up, 5 patients were operated less than 3 months before the study was activated, and 1 patient was non-compliant. Thus, a total of 40 questionnaires were completed and analyzed. All the candidates who agreed to fill out a QoL questionnaire also gave a full medical history and underwent a physical examination on the same day. The co-morbidity was defined according to the Charlson Co-morbidity Index.[64] An independent physician conducted all the interviews to avoid any bias that could stem from surgeon-patient interaction.

The development of the questionnaire, including its reliability and validity were described elsewhere.[65–67] Six relevant domains were identified by factor analysis: role of performance (6 items), physical function (7 items), vitality (7 items), pain (3 items), specific symptoms (7 items) and impact upon emotions (5 items). Table 28.3 summarizes the six categories of QoL, each category representing one domain. Internal consistency of each of

Table 28.3: Summary of domain questions in the skull base quality of life questionnaire

- Role of performance
- General performance
- Performance at work
- Performance at home
- Participation in social activities
- Communication with people
- Effect of health on performance
- Physical functioning
- Climbing stairs
- Leaning and standing
- Walking long distances
- Walking short distances
- Preferring to stay in bed
- Carrying out routine activities
- Reducing extent of physical activity because of disease
- Vitality
- Feeling weak
- Feeling tired
- Achieves what I desire
- Feeling enthusiastic
- Feeling motivated
- Feeling energetic
- Relationships with spouse
- Pain
- Experiencing pain
- Effect of pain on activity
- Use of painkillers
- Specific symptoms
- Change in appetite
- Altered sense of taste
- Altered sense of smell
- Altered appearance
- Nasal secretions
- Eye secretions
- Effect of surgery on vision
- Impact upon emotions
- Feeling tense
- Problems falling asleep
- Feeling worried or frustrated
- Feeling relaxed and calm
- Worrying about finances

the six domains was evaluated using Cornbach's alpha coefficient. Cornbach's alpha values for each domain were greater than 0.8. Construct validity demonstrated that the direction of differences for each domain was as hypothesized (paired *t* test; p < 0.05).

Forty of the 69 patients operated by us were enrolled in this study. The response rate was 98% (40 of 41 patients): For completing the questionnaire, after excluding the patients who died, who were lost to follow-up and who were operated less than 3 months before the study was activated. The tumors were malignant in 13 patients (32.5%) and benign in 27 (67.5%). There was no significant difference in age or sex between these two groups. The study population was divided into two groups according to the extent of the tumor:

1. The tumor is confined to the paranasal sinuses.
2. Intracranial extension of the tumor.

In the group of patients with benign tumors, 21 of 27 (78%) had intracranial extension of the tumor. In the group of patients with malignant tumors, 12 of 13 (92%) had intracranial involvement.

The study population was divided into subgroups as follows: age, gender, type of surgery (osteotomy A or B), time from surgery, type of tumor, perioperative radiotherapy and co-morbidity.

In the first section of the questionnaire, patients were asked to grade their overall postoperative QoL relative to their pre-operative QoL. Figures 28.24A to D show the overall results of 4 general questions relating to the effect of surgery on over all QoL, social activity, financial status and emotional state. The results show that 38% of the patients reported a significant improvement in overall QoL and 36% reported no change in QoL after surgical removal of their tumor. The minority of patients (26%) answered that the surgical procedure worsened their QoL. The scores of the social, financial and emotional state domains were lower relative to the overall QoL score.

In order to obtain estimates on the specific influence of the subcranial approach on various aspects of QoL, each patient was asked to answer 35 questions related to six distinct domains: Role of performance, physical function, vitality, pain, specific symptoms, and impact upon emotions. The domains of role of performance, physical function, vitality and impact upon emotions received lower scores than the overall QoL score. The domains of pain and specific symptoms had scores above the overall QoL.

In order to predict which of the patients may have poorer outcome after surgery, the study population was divided into seven subgroups according to demographic and clinical characteristics. The mean physical function score of patients younger than 60 years was significantly higher than that of older patients. Patients with benign tumors reported higher scores in the domains of role of performance, physical function, specific symptoms and impact upon emotions than patients with malignant tumors. Interestingly, both groups reported only a minor influence of the aspect of pain on their QoL.

Perioperative radiotherapy was associated with significantly lower scores in the domains of specific

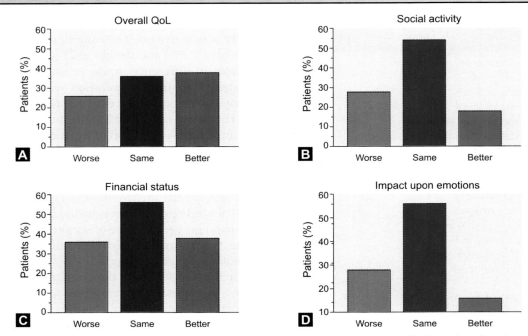

Figs 28.24A to D: The effect of surgery on different quality of life measures. (A) Overall quality of life. (B) Social activity. (C) Financial status. (D) Emotional state

symptoms and impact upon emotions. Type B surgery, which involves osteotomy and en bloc removal of the anterior and posterior frontal sinus wall, was also associated with lower scores in the impact upon emotions domain. As expected, patients with an additional illness reported lower scores of QoL in the physical function domain.

We prospectively evaluated the QoL of 20 more patients using the 35-item instrument in order to further test its utility and validity (Fig. 28.25). These patients were asked to complete the instrument before surgery and 5–6 months following surgery. The majority had malignant tumors (58%) and the rest had benign tumors (42%). The overall change in QoL was –16% (p < 0.03). The deterioration in QoL was –22% in the group of patients with malignancy, significantly more profound than the deterioration of –4.5% in the group with benign tumors. The preoperative QoL score of the two groups did not differ significantly (p = 0.4), but the QoL of the patients with malignancy was significantly poorer than that of the patients with benign tumors 5–6 months later (p = 0.027).

The overall results of this study show that the resection of tumors of the anterior skull base by the subcranial approach has a positive impact on the patients' QoL. Most of our patients (76%) reported that the surgical procedure improved or did not interfere with their overall QoL. The

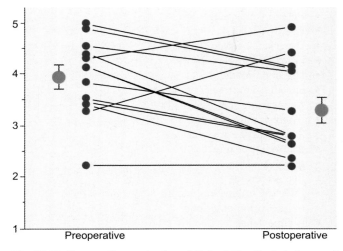

Fig. 28.25: Prospective evaluation of QoL of 13 patients before and after subcranial surgery. The red circles indicate Mean ± SE

relatively good scores recorded for the role of perfor-mance, pain and specific symptoms domains further demonstrate this positive impact of surgery on different aspects of QoL.

The stability of QoL following the first 6 months after surgery is an important issue of our study. We compared the QoL scores of patients operated 3–6, 6–24 and >24 months before the study was activated, in order to estimate the dynamic change in QoL following surgery. We have found that during the first 6 months after surgery there was a gradual improvement in QoL measures, while later no significant change in QoL was reported by the patients.

We recently reported a retrospective study of 175 skull-base operations performed without hair removal.[26] Our results showed that a skull-base operation without hair removal does not carry additional risk for wound infection and contamination when compared to the rates reported for identical procedures in which the hair was removed. Avoiding hair shaving may have contributed to the improved short-term QoL in our patients by sparing them additional psychological stress, by promoting the restoration of their self-image and by accelerating their return to normal life.

Further prospective, multi-center studies are required in order to assess more accurately the QoL measures of patients with various anterior skull base tumors. Comparative studies are essential in order to examine the impact of different surgical modalities with no clear survival advantage on patients QoL.

CONCLUSION

We routinely used the subcranial approach for tumors involving the anterior skull base. Wide exposure of the tumor area enables meticulous dissection, minimizes brain retraction and allows full control of blood loss with preservation of vital anatomical structures. There are well-established advantages of the extended subcranial approach, nevertheless we believe that it should be combined with complementary approaches in certain clinical situations, such as lesions involving the cavernous sinus or the carotid arteries, or massive intradural or invasion. An orbitozygomatic approach in addition to the subcranial approach may be used in case the tumor extends latero-posteriorly. An additional infratemporal fossa approach may be used if the tumor extends latero-inferiorly. A combined subcranial and midfacial degloving approach may offer improved exposure and excellent cosmetic results in cases of tumors involving the anterior fossa and the maxillary lateral walls or alveolar ridge. We choose to perform a formal maxillectomy using the transfacial or facial translocation approaches in cases of massive maxillary or orbital involvement by the tumor.

Reconstruction procedures for the management of anterior skull base tumor excisions vary widely. We reviewed our experience of skull base reconstruction after extirpation of tumors via the subcranial approach. The double layer fascia technique promises a simple and versatile means of skull base reconstruction after en bloc

resection of both malignant and benign tumors. The incidence and severity of perioperative complications associated with the double layer fascia lata technique is similar to, or lower than other reconstructive techniques. The findings of our study also indicate that free fascial grafts survive via local proliferation of a newly formed vascular layer embedded within the fascial sheath.

Finally, our work indicates that the overall QoL in the majority of patients after subcranial surgery can be classified as good, with significant improvement within 6 months following surgery. The financial and emotional QoL domains had the worse impact on the patients. Old age, malignancy, co-morbidity, radiotherapy and wide surgery were found to be negative prognostic factors for QoL measures. These findings can be applied for targeting medical resources, in order to improve QoL measures in this group of patients.

REFERENCES

1. Smith RR, Klopp CT, Williams JM. Surgical treatment of cancer of the frontal sinus and adjacent areas. *Cancer* 1954;7:991–994.
2. Ketcham AS, Wilkins RH, Van Buren JM, Smith RR. A combined intracranial approach to the paranasal sinuses. *Am J Surg* 1963;106:698–703.
3. Van Buren JM, Ommaya AK, Ketcham AS. Ten years' experience with radical combined craniofacial resection of malignant tumors of the paranasal sinuses. *J Neurosurg* 1968;28:341–350.
4. Derome PJ. The transbasal approach to tumors invading the base of the skull. In *Current Techniques in Operative Neurosurgery*, Schmidek MM, Sweet WH, (Eds). New York: Grune Stratton, 1977;223–245.
5. Jane JA, Parks Pobereskin LH. The supraorbital approach: Technical note. *Neurosurgery* 1982;11:537–542.
6. Jackson IT, Marsh WR, Hide TA. Treatment of tumors involving the anterior cranial fossa. *Head Neck Surg* 1984;6:901–913.
7. Johns ME, Kaplan MJ, Park TS. Supraorbital rim approach to the anterior skull base. *Laryngoscope* 1984;94:1137–1139.
8. Sundaresan N, Shah JP. Craniofacial resection for anterior skull base tumors. *Head Neck Surg* 1988;10:219–224.
9. Cheesman AD, Lund VJ, Howard DJ. Craniofacial resection for tumors of the nasal cavity and paranasal sinuses. *Head Neck Surg* 1986;8:429–435.
10. Al-Mefty O. The supraorbital pterional approach to skull base lesions. *Neurosurgery* 1987;21:474–477.
11. Persing JA, Jane JA, Levine PA. The versatile frontal sinus approach to the floor of the anterior cranial fossa: Technical note. *J Neurosurgery* 1990;72:513–516.
12. Jackson IT. Craniofacial osteotomies to facilitate resection of tumors of the skull base. In: Neurosurgery Update I, Wilkins RH, Rengachary S, (Eds). New York: *McGraw Hill International Book Co.* 1990;227–291.

13. Donald PJ. Skull base surgery combined results of treatment of malignant disease. *Skull Base Surg* 1992;2:76–79.

14. Sekhar LN, Nanda A, Sen CH, Snyderman CN, Janeka IP. The extended frontal approach to tumors of the anterior middle and posterior skull base. *J Neurosurg* 1992;76:198–206.

15. Raveh J, Schwere. Gesichtsschadelverletzungen: Eigene Erfahrungen und Modificationen. *Aktuel Probl ORL* 1979; 3:145–154.

16. Raveh J, Redle M, Markwalder T. Operative management of 194 cases of combined maxillo-facial-fronto-basal fractures: Principles and modifications. *Oral Maxillofac Surg* 1984;42: 555–564.

17. Raveh J, Vuillemin T. The surgical one stage management of combined cranio-maxillo-facial and fronto-basal fractures. Advantages of the subcranial approach in 374 cases. *J Craniomaxillofac Surg* 1988;16:160–172.

18. Raveh J, Vuillemin T, Sutter Franz. Subcranial management of 395 combined fronto-basal-midface fractures. *Arch Otolaryngol Head Neck Surg* 1989;114:1114–1122.

19. Raveh J, Laedrach K, Vuillemin T et al. Management of combined fronto-naso orbital/skull base fractures and telecanthus in 355 cases. *Arch Otolaryngol Head Neck Surg* 1992;118:605–614.

20. Raveh J, Vuillemin T. The subcranial-supraorbital temporal approach for tumor resection. *J Craniofac Surg* 1990;1:53–59.

21. Raveh J, Laedrach K, Speiser M et al. The subcranial approach for fronto-orbital and anteroposterior skull base tumor. *Arch Otolaryngol Head Neck Surg* 1993;119:385–393.

22. Neligan PC, Mulholland S, Irish J et al. Flap selection in cranial base reconstruction. *Plast Reconstr Surg* 1996;98:1159–1166.

23. Coleman JJ, III. Microvascular approach to function and appearance of large orbital maxillary defects. *Am J Surg* 1989;158:337–341.

24. Tachibana E, Saito K, Fukuta K et al. Evaluation of the healing process after dural reconstruction achieved using a free fascial graft. *J Neurosurg* 2002;96:280–286.

25. Hasegawa M, Torii S, Fukuta K et al. Reconstruction of the anterior cranial base with the galeal frontalis myofascial flap and the vascularized outer table calvarial bone graft. *Neurosurgery* 1995;36:725–731.

26. Gil Z, Cohen JT, Spektor S et al. The role of hair shaving in skull base surgery. *Otolaryngol Head Neck Surg* 2003;128: 43–47.

27. Gil Z, Cohen JT, Spektor S et al. Anterior skull base surgery without prophylactic airway diversion procedures. *Otolaryngol Head Neck Surg* 2003;128:681–685.

28. Fliss DM, Zucker G, Amir A et al. The subcranial approach for anterior skull base tumors. *Oper Tech Otolaryngol Head Neck Surg* 2000;11:238–253.

29. Fliss DM, Zucker G, Cohen A et al. Early outcome and complications of the extended subcranial approach to the anterior skull base. *Laryngoscope* 1999;109:153–160.

30. Fliss DM, Zucker G, Cohen JT et al. The subcranial approach for the treatment of cerebrospinal fluid rhinorrhea: A report of 10 cases. *J Oral Maxillofac Surg* 2001;59:1171–1175.

31. Fliss DM, Zucker G, Amir A et al. The combined subcranial and midfacial degloving technique for tumor resection: Report of three cases. *J Oral Maxillofac Surg* 2000;58:106–110.

32. Fliss DM, Zucker G, Spektor S, Amir A, Gatot A, Cohen JT. The combined subcranial pterional approach to the

anterolaterall skull base. *Oper Tech Otolaryngol Head Neck Surg* 2000;11:286–292.

33. Fliss DM, Gil Z, Spektor S et al. Skull base reconstruction after anterior subcranial tumor resection. *Neurosurg Focus* 2002;12:10.

34. Amir A, Gatot A, Zucker G et al. Harvesting of fascia lata sheaths: A rational approach. *Skull Base Surg* 2000;10:29–34.

35. Clayman GL, DeMonte F, Jaffe DM et al. Outcome and complications of extended cranial-base resection requiring microvascular free-tissue transfer. *Arch Otolaryngol Head Neck Surg* 1995;121:1253–1257.

36. Kiyokawa K, Tai Y, Inoue Y et al. Efficacy of temporal musculopericranial flap for reconstruction of the anterior base of the skull. *Scand J Plast Reconstr Surg Hand Surg* 2000; 34:43–53.

37. McCutcheon IE, Blacklock JB, Weber RS et al. Anterior transcranial (craniofacial) resection of tumors of the paranasal sinuses: Surgical technique and results. *Neurosurgery* 1996;38:471–479.

38. Nibu K, Sasaki T, Kawahara N et al. Complications of craniofacial surgery for tumors involving the anterior cranial base. *Neurosurgery* 1998;42:455–461.

39. Brockmeyer D, Gruber DP, Haller J, Shelton C, Walker ML. Pediatric skull base surgery. 2. Experience and outcomes in 55 patients. *Pediatr Neurosurg* 2003;38(1):9–15.

40. Steiner CC. Cephalometric for you and me. *Am J Orthod* 1953;39:729–755.

41. Riolo ML, Moyers RE JA Jr, Hunter WE. An atlas of craniofacial growth: Cephalometric standards from the University School Growth Study. The University of Michigen. Monograph 2, Craniofacial Growth Series. *Ann Arbor:* Center for Human Growth and Development. University of Michigan. 1974.

42. Gruber DP, Brockmeyer D. Pediatric skull base surgery. 1. Embryology and developmental anatomy. *Pediatr Neurosurg* 2003;38(1):2–8.

43. Bell W. Timing of treatment in growing patients. In *Surgical Correction of Dental Facial Deformities*, Bell W (Ed). Philadelphia: WB Saunders 1980.

44. Shapiro A, Zohar E, Hoppenstein D, Ifrach N, Jedeikin R, Fredman B. A comparison of three techniques for acute postoperative pain control following major abdominal surgery. *J Clin Anesth* 2003;15(5):345–350.

45. Gil Z, Fliss DM, Voskoboimik N et al. Two novel trans-locations, t(2. 4)(q35. q31) and t(X. 12)(q22. q24), as the only karyotypic abnormalities in a malignant peripheral nerve sheath tumor of the skull base. *Cancer Genet Cytogenet* 2003;145:139–143.

46. Gil Z, Fliss DM, Voskoboinik N, Leider-Trejo L, Spektor S, Yaron Y, Orr-Urtreger A. Cytogenetic analysis of three variants of clival chordoma. *Cancer Genet Cytogenet* 2004;154(2): 124–130.

47. Suarez C, Llorente JL, Fernandez De Leon R et al. Prognostic factors in sinonasal tumors involving the anterior skull base. *Head Neck* 2004;26:136–144.

48. Patel SG, Singh B, Polluri A et al. Craniofacial surgery for malignant skull base tumors: Report of an international collaborative study. *Cancer* 2003;98:1179–1187.

49. Jin Y, Mertens F, Arheden K et al. Karyotypic features of malignant tumors of the nasal cavity and paranasal sinuses. *Int J Cancer* 1995;60:637–641.

50. Jin YS, Higashi K, Mandahl N et al. Frequent rearrangement of chromosomal bands 1p22 and 11q13 in squamous cell carcinomas of the head and neck. *Genes Chromosomes Cancer* 1990;2:198–204.

51. Zaslav AL, Stamberg J, Steinberg BM et al. Cytogenetic analysis of head and neck carcinomas. *Cancer Genet Cytogenet* 1991;56:181–187.

52. Gollin SM, Janecka IP. Cytogenetics of cranial base tumors. *J Neurooncol* 1994;20:241–254.

53. Jin C, Jin Y, Wennerberg J et al. Nonrandom pattern of cytogenetic abnormalities in squamous cell carcinoma of the larynx. *Genes Chromosomes Cancer* 2000;28:66–76.

54. Tan PH, Lui WO, Ong P et al. Cytogenetic analysis of invasive breast cancer: A study of 27 Asian patients. *Cancer Genet Cytogenet* 2000;121:61–66.

55. Secker-Walker LM, Moorman AV, Bain BJ et al. Secondary acute leukemia and myelodysplastic syndrome with 11q23 abnormalities. EU Concerted Action 11q23 Workshop. *Leukemia* 1998;12:840–44.

56. Jin Y, Mertens F, Jin C et al. Nonrandom chromosome abnormalities in short-term cultured primary squamous cell carcinomas of the head and neck. *Cancer Res* 1995;55:3204–3210.

57. Mitelman F JB, Mertens F. Mitelman database of chromosome aberrations in cancer. In: Mitelman F, Johansson B, Mertens F, (Eds) http://cgap.nci.nih.gov/chromosomes 2003.

58. Gollin SM. Chromosomal alterations in squamous cell carcinomas of the head and neck: Window to the biology of disease. *Head Neck* 2001;23:238–253.

59. Fitzpatrick R, Fletcher A, Gore S, Jones D, Spiegelhalter D, Cox D. Quality of life measures in health care. I: Applications and issues in assessment. *BrMed J* 1992;305:1074–1077.

60. Portenoy RK. Quality of life issues in patients with head and neck cancer. In *Head and Neck Cancer*, LB Harrison (Ed). New York: Plenum Press 1995;218–231.

61. Gliklich RE, Goldsmith TA, Funk GF. Are head and neck specific quality of life measures necessary? *Head Neck* 1997;19:474–480.

62. Terrell JE, Nanavati KA, Esclamado RM, Bishop JK, Bradford CR, Wolf GT. Head and neck cancer-specific quality of life: Instrument validation. *Arch Otolaryngol Head Neck Surg* 1997;123:1125–1132.

63. Hassan SJ, Weymuller EA Jr. Assessment of quality of life in head and neck cancer patients. *Head Neck* 1993;15:485–496.

64. Singh B, Bhaya M, Stern J et al. Validation of the Charlson comorbidity index in patients with head and neck cancer: A multi-institutional study. *Laryngoscope* 1997;107:1469–1475.

65. Gil Z, Abergel A, Spektor S, Cohen JT, Khafif A, Shabtai E, Fliss DM. Quality of life following surgery for anterior skull base tumors. *Arch Otolaryngol Head Neck Surg* 2003;129(12):1303–1309.

66. Gil Z, Abergel A, Spektor S, Shabtai E, Khafif A, Fliss DM. Development of a cancer-specific anterior skull base quality-of-life questionnaire. *J Neurosurg* 2004;100(5):813–819.

67. Gil Z, Abergel A, Spektor S, Khafif A, Fliss DM. Patient, caregiver, and surgeon perceptions of quality of life following anterior skull base surgery. *Arch Otolaryngol Head Neck Surg* 2004;130(11):1276–1281.

Benign Tumors of the Nasal Cavity and Nasopharynx

Robin Youngs, Suchir Maitra

BENIGN TUMORS OF THE NASAL CAVITY

The clinical assessment of benign tumors of the nasal cavity takes the usual course of history, clinical examination and special investigation.

History

In the early stages, nasal neoplasia usually presents with unilateral nasal obstruction. Vascular neoplasms can also present with unilateral bloodstained discharge or frank epistaxis, although these features are more suggestive of a malignant neoplasm. As the neoplasm enlarges, particularly with anterior lesions the shape of the external nasal pyramid can be distorted. In the mid and posterior parts of the nasal cavity neoplasms can obstruct the outflow and ventilation of the paranasal sinuses, leading to symptoms of chronic sinusitis, such as unilateral purulent nasal discharge, postnasal discharge, headache and facial pain. With large lesions obstruction of the nasolacrimal duct can lead to symptoms of unilateral epiphora. Very large posterior lesions can also obstruct the eustachian tube with the formation of a secondary middle ear effusion and hence unilateral deafness.

Clinical Examination

Clinical examination begins with inspection of the facial features, looking for evidence of facial swelling or distortion. Next the nasal airway should be assessed for unilateral nasal obstruction. A nasal cavity neoplasm may be observed by examination with a Thudicum's speculum and headlight. Examination, however, is not complete without an assessment with a rigid or fiberoptic endoscope.

The use of a rigid Hopkin's rod type endoscope carries the advantage of a clear image suitable for photographic documentation. Although most rhinologists would use a 4 mm 0° endoscope, angled endoscopes (30°, 45° and 70°) can all be used. A flexible fiberoptic endoscope can also be used. Flexible endoscopes are slightly easier to insert and have the advantage of facilitating examination of the pharynx and larynx in addition.

Special Investigation

The cornerstone of assessment of nasal neoplasia is the use of radiological investigation. In the past the use of plain occipito-mental, occipito-frontal and lateral radiographs was common. Modern assessment, however, relies on the use of CT and MR. Using a combination of CT and MR an accurate three-dimensional picture of the nasal neoplasm can be obtained, used in the planning of surgical treatment. CT images show excellent bony definition, whereas MR has the ability to differentiate between tumor and surrounding inflammatory nasal and paranasal sinus disease.[1]

In order to confirm the diagnosis of a nasal neoplasm biopsy will also be necessary. This can usually be undertaken under local anesthetic in the outpatient setting. Care must, however, be taken in the biopsy of vascular tumors which should have undergone prior radiological assessment.

Classification

Benign tumors of the nasal cavity can be subdivided into epithelial and nonepithelial lesions (Table 29.1).

Table 29.1: Classification of benign tumors of the nasal cavity

Epithelial tumors
- Papillomas
  - Inverted papilloma
  - Squamous papilloma
- Adenomas
  - Papillary adenoma
  - Salivary gland—pleomorphic adenoma

Nonepithelial tumors
- Fibroma
- Hemangioma
- Nervous tissue
  - Gliomas and encephaloceles
  - Mengioma
  - Neurilemmoma
- Chondroma
- Osteoma
- Leiomyoma

EPITHELIAL TUMORS

Papillomas

Inverted Papilloma

Inverted papilloma is by far the most common benign epithelial neoplasm occurring in the nasal cavity and paranasal sinuses. Males predominate by a factor of 5:1, with the fifth decade being the commonest age of presentation.

Diagnosis: Diagnosis is made by histological analysis. The characteristic feature (Fig. 29.1) is the presence of invaginations of the epithelial lining with alternating

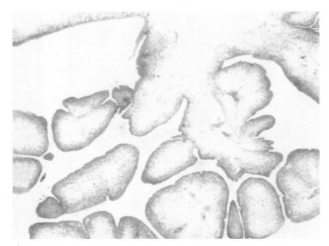

Fig. 29.1: Microscopic section of a nasal-inverted papilloma (hematoxylin and eosin)

stratified squamous epithelium and ciliated respiratory epithelium. These features give a characteristic 'heaped up' appearance. The underlying stroma is loose connective tissue with an inflammatory infiltrate similar to that of simple nasal polyps. The presence of mitotic figures in the epithelium of inverted papillomas has been linked to recurrence rate. Woodson, et al found that a greater incidence of mitotic figures in a histological section was related to a higher recurrence rate.[2]

Etiology: The cause of nasal inverted papilloma is unknown. The two most commonly proposed factors have been chronic inflammation and human papilloma virus infection (HPV). Ron et al studied the inflammatory cell component present in sinonasal papilloma and found that inflammatory cells were identified as a significant cell population in inverted papilloma.[3] They proposed a staging system based on inflammatory cells which may be of use in predicting recurrence or malignant transformation. Many authors have studied the occurrence of HPV in inverted papilloma with the results being inconclusive. Bernauer et al detected HPV DNA fragments in 7 out of 21 cases of inverted papilloma, including one case in which malignant transformation had occurred.[4] Zhou et al found a much higher rate of detection of HPV DNA, with 30 of 38 cases being positive for HPV.[5] They suggested that HPV played a role in the etiology of inverted papilloma. Interest has also been shown in the expression of the p53 gene in inverted papillomas. Franzmann, et al found overexpression of p53 in three out of five carcinomas arising from sinonasal papillomas, supporting the concept that p53 may have a role in the carcinogenic process in head and neck tumors.[6] Study of the cytokeratin profile of inverted papilloma has revealed increased expression of cytokeratin 5, typical for basal cells, and cytokeratin 13, typical for squamous epithelial cells, suggesting an origin from a cytokeratin 5 immunoreactive cell of the basal layer of mucosa.[7]

Malignant transformation: The potential for malignant transformation of sinonasal inverted papillomas was noted by Hyams in 1971, who found a 13% incidence of carcinomatous transformation or concurrent malignancy.[8] This high-figure may have reflected the tertiary referral nature of Hyams material, as most rhinologists observe a far lower incidence of malignant transformation. Indeed, a retrospective analysis of 86 cases of inverted papilloma failed to identify a single case of carcinoma.[2] It is likely that the true incidence of malignancy lies between these two extremes. A recent series of 53 cases revealed a malignant transformation rate of 9%.[9] When malignant transformation does occur it is to keratinizing or non-keratinizing squamous carcinoma. The histological features of malignant transformation are variable, and include carcinoma *in situ*, sharp transitions between carcinoma and papilloma, and early malignant change found in some papillomas.[10]

Clinical presentation: Macroscopically inverted papillomas have a polypoid appearance being usually more opaque and 'fleshy' than simple nasal polyps. The majority of inverted papillomas are unilateral, although bilateral cases can occur rarely.[8] The clinical features vary depending on the site of origin of the papilloma. Most tumors originate from the lateral nasal wall and present with unilateral nasal obstruction. Origin from any of the paranasal sinuses may occur with the maxillary sinus being most commonly affected (Fig. 29.2). When a papilloma arises primarily from the maxillary sinus symptoms normally occur only when the tumor passes through the maxillary ostium into the nasal cavity. As well as causing nasal obstruction, inverted papillomas can obstruct sinus outflow resulting in secondary infection of the paranasal sinuses. Tumors can thus present with unilateral purulent nasal discharge, headache and facial pain. Obstruction of the nasolacrimal duct can cause unilateral epiphora. Epistaxis is not a feature of inverted papillomas, and would be an indication that malignant transformation may have occurred.

Radiological features: The imaging modality of choice in inverted papilloma is CT, with MR used as an adjunctive investigation in select cases. The use of CT in axial and coronal planes allows the accurate localization of the tumor, shows bony changes and demonstrates anatomical considerations for surgical resection. CT findings are typically unilateral opacity of the nasal cavity and adjacent paranasal sinuses (Fig. 29.3). In longstanding cases, there may be erosion and expansion of adjacent bony structures. A recent study suggests that a lobulated appearance on CT is typical of inverted papilloma.[11] The value of MR is in distinguishing between tumor and secondary mucosal inflammation. The use of T2-weighted MR images which demonstrate mucosal involvement has been invaluable in the preoperative planning of surgery in inverted papilloma.

Management: The treatment of sinonasal inverted papilloma is surgical removal. Factors influencing the choice of surgical approach include the site of origin, extent and the high rate of local recurrence after removal. For many years the lateral rhinotomy operation, through an external incision, was the approach of choice for inverted papillomas. Through a lateral rhinotomy a medial maxillectomy removing the whole of the lateral nasal wall could be undertaken. The advent of endoscopic sinus surgery and high quality imaging has changed the approach to inverted papilloma treatment in recent years. For papillomas originating from the lateral nasal wall and the ethmoid sinuses an endoscopic approach to removal is now the treatment of choice,[12,13] giving comparable recurrence rates to open approaches.[14] In one series where aggressive endoscopic excision was performed a recurrence rate of 19% was observed.[15] The use of the microdebrider, a surgical instrument which removes tumor tissue, has also been useful in the treatment of inverted papilloma (Fig. 29.4). Recurrence rates are higher in inverted papillomas arising primarily in the frontal recess and maxillary sinus. These anatomical sites are less accessible

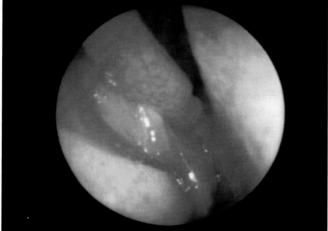

Fig. 29.2: Endoscopic view of inverted papilloma in the middle meatus originating from the maxillary sinus

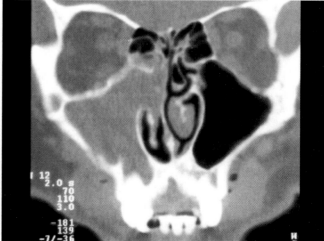

Fig. 29.3: Coronal CT scan of an inverted papilloma originating in the right maxillary antrum

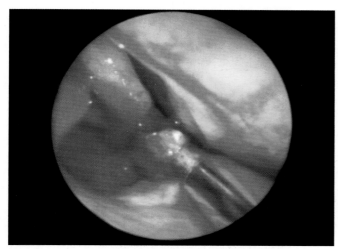

Fig. 29.4: Endoscopic removal of an inverted
papilloma with a microdebrider

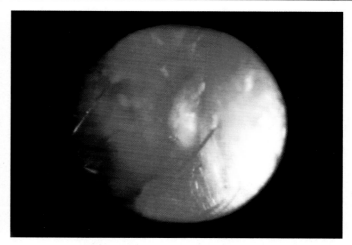

Fig. 29.5: Squamous papilloma of the nasal septum

with an endoscopic technique and an open approach may be required. For the maxillary sinus a Caldwell-Luc antrostomy can be combined with an endoscopic nasal approach to ensure complete removal of papilloma. Tumors arising from the anterior wall or floor of the maxillary sinus can be particularly difficult to view adequately. For tumors arising from the frontal recess or frontal sinus an external frontoethmoidectomy or osteoplastic flap approach is occasionally required.

Occasionally, a combined endoscopic and external approach to the frontal sinus can facilitate removal of inverted papilloma. A burr hole in the anterior wall of the frontal sinus can allow passage of an endoscope and thus visual control of removal of tumor from below.

Squamous Cell Papilloma

These lesions frequently occur on the anterior nasal septum and nasal vestibule, where they present with irritation and minor epistaxis (Fig. 29.5). Macroscopically, they are usually raised, papilliferous and arise from a broad base. Microscopically, they have a connective tissue core, with a squamous epithelial covering. Many may be caused by human papilloma virus (HPV) and it is not uncommon for these individuals to have viral warts elsewhere. Treatment is by surgical removal, which can be facilitated by laser therapy. Recurrence after removal, however, is very common.

Adenomas

Papillary Adenoma (Cylindric Papilloma)

These lesions, which are less frequent than inverted papilloma, occur usually on the lateral nasal wall.

Macroscopically, the lesion tends to be more friable than the inverted papilloma. Microscopically, the lesion is covered by ciliated respiratory epithelium, with a stroma containing cystic spaces containing mucus. Treatment is endoscopic surgical excision.

Minor Salivary Gland Tumors (Pleomorphic Adenoma)

These uncommon tumors occur most frequently on the nasal septum. They are usually discreet, lobulated swellings presenting with unilateral nasal obstruction. In a large series, Campagno and Wong reported 40 cases with an age range from 3 years to 82 years and no significant male/female predominance.[16] As in pleomorphic adenomas elsewhere the tumor is thought to arise from myoepithelial cells. Microscopically for diagnostic purposes both epithelial and mesenchymal elements should be present. The treatment is surgical excision. In the cases reported by Campagno and Wong, there were no instances of malignant transformation.

NON-EPITHELIAL TUMORS

Fibroma

These lesions usually present as a single pedunculated polypoid mass in the nasal cavity. Histologically, they consist of fibrous tissue and collagen, and may be the end stage of an inflammatory process rather than representing a true neoplasm.

Hemangioma

Capillary Hemangioma

This lesion commonly occurs on the anterior part of the nasal septum where it presents with frequent brisk epistaxis

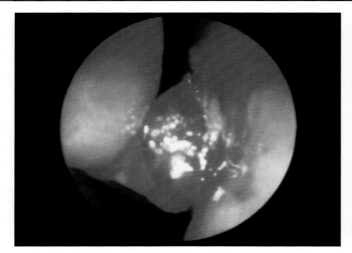

Fig. 29.6: Capillary hemangioma of the nasal septum

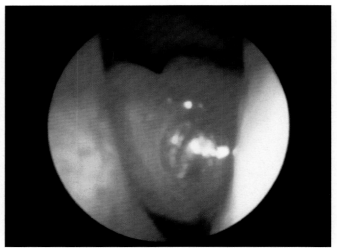

Fig. 29.7: A cavernous hemangioma arising from the left middle turbinate

(Fig. 29.6). The lesion is also often referred to as 'pyogenic granuloma' or 'bleeding polypus of the nasal septum'. Adults are most likely to be affected, including pregnant women, suggesting some hormonal influence. The lesion appears as a reddish, pedunculated mass which can bleed copiously even following the most gentle instrumentation. Microscopically, the lesion is composed of capillaries covered by frequently ulcerated epithelium. There is also acute and chronic inflammatory infiltrate. Treatment is by surgical removal which is usually curative.

Cavernous Hemangioma

The cavernous hemangioma is an uncommon neoplasm of blood vessels which usually presents within the bones of the nasal cavity, particularly the turbinates. Thus, endoscopically, the lesion often appears as a reddish enlargement of the inferior or middle turbinates (Fig. 29.7). Growth is slow and treatment is by surgical excision.

Benign Neoplasms Arising from Nervous Tissue

Gliomas and Encephaloceles

These are not true neoplasms but rather developmental anomalies. During normal intrauterine development a projection of dura between the developing facial bones and cartilage occurs through the foramen cecum. Failure of closure of the foramen cecum can result in trapped neurectodermal remnants. An encephalocele retains its connection with brain tissue, whereas a glioma remains isolated. By nature of their etiology these lesions typically occur in the superior part of the nasal cavity in infants and young children. They can often be seen externally as

widening of the nasal bridge. Adequate radiological assessment is vital before excisional surgery to quantify any intracranial connection. In this respect MR scanning with T2-weighted images to highlight cerebrospinal fluid (CSF) is the imaging modality of choice. Clearly, the danger of simple removal of these lesions is CSF fistula with possible meningitis. With modern endoscopic techniques these lesions can frequently be removed per nasally with direct repair of any resultant dural defect.

Meningioma

Most meningiomas presenting in the nasal cavity are extensions of intracranial tumors. Occasionally, however, a primary nasal meningioma occurs with no intracranial connection. The lesions usually present with unilateral nasal obstruction, with endoscopic examination revealing a polypoid mass which can fill the nasal cavity. As with all nasal neurogenic tumors adequate radiological assessment is essential in planning surgical removal (Fig. 29.8).

Neurilemmoma

These uncommon nasal tumors arise from Schwann's cells. They usually present as firm lobulated masses in the nasal cavity. Microscopically the appearance is of palisaded cells with Antoni A and B areas. Treatment is by surgical excision following radiological assessment (Fig. 29.9).

Chondroma

True chondromas of the nasal cavity are rare, and usually are found in the nasal septum and nasopharynx.[17] Some

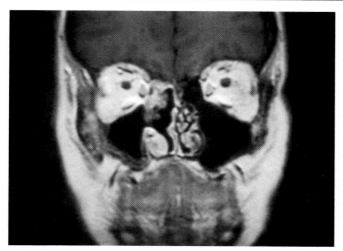

Fig. 29.8: MR scan showing postoperative appearance following endoscopic resection of nasal meningioma

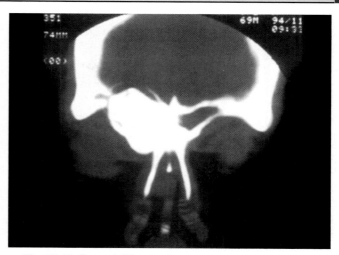

Fig. 29.10: Coronal CT scan showing a large frontoethmoidal osteoma obstructing frontal sinus outflow

of these tumors may actually be low-grade chondrosarcomas, and the histological distinction can be difficult.

Osteoma

Osteomas are not uncommon nasal and paranasal sinus tumors. They usually occur in middle age with a strong male predominance.[18] They are very slow growing and there has been some doubt as to whether they are true neoplasms. An alternative theory is that they arise from an isolated area of osteoneogenesis stimulated by an inflammatory or traumatic episode.[10] These tumors occur in the frontal, ethmoid, maxillary and sphenoid sinuses in decreasing frequency. Most nasal and paranasal osteomas are asymptomatic, and are often discovered as

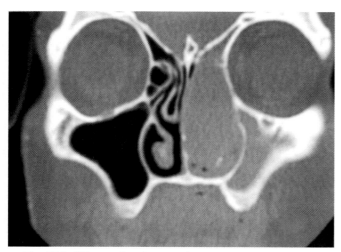

Fig. 29.9: CT scan showing complete opacity of the left nasal airway and paranasal sinuses due to a neuilemmoma

an incidental finding on sinus CT scans, where they appear as lobulated or spherical hard masses of bone. Headache and facial pain can occur due to secondary infection caused by obstruction to sinus outflow (Fig. 29.10). Asymptomatic patients may only need to be observed. When sinus outflow obstruction causes pain surgical treatment may be indicated. The surgical approach will depend on the anatomical location of the osteoma. If high-powered endonasal burrs are available intranasal endoscopic treatment may be possible. A combined external and endoscopic approach often gives good visualization.

Leiomyoma

This neoplasm, originating from smooth muscle, is extremely rare in the nasal cavity, with only a handful of reported cases.[19]

TUMORS OF THE NASOPHARYNX

Juvenile Nasopharyngeal Angiofibroma

Nasopharyngeal angiofibromas are rare benign tumor like lesions originating in the region of the nasopharynx and occurring almost exclusively in males. The term nasopharyngeal fibroma was introduced by Chaveau in 1906, and Friedberg in 1940 suggested the term angiofibroma.

Etiology

The etiology of the tumor is uncertain but its occurrence in adolescent males may have some relationship to high levels of male sex hormones. There have been reports of juvenile nasopharyngeal angiofibroma occurring

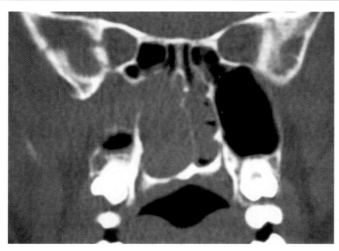

Fig. 29.11: Coronal CT scan showing a large nasopharyngeal angiofibroma originating from the right pterygopalatine fossa

inpatients with familial adenomatous polyposis suggesting it to be an extracolonic manifestation of adenomatous polyposis.[20]

Origin

The site of origin of the tumor is considered to be the junction of the sphenoidal process of the palatine bone, the horizontal ala of vomer and the root of the pterygoid process of the sphenoid bone at the superior margin of the sphenopalatine foramen. Lloyd et al after review of CT scans reported the possible site of origin to be at the pterygopalatine fossa (Figs 29.11 and 29.12), in the recess behind the sphenopalatine ganglion, at the exit aperture of the pterygoid canal.[21]

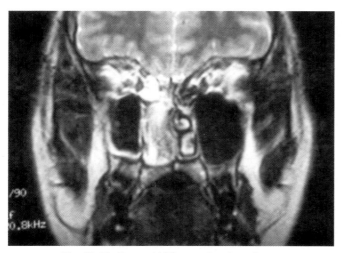

Fig. 29.12: Coronal MR scan showing a large nasopharyngeal angiofibroma

Background

Juvenile nasopharyngeal angiofibroma is a condition occurring almost exclusively in males. Very rare cases have been reported in females, however, doubt as to the histological diagnosis has been expressed in these cases.[22] The tumor commonly occurs in the age group 7–19 years with occasional patients presenting earlier or later. Incidence has been variously reported and ranges between 1:2000 and 1:15000.[23]

Histology

The tumor has vascular and stromal components with the blood vessels varying in size and shape. The muscular walls of the vessels display irregularly arranged smooth muscle which may be absent focally. These defects in the vessel walls preclude vasoconstriction thereby contributing to brisk bleeding following trauma.[24] The overlying epithelium can be either stratified squamous or respiratory in type.

Physical Characteristics

The tumor is reddish, frequently bilobed or dumb-bell shaped and firm in consistency having a tendency to bleed on touch. It is usually sharply-demarcated from its surrounding tissues as the tumors tend to displace rather than infiltrate surrounding soft tissues. An infiltrative pattern of growth is found only at its base at the mucosal attachments at the lateral nasal wall, nasopharynx, and septum.[25] The tumor can erode through bone infiltrating into nearby fissures and foramina in the nasopharynx and even into the intracranial cavity. Usually has a rich blood supply, most commonly from the internal maxillary artery, although feeding arteries from the internal carotid and contralateral external carotid may exist.

Routes of Spread

The tumor tends to grow inferiorly and anteriorly under the nasopharyngeal mucous membrane into the nasal cavity and the nasopharynx. It fills the nasal cavity and may deviate the septum to the opposite side. Straddling the sphenopalatine foramen the tumor grows laterally filling the pterygopalatine fossa resulting in anterior bowing of the posterior wall of the maxillary sinus. Further lateral extension occurs to the infratemporal fossa via the pterygomaxillary fissure. The tumor may invade the apex of the orbit through the inferior orbital fissure causing proptosis and also into the cheek resulting in a facial bulge.

Superior extension can occur to the middle cranial fossa through the superior orbital fissure. Posterior growth occurs along the pterygoid canal eroding or invading the base of the pterygoid process. Lloyd et al recognize two varieties of this extension. In the first, there is simple erosion of the pterygoid base and vaginal process of the sphenoid, but without invasion of the pterygoid base or the body of sphenoid, while in the second variety there is deep extension into the cancellous bone at the base of the pterygoid process often with extension and invasion of the diploe of the greater wing of the sphenoid and in some patients invasion of the middle cranial fossa.[21]

Recurrence

Juvenile nasopharyngeal angiofibromas are characterized by high recurrence rates following treatment. Gullane et al recorded a recurrence rate of 36% in 1992 while Lloyd et al reported a recurrence of 39.5% in 1999.[21] It appears that the principal determinant of recurrence is growth rate of the tumor along with incomplete excision at surgery. Total removal at surgery is difficult when there is deep invasion of the skull base, and invasion and expansion of the cancellous bone at the base of the pterygoid process is associated with a high recurrence rate.

Clinical Features

Nasopharyngeal angiofibromas presents most commonly with the symptoms of either nasal obstruction or epistaxis or both. Nasal obstruction is initially unilateral but as the tumor grows into the nasopharynx and also displaces the septum the obstruction may become bilateral. Epistaxis ranges from an occasional show, intermittent bleeding to severe hemorrhage. Focal absence of muscular wall in the tumor blood vessels contributes to the severe uncontrollable hemorrhage. Chronic or low-grade disseminated intravascular coagulopathy (DIG) with deranged clotting profile has been reported in patients with nasopharyngeal angiofibroma, and this may be contributory to impaired hemostasis in these patients.[26] Hyposmia and anosmia may occur from stasis of nasal secretions and headache may be due to sinus obstruction. Other symptoms include rhinolalia, deafness due to eustachian tube blockage, facial swelling, diplopia and trismus. Intracranial extension may present with headache and neurological signs.

Diagnosis

Adolescent males presenting with a history of epistaxis or nasal obstruction or both and the presence of a soft tissue mass in the nasopharynx point towards the diagnosis of a nasopharyngeal angiofibroma.

Diagnosis is confirmed by imaging studies. Biopsy of a juvenile nasopharyngeal angiofibroma is usually not necessary as imaging is sufficient to confirm the diagnosis. In addition, biopsy may lead to brisk epistaxis.

Radiology

Plain lateral views of the skull may show the anterior bowing of the posterior wall of the maxillary antrum giving rise to the so-called antral sign described by Holman and Miller.[21]

Diagnosis by CT scan is based on the site of origin of the lesion along with two features diagnostic of nasopharyngeal angiofibroma, namely a mass in the nose and pterygopalatine fossa and erosion of the bone behind the sphenopalatine foramen at the root of the pterygoid plate.[27] Contrast-enhanced CT scan shows diffuse enhancement of the tumor and helps to define bony anatomy better. CT scanning is considered more important than MRI preoperatively.

On MR scans juvenile nasopharyngeal angiofibroma presents signal voids due to its vascularity while strong enhancement is shown on gadolinium injection for the same reason. Gadolinium-enhanced MR is preferred inpatients presenting with intracranial extensions as it better defines soft tissue interfaces.[25] MR is particularly important in detecting tumor recurrence. Serial subtraction MR studies are used to show the precise size and extent of any residual tumor, record tumor growth or natural involution, and monitor the effects of radiotherapy.[27] Subtraction MR scan can be used for follow-up of patients with angio-fibroma but is used mostly to confirm a clinically suspected recurrence and monitor tumor behavior following treatment.[21]

Staging

Staging of nasopharyngeal angiofibromas is based on radiological findings and aims to allow accurate preoperative tumor assessment, evaluation for risk of tumor recurrence, appropriate surgical planning and comparing treatment results between hospitals. Various staging systems have been proposed over the years like that of Fisch, Sessions, and Chandler and more recently by Radkowski.[28] The staging systems are summarized in Table 29.2.

Treatment

The treatment of nasopharyngeal angiofibroma has undergone an evolution over time. Starting with surgical

Table 29.2: Staging of juvenile nasopharyngeal angiofibroma

Chandler et al	*Sessions et al*	*Radkowski et al*
1. Tumor confined to nasopharyngeal vault	1. a. Limited to nose and/or nasopharyngeal vault b. Extension into more than one sinus	1. a. Limited to nose and/or nasopharyngeal vault b. Extension into more than one sinus
2. Tumor extending into nasal cavity or sphenoid sinus	2. a. Minimal extension into pterygomaxillary fossa b. Full occupation of pterygomaxillary fossa with or without erosion of orbital bones c. Extension into infratemporal fossa with or without extension into cheek	2. a. Minimal extension into pterygomaxillary fossa b. Full occupation of pterygomaxillary fossa with or without erosion of orbital bones c. Extension into infratemporal fossa with or without extension into cheek or extension posterior to pterygoid plates
3. Tumor extending into antrum, ethmoid sinus, pterygomaxillary fossa, infratemporal fossa, orbit, and or cheek.	3. Intracranial extension	3. a. Erosion of skull base minimal intracranial extension b. Erosion of skull base-extensive intracranial extension with or without extension into cavernous sinus
4. Intracranial extension		

treatment, interest hovered around medical management and radiotherapy for a while before reverting back to surgery.

Medical management: Hormonal manipulation: Hormone preparations such as testosterone or oestrogen or a combination of both have been used for treating juvenile nasopharyngeal angiofibroma in the past. Flutamide, a testosterone receptor blocker has been used preoperatively to reduce tumor size.[29]

Radiotherapy: Radiotherapy is not usually used for primary treatment of nasopharyngeal angiofibromas owing to concerns regarding development of radiation induced malignancies of the head and neck and also malignant change in the angiofibromas. However, in 1984 Cummings et al reported success rates of 80% inpatients undergoing primary radiotherapy for juvenile nasopharyngeal angiofibroma with very low early and late radiotherapy induced complications.[30] Radiotherapy is usually reserved for patients presenting with intracranial extensions and unresectable lesions.

Surgical management: Surgical removal is the preferred method of treatment of juvenile nasopharyngeal angiofibroma. Many different surgical approaches have been described for removal of nasopharyngeal angiofibromas. The approach selected in an individual patient depends on the size and extent of the tumor.

Previously, lateral rhinotomy with medial maxillectomy was primarily used for exposure but more recently midfacial degloving is gaining popularity because of its use of intranasal and sublabial incisions, thereby avoiding facial scarring. However, wheremore exposure is needed lateral a lateral rhinotomy approach is still used. Other approaches which have been used are the transpalatal, transmaxillary and infratemporal fossa approaches. Presently endoscopic removal of tumor is gaining favor with surgeons. Surgery of juvenile nasopharyngeal angiofibroma can be associated with significant intraoperative hemorrhage and it is prudent to have cross-matched blood available prior to surgery. Preoperative embolization of the tumor has reduced the blood loss during surgery and transfusion may be unnecessary at times. Angiographic embolization is carried out 24–48 hours prior to surgery and may be undertaken with a variety of materials such as gel foam, polyvinyl alcohol, dextran microspheres and coils. Embolization of the tumor reduces the vascularity and also shrinks the tumor to a certain extent and may contribute to incomplete removal of tumors invading deeply into the sphenoid sinus, one of the main causes of recurrence.[27]

Endoscopic approaches are indicated for removal of angiofibromas limited to the nasal cavity, paranasal sinuses, pterygopalatine fossa, and medial infratemporal fossa.[25] With advances in the field of endoscopic surgery exclusive endoscopic resection has been carried out successfully in patients with minimal intracranial extension (Radkowski stage 3A).[31] More recently endoscopic laser assisted, image-guided surgical excision of juvenile nasopharyngeal angiofibroma has been undertaken carried out. Distinct advantages of this method of excision include diminished blood loss, superior cosmesis without altered facial growth, direct access to the skull base, with minimal morbidity, and ease of endoscopic follow-up.[32]

Follow-up after surgery of JNA is by regular clinical examination by endoscopy and MRI scans. Inpatients identified by CT scans to be at a high risk of recurrence, early imaging surveillance should be undertaken.[27]

REFERENCES

1. Rice D. Endoscopic approaches for sinonasal and naso-pharyngeal tumors. *Otolaryngol Clin North Am* 2001; 34(6):1087–1091.
2. Woodson GE, Robbins KT, Michaels L. Inverted papilloma. Considerations in treatment. *Arch Otolarygol* 1985; 111: 806–811.
3. Roh HJ, Procop GW, Batra PS, Citardi MJ, Lanza DC. Inflammation and the pathogenesis of inverted papilloma. *Am J Rhinol* 2004; 18:65–74.
4. Bernauer HS, Welkoborsky HJ, Tilling A, Amedee RG, Mann WJ. Inverted papilloma of the paranasal sinuses and the nasal cavity: DMA indices and HPV infection. *Am J Rhinol* 1997; 11:155–160.
5. Zhou Y, Hu M, Li Z. Human papilloma virus (HPV) and DNA test in inverted papillomas of the nasal cavities and paranasal sinuses. *Chin J Otorhinolaryngol* 1997; 32:345–347.
6. Franzmann MB, Buchwald C. Jacobsen GK, Lindeberg H. Expression of p53 in normal nasal mucosa and in sinonasal papillomas with and without associated carcinoma and the relation to human papillomavirus (HPV). *Cancer Letters* 1998; 128:161–164.
7. Plinkert PK, Ruck P, Baumann I, Scheffler B. Inverted papilloma of the nose and paranasal sinuses—diagnosis, surgical procedure and studies of cytokeratin profile. *Laryngo-Rhino-Otologie* 1997; 76:216–224.
8. Hyams VJ. Papillomas of the nasal cavity and paranasal sinuses. A clinicopathological study of 315 cases. *Ann Otol Rhinol Laryngol* 1971; 80:192–206.
9. Thorp MA, Oyarzabal-Amigo MF, du Plessis JH, Sellars SL. Inverted papilloma: A review of 53 cases. *Laryngoscope* 2001; 111:1401–1405.
10. Michaels L. Papilloma. In *Ear, Nose and Throat Histopathology*. London: Springer-Verlag 1987; 168.
11. Dammann F, Pereira P, Laniado M, Lowenheim H, Claussen CD. Inverted papilloma of the nasal cavity and paranasal sinuses: using CT for primary diagnosis and follow-up. *Am J Roentgenol* 1999; 172:543–548.
12. Rice D. Endonasal approaches for sinonasal and nasopharyngeal tumors. *Otolaryngol Clin North Am* 2001; 34:1087–1091.
13. Chee LW, Sethi DS. The endoscopic management of sinonasal inverted papillomas. *Clin Otol* 1999; 24:61–66.
14. Klimek T, Atai E, Schubert M, Glanz H. Inverted papilloma of the nasal cavity and paranasal sinuses: Clinical data, surgical strategy and recurrence rates. *Acta Oto Laryngol* 2000; 120: 267–272.
15. Schlosser RJ, Mason JC, Gross CW. Aggressive endoscopic resection of inverted papilloma: An update. *Otolaryngol Head Neck Surg* 2001; 125:49–53.
16. Campagno J, Wong RT. Intranasal mixed tumors (pleomorphic adenomas). A clinicopathologic study of 40 cases. *Am J Clin Path* 1977; 68:213–218.
17. Fu YS, Perzin KH: Nonepithelial tumors of the nasal cavity, paranasal sinuses and nasopharynx: A clinicopathologic study III. Cartilagenous tumors (chondroma, chondrosarcoma). *Cancer* 1974; 34:453–463.
18. Atallah N, Jay MM. Osteomas of the paranasal sinuses. *J Laryngol Otol* 1981; 95:291–309.
19. Fu YS, Perzin KH. Nonepithelial tumors of the nasal cavity, paranasal sinuses and nasopharynx: A clinicopathologic study IV. Smooth muscle tumors (leiomyoma, leiomyosarcoma). *Cancer* 1975; 35:1300–1308.
20. Giardello FM, Hamilton SR, Krush AJ, et al. Nasopharyngeal angiofibroma in patients with familial adenomatous polyposis. *Gastroenterology* 1993;105:1550–1552.
21. Lloyd G, Howard D, Phelps P, Cheesman A. Juvenile angiofibroma: The lessons of 20 years of modern imaging. *J Laryngol Otol* 1999; 113:127–134.
22. Michaels L. Angiofobroma. In *Ear, Nose and Throat Histopathology*, Michaels L. London: Springer-Verlag, 1987; 253.
23. Shaheen, OH. Angiofibroma. In *Scott Browns Otolaryngology*, Vol 5, 6th edn. London: Butterworth, 1997; 12/1–12-6.
24. Balogh K. The head and neck. In Pathology, Rubin E, Farber JL. (Eds). 3rd edn. Philadelphia: Lippincott-Raven, 1998; 1300–1334.
25. Carrau RL, Snyderman CH, Kassam AB, Jungreis CA. Endoscopic and endoscopic assisted surgery for juvenile angiofibroma, *Laryngoscope* 2001; 111:483–487.
26. Campbell B, Sandhu G, O'Donnell J, Howard D. Consumptive coagulopathy complicating juvenile angiofibroma. *J Laryngol Otol* 2004;118:835–839.
27. Lloyd G, Howard D, Lund VJ, Savy L. Radiology in focus: Imaging for juvenile angiofibroma. *J Laryngol Otol* 2000; 114:727–730.
28. Radkowski D, Mcgill T, Healy GB, Ohlms L, Jones DT. Angiofibroma: Changes in staging and treatment. *Arch Otolaryngol Head Neck Surg* 1996; 122:122–129.
29. Gates GA, Rice DH, Koopman CF Jr, Schuller DE. Flutamide induced regression of nasopharyngeal angiofibroma. *Laryngoscope* 1992; 102:641–644.
30. Cummings BJ, Blend R, Keane T et al. Primary radiation therapy for juvenile nasopharyngeal angiofibroma. *Laryngoscope* 1984; 94:1599–1605.
31. Metin OT, Taskin YO, Oguz O. Endoscopic surgery in treatment of juvenile nasopharyngeal angiofibroma. *Int J Paed Otorhinolaryngol* 2003; 67:1219–1225.
32. Mair EA, Battiata A, Casler JD. Endoscopic laser assisted excision of juvenile nasopharyngeal angiofibromas. *Arch Otolaryngol Head Neck Surg* 2003; 129:454–459.

CHAPTER 30

Microbiology and Medical Management of Bacterial Sinusitis

Itzhak Brook

The current principles of management of bacterial sinusitis include the accurate establishment of the diagnosis using clinical information, prescribing, and treating the patient with an antibiotic chosen for predicted probability of success and that reduces the potential of antimicrobial resistance. The growing resistance to antimicrobial agents of most respiratory tract bacterial pathogens has made the treatment of sinusitis more difficult. The upper respiratory tract including the nasopharynx serves as the reservoir for pathogenic bacteria that can cause respiratory infections including sinusitis.[1] Potential pathogens can relocate during a viral respiratory infection, from the nasopharynx into the sinus cavity, causing sinusitis.[2] The establishment of the correct microbiology of all forms of sinusitis is of primary importance as it can guide the adequate choice of antimicrobial therapy. This chapter summarizes the microbiology of acute and chronic sinusitis and the approaches to antimicrobial and adjuvant therapy.

The patern of sinusitis as well as other upper respiratory infections evolves in several phases (Fig. 30.1). The early stage often is viral that generally lasts up to 10 days and complete recovery occurs in most cases.[3] However, in a small number (about 0.5%) with viral sinusitis a secondary acute bacterial infection may develop. This is often caused by facultative aerobic bacteria (*Streptococcus pneumoniae*, *Haemophilus influenzae* and *Moraxella catarrhalis*). If resolution does not occur anaerobic bacteria of oral flora origin emerge over time. The dynamics of these bacterial changes were demonstrated by performing serial cultures in patients with maxillary sinusitis.[22]

Viral infection (usually rhinovirus, adenovirus, influenzae, and parainfluenzae viruses) is the most common predisposing factor for upper respiratory tract infections, including sinusitis.[3,4] Viral infection can also coexist with bacterial infection. The mechanism whereby

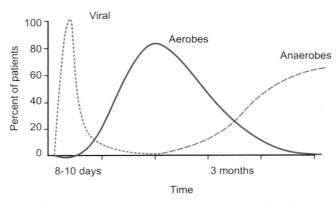

Fig. 30.1: The microbiological dynamics of sinusitis

viruses predispose to sinusitis may involve viral-bacterial synergy, induction of local inflammation that blocks the sinus ostia, increase of bacterial attachment to the epithelial cells, and disruption of the local immune defense.

MICROBIOLOGY OF ACUTE SINUSITIS

In about two-thirds of patients with bacterial maxillary sinusitis microorganisms can be isolated;[5] the methods used are direct puncture aspiration or surgery. The organisms thus recovered from children and adults with community-acquired acute purulent maxillary, frontal, and ethmoid sinusitis, are the common respiratory pathogens *S. pneumoniae*, *H. influenzae*, *M. catarrhalis* and beta-hemolytic streptococci (Table 30.1).[5–9] *Staphylococcus aureus* and *H. influenzae* are common pathogens in sphenoid sinusitis.[9]

The bacteria causing the infection in children are generally the same as those found in acute otitis media. Of 50 children with acute sinusitis *S. pneumoniae* was isolated in 28%, and *H. influenzae* and *M. catarrhalis* were both isolated in 19% of the aspirates.[7] Beta-lactamase-

Table 30.1: Microbiology of sinusitis[6,8,9,21]

Bacteria	Maxillary		Ethmoid		Frontal		Sphenoid	
	Acute	*Chronic* N = 66	*Acute* N = 26	*Chronic* N = 17	*Acute* N = 15	*Chronic* N = 13	*Acute* N = 16	*Chronic* N = 7
Aerobic								
S. aureus	4	14	15	24	–	15	56	14
S. pyogenes	2	8	8	6	3	–	6	–
S. pneumoniae	31	6	35	6	33	–	6	–
H. influenzae	21	5	27	6	40	15	12	14
M. catarrhalis	8	6	8	–	20	–	–	
Enterobacteriaceae	7	6	–	47	–	8	–	28
P. aeruginosa	2	3	–	6	–	8	6	14
Anaerobic								
Peptostreptococcus sp.	2	56	15	59	3	38	19	57
P. acnes		29	12	18	3	8	12	29
Fusobacterium sp.	2	17	4	47	3	31	6	54
Prevotella and Porphyromonas sp.	2	47	8	82	3	62	6	86
B. fragilis		6	–	–	–	15	–	–

Gwaltney, 2000; Brook et al. 1989, 2002, 2003.

producing strains of *H. influenzae* and *M. catarrhalis* were found in 20% and 27% of the patients, respectively. The infection is polymicrobial in about a third of the cases. Enteric organisms are recovered less often. Anaerobes are recovered from acute sinusitis associated with dental disease, mostly as an extension of the infection from the roots of the premolar or molar teeth.[10,11]

Pseudomonas aeruginosa and other aerobic gram-negative rods are often seen in sinusitis of nosocomial origin (especially in patients who have nasal tubes or catheters), sinusitis in patients using mechanical ventilation,[12] immunocompromised individuals, patients with HIV infection and those with cystic fibrosis.[13] Fungal sinusitis is common in immunocompromised or diabetic patients.[14]

We assessed the microbiology of nosocomial sinusitis in 20 mechanically ventilated children.[12] The study demonstrated the polymicrobial aerobic-anaerobic flora of nosocomial sinusitis in mechanically ventilated children. A total of 58 isolates (2.9/specimen), 30 aerobic or facultative and 28 anaerobic, were isolated. Aerobes only were present in 8 patients (40%), anaerobes only in 5 (25%), and mixed aerobic and anaerobic flora in 7 (35%). The predominant aerobes were *P. aeruginosa*, *S. aureus*, *Escherichia coli*, and *Klebsiella pneumoniae*. The predominant anaerobes were *Peptostreptococcus*, *Prevotella*, and *Fusobacterium* spp. Anaerobes were more commonly isolated from aspirate obtained after 18 days of mechanical ventilation (21 vs 7, P < 0.05).

MICROBIOLOGY OF CHRONIC SINUSITIS

Anaerobes were identified in chronic maxillary sinusitis whenever techniques for their cultivation were used.[15-18] The predominant isolates were pigmented *Prevotella*, *Fusobacterium*, and *Peptostreptococcus* spp. (Table 30.1). The most common aerobes were *S. aureus*, *M. catarrhalis* and *Haemophilus* spp. Aerobic and anaerobic beta-lactamase-producing bacteria (BLPB) were isolated from over a third of these patients.[15-19] These were *S. aureus*, *Haemophilus*, *Prevotella* and *Fusobacterium* spp. Nord[18] summarized 12 studies of chronic sinusitis, including 1090 patients (40 children). Anaerobes were recovered in 11 studies in 12–80% of the patients.

The microbiological features of chronic maxillary sinusitis that persist after sinus surgery is unique.[20] *P. aeruginosa* and gram-negative aerobic bacilli were more often isolated in the 33 patients who had surgery than in 75 patients who did not have surgery. Anaerobes were isolated more often in patients who did not have surgery than in those who did.

The importance of anerobes in chronic sinusitis is supported by the detection of antibodies (IgG) to two anerobic organisms commonly recovered from sinus aspirates (*Fusobacterium nucleatum* and *Prevotella intermedia*).[22] Antibody levels to these organisms declined in the patients who improved and were cured after therapy, but did not decrease in those who failed.

The transition from acute to chronic sinusitis was investigated by repeated endoscopic aspirations of sinus

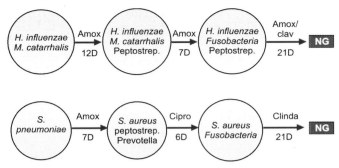

Fig. 30.2: Demonstration of the microbiological dynamics of sinusitis in two patients[23]

secretions in five patients with acute maxillary sinusitis who did not respond to therapy (Fig. 30.2).[23] Most bacteria found in the first culture were aerobic or facultative bacteria—*S. pneumoniae*, *H. influenzae* and *M. catarrhalis*. Failure to respond to therapy was associated with the recovery of resistant bacteria in subsequent aspirates. These included *F. nucleatum*, pigmented *Prevotella*, *Porphyromonas*, and *Peptostreptococcus spp*. Eradication of the infection was eventually achieved following administration of effective antimicrobials, and in three cases by surgical drainage too.

When chronicity develops, the aerobic and facultative species are gradually replaced by anaerobes. This transition may result from the selective pressure of antimicrobial agents that enable resistant organisms to survive, and from the development of conditions appropriate for anaerobic growth, which include the reduction in oxygen tension and an increase in acidity within the sinus. These are caused by the persistent edema and swelling, which reduces blood supply, and by the consumption of oxygen by the aerobic bacteria.[24] Other factors are the emergence over time or selection of anaerobes that possess virulence factors such as a capsule.[25]

Polymicrobial infection is common in chronic sinusitis, which is synergistic[26] and may be more difficult to eradicate with narrow-spectrum antimicrobial agents.

Discrepancies in the Recovery of Bacteria from Multiple Sinuses

There are differences in the distribution of organisms in a single patient who suffers from infections in multiple sinuses that emphasizes the importance of obtaining cultures from all infected sinuses. A recent study evaluated this phenomenon by studying the aerobic and anaerobic microbiology of acute and chronic sinusitis in patients with involvement of multiple sinuses. [27]

The evaluated patients (n = 155) had sinusitis of either the maxillary, ethmoid, or frontal sinuses (any combination) and organisms were recovered from 2–4 concomitantly infected sinuses. Similar aerobic, facultative, and anaerobic organisms were recovered from all the groups of patients. In patients who had organisms isolated from two sinuses and had acute sinusitis, 31 (56%) of the 55 isolates were found only in a single sinus, and 24 (44%) were recovered concomitantly from two sinuses. In those with chronic infection 31 (34%) of the 91 isolates were recovered only from a single sinus, and 60 (66%) were found concomitantly from two sinuses. Anaerobic bacteria were more often concomitantly isolated from two sinuses (50 of 70) than aerobic and facultative (10 of 21, $p < 0.05$). Similar findings were observed in patients who had organisms isolated from 3 or 4 sinuses. Beta-lactamase-producing bacteria were more often isolated from patients with chronic infection (58–83%) as compared to those with acute infections (32–43%). These findings illustrate that there are differences in the distribution of organisms in a single patients who suffers from infections in multiple sinuses and emphasizes the importance of obtaining cultures from all infected sinuses.

Bacteria in Acute Exacerbation of Chronic Sinusitis

Acute exacerbation of chronic sinusitis (AECS) represents a sudden worsening of the baseline chronic sinusitis with either worsening or new symptoms. Typically, the acute (not chronic) symptoms resolve completely between occurrences.[28] We evaluated the microbiology of maxillary AECS by performing repeated endoscopic aspirations in 7 patients over a period of 125 to 242 days.[29] Bacteria were recovered for all aspirates and the number of isolates varied between two and four. The aerobes isolated were *H. influenzae*, *S. pneumoniae*, *M. catarrhalis*, *S. aureus*, and *K. pneumoniae*. The anaerobes included pigmented *Prevotella* and *Porphyromonas*, *Peptostreptococcus*, and *Fusobacterium* spp., and *Propionibacterium acnes*. A change in the types of isolates was noted in all consecutive cultures obtained from the same patients, as different organisms emerged, and previously isolated bacteria were no longer found. An increase in antimicrobial resistance was noted in 6 instances. These findings illustrate the microbial dynamics of AECS where anaerobic and aerobic bacteria prevail, and highlights the importance of obtaining cultures from patients with AECS for guidance in selection of proper antimicrobial therapy.

Brook et al[30] compared the microbiology of maxillary AECS in 30 patients with the microbiology of chronic maxillary sinusitis in 32. The study illustrated the predominance of anaerobic bacteria and polymicrobial nature of both conditions (2.5–3 isolates/sinus). However, aerobic bacteria that are usually found in acute infections (e.g. *S. pneumoniae, H. influenzae,* and *M. catarrhalis)* emerged in some of the episodes of AECS.

MICROBIOLOGY OF NOSOCOMIAL RHINOSINUSITIS

Nosocomial sinusitis often develops in patients who require extended periods of intensive care (postoperative patients, burn victims, patients with severe trauma) involving prolonged endotracheal or nasogastric intubation.[31] Nasotracheal intubation places the patient at a substantially higher risk for nosocomial sinusitis than orotracheal intubation. Approximately 25% of patients requiring nasotracheal intubation for more than 5 days develop nosocomial sinusitis.[32] In contrast to community-acquired sinusitis, the pathogens are usually gram-negative enterics (*P. aeruginosa, K. pneumoniae,* Enterobacter species, *Proteus mirabilis, Serratia marcescens*) and gram-positive cocci (occasionally streptococci and staphylococci). Whether these organisms are actually pathogenic is unclear as their recovery may represent only colonization of an environment with impaired mucociliary transport and foreign body presence in the nasal cavity.

Evaluation of the microbiology of nosocomial sinusitis in nine children with neurologic impairment revealed anaerobic bacteria, always mixed with aerobic and facultative bacteria, in 6 (67%) sinus aspirates and aerobic bacteria only in 3 (33%).[33] There were 24 bacterial isolates, 12 aerobic or facultative and 12 anaerobic. The predominant aerobic isolates were *K. pneumoniae, Escherichia coli, S. aureus, Proteus mirabilis, P. aeruginosa, H. influenzae, M. catarrhalis,* and *S. pneumoniae* (1 each). The predominant anerobes were *Prevotella* spp., *Peptostreptococcus* spp., *F. nucleatum,* and *Bacteroides fragilis.* Organisms similar to those recovered from the sinuses were also found in the tracheostomy site and gastrostomy wound aspirates in five of seven instances. This study demonstrates the uniqueness of the microbiologic features of sinusitis in neurologically impaired children, in which, in addition to the organisms known to cause infection in children without neurologic impairment, facultative and anaerobic gram-negative organisms that can colonize other body sites are predominant.

ANTIMICROBIAL MANAGEMENT

Antimicrobial Resistance

Management of bacterial sinusitis is often a challenging endeavor in which selection of the most appropriate antimicrobial agents remains a key decision. This has become more difficult in recent years as all the predominant bacterial pathogens have gradually developed resistance to the commonly used antibiotics.

Three major mechanisms of resistance to penicillin occur:
- Porin channel blockage (e.g. used by *Pseudomonas spp.* to resist carbapenems).
- Production of the enzyme beta-lactamase (e.g. used by *H. influenzae* and *M. catarrhalis*).
- Alterations in the penicillin-binding protein (e.g. used by *S. pneumoniae*).

The increase in bacterial resistance to antibiotics is related to their frequent use. Previous therapy can increase the prevalence of BLPB. In a study of 26 children who had received a week of therapy with penicillin, 12% harboured BLPB in their oropharyngeal flora prior to therapy.[34] This increased to 46% at the conclusion of therapy, and the incidence was 27% after 3 months. The incidence of BLPB was high in siblings and parents of patients treated with penicillin, who probably acquired these organisms from the patient.[35] A greater prevalence of recovery of BLPB in the oropharynx of children occurs in the winter and a lower one in the summer.[36] These changes correlated with the intake of beta-lactam antibiotics. Monitoring the local variations in the rate of recovery of antimicrobial resistance may help the empirical choice of antimicrobial agents. The proper and judicious use of antimicrobials may control and reduce antimicrobial resistance.

Beta-lactamase Production

Bacterial resistance to the antibiotics commonly used for the treatment of sinusitis has consistently increased in recent years. Production of the enzyme beta-lactamase is one of the most important mechanisms of penicillin resistance. Several BLPB occur in sinusitis.

BLPB can be recovered from over a third of patients with sinusitis.[6,16] BLPB may not only survive penicillin therapy but in a polymicrobial infection they may also

Table 30.2: Microbiology and beta-lactamase detection in 4 patients with chronic maxillary sinusitis[30]

Organism	Patient no.			
	1	2	3	4
Staphylococcus aureus (BL +)		+		+
Streptococcus pneumoniae	+			
Peptostreptococcus spp	+			+
Propionibacterium acnes	+			
Fusobacterium spp (BL +)		+		+
Fusobacterium spp (BL –)		+		+
Prevotella spp (BL +)			+	
Prevotella spp (BL –)	+	+	+	
Bacteroides fragilis group (BL +)	+			+

'shield' other penicillin-susceptible bacteria from penicillin by releasing the free enzyme into their environment. The actual activity of the enzyme beta-lactamase and the phenomenon of 'shielding' were demonstrated recently in acutely and chronically inflamed sinus fluids.[30] BLPB were isolated in four of 10 acute sinusitis aspirates and in 10 of 13 chronic sinusitis aspirates (Table 30.2). The predominant BLPB isolated in acute sinusitis were *H. influenzae* and *M. catarrhalis*, and those found in chronic sinusitis were *Prevotella* and *Fusobacterium spp.*[37] Free beta-lactamase was detected in 86% of these aspirates, and was associated with persistence of penicillin susceptible pathogens.

S. Pneumoniae Resistance

S. pneumoniae uses a different mechanism of resistance to penicillin, through changes in penicillin-binding proteins. About half of the penicillin-resistant strains are currently intermediately resistant (minimal inhibitory concentration [MIC] of 0.1–1.0 mg/ml) and the rest are highly resistant (MIC > 2.0 mg/ml). A larger problem is multidrug-resistant pneumococci. Penicillin-resistant strains can also show resistance to other antimicrobial agents (including oral third-generation cephalosporins, trimethoprim-sulfamethoxazole (TMP/SMX), tetracyclines, and macrolides) but they are susceptible to vancomycin. Intermediately resistant *S. pneumoniae* are still susceptible *in vitro* to high concentrations of penicillin or amoxicillin.[38] Clindamycin and the oral second-generation cephalosporins, especially cefuroxime axetil and cefprozil, are also effective *in vitro* against over 95% of intermediately penicillin-resistant strains.[39]

Risk factors for the development of antimicrobial resistance include prior antibiotic exposure, day-care attendance, < 2 years of age, recent hospitalization and recurrent infection (especially at extreme ages).[40]

The variety of organisms involved in sinusitis, increasing levels of resistance to antibiotic agents and the phenomenon of beta-lactamase 'shielding' from antibiotic agents all contribute to the therapeutic challenges associated with the management of acute and chronic sinusitis.

Antimicrobial Agents

The antimicrobials most commonly used to treat acute sinusitis (Tables 30.3 and 30.4) include amoxicillin (with and without clavulanic acid), oral and parenteral cephalosporins, macrolides and TMP/SMX. Amoxicillin is safe and inexpensive, and when given in a high dose is still active against intermediately penicillin susceptible *S. pneumoniae*. However, the growing resistance of *H. influenzae* and *M. catarrhalis* to amoxicillin increases the risk that it will fail to clear the infection. However, the addition of clavulanic acid (a beta-lactamase inhibitor) to amoxicillin or the use of antimicrobial agents resistant to beta-lactamase activity is effective against resistant organisms.

The increase in resistance of *S. pneumoniae* to penicillin mandates an increase in the amount of amoxicillin (90 mg/kg/day in children and 4 g/day in adults). This requires the addition of an equal amount of amoxicillin to amoxicillin-clavulanic acid or the use of the newer formulation of this drug (given twice daily) that contains higher proportions of amoxicillin to the beta-lactamase inhibitor.

First-generation cephalosporins are not active against *H. influenzae* and many *S. pneumoniae* strains. The second-generation cephalosporins (cefuroxime-axetil, cefdinir, cefprozil and cefpodoxime) are more active against penicillin-resistant *Haemophilus* and *Moraxella* spp. and intermediately penicillin-resistant *S. pneumoniae*.[39]

Oral third-generation cephalosporins (cefixime and ceftibuten) are most active against penicillin-resistant *Haemophilus* and *Moraxella* spp., but are less effective against *S. pneumoniae* resistant to penicillin. Parenteral third-generation cephalosporins (cefotaxime or ceftriaxone) are active against beta-lactamase producing *H. influenzae* and *M. catarrhalis*, as well as over 90% of intermediately resistant *S. pneumoniae*.

TMP/SMX has lost efficacy against all major pathogens, including *S. pneumoniae* and Group A beta-hemolytic streptococci (GABHS). The sulfa component can cause hypersensitivity reactions.

Erythromycin is inactive against *H. influenzae* and some GABHS. Resistance of GABHS to erythromycin and other macrolides occurs in countries where these agents

Table 30.3: Antibiotics used for bacterial sinusitis (PO)

Antibiotic	Adult dosage	Pediatric dosage (mg/kg)	Duration of therapy for acute sinusitis (days)
Beta-lactams			
Cefprozil (Cefzil)	250–500 mg bid	7.5–15 bid	10
Cefuroxime axetil (Ceftin)	250–500 mg bid	10–15 bid	10
Cefpodoxime (Vantin)	200–400 mg bid	5 bid	10
Cefdinir (Omnicef)	300 mg bid	7 bid/14 qd	10
Amoxicillin (Amoxil, Trimox, Wymox)	500 mg tid or 875 mg bid	20–45 bid	14
Amoxicillin-clavulanate (Augmentin)	500 mg tid* or 875 mg or 2000 mg (XR) bid*	22.5 or 45 (ES600) bid	10
Ketolides			
Telithromycin (Ketek)	800 mg qd	NA	5
Macrolides			
Azithromycin (Zithromax)	250 mg qd	10 day 1, then 5 qd	3 or 5
Clarithromycin (Biaxin)	500 mg bid	7.5 bid	14
Fluoroquinolones			
Levofloxacin (Levaquin)	500 mg qd	NA	10
Gatifloxacin (Tequin)	500 mg qd	NA	10
Moxifloxacin (Avelox)	400 mg qd	NA	10
Others			
Clindamycin (Cleocin)	150–450 mg tid or qid	7.5 qid or 6 tid	10
TMP-SMX (Bactrim, Septra)	160 mg/800 mg bid	8–12 bid	10

*Based on amoxicillin component.
NA = not approved for patients < 18 years of age.

were overused (e.g. Japan, Finland, Spain, Taiwan and Turkey).[41] Cross-resistance of *S. pneumoniae* is common among all macrolides. Azithromycin has improved efficacy against aerobic gram-negative organisms (*H. influenzae* and *M. catarrhalis*), while clarithromycin is more efficient than erythromycin against aerobic gram-positive organisms.[42] Currently, however, increased resistance of *S. pneumoniae* has developed to all macrolides (up to 33%), and survival of azithromycin-susceptible *H. influenzae* in the middle ear and sinuses.[43] The persistence of the organism is believed to result from accumulation of azithromycin within the middle ear white cells only, and not in the middle ear fluid. Clindamycin is effective against aerobic gram-positive organisms, including penicillin-resistant *S. pneumoniae*; however, it is not active against aerobic gram-negative pathogens.[39] Vancomycin (a glycopeptide) is effective against penicillin-resistant *S. pneumoniae* and methicillin-resistant *S. aureus*. However, it has no efficacy against *H. influenzae* or *M. catarrhalis*. Telithromycin is effective against penicillin-resistant *S. pneumoniae* as well as *H. influenzae* or *M. catarrhalis*.

The older quinolones (i.e. ciprofloxacin, ofloxacin) are active against *H. influenzae* and *M. catarrhalis*, but have minimal activity against *S. pneumoniae*. The newer quinolones (e.g. levofloxacin, gatifloxacin, and moxifloxacin) are very effective against *S. pneumoniae*[35] but are currently not recommended for use in children because of the potential adverse effects on the cartilage.

PRINCIPLES OF ANTIMICROBIAL THERAPY

When selecting the empirical antimicrobial therapy for sinuses, a choice between narrow and broad spectrum antimicrobial agents must be made. In patient who fails to show significant improvement or shows signs of deterioration despite therapy, it is important to obtain a culture preferably through sinus puncture, as this may reveal the presence of resistant bacteria. Endoscopic culture is an alternative approach.[44] However, the specimen can become contaminated with nasal flora. Surgical drainage may be very important at that time. Culture of nasal pus or of sinus exudate obtained by rinsing through the sinus ostium can give unreliable information because of contamination by the resident

Table 30.4: *In vitro* efficacy of antimicrobial agents used in bacterial sinusitis therapy

Antimicrobial agent	S. pneumoniae		H. influenzae		M. catarrhalis	Anerobes		S. aureus
	Pen-S	Pen-IR	BL–	BL+	BL+	Pen-S	Pen-R	Pen-R§
Amoxicillin	+	+	+	–	–	+	–	–
Amoxicillin-clavulanate	+	+	+	+	+	+	+	+
Cephalexin (1st generation)	+	–	±	–	–	+	–	+
Cefactor (2nd generation)	±	–	+	±	±	+	–	+
Cefprozil (2nd generation)	+	+	+	±	+	+	–	+
Cefuroxime axetil (2nd generation)	+	+	+	+	+	+	–	+
Cefpodoxime (2nd generation)	+	±	+	+	+	+	–	+
Cefdinir (2nd generation)	+	±	+	+	+	+	–	+
Cefixime (3rd generation)	+	–	+	+	+	±	–	–
Ceftibuten (3rd generation)	+	–	+	+	+	±	–	–
Loracarbef	±	–	+	+	+	+	–	±
Ceftriaxone*	+	+	+	+	+	+	–	±
Erythromycin-sulfisoxazole	±	–	+	±	±	±	–	±
Trimethoprim-sulfamethoxazole	±	–	+	±	±	–	–	±
Erythromycin	+	±	±	–	±	±	–	±
Azithromycin	+	±	±	±	+	±	–	±
Clarithromycin	+	±	±	±	±	±	–	+
Telithromycin	+	+	+	+	+	+	-	+
Clindamycin	+	+	–	–	–	+	+	+
Quinolones								
Ciprofloxacin	±	±	+	+	+	±	–	±
Levofloxacin	+	–	+	+	+	±	–	+
Gatifloxacin	+	+	+	+	+	+	–	+
Moxifloxacin	+	+	+	+	+	+	±	+
Carbapenems*	+	+	+	+	+	+	+	+

BL– = beta-lactamase non-producers; BL+ = beta-lactamase producers; Pen-S = penicillin susceptible; Pen-R = penicillin resistance; Pen-IR = penicillin intermediate resistance.
+ = very susceptible; ± = minimal susceptibility; – = not susceptible.
*Available in parenteral form only; †Available (also) in parenteral form; ‡Imipenem-cilastatin, meropenem, ertapenem;§Methicillin susceptible.

bacterial nasal flora. Further antimicrobial therapy is based, whenever possible, on the results of the culture. Selection of the appropriate agent(s) is generally made on an empirical basis, and the agents should be effective against any potential organisms that may cause the infection.[23]

The goal of antimicrobial therapy is to eradicate the susceptible organisms in the sinus cavity. Although standard parameters of antimicrobial activity such as MIC and minimal bactericidal concentration are helpful, they do not provide information about the time course or rate of kill relative to concentration or whether post-antibiotic effects contribute to activity.[45] Antibiotics can be divided into two major groups: Those that exhibit concentration-dependent killing and prolonged persistent effects and those that exhibit time-dependent killing and minimal-

to-moderate persistent effects. With agents that fall into the former group the area under the concentration-time curve (AUC) (i.e. quinolones) and peak levels (aminoglycosides) are the major parameters that correlate with clinical efficacy. The ratio of peak concentration to MIC is a measure of potency that also indicates the efficacy of the drug in these agents. With drugs that exhibit time-dependent killing and minimal-to-moderate persistent effects, time above MIC is the major parameter determining efficacy. Beta-lactams and macrolides belong to this second group. Studies in otitis media show that there appears to be a relationship between the time above MIC in serum and in middle ear fluid (MEF) for beta-lactam antibiotics. It is predicted that to achieve at least 80–85% bacteriologic cure in otitis media, serum concentrations should exceed the MIC of pathogens for at least 40% of the dosing interval. For the same cure rate, the peak MEF to MIC ratio should be in the range of 3–6. If the MICs for pathogens are known, it will be possible to predict those agents for which adequate concentrations can be achieved.

Factors within the sinus cavity that can enable organisms to survive antimicrobial therapy are inadequate penetration of antimicrobial agents, high protein concentration (can bind antimicrobial agents), high content of enzymes that inactivate antimicrobial agents (i.e. beta-lactamase), decreased multiplication rate of organisms that interfere with the activity of bacteriostatic agents and reduction in pH and oxygen partial pressure, which reduces the efficacy of some anti-microbial agents (e.g. aminoglycosides and quinolones).[46]

Failure to attain clinical improvement on completion of appropriate antibiotic therapy should prompt consideration of bacterial resistance, non-compliance, or complicated sinusitis. Antimicrobial agents that achieve good intrasinus concentrations can, however, fail to eradicate the pathogen(s) if there is impairment of local defences (e.g. phagocytosis, ciliary motility) or the sinus environment.

Antimicrobial Therapy of Acute Sinusitis

A number of antimicrobials have been studied in the treatment of acute sinusitis, with the use of pre- and post-treatment aspirate cultures. Studied were ampicillin, amoxicillin, bacampicillin, cyclacillin, cefuroxime axetil, amoxycillin-clavulanic acid, loracarbef, levofloxacin, gatifloxacin, moxifloxacin, and gemifloxacin.[47] For a 10 days course of therapy, the success rate was a bacteriological cure over of 80–90%. Appropriate antibiotic therapy is of paramount importance, even though it is estimated that spontaneous recovery occurs in 48% of patients.[48]

Antimicrobial therapy is beneficial and effective in the prevention of septic complications.[48] The recommended length of therapy for acute sinusitis is at least 14 days, or 7 days beyond the resolution of symptoms, whichever is longer. However, no controlled studies have proved the length of therapy sufficient to resolve the infection.

Six expert panels recently presented reviews and rendered their recommendations how to diagnose and manage sinusitis within the last five years.[49–55] The recommendations of three of these guidelines are presented here, and a synthesis of all are presented at the end of the section.

The Sinus and Allergy Partnership published guidelines[51] are based on predicted bacterial efficacy rates from a mathematic modeling of acute sinusitis. These are based on pathogen distribution, resolution rates without treatment, and *in vitro* microbiologic efficacy. Antibiotics were placed into categories of expected clinical efficacy in adults and children with acute sinusitis.

For adults with mild disease or with moderate disease, bacterial efficacy rates are > 90% (gatifloxacin, levofloxacin, moxifloxacin, and amoxicillin clavulanate), 80 to 90% (high-dose amoxicillin, cefpodoxime proxetil, cefixime [based on *H. influenzae* and *M. catarrhalis* coverage only]), cefuroxime axetil and TMP/SMX, 70 to 80% (clindamycin [based on gram-positive coverage only], doxycycline, cefprozil, azithromycin, clarithromycin, and erythromycin), and 50 to 60% (cefaclor and loracarbef). The predicted spontaneous resolution rate in adults with acute sinusitis is 47%. Antibiotics were placed into a similar rank order of predicted efficacy in children except for the quinolones. Gatifloxacin, levofloxacin, and moxifloxacin are indicated for adults who are beta-lactam allergic or intolerant. Azithromycin, clarithromycin, erythromycin, or TMP/SMX are recommended if the patient has a history of hypersensitivity reaction to beta-lactams. Recommendations for initial therapy for those who have received antibiotics in the previous 4 to 6 weeks include amoxicillin/clavulanate, gatifloxacin, levofloxacin, moxifloxacin (in adults only), or combination therapy (amoxicillin or clindamycin [gram-positive coverage] plus cefpodoxime proxetil or cefixime [gram-negative coverage]). In 2004, the Sinus and Allergy Health Partnership published antimicrobial treatment guidelines for acute bacterial rhinosinusitis[55] that updated the original that was published in 2000.[51] The more recent guidelines largely reflected those of the original publication; the areas of significant update included diagnostic modalities, contemporary antibacterial susceptibility profiles, addition of newer antimicrobial agents as recommended therapy, and expansion of the various pharmacodymanic/pharmacokinetic principles and therapeutic outcomes model used to predict potential success of the individual agents.

The anti-infective agents recommended for use to treat pediatric and adult patients with mildly symptomatic sinusitis who had not been exposed to an antibiotic in the preceding 4–6 weeks were amoxicillin, amoxicilin-clavulanate, cefpodoxime, cefuroxime, and cefdinir. Treatment options for adult patients with mild sinusitis who had been exposed to an antibiotic in the previous 4–6 weeks and those adult patients with moderately symptomatic sinusitis were gatifloxacin, levofloxacin, moxifloxacin, amoxicillin-clavulanate, ceftriaxone, or a combination of either amoxicillin or clindamycin and either cefixime or rifampin. Treatment options for pediatric patients with mild sinusitis who had been exposed to an antibiotic in the previous 4–6 weeks and those pediatric patients with moderately symptomatic sinusitis were amoxicillin-clavulanate, cefpodoxime, cefuroxime, cefdinir, ceftriaxone, or a combination of either amoxicillin or clindamycin, and either cefixime or rifampin.

The Clinical Advisory Committee on Pediatric and Adult Sinusitis has developed guidelines of bacterial sinusitis, that were based primarily on expert opinion.[53] It was recommended to begin treatment with an inexpensive first-line agent (e.g. amoxicillin). Because of the increased resistance of *S. pneumoniae* the amoxicillin dose be doubled (up to 90 mg/kg/day in children; maximum of 4 g/day in adults). Second-line agents should be used in those who do not improve within 3–5 days and should also be considered for initial use when resistant pathogens are suspected.

The risk factors for infection with increased resistance include: recent use of antibiotic, resistance common in the community, failure of first-line agent, infection in spite of prophylactic treatment, smoker in family, child in daycare facility, age less than 2 years, patient history, allergy to penicillin or amoxicillin, frontal or sphenoidal sinusitis, complicated ethmoidal sinusitis, and presentation with protracted (> 30 days) symptoms. The second-line agents include agents with proven efficacy based on clinical and *in vitro* data against potential resistant pathogens. These agents include amoxicillin-clavulanate (containing high amoxicillin dose) and the second-generation cephalosporins with adequate *S. pneumoniae* and *H. influenzae* coverage (ceprozil, cefuroxime-axetil, cefpedoxime). For penicillin-allergic individuals, macrolides may be considered. If that approach fails, a combination of clindamycin plus a third-generation oral cephalosporin, or ceftriaxone (injectable), is an option. Fluoroquinolones with adequate *S. pneumoniae* coverage (gatifloxacin, moxifloxacin) can be used in adults.

The American Academy of Pediatrics Subcommittee on Management of Sinusitis recommended that when antibiotics are indicated these should be a high dose of amoxicillin or amoxicillin-clavulanate 90 mg/kg/day, cefuroxime, cefpodoxime, or cefdinir.[54] Azithromycin or clarithromycin are oindicated in penicillin allergic individuals.

A practical synthesis of all recomendations is the following: Amoxicillin can be appropriate for the initial treatment of acute uncomplicated mild sinusitis (Tables 30.3 to 30.6). However, antimicrobials that are more effective against the major bacterial pathogens (including those that are resistant to multiple antibiotics) may be indicated as initial therapy and for the re-treatment of those who have risk factors prompting a need for more effective antimicrobials (Table 30.5) and those who had failed amoxicillin therapy. These agents include: Amoxicillin and clavulanic acid, the newer quinolones (e.g. levofloxacin, gatifloxacin, moxifloxacin), telithromycin and some second- and third-generation cephalosporins (cefdinir, cefuroxime-axetil, and cefpodoxime proxetil).

These antimicrobials should be administered to patients where bacterial resistance is likely (i.e. recent

Table 30.5: Empirical antimicrobial therapy in acute bacterial sinusitis

Amoxicillin Therapy (High-dose)
- Mild illness
- No history of recurrent acute sinusitis
- During summer months
- When no recent antimicrobial therapy has been used
- When patient has had no recent contact with patient(s) on antimicrobial therapy
- When community experience shows high success rate of amoxicillin

Risk factors prompting a need for more effective antimicrobials*
Bacterial resistance is likely
- Antibiotic use in the past month, or close contact with a treated individual(s)
- Resistance common in community
- Failure of previous antimicrobial therapy
- Infection in spite of prophylactic treatment
- Child in day-care facility
- Winter season
- Smoker or smoker in family

Presence of moderate-to-severe infection
- Presentation with protracted (> 30 days) or moderate to severe symptoms
- Complicated ethmoidal sinusitis
- Frontal or sphenoidal sinusitis
- Patient history of recurrent acute sinusitis

Presence of co-morbidity and extremes of life
- Co-morbidity (i.e. chronic cardiac, hepatic or renal disease, diabetes)
- Immunocompromised patient
- Younger than 2 years of age or older than 55 years

Allergy to penicillin
- Allergy to penicillin or amoxicillin

* Amoxicillin and clavulanic acid, second- and third-generation cephalosporins, telithromycin, and the 'respiratory' quinolones.

antibiotic therapy, winter season, increased resistance in the community), the presence of a moderate to severe infection, the presence of co-morbidity (diabetes, chronic renal, hepatic or cardiac pathology), and when penicillin allergy is present (Tables 30.5 and 30.6). Agents that are less effective because of growing bacterial resistance may, however, be considered for patients with antimicrobial allergy. Thse include: the macrolides, TMP-SMX, tetracyclines, and clindamycin.

Antimicrobial Therapy of Chronic Sinusitis

Many of the pathogens found in chronically inflamed sinuses, are resistant to penicillins through the production of beta-lactamase.[56,57] These include both aerobic (*S. aureus*, *H. influenzae* and *M. catarrhalis*) and anaerobic isolates (*Bacteroides fragilis* and over half of the *Prevotella* and *Fusobacterium* spp.). Retrospective studies illustrate the superiority of therapy effective against both aerobic and anaerobic BLPB in chronic sinusitis.[46,58] Antimicrobials used for treatment of chronic sinusitis should be effective against both aerobic and anaerobic BLPB, as well as those resistant through other mechanisms. These agents include the combination of a penicillin (e.g. amoxicillin) and a beta-lactamase inhibitor (e.g. clavulanic acid), clindamycin, chloramphenicol, the combination of metronidazole and a macrolide, and the newer quinolones (e.g. trovafloxacin). All these agents (or similar ones) are available in oral and parenteral forms. Other effective antimicrobials are available only in parenteral form (e.g.

cefoxitin, cefotetan and cefmetazole). If aerobic gram-negative organisms, such as *P. aeruginosa*, are involved, parenteral therapy with an aminoglycosides, a fourth-generation cephalosporin (cefepime or ceftazidime) or oral or parenteral treatment with a fluoroquinolone (only in postpubertal patients) is added. Parenteral therapy with a carbapenem (i.e. imipenem, meropenem, ertapenem) is more expensive, but provides coverage for most potential pathogens, both anerobes and aerobes. Therapy is given for at least 21 days, and may be extended up to 10 weeks. Fungal sinusitis can be treated with surgical debridement of the affected sinuses and antifungal therapy.[14]

In contrast to acute sinusitis that is generally treated vigorously with antibiotics, surgical drainage is the mainstay of treatment of chronic sinusitis especially in patients who had not responded to medical therapy. Impaired drainage may contribute to the development of chronic sinusitis, and correction of the obstruction helps to alleviate the infection and prevent recurrence. The use of antimicrobial therapy alone without surgical drainage of collected pus may not result in clearance of the infection. The chronically inflamed sinus membranes with diminished vascularity may not allow for an adequate antibiotic level to accumulate in the infected tissue, even when the blood level is therapeutic. Furthermore, the reduction in the pH and oxygen tension within the inflamed sinus can interfere with the antimicrobial activity, which can result in bacterial survival despite a high antibiotic concentration.[39]

Table 30.6: Recommended antibacterial agents for initial treatment of acute sinusitis or after no improvement

Factors prompting more effective antibiotics	At diagnosis	Clinically treatment failure at 48–72 hours after starting treatment
No	High-dose amoxicillin	High-dose amoxicillin/clavulanate or a 'new' quinolone** or telithromycin** or cefuroxime or cefdinir or cefpodoxime proxetil
Yes	High-dose amoxicillin/ clavulanate or a 'new' quinolone** or telithromycin** or cefuroxime-axetil or cefdinir or cefpodoxime proxetil	High-dose amoxicillin/clavulanate or a 'new' quinolone** or telithromycin** or cefuroxime-axetil or cefdinir or cefpodoxime proxetil

** Not approved for children (< 18 years)

ADJUVANT THERAPIES

Acute Bacterial Sinusitis

Patients with a viral upper respiratory tract infection may receive benefit from symptomatic therapy, aimed at improving their quality of life during the acute illness. The use of normal saline as a spray or lavage can provide symptomatic improvement by liquefying secretions to encourage drainage. The short-term use (3 days) of topical α-adrenergic decongestants can also provide symptomatic relief, but its use should be restricted to older children and adults due to the potential for undesirable systemic effects in infants and young children. Topical glucocorticosteroids may also be useful in reducing nasal mucosal edema, mostly in those cases where a patient who has seasonal allergic rhinitis develops the complication of an acute upper respiratory tract infection. The antipyretic and analgesic effects of nonsteroidal anti-inflammatory agents can relieve or ameliorate the associated symptoms of fever, headache, generalized malaise, and facial tenderness. Until the clinical diagnosis of acute bacterial sinusitis is established, management of an upper respiratory tract infection should be only symptomatic. Furthermore, symptomatic care can be useful in the management of acute bacterial sinusitis as adjunctive therapy, but no adjunct has been shown essential in improving the outcome achieved by antimicrobial therapy or effective in preventing the development of acute bacterial sinusitis in persons who have a viral upper respiratory tract infection or allergic rhinitis.

Chronic Bacterial Sinusitis

Anti-inflammatories

Long-term, low-dose macrolide therapy represents one attempt at controlling the inflammation associated with chronic sinusitis. Medicines that have anti-inflammatory properties and are tolerated well are sought to help ease the reliance on systemic corticosteroids that affect both the number and function of inflammatory cells.[59] When used in a topical form, nasal steroid sprays have been shown to be safe and effective in reducing the symptoms of alleric rhinitis.[60] Their use in patients with chronic sinusitis can decrease the size of nasal polyps, and diminishing sinomucosal edema.[61] There are no set guidelines for duration of use, and side effects from long-term use are yet to be published and the use of oral steroids in the treatment of chronic sinusitis are only anectodal. The extended use of oral steroid may result in

serious side effects that include muscle wasting and osteoporosis. Because of the side effects, steroids are tapered and given in short courses that may span only 3–4 weeks.

Adjunctive Therapy

Adjunctive therapy is intended at promoting drainage of secretions and improving oxygenation to the obstructed sinus ostia. Multiple agents with different mechanisms of action are often administered. These include decongestants that are alpha-adrenergic agonists, that constrict the capacitance vessels and decrease mucosal edema. Topical therapy such as oxymetazoline or neosynephrine may be used in an acute setting, but overuse can cause a rebound effect and rhinitis medicamentosa. Systemic decongestants can be used for longer periods of time, but may cause insomnia and exacerbation of underlying systemic hypertension.

Antihistamines are used in patients with underlying allergic rhinitis. They can relieve symptoms of itching, rhinorrhea and sneezing in allergic patients, but in non-allergic patients they can cause thickening of secretions which may prevent needed drainage of the sinus ostia.

Guaifenesin (glyceryl guaicolate) given in a daily dose of 2400 mg, thins secretions thus facilitating drainage. Nasal saline irrigations are helpful in thinning secretions and may provide a mild benefit in nasal congestion. Hypertonic saline irrigations improve patient comfort and quality of life, decrease medication use and diminish the need for surgical therapy.[62]

Leukotriene inhibitors are systemic medications that block the receptor and/or production of leukotrienes, potent lipid mediators that increase eosinophil recruitment, goblet cell production, mucosal edema and airway remodeling. Their role in chronic sinusitis and nasal polyposis is not yet well established.[63,64]

REFERENCES

1. Faden H, Stanievich J, Brodsky L et al. Changes in the nasopharyngeal flora during otitis media of childhood. *Pediatr Infect Dis* 1990;9:623–626.
2. Del Beccaro MA, Mendelman PM. Inglis AF et al. Bacteriology of acute otitis media: A new perspective. *J Pediatr* 1992; 120:856–862.
3. Hamory BH, Sande MA, Sydnor A Jr et al. Etiology and antimicrobial therapy of acute maxillary sinusitis. *J Infect Dis* 1979;139:197–202.
4. Subausie MC, Jacoby DB, Richards SM, Proud D. Infection of a human respiratory epithelial cell line with rhinovirus: Induction of cytokine release and modulation of susceptibility to infection by cytokine exposure. *J Clin Invest* 1995;96: 549–557.

5. Evans RD Jr, Sydnor JB, Moore WEC et al. Sinusitis of the maxillary antrum. *N Engl J Med* 1975;293:735–739.

6. Wald ER, Milmore GJ, Bowen AD, Ledema-Medina J, Salamon N, Bluestone CD. Acute maxillary sinusitis in children. *N Engl J Med* 1981;304:749–754.

7. Wald ER, Guerra N, Byers C. Upper respiratory tract infections in young children: Duration of and frequency of complications. *Pediatrics* 1991;87:129–133.

8. Brook I. Bacteriology of acute and chronic frontal sinusitis. *Arch Otolaryngol Head Neck Surg* 2002;128:583–585.

9. Brook I. Bacteriology of acute and chronic sphenoid sinusitis. *Ann Otol Rhinol Laryngol* 2002;111:1002–1004.

10. Brook I, Frazier EH, Gher ME Jr. Microbiology of periapical abscesses and associated maxillary sinusitis. *J Periodontal* 1996;67:608–610.

11. Brook I, Friedman EM. Intracranial complications of sinusitis in children. A sequel of periapical abscess. *Ann Otol Rhinol Laryngol* 1982;91:41–43.

12. Brook I. Microbiology of nosocomial sinusitis in mechanically ventilated children. *Arch Otolaryngol Head Neck Surg* 1998; 124:35–38.

13. Shapiro ED, Milmoe GJ, Wald ER et al. Bacteriology of the maxillary sinuses in patients with cystic fibrosis. *J Infect Dis* 1982;146:589–593.

14. Decker CF. Sinusitis in the immunocompromised host. *Curr Infect Dis Rep* 1999;1:27–32.

15. Brook I. Bacteriological features of chronic sinusitis in children. *JAMA* 1981;246:967–991.

16. Mustafa E, Tahsin A, Mustafa O, Nedret K. Bacteriology of antrum in adults with chronic maxillary sinusitis. *Laryngoscope* 1994;104:321–324.

17. Finegold SM, Flynn MJ, Rose FV et al. Bacteriologic findings associated with chronic bacterial maxillary sinusitis in adults. *Clin Infect Dis* 2002;35:428–433.

18. Nord CE. The role of anaerobic bacteria in recurrent episodes of sinusitis and tonsillitis. *Clin Infect Dis* 1995;20:1512–1524.

19. Brook I. Bacteriology of chronic maxillary sinusitis in adults. *Ann Otol Rhinol Laryngol* 1989;98:426–428.

20. Brook I, Frazier EH. Correlation between microbiology and previous sinus surgery in patients with chronic maxillary sinusitis. *Ann Otol Rhinol Laryngol* 2001;110:148–151.

21. Brook I. Bacteriology of acute and chronic ethmoid sinusitis. Abstract of the 103 General Meeting of the American Society for Medical Microbiology. Washington DC. 2003;Absract D–138.

22. Brook I, Yocum P. Immune response to Fusobacterium Nucleatum and Prevotella Intermedia in patients with chronic maxillary sinusitis. *Ann Otol Rhinol Laryngol* 1999;108:293–295.

23. Brook I, Frazier EH, Foote PA. Microbiology of the transition from acute to chronic maxillary sinusitis. *J Med Microbiol* 1996;45:372–375.

24. Carenfelt C, Lundberg C. Purulent and non-purulent maxillary sinus secretions with respect to PO_2, PCO_2 and pH. *Acta Otolaryngol* 1977;84:138–144.

25. Brook I, Myhal LA, Dorsey CH. Encapsulation and pilus formation of Bacteroides spp. in normal flora abscesses and blood. *J Infect* 1992;24:252–257.

26. Brook I. Enhancement of growth or aerobic and facultative bacteria in mixed infections with *Bacteroides* species. *Infect Immun* 1985;50:929–931.

27. Brook I. Emergence and persistence of beta-lactamase-producing bacteria in the oropharynx following penicillin treatment. *Arch Otolaryngol Head Neck Surg* 1988;114:667–670.

28. Brook I. Discrepancies in the recovery of bacteria from multiple sinuses in acute and chronic sinusitis. *J Med Microbiol* 2004;53:879–885.

29. Clement PA, Bluestone CD, Gordts F et al. Management of rhinosinusitis in children: Consensus meeting, Brussels, Belgium, September 13. 1996. *Arch Otolaryngol Head Neck Surg* 1998;124:31–34.

30. Brook I, Foote PA, Frazier EH. Microbiology of acute exacerbation of chronic sinusitis. *Laryngoscope* 2004;114: 129–131.

31. Brook I. Bacteriology of chronic sinusitis and acute exacerbation of chronic sinusitis. The 7th Biennial Congress of the Anerobe Society of the Americas. July 19–21. 2004. Annapolis, Maryland. (Abstract # PH–34).

32. Bach A, Boehrer H, Schmidt H, Geiss HK. Nosocomial sinusitis in ventilated patients: Nasotracheal versus orotracheal intubation. *Anaesthesia* 1992;47:335–339.

33. Mevio E, Benazzo M, Quaglieri S, Mencherini S. Sinus infection in intensive care patients. *Rhinology* 1996;34:232–236.

34. Brook I, Shah K. Sinusitis in neurologically impaired children. *Otolaryngol Head Neck Surg* 1998;119:357–360.

35. Brook I. Emergence and persistence of beta-lactamase-producing bacteria in the oropharynx following penicillin treatment. *Arch Otolaryngol Head Neck Surg* 1988;114:667–670.

36. Brook I, Gober AE. Emergence of beta-lactamase-producing aerobic and anaerobic bacteria in oro-pharynx of children following penicillin chemotherapy. *Clin Pediatr* (Phila) 1984;23:338–341.

37. Brook I, Gober AE. Monthly changes in the rate of recovery of penicillin-resistant organisms from children. *Pediatr Infect Dis J* 1997;16:255–256.

38. Brook I, Yocum P, Frazier EH. Bacteriology and beta-lactamase activity in acute and chronic maxillary sinusitis. *Arch Otolaryngol Head Neck Surg* 1996;122:418–423.

39. Dominguez MA, Pallares R. Antibiotic resistance in respiratory pathogens. *Curr Opin Pulmonary Med* 1998;4: 173–179.

40. Fung-Tomc JC, Huczko E, Stickle T et al. Antibacterial activity of cefprozil compared with those of 13 oral cephems and 3 macrolides. *Antimicrob Agent Chemother* 1995;39:533–538.

41. McCracken GH Jr. Considerations in selecting an antibiotic for treatment of acute otitis media. *Pediatr Infect Dis J* 1994; 13:1054–1057.

42. Orden B, Perez Trallero E, Montes M, Martinez R. Erythromycin resistance of Streptococcus pyogenes in Madrid. *Pediatr Infect Dis J* 1998;17:470–473.

43. Spangler SK, Jacobs MR, Pankuch GA, Appelbaum PC. Susceptibility of 170 penicillin-susceptible and -resistant pneumococci to six oral cephalosporins, four quinolones, desacetylcefotaxime, Ro 23–9424 and RP 67829. *J Antimicrob Chemother* 1993;31:273–280.

44. Brook I, Gober AE. Microbiologic characteristics of persistent otitis media. *Arch Otolaryngol Head Neck Surg* 1998; 124: 1350–1352.

45. Brook I, Frazier EH, Foote PA. Microbiology of chronic maxillary sinusitis: Comparison between specimens obtained by sinus endoscopy and by surgical drainage. *J Med Microbiol* 1997;46:430–432.

46. Craig WA. Pharmacokinetic/pharmacodynamic parameters: Rationale for antibacterial dosing of mice and men. *Clin Infect Dis* 1998;26:1–10.

47. Carenfelt C, Eneroth CM, Lundberg C, Wretlind B. Evaluation of the antibiotic effect of treatment of maxillary sinusitis. *Scand J Infect Dis* 1975;7:259–264.

48. Gwaltney JM Jr. Acute community-acquired sinusitis. *Clin Infect Dis* 1996;23:209–225.

49. Wald ER, Chiponis D, Leclesma-Medina J. Comparative effectiveness of amoxicillin and amoxicillin–clavulanate potassium in acute paranasal sinus infection in children: A double-blind, placebo-controlled trial. *Pediatrics* 1998;77: 795–800.

50. Spector SL, Bernstein IL. Parameters for the diagnosis and management of sinusitis. *J Allergy Clin Immunol* 1998;102 (Suppl):S107–S144.

51. Williams JW Jr, Aguilar C, Makela M, Cornell J, Holleman D, Chiquette E, Simel DL. Antibiotics for acute maxillary sinusitis. 1: *Cochrane Database Syst Rev* 2000;(2):CD000243.

52. Sinus and Allergy Health Partnership. Antimicrobial treatment guidelines for acute bacterial rhinosinusitis. *Otolaryngol Head Neck Surg* 2000;123:S1–S32.

53. Benninger MS, Holzer SES, Lau J. Diagnosis and treatment of uncomplicated acute bacterial rhinosinusitis: Summary of the agency for health care policy and research evidence-based report. *Otolaryngol Head Neck Surg* 2000;122:1–7.

54. Brook I, Gooch III WM, Jenkins, SG et al. Medical management of acute bacterial sinusitis. Recommendations of a clinical advisory committee on pediatric and adult sinusitis. *Ann Otol Rhinol Laryngol* 2000;109:1–20.

55. Clinical Practice Guidelines: Managemement of Sinusitis. *Pediatrics* 2001;108:798–807.

56. Sinus and Allergy Health Partnership: Antimicrobial treatment guidelines for acute bacterial rhinosinusitis. *Otolaryngol Head and Neck Surg* 2004;130(Suppl. 1):1S–45S.

57. Sanders CV, Aldridge KE. Current antimicrobial therapy of anerobic infections. *Eur J Clin Microbiol* 1992;11:999–1011.

58. Brook I, Thompson DH, Frazier EH. Microbiology and management of chronic maxillary sinusitis. *Arch Otolaryngol Head Neck Surg* 1994;120:1317–1320.

59. Brook I, Yocum P. Management of chronic sinusitis in children. *J Laryngol Otol* 1995;109:1159–1162.

60. Schleimer RP. Glucocorticoids: Their mechanism of action and use in allergic diseases. In *Allergy: Principles and Practice*. Adhinson NF Jr, Yunginger JW, Busse WW (Eds) et al, 6th edn. St. Louis: *Mosby* 2003;912–914.

61. Nuutinen J, Ruoppi P, Suonpaa J. One dose beclomethasone dipropionate aerosol in the treatment of seasonal allergic rhinitis. A preliminary report. *Rhinology* 1987;25:121–127.

62. ChaltonR, Mackay I, Wilson R, Cole P. Double blind placebo controlled trial of betamethasone nasal drops for nasal polyposis. *Br Med J Clin Res Educ* 1985;291:788.

63. Brown SL, Graham SG. Nasal irrigations: Good or bad? *Curr Opin Otolaryngol Head Neck Surg* 2004;12:9–13.

64. Parnes SM, Chuma AV. Acute effects on anti-leukotrienes on sinonasal polyposis and sinusitis. *Ear Nose Throat J* 2000;79: 18–20.

CHAPTER 31

Headache and Facial Pain

William Nnuma, Adash Vasanath, Collin S Karmody

Acute pain serves to protect by calling attention to underlying disease and usually resolves with effective treatment. Chronic pain is classically defined as that lasting more than three months. It frequently has no obvious cause, seeming to represent a disease in and of itself. Chronic pain can be overwhelmingly distressing to the patient and is often exceedingly difficult to diagnose and treat.

At least 10% of the population in the USA complains of chronic or recurring headache and probably three times that number have taken medication for similar symptoms. The management of headache and facial pain costs over USD1 billion annually in the USA for medications and up to USD13 billion if the cost of lost workdays and reduced productivity are factored in (*Business Week August 26, 2002 p. 146*). Additionally although difficult to assess, the cost of alternative therapies probably equals or exceeds that of prescribed treatments.

This chapter addresses the common problems of headache and facial pain as they pertain to the otolaryngologist who plays a crucial role in diagnosing and treating these patients It is most important that both patients and physicians recognize that the management of headache and facial pain is best-handled by a multidisciplinary team that includes neurologists, otolaryngologists, dentists, anesthesiologists, neurosurgeons, nurses, physical therapists and psychologists. We must also recognize that many patients with headaches and facial pain seek relief in alternative remedies such as acupuncture, biofeedback, and meditation which indicates that our efforts are not always successful.

The public is extraordinarily gullible when it comes to the treatment of chronic pain but the efficacy of many of the leading remedies still remains unstudied. Advertisements in the lay and even the professional press, however, continue to bombard the public about the wonders of various treatments. The well-described phenomenon of rebound headache places an even greater burden on the practitioner who must be constantly aware of the possibility that after a while, medications might be the cause of continuing symptoms. The physician's role therefore must be both therapist and guidance counselor.

CLASSIFICATION OF HEADACHE AND FACIAL PAIN

The Classification of Headache and Facial Pain[1] by the International Headache Society (1989; 2004) lists more than 220 entities divided into three broad groups subdivided into fourteen sections. These are in turn subcategorized into individual entities. Here, we present a condensed categorization.

It must be noted that the same entity might have different names. Headaches and facial pains can be grouped into primary, secondary, and other (e.g. cranial neuralgias).[2,3]

- Primary headaches include such entities as migraine, tension-type headache and cluster headache.
- Secondary headaches are those for which specific causative factors can be demonstrated such as trauma, vascular disorders, infection, substances (use or withdrawal) and those attributed to disorders of the cranium, eyes, ears, nose, sinuses, teeth, mouth, or other facial structures.
- A recently-defined category consists of disturbances of homeostasis and psychiatric disorders.

Distinction between the different types of headaches carries diagnostic and therapeutic implications.

Abbreviated Classification of Headache

Migraine
- Migraine without aura
- Migraine with aura
- Basilar type migraine

- Complications of migraine
- Chronic migraine

Tension-type headache

- Episodic tension-type headache
- Chronic tension-type headache

Cluster headache and other trigeminal-autonomic cephalgias

- Cluster headache
- Paroxysmal hemicrania

Headache attributed to

- Head and/or neck trauma
  - Acute/chronic post-traumatic headache
- Cranial and/or cerebral vascular disorders
  - Vascular malformations
  - Arteritis
  - Carotid or vertebral artery pain
  - Arterial dissection
  - Cerebral venous thrombosis (CVT)
- Nonvascular, non-infectious intracranial disorder
  - Low cerebrospinal fluid pressure
  - Aseptic (non-infectious) meningitis
  - Intracranial neoplasm
- Abuse of a substance or its withdrawal
- Infection
  - Intracranial infection
    * Bacterial meningitis
    * Encephalitis
    * Brain abscess
    * Subdural empyema
    * AIDS
  - Systemic infection
- Disturbance of homeostasis
  - Hypoxia and/or hypercapnia
  - High altitude
  - Sleep apnea
  - Arterial hypertension

Disorder of the cranium, neck, eyes, ears, nose, sinuses, teeth, mouth or other facial or cranial structures.

- Neck
  - Cervicogenic headache
  - Craniocervical dystonia
- Refractive errors
- Otalgia
- Nose and sinuses
  - Acute rhinosinusitis
  - Mucosal contact point
- Teeth, jaws and related structures
  - Temporomandibular joint disease
- Psychiatric disorder
- Cranial neuralgias and central causes of facial pain
  - Trigeminal neuralgia
  - Glossopharyngeal neuralgia

- Occipital neuralgia
- Neck-tongue syndrome
- Cold stimulus headache

Facial Pain

Peripheral Causes

Disorders of the oral cavity

- Dental disease
  - Caries
  - Periodontal disease
  - Dental abscess
  - Atypical odontalgia
  - Neoplasms
- Diseases of the buccal mucosa
  - Ulcerations
  - Infections
  - Neoplasms
- Disorders of the temporomandibular joint
  - Myofascial disorders
  - Internal derangement of the temporo-mandibular joint

Disorders of the Sinonasal Complex

- Sinusitis
  - Infectious
  - Allergic
  - Combination of infectious and allergic
- Rhinitis
  - Allergic
  - Infectious
  - Combination of infectious and allergic
- Neoplasms
- Infections
  - Bacterial
  - Viral
    * Herpes zoster
    * Acute herpes zoster
    * Postherpetic neuralgia

Central Causes

Primary (Idiopathic)

- Cranial neuralgias
- Migraine
- Short-lasting unilateral neuralgiform headache/facial pain with conjunctival injection and tearing (?Sluder syndrome)

Secondary

- Intracranial neoplasms
- Multiple sclerosis
- Trauma
  - Acute
  - Chronic post-traumatic headache/facial pain
- Anesthesia dolorosa

Hypoxia causes headache within 24 hours of arterial PO_2 (PaO_2) < 70 mmHg. Hypercapnia (arterial PCO_2 >50 mm Hg) such as occurs with sleep apnea and vigorous exercise, causes relaxation of cerebrovascular smooth muscle which leads to increased intracranial pressure, and headache.

Sleep apnea induced headache requires polysomnographic documentation of a respiratory disturbance index of > 5. Diagnosis is based on the following characteristics. Headaches usually occur on awakening, more frequently than fifteen days per month, last more than 30 minutes, are bilateral and pressing, have no associated nausea, photo- or phonophobia. Headaches should subside within 72 hours after treatment of sleep apnea.

Clearly, morning headache is a nonspecific symptom and not diagnostic of sleep apnea. An increasingly important category is the headache associated with the use or withdrawal of various substances including analgesics and caffeine. A significant number of patients presenting with headaches, will have used analgesics/opioids for prolonged periods. Their symptoms will not improve unless the medications are withdrawn.

Headaches can be classified by the extent of associated disability as mild, moderate, and severe. Men and women have the same prevalence of headaches but women experience moderate and severe headaches almost twice as frequently as men, a phenomenon that is believed to be related to the estrogen cycle. Headaches usually begin in the second decade of life and the prevalence gradually decreases after the fourth decade (partly because of menopause). Headaches also tend to be familial, with up to 60% of sufferers having either one or both parents with similar symptoms.

Headaches might present as intermittent or continuous over a varied time frame.[2,3] An acute presentation usually lasts a few hours or days and is typically severe. Non-traumatic causes of acute headache include muscle-contraction headache (32%), migraine (22%), upper respiratory infection (12%), sinusitis (5%), hypertension (4%), gastroenteritis (3%), cerebral tumor (3%), cervical spine degeneration (2%), and others. Subacute headaches last for days to weeks, and can be caused by cerebral tumor, pseudotumor cerebri, ophthalmic zoster, temporal arteritis, and subdural hematoma. Cerebral tumors can obstruct the flow of CSF (as in posterior fossa tumors seen more commonly in children) causing headache without neurological symptoms. Adults more commonly present with cerebral hemispheric tumors that cause early neurologic symptoms. In addition to primary intracranial tumors, cerebral metastases (principally from breast and lung) can present similarly. Pseudotumor cerebri (benign intracranial hypertension) is caused by impaired absorption of CSF resulting in increased intracranial pressure. Often associated with obesity it is aggravated by sudden movements of the head, coughing, sneezing, straining, or bending over. Papilledema is usually present, and a lumbar puncture and MRI help to confirm the diagnosis. Chronic headaches may be experienced daily or intermittently over months or years, and have a strong female preponderance. The onset of headache was related to menarche in almost 30% of women. Daily headaches can be paroxysmal (cluster headache, paroxysmal hemicrania and stabbing headache), or more commonly non-paroxysmal. Chronic headache is thought to be related to abnormal functioning of extracranial muscles (tension-type headache) and arteries (migraine and cluster headache).[4] It has been shown that most patients with chronic headache have increased tightness of the neck and jaw muscles during an episode. Vasodilation can stretch the nerve fibers closely related to the vessel involved, triggering the pain.[5] This mechanism, particularly when it involves the frontal branch of the superficial temporal artery, is proposed in migraine and cluster headaches.[6,7]

Chronic headache can also be thought of as a continuum, where episodic tension-type headache and migraine mark the opposite ends of the spectrum with chronic tension-type headache and tension-type vascular headache falling between. Patients can present at any point in the continuum, and can progress along the spectrum overtime. Various trigger events have been identified in adult-onset chronic headache, such as, head, neck or back injury (29%), stress (17%), illness or surgery (14%), pregnancy or postpartum (12%), and estrogen therapy (9%).

It is important to recognize that long-term treatment of chronic headache with analgesics can be ineffective, and can even lead to progression of symptoms along the continuum. Analgesics do not target the underlying mechanisms, and overtime can even impair the efficacy of preventive treatment.

Cluster headaches (migrainous neuralgia or histaminic cephalagia) have typical presentations. They are less frequent than migraine and have a very strong male preponderance (14:1). Attacks tend to occur at night and can last from 15 minutes to 2 hours. They can occur once or twice per day, and in 85% of patients present in 'clusters' lasting from 2 weeks to 2 months, with remissions of 6 months to 1 year. Pain is intense, crushing, or burning. They are always unilateral, and can be localized to the retro-orbit, forehead, temple, or face. The acute headaches might be associated with ipsilateral autonomic symptoms such as rhinorrhea, tearing, sweating over the forehead, swelling and drooping of the upper eyelid and constriction of the pupil. Patients with cluster headaches typically pace the floor, while migraine sufferers prefer lying down in a darkroom during an episode. Alcohol and daytime napping are two of the more common triggers of cluster headaches. The treatment of cluster headaches focuses on avoidance of triggers as well as abortive and preventative pharmacologic agents similar to those used for migraine. Sumatriptan subcutaneous injection, oxygen inhalation and sublingual ergotamine are effective abortive therapies. Verapamil, prednisone and lithium can be used for prevention.

Paroxysmal hemicrania is a rare variant of cluster headache, consisting of similar headaches, but in greater frequency and lesser duration. Indomethacin is very effective in treatment of this type of headache.

MIGRAINE

Migraine is the French version of the Latin/Greek hemicrania (hemikrania). Migraine is one of the most frequent types of headache, affecting 10–15% of the population, and causes significant disability. It is a chronic paroxysmal disorder with symptom-free intervals. Migraine affects around 4% of children, 6% of men, and 18% of women, and are most common between the ages 25 and 55 years. Migraine affects women more than men (3 : 1). About 80% of such people have a family history of migraine, which suggests a possible genetic role.

Symptoms of Migraine

Although typically described as pain in the head migraine might present as pain in the face, neck or, in children, in the abdomen. There are two main types of migraine: Headache without aura (75%) and headache with aura (classical migraine) (25%).

Migraine without Aura (Common migraine)

The headache strikes suddenly, without warning and is usually described as severe throbbing pain,[8] frequently unilateral but about 30% of migraines occur on both sides. There might also be associated symptoms such as nausea, vomiting, diarrhea, photophobia, phonophobia, blurred vision, general malaise and even hemiparesis.[9] Activation of the sympathetic nervous system also leads to generalized vasoconstriction which causes concomitant facial pallor and coldness of the hands and feet. Patients usually retire to a dark quiet room and avoid all personal contact. Attacks can last for 4 to 72 hours.

It should be noted that the pain of migraine might also (and sometimes only) involve other areas such as the face and jaws.

Migraine with Aura (Classic migraine)

These patients sense the onset of an attack because symptoms (called auras) develop before the migraine symptoms. This is frequently a visual disturbance such as blind spots (scotomas); geometric patterns or flashing, colorful lights; or loss of vision on one side (hemianopias). Occasionally, the symptoms can be more severe—there may be a tingling around the mouth or in one arm, difficulty in speaking, or weakness in an arm or leg. Auras usually last less than an hour. Some patients get the aura without the subsequent headache. This is more common in the elderly.

Migraine Triggers

In some patients attacks of migraine are triggered by one or more factors such as stress, certain foods, menstruation, flashing lights, weather, etc.

The cause of migraine is not fully understood but involves the balance between the body processes that stimulate the nervous system and those that relax it. For instance the level of serotonin in the brain drops during a migraine and the majority of migrainous women can relate their headaches to their menstrual period.

Unfortunately, the pathophysiology of migraine is much more complex. Three concomitant mechanisms are proposed for the pathogenesis of the migraine headache: Extracranial arterial vasodilatation, extracranial neurogenic inflammation, and decreased inhibition of central pain transmission. The popular explanation for migraine attacks is that vasoconstriction, which primarily involves the frontal branch of the superficial temporal artery, causes the characteristic pain in the temple and supposedly the aura, and is followed by vasodilatation that causes the headache.[4-6]

Neurogenic inflammation is mediated by various substances (neurokinin A, substance P, and calcitonin gene-related peptide) that are released upon activation of the primary sensory nerve fibers involved in pain transmission. It has also been shown that neurogenic inflammation decreases the local pain threshold. Enkephalin, an endogenous opioid that inhibits pain transmission in the central nervous system, is decreased during a migraine headache. This also supports a central mechanism for further decrease of the pain threshold.

Migraine aura is now thought to be caused by a spreading wave of cortical excitation and depression. Cerebral blood flow studies have demonstrated increased flow in the cingulate, visual, and auditory cortices during a migraine headache. Photophobia and phonophobia are related to involvement of the visual and auditory cortices.

Management of Migraine

Management of migraine involves avoidance of triggers[12] (not always successful), as well as abortive and preventive pharmacological therapy. Effective treatment can decrease the recurrence of headache and reduce the associated symptoms.

Abortive Treatment

Effective abortive treatment is always indicated because of the incapacitating nature of the headache and also because ineffective treatment can lead to progression of the condition, and eventually to chronic migraine. Analgesics, anti-inflammatory agents and vasoconstrictors can be used for abortive treatment. Vasoconstrictors and anti-inflammatory medications address the underlying mechanisms of neurogenic inflammation and arterial inflammation, and are thus more specific therapies. Common analgesics include acetaminophen and opioids. The latter should be used with caution, because they are potentially addictive and migraine is a chronic condition. Indomethacin, in addition to being a potent analgesic, is also a constrictor of the cranial arteries which sets it apart from the other non-steroidal anti-inflammatory medications. Three types of vasoconstrictors are used in the treatment of migraine: caffeine, sympathomimetics and serotoninergics (selective or non-selective). Caffeine is long-acting and hence should not be used more often than 2 days per week. The potency of caffeine is increased when it is combined with an analgesic. Sympathomimetic vasoconstrictors include topical phenylephrine, and isometheptene (indirectly acting). Serotoninergic vasoconstrictors are more potent than the sympathomimetics and include the ergots and triptans. Ergotamine which was introduced for the treatment of migraine in 1926, is a potent constrictor of

extracranial arteries, and also inhibits neurogenic inflammation. Dihydroergotamine, a derivative of ergotamine, is available for parenteral administration and as a nasal spray. The ergots are long-acting and can maintain vasoconstriction for up to 3 days. This limits the frequency of their use to about once per week on average. Triptans are more selective (serotonin 1B, 1D and 1F receptors) than the ergots and therefore have fewer side effects. Ergots also stimulate serotonin 1A receptors and dopaminergic receptors (causing nausea and vomiting), and have an affinity for serotonin 2A and alpha-adrenergic receptors (causing coronary artery and peripheral vasoconstriction). Triptans[10] can also be used more frequently than ergots because of their shorter half-lives. The sensory phenomena associated with migraine can be treated symptomatically, such as lying in a dark and quiet room with the head elevated, using a cold forehead compress or applying pressure to the temples. Anti-emetics (metoclopramide) helps to control gastrointestinal symptoms.

Preventive Treatment

Preventive treatment should be initiated once effective abortive treatment has been established.

Preventive treatment aims at decreasing the frequency of the headaches and involves daily medication. It is usually prescribed when headaches occur more often than three or four times a month. This strategy is used for at least 6 months, after which medication is tapered to a maintenance level or completely withdrawn.

Propranolol (a beta-blocker) prevents the dilation of extracranial arteries. Amitriptyline potentiates the effects of serotonin through a postsynaptic mechanism. Serotonin increases pain thresholds in the central nervous system by inhibiting the transmission of pain signals. Verapamil is also thought to interrupt synaptic transmission (a calcium-dependent process), thereby increasing pain thresholds. Divalproex sodium may also inhibit central pain transmission, but through potentiation of the GABA-ergic inhibitory system.

The choice of medication depends on the features of the headache as well as concomitant conditions. Beta-blockers are most effective in headaches of relatively low frequency but of high intensity but might have side effects that include fatigue, depression, insomnia, and impotence. Beta-blockers are contraindicated in sinus bradycardia, atrioventricular block, congestive heart failure, obstructive pulmonary disease (asthma) and diabetes mellitus. Amitriptyline is more effective when the headaches occur frequently but are not so intense.

It is long-acting can be taken once daily at bedtime (because of sedation). Amitryptiline is contraindicated in glaucoma, prostate hypertrophy, epilepsy, and cardiac disease. Verapamil is the medication of choice when headaches occur mostly during the night and awaken the patient. Verapamil[11] can cause constipation, and is contraindicated in atrioventricular block and sick-sinus syndrome (as it slows atrioventricular conduction). Divalproex sodium tends to be mood stabilizing, but is teratogenic and is contraindicated in liver disease. Preventive medications should be attempted as a single agent, with the addition of another agent as necessary.[13] Amitriptyline with a beta-blocker is a good combination for multi-agent treatment.

Causes of Pain in the Head and Face

The reader is referred to other sections of this book for a more comprehensive discussion of otalgia. This section discusses only a few entities around the ear that might also cause pain in the head and face.

Viral Cranial Neuropathy

Ramsay-Hunt syndrome[14,29] (Herpes zoster oticus) is a viral polycranial neuropathy, with a pathognomic presentation of otalgia, facial palsy and vesicular rash of the pinna, external auditory canal, and tympanic membrane. This entity is secondary to reactivation of latent varicella zoster virus that remains dormant in the sensory ganglion of the facial nerve.[15] It is also important to note that all cranial nerves can be affected. Otalgia may be due to sensation from the vesicles themselves or from irritation and inflammation of the affected cranial nerves. Some patients can have postherpetic neuralgia for many months even after resolution of the disease. Involvement of the vestibulocochlear nerve (or direct labyrinthine involvement) can also cause hearing loss, vertigo and tinnitus. Idiopathic facial paralysis (Bell's palsy) is also considered to be associated with herpes virus infection and some patients present with otalgia prior to onset of facial weakness. Prognosis for recovery of facial nerve function is better in Bell's palsy than it is in herpes zoster oticus.[30]

Relapsing Polychondritis

This chronic autoimmune disease leads to recurrent inflammation of cartilage that causes chronic fibrosis. Auricular cartilage is particularly prone because it has a high concentration of glycosaminoglycans.[16] Other structures that have high proteoglycan content (eyes, heart and inner ear) can also be involved. In relapsing polychondritis the lobule is spared which distinguishes it from infective auricular cellulitis. It is important to note that up to 50% of patients with relapsing polychondritis can have airway involvement (presenting with dysphonia, dyspnea and stridor) and an associated high mortality rate.[17,18]

THE EYE AND HEADACHES

Headache might be an indicator of eye problems and anyone suffering from constant headache should consult an ophthalmologist.

Many eye problems can cause headache. Squinting and overworking the eye muscles in an attempt to better focus vision can cause headache. Squinting can be secondary to astigmatism, hyperopia or presbyopia. Most of these conditions can be corrected with prescription glasses. Glaucoma, particularly acute closed angle glaucoma, can cause severe pain, blurred vision, watering of the eyes, nausea, and vomiting and headache. This type of glaucoma needs prompt medical attention.

Ophthalmic zoster (herpes zoster ophthalmicus) caused by reactivation of the latent varicella zoster virus, classically presents in the elderly and immunocompromised patients, as unilateral pain in the forehead and anterior vertex. The pain usually resolves in 1–4 weeks, but may persist for months or years (postherpetic neuralgia).

Cranial Neuralgias and Headaches Associated with Cranial Vascular Disorders

Trigeminal Neuralgia

Trigeminal neuralgia (tic doulourex) is the most common facial neuralgia and usually affects patients in middle and late age. Patients experience paroxysmal pain in the distribution of the divisions of the trigeminal nerve (second and third division involvement is more common), either alone or in combination.[21] The pain may be triggered by various stimuli, such as yawning, shaving, brushing teeth, talking, eating or even a light touch. Neuralgic pain is typically described as a lancinating, electric shock-like, shooting pain lasting for several seconds to minutes. The term tic arises from the fact that patients tend to wince during the paroxysms of pain. Attacks can occur repetitively, and lingering facial pain is possible after multiple attacks. This disorder is episodic,[22] with relapses and remissions over many years. Remissions may last for months to years.

Trigeminal neuralgia can be classified as primary (idiopathic) or secondary to lesions of the gasserian ganglion sensory root of root entry zone in the pons. Patients with primary trigeminal neuralgia have negative physical findings, and normal sensory and motor functions. EMG and nerve conduction studies are typically normal in primary disease.

The cause of primary trigeminal neuralgia is debatable:[23] Some consider the cause to be vascular compression of the trigeminal roots, while others postulate segmental demyelination and neurovascular changes in the gasserian ganglion as contributing to the symptoms. Secondary trigeminal neuralgia may have associated physical findings due to intracranial masses, basilar artery aneurysm, pontine infarcts, demyelinating disease or other infiltrating lesions. Bilateral trigeminal neuralgia can be seen in demyelinating disease.

Carbamazepine (600–1200 mg/day) is an effective treatment, giving relief in approximately 75–80% of patients. Approximately, half of these patients become resistant to this drug over a period of years. Once complete relief has been obtained, carbamazepine can[31] be tapered slowly to check for remission. Phenytoin, baclofen, valproic acid, clonazepam, and gabapentin can also be used alone, or in combination with carbamazepine or each other. For pain refractory to medical therapy, invasive procedures such as percutaneous radiofrequency thermocoagulation, microvascular decompression and stereotactic radiosurgery with gamma knife are some options.[24] Percutaneous radiofrequency thermocoagulation[24] offers effective pain relief (in up to 95% of patients) and can be repeated but possible complications such as injury to the carotid artery and adjacent cranial nerves as well as anesthesia dolorosa (sensation of pain in a region of numbness)[26,27] should be considered. Decompression of vascular loops in the posterior fossa offers pain relief in 70% of patients, but has a 1–2% mortality rate and a risk of injury to adjacent cranial nerves. Stereotactic radiosurgery has a similar efficacy, but up to 10% of patients can develop new or increased facial paresthesias or numbness.[25]

Glossopharyngeal Neuralgia

Glossopharyngeal neuralgia has very similar pain characteristics to trigeminal neuralgia, but is localized to the distribution of the glossopharyngeal nerve. Patients experience a paroxysmal, lancinating pain in the throat, posterior third of the tongue, tonsillar region, nasopharynx, larynx, and ear. Triggers include swallowing, chewing, laughing, yawning and talking.[28] Bradycardia and syncope can also be associated with an attack. Clinical exam of affected patients is typically normal. While no specific etiology has been determined, there is some evidence to suggest the presence of microvascular compression. Treatment is similar to trigeminal neuralgia. If medical therapy has failed, surgical options include intracranial sectioning of the glossopharyngeal nerve and the upper rootlets of the vagus nerve, or microvascular decompression of the root entry zone.

Geniculate Neuralgia (Nervus Intermedius Neuralgia of Hunt)

Geniculate neuralgia is a very rare pain syndrome involving the pinna of the ear and the auditory canal. This has been related to a neuralagia of the geniculate ganglion and nervus intermedius. There is no clear etiology in most cases. In addition to the classic attacks of pain (similar to other neuralgias), associated abnormalities of lacrimation, salivation and taste can be involved. Light touch within the posterior aspect of the auditory canal can trigger the pain. Some patients respond to carbamazepine, and there are some reports of relief with excision of the nervus intermedius and geniculate ganglion.

Occipital Neuralgia

This paroxysmal disorder occurs in the distribution of the occipital nerves and may occasionally be associated with sensory loss. Percussion of the involved nerve as it exits the trapezius muscle can reproduce the pain. Although this condition frequently has no inciting event, trauma to the occipital region can sometimes be an initiating factor. Carbamazepine is effective in some patients, although others may obtain temporary benefit from local anesthetic injections (alone or in combination with a corticosteroid). Sectioning of the nerve is not advised as this can lead to formation of a neuroma or cause anesthesia dolorosa.

Atypical Facial Pain

Facial pain presenting in patients without identifiable causes after extensive investigation is described as atypical facial pain. Patients tend to be middle-aged females who describe a poorly localized deep, intense and constant burning or aching pain. Symptoms can be unilateral or bilateral, with associated symptoms of paresthesia, numbness and tenderness. Unlike the neuralgias noted above, there are no particular anatomic patterns and no identifiable triggers to these symptoms. There is, however, a high incidence of anxiety and depression in these patients.

Treatment consists of tricyclic antidepressants, monoamine oxidase inhibitors as well as benzodiazepines.

Headaches in Strokes and Cerebrovascular Accidents

Headaches may precede TIAs and CVAs by days or weeks and might take the form of a migraine or tension-type headache. This type of headache has been reported in up to 18% of patients and are more prominent in larger strokes or strokes in the posterior cranial fossa (secondary to edema and mass effect leading to obstruction of ventricular flow, causing hydrocephalus). Treatment consists of simple analgesics, as narcotics should be avoided to keep the patient alert. The majority of patients complain of progressive ipsilateral headache at the onset of intracerebral hemorrhage (ICH) particularly when it involves the cerebral hemispheres, cerebellum or locations near meningeal surfaces. Dizziness and vomiting can be associated symptoms.

Treatment, once again involves non-sedating analgesics and measures to reduce intracranial pressure (mannitol, hyperventilation, and evacuation of the hematoma where appropriate).

Subarachnoid Hemorrhage (SAH)

The classic description of the headache of an SAH, is a sudden onset of excruciating pain building in intensity over seconds, that patients report as 'the worst headache of my life.' Focal at onset, the pain quickly generalizes and can be associated with nuchal rigidity, photophobia, and vomiting. Loss of consciousness and focal neurologic deficits can also occur in severe bleeds. Diagnosis is usually made on unenhanced CT scan with or without a lumbar puncture. Angiography or MRA can further confirm the presence of a ruptured saccular aneurysm of AVM. Treatment of the headache consists of analgesics, without compromising the neurological status of the patient. Surgical intervention is sometimes necessary to seal an aneurysm.

Benign Thunderclap Headache (BTH)

This is a separate entity but with similar symptoms to headaches with SAH; BTH can be precipitated by activity and last from an hour to many days, and in rare cases, up to 4 weeks. There might be associated transient focal neurological deficits, and reversible segmental vasoconstriction may be seen on angiography.

Cerebral Venous Thrombosis

About 70–88% of patients with CVT present with a global headache. Frequently there might be associated papilledema, transient visual changes, focal or generalized seizures, vomiting, lethargy, and even obtundation. Various focal neurological deficits may be seen depending on the location of the thrombosed vein.

Pseudotumor cerebri (benign intracranial hypertension) may also present with headache, transient visual changes, papilledema and sixth nerve palsy.

Treatment of CVT consists of reducing intracranial pressure by the use of mannitol, other diuretics, ventricular drains, repeated lumbar punctures, corticosteroids and anticoagulants or thrombolytic agents for selected cases.

Carotid and Vertebral Artery Dissection

Dissection of the carotid and vertebral arteries is usually secondary to trauma, but can also occur spontaneously in patients with fibromuscular dysplasia, cystic medial necrosis, Ehlers-Danlos' syndrome, Marfan's syndrome, osteogenesis imperfecta type I, and polycystic kidney disease. A constant ache or a throbbing, sharp pain is usually the initial manifestation of a carotid artery dissection. This pain may be localized to the ipsilateral face, particularly the orbit, frontotemporal region and angle of the mandible or high neck. Horner' syndrome (oculosympathetic palsy), delayed focal cerebral ischemic events (ipsilateral amaurosis fugax, hemispheric signs), or lower cranial nerve palsies can also be associated findings.

In vertebral artery dissection, patients experience pain in the back of the head and neck that may be bilateral, throbbing and sharp in nature. Associated ischemic events involve the brainstem (particularly the lateral medulla) and the cerebral and cerebellar hemispheres.

Conventional angiography is the gold-standard for diagnosis, and treatment consists of anticoagulation (to prevent emoblization) and surgery (in patients with continued cerebral ischemic events despite anticoagulation).

Temporal Arteritis (Giant Cell Arteritis)

This is a chronic vasculitis of medium and large-sized vessels typically involving the cranial branches of arteries originating from the aortic arch is more frequent in the elderly.[32] Approximately half of the patients with temporal arteritis also have symptoms of polymyalgia rheumatica. Headache is a common presenting symptom.

The headache can be throbbing or non-throbbing, unilateral or bilateral. Transient (Amaurosis fugax) or permanent loss of vision can be the first manifestation of the disease. Diplopia and jaw claudication may also occur. There can also be associated systemic symptoms of low grade fever, weight loss and malaise.

On examination, the affected vessels (frontal and parietal branches of the superficial temporal artery, or the occipital, postauricular or facial arteries) may be tender, thickened, and pulseless. Fundoscopic findings include optic neuritis, with slight pallor and edema of the disk and scattered cotton-wool patches. The sedimentation rate is almost always elevated. Biopsy of the involved vessel confirms the diagnosis showing infiltration of the vessel wall with inflammatory cells and giant cells, intimal proliferation, and thrombosis.

This is a medical emergency and treatment with high doses of prednisone (over 60 mg) should be given immediately even before a histologic diagnosis is obtained. The corticosteroid is then tapered to a maintenance level for several months.

Pharmacological Management of Head and Neck Pain

Worldwide, headaches and facial pain collectively account for most of the prescription and non-prescription drugs used by the general population.

Nonopioids

This class of medications includes nonsteroidal anti-inflammatory drugs (NSAIDs), APAP and Tramadol. NSAIDs are recommended for the initial pain with an inflammatory component or for musculoskeletal pain. They are cyclo-oxygenase (COX) inhibitors, thereby inhibiting the production of prostaglandins, and thromboxanes. Prostaglandins trigger nociceptive impulses that lower the brain's threshold of pain intensity. APAP and NSAIDs have a dose ceiling effect, although this sometimes cannot be determined because of the gastrointestinal side effects (dyspepsia, erosions and ulcerations) at higher doses. Aspirin (ASA) inhibits COX irreversibly and non-specifically, while ibuprofen and COX-2 specific agents are selective inhibitors. All NSAIDs shunt the arachidonic pathway toward leukotriene synthesis, and may precipitate reactions in patients who have increased tissue responses (bronchospasm and anaphylaxis) from increased leukotriene levels. Compared to other NSAIDs, ASA has less analgesic efficacy and a greater incidence of side

effects. It is important to note that an unsatisfactory response with one NSAID does not preclude the use of another.

Acetaminophen interrupts the influence of prostaglandins within CNS pathways, but its mechanism of action is poorly defined. Acetaminophen is almost as active as ASA in inhibiting COX within the CNS, but has little effect on peripheral prostaglandin synthesis. It therefore lacks an anti-inflammatory effect and lacks peripheral side effects (GI disturbance, etc). Its major side effect is hepatoxicity secondary to a metabolite that is not adequately conjugated in very high doses, or in patients with primary liver dysfunction, or receiving hepatotoxic medications.

Tramadol is a central analgesic with binary action (CABA). It binds weakly to muopioid receptors and inhibits the reuptake of norepinephrine and serotonin. Nausea, vomiting and dizziness are possible side effects. Tramadol should be used with caution in patients with a history of seizure disorder. Acetaminophen/tramadol combination formulations offer pain control comparable to acetaminophen/codeine, while having a lesser incidence of somnolence and constipation.

Opioids

These drugs are agonists at mu and/or kappa opioid receptors. Unlike non-opioids, there is no ceiling effect, and the analgesic efficacy is essentially unlimited. Side effects at higher doses include sedation, respiratory depression, dependence, nausea, miosis, and constipation. Patients can also develop tolerance to most opioids after prolonged use (except for constipation and miosis). All traditional opioids have similar efficacy. Thus, at equipotent doses, opioids will provide the same degree of pain relief. It is a common misconception that pain unresponsive to codeine will respond to oxycodone, meperidine, or morphine. There is some genetic predisposition for poor analgesia in some patients receiving certain opioids. About 10% of codeine is converted to morphine by cytochrome P450 CYP2D6, and 7% of the Caucasian population metabolizes codeine and hyrdrocodone poorly. Therefore, in these individuals, analgesia from codeine, oxycodone, or hydrocodone will be less than expected in the general population.

Adjunctive Therapy

Certain agents such as local anesthetics and GABA-ergic drugs can be used to complement the opioid and nonopioid agents. Benzodiazepines such as ativan are useful when patients experience associated symptoms of muscle spasm, sleep disturbance, and anxiety. Longer acting local anesthetics such as marcaine also have use in a multimodal treatment approach to various headaches and facial pain syndromes.

FACIAL PAIN

The terms headaches and facial pain are often used interchangeably. Differentiation between the two is difficult but necessary since it is of great help in diagnosis. By definition, facial pain is localized to the area limited by the forehead superiorly, the masseter regions laterally and the chin inferiorly. Headaches classically present in the vertex, parietal, temporal, occipital and retro-orbital areas. The frontal area is common to both headaches and facial pain.

Misdiagnosis and multiple failed treatments are common in patients with chronic facial pain. They often carry multiple diagnoses, managed by multiple disciplines.

The majority of facial pain is dental in origin, or caused by disorders of the temporomandibular joint and the associated muscles of mastication.

Dental Causes

When considering pain of dental origin one must keep in mind the phenomenon of referred pain. As all teeth and gingiva are innervated by the fifth cranial nerve, pain arising from these structures might be referred to any sensory distribution of the nerve, including the meninges. Atypical odontalgia (persistent pain in apparently normal teeth) is a real entity that might have its source at points distant from the teeth. Atypical facial pain is more frequent in women aged 40–50 years and present in a molar or bicuspid. Pain of dental origin might be caused by infection of the pulp or gingiva separately or in combination. Pain from pulp, mucosa, bone, etc. tends to be poorly localized but can usually be precisely pinpointed by percussion of the teeth.

Caries causes the dentin to be sensitive to thermal stimuli initially. With progression of infection the pulp becomes involved. Pulpitis is the most common cause of pain of dental origin. Pulpalgia is frequently difficult to localize because of its tendency to radiate to other teeth, the maxilla, mandible, the face and head. Eventually infection spreads to the apex of the tooth with the formation of an apical abscess at which point the pain becomes well-localized to the involved tooth and its adjacent gingiva.

Periodontal disease involves the alveolar bone, periodontal ligament and keratinizing gingiva. Pain might also result from uninflamed exposed dental roots in an atrophic jaw while pain from third molars frequently radiate to ear.

Treatment

All dental infection demands attention by a dentist but treatment with antibiotics can be initiated by a physician who should be aware of the possibility of dental infections to spread sometimes rapidly, to adjacent soft tissue.

Craniomandibular Disorders

The temporomandibular joint (TMJ) is susceptible to all the conditions that affect other joints. Although treatment is often similar to that used in other joints there are some variations.

Craniomandibular disorders (CMD) is a term that encompasses clinical problems involving the muscles of mastication, the TMJ or both. Included under this heading are TMJ arthropathies and the myofacial pain syndrome. CMD usually begins around the third to fifth decades, and has a 5:1 female to male ratio. Several theories have been postulated to explain the development of CMD. The tooth-muscle theory asserts that occlusal disharmony alters proprioception and causes muscle discoordination and spasm. The psychophysiologic theory claims that myospasm and muscle overactivity are the result of bruxism which is a manifestation of stress. Others feel the cause is multifactorial and frequently the result of macro- or microtrauma.

Some experts believe that increased stress causes bruxism, clenching, and even excessive gum-chewing. These lead to muscular overuse, fatigue and spasm, and pain.

The Myofacial Pain Syndrome

This is the most common cause of CMD. Friction describes the syndrome as a disorder in the regional musculature with trigger points in muscle bands that causes pain referred to the face. A vicious cycle develops. To reduce the pain, muscle stretching is avoided and the muscles of mastication are held in a contracted, shortened state. The accompanying episodes of myospasms can cause the TMJ to be in an abnormal position, frequently resulting in arthralgias. Trigger points develop in areas of maximal skeletal muscle tension. Patients complain of a dull, usually unilateral preauricular pain that may be exacerbated by stimulation of the trigger points. Patients might also present with a variety of aural symptoms: otalgia, tinnitus, aural fullness, vertigo, etc. Patients with nocturnal bruxism experience their worst pain in the morning while those with stress related jaw clenching have increasing pain throughout the day. Physical examination will identify 2–5 mm trigger points within hard palpable bands of muscle. Manipulation of these points triggers a sharp pain that is referred to as a 'positive jump sign'. Short-term relief may be obtained by cutaneous counterstimulation with fluorimethane spray (coolant spray), diathermy, transcutaneous electrical nerve stimulation, or injections of local anesthetic and corticosteroids. Muscle relaxants like baclofen and clonazepam (antispasmodics with central analgesic properties) and NSAIDs may also be used for short-term relief. Long-term relief can be by passive and active muscle stretching, postural rehabilitation, and correction of underlying contributing factors.

The treatment of myofascial pain is divided into four phases. The first phase of treatment is initiated on diagnosis, and consists of educating the patient about muscle fatigue and spasm as causes of pain and dysfunction. Emphasis is placed on the avoidance of clenching and the use of a soft diet. NSAIDs, with or without a muscle relaxant are prescribed. The most frequently used agents are diazepam and ibuprofen. One half of the patients will obtain significant relief in 2–4 weeks

Phase II therapy is initiated if phase I fails. Medications are continued, but a bite appliance (splint) is added. This helps to prevent muscle overuse such as bruxism. The appliance is usually worn at night, but can also be worn during the day if necessary. The appliance must not be worn constantly, as the posterior teeth may be displaced. An additional 25% of patients will receive relief with this therapy. Once relief is obtained, medications can be discontinued. If the patient remains asymptomatic, the appliance is discontinued but can be resumed at night, if symptoms recur.

If phase II therapy fails, physical therapy of the muscle groups, including ultrasonic therapy, electric stimulation or biofeedback can be useful. No one form of treatment is superior. Another 15% of patients will find relief within four weeks. If phase III therapy fails, psychological counseling is advised to identify stressors, and patients are referred to a TMJ center. More recently intramuscular injections of botulinum A have been successful in relieving the symptoms of masticatory muscle hyperactivity.

Internal Derangement of the Temporomandibular Joint

The temporomandibular joint is a complex bichambered joint with superior and inferior chambers separated by a tough fibrocartilaginous articular disk (meniscus) which is attached to the joint capsule and the capsular ligaments.[19] This joint architecture which is similar to that of the knee, allows the condyle of the mandible to both rotate and glide. Several ligaments hold the mandible in position: Medial and lateral capsular ligaments, and the posteriorly placed meniscotemporomandibular frenum (retrodiscal pad). The stylo- and sphenomandibular ligaments and the muscles of mastication also contribute. The articular disk and condyle are considered to be functionally one continuous anatomical structure. As the lateral and medial ligaments and the retrodiscal pad are connected to the disk and the condyle, disorders of the disk are sometimes caused by pathologic changes in the ligamentous attachments.

Internal derangement of the TMJ is usually caused by anterior displacement of the articular disk secondary to tearing of its ligamentous attachments.[20] The disk is pulled anteromedially by the lateral pterygoid muscle. On opening the jaw the condyle slides forward and suddenly rides over the displaced disk often resulting in a palpable or audible click which might or might not cause pain and the jaw might even become locked in an open position. Further disintegration or displacement of the disk causes degeneration of the articular surfaces.

Patients complain of dull preauricular aching (otalgia) often exacerbated by chewing. Clinically, there is tenderness over the joint, decreased range of mandibular motion, palpable crepitation and palpable, and/or an audible click. Although MRI provides the best assessment of the position and morphology of the intrarticular disk it has recently been shown that there is poor correlation between symptoms attributed to the TMJ and positive findings on MRI. The diagnosis therefore remains primarily clinical. Arthroscopy is reserved for those who are also surgical candidates.

While pharmacotherapy with NSAIDs and muscle relaxants provides short-term relief, the basic treatment for internal derangements of the TMJ is the use of orthotic appliances and physical therapy. Malocclusions should be corrected and all stressful situations should be addressed. Surgery is reserved for more advanced cases but might even exacerbate symptoms Early treatment of the internal derangement is imperative, as progression of disease leads to a less favorable prognosis. Therapy for type I and type II derangements is similar to that for myofascial disorders. NSAIDs and muscle relaxers (valium) are prescribed as is a soft diet and jaw rest. Failure of these methods requires the addition of a splint to attempt the repositioning of the condyle into a more favorable position relative to the disk. Clicking is usually not eliminated, but it may be reduced. If repositioning with a splint fails, arthoscopic or open surgical repair is recommended. The purpose of these procedures is to remove adhesions and to reposition the disk into a favorable position. A type III derangement requires earlier and more aggressive therapy.

Neoplastic Causes of Facial Pain

Perhaps the most feared cause of facial pain is an occult neoplasm. Huntley[33] reporting on a series of 8 patients with facial pain who were ultimately diagnosed with malignancies found that a correct diagnosis was only made after the patients had seen 3 to 11 different physicians and 3–48 months had elapsed. Neoplasm might be in the paranasal sinuses, nasopharynx, parpapharyngeal space, infratemporal fossa, or the intracranial cavity without displaying any obvious external signs. A careful history and complete physical examination will help in earlier diagnosis. Significant signs and symptoms that point to underlying neoplasms include facial swelling, oral cavity swelling, trismus, hearing loss/ear blockage, nausea, lethargy, and weight loss.

All patients with facial pain need a careful history[34] and a complete examination of the head and neck. Specific questions should be asked about nasal congestion or drainage, epistaxis, facial pressure, aural pressure or change in hearing, otalgia, oral pain, difficulty chewing or talking, dysphagia or odynophagia, changes in voice, weight loss, poor appetite, or energy level. A history of tobacco and alcohol use should be elicited from all patients. Clinical evidence of a mass lesion, swelling, middle ear effusion, trismus, cervical lymphadenopathy, abnormal neurological findings or weight loss should raise suspicion and warrant intensive diagnostic work-up and appropriate consultation.

Sinonasal Facial Pain

Disease of the paranasal sinus should always be considered as a cause for facial pain.[37] Understanding the anatomy of the nose and sinuses and their afferent innervation helps in the evaluation of facial pain.

Headache from paranasal sinus disease is most often a deep, dull, aching, pulsatile or non-pulsatile pain. The pain of acute maxillary sinusitis usually localizes over the cheek and radiates to the upper teeth, while pain in acute ethmoiditis is located in the nasion and retro-orbit with possible radiation to the temporal area. In acute frontal sinusitis, headache is located directly over the forehead with radiation to the vertex or retro-orbit.

Acute sphenoiditis localizes to the occipital, vertex, frontal, and retro-orbital areas. There is therefore a significant amount of overlap between symptoms. Chronic sinusitis does not usually cause headache or facial pain, unless when relapsing into an acute phase. Some studies have shown poor correlation between patient-based reports of sinus pain/pressure and findings on CT scans, while others have demonstrated poor correlation between the severity of pain and the extent/location of mucosal disease.

The turbinates, ostia, septum, and naso-frontal duct are the most pain-sensitive areas and are responsible for most of the pain from the nasal and paranasal structures. The mucosal lining of the sinuses, however, has low sensitivity to pain. Most sinonasal pain is referred to distant locations. For instance the inferior turbinate refers pain to the maxillary teeth, zygoma and eye while the middle turbinate refers to the temple, zygoma, eye, and forehead. The afferent fibers of the sinonasal mucosa terminate in the sensory nucleus of the trigeminal nerve close to the afferent fibers that innervate the skin. This could explain referral of pain to the skin.

Mechanical and chemical stimuli can affect the sinonasal mucosa resulting in pain. Rhinitis (allergic or vasomotor), nasal polyps, anatomical abnormalities (such as bony spurs) with contact points between opposing mucosal surfaces, intranasal tumors, trauma, septal hematoma, and inflammation and engorgement of the turbinates, ostia and naso-frontal duct can cause rhinogenic headache.

Some authors have also divided facial pain into neuralgiform and non-neuralgiform types. Neuralgiform types include typical trigeminal neuralgia (attacks of not more than 2 minutes, and with pain-free intervals), and atypical trigeminal neuralgia (attacks of several minutes, or brief pain paroxysms with interval pain). Non-neuralgiform pain is either constant or occurs with periods of pain lasting hours or days.

The proper diagnosis depends on thorough understanding of the nature, site, frequency and symptoms associated with the pain. A complete clinical evaluation should start with a thorough history evaluating the character and site of the pain, and precipitating or alleviating factors. Signs such as nasal drainage, congestion and response to medical treatment should also be ascertained. Physical examination should include nasal endoscopy with rigid telescopes. Imaging with CT scan may be required for a definitive diagnosis.

Patient Management

When evaluating a patient with facial pain, evidence of sinusitis, dental disease or TMJ problems does not necessarily explain the patient's symptoms as these conditions occur frequently in the general public. Indeed several potential causes of facial pain seemingly might coexist in one patient. The presence of sinus or oral cavity disease warrants surgical intervention only if the process is causing clinically identifiable symptoms as many patients with facial pain have undergone numerous operative procedures without resolution of their pain.

These patients require a sympathetic physician because perhaps the easiest way of helping is by listening to them. The benefits from this are two-fold. Patients with facial pain have frequently seen many physicians and have had their problem minimized, dismissed or misdiagnosed. Simply taking the time to patiently listen to their concerns and express understanding may go a long way toward successful treatment evaluation.

Secondly, many of the diagnoses listed above can be made by taking a careful history, that explore the character of the pain, exacerbating factors, associated symptoms, and details of the past medical history.

The physical examination must include a complete otolaryngologic and neurological check-up. Careful evaluation should point to a specific diagnosis. Ancillary tests or assistance from one or more consultants may be required to confirm the diagnosis. The term idiopathic facial pain should be avoided until all potential causes have been thoroughly investigated.

A vast array of treatment modalities is available to manage facial pain.[34] Treatment goals include: Reduction[35] of pain, improvement in functional capacity, elimination of dependence on pain medication, and acknowledgement of the behavioral and psychiatric aspects of the illness. Occasionally an, enlightened physician might be able to address all of these needs but more frequently a multidisciplinary approach is required. The otolaryngologist can and should play a central role in the overall management of these patients. Finally, counseling may help the patient appreciate the behavioral and psychiatric aspects of the disease.

Regional Anesthesia Therapy

Head and neck regional anesthesia provides the practitioner the option of managing acute and chronic pain. The dermatomes are well-defined with good options for approaching and blocking the majority of the peripheral nerves in this region.

Carefully administered in selected patients, nerve blocks can be very effective in the management of acute and chronic head and neck pain. For office-based therapy, 1–2% lidocaine or 2–3% mepivacaine are effective in producing rapid short duration regional anesthesia. With the addition of epinephrine 1:100,000 or 1:200,000, a degree of hemostasis can be obtained and anesthesia prolonged. Because of bupivacaine's longer onset time, this agent is often injected later after the initial block has been assured to provide sustained anesthesia. Reinforcement of the block using 0.5% bupivacaine can provide anesthesia for longer procedures.

Blockade of the sympathetic nerves can be achieved[36] by using concentrations of local anesthetic below that required for sensory and motorloss. Thus, selective block of unmyelinated C fibers and A delta fibers, can be achieved without significant impairment of motor function. Typically, 0.25% bupivacaine is used for diagnostic and therapeutic blocks for pain that is sympathetically mediated. Often sympathetic blockade significantly outlasts the pharmacologic action of the local anesthetic. Neurolytic blocks can be produced by the use of alcohol, phenol, cryotherapy (− 70°C) or thermocoagulation (70°C).

Local anesthesia toxicity occurs when a large volume of concentrated local anesthetic is used. Toxicity can be avoided by using the lowest concentration of anesthetic that will produce the required effect and pre-injection calculation of the maximum volume of that the patient may receive. This is especially important in children, where drug toxicity can be life-threatening.

Neurolytic agents may also produce significant complications such as neuritis and vascular compromise.

The reader is strongly encouraged to review the technical details on the performance of regional anesthesia of the head and neck.

Some of these blocks include, blocks of the cervical plexus, occipital nerve, trigeminal nerve (orbital blocks [supratrochlear, supraorbital, retrobulbar], second and third division trigeminal [intra/extraoral maxillary and mandibular, infraorbital nerve, nasopalatine, greater/lesser palatine nerve, sphenopalatine], glossopharyngeal, stellate ganglion, and cervicothoracic ganglion sympathetic chain, among others.

Selective nerve blocks of the head and neck is an effective method of obtaining regional anesthesia which can be used as both a diagnostic and therapeutic tool in the management of many chronic pain conditions such as headache, postherpetic neuralgia and the pain of cancer. Gamma-knife surgery offers a unique approach to the management of refractory trigeminal neuralgia. The close proximity of so many critical structures to these nerves, demands a thorough understanding of the anatomical basis of these nerve blocks. Appropriate patient selection, careful monitoring, proper injection technique, knowledge of the pharmacokinetics and pharmacodynamics of local anesthetics and vasoconstrictors, possible drug interactions, and recommended doses will ensure safe and successful application of head and neck nerve blockade.

REFERENCES

1. The International Classification of Headache Disorders. *Cephalalgia* 2004;24:Suppl. 1.
2. Silberstein SD, Gordon CD, Hamel RL, Swidan S, Saper J (Eds). *Handbook of Headache Management: A Practical Guide to Diagnosis and Treatment of Head, Neck and Facial Pain*. 2nd edn. Philadelphia: Lippincott Williams and Wilkins 1999.
3. Wolff HG, Lipton RB, Dalessio DJ, Silberstein SD (Eds). *Wolfe's Headache and Other Head Pain*. 7th edn. New York: Oxford University Press, 2001.
4. Iversen HK, Nielsen TH, Olesen J, Tfelt-Hansen P. Arterial responses during migraine headache. *Lancet* 1990;336:837–839.
5. Goadsby PJ, Edvinsson L, Ekman R. Vasoactive peptide release in the extracerebral circulation of human during migraine headache. *Ann Neurol* 1990;28:183–187.
6. Sanchez del Rio M, Bakker D, Wu O et al. Perfusion weighted imaging during migraine: Spontaneous visual aura and headache. *Cephalalgia* 1999;19:701–707.
7. Spierings ELH. Angiographic changes suggestive of vasospasm in migraine complicated by stroke. *Headache* 1990;30:727–728.
8. Spierings ELH. Recent advances in the understanding of migraine. *Headache* 1988;28:655–658.
9. Palmer JE, Chronicle EP, Rolan P, Mulleners WM. Cortical hyperexcitability is cortical under-inhibition: Evidence from a novel functional test of migraine patients. *Cephalalgia* 2000;20:525–532.
10. Spierings ELH. The (suma)triptan history revisited (letter). *Headache* 2000;40:766–767.
11. Solomon GD, Steel JG, Spaccavento LJ. Verapamil prophylaxis of migraine. A double-blind, placebo-controlled study. *JAMA* 1983;250:2500–2502.
12. Spierings ELH. *Management of Migraine*. Boston: Butterworth-Heinemann 1996.
13. Savitz SI, Caplan LR. Vertebrobasilar disease. *N Engl J Med* 2005;352(25):2618–2626.
14. McDonald JS, Pensak MP, Phero JC. Differential diagnosis of chronic facial, head and neck pain conditions (Pt 1). *Am J Otol* 1990;119(4):299–303.
15. Heft MW: Orofacial pain. *Clin Geriatric Med* 1992;8(3):557–568.
16. Rhodus NL, Fricton J, Carlson P, Messner R. Oral symptoms associated with fibromyalgia syndrome. *J Rheumatol* 2003;30:1841–1845.
17. Friction JR, Kroening R, Haley D, Siegart R. Myofacial pain syndrome of the head and neck: Review of clinical characteristics of 164 patients. *Oral Surg Oral Med Oral Pathol* 1982;60:(6)615–623.
18. Tuz HH, Onder EM, Kisnisci RS. Prevalence of otologic complaints inpatients with temporomandibular disorder. *Am J Orthod Dentofacial Orthop* 2003;123(6):620–623.
19. Emshoff R, Brandlmaier I, Gerhard S, Strobl H, Bertram S, Rudisch A. Magnetic resonance imaging predictors of temporomandibular joint pain. *J Am Dent Assoc* 2003;134(6):705–714.
20. Levine HL. Otorhinolaryngologic causes of headache. *Med Clin North Am* 1991;75(3):677–692.
21. Rothman KS, Monson RR. Epidemiology of trigeminal neuralgia. *J Chron Dis* 1973;26:3–12.
22. Donlon WC, Jacobson AL, Truta MP. Neuralgias. *Otolaryngol Clin North Am* 1989;22(6):1145–1158.
23. Dalessio DJ. Diagnosis and treatment of cranial neuralgias. *Med Clin North Am* 1991;75(3):605–615.
24. North RB, Kidd DH, Piantadosi S, Carson BS. Percutaneous retrogasserian glycerol rhizotomy – predictors of success and failure in treatment of trigeminal neuralgia. *J Neurosurg* 1990;72:851–856.
25. Young JN, Wilkins RH. Partial sensory trigeminal rhizotomy at the pons for trigeminal neuralgia. *J Neurosurg* 1993;79:680–687.
26. Linskey ME, Jho HD, Janetta PJ. Microvascular decompression for trigeminal neuralgia caused by vertebrobasilar compression. *J Neurosurg* 1994;81:1–9.
27. Moorley TP. Case against microvascular decompression in treatment of trigeminal neuralgia. *Arch Neurol* 1985;42:801.
28. Mairs AP, Stewart TJ. Surgical treatment of glossopharyngeal neuralgia via the pharyngeal approach. *J Laryngol Otol* 1990;104:12–16.
29. Pappagallo M, Campbell JN. Chronic opioid therapy as alternative treatment for post-herpetic neuralgia. *Ann Neurol* 1994;835:54–56.
30. Max MB. Treatment of postherpetic neuralgia—antidepressants. *Ann Neurol* 1994;835:50–53.
31. Epstein JB, Marcoe JH. Topical application of capsaicin for treatment of oral neuropathic pain and trigeminal neuralgia. *Oral Surg Oral Med Oral Pathol* 1994;77:135–140.
32. Berlit P. Clinical and laboratory findings with giant cell arteritis. *J Neurol Sci* 1992;111(1):1–12.
33. Huntley TA, Wiesenfeld D. Delayed diagnosis of the cause of facial pain in patients with neoplastic disease—a report of eight cases. *J Oral Maxillofac Surg* 1994;52:81–85.
34. Cooper BC, Cooper DL. Multidisciplinary approach to the differential diagnosis of facial head and neck pain. *J Prosthet Dent* 1991;66(1):12–21.
35. Phero JC, Dionne RA. Pharmacological management of head and neck pain. *Oto Clin N Am* 2003;36:1171–1186.
36. Rosenberg M, Phero JC. Regional anesthesia and invasive techniques to manage head and neck pain. *Oto Clin N Am* 2003;36:1201–1220.
37. Holbrook EH, Brown CL, Lyden ER, Leopold DA. Lack of significant correlation between rhinosinusitis symptoms and specific regions of sinus computer tomography scans. *Am J Rhinol* 2005;19(4):382–387.

FACIAL PLASTICS

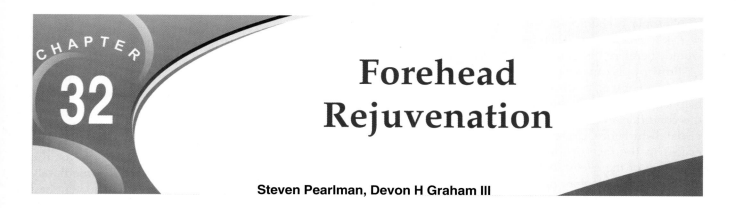

Forehead Rejuvenation

Steven Pearlman, Devon H Graham III

Browlift surgery restores a youthful look to the upper one-third of the face. Facial rejuvenation is classically thought of as cervicofacial rhytidectomy accompanied by blepharoplasty.[1] Facelift surgery only addresses the lower two-thirds of the face. However, aging of the face occurs in a symmetrical fashion. Changes in the forehead and eyebrow position are frequently ignored. Browlift not only transforms eyebrow position and shape but can also affect forehead rhytids and upper eyelid ptosis. Until 1992, the coronal browlift was the primary technique for forehead rejuvenation.[2,3] Since then, however, treatment for the aging forehead has undergone widespread changes. Application of endoscopic surgical techniques has made this procedure far more acceptable to patients by minimizing surgical morbidity and healing time (Table 32.1).

The primary surgical technique used by the authors for forehead rejuvenation is endoscopic browlift. The indications for endoscopic browlift are the same as for any open technique and include patients with generalized brow ptosis and forehead rhytids. Correction of eyebrow and associated eyelid skin psuedo-ptosis, as well as brow asymmetry and lateral canthus malposition are the primary surgical objectives. Furrows in the glabella, horizontal forehead rhytids, and lines across the radix of the nose can all be addressed surgically or non-surgically with the use of Botox.

Table 32.1: Indications for forehead rejuvenation

1. Correction of eyebrow ptosis
2. Indirect removal of excess eyelid skin
3. Correction of eyebrow asymmetry
4. Correction of lateral canthal malposition
5. Elimination of glabellar frown lines
6. Reduction of horizontal forehead lines
7. Reduction of lines at the nasal radix
8. Balance facelift surgery to prevent 'bunching' lines
9. Skin resurfacing for texture and color changes

Generally, the most favorable candidates for endoscopic browlift are relatively thin-skinned individuals with average or deep-set eyes. More difficult and less favorable are patients who have thick, heavy sebaceous skin with marked brow ptosis or patients who have complete paralysis of the frontal branch of the facial nerve. These patients exhibit no frontalis muscle tone at all and usually require some skin excision in conjunction with a suspension or reanimation procedure. Additionally, patients with a pre-existing high frontal hairline, where brow elevation is needed, are not ideal candidates as this technique does move the hairline somewhat superiorly in relation to the skull. The relationship between the brows and the hairline, however, remains relatively constant as opposed to the traditional coronal technique.

Other techniques for browlift surgery are necessary for patients with very high frontal hairlines. For these patients, a pretrichial or trichophytic 'in the hairline' modification of the traditional coronal browlift has been developed.[4] Adjunctive technique have also arisen that can minimize aging effects on the brow. Botox and direct excision of glabellar musculature treats dynamic lines that have become equated with a stern, maturing face. Facial skin resurfacing has also improved with a variety of lasers to smooth the skin to complement surgical or chemical Botox rejuvenation.

Facial aging occurs as a result of the effects of gravity, loss of support from reduced elastic tissue and collagen changes within the dermis and dynamic rhytids from hyperactive muscular activity. This may first become apparent as excess skin in the upper eyelids. Patients often present with this complaint. Evaluation of the entire upper third of the face is necessary to determine the true cause, rather than focusing on the eyelids alone. Another manifestation of true brow ptosis is lateral hooding of the skin, often perceived as extension of excess upper eyelid skin. However, excision of skin during upper blepharoplasty should not extend beyond the orbital rim or risk a visible scar.[5] Therefore, lateral eyelid hooding would, therefore, be better treated by browlift surgery.

Brow ptosis can even cause superolateral visual field defects, typically thought to be due to upper blepharochalasis. Browlift may be more appropriate in this condition, even for medically indicated treatment of visual disturbance. Upper blepharoplasty to correct skin excess in the face of low eyebrows can cause more crowding of the eyelid/brow complex. Following skin excision during blepharoplasty, approximately 20 mm of skin should remain between the inferior edge of the brow and the eyelashes to retain normal upper eyelid function.[6] Removing hooded skin via blepharoplasty in the face of a low brow may worsen brow ptosis causing incarceration of the brow, possibly pulling it more inferiorly.[7]

FOREHEAD ANATOMY

Understanding the anatomy for surgical dissection is often distinguished from that encountered in the gross anatomy lab. The same principle must be altered to facilitate anatomic findings encountered during the endoscopic approach to the brow as well. Through the endoscope, familiar structures are viewed in an unfamiliar manner; therefore, a thorough grasp of the anatomy and the fascial planes is indispensable.

Scalp and Forehead Musculature

The scalp consists of the skin, subcutaneous tissue, aponeurosis or galea, loose areolar tissue, and periosteum (S-C-A-L-P). These layers continue into the forehead. The galea is a tendinous inelastic sheet that connects the frontalis muscle to the occipitalis muscle and merges laterally with the temporoparietal fascia (TPF), which is continuous with the superficial musculoaponeurotic system (SMAS) in the lower face. The frontalis muscle originates from the galea and inserts in the forehead skin and acts as the primary elevator of the brow. Motor nerve supply to the frontalis muscle is via the frontal branch of the facial nerve. During the subperiosteal endoscopic forehead lift, the frontalis muscle is not usually visualized. The depressor muscles of the brow include the paired corrugator supercilli, the orbicularis oculi, depressor supercilli and the procerus muscles. The corrugator supercilli muscles are the primary muscle responsible for the often deep vertical rhytids of the glabella that trouble most patients. The procerus muscle, originating from the nasal bones, produces the transverse rhytids in the nasion.

Fascia

During an endoscopic browlift, the dissection crosses several fascial planes. Endoscopic browlift is performed in two different planes. Laterally, over the temporalis muscle, the dissection is supraperiosteal. Medially, over the forehead, elevation is performed in a subperiosteal plane. The fascial planes are described in the order in which they are encountered during the procedure. The superficial temporal fascia, also known as the temporoparietal fascia (TPF), is located immediately beneath the skin and subcutaneous fat of the temporal area. The temporal artery and vein course superiorly within this fascial layer. Medially, over the forehead, the TPF merges with the galea. The TPF is continuous with the SMAS in the lower face. Beneath the TPF is the deep temporal fascia or true temporalis fascia. Dissection in the temporal region occurs on top of the deep temporal fascia and, therefore, below the TPF. If identification of the plane is necessary, it is sometimes helpful to nick the deep temporal fascia, exposing a small area of the temporalis muscle to confirm that dissection will then be carried anteriorly in the proper plane. The deep temporal fascia splits at the level of the supraorbital ridge to become the intermediate temporal fascia and the deep temporal fascia with the intermediate fat pad in between (Fig. 32.1). The intermediate temporal fascia attaches to the superior edge of the zygomatic arch laterally and the deep temporal fascia attaches medially. Deep to the deep temporal fascia is the deep temporal fat pad. Dissection should be right on top

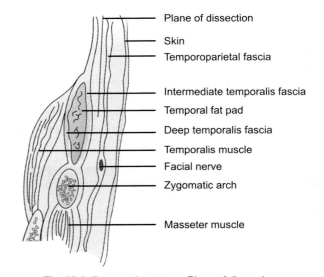

Fig. 32.1: Temporal anatomy: Plane of dissection in the temporal area, right side of the face

of this layer to protect the facial nerve. However, violation of the fascial covering of the deep temporal fat pad can result in atrophy of the fat and cause temporal wasting.

Sensory and Motor Nerves in the Forehead

The facial nerve (VII) supplies all of the muscles of facial expression, including the centrally located corrugator and procerus muscles. The branches of the trigeminal nerve (V) provide sensation. The supratrochlear and supraorbital branches of V_1 emerge from the skull deep to the eyebrow. They are visualized during dissection and should be preserved when corrugator resection is performed. These nerves typically exit from the supraorbital notch or foramen. In up to 10% of cases, one or both of these nerves may arise from a true foramen 1 to 2 cm superior to the orbital rim, which puts the nerves at risk for transection if blind non-endoscopic-assisted dissection is performed. The notch is usually palpable and marked preoperatively to denote the origin of the supraorbital nerve. To facilitate finding the notch, place the index, middle, and ring fingers over the root of nose from above: The notch should be just lateral to the fingers on either side.

The temporal branch of the facial nerve crosses the zygomatic arch halfway between the lateral canthus and the root of auricular helix within the TPF. Sabini et al described a more accurate means of identifying the precise location of the frontal branch of the facial nerve during endoscopic forehead surgery.[9] A series of bridging vessels, including one larger sentinel vein, are encountered between the deep temporal fascia and the TPF during the dissection in the temporal region. These bridging vessels were shown to point to the frontal branch of the nerve as it coursed through the TPF.

AESTHETIC EVALUATION OF THE FOREHEAD

The upper face should be evaluated for eyebrow position and shape. The amount of excess skin and soft tissue of the eyelids and the extent of lateral hooding is important. The presence of dynamic or static rhytids present in the glabella, across the nose, in the forehead and the crow's feet area must be assessed. The brow should be in balance with the remainder of the face. In patients considering facelift surgery, which addresses the lower half to two-thirds of the face, a browlift may be necessary to eliminate transition 'lines' and new furrows which may appear from the lateral canthi to above the ears.

The 'classic' eyebrow is club-shaped and tapers laterally with its medial origin along a vertical line drawn through the nasal alar-facial junction. The lateral extent is along a line drawn from the nasal alar-facial junction through the lateral canthus. Both the medial and lateral brow should be at the same horizontal position, typically at or just above the bony orbital rim. Generally, in women, the brow should arc delicately above the orbital rim with its highest point between the lateral limbus and the lateral orbital rim. More medial elevation tends to create an unnatural, surprised look. The male brow should rest on the superior orbital rim and is more horizontal. Robyn Cosio, an aesthetician internationally known for brow shaping described a 'pencil trick' for brow shaping[10] (Figs 32.2A to C).

The height of the brow is not the only concern in forehead rejuvenation: shape is important as well. If the shape is pleasing, eyebrows do not necessarily need to be high. Any current fashion magazine corroborates this. Low, full eyebrows are as prevalent as high, tapered ones (Figs 32.3A and B). During patient evaluation, we may ask

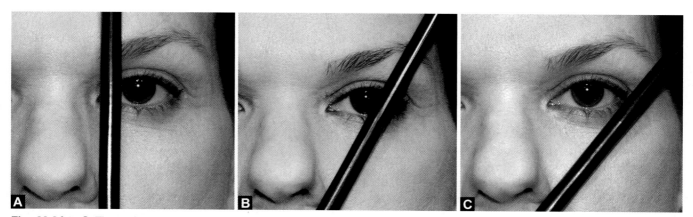

Figs 32.2A to C: The perfect brow begins just inside the corner of the nasal ala. Hold a brow stick. (A) Pencil or ruler perpendicular from the side of the ala, that is where the eyebrow should begin. (B) The stick is then angled laterally from the center of the bottom lip past the nasal ala to the outside of the pupil. Where it meets the brow should be the peak. (C) The lateral extent is determined from the same origin angling the ruler past the lateral canthus

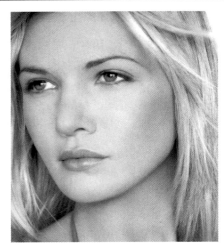

Fig. 32.3A: Fashion model showing aesthetically pleasing brow shape and position; note that it does not need to be placed high

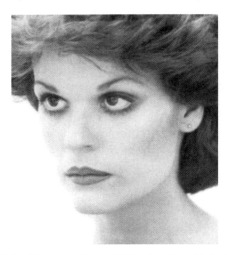

Fig. 32.3B: Fashion model from 1980s showing a higher brow: This is what many of our current patients identify with as their goal

for old photographs to compare brow height and shape, and then compare them to both the present brow position and the patient's desires. Patients frequently identify with aesthetics from when they were in their 20s and 30s when brow height trends were different. Familiarity with those trends will aid in planning.

The presence of glabellar frown lines occurs primarily from action of the corrugator muscles with contributions from the orbicularis oculi and depressor supercilli muscles.[11] Horizontal forehead lines are a result of hyperactive frontalis muscles. These muscles were traditionally incised during open browlift surgery; however, it has become unnecessary and counterproductive to perform this maneuver during an endoscopic lift.[12] Deep horizontal forehead lines result from the natural

tendency to hold the brow upward, relieving secondary heaviness of the upper eyelids. Surgical elevation of the brow reduces this propensity.

PATIENT SELECTION

As with any facial plastic surgery procedure, patient selection is critical. Patient evaluation should begin with a thorough history and physical examination. In the history, we typically elicit complaints about droopy eyelids and the appearance of weariness. The angry countenance of glabellar in-frowning is also a frequent concern of the patient. Botulinum toxin injections are very effective for this; however, the endoscopic approach with partial resection of the corrugator supercilli and procerus muscles yields lasting result. Physical examination of the periorbital area should evaluate for eyelid blepharochalasis, brow ptosis, eyelid position and muscular hyperfunction.

When examining a patient for aging upper face, the patient should be seated in front of a mirror facing forward with the head level, using the Frankfort horizontal plane. The patient is instructed to close his or her eyes and relaxes the forehead for a full 15 to 20 seconds. Next, the patient opens the eyes just enough to look straightforward without raising the brows. In this manner, the level of the brows can be evaluated in repose without the effects of exaggerated muscle contraction. The shape and position of the brows as they relate to the underlying orbit is then evaluated and compared with the classic brow. Again, it is important to compare the patient's brow with the shape that they desire, which may be from old photographs of themselves or the fashion era that they tend to identify with. In most cases involving the aging upper face, the eyebrow fat pad, which is designed to lie on and cushion the orbital rim, is ptotic, resting to various degrees on the upper eyelid. A common mistake is to overlook brow position and simply address hooded eyelids as upper lid dermatochalasis. By performing an upper lid blepharoplasty without repositioning and fixating the brows, the natural spaces between the lateral canthus and lid crease as well as the lid crease and brow may be shortened, sometimes markedly, leaving an abnormal appearance due to an even lower brow position.

SELECTION OF BROWLIFT TECHNIQUE

Until the introduction of the endoscopic browlift, the coronal lift had been the gold standard for upper facial rejuvenation. This technique relies on a long incision within the scalp, several centimeters behind the hairline following its shape. The dissection is in a sub-galeal plane and the corrugator muscles are directly excised while the frontalis muscle is scored. For most authors, the endoscopic browlift has all but replaced this classically described procedure.[13-15] Other surgical options include mid-forehead, direct and trichophytic browlifts. The direct browlift is rarely used, except in patients with unilateral facial paralysis. The mid-forehead browlift is usually reserved for males with high hairlines. With this procedure, the surgical incision is placed in existing forehead creases; however, the scars take many months to heal.[12] Males with high hairlines, could be offered minimal incision endoscopic browlift. This would avoid creating a scar across the middle of the forehead. Open browlift techniques rely on skin resection and tension to provide brow fixation and elevation. Endoscopic browlift surgery relies on skin retraction and full brow release to maintain brow position.[16] The advantages and disadvantages of open versus endoscopic techniques are outlined in Table 32.2.

One of the significant advantages of the endoscopic browlift technique is patient acceptance. Patients are willing to tolerate long incisions around the ear for rejuvenation of the lower face, yet demonstrate much trepidation at the thought of an incision across the top of their head for forehead rejuvenation. Patient rate of acceptance for forehead rejuvenation is much higher for endoscopic browlift via 4 to 5 small incisions than for open browlift.[14] Early complaints of the endoscopic technique were early relapse or over-correction. These issues are addressed by more complete elevation and separation of the periorbital periosteum. The only remaining controversy over browlift surgery is the method of fixation.

Endoscopic Browlift: Surgical Technique

Once an appropriate candidate for endoscopic brow and forehead lifting is selected, standard patient preparation and preoperative precautions are undertaken. A useful adjunct to surgery is injection of botulinum toxin A to the central brow and glabella depressor muscles 2 weeks before the surgical procedure. This allows not only excellent aesthetic improvement but also redraping and reattachment of the elevated periosteum unencumbered by depressor muscle action pulling the brows downward.[17] In addition, the corrugator supercilli muscles can be partially resected during the surgical procedure.

Surgical Dissection

The procedure begins in the holding area prior to administration of anesthetic. The patient is examined in the sitting position and the brow position is assessed. The planned vectors of pull are determined and marked on the patient's forehead and temporal area. In women, the vectors are typically more superior and lateral; whereas, in men, the emphasis is on a slightly more lateral than superior vector. The paramedian incisions in women are made directly above the desired peak of the brow, between the lateral limbus and canthus (Fig. 32.4). These markings are performed with the patient in the upright position, allowing gravity its full effect. The supraorbital nerves are also marked as palpated from their notch, as well as a half circle 2 cm in diameter around the nerve origin for later endoscopic dissection. If concomitant blepharoplasty is to be performed, the lower limb of the blepharoplasty incision corresponding to the existing lid crease is marked at this time. Additional preoperative marking includes the glabellar in-frowning lines and the frontal branch of the facial nerve if desired.

The patient is then brought to the operating suite where the equipment is arranged for proper visualization and function. Intravenous analgesics are administered, followed by infiltrative local anesthesia using nerve and field blocks. Approximately 15 to 20 minutes is allowed for complete anesthesia and vasoconstriction. One central

Table 32.2: Open coronal versus endoscopic browlift*	
Coronal browlift	*Endoscopic browlift*
Advantages	**Advantages**
Easy to perform	Accurate preservation of sensory nerves
Accurate muscle dissection	Selective resection of muscles
Versatile incision: At or behind hairline	High patient acceptance
Good for high hairline (tricophytic)	Minimal alopecia
Disadvantages	Minimal stretch back
Long scar	Accurate control of brow position
Scar alopecia	Less recovery time
Stretch-back with recurrent ptosis	Less blood loss
Brow numbness and paresthesias	Shorter procedure
Longer recovery	Applicable to male pattern baldness
Greater blood loss	**Disadvantages**
Longer procedure	More difficult to perform
Poor for high or thin hairline (coronal approach)	Requires more expensive equipment
	May raise forehead

*Adapted from Ramirez.

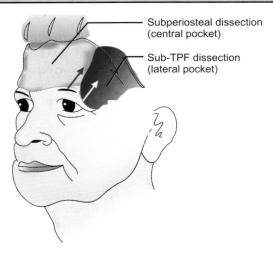

Fig. 32.4: Incisions and planes for undermining. The central, paramedian and temporal incisions are indicated. The central forehead is undermined in a subperiosteal plane and the temporal region beneath the temporal parietal fascia (Permission awaited)

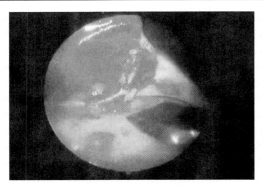

Fig. 32.5A: Supraorbital nerve exiting the supraorbital foramen

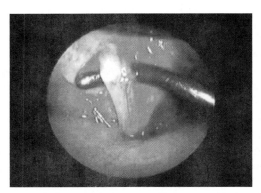

Fig. 32.5B: Supraorbital nerve exiting supraorbital notch

and two paramedian vertical incisions are made 1–1.5 cm in length, approximately 1.5 cm posterior to the anterior hairline corresponding to the desired vectors of pull. The central incision may or may not be necessary, depending on the desire for central brow elevation and fixation. The incisions are made with a No. 15 blade through all layers down to the skull. The periosteum is then elevated carefully in the region of the incision using a small sharp periosteal elevator, with care taken not to fray or damage the periosteum. Complete continuity of the periosteum around this incision is necessary, as this will be vitally important when it is time to place the suspension sutures. Elevation then proceeds blindly using endoscopic dissectors in the subperiosteal plane to a level approximately 1.5–2 cm above the orbital rims inferiorly (as marked preoperatively), to the temporal lines laterally, and approximately 2–3 cm posteriorly. At this point, the 30° endoscope with sheath is introduced and the dissection proceeds inferiorly under direct vision. The visualized optic cavity should be almost bloodless, with excellent contrast between the underlying bone and overlying periosteum. The advantage of the subperiosteal dissection plane is the whiteness of the frontal bone creating an excellent optical cavity.

Attention is directed to the region of the supraorbital neurovascular bundles. Care must be taken when dissecting toward this area, as in 10% of patients the neurovascular bundle exits through a true foramen as opposed to a supraorbital notch (Figs 32.5A and B). If corrugator and procerus resections are performed, the neurovascular bundle can be delineated by blunt dissection parallel to the fibers using a small pick. A temporary

transcutaneous stitch can be placed in the medial brow and lifted by an assistant to open the pocket of dissection. Alternatively, the assistant controls the endoscope while the surgeon holds and elevates the eyebrow with the non-dominant hand, while using the elevator with the other. If indicated, the corrugator supercilli and procerus muscles are resected and cauterized to maintain hemostasis. Electrocautery or careful use of CO_2 laser may be used. Additionally, orbicularis oculi myotomies may be performed by making multiple radial incisions in the muscle deep to the brow with a scissors or Colorado tip cautery, with caution to avoid the frontal branch of the facial nerve. Unilateral orbicularis myotomies may be used on a depressed brow to allow for increased single-brow elevation in patients with asymmetrical brows. Once the neurovascular bundles have been located, dissection is continued medially and laterally to these nerves continuing inferiorly over the orbital rim releasing the periosteum at the arcus marginalis. A gentle prying maneuver causes the periosteum to separate, revealing the overlying brow fat pad or ROOF (retro-orbicularis oculi fat pad). It is critical that periosteal separation be performed at the arcus marginalis, which lies below the level of the eyebrows. Only by a complete release at this level can the periosteum be elevated and re-suspended as a bipedicled flap. This release is the key step for longevity of surgical results. In patients with very heavy brows and thick corrugator musculature, the muscle may be divided and a portion removed if warranted.

After dissection is completed in the central pocket, attention is turned to elevation of the temporal pockets bilaterally. These will then be connected to the central optical cavity for completion of the elevation. The temporal pocket lies over the temporalis muscle and is bordered by the cephalic edge of the zygomatic arch inferiorly, the orbital rim anteriorly, and the temporal line superiorly. Temporal pocket access is obtained through a 1.5–2 cm incision within the hairline of the temporal tuft corresponding to the superior and lateral vector of pull desired for the brow. If a midface lift is planned in addition, this incision is extended to 3–4 cm. The incision is made through the skin, subcutaneous tissues, and TPF. The incisions should be beveled according to the directions of hair growth to preserve the follicular units and minimize alopecia. The dissection proceeds inferiorly in the plane deep to the TPF and above the deep temporal fascia covering the temporalis muscle. This dissection is performed carefully using a blunt endoscopic dissector under direct visualization using the 30° endoscope. Respect for the plane of dissection is important to protect the frontal branch of the facial nerve.

In a standard brow and forehead lift, the inferior dissection is complete at a level just superior to the zygomatic arch approximating a horizontal line from the lateral canthus, which usually corresponds to the level of the sentinal vein. The temporal pocket is then joined to the central pocket under direct visualization by sharp and blunt dissection of the temporal line attachments consisting of periosteum, galea, and temporal fascias. The dissection to join the temporal and central pockets should proceed in a lateral to medial direction to maintain the proper plane. Once the two pockets have been joined superiorly, the dissection proceeds inferiorly, elevating the temporal attachments. Elevation is carried inferiorly to the area of the lateral orbital rim where dense connected tissue attachments to the bone are encountered. This conjoined tendon is sharply elevated in the subperiosteal plane using an endoscopic dissector, scissors, or endoscopic knife. Once this dissection has been completed, the contralateral side is performed in the same manner. At this point, the entire forehead-brow complex will be quite mobile and can be slid superiorly and inferiorly over the underlying bone.

BROW FIXATION

After the entire elevation has been completed, the TPF is suspended through the temporal incision to the deep temporal fascia using a heavy absorbable suture. Maximal support and elevation in this area should be obtained, as this region cannot be over-corrected. After this has been completed bilaterally, suspension in the central region is begun. There are multiple approaches to fixation of the forehead, both permanent and temporary (Table 32.3). The method of fixation reflects the surgeon's preference and should be based on patient comfort, surgical ease, and cost. Complete surgical release of the entire forehead–brow complex is more significant than the method of suspension (Fig. 32.6A to C).

Healing with re-adhesion of the periosteum is necessary to prevent recurrent ptosis of the brow following

Table 32.3: Endoscopic brow fixation techniques

1. Temporary fixation
   a. External bolster fixation
   b. External (removable) surgical screws
2. Long-term fixation
   a. Buried spanning sutures
   b. Absorbable screws
   c. Tissue adhesives
   d. Endotine device
3. Permanent fixation
   a. Internal screws
   b. Internal Mitek anchor
   c. Cortical bone tunnels

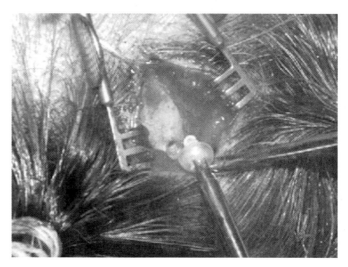

Fig. 32.6A: Absorbable screw is placed in outer table of skull

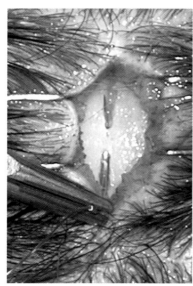

Fig. 32.6B: Cortical bone tunnel with suture being passed for brow fixation

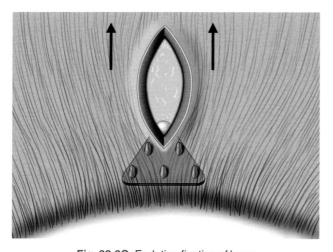

Fig. 32.6C: Endotine fixation of brow

surgery. Conflicting studies exist about the length of time required for the elevated periosteum to completely reattach. Romo[18] in a clinical study compared temporary to permanent fixation and concluded that the latter is superior. In an animal laboratory study, Brodner[19] found periosteal re-adhesion to be complete by the seventh postoperative day, indicating that long-term suspension might not be necessary. Most authors believe that complete release is more important than the actual suspension technique employed.[1,14,16]

Once the brow is fully released, fixation is performed to maintain brow position during healing and periosteum re-adherence. Two of the earliest methods for brow fixation

are temporary. These include external bolsters and removable screws placed into the outer table of the skull.[16] These fixation screws are used in the paramedian incisions to give maximal elevation at the desired brow peak (see section on brow aesthetics). The amount of desired elevation is measured preoperatively and marked in the skull right after the scalp incision is made. The screw is placed 20% beyond the desired elevation to compensate for postoperative stretch-back. The scalp is then fixed to the screws by placing the external scalp staples right behind the screw. Some surgeons use buried sutures placed from the galea around the screw as well. There should be no tension on the closure, indicating a complete release. The screws are removed at the same time as the scalp staples, approximately 8 to 10 days postoperatively. Screws are available with thread stops at 4 mm to prevent any possibility of skull penetration.

Long-term suspension is used when the surgeon desires more time for scalp adhesion. One such technique is buried spanning sutures. Use of absorbable screws is one of the most common methods.[1] These screws are placed in a similar fashion to the removable ones, but are preferred by many to eliminate screws emanating from the scalp following surgery and the need for later removal. A third method for long-term fixation is with fibrin glue. Marchac et al[13] found that fibrin glue could replace skull-anchoring devices. Two commercially available forms of fibrin glue are now approved for use in the USA.

Short titanium surgical screws or Mitek anchors achieve permanent fixation of the brow.[18] Hardware of any type can also be avoided by creation of cortical tunnels.[20] The outer table of the skull can be drilled to a depth of 3–4 mm crafting a bone tunnel for passage of permanent suspension sutures. The very small chance for transgressing the skull with the burr is eliminated by the use of a tunnel drill system created by Sykes.[21]

Final adjustments may be made in brow height by elevating the patient to an upright position. Central fixation may be desired if there is significant ptosis of the medial brow as well. All incisions are closed with skin staples. A soft pressure dressing may be used, which is removed on the first postoperative day (Figs 32.7A to F).

TRICHOPHYTIC BROWLIFT IN THE HAIRLINE

For patients with high foreheads, endoscopic browlift can further elevate the hairline in relation to the skull. This elevation may be minimal since eventual brow position can better be controlled by selective release and elevation. However, if no ascent or even lowering of the brow is

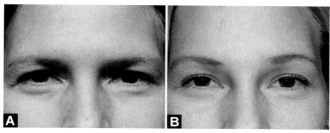

Figs 32.7A and B: Young patient with low brow, ideal for endoscopic browlift

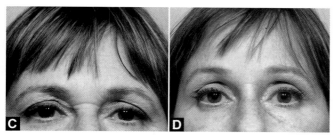

Figs 32.7C to D: Patient with significant medial and lateral brow ptosis with hooding, pre- and post-endobrow lift

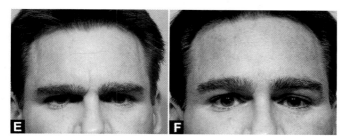

Figs 32.7E and F: Male with ptotic brow pre- and post-endobrow lift

desired, the trichophytic browlift[4] is our preferred technique. Elevation is similar to the traditional coronal lift with changes in the incision. An irregular incision is made within the anterior hairline. However, contrary to traditional teaching, the scalpel is beveled inferiorly to leave hair follicles at the distal edge. The desired amount of elevation is achieved by resecting forehead skin. The elevated forehead skin is thinned and sutured over the buried hair follicles. This hair then grows through the scar providing natural camouflage.

BOTOX FOREHEAD REJUVENATION

Botox has been shown to be helpful in temporarily immobilizing the brow depressors in endoscopic browlift, possibly aiding periosteal adhesion.[17] Even before the application of Botox to browlift surgery, it has been used for treatment of dynamic rhytids of the forehead.[22] There are three 'regions' of the forehead that can be smoothened by the use of Botox immobilization. Vertical glabellar furrows can be reduced by injection into the corrugator muscle with secondary effects on horizontal nasal lines by procerus injection. Horizontal lines from hyperactive frontalis muscles are reduced by forehead injection. Use of Botox in very ptotic brows, however, can lead to excess upper eyelid heaviness and even exacerbate visual disturbance. In such a case, Botox should be avoided; browlift is the best treatment. Lastly, crow's feet are diminished by injection into the orbicularis oculi muscles lateral to the orbital rim.

Observation of the effects on brow position from Botox treatments led to the minimally invasive procedure called chemical browlift. Frankel found that treatment of the brow depressors could elevate the medial brow and increase inter-brow distance.[23] Ahn et al further refined this technique yielding lateral brow elevation by injection of the lateral orbicularis muscle, leaving unopposed frontalis elevation.[24] The brow was elevated to an average of 1 mm in the mid-pupillary line and 4 mm at the lateral canthus. These latter results are not consistent between patients but more closely follow aesthetic desired for eyebrow position and shape. Therefore, a chemical Botox browlift may be used to temporarily raise the brow and to indicate potential improvement from a more permanent surgical browlift.

Complications

Following surgical forehead rejuvenation, there usually will be some temporary numbness over the forehead. This numbness is rarely over the entire distribution of the supraorbital nerve and typically resolves within 2 to 6 months in the forehead and 9 to 12 months at the crown. During recovery of sensation, paresthesias and itching are common. There may also be alopecia along the incisions if tension is placed during suspension. Since the incisions for the endoscopic browlift are short, this can be covered with the surrounding hair. Hair growth generally returns in about 3 months. Transient frontal nerve palsy is uncommon. If the proper surgical dissection planes have been respected, palsy is then felt to be a result of either thermal trauma secondary to electrocautery or overzealous temporal pocket elevation with nerve stretching. An abnormal brow position may occur, which is initially treated with massage. If this does not achieve the desired result, releasing of the tissue may be necessary. Hematomas in the forehead or scalp may occur. However, respect for proper dissection planes, the use of a closed-suction drain, compression dressings or fibrin glue will minimize these.

CONCLUSION

Evaluation and treatment of the aging forehead is important in facial rejuvenation. There are a number surgical and non-surgical options available. The advent of endoscopic browlift surgery has significantly enhanced the ability to revitalize the forehead through minimal incisions with negligible surgical morbidity. Every patient presenting for eyelid as well as forehead rejuvenation should be evaluated for contributions from brow ptosis to the maturing upper face. The aging forehead can be treated in a stepwise manner. Dynamic furrows of the forehead can be treated with Botox injections. Surgical brow elevation is best performed through the endoscopic approach. In patients with a high hairline, the pre- trichial, (in the hairline browlift), is the preferred technique. In men, the endoscopic technique minimizes incisions to allow treatment of patients with receding hairlines and the risk of an exposed incision. Therefore, a more precise treatment can be offered to patients, directed at the specific cause for the aging forehead.

REFERENCES

1. Quatela VC, Graham HD, Sabini P. Rejuvenation of the brow and midface. In *Facial Plastic and Reconstructive Surgery*, eds Papel ID, Frodel J, Park SS, Holt GR, Sykes JM, Larrabee WF, Toriumi D, Nachlas N, 2nd edn. New York: Thieme 2002; 171–184.
2. Core GB, Vasconez LO, Askren C et al. Coronal facelift with endoscopic techniques. *Plast Surg For* 1992;15:227.
3. Liang M, Narayanan K. Endoscopic ablation of the frontalis and corrugator muscles: A clinical study. *Plast Surg For* 1992; 15:58.
4. Flemming RW, Mayer TG. Open versus closed browlifting. *Clin Fac Plast Surg* 2000; 8(3):361–77.
5. Delgado JA, Jacobs JL, Baylis HI, Goldberg RA. Blepharoplasty and periorbital surgery. *Clin Fac Plast Surg* 1998; 6(1):41–58.
6. Baylis HI, Goldberg RA, Kerivan KM, Jacobs JL. Blepharoplasty and periorbital surgery. *Dermatol Clin* 1997; 15(4):635–647.
7. Koch RJ, Troell RJ, Goode RL. Contemporary management of the aging brow and forehead. *Laryngoscope* 1997; 107:710–715.
8. Isse NG. Endoscopic facial rejuvenation. *Clin Plast Surg* 1997; 24(2):213–231.
9. Sabini P, Wayne I, Quatela VC. Anatomic guides to precisely locating the frontal branch of the facial nerve. Spring meeting of the American Academy of Facial Plastic and Reconstructive Surgery, Orlando, Florida, May 2000.
10. Cosio R. *The Eyebrow*. New York: Harper Collins, 2000.
11. Sykes JM. Applied anatomy of the forehead and brow. *Clin Fac Plast Surg* 1997; 4(2):99–112.
12. Becker FF, Johnson CM, Mandel LM. Surgical management of the upper third of the aging face. In *Otolaryngology–Head and Neck Surgery*, Cummings CW, Fredrickson JM, Harker LA, Krause CJ, Richardson, MA, Schuller, DE. (Eds). St. Louis: Mosby, 1998; 660–675.
13. Marchac D, Ascherman J, Arnaud E. Fibrin glue fixation in forehead endoscopy: Evaluation of our experience with 206 cases. *Plast and Reconstr Surg* 1997; 100(3):704–714.
14. Ramirez OM. Why I prefer the endoscopic forehead lift. *Plast and Recon Surg* 1997; 100(4):1033–1046.
15. Koch RJ. Endoscopic browlift is the preferred approach for rejuvenation of the upper third of the face. *Arch Otolaryngol Head and Neck Surg* 2001; 127:87–92.
16. Rohrich RJ, Beran SJ. Evolving fixation methods in endoscopically assisted forehead rejuvenation: Controversies and rationale. *Plast and Reconstr Surg* 1997; 100(6):1575–1582.
17. Dyer WK, Yung RT. Botulinum toxin–assisted brow lift. *Clin Fac Plast Surg* 2000; 8(3):343–354.
18. Romo T, Sclafani AP, Yung RT. Endoscopic foreheadplasty: Temporary vs. permanent fixation. *Aest Plast Surg* 1999; 23:388–394.
19. Brodner DC, Downs JC, Graham HD. Periosteal readhesion after brow-lift in New Zealand white rabbits. *Arch Facial Plast Surg* 2002; 4:248–251.
20. Newman JP, LaFerriere KA, Koch RJ, Nishioka GJ, Goode RL. Transcalvarial suture fixation for endoscopic brow and forehead lifts. *Arch Otolaryngol Head and Neck Surg* 1997; 123:313–317.
21. Medtronic Xomed Cor, Web publication: http://www.xomed.com/Adobe/st_endobrowlift.pdf. Jacksonville, FL.
22. Blitzer A, Binder WJ. Cosmetic uses of botulinum neurotoxin type A. *Arch Facial Plast Surg* 2002; 4:214–220.
23. Frankel AS, Kamer FM. Chemical browlift. *Arch Otolayngol Head and Neck Surg* 1998; 124(3):321–323.
24. Ahn MS, Catten M, Maas CS. Temporal brow lift using botulinum toxin A. *Plast and Reconstr Surg* 2000; 105(3): 1129–1135.

CHAPTER 33

Mandible Fractures

Brian E Emery

The mandible is the second most commonly fractured facial bone and the most common requiring treatment. Complications and infections exceed other facial fractures.[1] The higher infection rate may be because all mandible fractures can be considered open because of the tightly adherent mucosa. Open fractures have been demonstrated as having a higher rate of infection in orthopedic literature.[2]

The management of mandible fractures is directed by principles developed in both orthopedics and dentistry. These principles include the reduction of the fracture site to its correct anatomical position, restoration of the premorbid occlusion, rigid immobilization of the fracture to facilitate healing, optimal and early restoration of function, and prevention of infection and subsequent non-union or malunion of the fracture.[3]

The etiology of mandible fractures is socioculturally dependant as most series in the USA reveal assault as the primary cause[4-9] while two series of mandible fractures from Europe revealed that the majority were from motor vehicle accidents.[10,11] A common presentation in the USA is a male without insurance who was assaulted and is referred to multiple facilities over several days, delaying care.[6,7]

EVALUATION

Patients who have suffered facial trauma often sustain other injuries.[6] The Advanced Trauma Life Support (ATLS) protocol is followed and life-threatening injuries are stabilized first. An evaluation of the cervical spine is required prior to addressing a fracture of the mandible as the neck may be manipulated during reduction or fixation.

Patients with mandible fractures frequently complain of malocclusion, pain, trismus, and paresthesias.

Perceived malocclusion may be related to muscle spasm, chipped teeth, or injury to the trigeminal nerve. Overall, fractures at the angle are the most common, while the remaining fractures are divided among the body, symphysis, and condylar region.[12] Weak spots in the mandible such as the third molar, condylar neck, and mental foramen/socket of canine suggest why these sites are common sites of fracture.

Past medical history, past surgical history, medications, allergies, and social history must be obtained prior to proceeding with treatment. Specifically, intravenous drug abuse,[13] alcoholism, seizures, HIV status[14] and nutritional concerns are common in this population and impact treatment options and outcome.[15] A higher incidence of complications is seen in alcoholics (16%), non-IV drug users (19%), and IV drug users (30%), as compared to those without a history of substance abuse (6.2%).[8] Direct questions about prior facial trauma, prior orthodontic treatment, premorbid occlusion, and dentures should be asked.

Examination

After the patient is stabilized, a comprehensive evaluation for any facial injury is undertaken. An overview is made of the face as a patient with an overlying soft tissue injury may have an underlying bony injury. Trismus as a result of the injury (inter-incisal distance < 40 mm) may make the oral examination difficult. The presence of trismus does not necessarily suggest a mandible fracture, as trismus may be present due to spasm or splinting or from a depressed zygomatic arch fracture. The oral cavity is examined for loose or missing teeth as they pose an aspiration risk.

The teeth and occlusal relationships are examined in detail. The dental numbering system is used to identify dental pathology and to describe the site of the fracture. Mucosal lacerations are identified and may suggest an underlying fracture. The mandible is palpated for the presence of tenderness, step-offs, or mobility. A comprehensive head and neck and neurological exam is performed with specific attention to cranial nerves V and VII.

Radiologic Assessment

The preferred radiologic assessment of a potential mandible fracture includes a panorex, mandible series, and reverse Towne's view. In addition to defining the bony anatomy, the dental roots are assessed with these studies. CT scans are frequently obtained to assess trauma to the head, upper third of the face and midface and often identify fractures of the mandible. If however, the fracture is in the plane of the CT scan, the fracture may be missed. A high index of suspicion should be maintained if a fracture is suspected but not seen on CT scan, and plain films should be obtained (Figs 33.1A and B). CT scans do however provide the most reliable and important details of condylar fracture[16] (Figs 33.2A and B).

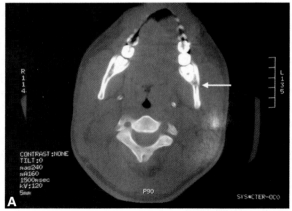

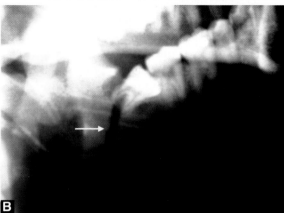

Figs 33.1A and B: (A) Although the fracture at the angle is identified by this axial CT scan. (B) It is more clearly seen on this plain film

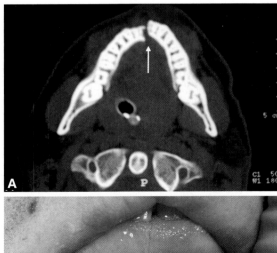

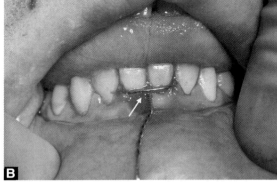

Figs 33.2A and B: (A) A displaced fracture is identified at the parasymphyseal region (white arrow). (B) A circumdental bridle wire is frequently utilized to aid in reduction (white arrow)

Time Until Treatment

Delay in treatment may be caused by a delay in presentation related to social issues such as alcohol or drug abuse.[17] This delay can result in an increased infection rate for both closed reduction and open reduction with internal fixation[7] and may be the central factor in placing a patient at increased risk of developing a bone infection or a non-union.[17] Treatment within 12 hours[18,19] or 24 hours[20] has been recommended while a higher incidence of non-union in those receiving delayed treatment of greater than 5 days has been reported.[21] Others have not observed a difference in infection rate for those treated 1–16 days after injury.[8,15,22–24]

This controversy about whether a delay in treatment contributes to the complication rate suggests that other factors such as type of injury, dental status, medical status, operative experience, adequacy of reduction, or fixation might be at play.[17]

TREATMENT

The goals of treatment are to effect rapid healing by anatomic reduction with reestablishment of premorbid occlusion and function with minimal disability and complications.[3] Reliable, healthy individuals with normal occlusion and non-displaced fragments may require only a soft diet.[25] Simple or compound fractures treated within 72 hours should heal uneventfully treated either open or closed in a compliant patient.[26]

Healing of bone or soft tissue may be by primary or secondary intention. Soft tissue wounds that are allowed to heal by secondary intention take longer to heal and are more liable to complications and have less satisfactory results. This can also be said of bone.[20,27] The use of maxillomandibular fixation with or without wire osteosynthesis has in the past been the standard for treatment of most mandible fractures. Mandibular fractures that are treated with maxillomandibular fixation alone heal by secondary intention, as there is some interfragmentary motion with muscle activity. Mandible fractures treated with rigid internal fixation heal by primary intention. Earlier, the primary concern was the reduction and stabilization of fracture segments, while preserving maximal periosteal blood supply. Over the last 15–20 years, the treatment of patients with mandible fractures has been altered by the introduction of rigid internal fixation. Maxillomandibular fixation remains the appropriate treatment for nondisplaced, stable fractures and most condylar fractures.[15] However, rigid fixation seems appropriate in the treatment of the majority of other fractures and is the standard method of fracture treatment.[28] Patients not amenable to the use of maxillomandibular fixation include edentulous and partially edentulous patients, those with infected fractures and those not able to tolerate maxillomandibular fixation for medical or social reasons. Closed reduction with maxillomandibular fixation delays functional rehabilitation and therefore is not without morbidity. Complications of maxillomandibular fixation include weight loss, poor hygiene, loss of function, and vocational, social and communication issues. Patients routinely stop working during the first week of maxillomandibular fixation, while the majority stays away from work during the entire maxillomandibular fixation period.[29]

The benefits of rigid and semirigid fixation over closed reduction and maxillomandibular fixation remains controversial. The proposed advantages of internal fixation include more accurate and stable reduction, elimination of the need for prolonged maxillomandibular fixation, quicker rehabilitation, and return to work. The rate of recovery of normal jaw function and normal body weight is significantly greater when fixation is with miniplates than in intermaxillary fixation.[20]

Factors that are thought to contribute to treatment failure regardless of the technique used[7] include location of the fracture, multiple fractures,[8] poor patient compliance, length of time from the trauma to the repair, antibiotic choice and operator skill and experience. Although some studies have suggested that rigid internal fixation results in a lower rate of complications when compared with closed reduction or open reduction with wire fixation,[30] other studies comparative analysis did not reveal a significant difference in treatment results,[11,31] while other studies, results favor closed reduction.[15,26] In one study that showed no significant difference in the postoperative complication rates in the two groups, the types of complications in the two groups were different. Patients treated with rigid internal fixation had a higher level of malocclusion and transient facial palsy. Although the two treatment modalities have similar outcome and complications, rigid internal fixation offers advantages for the indigent and transient population that most frequently suffer mandible fractures, as non-compliant patients who prematurely released their maxillomandibular fixation had the highest complication rate of 28%.[15] The use of rigid fixation eliminates the risks associated with premature removal of maxillomandibular fixation by the patient.[14]

Rigid internal fixation is technically challenging. Evaluation of ORIF in the teaching laboratory using lag screw fixation of a symphyseal fracture revealed that only 39% were fixed effectively without anatomic morbidity.[32] In addition, 76% of all mandible fractures not using a lag screw technique in another group were effectively treated without anatomic morbidity. In this group, 24% of the fractures were treated with methods that would have resulted in clinical failure during function.

Open reduction with internal fixation may be more cost effective overall because of costs related to managing complications than open reduction with non-rigid techniques despite an initial cost savings[6] while others have suggested otherwise.[33] A British study that compared maxillomandibular fixation with miniplate osteosynthesis demonstrated cost savings with miniplate osteosynthesis related to costs from longer hospitalization, increased ICU stay and greater number of outpatient visits with maxillomandibular fixation.[26] However, other studies suggest longer hospitalization after treatment with open reduction with internal fixation versus maxillomandibular fixation alone.[34] Comparative studies evaluating costs do not always factor in related issues such as an earlier return to work or school and functional or aesthetic results.[34]

MAXILLOMANDIBULAR FIXATION

Appropriately tight arch bars are the key initial step to a favorable treatment outcome. This is a tedious step the surgeon should not compromised on this. It is best performed with a capable assistant but may be performed by an individual (Table 33.1). If the premorbid occlusion is not obtainable after arch bar placement, the fracture line may need to be opened, the fracture reduced, and the occlusion established. On occasion, the arch bars may inhibit the reduction of the fracture. In such cases, the arch bar should be loosened, the reduction established, and the arch bar re-tightened.

Table 33.1: Technique of maxillomandibular fixation
• Usually general anesthesia with nasal intubation (can be performed under local anesthesia with sedation).
• Use head light and bite block as needed.
• Re-examine under anesthesia.
• Re-evaluate integrity of teeth.
• Brush teeth with chlorhexidine
• Circumdental bridle wire as needed at fracture line to assist with reduction (Fig. 33.3)
• Size arch bars using all reliable teeth
• Circumdental 24-gauge wire from the canines distally
• Orient bars carefully.
• The circumdental wire is placed inferior in relation to the arch bar, placed distally in the mandible, and superiorly in relation to the arch bar, placed distally in the maxilla.
• Tighten wire clockwise from canine distally, alternating sides. Tightly adapt arch bar against central and lateral incisors.
• Consider 26-gauge wire mesial to the canines after arch bars are in place.
• Seat condyles
• Medialize the angles with digital pressure. This counteracts the tendency to splay the lingual cortex outward at the symphysis.
• Establish premorbid occlusion.
• Use 24-gauge wire for maxillomandibular fixation using one opposing hook in each dental arch, minimum of three wires on each side.

We prefer 24-gauge wire as single loops on opposing hooks; 26-gauge wire or elastics can also be considered. Maxillomandibular fixation wires should not be placed more mesial or distal to the last secured tooth. One should be aware that any tension from the maxillomandibular fixation wires or elastics directly on teeth will move teeth in the same fashion that orthodontic appliances do so. This is particularly of concern at the incisors. A minimum of three loops should be placed on each side. The circumdental wires and intermaxillary fixation wires should be trimmed and turned clockwise in order to avoid soft tissue irritation.

Technique of Fixation

Approach

An intraoral approach is appropriate for fractures mesial to the angle and for minimally displaced and non-comminuted fractures at the angle. Lacerations may provide adequate exposure when present. The intended incision site is infiltrated with 1% lidocaine with epinephrine 1:100,000. The initial incision is made sharply with a 15 blade perpendicular to the mucosa overlying the fracture. Care should be taken to provide an adequate mucosal cuff for closure to avoid the loss of sulcus. The soft tissue may then be incised with cautery but the periosteum is incised sharply. The periosteum is elevated to the inferior border of the mandible. The soft tissue envelope is maintained superiorly at the alveolus. Only adequate soft tissue is elevated in order to expose the fracture line and place the fixation. Any debris is removed from the fracture line and the wound is irrigated vigorously. All fracture sites are exposed prior to reduction or fixation.

Fracture Reduction

After all fractures are exposed, they can then be reduced. Options for reduction include digital manipulation, manual reduction with clamps, monocortical holes approximated with a modified towel clamp (Fig. 33.3A) and monocortical screws approximated with 24 gauge wire (Fig. 33.3B). If the fracture is not reducible, the maxillomandibular fixation wires are cut and the reduction is reassessed. If the fracture is still not reducible, selected circumdental wires adjacent to the fracture line are loosened or removed. Comminuted fractures with missing teeth may be difficult to reduce accurately. In order to obtain premorbid occlusion in those cases, the fabrication of a dental splint should be considered.

Fixation

After fracture reduction, the fractures are fixated. Factors which appear to contribute to ultimate plate stability include the quality of the bone in which the screws are placed, bicortical screw placement, diameter of the screw and the dynamic load placed on the fracture.[35] Plates are carefully adapted to the outer cortex and are bent a little more to encourage lingual contact. Precision in plate bending and adaptation is critical for all plates, especially those larger than 2 mm. A low speed drill while irrigating with saline is preferable for monocortical hole placement and necessary for bicortical hole placement.[19] A hole adjacent to the fracture line is made first taking care to avoid placing the hole close to the fracture line. A common mistake is to place the first hole that is drilled inappropriately too far from the fracture line, bringing the second hole too close to the fracture line. The screw is placed snugly into the first hole and the second hole is made and the screw is placed. The distal screws are then placed. The distal holes are always drilled neutrally, while the holes adjacent to the fracture line may be placed in neutral or compression mode. All screws are then firmly tightened. Bicortical holes are placed below the inferior alveolar nerve, and monocortical holes are placed between tooth roots. A depth gauge is required to identify the appropriate length of screw to capture the lingual cortex when a bicortical screw is placed.

Multiple options are available for fixation. Each option has advantages and disadvantages. Two plates are commonly positioned in a fashion to neutralize the compressive forces at the inferior border of the mandible and tension at the superior border (Figs 33.3A to D). Options include rigid fixation at the inferior border using plates held in position with bicortical screws 2.3 mm or larger in size, with or without a monocortical tension band plate placed superiorly. The arch bar may be used as a tension band. Other options include the use of 1.7 or 2.0 miniplates using either bicortical or monocortical screws. The use of miniplates has been described by multiple authors[20,36–39] including Champy, who identified ideal lines of osteosynthesis, which are used to overcome the displacing forces on the mandible. By placing the plates at the most biomechanically favorable sites, the thickness of the plate can be kept to a minimum. The Champy technique, when used between the mental foramina uses two miniplates: One is fixed at the inferior border and the second is fixed 5 mm above the first, at least 5 mm below the level of the alveolar processes. A single subapical plate is adequate in the body and the synthesis should be placed higher as the fracture proceeds more distally.[19] Semirigid 1.7 or 2.0 mm miniplates are easy to insert and adapt due to the smaller size and improved malleability of the plate. Additional advantages of miniplate fixation are the use of an intraoral approach without exposed scar or risk to the facial nerve, decreased OR time, preservation of blood supply, and less likely alteration of occlusion.[19] Raveh does not feel

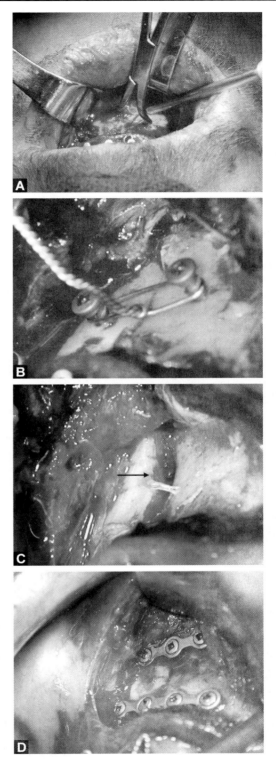

Figs 33.3A to D: (A) The creation of monocortical holes and the placement of a modified towel clamp; (B) Or Screws and a wire; (C) Useful in the reduction of a displaced fracture; (D) The screws and wires are removed after fixation

that miniplate fixation offers adequate stabilization to eliminate maxillomandibular fixation.[40]

Clinically, the results obtained from the use of miniplates for semirigid fixation seems comparable to rigid fixation in most circumstances. There are however, circumstances when rigid fixation may be more appropriate, such as in angle fractures, comminuted fractures, infected fractures and 'severe' fractures. [28,41, 42]

The wound is irrigated generously with saline. Prior to closing the incision, the maxillomandibular fixation wires are cut and premorbid, reproducible occlusion is verified. With the index finger under the symphysis, the mandible is repeatedly opened and closed. The occlusion should be easily established and not forced (Figs 33.4A and B). If the premorbid occlusion is not established, re-evaluation of the reduction and fixation is undertaken. Condyle position is verified. Removal and replacement of the fixation may be required. The mucosa is closed with 3-0 chromic catgut. A single layer mucosal closure is adequate if muscle is incorporated with the suture; two-layer closure is also acceptable.

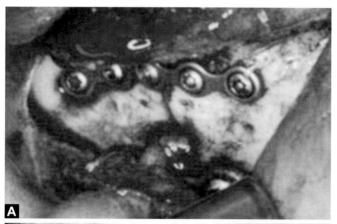

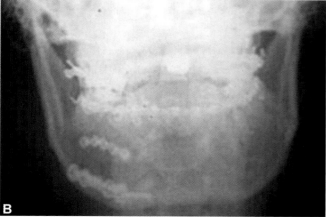

Figs 33.4A and B: Two monocortical miniplates are often used mesial to the angle. Plate position is verified radiologically

Compression Synthesis Versus Non-compression Synthesis

The use of compression plates as described by Bagby and Janes is based on the spherical gliding principle. The screw glides down the inclined plane of the specially designed plate and creates compression at the bone-bone interface. The advantages of compression include a direct benefit of compression, with indirect benefits of the close approximation of bone decreasing the fracture gap, and better immobilization.[43] Close approximation of fragments result in many points of bony contact and thus encourages osteogenesis by induction. Fractures treated with compression plates show evidence of primary bone healing without any sign of fibrous tissue or cartilage during the healing process.[44]

Compression is a relatively new concept in the treatment of mandible fractures and its use is controversial. The treatment of mandibular fractures by means of compression osteosynthesis has been shown to produce good results in 83% of patients[10] while the complication rate compares favorably with other techniques.[5] The complications encountered being either soft tissue infections or minor malocclusions. The relatively low rate of complications can be further reduced by patient selection and meticulous performance of the technique. Champy argued that it was impossible to measure the force of compression and that compression may result in bone necrosis.[19] It has been suggested that inferior border dynamic compression plating is fraught with complications such as paresthesias, root injury, and less than anatomic reduction.[5]

It appears that the use of compression may be appropriate when there is adequate bony buttressing, and non-compression plates should be used when there is not. Where interfragmentary compression is uncertain (thin areas of the mandibular bone at the angle and proximal part of the body, atrophic edentulous mandibles, after extraction of a tooth from the fracture line, irregularity of the fracture line, and even a slight degree of comminution) a compression technique may not be suitable; the use of lag screws at the symphysis can be considered in experienced hands.

Postoperative Maxillomandibular Fixation

Concerns about postoperative maxillomandibular fixation include airway issues, inadequate nutrition, poor oral hygiene in a frequently already compromised patient, insomnia, difficulty phonating, vocational issues, social embarrassment and range of motion difficulty.

Rigid fixation without maxillomandibular fixation resolves most of these problems.

Current trends support early mobilization. Selected patients (no comminution, no ramus fracture, no condyle fracture, and no alveolar or dental fracture) may immediately be released from maxillomandibular fixation after rigid fixation. Intuitively, however, it might seem appropriate to rest or splint the soft tissues afterward similar to using a cast or a splint after a long bone fracture. Postoperative maxillomandibular fixation helps stabilize the occlusion, allows reattachment of the soft tissue drape and promotes initial primary bone healing without tension.[45] Maxillomandibular fixation also confirms to the patient that they must modify their behavior and be compliant with a blenderized diet. No difference in relation to trismus, oral hygiene and weight loss was noted after 2 weeks maxillomandibular fixation versus immediate mobilization. A variable length of maxillomandibular fixation based on the type and size of plates used has been advocated (Table 33.2).[5]

In addition to the alteration in the length of maxillomandibular fixation based on the type of fixation used, the required length of maxillomandibular fixation can be altered based on the age of the patient.[46] In patients treated with maxillomandibular fixation alone, most fractures in children need only 2 weeks of immobilization, 75% of young healthy adults need 3–4 weeks, and the elderly need 5 weeks or more. The rate of healing is similar at different anatomical sites except for the ramus where healing appears to be quicker.

Postoperative Care

Patients are generally discharged within 48 hours of surgery (Table 33.3) after nutritional and oral hygiene techniques are mastered. Postoperative X-rays are routinely obtained to ensure bony alignment, plate position and to provide documentation for medicolegal reasons.[8,33,47] Compliance in the post-operative period is critical for a favorable outcome, but unfortunately it is difficult to achieve in this population. Seventeen percent of patients are frequently lost to follow-up as early as 1 week.[6] Many patients in this group remove their maxillomandibular fixation prematurely resulting in a complication rate of 29%[6] while a third do not return to have their arch bars removed at all.[8] Patients are reminded that the masticatory forces are strong and they should not 'test' the arch bars by trying to open the mouth. Weekly evaluations are critical to ensure tight maxillomandibular fixation when used and to identify infections at an early stage.

Table 33.2: Length of maxillomandibular fixation (MMF) based on the size of the plates (Lazow 1993)

- MMF for 1 week with dynamic compression plates, eccentric dynamic compression plates, or reconstruction plates.
- MMF for 2 weeks with 2.0 mm miniplates
- MMF for 3 weeks with 1.7 mm miniplates

Table 33.3: Postoperative care

- Dental wax to protect soft tissue from wires
- Water pic or syringe with red rubber catheter for oral hygiene
- Liquidized diet (syringe with red rubber catheter with training)
- Liquid pain medication and liquid penicillin or clindamycin for one week postoperatively
- Examine/tighten arch bars at weekly intervals. Length of maxillomandibular fixation is 2–6 weeks
- Soft diet for a total of 6 weeks
- Postoperative dental evaluation within 6 weeks
- Follow-up at monthly intervals for an additional 2 months after arch bars are removed

Arch bars are generally removed in the office under local anesthesia after 6 weeks. Uncommonly, they are removed in the operating room in young patients or in patients who cannot tolerate removal in the office.

Various devices are available to aid the patient in the rehabilitation of the jaw after the removal of maxillomandibular fixation. A physiotherapist is consulted for evaluation and treatment if necessary. The physiotherapy technique is generally continued for 2–4 months or until an opening over 40 mm is achieved.

Antibiotics

Fractures associated with tooth-bearing segments of the mandible are classified as Class III contaminated wounds. Patients who are treated in a delayed fashion or who present with evidence of infection at the fracture are classified as class IV infected wounds. The risk of infection of Class III wounds is 22–50% without antibiotic coverage but is reduced to 10% with prophylactic antibiotic use.[48,49] In a series that included all facial fractures, only mandible fractures became infected.[50] The benefit of perioperative antibiotics in preventing infection when treating mandible fractures has been established.[23,50,51] A controlled study showed a decrease in the incidence of postoperative infections from 42.2% in the group that did not receive any antibiotics to 8.9% in the group that received

Cefazolin 1 hour preoperatively and a single second dose 8 hours later. The early use of appropriate antibiotics in patients also appears to remove any increased risk that a delay in treatment might have.[50] The intravenous administration of appropriate antibiotic coverage preoperatively, perioperatively and postoperatively for 12 hours is supported by current data and the oral administration of antibiotics after that time may be unnecessary.[49] This information however, is based on 'uncomplicated' fractures of the mandible in a group that was healthy with non-comminuted fractures with no infection on presentation, and no associated systemic or midfacial injuries. The use of postoperative antibiotics for at least 5 days continued.[6,7,23]

Experience

Rigid fixation techniques are technically demanding. It has reasonably been suggested[24] that complications might decrease with experience or specialized training;[51] however, an *in vitro* rigid internal fixation lab demonstrated a high complication rate of 24%.[52] Experience has not always been shown to reduce the complication rate significantly. In a clinical study, experience actually appeared to negatively impact the complication rate concerning marginal mandibular injury as there was a higher incidence of transient postoperative facial nerve palsy after experience was achieved.[13] This was thought to be due to greater soft tissue retraction to permit the placement of larger bone plates. Others have shown an overall downward trend in the complication rate (such as infections) as surgeon experience increased.[24] Fewer occlusal discrepancies have been noted with operator experience. This improvement in occlusal relationships was probably due to the use of arch bars instead of Ivy loops,[6] and the knowledge that precise contouring of the plate was required.

Complications

Paresthesias

After open reduction and internal fixation of fractures of the body and angle, the frequency of hypoesthesia is as high as 91% in the immediate postoperative stage, but diminishes during follow-up to a 47% incidence of some sensory disturbance.[53] In the majority of cases, the patients claim to have normal sensation. An 8% incidence of iatrogenic injury is associated with fractures near the mental foramen[20] while others report no iatrogenic injuries.[5] Interestingly, control groups treated with maxillomandibular fixation alone have an incidence of sensory disturbance of 4%. Postoperative hypoesthesia

was significantly more likely in an edentulous group compared to a fully dental group, especially when a compression plate was used[53] and may or may not be affected by fracture displacement.[11,54]

Wound Dehiscence/Exposed Plates

Wound dehiscence is reported to occur in 12% of cases and usually appears quite early, within 3-10 days after surgery.[20] Interestingly, wound dehiscence occurred in 6% of those cases treated with maxillomandibular fixation alone. Possible explanations for wound dehiscence include treatment delay, preexisting mucosal tears, and poor oral hygiene. Wound breakdowns in the posterior region were encountered more frequently, attributing this to a single layer closure.[20] In general, wound dehiscence and plate exposure is successfully treated with oral irrigation.

Malocclusion

The incidence of malocclusion is as high as 18% in patients treated with rigid internal fixation.[41] The incidence of malocclusion is comparable for fractures treated with miniplate semirigid fixation with maxillomandibular fixation alone, 4.8–5.7% for the miniplate group[19,20] and 4% for the maxillomandibular fixation group. Malocclusion was seen significantly more often when two osteosynthesis (26%) rather than one (8.5%) had been performed.[54]

Minor occlusal discrepancy can be altered with training elastics.[42] This of course does not correct the skeletal abnormality but corrects the occlusion by orthodontic means. Minor malocclusions may also be treated successfully with minimal grinding of the teeth by a dentist. The correction of large occlusal discrepancies should not be attempted with elastics. Large occlusal discrepancies should be evaluated carefully and consideration should be given to removing and readapting the bone plate. Malocclusions identified immediately postoperatively should be avoided by releasing the maxillomandibular fixation at the end of the procedure and verifying the occlusion. If however, a malocclusion is recognized immediately after surgery, verification of condyle position in the fossa should be demonstrated and the fracture line should be examined and possibly revised.

Controversies

Stress Shielding

Physiologic stresses can stimulate osteogenic cells, while lack of physiologic stimulation may lead to bone loss.[19,37]

This phenomenon is referred to as stress shielding. In long bones, resorption of bone underneath a fixation plate and redistribution of stresses resulting from the plate have been described.[55]

Stress shielding in an animal model has been evaluated by examining the structural properties of mandibular bone following application of a bone plate.[56] Although bone strain inferior to the plates was reduced, long-term placement of bone plates and the resulting stress shielding were not found to result in structural changes in the mandibular corpus. The role of this stress shielding in the mandible is thought by some to be insignificant,[57] but is currently not completely understood.[58]

Teeth in Line of Fracture

The disposition of teeth in the line of fracture is controversial and should be individualized. The presence of a tooth in the line of fracture creates a compound fracture and whether it is removed is usually irrelevant.[17] It seems that a healthy tooth in the line of a fracture provides good support when the fracture is reduced while its extraction makes the fracture more unstable (Fig. 33.5) and the reduction more difficult. Teeth with caries, periodontal disease, or root fractures should be extracted.[59]

A body of literature supports leaving a tooth in place in the line of fracture,[22,35] while one of the same authors provides support for extracting the tooth.[14] The high infection rate associated with the extraction of the third molar may be related to a loss of bony buttressing when the tooth is removed. In these cases more rigid fixation

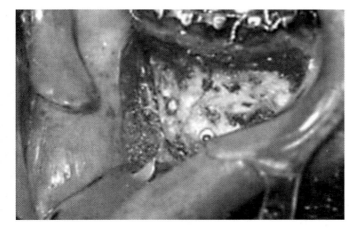

Fig. 33.5: The use of two lag screws is a quick, low-cost alternative to address a fracture at the symphysis for surgeons who have experience with this technique

with a reconstructive plate may be appropriate, as it has been demonstrated that dental extraction did not increase the infection rate when more rigid forms of internal fixation were used.[42] However, no clear relationship between infection and removal or retention of teeth in the line of fracture in open or closed reductions has been found.[23] In one study, all patients with complications had a tooth in the line of the fracture while an equal number had the tooth extracted or left in place.[8] This would suggest that the tooth in the line of the fracture is the most important issue, and addressing it is secondary. The extraction of a tooth from the fracture line before reduction and osteosynthesis allows an increase of oral contamination, and reduces the stability.[54] The plan that we prefer is to leave the tooth in place until the osteosynthesis is complete and then consider extraction.

SUBCONDYLAR/CONDYLAR FRACTURES

The incidence of condylar process fractures among all mandibular fractures is high, possibly 25–50%.[9] Patients with repeatable premorbid occlusion are treated with a soft diet and followed-up closely. Although there are controversies about the treatment of subcondylar fractures, most authors routinely treat subcondylar fractures in a closed fashion with 2 weeks of maxillomandibular fixation.[28,33] There is no obvious relationship between the severity of fracture displacement and the outcome of closed treatment.[60] Closed techniques are advocated except for the absolute indications as outlined by Zide and Kent.[61] These absolute indications for open reduction are proposed as displacement of the proximal segment into the middle cranial fossa, lateral extra-articular displacement of the proximal segment, bilateral subcondylar fractures with non-reproducible occlusion, and multiple fragmented mandibular fractures in association with multiple complex craniofacial fractures. Relative indications, which should be assessed in a benefit/risk ratio include: Bilateral or unilateral condylar fractures with crushed midfacial fractures, comminuted symphysis fractures and condyle fractures with associated tooth loss, displaced condyle fractures in mentally retarded or medically compromised adults with clinical evidence of open bite or retrusion, and edentulous or partially edentulous mandibles with posterior bite collapse and displaced condyles.[62] Although there is evidence to suggest that at least one fracture should be treated open when there are bilateral fractures, such treatment may increase the displacement of the other side.[60] The absolute indications for conservative treatment

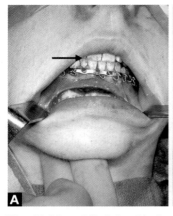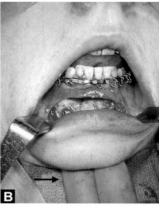

Figs 33.6A and B: It is critical to verify premorbid occlusion after fixation. The MMF is released and light digital pressure (white arrow) is used to establish the occlusion (black arrow)

Table 33.4: Consensus treatment opinions of subcondylar fractures based on displacement and occlusion (Baker 1998)

Displacement	Occlusion	Majority opinion
Slight	Normal	No IMF
Slight	Altered	IMF
Displaced	Altered	IMF
Dislocated	Altered	53% IMF, 26% Open fixation
Intracapsular/ Comminuted	Altered	IMF

include intracapsular fractures (Figs 33.6A and B), fractures in children below 12 years, and fractures without dislocation of the condylar head. Without an absolute indication for open treatment, consideration should be given to delaying treatment for 5 days to reassess function, in particular occlusion. If function is poor, treatment should be considered.[60] While guidelines for the treatment of these extreme cases exist, there are a wide range of fractures that do not fit either absolute indication. The obvious problem is selecting group of patients in whom the open procedure is more likely to yield superior results. A concern with fixation is the difficulty in achieving absolute reduction, which may result in fixation of the condylar head in a non-physiologic position. Exact reduction of the fracture borders may be secondary to the correct physiologic relation of the condyle in the articular fossa.[90]

A questionnaire was used to determine consensus treatments advocated by a group of experts in the field of facial trauma.[63] For the most part, there was a strong overall consensus in the evaluation and treatment of subcondylar fractures in general except for the treatment of dislocated fractures, where opinion diverged (Table 33.4). A panorex was requested in 95% of patients to radiologically evaluate the condyle. Few surgeons believed that malocclusion was a prevalent problem as a consequence of unilateral condylar fractures. Fifty-seven percent of those questioned had a preference for open reduction internal fixation to treat dislocated fractures and cited anatomical reduction and fixation, occlusal stability and early restoration of function as justification. Those who preferred closed treatment cited reduction in morbidity in general, equally good results and absence of surgical complications as reasons for closed therapy.

There is a limited body of literature that directly compares open and closed techniques.[64] Limitations in randomization make interpretation of these studies especially difficult. Because of these difficulties in randomization, there appears to be no difference in clinical outcome when closed versus open techniques are used;[65] however there may be some benefits achieved when an open technique is used for significantly dislocated fractures. Dislocated subcondylar fractures treated conservatively may incur complications that could have been significantly reduced if open reduction had been performed, as closed reduction techniques rarely achieve accurate reduction. Continued fracture malalignment leads to condylar head displacement and shortening of the posterior mandibular height.[16] One study showed a 39% complication rate in a non-surgical group and only 4% in the surgical group supporting an open treatment in mid to low subcondylar fractures with displacement.[66] In this study, patients with severely dislocated fractures were treated using an open technique introducing this as a confounding variable. However, there were no significant differences in clinical outcomes, possibly suggesting that an open technique is advocated in severely dislocated fractures. A 15-year follow-up on a group of children, teenagers, and adults that were treated with maxillomandibular fixation has been reviewed. This study revealed that there was a subjective and objective progression of anatomical and functional alterations of the temporomandibular joint as the age group increased. However, even in adults, the dysfunction was not considered serious by the patient.[67] Interestingly, the reported symptoms and clinical signs were similar at the 6-month and 15-year follow-up for most subjects in all age groups. They concluded that in cases of condylar fractures, signs and symptoms of dysfunction may be expected based on degree of displacement of the condylar head. They also suggested that an open reduction in older patients might be useful in preventing dysfunctional problems.

Efforts at basing the treatment on the angle of displacement from the glenoid fossa have been described[57,68] but have been met with resistance in part due to further changes after the placement of the maxillomandibular fixation.[69] The degree of dislocation or angulation of the condyle and the number of complications have not been correlated. Uprighting of the fractured condylar process may occur with manipulation, but may result in distraction of the condyle from the ramus. Radiographic superiority with open reduction and with osteosynthesis has not correlated with clinical superiority.[65]

In addition to the indications outlined by Zide and Kent, we advocate open reduction in cases where the condyle is displaced out of the glenoid fossa in order to help avoid late complications such as malocclusion, ankylosis and temporomandibular joint dysfunction. At present, however there are no sufficient long-term data to support open reduction to prevent future joint problems. In fact, arthritic changes including remodeling can occur with both open and closed reduction techniques in the same degree of frequency.[61]

Open reduction internal fixation of dislocated subcondylar fractures is not an easy procedure and some of the surgical methods described are technically difficult as indicated by the high complication rates in some studies. The application of plates and screws frequently necessitates a preauricular and submandibular or retromandibular approach. Factors that should be considered when designing a treatment plan for subcondylar fractures includes the degree of displacement of the fractured segments particularly in relation to the articular fossa, the level of the fracture, the age of the patient, and the presence of other facial fractures. The experience of the surgeon with open techniques is a critical consideration.[65] The initial step in the open reduction of subcondylar fractures is the placement of the patient into maxillomandibular fixation with elastics. We advocate 2 weeks of training elastics and 1 week of bedtime elastics. This guideline is adjusted based on the patient's occlusion. Post-treatment physiotherapy for 4–5 weeks is a critical portion of the treatment in all cases.[40]

The cost of an open procedure in the treatment of subcondylar fractures is greater than that of a closed procedure.[70] However, it may be better to treat severely displaced fractures by an open reduction if a fair percentage treated by closed reduction may subsequently need additional treatment for functional or occlusal problems. This subsequent treatment may actually cost more and produce a less ideal result.

EDENTULOUS MANDIBLE FRACTURES

The treatment of the edentulous mandible presents the surgeon with a paradox. The anatomic result need not be exact because minor irregularities in the mandible can be masked by the fabrication of new dentures. However, the lack of teeth makes fracture reduction more difficult because maxillomandibular fixation can not be used to assist in reduction of the bony segments.[71] In the Second Chalmers J. Lyons Academy Study of Fractures of the Edentulous Mandible, 26.3% of patients treated by closed reduction developed problems with union. This rate was unfavorable as compared to internal fixation using an external approach. Rigid internal fixation with intraoral approach was not as successful resulting in a higher complication rate.

The treatment of an edentulous atrophic mandible fracture is challenging as complications have been seen with both closed and open techniques. In addition to the difficulties encountered because of the older patients who these fractures tend to occur in (decreased osteogenesis, increased operative risk, local factors relating to atrophic, dense cortical bone and inadequate blood supply) these cases are difficult because they are uncommon. In one series, 56% of the surgeons involved performed only a single case in 3 years.[71] Traditionally, closed techniques using splints or the patient's dentures have been used to treat fractures of the edentulous mandible. In general, conservative closed management of edentulous mandible fractures requires less operating time than an open reduction and fixation procedure. Conservative management too may not require the use of general anesthesia. The avoidance of general anesthesia in this older population may be desirable.[72] Anatomic alignment and fixation of edentulous mandible fractures is consistent with the basic principles of facial fracture repair. The controversy in management is weighing the risks and benefits of more aggressive treatment for the patient.[73] The surgeon must critically evaluate the risks and benefits in each case.

The amount of displacement of the fractured segments determines whether conservative management is an option. Conservative management provides a viable option when the fracture segments are not grossly displaced (Fig. 33.7). Unfortunately, the fractures are displaced in 89% of cases.[71] A significantly displaced edentulous fracture is not amenable to conservative treatment and open reduction with internal fixation should be considered. Heavy plates onto the contralateral side with at least 3 bicortical screws on each side should be considered as use of 2 mm screws may not provide sufficient stabilization in edentulous fractures, as the plates may bend and break (Figs 33.8A to D). An external

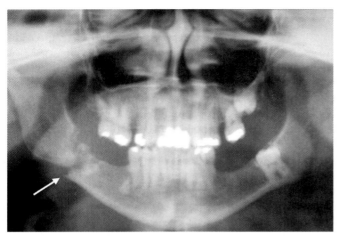

Fig. 33.7: The instability that can be created by the extraction of a molar tooth is identified by this fracture, caused by the extraction of a tooth (arrow). The molar tooth on the contralateral side illustrates the root extension to the inferior border

approach with minimal periosteal stripping should be used. Consideration may be given to placing the plates on top of the periosteum in order to theoretically preserve a tenuous blood supply. The option of immediate bone grafting can also be considered but again the morbidity of harvesting a bone graft is raised in these populations.

INFECTED OR COMMINUTED FRACTURES

The treatment of infected or comminuted fractures is based on two differing treatment philosophies:
1. Closed reduction and leaving the periosteal attachments to the bony fragments intact, allowing for ultimate healing.
2. Exposure of the fractures, reduction and absolute rigid fixation.

It is hypothesized that the majority of infected fractures are due to inadequate immobilization of comminuted fragments and subsequent infection rather

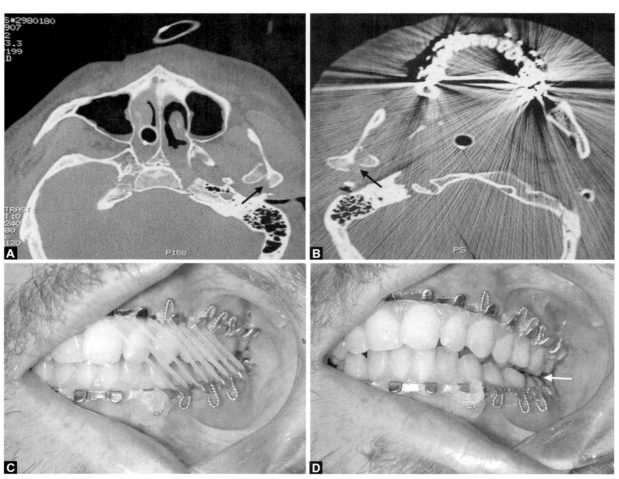

Figs 33.8A to D: (A) Bilateral condylar head fractures are identified by this axial CT scan. (B) Training elastics. (C and D) A critical part of treatment for the open bite deformity

than to initial loss of bone. Stability on both sides of the comminution is probably as important as concern about maintaining periosteal attachments (and thus blood supply) to bony fragments. With rigid fixation, an extraoral approach is usually used, reserving an intraoral approach for very anterior fractures with minimal inferior displacement. Success with rigid fixation has been achieved using three 2.7 mm screws into the two stable segments. Although the placement of three screws may be adequate,[1,42] the use of four screws in each fragment may be more biomechanically favorable. Additional screws can be placed in the comminuted fragments for stabilization, or the segments may be reduced and left in position.[74] The fabrication of lingual splints is frequently required in the treatment of comminuted fractures. A limited experience when the ramus is comminuted suggests that 2.0 miniplates may be used (Figs 33.9A and B). The fragments are often held in place with wire prior to application of the plate. Patients treated with rigid fixation may be mobilized immediately, although a higher infection rate has been reported in this group.[74] We prefer a short course of immobilization in order to rest the soft tissues and to possibly decrease the infection rate.

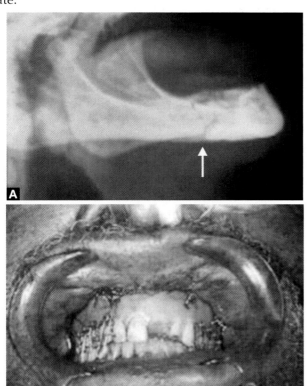

Figs 33.9A and B: (A) A nondisplaced fracture of the edentulous mandible; (B) may be treated with closed reduction, by using the patient's dentures

Fractures at the Angle

A large part of this chapter is dedicated to the management of fractures at the angle. Angle fractures are frequently cited as the most common and have the highest incidence of complications.[8,24] The frequent involvement of the angle in jaw fractures can be attributed to its thin cross-sectional bone area and the presence of the third molar tooth socket.[12] Although selection of approach, plates, technique and concern about teeth in the fracture line are issues in all mandible fractures, these issues are highlighted at the angle.

It appears that biomechanically, the forces exerted by the muscles of mastication have a greater influence on the angle than in other regions of the mandible.[75] The superior border is generally a zone of tension when an occlusal load is placed on the anterior teeth. During the same maneuver, the inferior border is a zone of compression. In summation, these forces result in separation at the superior border with overriding at the inferior border.[39] These complex resultant forces cause loosening of hardware and the bending of soft plates and probably contribute to the higher infection rate.[76]

The presence of the third molar also adds a level of complexity in that the third molar makes fractures here more frequent, creates a compound fracture intraorally, inhibits subsequent bone contact, can inhibit reduction, alters the vascularity of the fracture site and can be a source of infection. Plate and screw fixation of fractures at the angle of the mandible pose unique problems.[75] The angle is the most difficult area of the mandible in which to approach the inferior border transorally. The inferior border of the angle is thin and not well buttressed for treatment with compression. Frequently, the fractures in this region are oblique, again suggesting that compression is not appropriate.

Rigid versus Non-rigid Techniques

A displaced fracture at the angle can rarely be satisfactorily reduced with maxillomandibular fixation alone (Figs 33.10A to C).[54] In such cases, more than for other fractures of the mandibular body, open reduction and osteosynthesis are indicated. Unfortunately, experienced surgeons were able to achieve successful fixation at the angle only 71% of the time in a teaching laboratory using dry specimens.[32]

Closed reduction has been reported as having a more favorable infection rate (0%) as compared to wire osteosynthesis (20%) and rigid internal fixation (6.3%).[6,15] Other reports suggest that angle fractures treated with

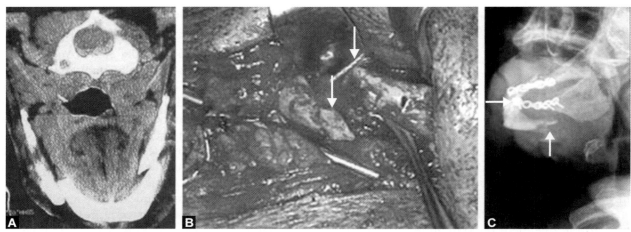

Figs 33.10A to C: (A) The edentulous mandible frequently is fractured at the bilateral body. (B) The atrophic, displaced edges are identified. (C) The use of 2.0 mm plates did not provide enough stability, resulting in displacement of the fracture (C, large arrow), and loosening of the hardware (C, small arrow)

non-rigid (wire or small plate) fixation techniques or maxillomandibular fixation alone have a high incidence of complications at 17%, most commonly infections,[8] while techniques using a reconstruction plate showed an infection rate of 7.5%. Dodson reported no differences in treatment results between non-rigid and rigid techniques although there was a bias toward non-rigid therapy. Factors that may contribute to failure with the use of plates are poor patient compliance, length of time from trauma to repair, location of the fracture, and choice of antibiotic.[7]

Approach and Choice of Plate

This choice of approach should take into account the periosteal blood supply and healing of the fracture site. Less hardware requires less stripping and creates better vascularization. However, at times visualization of as much of the fracture line as is possible is important for optimal reduction. Angle fractures may be approached intraorally with percutaneous screw placement for selected non-displaced or minimally displaced fractures. The incision is made over the external oblique line, beginning from the first molar tooth to halfway up the ascending ramus on the buccal side. Care is taken not to create a mucosal incision that is too far medial so that the incision does not retract lingually. If a third molar requires extraction it is usually performed after fixation. In those cases, the initial incision includes the mucosa of the split socket. It is technically demanding to place a 2.7 mm plate through an intraoral incision and this size of plate should be considered only if the surgeon is very experienced. Attempts at using smaller plates using the intraoral

approach have met with varying degrees of success.[22,77] There is a slightly increased incidence of infection in angle fractures plated intraorally: however, this difference was not statistically significant.[7] An extraoral approach is chosen when the fragments are severely displaced, in the treatment of older fractures and where anatomic limitations precluded precise and accurate plate placement intraorally.[35] Ellis demonstrated that the external approach with rigid fixation and using a reconstruction plate offered the lowest complication rate of 7.5% versus all other techniques tried.[42] However, there are several disadvantages to this method. The external incision requires increased operating time, risk of damage to the facial nerve (1.2%) and hypertrophic scarring.[54] Ellis exposed the entire mandibular ramus and body to the mental foramen using a subperiosteal dissection. This degree of exposure was required to permit the placement of three screws on each side of the fracture line. He recommended not placing the screws any closer than 7 mm to the fracture line.

The external approach is similar to the approach taken for a submandibular gland resection. The initial incision is designed approximately 2 fingerbreadths below the inferior aspect of the mandible. The intended incision is marked with a surgical marker and infiltrated with epinephrine 1:100,000 for hemostasis. The neck is propped up so that the corner of the mouth is visualized in the operative field. The incision is carried through the skin and platysma. The inferior most border of the submandibular gland is identified and the submandibular fascia is incised. A wide layer of fascia is elevated to ensure preservation of the marginal branch of the facial nerve. This plane is followed to the inferior border of the mandible, which is sharply incised and the periosteum elevated. Care is taken to avoid entrance into the oral cavity. A suction drain is selected when the integrity of the mucosa has not been violated. A passive drain is chosen otherwise. The wound is closed in three layers (platysma, subcutaneous tissue, skin). A compressive dressing is optional.

A study comparing identical plates and screws except for size showed that 2.7 mm diameter screws with 2.0 mm thick plates held greater functional loads than 2.4 mm diameter screws with 1.6 mm thick plates.[75] Ellis published multiple papers on the treatment of angle fractures, using plates of various sizes. He used plating systems with varying amounts of biomechanical rigidity and load-carrying capacity. These studies included relative extremes of fixation including reconstruction plates. Direct comparisons are available concerning functional loading, however different approaches were used. The type and incidence of complications is related to the size of the plate and whether compression or non-compression is used. The use of the reconstruction plate produced the lowest infection rate but more malocclusions are seen in this group than with other methods.[42] Contouring the reconstruction plate to the mandible is tedious and must be performed without compromise. Any errors in contouring of the plate will result in an alteration in occlusion. The large bone plate can also 'take the patient out of maxillomandibular fixation' and therefore tight maxillomandibular fixation is required. The successful use of a single large non-compression plate adds credence to the concept that absolute stability is a critical step in the treatment of mandible fractures. The use of two 2.0 mm compression miniplates has been examined.[77] There was a high infection rate of 29%. One proposed reason for the high rate of infection was the lack of rigidity offered by the two small miniplates. An additional study using two 2.4 mm screws was performed to offer increased rigidity, but the infection rate remained high at 32%.[77]

Champy identified two lines of osteosynthesis at the mandibular angle. In addition to the external oblique line, a second line is located at the level of the dento-alveolar junction and anterior to the canal of the inferior alveolar nerve. At the angle, a miniplate is placed as high as possible along the oblique line and an additional plate is placed subapically as a tension band. Studies by,[39] which show splaying at the inferior border of the angle when axial loading is done at the molar area suggest why poorer results are obtained when a single miniplate is used. Two miniplates fixed along the dual lines of osteosynthesis at

the angle overcomes this effect. The placement of six screws as compared to four increases the load-bearing capacity of the hardware.[78]

The use of one monocortical miniplate versus two monocortical miniplates in the treatment of angle fractures has been investigated (Table 33.5). The complication rate in the double miniplate group was very low and 'the lowest reported of any plating technique'. The advantages of miniplates include the avoidance of

Table 33.5: Single and double monocortical fixation with and without MMF at the angle (Levy 1991)

Rate	*Complication*
Single 2.0 monocortical plate, no MMF	22%
Single 2.0 monocortical plate, with MMF	30%
Double 2.0 monocortical plates, no MMF	0%
Double 2.0 monocortical plates, with MMF	7.1%

an external incision, eliminating the potential for inferior alveolar and marginal mandibular nerve damage, and simultaneous surveillance of fracture line reduction and occlusal relationships.

Compression and Angle Fractures

According to the classic AO technique, additional stability of the fracture is achieved by using interfragmentary compression.[44] Compression osteosynthesis can be used successfully in angle fractures when there is good bone contact of the fracture ends. However, owing to the form of the mandibular angle and the presence of third molars, fractures of this region are often oblique and/or irregular. This makes precise reduction difficult.[43] In compression osteosynthesis, the resulting force vectors can be particularly unfavorable, causing asymmetrical force distribution at the fracture site. Additionally, the small cross-sectional bone area in this region may not constitute a contact between segments large enough for technically sound compression osteosynthesis. Dynamic compression plating should probably be avoided in the angular region if prospects of achieving interfragmentary compression are uncertain, which they appear to be in many cases.[54] The AO/ASIF recommends the application of two compression bone plates for angle fractures, one along the superior border and one along the inferior border of the buccal cortex. Experimental studies have suggested that rigid fixation with an AO dynamic compression plate is based on the rigidity of the thick plate itself rather than on the compressive force.[24] Thus, the need for additional interfragmentary compression would seem questionable.

In a series that examined the use of compression plates in the management of mandible fractures, the angle had the highest complication rate.[35] Studies by Ellis reveal a 29% infection rate with compression when MMF is not used, and a 28% infection rate without compression at the angle when MMF is not used. This might suggest that the use of compression is not the primary problem.

One explanation for a higher complication rate with compression is that the holes in a straight compression plate offer limited possibilities for positioning the screws in relation to the course of the fracture line. Placing a screw in an unfavorable site, for example, directly in the fracture line could occur more easily. The angular region especially with a lack of space for the plate may be prone to such error.

Use of a solitary lag screw at the angle produces an infection rate of 13%.[79] Lag screw fixation at the angle is technically challenging. The same factors that make the use of compression techniques difficult also make lag screw placement difficult (Figs 33.11A to D and 33.12A and B).

COMPLICATIONS IN ANGLE FRACTURES

Infection

The incidence of infection is 7–13% in fractures of the mandible, with the highest rate seen at the angle. In a series of 214 cases, only one infection occurred outside of the proximal body or the angle.[24] A possible explanation for the increased incidence of infection in the angle/body region of the mandible is that in this region greater forces are developed from mandibular function, which may overcome the rigidity of the compression plate.[35] When this occurs, and sufficient bony callus has not formed the resultant mobility at the fracture site may result in infection. The main reason for infection at the angle in a rigid fixation group was the failure to achieve stable fixation in multiple studies[6,32,53] (Figs 33.13A to C).

Studies on miniplates however, suggest that it is unlikely that fracture instability is a major reason for the development of infections.[22] One might assume that two non-compression miniplates are less rigid than two

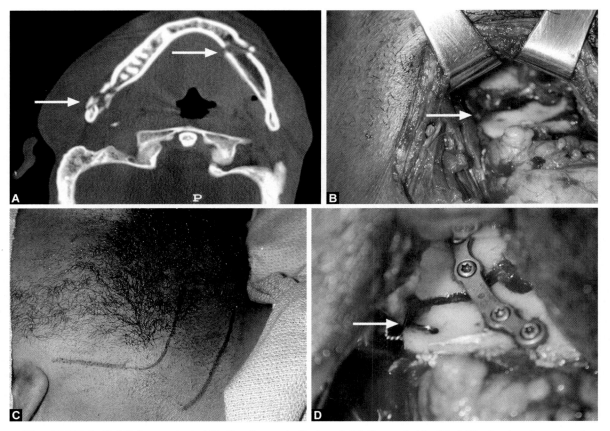

Figs 33.11A to D: (A) A comminuted (A, Small arrow), displaced. (B) Ramus is identified. The fracture is exposed by an external approach. (C) A combination of wires (arrow). (D) Plates may be used under these circumstances

mandibular compression bone plates. In spite of this difference in rigidity, the rate of infection and the severity of the complications actually decreased with double miniplate non-compression fixation. In addition to fracture stability, other factors such as the extent of traumatic disruption of blood supply to the fracture and surgical disruption of blood supply to the fracture, teeth in the fracture line, removal versus leaving teeth in the fracture line, use of compression versus non-compression, the nutritional status of the patients, their compliance, oral hygiene and abuse of substances and other factors may or may not be important in treatment outcome. The generous stripping of periosteum from the lateral surface of the mandible to obtain the necessary exposure to plate the angle fracture must rob the already traumatized cortical bone of a significant source of its blood supply. Since this is a constant factor in the treatment using both miniplates and compression, it may be the most important factor.[22] However, the disruption of the blood supply caused by the fixation devices may be an important concern.

Signs and symptoms of infection generally include pain, swelling, erythema and purulent discharge.

Infections that occur within 6 weeks are treated with incision and drainage in the clinic and the patient is placed on oral antibiotics and irrigations. This treatment is generally maintained as long as possible to overcome the infection or to obtain osseous healing along the lingual cortex. However, most early infections became chronic and require plate removal later.[22] If swelling and drainage persists for more than two additional weeks, surgical exploration of the fracture is performed.[42] Some suggest that in all cases of infected fractures that use fixation materials the osteosynthesis material should be removed. In most cases, all of the hardware is removed if any of the hardware is taken out, even if only one of the plates is loose. If the fracture site is mobile, the patient is also placed into maxillomandibular fixation. The need for secondary application of a reconstruction plate with or without a bone graft from the iliac crest is low.[41]

Patients who develop postoperative swelling greater than 6 weeks after their surgery initially respond to oral antibiotics, but recur on discontinuation of the antibiotic.[77] These patients are treated with removal of their hardware and any sequestra, and most are routinely found to be healed and do not require any additional treatment.

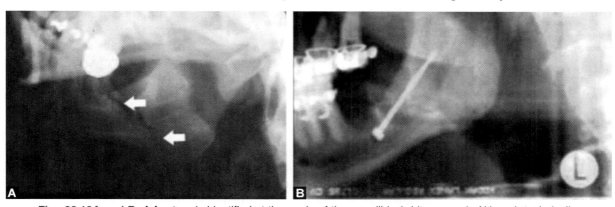

Figs 33.12A and B: A fracture is identified at the angle of the mandible (white arrows). Although technically challenging, a single lag screw may be used successfully by experienced surgeons

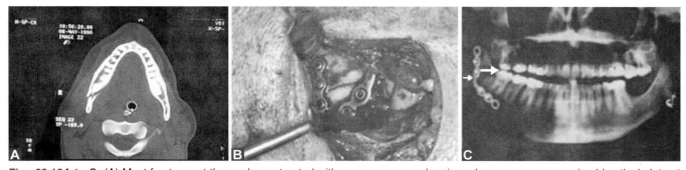

Figs 33.13A to C: (A) Most fractures at the angle are treated with an open approach using a large, non-compression bicortical plate at the inferior border. (B) A monocortical miniplate subapically. (C) A single miniplate may not provide adequate stability resulting in a broken plate (Small arrow) and a premature contact (C, Large arrow)

Infections that occur after 6 weeks are most commonly localized to the area of the superior bone plate and large collections of purulence are uncommon. These patients tend to present with less swelling, less trismus and clearer drainage than those infections that occur earlier than 6 weeks. Those that are not healed frequently respond to 2–4 weeks of additional maxillomandibular fixation. Osseous union occurs on the lingual side where less disruption of the blood supply has occurred.

ADVANCES IN SURGICAL TECHNIQUES

Maxillomandibular Fixation Screws

The benefits of the use of maxillomandibular fixation screws instead of arch bars for maxillomandibular fixation includes decreased operative time, decreased cost, lower risks for percutaneous and mucosal wire punctures and ease of use (Fig. 33.14). This theoretically

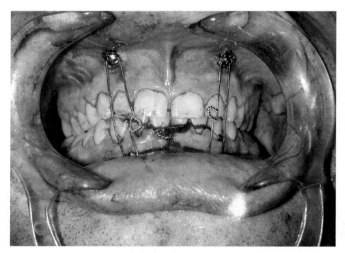

Fig. 33.14: The development of MMF screws illustrated here saves time and may decrease the risk of blood born disease transmission to the surgeon

reduces the risk of blood-borne disease transmission such as HIV and hepatitis B to the surgeon. This technique is not appropriate for comminuted fractures or multiple anterior mandibular arch fractures with floating segments. Malocclusion rates of 4.4% are comparable to other series treated with arch bars.[80]

Endoscopic Approach to the Subcondylar Fracture

The traditional indications for the open reduction of subcondylar fractures are limited by the risks associated with the open technique. If these risks were reduced, a shift in the risk-benefit ratio in favor of surgical

intervention may lead to a reassessment of the indications for surgery.[81] Advantages of an endoscopic approach include reduced soft tissue trauma attributable to the limited exposure of bone in the condylar region. Endoscopic management of subcondylar fractures has generated the largest number of reports in the facial trauma literature as compared to other anatomic sites,[82-85] although a panel of facial trauma surgeons suggested that the use of an endoscope was used least in this site. As many as 30% of surgeons feel that this technique offers nothing more than a good light source that did not aid in the case.[86] The endoscopy assisted technique is least useable in the situation in which it is probably most indicated, severely dislocated or comminuted fractures.[82,87] Although reports demonstrate the successful use of this technique, endoscopic repair of subcondylar fractures is a technically demanding procedure. The difficulty with the technique concerns the basics of open reduction and internal fixation. It is difficult to reduce the fracture and hold the fragments in position while applying the plate and screws. There is also a steep learning curve with this technique and the use of this technique often requires increased operating time.[16,82,87] Lack of accompanying instrumentation, such as proper drills is a significant problem. If proper accompanying instrumentation were to be developed, endoscopes could become an integral component in the management of craniofacial trauma.[86] Efforts have been directed toward the development of such an endoscope/special channel combination.

Resorbable Plates

Clear benefits of resorbable plates are lacking in the treatment of mandibular fractures.[88] One potential beneficial application would be in the treatment of pediatric mandible fractures. This application has not been evaluated in detail.

Locking Screws

Contouring larger 2.3 and 2.7 mm plates in the treatment of mandible fractures is sometimes difficult and potentially time consuming. Plate and screw systems have been introduced that 'lock' the screw into the plate. An advantage of a locking plate is that it becomes unnecessary for the plate to have intimate contact with the underlying bone, making plate adaptation easier.[89] This is an advantage for large plates but contouring miniplates is not a problem. Some benefit may be lost in that the screw must be centered and placed at 90° in order to lock. A disadvantage is that locking screws are more expensive.

Summary

The successful treatment of mandible fractures is predicated on appropriate reduction and stabilization in order to facilitate bone healing. The restoration of premorbid occlusal relationships and masticatory function is necessary for a good outcome. The best treatment options would combine techniques that provide ease of access, ease of application, low expense, provide stabilization of the fracture line, and permit immediate mobilization with no complications. The ultimate plan must factor in the fracture, the patient, and the experience and comfort level of the surgeon with various techniques (Stone 1993).[15] It is critical to be versed in more than one treatment modality so that the appropriate treatment is rendered, rather than tailoring a single mode of treatment to every fracture.

ACKNOWLEDGMENT

Special thanks to Damion Dzambo for assistance in manuscript preparation.

REFERENCES

1. Koury M, Ellis E. Rigid internal fixation for the treatment of infected mandibular fractures. *J Oral Maxillofac Surg* 1992; 50:434–443.
2. Towers AG. Wound infection in an orthopaedic hospital. *Lancet* 1965; 2:379–381.
3. Reitzik M, Schoorl W. Bone repair in the mandible: A histologic and biometric comparison between rigid and semirigid fixation. *J Oral Maxillofac Surg* 1983; 41:215–218.
4. Ellis E III, Moos KF, El-Attar A. Ten years of mandibular fractures: An analysis of 2,137 cases. *Oral Surg* 1985; 59:120–229.
5. Lazow SK. The mandible fracture: A treatment protocol. *J Cranio-Maxillofac Trauma* 1993; 2:24–30.
6. Dodson TB, Perrott DH, Kaban LB, Gordon NC. Fixation of mandibular fractures: A comparative analysis of rigid internal fixation and standard fixation techniques. *J Oral Maxillofac Surg* 1990; 48:362–366.
7. Theriot BA, Van Sickels JE, Triplett RG, Nishioka GJ. Intraosseous wire fixation versus rigid osseous fixation of mandibular fractures: A preliminary report. *J Oral Maxillofac Surg* 1987; 45:577–582.
8. Passed LA, Ellis E III, Sinn DP. Complications of nongrid fixation of mandibular angle fractures. *J Oral Maxillofac Surg* 1993; 1:382–384.
9. Silvennoinen U, Iizuka T, Lindqvist C, Oikarinen K. Different patterns of condylar fractures: An analysis of 382 patients in a 3-year period. *J Oral Maxillofac Surg* 1992; 50:1032–1037.
10. Peled M, Laufer D, Helman J, Gutman D. Treatment of mandibular fractures by means of compression osteosynthesis. *J Oral Maxillofac Surg* 1989; 47:566–569.
11. Bochlogyros PN. A retrospective study of 1,521 mandibular fractures. *J Oral Maxillofac Surg* 1985; 43:597–599.
12. Mathog RH, Toma V, Dayman L, Wolf S. Nonunion of the mandible: An analysis of contributing factors. *J Oral Maxillofac Surg* 2000; 58:746–752.
13. Kearns GJ, Perrott DH, Kaban LB. Rigid fixation of mandibular fractures: Does operator experience reduce complications? *J Oral Maxillofac Surg* 1994; 52:226–231.
14. Ellis E III, Sinn DP. Treatment of mandibular angle fractures using two 2.4 mm dynamic compression plates. *J Oral Maxillofac Surg* 1993b; 51:969–973.
15. Stone I, Dodson T. Risk factors for infection following operative treatment of mandibular fractures: A multivariate analysis. *Plast Reconstruct Surg* 1993; 91:64–68.
16. Lee C, Mueller RV, Lee K, Mathes SJ. Endoscopic subcondylar fracture repair: Functional, aesthetic, and radiographic outcomes. *Plast Reconstruct Surg* 1998; 102:1434–1445.
17. Maloney PL, Welch TB, Doku HC. Early immobilization of mandibular fractures: A retrospective study. *J Oral Maxillofac Surg* 1991; 49:698–703.
18. Anderson T, Alpert B. Experience with rigid fixation of mandibular fractures and immediate function. *J Oral Maxillofac Surg* 1992; 50:555–556.
19. Champy M, Lodde JP, Schmitt R, Jaeger JH, Muster D. Mandibular osteosynthesis by miniature sere-wed plates via a buccal approach. *J Maxillofac Surg* 1978; 6:14–21.
20. Cawood JI. Small plate osteosynthesis of mandibular fractures. *Br J Oral Maxillofac Surg* 1985; 23:77–91.
21. Mathog RH, Rosenberg Z. Complications in the treatment of facial fractures. *Otolaryngol Clin of N Am* 1976; 9:533–552.
22. Ellis E III, Walker L. Treatment of mandibular angle fractures using two noncompression miniplates. *J Oral Maxillofac Surg* 1994; 52:1032–1036.
23. Zallen RD, Curry JT. A study of antibiotic usage in compound mandibular fractures. *J Oral Surg* 1975; 33:431–434.
24. Iizuka T, Lindqvist C, Hallikainen D, Paukku P. Infection after rigid internal fixation of mandibular fractures: A clinical and radiologic study. *J Oral Maxillofac Surg* 1991a; 49:585–593.
25. Maw RB. A new look at maxillomandibular fixation of mandibular fractures. *J Oral Surg* 1981; 39:187–190.
26. Brown JS, Grew N, Taylor C, Millar BG. Intermaxillary fixation compared to miniplate osteosynthesis in the management of the fractured mandible: An audit. *Br J Oral Maxillofac Surg* 1991; 29:308–311.
27. Tu HK, Tenhulzen D. Compression osteosynthesis of mandibular fractures: A retrospective study. *J Oral Maxillofac Surg* 1985; 43:585–589.
28. Joos U, Meyer U, Tkotz T, Weingart D. Use of a mandibular fracture score to predict the development of complications. *J Oral Maxillofac Surg* 1999; 57:2–7.
29. Kahnberg KE. Conservative treatment of uncomplicated mandibular fractures. *Swed Dent J* 1981; 5:15–20.
30. Luhr HG. Compression plate osteosynthesis through the Luhr system. *Oral Maxillofac Traumatol* 1982; 1:332.
31. Assael LA. Evaluation of rigid internal fixation of mandible fractures performed in the teaching laboratory. *J Oral Maxillofac Surg* 1993; 51:1315–1319.
32. Schmidt BL, Kearns G, Gordon N, Kaban LB. A financial analysis of maxillomandibular fixation versus rigid internal

fixation for treatment of mandibular fractures. *J Oral Maxillofac Surg* 2000; 58:1206–1210.

33. El-Degwi A, Mathog RH. Mandible fractures - Medical and economic considerations. *Otolaryngol Head Neck Surg* 1993; 108:213–219.

34. Ardary WC. Prospective clinical evaluation of the use of compression plates and screws in the management of mandible fractures. *J Oral Maxillofac Surg* 1989; 47:1150–5113.

35. Valentine J, Levy FE, Marentette LJ. Intraoral monocortical miniplating of mandible fractures. *Arch Otolaryngol - Head Neck Surg* 1994; 120:605–612.

36. Worthington P, Champy M. Monocortical miniplate osteosynthesis. *Otolaryngol Clin of N Am* 1987; 20:607–620.

37. Michelet FX, Deymes J, Dessus B. Osteosynthesis with miniaturized screwed plates in maxillo-facial surgery. *J Maxillo-Facial Surg* 1973; 1:79–84.

38. Kroon F, Mathisson M, Cordey JR, Rahn BA. The use of miniplates in mandibular fractures: An in vitro study. *J Cranio-Maxillofacial Surg* 1991; 19:199–204.

39. Raveh J, Vuillemin T, Ladrach K, Roux M, Sutter F. Plate osteosynthesis of 367 mandibular fractures: The unrestricted indication for the intraoral approach. *J Cranio-Maxillofacial Surg* 1987; 15:244–253.

40. Iizuka T, Lindqvist C. Rigid internal fixation of mandibular fractures. An analysis of 270 fractures treated using the AO/ASIF method. *Intl J Oral Maxillofac Surg* 1992; 21:65–69.

41. Ellis E III. Treatment of mandibular angle fractures using the AO reconstruction plate. *J Oral Maxillofac Surg* 1993a; 51: 250–254.

42. Bagby GW, Janes JM. The effect of compression on the rate of fracture healing using a special plate. *Am J Surg* 1958; 95: 761–771.

43. Perren SM, Huggler A, Russenberger M. The reaction of cortical bone to compression. *Acta Orthoped Scand* 1969; 125 (Suppl):19–28.

44. Kaplan BA, Hoard MA, Park SS. Immediate mobilization following fixation of mandible fractures: A prospective, randomized study. *Laryngoscope* 2001; 111:1520–1524.

45. Amaratunga NA. The relation of age to the immobilization period required for healing of mandibular fractures. *J Oral Maxillofac Surg* 1987; 45:111–113.

46. Levy FE, Smith RW, Odland RM, Marentette LJ. Monocortical miniplate fixation of mandibular angle fractures. *Arch Otolaryngol - Head Neck Surg* 1991; 117:149–154.

47. Paradisi F, Corti G. Which prophylactic regimen for which surgical procedure? *Am J Surg* 1992; 164 (Suppl):2–5.

48. Abubaker AO, Rollert MK. Postoperative antibiotic prophylaxis in mandibular fractures: A preliminary randomized, double-blind, and placebo-controlled clinical study. *J Oral Maxillofac Surg* 2001; 59:1415–1419.

49. Chole RA, Yee J. Antibiotic prophylaxis for facial fractures: A prospective, if randomized clinical trial. *Arch Otolaryngol Head Neck Surg* 1987; 113:1055–1057.

50. Morgan CE, Hicks JN, Eby TL, Borton TE. Repair of mandibular fractures: Plating vs. traditional techniques. *Otolaryngol - Head Neck Surg* 1992; 106:249.

51. Assael L, Rogerson K, Shafer D. Evaluation of 2.4 mm low contact plates in a mandibular fracture model. *J Dent Res* 1992; 71:119.

52. Iizuka T, Lindqvist C. Sensory disturbances associated with rigid internal fixation of mandibular fractures. *J Oral and Maxillofac Surg* 1991b; 49:1264–1268.

53. Iizuka T, Lindqvist C. Rigid internal fixation of fractures in the angular region of the mandible: An analysis of factors contributing to different complications. *Plastic Reconstruct Surg* 1993; 91:265–271.

54. Mayor MB. Bone remodeling in response to local mechanics. *Bull Hosp Joint Disorder Orthoped Ins* 1983; 43:100–102.

55. Dechow PC, Ellis E III, Throckmorton GS. Structural properties of mandibular bone following application of a bone plate. *J Oral Maxillofac Surg* 1995; 53:1044–1051.

56. Klotch DW, Lundy LB. Condylar neck fractures of the mandible. *Otolaryngol Clin North Am* 1991; 24:181–194.

57. Throckmorton GS, Ellis E III, Winkler AJ, Dechow PC. Bone strain following application of a rigid bone plate: An *in vitro* study in human mandibles. *J Oral Maxillofac Surg* 1992; 50:1066–1073.

58. Thaller SR, Mabourakh S. Pediatric mandibular fractures. *Ann Plast Surg* 1991; 26:511–513.

59. Hammond M, Stassen L. Mandibular condyle fractures: A Consensus. *Br J Oral Maxillofac Surg* 1999; 37:87–89.

60. Zide MF, Kent JN. Indications for open reduction of mandibular condyle fractures. *J Oral Maxillofac Surg* 1983; 41:89–98.

61. Zide MF. Open reduction of mandibular condyle fractures: Indications and technique. *Clin Plast Surg* 1989; 16:69–76.

62. Baker AW, McMahon J, Moos KF. Current consensus on the management of fractures of the mandibular condyle. *Int J Oral Maxillofac Surg* 1998; 27:258–266.

63. Worsaee N, Thorn JJ. Surgical versus nonsurgical treatment of unilateral dislocated low subcondylar fractures: A clinical study of 52 cases. *J Oral Maxillofac Surg* 1994; 52:353–360.

64. Konstantinovic VS, Dimitrijevic B. Surgical versus conservative treatment of unilateral condylar process fractures: Clinical and radiographic evaluation of 80 patients. *J Oral Maxillofac Surg* 1992; 50:349–353.

65. Takenoshita Y, Ishibashi H, Oka M. Comparison of functional recovery after nonsurgical and surgical treatment of condylar fractures. *J Oral Maxillofac Surg* 1990; 48:1191–1195.

66. Dahlstrom L, Kahnberf K, Lindahl L. 1 to 5 years follow-up on condylar fractures. *Intl J Oral Maxillofac Surg* 1989; 18: 18–23.

67. Kleinheinz J, Anastassov GE, Joos U. Indications for treatment of subcondylar mandibular fractures. *J Cranio-Maxillofac Trauma* 1999; 5:17–26.

68. Ellis E III, Palmieri C, Throckmorton G. Further displacement of condylar fractures after closed treatment. *J Oral Maxillofac Surg* 1999; 57:1307–1316.

69. Hall MB. Condylar fractures: Surgical management. *J Oral Maxillofac Surg* 1994; 52:1189–1192.

70. Bruce RA, Ellis E III. The second Chalmers J. Lyons Academy study of fractures of the edentulous mandible. *J Oral Maxillofac Surg* 1993; 51:904–911.

71. Barber HD. Conservative management of the fractured atrophic edentulous mandible. *J Oral Maxillofac Surg* 2001; 59:789–791.

72. Marciani RD. Invasive management of the fractured atrophic edentulous mandible. *J Oral Maxillofac Surg* 2001; 59: 792–795.

73. Smith BR, Johnson JV. Rigid fixation of comminuted mandibular fractures. *J Oral Maxillofac Surg* 1993; 51:1320–1326.

74. Assael LA. Treatment of mandibular angle fractures: Plate and screw fixation. *J Oral Maxillofac Surg* 1994; 52:757–761.

75. Rudderman R. Biomechanics of the facial skeleton. *Clin Plast Surg* 1992; 19:11–29.

76. Ellis E III, Karas N. Treatment of mandibular angle fractures using two mini dynamic compression plates. *J Oral Maxillofac Surg* 1992; 50:958–963.

77. Haug RH. The effects of screw number and length on two methods of tension band plating. *J Oral Maxillofac Surg* 1993; 51:159–162.

78. Ellis E III, Ghali GE. Lag screw fixation of mandibular fractures. *J Oral Maxillofac Surg* 1991; 49:234–243.

79. Vartanian AJ, Alvi A. Bone-screw mandible fixation: An intraoperative alternative to arch bars. *Otolaryngol - Head Neck Surg* 2000; 123:718–721.

80. Antonyshyn O. Endoscopic subcondylar fracture repair: Functional, aesthetic and radiographic outcomes. *Plast Reconstruct Surg* 1998; 102:1444–1445.

81. Lauer G, Schmelzeisen R. Endoscope-assisted fixation of mandibular condylar process fractures. *J Oral Maxillofac Surg* 1999; 57:36–39.

82. Troulis MJ, Kaban LB. Endoscopic approach to the ramus/condyle unit: Clinical applications. *J Oral Maxillofac Surg* 2001; 59:503–509.

83. Chen CT, Lai JP, Tung TC, Chen YR. Endoscopically assisted mandibular subcondylar fracture repair. *Plast Reconstruct Surg* 1999; 103:60–65.

84. Jacobovicz J, Lee C, Trabulsy PP. Endoscopic repair of mandibular subcondylar fractures. *Plast Reconstruct Surg* 1998; 101:437–441.

85. Barone CM, Boschert MT, Jimenez DF. Usefulness of endoscopy in craniofacial trauma. *J Cranio-Maxillofac Trauma* 1998; 4:36–41.

86. Betts NJ. Discussion: Endoscope-assisted fixation of mandibular condylar process fractures. *J Oral & Maxillofac Surg* 1999; 57:39–40.

87. Kim YK, Kirn SG. Treatment of mandible fractures using bioabsorbable plates. *Plast Reconstruct Surg* 2002; 110:25–33.

88. Ellis E III, Graham J. Use of a 2.0 mm locking plate/screw system for mandibular fracture surgery. *J Oral Maxillofac Surg* 2002; 60:642–646.

89. Raveh J, Vuillemin T, Ladrach K. Open reduction of the dislocated, fractured condylar process: Indications and surgical procedures. *J Oral Maxillofac Surg* 1989; 47:120–127.

Asian Rhinoplasty

Samuel M Lam, Edward W Chang

Asian rhinoplasty constitutes an entirely different surgical endeavor from Western aesthetic rhinoplasty. First, the Asian nose and overall facial morphologic features differ markedly from that of the Caucasian not only in terms of appearance but also in the underlying anatomic structure. Second, the aesthetic objectives for Asian rhinoplasty are almost entirely contrary to those for Western rhinoplasty in that augmentation rather than reduction is the primary goal. Based on these two principles, operative strategies that rely on traditional Western techniques will fall short of the aesthetic target that the Asian patient desires to attain. This chapter will try to explain exactly how the Asian nose differs from that of the Caucasian, what the aesthetic goal of Asian rhinoplasty is, and elaborate upon the various surgical approaches that can help achieve those objectives.

ANATOMY

The Asian nose exhibits fundamentally different anatomic features from those of the Caucasian. The nasal dorsum tends to be shallower and less well-defined, a characteristic that can be exacerbated by a broad epicanthal fold of the eye (see related chapter on Asian Blepharoplasty). In addition, the bony orbital shelf tends to be less recessed and the eyelid fuller in appearance due to the abundant adipose tissue and lack of a supra-tarsal crease. The combined effect of the neighboring midfacial attributes is to render the already flattened nose even more flat and to impart an overall washed-out appearance.

The nose itself also exhibits unique properties that will guide surgical management. The overlying skin envelope is generally much thicker than is evident in most Caucasian noses. Similarly, the remaining facial skin also shares this feature of increased dermal depth by virtue of the rich collagen layer, which combined with the

greater pigmentation provides a more impervious barrier to solar rays. The underlying cartilage of the nasal tip is relatively weaker and less abundant than in the Caucasian. In particular, septal cartilage supply for tip and dorsal grafting is often insufficient to meet these aesthetic requirements. Functionally, speaking, the wider expanse of the nasal dorsum and the relatively straight orientation of the Asian septum make nasal obstruction less likely. The wide divergence of the upper lateral cartilage-septal junction (that defines the internal nasal valve) makes internal-valve compromise quite infrequent in the Asian nose. Typically, hypertrophied turbinates can impede airflow due to an allergic or non-allergic cause. External valve collapse is typically a result of prior nasal surgery that leads to dynamic collapse or nasal stricture.

In addition, the nasal base is quite different from the leptorrhine nose as well. The premaxillary component tends to be deficient which leads to a more simian-appearing, acute nasolabial angle. Premaxillary augmentation helps to ameliorate this by opening up this closed angle. The alar-base can also be excessively flared, making the nose appear even flatter. Proper alar-base reduction can reduce this unsightly flare and lend refinement to the principal augmentation effort. Some bulbosity of the nasal tip can also be eliminated in select patients who exhibit this quality. All these adjunctive rhinoplasty techniques are discussed in this chapter.

SILICONE NASAL AUGMENTATION

Based on these different anatomic constituent elements and the desired goal to augment the nose to a more elevated level, a unique strategy suitable for the Asian nose must be devised. Although silicone as augmentation material has been frowned upon in the West, it has a long legacy of safety in the East.[1] Silicone nasal augmentation has become the principal method for Asian rhinoplasty (Figs 34.1A to H). A precise surgical method and particular type and configuration of silicone must be used to achieve the optimal aesthetic result and to ensure maximal safety.

In the past, various augmentation materials were used in South Asia, most of which were incompatible with rhinoplasty. The substances were typically too indurated in nature or poorly tolerated by the recipient soft tissue to achieve a reasonable measure of safety. Even silicone in the past was formulated in a much harder form than today's softer, more pliable version. Besides concern for safety, use of hard materials also feels unnatural, as the tip loses natural sway and resilience. Over-augmentation of the nose also proved to be a troublesome problem both in terms of the artificially unaesthetic appearance of the

nose as well as complications that arose. Similarly, a large L-shaped strut that rests on the nasal spine is a dangerous configuration, as it tends to apply undue force along the nasal tip tissue.[2]

Most complications that should arise occur along the nasal tip and can be mostly attributed to improper selection of implant and poor technique. Again, over-augmentation, particularly with indurated materials, can cause excessive pressure on the nasal-tip skin envelope that predisposes to eventual extrusion, or worse yet, frank cutaneous necrosis. At the time of surgery, if the skin envelope appears to be under tension or exhibits some blanching, the surgeon should rethink the size of the implant that has been inserted. A very large columellar segment (as in an L-shaped implant) can lead to similar problems. In addition, an exaggerated L-shape can also favor implant extrusion, which most likely occurs along

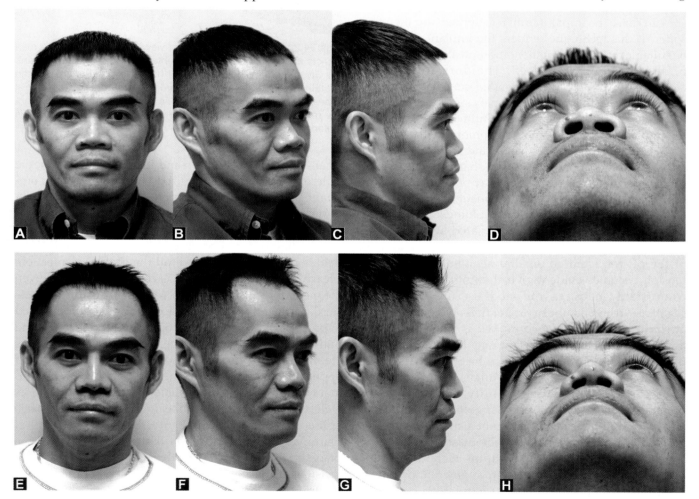

Figs 34.1A to H: (A to D) Preoperative photographs. (E to H) Postoperative photographs: This series of photographs show the benefit of a silicone dorsal/tip implant on the rather feminine appearing nose on the preoperative lateral view. In addition, the wide girth of the alar base was reduced using the technique for alar-base reduction discussed in the text

the incision line. An L-shaped implant is safe if it does not extend more than 50% of the entire columellar length. Projection is achieved by virtue of the cantilever effect of the dorsal component rather than as a tent-pole mechanism of the nasal spine.[2] Precise technique will be further elaborated in detail.

Another problem associated with nasal implants is the risk of mobility and displacement. However, fixation of the implant under the nasal-bone periosteum renders the implant immobile and makes mobility of the implant unlikely. Other surgical and postoperative advice will be offered later in the text.

Surgical Technique

The silicone implant should be soft and pliable. Harder implants are absolutely discouraged for reasons given earlier. If the surgeon is in possession of a harder implant, she can carve the implant until it is thinner and therefore softer. If this technique renders the implant too thin to be suitable for proper augmentation, an alternative brand of silicone should be used. The dorsal (or distal) component should have a rounded concavity that will approximate to the relatively convex surface of the nasal dorsum. This curvature permits intimate apposition of the implant to the dorsum and promotes better fixation than a flatter design (Figs 34.2A and B). The tip of the implant should also not be overly sharp so that the risk of extrusion or of unnatural appearance will be minimized. The columellar component must also not be so long as to pass 50% of the total columellar length. The authors use an implant that has a flared, wedge-shaped design in the columellar region that permits advancement of the oft-retracted columellar segment. However, if tension becomes evident or if the implant fails to rest comfortably between the medial crura, the excess segment is trimmed until a proper fit is obtained. Another attribute that is often overlooked is the color of the implant. A transparent implant may be visible through the nasal skin, particularly when bright or harsh light strikes the nose from an oblique angle, such as on stage. Therefore, a semiopaque to fully opaque color is preferable. The two most popular colors are white and flesh-tone, but the exact color is not a critical factor.

Unlike traditional Western rhinoplasty that may take several hours to accomplish with intravenous sedation or full general anesthesia, Asian augmentation rhinoplasty using a silicone alloplast is relatively straightforward and does not necessarily require the same level of patient anesthesia. Besides, a short-acting intravenous anesthetic that can be used to mitigate the discomfort of

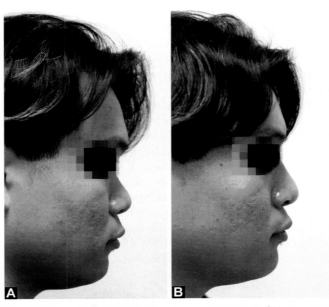

Figs 34.2A and B: (A) This lateral view of a young Chinese man depicts the benefit of nasal augmentation with a silicone implant. (B) Given the very deep recess of his nasofrontal angle, he can sustain a proportionately large implant without the unnatural appearance of blunting this angle. The patient also exhibits a simian-like retrusion of his premaxilla but did not endeavor to have this feature altered

local-anesthesia infiltration and induce related amnesia, little other sedative is required. Therefore, in the compliant patient, this type of procedure can be typically undertaken in the office that is outfitted with proper surgical instrumentation and ancillary equipment.

The first order of business is to ensure that a sterile field is present in order to limit the chance of infection. Clearly, the intranasal tissue is contaminated, and even the most diligent preparation will fail to ensure absolute sterility. Nevertheless, a povidone-iodine solution is used to prepare the external nasal tissue and the surrounding midface using a gauze sponge. The internal vestibule is cleaned with povidone-iodine on a cotton-tipped applicator. A surgical marking pen (Fig. 34.3) is used to mark the nasal bone-upper lateral cartilage junction as well as the midline; 1% lidocaine mixed with 1:50,000 epinephrine is infiltrated into the limited, bilateral marginal incisions and nasal tissue (in the sub-SMAS) plane up to the nasal bones through the same marginal incisions. Typically, 1–2 cc is required for complete nasal infiltration. The bony nasal dorsum (as delineated by the aforementioned external surgical marking) should be directly infiltrated transcutaneously in order to hydrodissect the periosteum of the underlying nasal

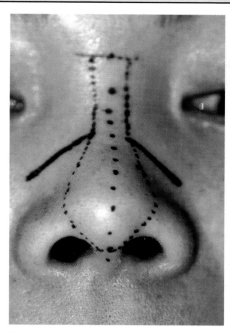

Fig. 34.3: Surgical markings that indicate the nasal midline, the proposed dissection pocket, and the upper extent of the implant that should rest halfway between the glabella and the sellion. The caudal border of the nasal bones is also marked out to determine where the subperiosteal plane should be entered

bone. By doing so, subperiosteal dissection will be facilitated, that will in turn ensure implant fixation.

After ten minutes (to allow for maximal hemostasis and time for onset of the anesthesia) the actual procedure may begin. During this interval, the sterilized implant should be placed along the external nasal dorsum to ensure that it is of adequate height. As the patient is supine and may also lack a supratarsal fold, the desired radix may be difficult to ascertain. Therefore, the authors have devised a reliable method to ensure a reproducibly suitable dorsal height. The implant generally should rest halfway between the sellion (the deepest concavity) and the superior protuberance or glabella.[3] A telltale sign of a poor rhinoplasty is overaugmentation in this region in which the nasofrontal angle is blunted or entirely effaced. Therefore, attention should be paid to ensure that a sharp, natural nasofrontal angle is maintained. Accordingly, a patient with a very deep recessed sellion can tolerate a larger implant than an individual who possesses a shallower angle. Also, the cheekbone height is another indicator for how high the dorsum can be elevated and still retain a natural appearance. For a very flat cheek contour, the nasal dorsum should not be excessively augmented. Malar prominence is a sign of masculinity in the East Asia and is considered aesthetically

unfavorable. Therefore, malar augmentation to achieve facial harmony is rarely an option. In fact, malar-bone reduction procedures are in vogue throughout Asia, particularly in the Korean peninsula.[4]

In order to ensure symmetry, the marginal incision is made bilaterally, and dissection is carried out upward from both marginal incisions. The extent of the incision is more abbreviated than the traditional marginal incision used for endonasal delivery rhinoplasty or external rhinoplasty. The incision should basically fall only within the height of the vestibular recess with about the same distance that traverses medial to the dome as lateral to this point. Dissection is carried out with a pair of fine, sharp scissors in a sub-SMAS plane (Figs 34.4 to 34.6), i.e., supraperi-chondrial but below the SMAS/muscular sling just as in standard Western rhinoplasty. Again, the same dissection should be carried out upwards in this plane from both marginal incisions up toward the nasal bone and terminating at that point. The amount of dissection should be generous enough to open up most of the columella, the entire lobule, nasal tip, and the medial portion of the upper lateral cartilage in order to accommodate the implant. It is not absolutely critical to dissect a precise glove-in-hand pocket in the nasal tip region. However, a narrower, more confined space should be attempted over the nasal-bone region to ensure a tight subperiosteal fixation pocket.

When the nasal bones are reached (as indicated by the external line of demarcation drawn with the marking pen), the scissors should be withdrawn and a sharp, Joseph periosteal elevator inserted into the nose through either marginal incision, in order to undertake the subperiosteal dissection. The non-dominant hand is placed along the radix of the nose to provide proper

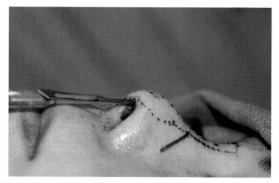

Fig. 34.4: A no. 15 Bard-Parker blade is used to incise only along the clinical dome with equal length medial to the dome as lateral to it. The incision should end approximately where the lower lateral cartilage begins to arch superiorly away from the caudal border of the nostril rim. Both nostrils are incised and dissected in order to ensure symmetrical dissection

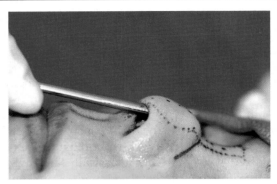

Fig. 34.5: A pair of dissecting scissors is used to dissect in a sub-SMAS, supraperichondrial plane along the outlined pocket up to the caudal border of the nasal bones. Both marginal incisions are used for dissection to ensure that a symmetrical pocket is fashioned. The dissection should also include the anterior aspect of the columella: Passing the scissor tips across through to the other marginal incision ensures that the columella is sufficiently dissected

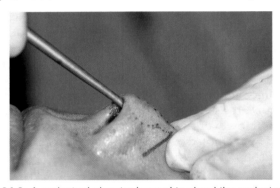

Fig. 34.6: A periosteal elevator is used to shred the periosteum in the midline up to the marked superior extent of where the implant should terminate. Care should be taken to stay relatively narrow in the midline so that an overly wide dissection pocket is not created. Although a wide-tip pocket is permitted (and encouraged), a narrower dorsal pocket should be fashioned to maintain the implant in the midline

countertraction, as the elevator is maneuvered firmly over the nasal bones to lift and scrape the periosteum of the nasal bones, all the while to remain in the midline and to stay relatively confined to a diameter just greater than the width of the implant. Some authors have stated that actual elevation of the periosteum is not feasible but that sharply shredding the periosteum is sufficient to promote periosteal growth around the implant for proper stability. Nevertheless, periosteal dissection is absolutely essential to avoid the complication of implant mobility.

Bayonet forceps or straight forceps with teeth should be used to guide the implant into the created pocket using either marginal incision. With the patient in supine position, the surgeon should carefully evaluate the superior termination of the implant (Fig. 34.7), its height and effect on the lobule and columella. If the nasofrontal

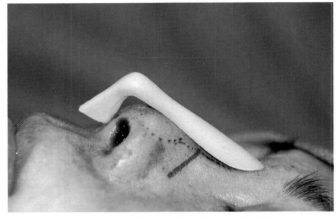

Fig. 34.7: The implant is placed along the dorsum to verify the height of the implant

angle appears blunted, the dorsum too high, the tip overly projected, or the columella improperly distended, the implant should be removed and recontoured using a No.10 Bard-Parker blade until the desired configuration is achieved. Conservative resection should be followed, as further resections can be undertaken for additional refinement. The anterior aspect of the dorsal implant is most easily trimmed to achieve the desired dorsal height (Figs 34.8 to 34.10), and any minor surface irregularities along the implant that arise due to imprecise carving are generally camouflaged by the thick skin envelope. If the implant does not seem to fit readily into the pocket, a wider dissection may need to be undertaken in order to achieve adequate space to accommodate the implant. A small dorsal hump can be effectively camouflaged with an implant, but a larger convexity (a feature found more prevalently in the Japanese race) often requires dorsal rasping in order to avoid a seesaw effect over this prominence. As the open-roof deformity created by the

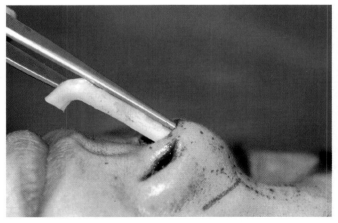

Fig. 34.8: The implant is inserted through either marginal incision using a pair of Debakey forceps

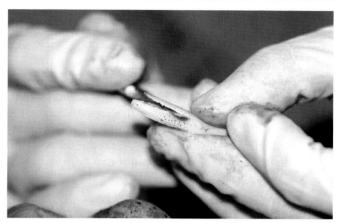

Fig. 34.9: The implant is then shaved down with a No.10 Bard-Parker blade until it is of the right size and configuration according to aesthetic judgment. Often, the implant must be removed, reshaved, and replaced several times before a satisfactory contour and shape is achieved

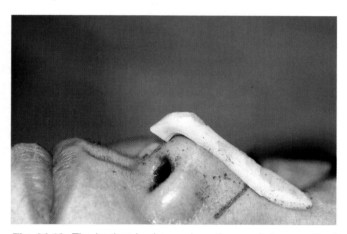

Fig. 34.10: The implant is shown along the nasal dorsum after it has been completely shaved and trimmed to the appropriate aesthetic dimensions. After the implant is inserted and confirmed to be in the midline, the marginal incisions are closed with interrupted 5-0 chromic sutures. Only Benzoin and 1/2″ brown Micropore tape are applied at the end of the procedure in the standard rhinoplasty method

rasping is camouflaged with the implant, osteotomies are usually not indicated.

When the implant is properly seated in the pocket, the patient can be asked to examine the height of the dorsum and shape of the lobule using a handheld mirror to ensure that the nasal proportions are to his or her specifications. The two marginal incisions can then be closed using a 5-0 chromic suture with a P-3 needle in an interrupted fashion. Because of the short incision, generally two sutures are adequate to close each side of nose. Benzoin is applied to the external nose and 1″ brown-toned Micropore tape is fitted along the dorsum

and tip as in a standard Western rhinoplasty. A nasal splint is generally unnecessary, as the nasal-bone attachments have not been violated.

ADJUNCTIVE PROCEDURES

Besides dorsal augmentation with a silicone alloplast, three different adjunctive procedures can be incorporated to achieve the optimal aesthetic result: Premaxillary augmentation, alar-base reduction, and cephalic trimming of the lower lateral cartilage.

As the premaxillary component is often deficient in the Asian patient, an acute nasolabial angle is often present. This appearance may be deemed unfavorable to the patient and is most evident on inspection of the lateral view. Although many alloplasts have been recommended in this area, alloplasts may not be as safe a choice as autogenous augmentation. The reader is reminded that the dorsal silicone alloplast should not extend past approximately 50% of the columellar length. Both septal and auricular cartilage provides suitable grafting material for premaxillary augmentation. As auricular cartilage is easier to harvest in the office setting and is often more plentiful than septal cartilage in the Asian patient, the ear is preferred as the chief augmentation material in the premaxillary region. On the other hand, if the patient is in an ambulatory surgical facility with deeper sedation, then septal harvesting may be opted. Although the authors typically rely on a preauricular incision for graft harvesting in the Caucasian patient, the risks of scarring and a hypopigmented, visible incision line make post-auricular approach more suitable for the Asian patient. In addition, wound closure should be obtained with a running, monofilament suture, e.g., 5-0 nylon, to mini-mize any exuberant scarring. The premaxillary pocket is created along the medial nasal sill and dissected using fine sharp scissors down to the premaxilla. Morselized auricular cartilage can then be used to fill this recipient pocket until the desired amount of augmentation is achieved. The incision is then closed with a 5-0 chromic suture. The reader is reminded to bolster the ear donor site for several days to avoid hematoma and related auricular deformity.

Alar-base reduction can complement and balance augmentation rhinoplasty using a silicone implant. Alar-base resection should be undertaken only after the silicone implant has been inserted, and the position and height confirmed to be favorable. Carrying out augmen-tation rhinoplasty after alar-base reduction can disturb the delicate sutures that are placed along the alar margin when the implant is being manipulated. Wedge resections can be resected along the alar rim to achieve this aesthetic result, being careful not to over- resect tissue or to place undue tension on the wound closure. For further refinement, a 3-0 nylon is used to cinch the alar base further inward. The suture is passed upward through the free margin of the resected ala and then down across the nasal root to exit through the contralateral alar defect. Again, the suture is passed upward to draw the free segment down toward the nasal base and passed back to the original side. The suture is then tightened with a surgeon's knot until the precise amount of alar translocation is achieved before completing the remaining suture throws. At times, the alar segment may appear excessively bowed outward after drawing the base inward. Additional wedge resections can be undertaken to reduce this flare, being careful not to transect the cinching suture. The alar incisions are then closed with 6-0 nylon suture. Generally, the alar margin is not as predisposed toward unsightly scarring as the medial upper eyelid and the postauricular region in the Asian patient. Nevertheless, use of prophylactic injection of 0.1 cc of triamcinolone 10 mg/cc may prove helpful and is routinely implemented in the authors' practices. The sutures may be safely removed after 7 days.

Another simple technique that complements allo-plastic augmentation of the nose is non-delivery cephalic resection of the lower lateral cartilages. This technique does not represent any departure from the known method that is reported in standard Western rhinoplasty textbooks. Resection of the cephalic border of the lower lateral cartilage can be most easily undertaken prior to augmentation rhinoplasty with the silicone implant when the native tissue has been relatively undisturbed. Briefly, the authors advocate a simple cartilage-splitting technique along the proposed excision line rather than a retrograde technique starting from the intercartilaginous incision.

Postoperative Care

In the postoperative setting, the patient is asked not to shower for one week but only to wash the hair, face, and body separately so as not to dampen the adhesive dressing affixed to the nasal dorsum, which would prematurely fall off if it should become wet. Accordingly, ice packs are not recommended for rhinoplasty for the same reason, as the condensation around the ice pack will also serve to undermine the adhesive qualities of the dressing. The nasal-tape dressing will assist to keep edema to a minimum and also to maintain the orientation of the implant.

More important than any other aspect of post-operative care is proper nocturnal head positioning. Early implant displacement can be avoided by keeping the head in a relatively straight position, held in place with bilateral sandbags or equivalently heavy props.[3] Displacement at night is common: if this should occur, the implant must be removed and reinserted after the dorsal pocket is reconfigured. For minor displacements or mild mobility of the implant, bilateral digital pressure along the sides of the nasal dorsum can help maintain the implant's position.

Complications

If the described implant type is used and the proper surgical technique is followed, complications remain relatively rare.[5,6] As mentioned, early displacement may be an irritant but can be avoided if proper postoperative care is observed. Displacement can also occur due to poor surgical technique in which an asymmetric pocket was created or the implant was inserted askew into the pocket. The right-handed surgeon should be particularly mindful of placing the implant from a right-superior to left-inferior position; the converse is true for the left-handed surgeon.

Infection is rarely encountered if proper sterile technique is respected and a short five-day course of perioperative antibiotic regimen is prescribed. Generally, an anti-staphlyococcal medication, e.g. cephalexin, is begun the night prior to surgery. If an infection should arise, a dose of intravenous antibiotics and/or a course of broad spectrum oral antibiotics should be administered. The patient must be carefully followed for worsening of this condition. If no improvement in the condition is noted after 1 to 2 days or if frank abscess develops, the implant should be promptly removed. The patient should remain without attempted reinsertion for several weeks to months until all signs of infection have completely dissipated and the patient has been symptom-free for several weeks.

Extrusion of the implant typically occurs along the incision line, and this can be addressed by trimming the implant and/or by redissecting the pocket to accommodate the implant. A limited columellar segment usually minimizes the risk of this possibility. Fortunately, cutaneous tip necrosis is unheard of if the right implant and technique are used. However, if this complication should arise, the implant obviously must be promptly removed and the wound dressed with wet-to-dry dressings until complete closure. Besides frank necrosis, the most ominous complication that can occur with silicone implantation is extreme capsular contraction around the implant that leads to an unnatural, upward rotation of the nasal tip so that the nose appears porcine in appearance. Use of a longer implant can at times buttress against this complication if it begins to manifest.[3] Fortunately, this problem remains quite rare but is typically encountered in the patient with repeated bouts of infection or multiple rhinoplasties.

SUMMARY

Asian rhinoplasty is fundamentally different from Caucasian rhinoplasty. Use of Western techniques often fails to achieve the desired aesthetic result in Asian patients. Accordingly, silicone augmentation if properly executed with the correct material, can lead to a rapid, reliable, reproducible, and reversible result.

REFERENCES

1. Deva AK, Merten S, Chang L. Silicone in nasal augmentation rhinoplasty: A decade of clinical experience. *Plast Reconstr Surg* 1998; 102:1230–1237.
2. McCurdy, JA. The Asian nose: Augmentation rhinoplasty with L-shaped silicone implants. *Facial Plast Surg* 2002; 18:245–252.
3. Lam SM, Kim YK. Augmentation rhinoplasty of the Asian nose with the "bird" silicone implant. *Ann Plast Surg* 2003; 51:249.
4. McCurdy JA Jr., Lam SM. *Cosmetic surgery of the Asian face.* 2nd edn. New York: Thieme Medical Publishers, 2004.
5. Hinga, Y. Complications of augmentation rhinoplasty in the Japanese. *Ann Plast Surg* 1980; 4:495–499.
6. Ham KS, Chung SC, Lee SH. Complications of oriental augmentation rhinoplasty. *Ann Acad Med Singapore* 1983; 12:406–462.

Asian Blepharoplasty

Edward W Chang, Samuel M Lam

The Asian eyelid differs markedly from that of the Caucasian in many fundamental respects: surgical techniques and aesthetic objectives have been tailored to these unique constraints. The history of the 'double eyelid' procedure dates back to late nineteenth-century Japan. In 1896, the Japanese surgeon Mikamo was the first to report a technique to create a supratarsal fold in a patient born with the unilateral absence of such a fold.[1] Since that time, it has been widely recognized that approximately 50% of the Asian population is born without a supratarsal fold. The presence of a supratarsal fold is not meant to imply that the patient exhibits a Western or Caucasian eyelid. Instead, this feature represents a variation that is common across different Asian ethnicities.[2] In the 1980s, Westernization techniques of the Asian eyelid were common, in which a very high supratarsal fold was created and considerable orbital fat was removed. This type of surgical intervention was not based on any cultural sensitivity, and true Westernization procedures often left the patient looking unnatural.[3,4]

Since that time, surgical techniques have been modified somewhat to preserve ethnicity through more conservative operative measures, e.g., a lower lid crease is preferred and only partial removal of orbital fat is undertaken.[5] Currently, Asian patients who desire eyelid surgery rarely seek to erase their ethnic identity completely but favor more subtle and natural enhancement of their eyes.[4,6]

Asian eyelids that lack a supratarsal fold are quite dissimilar to the Caucasian upper lid (Fig. 35.1). Unlike the Caucasian eyelid, the levator does not insert into the overlying dermis in the single eyelid configuration of the Asian. Further, significant adipose tissue lends even greater fullness to the upper eyelid (Stewart, 2002: missing reference). Sometimes this fullness in the upper eyelid imparts a tired or sleepy look that may belie the

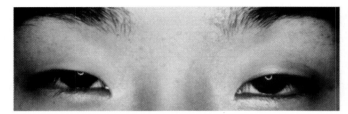

Fig. 35.1: An Asian with no significant supratarsal fold

patient's true temperament or disposition. This condition has been referred to as pseudoptosis orientalis.[7] The epicanthal fold, present in 40–90% of Asians, constitutes another significant anatomic difference. The epicanthus is a web-like fold that drapes over the medial aspect of the eye and obscures the typically exposed caruncle or lacrimal lake. This anatomic feature is attributed to a vertical shortage and a horizontal redundancy of the skin-orbicularis complex situated at the medial aspect of the upper eyelid.[7] A heavy epicanthal fold can make an already broad and flat nasal dorsum appear even more exaggerated and further make the palpebral aperture appear even narrower. Accordingly, various advancement techniques have been advocated to eliminate or reduce this fold.[7-9] However, often patients desire to retain this attribute so as not to lose their ethnicity.

TECHNIQUES

Asian blepharoplasty or 'double-eyelid' blepharoplasty represents the most popular cosmetic surgery in the Asian population today. Innumerable permutations exist of the double-eyelid procedure, but the principal techniques can be broadly classified into three categories: The suture, partial-incision, and full-incision methods. Mikamo's original thesis described the suture method for creation of a supratarsal crease, which Boo-Chai refined a half century later in 1963.[10] Incision-based methods arose to challenge the suture technique and contended that suturing alone failed to achieve a permanent adhesion and also could not address the excessive fat, skin or muscle that often predominates. The suture technique offers the advantage of technical ease, reversibility, and shorter operative time but may lack permanence by many reports.[11] Conversely, the full incision method requires more technical expertise and operative time, and is practically irreversible.[3-6] With the added labor, the full incision risks prolonged edema and potential unsightly scar formation. The lid crease will look unnaturally full and therefore higher than it will in its final appearance due to edema that can persist for several weeks, as opposed to minimal to no edema with the suture method.[12,13]

Scar formation is most commonly encountered along the medial incision and can be prophylactically addressed with 0.1 cc of triamcinolone acetonide in this area at the time of surgery.[6] The partial incision technique offers the balance between the suture and the full incision methods. Only a third of the entire eyelid length is incised along its central aspect to achieve a permanent lid crease. This technique offers less postoperative edema, risk of scarring, and technical labor than the full incision method. It also permits correction of a full upper lid by resection of the middle fat compartment, which is the only adipose bed to be addressed even with a full incision. However, if redundant skin is present, the partial incision cannot readily manage this problem. Further, if a prominent epicanthal fold is the object of scrutiny, the abbreviated incision fails to allow intervention in this region. In reviewing the anatomy, the bony architecture of the midface differs somewhat between the Caucasian and Asian races, in that the latter typically has a shallower orbit and midfacial bone structure. Combined with a full upper eyelid, narrower palpebral fissure, and flatter bony nasal bridge, the overall impression of the Asian face is that it lacks central projection vis-à-vis that of the Caucasian. Both pre- and postaponeurotic adipose can be in abundance, which contribute to the full lid appearance. The excess pre-aponeurotic adipose component is attributed to the lack of a levator attachment to the overlying skin, which permits the pre-aponeurotic fat to descend toward the ciliary margin. A minimal fusion of the orbital septum to the levator exists which encourages further prolapse of fat. The levator has a variable insertion into the upper-lid skin, and some anatomic studies suggest that the tarsus rather than the levator actually inserts into the skin.[14] Some authors contend that a septal-aponeurotic sling defines the level of the fold. The lower height of the sling in the Asian allows the fat to reside in a more dependent position in the eyelid, which contributes to a smaller fold, and a fuller upper eyelid. The objectives of surgery include creating a supratarsal fold which lies at a natural height of 6 to 10 mm above the lash line, debulking the pretarsal soft tissue, and correcting the epicanthal fold as desired. Part of the preoperative consultation entails determining what the aesthetically desirable lid-crease height is. A classification scheme that divides the proposed lid height into small, medium, and large has been devised. Generally, a small fold lies 6 to 7 mm above the lash line; a medium fold at 8 mm; and a large fold at 9 to 10 mm. The large fold is designed to impart a more Westernized appearance to the upper eyelid and a concomitant amount of fat debulking and skin excision are usually incorporated into this procedure to achieve that objective.

The shape of the new eyelid may be defined as either round or oval, but these surgical options rely on a full incision to modulate these subtle differences. The 'round' eyelid imparts a more Caucasian appearance but is a natural attribute of many Asian eyelids. This configuration is designed by lowering the lateral aspect of the proposed incision by approximately 2 mm as the lateral orbital rim is approached. In making a more oval eyelid, the incision level falls 2 mm from its straight course at the mid-palpebral level as it approaches the medial canthus. Also, the surgeon should consult the patient about the epicanthal fold. The fold can terminate at the medial canthus, the so-called 'inside fold', in which the lid crease and the ciliary margin join at the medial canthus. Alternatively, the fold can end more medially and remain distinctly apart from the medial termination of the ciliary margin — the so-called 'outside' fold.[7] As the termination of the 'outside' fold ends medial to the medial canthus (at the punctum), the intervening skin bridge can be advanced medially to efface the epicanthal fold. This technique is the least invasive method of epicanthoplasty. In addition, a modified half Z-plasty can be used for more significant skin advancements, whereas the W-plasty is reserved for significant epicanthal transposition (and is rarely indicated).[8,9] With these more aggressive techniques, the chance for epicanthal webbing increases significantly, and the reader is reminded that prophylactic usage of triamcinolone is warranted to minimize this complication. Again, with the full incision method precise adjustments may be made to the medial fold (i.e. making an inside versus an outside fold) and to the shape of the eye (i.e. a round or oval configuration): An oval-shaped eye naturally works with an inside fold (less Western), and a round-shaped eye is balanced with an outside fold. It is important for the surgeon to understand that the height of the incision is not necessarily the height of the fold in the blepharoplasty for Asians. In Korean patients, 1.5 mm of pretarsal exposure in women was reported to be prevalent in an anthropometric study.[15] Most people in Korea agree that pretarsal exposure greater than 3 mm is unacceptable. In the Caucasian eyelid, the pretarsal exposure is the same as the height of the fold, but in Asians it is much less: Hence much less skin needs to be excised. The pretarsal exposure bed is according to the height of the incision from the ciliary border but it also changes with the amount of pretarsal tissue, height of fixation, levator function, etc.[4]

DEBULKING

Debulking of the upper eyelid can be accomplished through many techniques. Flowers remove the pretarsal fat, residual connective tissue, and pretarsal orbicularis-oculi muscle to a degree that may seem excessive. Boo-Chai partially clears the pre-aponeurotic fat to thin the eyelid. Nevertheless, an important point is fixation of the lower skin-muscle flap to the levator with appropriate tension to permit elevation when the levator is activated. This technique allows for smooth union of the pretarsal skin flap to the tarsus yielding a flat, smooth pretarsal skin surface. However, excessive tension on the lower-lid flap may cause undue eyelash eversion, leading to an unnatural appearance, and worse, corneal exposure. The desired tension on the lower skin flap is adjusted to incipient eyelash eversion, in which the eyelashes are directed just perpendicular to the skin surface. Removal of excessive fat will result in hollowed appearance to the Asian eye that will look unnatural and for the more mature patient, excessively aged. As a general rule of thumb, only half of the exposed fat should ever be removed, and a more conservative amount is recommended in equivocal cases or in patients with already thin eyelids. Fixation sutures that will maintain the supratarsal fold can be set either externally or internally. External-fixation sutures that hold the levator to the overlying skin are meant to be removed after a couple of weeks, as they pass through the external skin. Internal fixation is achieved by placing a suture that incorporates the dermis and the levator only (but not the epidermis) in a buried fashion so that it can be maintained permanently (unless it should extrude). Females typically present to the physician during adolescence or in their early 20s. Males, on the other hand, are generally slightly older in their late 20s or early 30s. It is common practice

for women to tape their eyelids to create a temporary fold as part of their daily makeup routine. In addition, there exists a subset of patients who are older and desire rejuvenation to eliminate ptotic, redundant upper-eyelid skin. It is important that the patient and parent alike fully comprehend the risks, benefits, limitations, and alternatives of the procedure before choosing to proceed. In particular, the potential for asymmetry should be underscored because perfect symmetry is an elusive goal. If the patient is an adolescent, personal motivation and psychological maturity must be properly assessed before deciding to undertake the procedure. Standard photographic documentation, as in any other facial plastic procedure, is mandatory.

In the preoperative analysis, upper-eyelid position must be assessed in conjunction with brow movement, particularly in the older patient with true blepharo- or brow-ptosis. The absence of the pretarsal fold should be noted as well as any asymmetries that exist, and these anatomic subtleties pointed out to the patient. Brow position and any excess soft tissue including skin, muscle, and fat should be noted. Desired lid-crease height should be discussed with the patient, and dialogue can be facilitated by using an open paperclip or equivalent device that is gently pressed into the upper lid to create the proposed fold while the patient checks the appearance in a mirror. The patient should also be offered the option of addressing the epicanthal fold if so desired. If the surgeon is comfortable with different techniques, the proper choice of surgical method can also be discussed with the patient based on the perceived advantages and disadvantages of each technique.

The partial-incision technique is explained here in detail as the authors have significant experience in this area. The procedure can be done under local anesthesia with or without mild sedation. A brief-acting sedative may be used: this is the only uncomfortable part of the procedure. It is crucial that the patient be able to respond to commands during the procedure, as the level of the eyelid must be ascertained intraoperatively and any asymmetries corrected at the time of surgery. After the lid height is confirmed with the patient in an upright position, the patient is placed supine for lid marking. To recreate the position that the lid assumes when the patient is upright, the lid should be tensed until incipient eyelash eversion. The lid height should then be marked at the desired height with the lid under this tension, e.g., if lid height of 8 mm is desired, then that measurement should be taken with the patient supine and the lid under the prescribed tension. The crease should measure approximately 1.5 cm in length and begin at the medial limbus of the iris. Castroviejo calipers are a refined instrument to achieve the most studied symmetry, and measure-ments should be confirmed several times (both by calipers and by visual assessment) before commencement of the procedure. The distance from the medial canthus, the lid crease height, and the incision length should all be verified for symmetry. A total of 0.3 cc of 1% lidocaine with 1:50,000 epinephrine is infiltrated into the central aspect of each incision, and ten minutes are allowed to transpire before incision time to permit maximal hemostasis and full effect of the anesthesia. A Bard-Parker no. 15 blade is used to incise the skin and orbicularis-oculi muscle over both eyelids, and hemostasis is achie-ved using pinpoint needle cautery before proceeding. Attention is then turned to one eyelid, and a small wedge of orbital septum is incised to permit visualization and removal of the pre-aponeurotic middle fat pad. As the fat is identified, the remaining septum is incised along the entire length of the incision. As the fat prolapses forward, the surgeon can assess how much to remove. In order to maintain symmetry, the contralateral lid is addressed in the same fashion until the fat is exposed. With both fat pads exposed, half of the orbital fat is clamped on one side and removed. Hemostasis is achieved with electrocautery. The excised fat pad is laid adjacent to the fat pad on the other side and used as a gauge of how much fat should be removed from the contralateral bed. Under the fat pad should lie the glistening white levator aponeurosis. The levator is pierced superiorly to inferiorly with a 7-0 nylon suture (outfitted with a P-1 needle) and then passed through the dermal/epidermal edge of the inferior skin flap without actually traversing the entire thickness of the epidermis. This is a critical aspect as the needle must pass through the full thickness of the dermis and almost through the cornified layer of the epidermis but still remained buried. The lower skin edge is pulled upward until eyelash eversion is just noted. This suture is placed at the center of the incision, and the patient is asked to open his or her eyes to confirm appropriate lid height. The contralateral side is then addressed in a similar fashion and alternating sutures with 7-0 nylon are placed until a total of 5 to 6 sutures have been placed. The skin edges can then be approximated using 2 to 3 interrupted sutures. These skin sutures can be removed on the fourth postoperative day (Figs 35.2A and B, 35.3A and B).

Suture techniques have also been used with success in a patient intolerant of any recovery period, without need for fat removal, and cognizant of the risk for impermanence. Originally the use of silk sutures was described, but currently most authors prefer a mono-

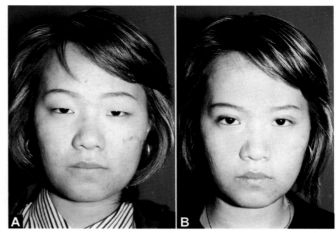

Figs 35.2A and B: Preoperative and postoperative frontal views

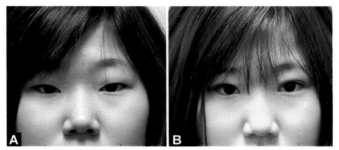

Figs 35.3A and B: Preoperative and postoperative frontal views

filament of 6-0 to 7-0 in size. However, some authors have suggested that the use of silk may engender a favorable tissue fibrosis that contributes to greater permanence of the lid adhesion. Just as in the partial-incision technique, the full length of eyelid does not need to be fixated to achieve complete crease adhesion. The exact same marked-line length and configuration described above for the partial-incision method can be used here. However, only half of the total drawn line is taken with each double-armed suture. Therefore, two sutures are required to fix each lid crease. The sutures are passed through-and-through from conjunctiva through the epidermis using double-armed sutures. The distance between the conjunctival sutures should be small whereas the distance between the epidermal sutures should be wide, i.e. each needle should be driven through asym-metrically with very close entry points and very widely spaced exit points. The exit points should be at one end of the marked line and the other at the halfway point. One needle is then driven through the epidermis under the skin to exit exactly at the other epidermal exit point without cutting the other suture. The two ends are then sawed back and forth so that the conjunctival suture

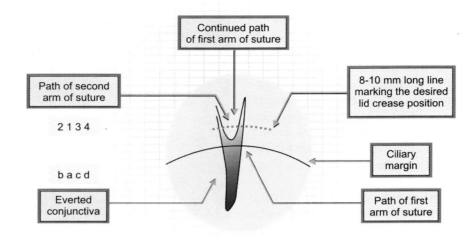

Fig. 35.4: Double-eyelid procedure

becomes progressively more buried in the conjunctiva rather than remain exposed to the cornea. The knot is then tied down, and the suture ends trimmed very close. The same technique is used to fix the remaining half of the marked line, and the same two sutures are undertaken on the other side to fix the contralateral lid.

Asian women and men in Asia, and particularly in Southeast Asia, are increasingly opting for plastic surgery. In literature a number of techniques for the creation of the double eyelid have been discussed. The technique chosen is based on surgeon preference, opinion and experience. Cultural sensitivity, anatomic knowledge, and technical expertise should guide every surgical effort. Despite misconceptions of the double-eyelid procedure as a method of fashioning a foreign 'Western' visage, the surgery more rightly represents an established technique that can achieve enhancement of the Asian eye within a purely Oriental context (Fig. 35.4).

REFERENCES

1. Sergile SL, Obata K. Mikamo's double-eyelid operation: The advance of Japanese aesthetic surgery. *Plast Reconstr Surg* 1997; 99:662.
2. Fernandez LR. Double eyelid operation in the Oriental in Hawaii. *Plast Reconstruct Surg* 1960; 25:257–264.
3. Fernandez LR. The East Asian eyelid: Open technique. *Clinic Plastic Surg* 1993; 20:247.
4. Yoon KC, Park S. Systematic approach in selective tissue removal and blepharoplasty for young Asians. *Plast Reconstruct Surg* 1998; 102(2):502–508.
5. Chen WP. Asian blepharoplasty: Update on anatomy and techniques. *Ophthalmol Plast Reconstruct Surg* 1987; 3(3): 135–140.
6. McCurdy JA. Double eyelid operation: External approach. *Facial Plast Surg Clin North Am* 1996a; 4(1):7–23.
7. McCurdy JA. Management of the epicanthal fold. *Facial Plast Surg Clin North Am* 1996b; 4(1):25–33.
8. Park JI. Z-Epicanthoplasty in Asian Eyelids. *Plast Reconstr Surg* 1996; 98:602–609.
9. Matsunaga RS. Westernization of the Asian eyelid. *Arch Otolaryngol* 1985; 111:149–153.
10. Boo-Chai K. Plastic construction of the superior palpebral fold. *Plast Reconstruct Surg* 1963; 31:74.
11. Choi AK. Oriental blepharoplasty: Nonincisional suture technique versus conventional incisional technique. *Facial Plast Surg* 1994; 10:67.
12. Yang H-H, Peterson RL. Asian blepharoplasty: Suture technique. *Facial Plast Surg Clin North Am* 1996; 4(1):35–40.
13. Homma K, Mutou Y, Mutou H, Ezoe K, Fujita T. Intradermal stitch blepharoplasty for orientals: Does it disappear? *Aesthetic Plast Surg* 2000; 24:289–291.
14. Jeong S, Lemke BN, Dortzbach RK, Park YG, Kang HK. The Asian upper eyelid: An anatomical study with comparison to the Caucasian eyelid. *Arch Ophthalmol* 1999; 117(7):907–912.
15. Park JS, Han KS, Yoon JK, Cho YJ. Study on the beauty sense for the eyes in Korean. *Kor J Plast Reconstruct Surg* 1990; 17:196.

The Use of Botulinum Toxin in the Head and Neck

Moshe Ephrat

Perhaps there has never been a product of nature that has had such a chequered career: from its known properties of being the most toxic substance to use in biological warfare and now with expanding use in all aspects of medicine. This protein, botulinum toxin (BTX), is commonly used in otolaryngology.

HISTORY OF *CLOSTRIDIUM BOTULINUM*

The German physician, health officer and poet Justinus Kerner first published an accurate description of the autonomic effects of BTX and the first clinical descriptions of food-borne botulism in 1817. He believed that a toxic substance in sausages was responsible for the clinical features of botulism. In 1822, he reviewed 155 poisoned patients and described their autonomic dysfunctions: 'The tear fluid disappears, the gullet becomes a dead and motionless tube; in all mucous cavities of the human machine the secretion of the normal mucus stands still, from the largest, the stomach, to the tear duct and the excretory ducts of the lingual glands. No saliva is secreted. No drop of wetness is felt in the mouth…'[1]

The Greek word for sausage is *botulus*, and botulism has been referred to the illness caused by eating spoilt sausages. This was known well before the actual toxin was described. In 1895, van Ermengem was called upon to investigate an episode of lethal food poisoning in Ellezelles, Belgium, where people had eaten uncooked ham at a wake. They displayed the same autonomic features that Justinus Kerner described in 1822. They suffered from nausea, paralytic ileus, postural hypotension, dry mouth, and no fever. After examining the autopsy specimens and the spoilt meat, van Ermengem described *Clostridium botulinum* and its exotoxins.[2]

For use as a biological weapon, the exotoxins were isolated. The United States government had begun research on the protection of its military from such uses in World War II. This research eventually resulted in the purification of BTX. When the threat to the United States military was over after the war had ended, the purified toxin was made available to other researchers who determined its mechanism of action.

In the 1960s, research in the use of Botox for human ailments began when Dr Alan Scott, an ophthalmologist treating strabismus with surgery, came into contact with a toxicologist, Dr Edward Schantz, who introduced him to his purified toxin and the possibility of its use to weaken hyperdynamic muscle. In 1980, their research led to the first published report of the use of Botox in humans for the non-surgical treatment of strabismus.[3]

The Food and Drug Administration (FDA) gave full approval for the use of Botox in strabismus, blepharospasm, and certain hemifacial spasms, in 1989. Its clinical use, however, was expanding rapidly in all facets of medicine; research proved its benefit in larger muscle groups as well as its use in improving facial wrinkles. In 1989, Dr Jean and Alastair Carruthers realized its benefits in the treatment of frown lines. Their blepharospasm patients treated with Botox had improved glabellar vertical creases. This led to their 1992 publication on the treatment of glabellar lines with Botox. By early 2003 FDA approval had included cervical dystonia as well as cosmetic treatment of glabellar wrinkles.[4]

DEFINING BOTULINUM TOXIN

The anerobic, gram-positive bacillus, *Clostridium botulinum*, produces BTX. This bacterium is found in soil, pond and lake sediments and is spore forming. There are seven different neurotoxins which are produced by

C. botulinum, designated as types A, B, C1, C2, D, E, F, and G. All are proteases with similar properties and similar structure, composed of a light chain linked by a disulfide bond to a heavy chain.[5]

Two serotypes are commercially available in the USA: Type A and type B. Botulinum toxin type A (BTX-A) is the most studied of the seven serotypes (Botox, Allergan Inc, Irvine California); it is approved by the FDA for use in the US for strabismus, blepharospasm, cervical dystonia, glabellar lines and VII nerve dysfunction. Subsequently, another botulinum toxin type A complex (Dysport, Ipsen) was approved in the United Kingdom in 1991; however, it is not available in the US.

Botulinum toxin type B (BTX-B) is also produced in the US (MyoBloc; Elan Pharmaceuticals, South San Francisco, California). BTX-B received FDA approval in January 2001 for use in patients with cervical dystonia. These two preparations have distinctly different sites of action and are antigenically different. They also have sufficiently different doses, efficacy and safety profiles and therefore, should not be considered equivalents comparable by dose ratios.

MECHANISM OF ACTION

Botulinum toxin interferes with the release of the neurotransmitter acetylcholine (ACh) from presynaptic nerve endings, resulting in temporary chemical denervation and muscular paralysis. The majority of commercial development of BTX for clinical use has been based on BTX-A. Clinical studies have found that BTX-A is more potent (less number of units needed per patient per session) than BTX-B.[6]

ACh is the major neurotransmitter involved in skeletal muscle contraction. The action of ACh in skeletal muscle occurs at the neuromuscular junction. ACh enters the synapse at this junction through its calcium-activated release from the presynaptic membrane. It then binds to receptors on the postsynaptic muscle membrane. These postsynaptic receptors then initiate the propagation of an action potential along the cell membrane of the skeletal muscle and ultimately skeletal contraction. It is the exocytosis of ACh from the presynaptic membrane, which is blocked by BTX-A and BTX-B.

Chemodenervation with BTX occurs through a three-step process. First, it is bound irreversibly to peripheral cholinergic nerve terminals. The toxin is then internalized through receptor-mediated endocytosis to the cytosol of the presynaptic nerve terminal. Lastly, the toxin is a protease that cleaves one of the essential proteins required for the release of ACh. These proteins include the vesicle-associated membrane protein (VAMP), synaptosome-associated protein (SNAP-25) and syntaxin. It is at this stage that the two serotypes differ. BTX-A targets SNAP-25 and BTX-B cleaves VAMP.[2,5,7]

When injected intramuscularly at localized therapeutic doses, BTX produces partial chemical denervation of the muscle resulting in a localized reduction in muscle activity. Recovery takes place after two phases. First accessory terminals sprout from the axon and stimulate muscle. One month later the main terminal begins to release ACh, possibly through synthesis of new SNAP-25 in the case of BTX-A.[6] After approximately three months recovery is complete and this correlates well with the duration of effect found clinically. In addition the muscle may atrophy, axonal sprouting may occur, and extrajunctional ACh may develop. There is evidence that reinnervation of the muscle may occur, thus slowly reversing muscle denervation produced by BTX (Botox Cosmetic Package Insert, Allergan). This explains the temporary effects seen clinically.

SAFETY AND ANTIGENICITY

Since the mechanism of action of BTX-A is very specific, side effects are uncommon and systemic effects are rare. The most common side effect may be considered muscle weakness in an undesired area or when weakness is greater than intended. In order to discuss toxicity one must understand the way in which BTX-A is supplied and dosed.

In the USA, BTX-A is supplied in 100 U vials of vacuum dried, purified crystalline toxin. A unit is defined in terms of its biological potency. The median lethal dose (LD50) has been determined in several animal species, but not humans. One (mouse) unit of BTX-A equals the LD50 for a 20 g Swiss-Webster mouse. The sensitivity of BTX-A varies among species. The LD50 of monkeys is determined to be 39 U/kg. Based on these findings involving primates, a human LD50 is estimated to be about 3000 units for a 70 kg adult (The doses used for cosmetic purposes are less than 100 units and 60–400 units in a single session for larger muscle groups). There have been no reported deaths resulting from overdose of BTX-A; however, antibody is available to treat massive overdose.[8]

As mentioned earlier, the most common adverse effects are either excessive weakness of the treated muscle or local diffusion of the neurotoxin from the injection site causing unwanted weakness of adjacent muscles.

For instance, ptosis may occur when treating blepharospasm or glabellar lines due to the levator muscle being affected. These adverse effects are usually mild and transient. The unintended weakening of local muscles is usually related to diffusion of toxin and accurate site of injection. Limiting the dose and volume of injection can minimize this. Electromyography has been described and used to more precisely treat certain muscle groups.[8]

Immunoresistance[27] has been reported in 3–5% of patients treated for cervical dystonia. This is possibly due to antibody formation to a specific protein in BTX. All BTX serotypes contain a neurotoxin protein and one or more non-toxin proteins. The neurotoxin protein is the active component and the other proteins protect it from degradation. Patients may develop antibodies to either of these proteins. Antibodies against the neurotoxin protein[28] will neutralize or interfere with the toxin's activity.[29] The incidence of neutralizing antibodies and immunoresistance is thought to be influenced by the patient's genetic characteristics and overall exposure to the neurotoxin complex protein. Overall exposure relates to protein load per effective dose, frequency of exposure and dosing experience.

Higher amounts of protein antigen exposure are usually associated with a higher probability of antibody formation.[9] This is supported by both ophthalmic and neurological literature. In a retrospective observation, it was noted that the mean dose of BTX-A when treating an episode of cervical dystonia was 150–300 U, while for blepharospasm it is 15–80 U. Clinically, antibody formation is a significant problem in cervical dystonia, while it is very uncommon in blepharospasm. This is believed to be due to higher doses of antigen per treatment in cervical dystonia.[10]

Since more frequent injections of protein antigen have been shown to increase the immunological response, it may also increase the risk of antibody formation. In fact, Greene et al recommend waiting as long as possible between treatment injections, avoiding booster injections and using the smallest possible amount of toxin.[11] The original BTX-A available from Allergan prior to December 1997 contained 25 ng of neurotoxin complex protein per 100 U. However, since December 1997 Allergan has decreased the protein load to 5 ng per 100 U.[12] Most of the data regarding resistance is with the old batch of BTX-A. The new batch is expected to have less antigenicity.

Furthermore, resistance to BTX-A does not necessitate resistance to BTX-B. While clinical effects of the two serotypes are similar, their target proteins are different.

As mentioned earlier, BTX-A cleaves SNAP-25, while BTX-B targets VAMP. Types A and B are distinct antigenically as well, that is, neutralizing antibodies to BTX-A do not protect against the effects of BTX-B.

Contraindications include infection at the injection site, pregnancy, active nursing, and pre-existing neuromuscular conditions. Patients with neuromuscular disorders (e.g. amylotrophic lateral sclerosis, myasthenia gravis or Lambert-Eaton syndrome) may be at increased risk of clinically significant systemic effects.

RECONSTITUTION

Botulinum type A produced by Allergan for the US is supplied in a lyophilized form in 100 U vials. It is reconstituted with a desired amount of preservative-free sterile saline. The amount of saline added determines the final concentration of the injected solution. Higher concentrations and therefore smaller volumes tend to keep the toxin and its effect in a more localized distribution, while smaller doses in higher volumes tend to give a more widespread effect with increasing likelihood of undesired muscle weakness. The volume of dilution ranges from 1–8 ml per 100 U vial.[13] Most physicians prefer to use a concentration of 2–4 ml per vial.

The toxin is thought to easily denature and is drawn into the vial by vacuum and is not agitated. Package insert indicates that prior to reconstituting BTX-A should be stored in a freezer at or below –5°C. After reconstitution it should be stored in a refrigerator at 2–8°C for up to 4 hours. Injections are performed with a 30-guage needle and 1 cc syringe. Clinical effects of BTX are usually seen within 1 week and will last about 3–5 months.

COSMETIC USES

Injection of BTX-A for cosmetic purposes has become the most common aesthetic procedure performed in the US.[30] The use of BTX-A for the treatment of glabellar lines was FDA approved in the USA in 2002. In 2001, injections of BTX were the most common nonsurgical cosmetic procedure performed with over 1.6 million treatments compared to only 65,000 in 1997.[14]

When treating patients for facial wrinkles it is imperative to obtain pretreatment and post-treatment photos in both relaxed and maximum contraction of the proposed treatment site. One must point out any visible pretreatment asymmetries that the patient may not realize are present.

Glabella BTX

It can be used to treat horizontal and vertical glabellar lines. These lines are produced secondary to hyperdynamic local musculature. The muscles that control a frown include corrugator and obicularis (medialize the brow and result in vertical lines) as well as the procerus and depressor supercilii (brow depressors and result in horizontal lines).

The BTX-A is reconstituted with 2.5 ml of non-preserved sterile saline. This will result in 40 U/ml or 4 U per 0.1 ml. The injections sites for the glabella include one to the procerus and two to each corrugator. The procerus injection is at a point in the midline just below the level of the medial brows. The next injections are at a vertical line from the medial canthus and one at the mid-pupillary line. They are injected at a level above the orbital rim and usually 1 cm above the eyebrow. Digital pressure with one's thumb at border of the supraorbital ridge may help prevent ptosis. Higher volume injections have a greater chance of diffusing downward and affecting the levator muscle resulting in ptosis. Each injection is of 4 U (0.1 ml) of BTX-A is used, resulting in a total of 20 U for this region. Some patients may require more BTX-A; however, this is a good starting point. The patient is then seen after 1–2 weeks and any areas that did not 'take' would then get a 'touch up'.

Complications may include local bruising, erythema, eyelid ptosis, and diplopia. Patients are reminded not to take aspirin and non-steroids to minimize chances of bruising. Diplopia may occur and is due to injections being placed too close to the bony orbital rim resulting in diffusion of toxin to a periocular muscle. Eyelid ptosis can occur if the toxin is injected too close to the superior orbital rim and migrates to the levator muscle. If ptosis does occur, it may be treated with alpha-adrenergic agonist eyedrops to the affected side (apraclonidine 0.5% or phenylepherine 2.5%). These drops cause contraction of Muller's muscle and will result in 1 to 2 mm elevation of the eyelash margin, making the patient more symmetrical. A dosage of 1–2 drops three times a day is used until the ptosis resolves (usually within four weeks).

Forehead

Forehead horizontal lines are due to hyperdynamic frontalis. This area may be treated with serial injections horizontally across the forehead at least 2.5 cm above the eyebrows. Sites are usually at vertical lines drawn from the medial and lateral canthi of the eyes. This results in four injection sites each getting 4 U (0.1 ml). For wider brows a fifth injection may be placed. One must realize that the frontalis is the brow elevator and therefore should not be treated without treating the glabella as well (brow depressors). Otherwise, the brow depressors will go unopposed and brow ptosis will result.

One must be careful to ensure that the lateral fibers of the frontalis muscle are adequately injected otherwise persistent lateral movement will result in a surprised or peaked eyebrow appearance. If this is noticed on follow-up evaluation it may be remedied by injecting a small amount into the frontalis, which is still active. Asymmetries may also be handled in this manner.

Crow's Feet

When squinting or smiling contraction of the lateral obicularis muscle results in crow's feet in the lateral canthal area. Crow's feet can be one of the earliest signs of aging. This is easily treated with BTX and experience shows significant patient satisfaction. Treatment involves two to three injections of 4 U each per side. One must palpate the lateral orbital rim and be sure to inject at least 1 cm lateral to this margin. This will prevent unwanted weakening of one of the lateral rectus muscle and the resultant diplopia. Injections are delivered very superficially in the intradermal plane. Treatments in this area carry a greater risk for bruising, and patients are notified of this.

Besides diplopia there have been reports of lip ptosis as well as drooping of the lateral aspect of the mouth due to inadvertent toxin effect on the zygomaticus major muscle. This muscle is adjacent to the obicularis and contributes to the medial and inferior crow's feet rhytides.[15,16]

Treatment of the Lower Third of the Face

Injections to the lower third of the face need to be given with extreme care and using small doses. Complications may include facial asymmetry. Areas include upper lip vertical rhytides, nasolabial folds, mentalis, and platysma.

SPASMODIC DYSPHONIA

This central neurological disorder results in spasms of the vocal cords. There are two types, adductor (causing glottal closing) and abductor (causing glottal opening) dysphonia. Patients with the adductor type have a strangled voice and breaks in pitch, while those with abductor type have a breathy voice.

In adductor dysphonia BTX-A is injected into the thyroarytenoid muscle to reduce the spasm. In abductor dysphonia the posterior cricoarytenoid muscle is injected. Bilateral posterior cricoarytenoid muscle treatments may be done, however not simultaneously, so as to avoid airway obstruction. Two weeks after one side is treated the patient returns for flexible laryngoscopy to confirm weakened but adequate abduction of the treated side. If adequate abduction is absent, then the contralateral treatment is avoided.

Patients with adductor spasmodic dysphonia show better response to treatment and report improvements in speech lasting about 3–4 months with each injection. Blitzer et al report excellent results with doses of 1 U bilaterally.[17] Abductor spasmodic dysphonia treatment tends to last a shorter time; this is probably because only a small dose may be used so there are no airway complications. These patients were treated with 3.75 U to one posterior cricoarytenoid muscle and re-evaluated in 2 weeks. If they are still symptomatic and have no respiratory complaints then the contralateral muscle is injected.

Complications of BTX-A treatments to the larynx are secondary to its diffusion and unintended effect on local muscles. Electromyography has been used to minimize complications by directing the physician to the appropriate muscle tissue and allowing the use of the smallest dose and volume of BTX-A. These may include breathiness, coughing on liquids, and stridor.

ESOPHAGEAL DISORDERS

Cricopharyngeal spasm could cause dysphagia and is know to complicate recovery of tracheoesophageal speech after laryngectomy.[18] Botulinum toxin injections to the cricopharyngeus muscle have been shown to alleviate dysphagia due to cricopharyngeal spasm in 70–100% of patients.[19,20] The cricopharyngeus can be approached both percutaneously through electromyographic guidance as well as endoscopically.

FACIAL DYSTONIAS

Facial dystonias are also treatable using BTX-A. Blepharospasm, hemifacial spasm, and the synkinesis seen with facial nerve recovery after paresis have all been helped with chemodenervation. When treating facial dystonias one must be aware of post-treatment facial asymmetry, ptosis, and diplopia.

HEADACHE

The first evidence of BTX-A being beneficial in patients with headaches was as a side effect of patients being treated for facial lines. This led to two randomized and controlled studies that showed the efficacy of this treatment for migraine headaches. These studies showed a significant reduction in the intensity and frequency of the attacks. Doses totaling as low as 25 U were effective and were administered into three pericranial muscle groups: frontalis, temporalis, and glabella.[21,22] Adverse events included blepharoptosis and diplopia.

FREY'S SYNDROME

The peripheral parasympathetic nervous system also uses ACh as a neurotransmitter and the use of BTX-A has proved successful in the treatment of gustatory sweating. Intracutaneous injections of BTX-A have been reported to be up to 100% effective, and lasts for at least 6 months; severity is reduced when compared to initial disease. Overtime repeat injections become unnecessary possibly due to sweat gland atrophy from chronic denervation.[23]

HYPERHIDROSIS

Primary hyperhidrosis is a chronic idiopathic disorder that can affect the axilla, palms, feet, and face. The profuse sweating may result in medical complications such as infection and skin maceration. Several therapies are available for the treatment of primary hyperhidrosis. These include topical aluminum chloride, systemic anticholinergics and direct surgical sympathectomy. Some of these treatments are short-lived and others have side effects, which may not be acceptable. Sympathectomy has its significant surgical risks and there have been reports of compensatory hyperhidrosis in other areas of the body after this method of treatment.[24,25]

Innervation of both the neuromuscular junction and the eccrine sweat glands use acetylcholine as the neurotransmitter. This is why BTX-A has been effective at treating both dynamic facial wrinkles and focal hyperhidrosis.

A 5–10 U injection of BTX-A intradermally produces an anhidrotic area of about 1.5 cm^2 within 6 days and lasts approximately 6 months. Naumann et al reported on a multicenter randomized clinical trial which was placebo controlled in Europe. Patients with axillary hyperhidrosis were given 50 U of BTX-A to each axilla with a 94% response by 4 weeks. The proportion of responders was significantly higher in the BTX-A group than the placebo group.[26]

When treating the palms or axilla a Minor starch iodine test is performed prior to treatment to determine the exact treatment area. Fifty U of BTX-A is then evenly distributed intradermally to each axilla or palm.

The average interval between retreatment should be about 6 months. Patients who play musical instruments or who require fine motor movements of their hands should be cautioned as transient (brief) grip weakness may occur after palmar treatment.

REFERENCES

1. Erbguth F. Botulinum toxin—a historical note. *Lancet* 1998; 351:1820–1830.
2. Blitzer A, Lucian S. Botulinum toxin: Basic science and clinical uses in otolaryngology. *Laryngoscope* 2001; 111:218–226.
3. Scott AB. Botulinum toxin injection into extraocular muscles as an alternative to strabismus surgery. *Ophthalmology* 1980; 87:1044–1049.
4. Carruthers JDA, Carruthers JA. Treatment of glabellar frown lines with *C botulinum* A exotoxins. *J Dermatol Surg Oncol* 1992; 18:17–21.
5. Brin MF. Botulinum toxin therapy: Chemistry, pharmacology, toxicity, and immunology. *Muscle Nerve* 1997; Suppl 6: S146–168.
6. Sloop RR, Cole BA, Escutin RO. Human response to botulinum toxin injection: Type A compared with type B. *Neurology* 1997; 49:189–194.
7. Setler P. The biochemistry of botulinum toxin type B. *Neurology* 2000; 55(suppl 5):22–28.
8. Childers MK, Wilson DJ, Simison D. Key facts. In *Use of botulinum toxin type A in pain management: A clinician's guide.* Columbia: Academic Information Systems 1999; 4–5.
9. Goschel H, Wohlfarth K, Frevert J et al. Botulinum A toxin therapy: Neutralizing and nonneutralizing antibodies— therapeutic consequences. *Exp Neurol* 1997; 147:96–102.
10. Brodic G, Johnson E, Goodnough M et al. Botulinum toxin therapy, immunologic resistance, and problems with available materials. *Neurology* 1996; 46:26–29.
11. Greene P, Fahn S, Diamond B. Development of resistance to botulinum toxin type A in patients with torticollis. *Mov Disord* 1994; 9:213–217.
12. Allergan Publication. Immunological considerations in botulinum neurotoxin therapy. March 2001.
13. Klein AW. Dilution and storage of botulinum toxin. *Dermatol Surg* 1998; 24:1179.
14. American Society for Aesthetic Plastic Surgery statistics on cosmetic surgery. www.surgery.org.
15. Garcia A and Fulton JE. Cosmetic denervation of the muscles of facial expression with botulinum toxin: A dose–response study. *Dermatol Surg* 1996; 22:39.
16. Matarasso SL, Matarasso A. Treatment guidelines for botulinum toxin type A for the periocular region and a report on partial upper lip ptosis following injections to the lateral canthal rhytids. *Plast Reconstr Surg* 2001; 108:208–214.
17. Blitzer A, Brin MF, Stewart CF. Botulinum toxin management of spasmodic dysphonia (laryngeal dystonia): A 12-year experience in more than 900 patients. *Laryngoscope* 1998; 108:1435–1441.
18. Zormeier MM, Meleca RJ, Simpson ML et al. Botulinum toxin injection to improve tracheoesophageal speech after total laryngectomy. *Otolaryngol Head Neck Surg* 1999; 120:314–319.
19. Ahsan SF, Meleca RJ, Dworkin JP. Botulinum toxin injection of the cricopharyngeal muscle for the treatment of dysphagia. *Otolaryngol Head Neck Surg* 2000; 122:691–695.
20. Blitzer A, Brin MF. Use of botulinum toxin for diagnosis and management of cricopharyngeal achalasia. *Otolaryngol Head Neck Surg* 1997; 116:328–330.
21. Brin MF, Swope DM, O'Brian C et al. Botox for migraine: Double-blind, placebo-controlled region-specific evaluation. *Cephalalgia* 2000; 20:421–422.
22. Silberstein S, Mathew N, Saper J et al. Botulinum toxin A as a migraine preventive treatment. *Headache* 2000; 40:445–450.
23. Laccourreye O, Akl E, Gutierrez-Fonseca R et al. Recurrent gustatory seating (Frey's syndrome) after intracutaneous injection of botulinum toxin type A: Incidence, management and outcome. *Arch Otolarngol Head Neck Surg* 1999; 125(3): 283–286.
24. Stolman LP. Treatment of hyperhidrosis. *Dermatol Clin* 1998; 16:863–867.
25. Herbst F, Plas EG, Fugger R, Fritsch A. Endoscopic thoracic sympathectomy for primary hyperhidrosis of the upper limbs: A critical analysis and long-term results of 480 operations. *Ann Surg* 1994; 220:86–90.
26. Naumann N, Lowe NJ. Botulinum toxin type A in treatment of bilateral primary axillary hyperhidrosis: Randomized, parallel group, double blind, placebo controlled trial. *Br Med J* 2001; 323:1–4.
27. Jakovic J, Schwartz K. Response and immunoresistance to botulinum toxin injections. *Neurology* 1995; 45:1743–1746.
28. Sakaguchi G. *Clostridium botulinum* toxins. *Pharmacol Ther* 1983; 19:165–194.
29. Siegel LS. Evaluation of neutralizing antibodies to type A, B, E, and F botulinum toxins in sera from human recipients of botulinum pentavalent (ABCDE) toxoid. *J Clin Microbiol* 1989; 27:1906–1908.
30. Yin S, Stucker FJ, Nathan CA. Clinical application of botulinum toxin in otolaryngology head and neck practice (brief review). *J La State Med Soc* 2001; 153(2):92–97.

Transconjunctival Lower Lid Blepharoplasty

Mathew Karen

Transconjunctival lower lid blepharoplasty has gained much popularity in the facial cosmetic surgery field within the last ten years. Originally described in the 1920s in France and revisited by Baylis in the late 1980s, it has now become a procedure of choice for many renowned facial plastic surgeons.[1]

In the mid 1980s, the transconjunctival approach was instituted as a method to repair malar complex fractures. Together with a lateral cantholysis, exposure for fracture repair was unprecedented. External incisions were not needed and therefore the risk of ectropion was virtually eliminated. This technique paved the way to approach lower lid blepharoplasty through the transconjunctival incision.[2]

Transcutaneous lower lid blepharoplasty, a surgically sound procedure to remove psuedoherniated orbital fat as well as excess skin and muscle, has been the gold standard approach for the lower lid. Wide exposure is easily achieved, and skin/muscle can be addressed through the same incision. However, a known, common and dreaded complication, lid malposition/ectropion, is a significant concern. Transconjunctival lower lid blepharoplasty virtually eliminates this risk. Exposure to all three fat pads is excellent. Excess skin is addressed through a 'pinch' excision. The anterior lamella (muscle sling) is not violated; therefore ectropion is avoided. Combining this approach with chemo-exfoliation, the lower lid is tightened, rejuvenating a patient's appearance and enhancing the overall result. Chemical peeling can be undertaken at the same operative session. Since the skin/muscle is left intact (no flap elevation) full-thickness skin injury due to chemical burn is not seen.[2]

This chapter will focus on giving an overview of the transconjunctival approach to lower lid blepharoplasty and will explain the surgical anatomy of the lower lid,

the transconjunctival technique and its complications, and proper selection of patient.

SURGICAL ANATOMY OF THE LOWER LID

The lower lid comprises various anatomic layers. These mimic that of the upper lid. A clear knowledge and understanding of these anatomic relationships are paramount when attempting transconjunctival lower lid blepharoplasty.

Transconjunctival blepharoplasty approaches the orbital fat posteriorly, through the posterior lamella. Therefore, anatomic relationships are reversed from the traditional techniques. The posterior lamella consists of the conjunctiva, the capsulopalpebral fascia, the posterior septum, and the tarsus.[3]

In the sagittal plane, the tarsal plate is found in the superior aspect of the lower lid just deep to the conjunctiva, running medial to lateral across the entire lid. Its superior/inferior dimension is 4 mm, less than half its upper lid counterpart. Below the tarsus, capsulopalpebral fascia extends to the orbital septum, which divides to surround the orbital fat. The septum is confluent with the periorbita and periosteum of the orbit. It is through the posterior orbital septum that the transconjunctival blepharoplasty technique approaches orbital fat. This technique preserves the anterior lamella. The anterior lamella consists of the anterior septum, orbicularis oculi muscle, and eyelid skin and is the outermost layer in posterior to anterior dimensions in the sagittal plane.[3]

In the coronal plane, there exist important anatomic considerations as well. The orbital fat is located in three distinct regions from medial to lateral. Medially, there is a small pale fat pad. The central fat pad lies lateral to this and is separated from the medial fat pad by the inferior oblique muscle. A fascial arcuate expansion from the inferior oblique separates the central fat pad from the lateral fat pad. It is these fatty deposits that are addressed in lower lid blepharoplasty. The inferior oblique muscle is an important landmark and must be identified in order to preserve its function.

These anatomic relationships are constant. Once mastered, transconjunctival lower lid blepharoplasty is quite successful in rejuvenating the lower lid.

PATIENT SELECTION

Proper patient selection is critical in order to achieve the desired result. Certain patients are ideal candidates for transconjunctival lower lid blepharoplasty: those with familial, hereditary, dermatochalasis show excellent results after surgery. These patients are usually young (15–40 years of age), and on examination only demonstrate psuedoherniation of orbital fat. Patients aged 40–55 years with psuedoherniation of fat and minimal skin excess also show excellent results. Transconjunctival lower lid blepharoplasty combined with either pinch excision or chemical peel will also show excellent results. Patients undergoing revision lower lid blepharoplasty are likewise good candidates for the transconjunctival approach. Residual or recurrent fat herniation is easily addressed. This technique can also improve mild lid malpositions in patients with rounding and/or scleral show preoperatively. Patients with lower lid laxity preoperatively could be protected from lid malposition if transconjunctival lower lid blepharoplasty were performed. Finally, patients who request no external scarring as well as dark-skinned patients are also possible candidates.[2]

SURGICAL TECHNIQUE

Transconjunctival lower lid blepharoplasty is usually performed in conjunction with other rejunvenative procedures[5] (upper lid, brow lift, rhytidectomy). When done as a single procedure, transconjunctival lower lid blepharoplasty can be performed in the office under local anesthesia and oral sedation. One milligram of xanax, given 20 minutes preoperatively, relaxes the patient; 1–2 drops of 0.5% topical tetracaine ophthalmic solution is then placed on the conjunctiva. The upper face is then prepped with a 5% betadine eye solution. The lower lid is then retracted with a small Desmarre's retractor and 1% with 1/100,000 epinephrine local anesthesia is used to anesthetize the conjunctiva from the punctum medially

to the lateral canthus. After waiting approximately ten minutes for the vasoconstrictive properties to take effect, needle tip cautery is used to open the conjunctiva from lateral to medial, stopping 4 mm before the level of the inferior punctum. This incision is located approximately 5 mm inferior to the tarsal plate. Once the conjunctiva is opened a 5/0 silk suture is used to retract the conjunctiva cephalad, in order to protect the cornea. This suture is clamped and placed over the eye on forehead. Dissection then turns laterally and the lower lid retractors are opened visualizing the orbital septum. Light pressure on the globe will allow the surgeon to see the fat bulging. A small nick is made in the septum and the fat is teased out gently. The base of the fat pad is injected with local anesthetic and is then cauterized with a bipolar instrument to prevent heat transmission posteriorly in the orbit. One must be careful not to forcibly remove fat, but only remove what comes easily. The fat pad stump is carefully examined for bleeding and is then allowed to retract into its bed.

The central fat pad is approached in same manner. Small fascial attachment separate the lateral and central fat pads. Once the fascia is divided the septum is seen and opened allowing the central fat pad to be teased out. Again, this is helped by lightly pressing on the globe. After injecting the base of the fat pad with anesthetic it is cauterized at the two poles and excised. The stump is inspected for bleeding and after hemostasis is achieved, the pad is allowed to retract into its bed. Finally, the medial fat pad is approached. The medial fat pad is separated from the central fat pad by the inferior oblique muscle. This muscle is identified and medial dissection through the capsulopalpebral fascia allows you to view the septum. The medial fat pads usually lies in the most medial aspect of your incision. Light global pressure allows you to see it bulge. The orbital septum is opened and a more pale fat pad is encountered. It is carefully teased outward, injected, cauterized, and excised. After achieving hemostasis the pad is allowed to retract. This completes the fat pad treatment. The conjunctival suture is removed and the conjunctiva is placed in its normal anatomic position. The lower lid is repositioned as well. There is no need to close the conjunctival incision. The removed fat is placed on a side table for comparison with the other side.

The surgeon can now address the external lower lid deformities. Pinch excision of skin will address the excess lower lid skin problem: the skin alone is removed, thereby preserving the anterior lamella and preventing various forms of ectropion. Thereafter 1% lidocaine with

1/100,000 epinephrine is injected below the lash line. A straight hemostat is used to pinch 1–2 mm of skin at the lower lid crease. Once removed the excess skin is tented outwards. It is excised with small scissors. Up to five simple 6/0 prolene sutures are evenly placed across the excision line to hold the skin in place.

If only fine rhytids are present on the lower lid skin, a concomitant 35% trichloroacetic acid peel can be applied to the skin. This will tighten the skin and efface these fine lines. This is a safe and effective procedure; the anterior lamella is preserved and therefore the blood supply is not violated.

COMPLICATIONS

As with all surgical procedures transconjunctival lower lid blepharoplasty too carries risks and complications. However, it has gained popularity because risks are relatively few. The most common complication stemming from transcutaneous lower lid blepharoplasty, lid malposition, is avoided.[4] In the transconjunctival approach the anterior lamella is kept intact thereby preventing scar formation and lower lid malposition. Even when pinch excision is additionally performed to address excess skin the orbicularis muscle is preserved. Its anatomic position relative to the orbital septum is not disrupted; therefore citrical scarring is avoided. The author therefore advocates a posterior septal approach to orbital fat.

The most common complication resulting from transconjunctival lower lid blepharoplasty is inadequate fat removal (often by an overly conservative surgeon). The approach affords excellent exposure and is not the cause. Other minor complications include excess lower lid skin and/or excessive wrinkling postoperatively. These problems are addressed by performing either a pinch excision of skin or chemical peel concurrently with transconjunctival blepharoplasty.[3]

Major complications seen with all types of blepharoplasty are postoperative hematoma, blindness, injury to ocular musculature, and infection; these may need to be addressed with each patient preoperatively.

CONCLUSION

Eyelid surgery can be an important part of the rejuvenation process for many individuals. In order to obtain a superior, repeatable result the blepharoplasty surgeon must master the surgical anatomy. Once the surgeon is comfortable, a successful outcome is routinely encountered.

When performing aesthetic surgery, procedures must be chosen that offer superior results with a minimal risks of complications. Lower lid transconjunctival blepharoplasty affords the surgeon a direct approach to the orbital fat without violating the anterior lamella, thereby avoiding lid malposition, the most common complication of transcutaneous lower lid blepharoplasty; however, in transconjunctival lower lid blepharoplasty it is virtually unseen.

Transconjunctival lower lid blepharoplasty is an excellent means to rejuvenate the lower lid. On selected patients excellent results are routine. Performed with care and meticulous technique, longlasting desirable outcomes are the norm. Over the last decade, this approach has gained favor with many facial plastic surgeons.

REFERENCES

1. Baylis HI, Long JA, Groth MJ. Transconjunctival lower eyelid blepharoplasty—Technique and complications. *Ophthalmology* 1989; 96(7):1027–1032.
2. Perkins SW, Dyer II WK, Simo F. Transconjunctival approach to lower eyelid blepharoplasty – Experience, indications, and techniques in 300 patients. *Arch Otolaryngol Head Neck Surg* 1994; 120:172–177.
3. Waldman SR. Transconjunctival blepharoplasty: Minimizing the risks of lower lid blepharoplasty. *Facial Plastic Surg* 1994; 10:27–41.
4. Palmer III FR, Rice DH, Churukian MM. Transconjunctival blepharoplasty—Complications and their avoidance: A retrospective analysis and review of the literature. *Arch Otolaryngol Head Neck Surg* 1993; 119:993–999.
5. Zarem HA, Resnick JI. Operative technique for transconjunctival lower blepharoplasty. *Clin Plastic Surg* 1992; 19:351–356.

CHAPTER 38

Facial Contouring—Malar and Chin Augmentation

Edward W Chang, Edward H Farrior

While patients seeking advice about facial cosmetic surgery often focus on structures such as the nose, the eyes, and the laxity of their skin, the facial plastic surgeon's assessment frequently identifies areas of the face that could be surgically modified to improve overall appearance and harmony. When considering facial augmentation, the surgeon contemplates the face not just as bony protuberances, but rather as three-dimensional prominences consisting of soft tissue components and bone. Additionally, areas such as the chin are considered in relationship to other structures, like the nose. The smaller the chin, the larger the nose appears. Augmenting the chin thus gives the nose a diminished appearance (Fig. 38.1).

These relationships are critical to facial balance. The profile of a patient can be significantly altered with facial contouring. This, in turn, has a significant effect on overall facial aesthetics. The goal of facial contouring is to produce a natural appearance of youth and beauty by enhancing or restoring structure, and creating the smooth

facial contour that tends to degrade with age. Several surgical options exist for the augmentation of the face. Alloplastic implants, autogenous grafts and bony osteotomies represent the currently accepted methods of augmentation. Alloplastic facial implants offer the reconstructive surgeon many advantages over autogenous tissue, including availability of material and simplification of operative procedure. Care must be taken to choose the proper implant characteristics for the desired aesthetic result, since each synthetic material has unique properties. With all implant types and materials, careful surgical technique is essential in minimizing the risks of extrusion and infection.

ANALYSIS

The components of the face profoundly influencing facial beauty are the malar–midface region, the nose, and the chin. Facial aesthetics are determined by the size, shape, and position of these individual features. Although it is important to evaluate soft tissue contours, the skeletal structures support the soft tissues, and proper proportions of the skeletal areas help determine a more complete facial aesthetic. Therefore, proper movement or augmentation of the underlying skeletal structures will yield a pleasing soft tissue contour.[1] Three-dimensional CT reconstructions are currently available and greatly assist the evaluation of the bony structures, and also allow for custom-fabricated implants.

The preoperative consultation should include a complete history and physical (including dental) evaluation, along with standard facial photographs. The patient should be evaluated from at least six angles, including frontal, right/left lateral, right/left oblique, and basal views. Additionally, analysis of the frontal view with the patient smiling is crucial to evaluate skeletal

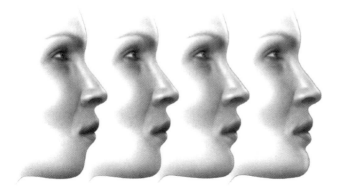

Fig. 38.1: The position of the chin has a profound influence on the perceived projection of the nose. As the chin position alone is changed, notice the effect on nasal projection

deformities. The smiling AP view will help define maxillary excess or deficiencies (Fig. 38.2C). It is normal to have 0–3 mm of maxillary teeth to be visible in repose. Beyond this point, maxillary vertical excess is suspected. In the lateral view, nasal ptosis and lip incompetence can be seen (Fig. 38.2D). It is standard to divide the face into horizontal thirds, from the hairline to the glabella, the glabella to the subnasale (where the nasal columella meets the upper lip), and subnasale to the menton. Vertically, the face is divided into fifths. The eyes and the nose are generally equal to a fifth (Fig. 38.2A). There are alternative ways to evaluate the face, especially if the hairline is missing. The lower two-thirds of the face is evaluated alone, from the nasal starting point called nasion to the chin. The midface is 43% of this region and the lower third comprises the rest (Fig. 38.2B). Assess asymmetry in the transverse dimension by using standard photographs on frontal view. Asymmetry may exist for various reasons, and it is crucial to appreciate asymmetry preoperatively. Asymmetry in the chin can be corrected easily with an offset (transverse) genioplasty. The overall face is also considered, mindful that a youthful face has qualities such as smooth, full cheeks, and symmetric contours. The malar area and chin should also be assessed to determine if they are in harmony with the remainder of the face.

The malar eminence is evaluated in context of other facial features, including overall facial form, chin position, and nasal projection. One method of analyzing the malar involves the use of anatomical landmarks and reference lines. A line is formed from the outer canthus of the eye to the ipsilateral oral commissure. Another line is created from the superior tragus to the ipsilateral nasal alar. The intersection of these lines represents the ideal location for the most prominent point of the malar complex, which is thought to be the most important aspect of the oblique view.[2] The malar prominence should be about one-third of the distance down the line drawn from the lateral canthus to the oral commissure.[3] Malar deficiency can also be divided into an anteromedial, posterolateral, or a combination of these areas. The dividing vertical line is made perpendicular to the Frankfurt horizontal, at the lateral canthus. The anteromedial segment includes part of the infraorbital rim, and the anterior buttress formed by the zygoma. The posterolateral segment is made up of the zygomatic arch and some of the malar eminence and the lateral orbital rim.[4] This analysis helps determine the treatment plan that conjoins the surgeon's conception of facial beauty with the desires of the patient. The facial plastic surgeon should also be aware that facial defects vary among patients and may differ from one side of the face to the other. Any facial asymmetries should be brought to the patient's attention and documented in written and photographic form. The surgeon should carefully analyze and identify patterns of mid-face and chin deficiencies in order to choose the most appropriate technique and augmentation.

Terino (1999) has described five zones of facial contouring:[5]

- *Zone 1*: This includes the major portion of the malar bone and the first third of the zygomatic arch. Projection of the malar eminence—creating a high, sharp, angular appearance—is produced when this region is augmented.

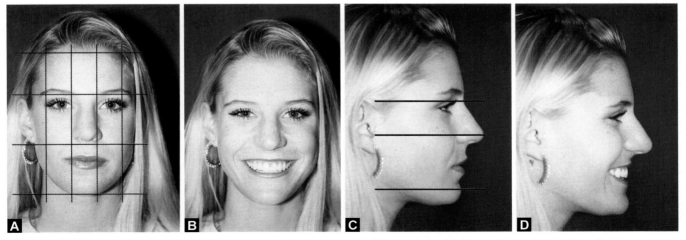

Figs 38.2A to D: (A) Standard horizontal thirds and vertical fifths analysis. (B) Alternative analysis of Powell, where the mid face is 43% and the lower third is approximately 57%. (C) A smiling AP view to access vertical maxillary excess. (D) A smiling lateral to access lip incompetence and nasal tip movement

- *Zone 2:* The middle third of the zygomatic arch constitutes zone 2. When this area is augmented with zone 1, the upper third of the face appears broader, as the cheekbone is accentuated laterally.
- *Zone 3:* This lies between the infraorbital foramen and the nasal bone. Augmentation of the paranasal area creates medial fullness in the infraorbital region.
- *Zone 4:* The posterior third of the zygomatic arch comprises zone 4. Augmentation in this area should be avoided because it creates an unnatural appearance and places branches of the facial nerve at risk.
- *Zone 5:* This is the submalar triangle.

The reasons for facial augmentation and contouring are:

- Post-traumatic reconstruction
- Congenital deformities
- Midface, and/or chin hypoplasia
- Facial senescense with atrophy and soft tissue ptosis
- Facial disharmony, long narrow face or a round full face
- Unbalanced aesthetic triangle

The goals of augmentation are:

- To reconstruct surgically or traumatically created tissue voids
- To restore bulk to ptotic tissues in order to rejuvenate soft tissue folds or rhytides
- To augment the face for cosmetic enhancement

When facial analysis identifies a patient's profile with facial disharmony in the lower third of the face, one must determine whether there is an underlying occlusal and skeletal deformity or if the mentum is merely poorly projected or over projected. When the poor projection is skeletal in nature, the situation is considered an Angle's Class II skeletal deformity. The Angle skeletal classification is based on the position of the first molar (Fig. 38.3).

In retrognathia, the mesiobuccal cusp of the maxillary first molar is mesial (or anterior to) the buccal groove of the mandibular first molar. If only hypoplasia of the mandible exists, the term micrognathia is more accurate and should be used. When there is no skeletal malformation, the terms for a recessed chin include retrogenia, microgenia, retruded chin, hypoplastic mentum, and horizontal mandibular hypoplasia. In chin augmentation, genioplasty usually implies an osseous movement, whereas mentoplasty suggests the use of an alloplastic implant. However, the two terms are currently used synonymously.

For a genioplasty, dental occlusion and skeletal structures are evaluated using preoperative photography as well as a lateral cephalometric soft-tissue study and panoramic radiographs. Dental models should be fabricated, and are extremely important in the work-up. Functional and cosmetic goals should be discussed with the patient. For patients undergoing sliding genioplasty, complete cephalometric tracings and measurements should be generated. Cephalometric evaluation includes measurements of sella-nasion-subspinale A-point of the maxilla (S-N-A) and sella-nasion-supramentale B-point of the mandible (S-N-B) angles to provide information on the sagittal relationship between the anterior skull base and the maxilla and mandible, respectively (Fig. 38.4).[6] The soft-tissue and lip-profile yields a tremendous amount of information on the chin projection. As with the midface, the evaluation of the chin prominence can be accomplished many different ways. In Burstone's analysis, a vertical line tangential to the subnasale and pogonion is used as a reference plane. Ideally, the upper

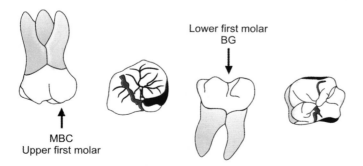

Fig. 38.3: The Angle skeletal classification is based on the position of the first molar

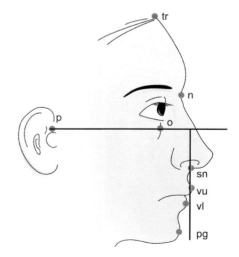

Fig. 38.4: Cephalometric evaluation is based on tracings and measurements of these points

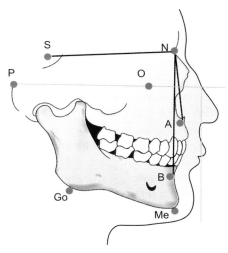

Fig. 38.5: One of the methods of evaluation

lip lies 3.5 mm anterior, and the lower lip lies 2.2 mm anterior to this line. Ricketts draws a vertical line tangential to the nasal tip and pogonion. The upper lip should rest 4 mm behind this line, and the lower lip 2 mm. Gonzalez-Ulloa uses the Frankfurt plane and a line designated as the zero-degree meridian. The Frankfurt plane is a horizontal line from the upper external auditory canal to the infraorbital rim. The zero-degree meridian is perpendicular to the Frankfurt plane and is started at nasion. If the chin is behind the zero-degree meridian, it is considered retruded.[1] Another method drops a line perpendicular to the Frankfurt plane through sub nasale. The upper lip should be at this vertical ± 2 mm, the lower lip behind this line by 2 mm ± 2 mm, and the chin should be 4 mm posterior (Fig. 38.5). Deficits that are measured in this manner can be used to determine osteotomy movements, since bony advance-ment in this area usually yields an equivalent movement of the soft tissue.[7]

Determine the vertical height of the face, by employing the method described by Powell and Humphreys.[8] Use this information to advise the patient of the choices available for obtaining the best result. If a skeletal abnormality exists, one must suggest orthodontic realignment and orthognathic surgery as a surgically alternative. When the patient desires a purely cosmetic correction, discuss options of alloplastic implant augmentation versus a sliding genioplasty. If the deformity is addressable by either of these treatment options, recommendations are based on the severity of the deformity and concomitant facial procedures being considered.[9]

In addition to the analysis of the facial contours, the character of the overlying skin and soft tissue should be assessed. The thickness and quality of soft tissue influences implant size and positioning.

Detailed preoperative counseling allows the surgeon and the patient to discuss and evaluate the desired changes. Computer imaging is often a useful teaching tool and helps discussion. It is important to emphasize to the patient that a digitally altered image may not be representative of the actual surgical changes.[3]

IMPLANTS

Alloplastic materials such as ivory, acrylic, and precious metals have been used in the past, but are now primarily of historic interest. Other materials such as silicone, polytetrafluoroethylene and polyamide mesh have been popular as well.[10] New materials for implants are now in use, including softer ones (Soft form II, Collagen Corp., Palo Alto, CA and Adventa, Atrium Medical Corp., Hudson, NH) and harder ones (Medpor, Porex, Fairburn, GA). Each has specific benefits as well as disadvantages.

Several general qualities contribute to the biocompatibility of an implant, the most important being the risk of a chronic inflammatory response or foreign body reaction. Lack of immunogenicity and carcinogenicity are also favorable implant characteristics.[11] Implant material must be non-degradable and should be amenable to contouring.[12]

Alloplastic implants have been used for centuries in cosmetic and reconstructive surgery. Implants placed in the cheek and malar area are used in aesthetic and reconstructive practices to achieve symmetry and balance. Autogenous grafts, as well as bony osteomies have also been a part of the surgeon's armamentarium. The most convincing argument with grafts and osteotomies used for facial augmentation is that they are autogenous, and do not cause a foreign body reaction.

Alloplastic Implants

Alloplastic implants offer many advantages over reconstruction using autogenous tissue, including availability of material and less operative time required. When insufficient autogenous material is available or donor site morbidity is of concern, alloplastic implants can provide the augmentation without the need for patient tissue harvest. The wide variety of compositions of synthetic materials allows the surgeon to choose a specific combination which best suits the patient.

The success of synthetic implants depends upon the interaction between implant material and host reaction, and this biocompatibility hinges on numerous factors, including the characteristics of the material, the proposed location and function of the implant, and the handling of the implant by the surgeon. The ideal implant material has not been discovered, but implant materials should be non-toxic, non-carcinogenic, and should not elicit an inflammatory reaction.[13] Cost should not be a limiting factor. Advances in surgery such as sterile and 'no-touch' operative techniques as well as broad spectrum antibiotics have reduced the incidence of implant infection.[14]

Implant Materials

The wide range of implantable synthetic materials can be divided into three categories:
- Non-carbon-based polymers
- Carbon-based polymers (including aliphatic polyesters and acrylics)
- Calcium phosphate ceramics.

Each of these materials differs in strength, flexibility, durability, resistance to infection, and tissue in-growth.[13]

Non-carbon-based Polymers

Silicon can be polymerized into silicone, which can exist either as a liquid (i.e., silicone 'gel') or vulcanized into solid rubber, the most common form for facial implants. Silicone can be commercially preformed or carved into custom shapes, and is also available in 'room temperature vulcanized' form, or RTV silicone, which, upon mixing, can be molded or implanted before it hardens. The material is highly resistant to degradation, and because of its silicon-oxygen bonds has a high degree of chemical inertness. In solid form, silicone has not caused significant clinical toxicity or allergic reactions. However, in the liquid or gel form, silicone is not as inert and can incite a chronic inflammatory reaction. The body reacts to silicone implants by forming a capsule without in-growth of tissue, and this capsule usually remains stable throughout the life of the implant. An advantage over the porous or textured implants, is that the encapsulation of the silicone implant allows for it to be removed with greater ease.

Silicone was first reported for use in facial implants in 1953 by Brown, and since then silicone (dimethylsiloxane) has been used in the augmentation of frontal, zygomatic, nasal, chin, parasymphyseal, paranasal, orbital, maxillary, malar, nasal dorsum, ear, and mandibular deficiencies.[15] Because silicone has 'memory', adaptation to bone contour must be passive, since bending may lead to extrusion or bone resorption.[11] These implants can be easily fixed with a screw or a suture to adjacent tissues. When silicone implants are fixed against a bony surface in their solid form, long-term stability is very high.[16] Porous silicone implants and silicone bonded to Dacron have been used to enhance stability. The use of porous silicone implants should be limited to areas of minimal or no tissue stress, because when subjected to continual mechanical loading, silicone has a tendency to fragment and deteriorate.[14]

Silicone implants retain their strength and flexibility though a wide range of temperatures and can easily be sterilized using steam autoclave or irradiation without damaging the material.[13]

One complication of silicone implants is extrusion: rates are as high as 5%. Care must be taken to place the implant under a thick, well-vascularized flap without tension, and be wary of placing an implant under previously irradiated or scarred tissue. In a 5-year retrospective study, silastic malar implants were found to be safe and effective in treating malar hypoplasia and facial asymmetry.[14]

Silicone implants are popular because of their cost and comfort.

Carbon-based Polymers

Carbon-based polymers have been used in various forms for decades and include polytetrafluoroethylene (PTFE), polyethylene (PE), aliphatic polyesters, and acrylics. PTFE, an ethylene monomer with four fluorine moieties attached, is a spongy material and was originally introduced in the 1980s as Proplast (Formly Vitek, Houston, Texas) The original Proplast (Proplast I) was black and consisted of Teflon (PTFE) and graphite, and was replaced by Proplast II, which, is a white material composed of Teflon and aluminum oxide. It is a porous material with pore sizes of 50–400 μm in diameter, allowing fibrovascular tissue in-growth. Proplast was discontinued after its recall by the Food and Drug Administration (FDA). This was due to a high number of failures seen in temporomandibular joint reconstructions when used as a glenoid fossa replacement. In this setting, repetitive mechanical forces led to the breakdown of the implant material and cause subsequent inflammatory foreign body reaction. Proplast is no longer manufactured in the USA.[13]

PTFE has been re-introduced by Gore and associates (Flagstaff, Arizona) as Gore-Tex, an expanded microporous polymer of PTFE (e-PTFE) that has proven very useful in the augmentation of many soft tissue and bone defects. Easily cut or shaped for facial contour augmentation, Gore-Tex is available in a variety of preformed implants, blocks, 1, 2, and 4 mm sheets, and strands. Pore sizes range from 10 to 30 microns, and allow for limited fibrovascular in-growth. Gore-Tex generally forms a fibrous capsule, which facilitates easy removal in the event of infection or revision. Expanded polytetrafluoroethylene (e-PTFE) is by far the most commonly used synthetic implantable material for soft tissue augmentation.[17] In facial plastic applications, it is marketed as Soft-Form or Gore-Tex subcutaneous augmentation material (SAM), and has been used extensively for nasolabial fold and lip augmentation, because the material is well-tolerated and easily placed. The recipient pocket should be made to fit the implant snugly. To promote tissue stabilization of the implant, Soft-Form (Collagen Corp, Palo Alto, CA) was made into a tubular form, providing an avenue for tissue in-growth. Complaints of this product included implant firmness and visibility. On removal, there was evidence of contraction of the material.[12] It has currently undergone modifications, and has been released as Soft form II. Reports of less contracture and increased pliability should make it more acceptable to the patient and the surgeon.

Polyethylene is a porous material with high tensile strength. Since the 1940s, polyethylene has been used as a bone and cartilage substitute in its ultrahigh molecular weight form. The modern version is high density polyethylene (HDPE), and is similar to PTFE because it is non-resorbable and highly biocompatible, with no tendency for chronic inflammatory reaction. HDPE currently is produced as mesh (Marlex, Prolene) and solid implants (Medpor). Its pore sizes are 125–250 μm, and this porosity allows for some soft tissue and vascular in-growth. It produces a minimal tissue response and results in a thin fibrous capsule with insignificant contraction. As compared to Gore-Tex, Medpor implants are believed to cause fewer infections, in part because of the pore size of HDPE, which allows for macrophages to traverse the implant and engulf bacteria. Also the increased stability from host tissue in-growth of the implant is believed to help decrease the infection and extrusion rate. This material can be carved or contoured to a degree. The contouring is made easier by heating the material in a warm water bath. HDPE implants offer an excellent alternative to autogenous and other alloplastic materials in midfacial, chin, and mandibular reconstruction. The disadvantages include its rigid nature and the difficulty in contouring it to the surface of complex skeletal structures.[18]

The aliphatic polyesters are resorbable carbon-based polymers. They have been used as suture material and currently are being marketed as resorbable plates and screws. They maintain their strength for 6–8 weeks and are reported to be completely resorbed at one year. Nylamid, a polyamide mesh, has been used in facial augmentation with good short-term results, but some hydrolytic decomposition was observed with resultant volumetric loss. The aliphatic polyesters currently are among the most commonly used polymers in surgery.[15]

Mersilene mesh (Ethicon Inc, Somerville, NJ) is a softer material composed of nonabsorbable polyester fiber sheeting that can be folded and constructed into an appropriate implant. It has been in use for over fifty years and was first introduced for hernia repair. Unlike Supramid (Ethicon, Inc.), polyamide nylon mesh Mersilene does not degrade, and is cut easily without fraying or shrinking. Johnson described its use as chin augmentation material. Perkins has reported excellent long-term aesthetic results with this material.[19]

Acrylics are derived from polymerized esters of either acrylic or methyl acrylic acids. Polymethylmethacrylate (PMMA) resin is a polymer commonly used as bone cement, and is fabricated by mixing a liquid monomer with a powdered polymer in an exothermic reaction, forming rigid plastic. Because of the exothermic reaction, there is a potential for damage to the surrounding tissues from the material's high cure temperatures (as high as 80°C), and thus cool irrigation must be applied after placement of the material. Models can also be made preoperatively, and an implant can be fabricated preoperatively, sterilized, and used in the operating room, avoiding potential surrounding tissue damage by the exothermic reaction. Once solidified, PMMA forms an impervious, non-degradable material with encapsulation. The disadvantages of PMMA are that its odor is difficult to tolerate and its fumes are teratogenic.[11] Another disadvantage is its high bacterial adhesion properties, predisposing it to infection. Although used in the setting of infected mandible fractures and reconstructions in the form of antibiotic-impregnated beads, methylmethacrylate, as a structural implant, is very poorly tolerated in close contact with oral cavity, sinuses, or active infection.[11] The material has been used frequently in cranioplasty procedures for full-thickness skull defects, but because of the hardness of this material, it is not often used as a soft tissue implant.

A similar material, hard tissue replacement (HTR, Biomet, Inc., Warsaw, IN), is a composite of PMMA and polyhydroxyethylmethacrylate. HTR has interconnected pores, is hydrophilic, and has a calcium hydroxide coat believed to promote tissue in growth.[15] It has been used in dentistry, and is currently available as a preformed implant, which can be custom-made from a CT scan of the patient's defect. It is useful in the replacement of large full-thickness defects in the cranium and other regions. Scant data exist documenting its use in malar and chin augmentation.

Another composite material is Artecoll, which consists of PMMA microspheres 20–40 μm in diameter suspended in atelocollagen. The microspheres cause fibroblasts to be stimulated. Although indications include rhydids, lip, chin, and malar augmentation; this material has not gained much support for its use.[12]

Calcium Phosphate Ceramics

Hydroxyapatite (HA) is a calcium phosphate salt, the principal inorganic compound in bone matrix. Their biocompatibility is excellent, and they appear to bond to bone by natural cementing mechanisms. This material is osteoconductive and allows for tissue in-growth without the formation of a fibrous capsule, but it is not osteoinductive (osteogenic ability in the absence of inductive growth factors).[13]

There are two forms of HA, a harder ceramic form and a non-ceramic form. Ceramic HA can be produced synthetically in a dense form (in which it originally was used in alveolar ridge augmentation), but this dense form of HA was found to be difficult to shape and prone to migration and extrusion. Porous forms of ceramic HA, based on the calcium carbonate structure of marine corals, have been more successful. Their porosity permits fibrovascular and osseous in-growth. Both porous and dense ceramic forms can be used for implantation. Block forms have been used as interpositional grafts in facial osteotomies. However, HA implants cannot tolerate significant load-bearing and have a tendency to crack and fracture. HA also comes in powder and liquid forms, which are mixed intraoperatively to form a non-ceramic HA without the production of heat (Bone Source HAC, Leibinger, Dallas, TX). It does not tolerate movement or shear forces, particularly while hardening, and this is generally used in non-stress bearing craniofacial applications. Constantino has extensively researched the use of non-ceramic HA, and it has been cleared for clinical use in aesthetic facial contouring.[13]

AUTOGENOUS GRAFTS

When available, autogenous grafts are the most favored implants. The malar area has had much more success

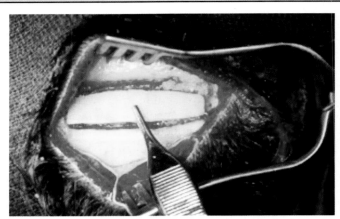
Fig. 38.6: Split calvarial bone graft is easily obtainable, and is an excellent graft for facial augmentation

with autogenous grafts, in contrast to the chin augmentation. Autografts such as iliac crest and rib cartilage have been used more frequently for chin augmentation in the past. Nasal bone and cartilage have been used as well. Unfortunately, their use appears to be associated with an increased rate of infection, even after as many as 40 years.[20] Many other autologous materials have been suggested (fascia lata, dermal-fat grafts), although fascia is often too thin to provide significant bulk. Dermal-fat grafts can be used successfully, especially if skin excision is already planned; careful and thorough removal of all epidermis is necessary to prevent epidermal inclusion cyst development. Split calvarial bone has proven to be an excellent graft material for facial contouring. Although another surgical site is necessary, the harvest is not technically demanding and there is minimal morbidity associated with obtaining the graft (Fig. 38.6). From the parietal area a good amount of bone may be harvested for use in the augmentation of the facial skeleton.

OSTEOTOMY

Bony osteotomies can be used to modify the facial skeletal structure (Figs 38.7 to 38.9). The cut segments of bone can be moved to a new position and rigidly fixated. This can be performed alone, as in the sliding genioplasty, or used along with placement of autologous bone grafts in areas such as the malar eminence. The osteotomy is more technically demanding, and is more time consuming, but yields excellent cosmetic results.

Malar Augmentation

Prominent malar eminences are a hallmark of beauty in many cultures, and is an important component of the

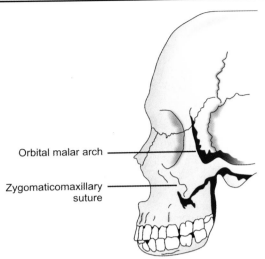

Fig. 38.7: Bone landmarks of the malar region

Orbital malar arch

Zygomaticomaxillary suture

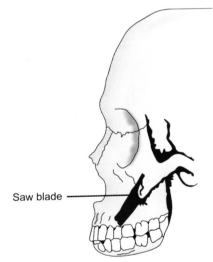

Fig. 38.8: Location of osteotomy

Saw blade

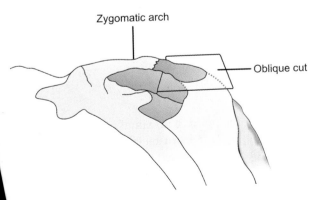

Fig. 38.9: Inferior view of the osteotomy

Zygomatic arch

Oblique cut

Western concept of facial youth and beauty. Individuals with strong high cheek bones convey a healthy and youthful look, although it is important to note ethnic differences, with Asians having a flatter and widened midface, compared to people of European descent.[21] A hypoplastic flat malar area can make the face appear tired and aged. Aside from the skeletal deficit in this area, aging results in atrophy and ptosis of the soft tissues overlying the zygoma. Deficiencies in the malar region can be secondary to trauma, congenital defects, inherited ethnic bony structure, and aging.

Midface augmentation helps counterbalance unfavorable facial topography by providing more angulation and lift to the face, rejuvenating the appearance. Patients may not be aware of the contribution the midface makes to overall facial harmony; instead, they may tend to focus on concerns regarding the nose, eyes, or redundant or ptotic facial skin. The facial plastic surgeon should educate patients by describing how malar and submalar augmentation serves to efface the melolabial folds, and provide elegance to the midfacial area. In patients who lack the supporting skeletal substructure, soft tissue repositioning alone does not provide sufficient rejuvenation in the midface region.

Malar deficiencies or asymmetries can be corrected by osteotomies or implants, and these implants can be composed of autogenous or synthetic materials. Patients with midface hypoplasia, gain aesthetic benefit from improved facial contour. This augmentation may be performed in conjunction with a maxillary advancement procedure. Some patients may request facial augmentation to produce a dramatic high and sharp cheek contour. As in chin augmentation, a malar–submalar implant often enhances the result of a rhytidectomy or rhinoplasty by further improving facial balance and harmony.

Originally, malar augmentation was described for the purpose of craniofacial reconstruction. The reconstruction was done for patients who had craniofacial syndromes with zygomatic aplasia. Split calvarium, rib, and iliac crest were harvested as autogenous bone grafts, and osteotomies were sometimes necessary to achieve appropriate contouring.[22] Since then, there have been numerous variations to this technique. Due to potential donor site morbidity and an increase in operative time, other alternatives have been introduced. Gonzalez-Ulloa and Hinderer were among the first surgeons to describe malar augmentation with alloplastic materials. Malar augmentation has developed as an important aesthetic procedure, since poor malar prominence detracts from

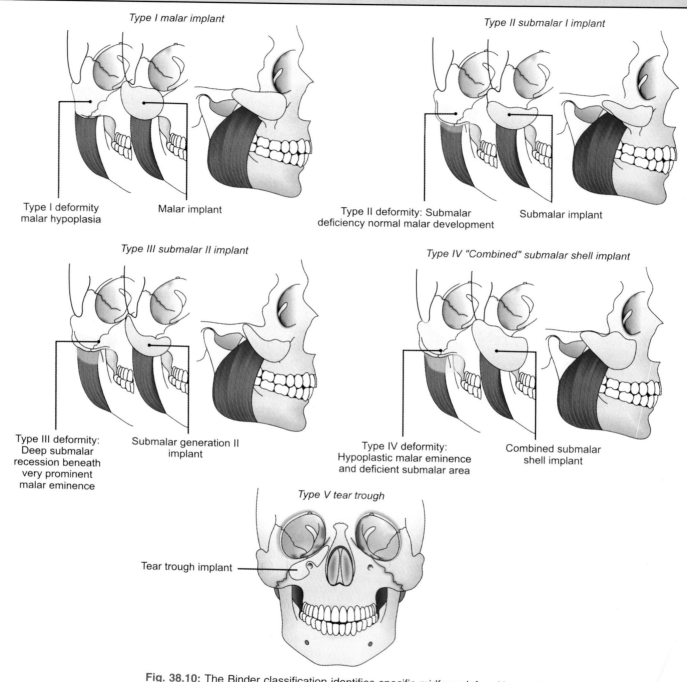

Fig. 38.10: The Binder classification identifies specific midface deformities, and suggests the type of implant to address the defect

the overall facial appearance. Several authors have described techniques to characterize the types of malar deficiency, and ways to determine the appropriate implant size. Binder correlated midfacial deficiencies with specific implant designs (Fig. 38.10).[23] A patient may demonstrate a lack of anterior projection of the malar eminence, or the point of maximal projection ma[ ] far medially; both disrupt facial harmony and disproportionately widened midface. Hinderer of analysis indicated that the implant be pl[ ] upper outer quadrant as delineated by the lines.

Relevant Anatomy

Binder (2002) created a classification of midfacial deformities, as follows (Fig. 38.10): [23]

- *Type I deformity:* This deformity occurs in a patient with adequate midfacial fullness but insufficient malar skeletal development. A malar implant corrects this by augmenting the zygoma and creating a higher arched and more projecting cheekbone.
- *Type II deformity:* Atrophy of the midfacial soft tissues in the submalar area with adequate malar development is seen in type II deformity. Patients with this deformity have wide or flat faces and benefit from the placement of a submalar implant.
- *Type III deformity:* This deformity is seen in patients with prominent malar eminences and thin skin. A skeleton-like appearance results from the sudden transition to a hollowed submalar region. A submalar implant may be used to soften the transition and to provide anterior projection to the deficient submalar area.
- *Type IV deformity:* A combination of malar hypoplasia and submalar soft-tissue deficiency creates a volume-deficient face, known as the type IV deformity. Placement of a combined malar–submalar implant provides correction.
- *Type V deformity:* In the type V, tear-trough deformity, a pronounced nasojugal fold may be effaced by placement of a Silastic or Gore-Tex implant.

Alloplastic Implant Placement

Generally, facial implants have the advantage of being placed in areas of good blood supply. In situations where vascular compromise may exist, one must weigh the benefits of implantation versus the risks. Areas with poor vasculature supply are seen in radiation damage, prior surgical scarring, facial trauma, and excessively thin skin. Patients with significant facial asymmetry, or extremely prominent bone structure may also have skin with less than ideal blood supply. [14] It is important to keep the implant uncontaminated throughout its placement, and many surgeons elect to use a no-touch technique in which the implant does not come in contact with gloved hands, skin, or oral mucosa. [14] Rinsing the pocket thoroughly and changing surgical gloves just before placing the implant may also serve to decrease the bacterial contamination load. Alloplastic implant materials lessen the bacterial load needed for a clinically significant infection. Antibiotics should be given intravenously in the perioperative period followed by an oral course postoperatively.

Malar implants can be placed through any of several approaches: Commonly the intraoral, subciliary,

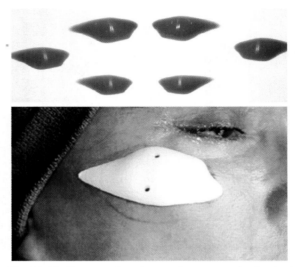

Fig. 38.11: Sizer used to choose the correct size implant

rhytidectomy, and transconjunctival approaches. Malar implants can be placed as through a facelift incision or coronal incision by dissecting down to the level of the zygoma. Subciliary incisions also may be used but add the risk of ectropion to the procedure. [3]

The following describes a technique for intraoral placement of malar and/or submalar implants. [24] The intraoral approach has the advantage of leaving no visible scar and can be performed under local anesthesia. Theoretically, an increase in the risk of infection exists from introducing the implant through the mouth. Clinically, this has not been the case. [11]

Once the appropriate implant is chosen, it is placed on the skin overlying the malar-submalar area (Fig. 38.11). During the preoperative analysis the optimal area of augmentation is determined. The edges of the prosthesis are outlined on the skin (Fig. 38.12). The procedure can

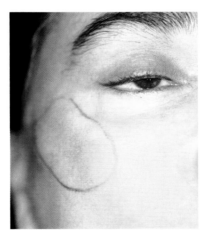

Fig. 38.12: Outline is marked on the face

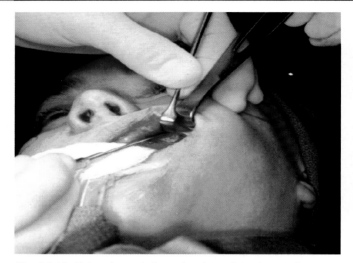

Fig. 38.13: Subperiosteal dissection through an intraoral access

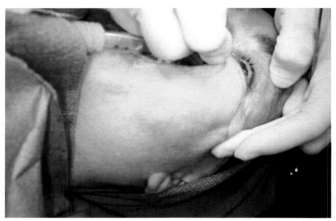

Fig. 38.14: The surgeon's free hand constantly palpates as the internal dissection is completed

be completed with the patient under general anesthesia or local anesthesia with sedation. Injection of 0.25% bupivacaine with epinephrine (1:200,000) mixed in equal part with 1% lidocaine with epinephrine (1:100,000) can reduce operative bleeding and provide long-lasting anesthesia. Hemostasis is required to provide accurate visualization and proper implant placement.

The intraoral approach begins with an upper buccal sulcus incision, leaving an adequate cuff of tissue for closure. The incision in the mucosa should be inferior and anterior to the parotid duct, in the area of the canine fossa (Fig. 38.13). Divide the muscle down to the periosteum and maintain hemostasis with bipolar cautery. The safest plane of dissection in the face is the subperiosteal plane, which is directly on bone. Dissection in this plane provides the greatest amount of protection for the facial nerve, prevents unnecessary bleeding, and maximizes the amount of soft tissue coverage of the implant. As the dissection proceeds superolaterally, the infraorbital foramen and nerve is identified to avoid accidental injury. The free hands constantly supports and palpates the internal dissection, limiting the pocket formation (Fig. 38.14). The dissection should elevate the periosteum off of the zygoma, creating a snug pocket. The size of the pocket should be such that it can accommodate passive placement of the implant because a pocket that is too small pushes the implant in the opposite direction, leading to possible extrusion. Binder et al (2002) report that 4 mm of projection is the most commonly used thickness of malar implant.[23] Others feel the standard implant size gives a 6 mm projection, using 4 mm implant in the patient with a thin skin covering,

and a larger 8 mm implant for severe malar hypoplasia.[3] For the submalar or combined malar–submalar implant, create a pocket by elevating the soft tissue that overlies the masseter muscle. The tendons of the masseter are characteristically glistening white and should be kept intact to provide support for the implant. Place the submalar implant below the zygoma and zygomatic arch, overlying the masseter tendon, or position it more superiorly over bone. The pocket should be irrigated and the implant soaked in bacitracin antibiotic solution prior to placement. The incision is closed in two layers using 3-0 chromic sutures.

Not all surgeons agree on the need for fixation, and several recent articles emphasize creation of a precise pocket over suture fixation. A freer elevator can be used to assist in positioning. Manipulation of the implant into position can be facilitated by using a stabilizing suture (Figs 38.15 and 38.16). Confirm proper placement by

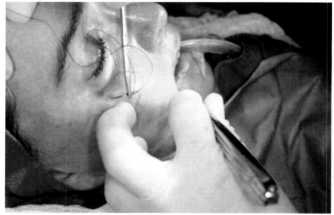

Fig. 38.15: A stabilization suture is used to help in implant placement

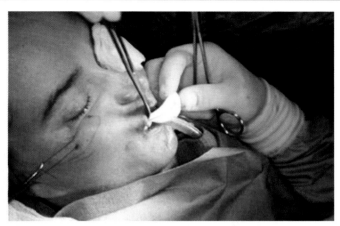

Fig. 38.16: The suture is used to pull the implant into position

passing an elevator over and under to the implant to ensure that no folding has occurred. Inspect and simultaneously palpate the implants from the head of the bed to check for symmetry. The implant can be held in place by a tight pocket of periosteum, or secured with non-absorbable sutures or alternatively, a single screw can be placed at the inferomedial extent of the implant to prevent migration.[16] If transcutaneous fixation is desired, pass a long Keith needle suture through the lateralmost aspect of the implant and then exit transcutaneously. Then, gently tie the suture over a dental roll bolster (Fig. 38.17).

Recently designed facial implants have been very successful, based in part on their anatomic conformability to the facial skeleton. The projecting contour of the bone

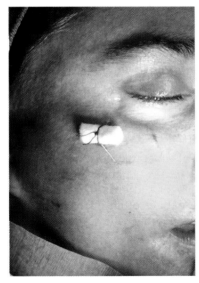

Fig. 38.17: The same suture is used to stabilize the implant with a tie over the bolster

is accommodated by the posterior surface of the implant as it molds over the surface.

The subciliary approach can be used when malar-submalar augmentation is performed in conjunction with a lower lid blepharoplasty that requires skin excision. After a skin-muscle flap is elevated, an incision is made in the orbital septum. The periosteum then is incised just below the prominence of the infraorbital rim. A precise subperiosteal pocket is created, into which the implant is placed. The cheek flap is re-draped, and the blepharoplasty is completed. Implant placement is performed prior to the blepharoplasty because it often reduces the amount of skin that needs to be excised. This technique is used less commonly because of possible problems with lid malposition and ectropion.[21]

The rhytidectomy approach is the most difficult of all the techniques and is infrequently used. The superficial musculoaponeurotic system (SMAS) may be penetrated just medial to the zygomatic eminence down to the level of bone with a blunt elevator. The malar pocket is created by a retrograde dissection.

The transconjunctival approach too is infrequently used. For implant placement, a lateral canthotomy is needed to accommodate the implant size. To keep the integrity of the lower lid, a suture suspension of the lateral canthal tendon is also performed.

The patient should maintain head elevation for 24–48 hours, and ice packs or cold compresses should be applied for the first 24 hours; oral antibiotics are continued for 5 days. The patient should take a soft diet for the first week, and avoid strenuous activity for two to three weeks.

The surgeon should evaluate the patient within the first 12–24 hours to check for any facial asymmetry that may develop secondary to hematoma or seroma. If placed for fixation, bolsters, and sutures can be removed on the third postoperative day.

Common complications include implant malposition, asymmetric placement, or placing an inappropriate size. Improper positioning of the implant is the most common complication, followed by improper implant size.[25] In addition, the implant may become exposed or extruded. The patient may develop a hematoma or seroma, which may require only surgical drainage, or the patient may develop an infection around the implant, which may require its removal. After resolution of the process, an implant may be reinserted in 6–8 weeks. Problems with local tissue reactions and capsule formation causing abnormal ridging and projections too may necessitate removal. Re-implantation should be avoided in these situations.

Facial nerve injury is rare and transient. The infraorbital nerve is often stretched during the dissection and transient paresthesias may result. Numbness may last up 6 months. It may persist if the implant impinges on the nerve. Persistent cheek pain, sometimes caused by traumatic neuroma formation, may require removal of the implants. Incisions that divide the zygomaticus muscles may cause transient or even permanent partial muscle weakness. The patient's smile may be altered as normal lip elevation may be hindered.

Placement of malar-submalar implants via a subciliary or transconjunctival approach may be complicated by lower eyelid malposition or ectropion.

Unlike the findings of bone erosion associated with silastic chin implants, malar and submalar implants maintain facial contour without compromise to the underlying skeleton.[21]

Malar and submalar augmentation with alloplastic implants can be used to enhance and restore facial harmony and balance. Defects that have developed as a result of aging or trauma as well as congenital defects may be addressed. Strong skeletal contours enhance beauty. Re-draping, reshaping, and redistributing the soft tissue over a strong facial skeleton enhance restoration and rejuvenation of the face. Successful malar and submalar augmentation results from proper patient and implant selection as well as appropriate facial analysis and surgical technique. Alloplastic facial augmentation produces reliable, durable, and predictable results with little morbidity and high patient satisfaction. Alloplastic facial augmentation produces permanent and effective three-dimensional changes in facial contour with low risk and minimal morbidity.

Malar Osteotomy

The osteotomies are placed at the junction of the zygomatic arch and the zygomatic process of the maxilla. In addition to these important landmarks, the surgeon must be aware of the close proximity of the infraorbital foramen and nerve. A standard intraoral incision at the canine fossae region allows for visualization of these structures. Dissection should be subperiosteal, as in the placement of the alloplastic malar implant. The decision whether to include any of the anterior buttress in the oblique sagittal cut, or if it should be completely lateral to the zygomaticomaxillary suture line, should be made preoperatively at the time of facial analysis. The osteotomy is made with a sagittal or reciprocating saw, starting inferiorly and extending superiorly to the notch made by the zygoma and the lateral orbital rim. Once the cut is made a bone graft is wedged

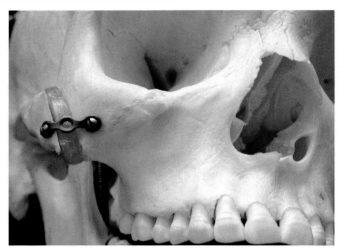

Fig. 38.18: Malar osteotomy location with interpositional graft

between the osteotomy. Although, alloplastic materials can be used as a spacer, it defeats one of the benefits of this procedure, which is to achieve augmentation with the patient's own tissues. The degree of the augmentation can be adjusted by the thickness of the graft. The graft usually measures 5 to 8 mm on each side. There is enough tension between the proximal and distal fragments to keep the graft stable. If any question of stability exists, rigid fixation may be accomplished with microplates and screws (Fig. 38.18). Because the patients' own arch is used, an anatomic result with a natural appearance is the expected result. Thus, symmetry and predictability make this surgical option appealing.[4]

With this type of surgery the potential complications include bleeding and nerve damage. Powell et al (1988), reported only transient paresthesia as the only sequelae from his series of patients.[4]

Chin Augmentation

In the mid 1940s, surgeons began to use bony osteotomy techniques to address the retruded mentum.[26] Currently, the sliding genioplasty is performed by several surgical subspecialties.[27]

Correction of poor projection of the mentum is desirable in approximately 20% of patients undergoing rhinoplasty and about 25% of patients having a rhytidectomy. However, the patient often must be educated that this deficiency exists and that, with surgery, an overall balanced cosmetic result may be achieved.

Surgical goals include creating an aesthetically pleasing facial contour and establishing proportionate facial height. This may entail reduction of a prominent chin or augmentation of a poorly projected chin.

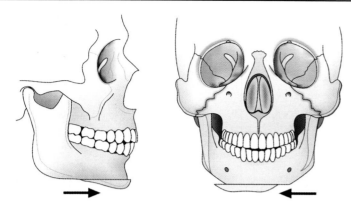

Fig. 38.19: Versatility of the sliding genioplasty; treats abnormalities in three dimensions

Ideally, the augmentation procedure should be performed with minimal morbidity. In general alloplastic implants are not technically demanding and have a low complication rate. Furthermore, these implants may be placed easily under local anesthesia. This is an accepted technique for correction of chins with only mild-to-moderate microgenia and a shallow labiomental fold.[28,29]

The sliding genioplasty has been reported to have similar rates of success.[9] Additionally, this technique can address abnormalities in three dimensions of asymmetry, including vertical microgenia with and without retrogenia, vertical macrogenia with retrogenia, and prognathia), making it a more versatile procedure[28,29] (Fig. 38.19).

Relevant Anatomy

In the case of augmentation, the depth of the labiomental fold may dictate the technique to be used. Alloplastic implants tend to deepen the sulcus, which may be particularly unattractive in female patients. With osseous genioplasty, the fold generally increases with advancements and/or vertical shortening and becomes more effaced with vertical lengthening.[28,29]

The surgeon should always be cognizant of the location of the mental foramen. The mental foramen lies on the same vertical line defined by the pupil, infraorbital foramen and the second bicuspid tooth.

The mentalis muscle elevates and protrudes the chin. It attaches the chin to an area just beneath the tooth roots. An intraoral incision will transect this muscle. It is important to reestablish this muscle otherwise chin ptosis may ensue.

When considering a mandible reduction or a sliding osteotomy, carefully evaluate the teeth and the height of the mandible prior to surgery. Having long teeth with a short mandibular height is a relative contraindication for an osseous genioplasty or an aggressive bony reduction.

Once deficiencies have been measured, plan the movement. The literature shows the ratio of correlation from bone to soft tissue movement is 1:0.6–1. More recent studies show the ratio to be about 1:0.9 for horizontal movements up to 8 mm.[7] Beyond this length, muscular and soft-tissue forces are thought to cause resorption. Also, literature reports less predictability in vertical movements. With alloplastic implants, on the other hand, preoperative measurements usually allow an accurate size to be implanted.

Alloplastic Augmentation

For alloplastic augmentation, surgical approach options include a submental or an intraoral sulcus approach. A submental incision allows for other adjunctive procedures, such as cervical liposuction and effacement of platysmal banding, to be performed through it. On the other hand, an intraoral incision precludes a facial scar.

Once the appropriate implant is chosen, it is placed on the skin overlying the chin area. During the preoperative analysis the optimal area of augmentation is determined. The edges of the prosthesis are outlined on the skin. The midline of the implant should come marked if; it is not do so (Fig. 38.20). The procedure can be completed with the patient under general anesthesia or local anesthesia with sedation. Injection of 0.25% bupivacaine with epinephrine (1:200,000) mixed in equal part with 1% lidocaine with epinephrine (1:100,000) can reduce operative bleeding and provide long-lasting anesthesia. Hemostasis is required to provide accurate visualization and proper implant placement. As with the malar implant placement perioperative and post-operative antibiotics should be administered.

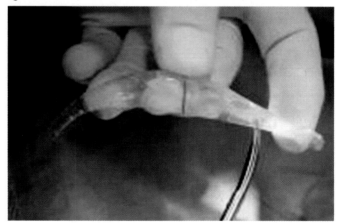

Fig. 38.20: Make sure implant has the midline marked

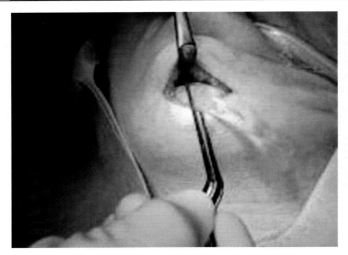

Fig. 38.21: Place the lateral ends of the implant subperiosteally

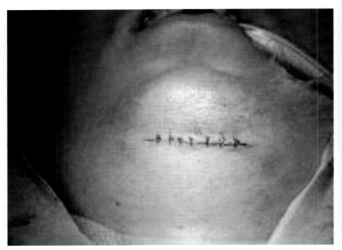

Fig. 38.23: Submental incision closed with interrupted sutures

With either approach, carry the dissection down to the level of the periosteum. Take care to preserve and not traumatize the mental nerves. Mark the midline with a suture in the soft tissue, and place the lateral third of the implant subperiosteally (Fig. 38.21). The pocket should be irrigated and the implant soaked in bacitracin antibiotic solution prior to placement.

Once the implant is in proper position and the mid line of the implant matches that of the soft tissue (Fig. 38.22), close the soft tissue in layers with 3-0 resorbable sutures (Fig. 38.23). Re-drape the soft tissue with tape (Fig. 38.24) and schedule a follow-up visit with the patient within one week of surgery (Fig. 38.25A and B). The patient should be on a soft diet for one week and avoid strenuous exercise for two weeks. The procedure takes about 15 minutes.

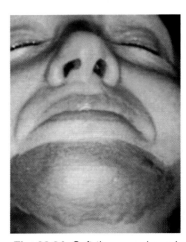

Fig. 38.24: Soft tissue re-draped with tape dressing

SLIDING GENIOPLASTY

A patient undergoing sliding genioplasty is admitted into the hospital only if orthognathic surgery is performed. Otherwise, the procedure can be performed in an outpatient setting even when concomitant procedures, such as rhinoplasty or liposuction, are performed. The sliding genioplasty also can be performed under local anesthesia or in an outpatient setting with good results; however, general anesthesia is most commonly used with this procedure. Patients are more comfortable, and the airway is better protected under general anesthesia. Unless a rhinoplasty is performed concurrently, nasotracheal intubation is preferred.

Injection of 0.25% bupivacaine with epinephrine (1:200,000) mixed in equal part with 1% lidocaine with

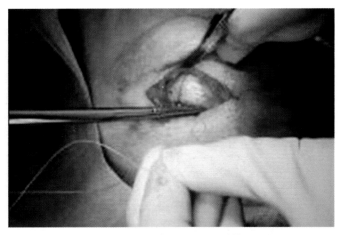

Fig. 38.22: Match the implant midline with that made in the soft tissue

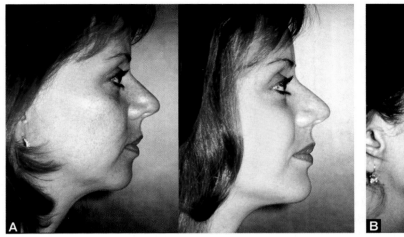
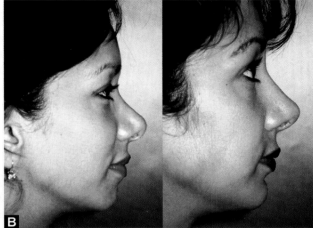

Figs 38.25A and B: Preoperative and postoperative photographs of two patients with alloplastic chin implants

epinephrine (1:100,000) locally in the mental foramen region, can reduce operative bleeding and provide long-lasting anesthesia. Perioperative and postoperative antibiotics should be administered. Access is through the gingivolabial sulcus incision. It is crucial to leave an adequate cuff of mucosa along with a good part of the mentalis muscle for later resuspension; this technique helps prevent lower-lip ptosis[29] (Figs 38.26A and B).

The foramina of the nerve are generally found between the first and second premolar teeth at the level of the origin of the mentalis muscle or 2–4 mm below the level of the bicuspid teeth apices. The foramina are situated deep to the mid-portion of the depressor anguli oris.[31] Dissect inferolaterally to allow for a longer osteotomy preventing unsightly mandibular notching. Leave the periosteum at the inferior rim intact. Align the skeletal midline with the overlying soft-tissue corollary. Use a sagittal saw with a 30° bend to facilitate an even cut while minimizing soft tissue trauma (Figs 38.27A and B).

Perform double osteotomies in the same manner. Plan asymmetric cuts well in advance. Fixation can be achieved with wires or plates (Figs 38.28A and B).

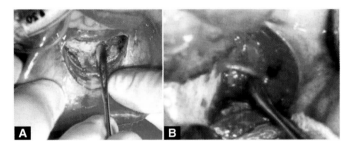

Figs 38.27A and B: Subperiosteal dissection is carried out laterally to identify the mental nerve

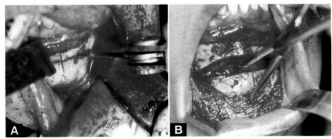

Figs 38.26A and B: Lateral cuts should be 4–5 mm below the foramina to compensate for the path of the inferior alveolar nerve. Bone forceps help mobilize the distal segment

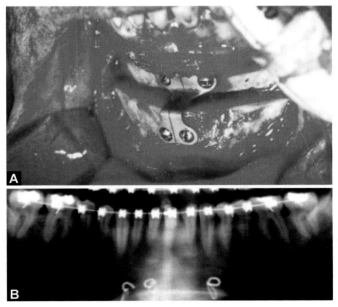

Figs 38.28A and B: Fixation can be done with preformed plates or with wires

Wire fixation may lead to increased resorption due to greater periosteal dissection and a possible drop of the anterior segment from muscle pull. Considerable success has been achieved using a single, 4-hole, titanium plate with 12 mm screws for males and 10 mm screws for females. Each plate is marked with the amount of movement obtained on the face of the plate.

Closure is accomplished in multiple layers. Re-suspend the mentalis with 3-0 interrupted buried Vicryl sutures and close the mucosa with a running 3-0 chromic suture.

Re-drape the skin at the level of the labiomental fold with Mastisol (Ferndale Laboratories, Ferndale, MI) and Steri-Strip tape. Advise patients to stay on a soft diet and to rinse frequently with saline solution until the first postoperative visit. Strenuous activity should be avoid, and physical contact to the chin should be delayed for four weeks. The surgical time for the osseous genioplasty procedure ranges from 15 to 105 minutes, with an average surgical time of about 45 minutes.[9] The alloplastic implantation is roughly 25% shorter in operative time.

Schedule a follow-up visit with the patient on post-operative days 7 and 14. Each of the procedures described has its own unique advantages, disadvantages, and complications.

Alloplastic mentoplasty may cause bone resorption, infection, extrusion, dehiscence, overprojection or underprojection, asymmetry, displacement, capsular contraction, lower-lip retraction, and chin ptosis.[32] Studies have shown that resorption occurs to some extent in many, if not all, patients. One study showed up to 5 mm of resorption at 48 months after surgery. Resorption has been attributed to subperiosteal placement of the implant. Tension in the soft-tissue pocket due to pressure from the overlying skin or mentalis musculature has been thought to cause this pressure resorption. The overall soft-tissue profile, however, is usually not affected by this bone resorption. Reporting evidence to the contrary, a study on adult hounds showed no significant difference between supraperiosteal and subperiosteal placement of silastic implants.[33]

Osseous genioplasty too could have complications. Mental nerve injury, malunion, non-union, irregularities, step-type deformities, lip drop, and overcorrection or undercorrection have been reported.[34] Note that undercorrection is better accepted than overcorrection in which the chin placed forward to the lower lip can yield a disharmonious profile.

Whether an alloplastic implant or an osseous implant is used, more than 90% of patients are satisfied with their

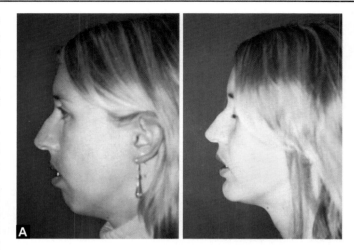

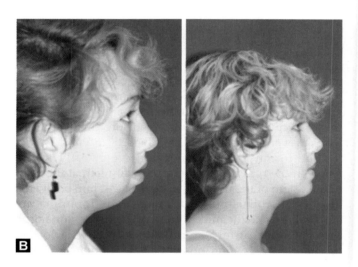

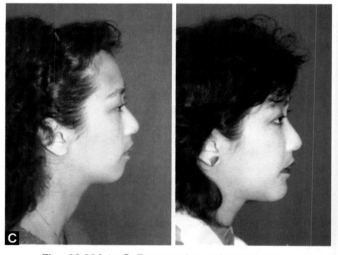

Figs 38.29A to C: Preoperative and postoperative photographs of a patient with a sliding genioplasty

results.[34] Complications observed with genioplasty are minimal, and benefits are readily evident to both patient and surgeon.[9]

In addressing the underprojected chin, alloplastic implants and sliding genioplasty are generally considered equally acceptable (Figs 38.29A to C). The benefits of sliding genioplasty include its versatility in correcting chin abnormalities in every dimension and its relative ease of use. For the mild to moderate deficiency of the chin, alloplastic implantation is simple, easy to place, and requires only short operative time. Excellent results are obtained, surgical time is acceptable, and patient satisfaction achieved with both alloplastic implants and sliding genioplasty.[30]

CONCLUSION

Facial analysis allows the surgeon to evaluate the proportions of facial structures, with the nose, malar, and chin regions contributing the most balance to the face. Skeletal asymmetries or deficiencies, as well as soft tissue changes, may result in suboptimal aesthetic situations. Facial contouring enables the surgeon to change this through augmentation. Alloplastic implants, autogenous grafts and osteotomies are the techniques used for facial augmentation. Each method has its own advantages and disadvantages, and these should be balanced with the desires of the patient, along with the experience of the surgeon to achieve harmonious and cosmetically pleasing aesthetic results.

ACKNOWLEDGMENT

Acknowledgment and thanks to Nelson Powell, MD for many of the figures in this chapter.

REFERENCES

1. Gonzalez-Ulloa M. Building out the malar prominences as an addition to rhytidectomy. *Plast Reconstr Surg* 1974; 53:293.
2. Hinderer U. Profileplasty. *Int Macro J Aesth Plast Surg* 1971; 1:12.
3. Schoenrock LD. Correction of subcutaneous and subperiosteal facial defects with expanded polytetrafluoroethylene (Gore-Tex). In *The art of alloplastic facial contouring*, Terino EO, Flowers RS (Eds). Baltimore: Mosby Inc, 2000; 209–219.
4. Powell NB, Riley RW, Laub DR. A new approach to evaluation and surgery of the malar complex. *Ann Plast Surg* 1988; 20(3):206–214.
5. Terino EO. Facial contouring with alloplastic implants: Aesthetic surgery that creates three dimensions. *Facial Plast Surg Clin North Am* 1999; 7:55–83.
6. Grayson BH. Cephalometric analysis for the surgeon. *Clin Plast Surg* 1989; 16(4):633–644.
7. Van Sickels JE, Smith CV, Tiner BD, Jones DL. Hard and soft tissue predictability with advancement genioplasties. *Oral Surg Oral Med Oral Pathol* 1994; 77(3):218–221.
8. Powell N, Humphreys B. Proportions of the aesthetic face. New York: Thieme-Stratton, 1984.
9. Chang EW, Lam SM, Karen M, Donlevy JL. Sliding genioplasty for correction of chin abnormalities. *Arch Facial Plast Surg* 2001; 3(1):8–15.
10. Stucker FJ, Hirokawa RH, Bryarly RC. Technical aspects of facial contouring using polyamide mesh. *Otolaryngol Clin North Am* 1982; 15:123–131.
11. Rubin JP, Yaremchuk MJ. Complications and toxicities of implantable biomaterials used in facial reconstructive and aesthetic surgery: A comprehensive review of the literature. *Plast Reconstr Surg* 1997; 100(5):1336–1353.
12. Min SA, Monhian N, Maas CS. Soft tissue augmentation. *Facial Plast Surg Clin North Am* 1999; 7:35–41.
13. Gavindaraj S, Costantino PD, Friedman CD. Skeletal implants in aesthetic facial surgery. *Facial Plast Surg* 1999; 15(1):73–81.
14. Metzinger SE, McCollough EG, Campbell JP, Rousso DE. Malar augmentation: A 5-year retrospective review of the silastic midfacial malar implant. *Arch Otolaryngol Head Neck Surg* 1999; 125(9):980–987.
15. Cox AJ III, Wang TD. Skeletal implants in aesthetic facial surgery. *Facial Plast Surg* 1999; 15(1):3–12.
16. Goldman ND, Alsarraf R, Nishioka G, Larrabee WF Jr. Malar augmentation with self-drilling single-screw fixation. *Arch Facial Plast Surg* 2000; 2(3):222-225.
17. Ramirez AL, Monhian N, Maas CS. Current concepts in soft tissue augmentation. *Facial Plast Surg Clin North Am* 2000; 8:235–250.
18. Frodel JL, Lee S. The use of high-density polyethylene implants in facial deformities. *Arch Otolaryngol Head Neck Surg* 1998; 124(11):19–23.
19. Gross EJ, Hamilton MM, Ackermann K, Perkins SW. Mersilene mesh chin augmentation. A 14-year experience. *Arch Facial Plast Surg* 1999; 1(3):183–189; discussion 190.
20. Kelly JP, Malik S, Stucki-McCormick SU. Tender swelling of the chin 40 years after genioplasty [clinical conference]. *J Oral Maxillofac Surg* 2000; 58(2):203–206.
21. Constantinides MS, Galli SK, Miller PJ, Adamson PA. Malar, submalar, and midfacial implants. *Facial Plast Surg* 2000; 16(1):35–44.
22. Tessier P. The definitive plastic surgery treatment of severe facial deformities of craniofacial dysostosis: Crouzon's and Alpert's disease. *Plast Reconstr Surg* 1971; 48:419–442.
23. Binder JB. *Aesthetic facial implants, facial plastic and reconstructive surgery*, np, 2nd edn, 2002; 276–298.
24. Jabaley ME, Hoopes JE, Cochran CC. Transoral silastic augmentation of the malar region. *Br J Plast Surg* 1974; 27: 98–102.
25. Wilkinson TS. Complications in aesthetic malar augmentation. *Plast Reconstr Surg* 1983; 71:643–647.
26. Gilles HD, Millard DR Jr. *The principles and art of plastic surgery*. Philadelphia: Lippincott Williams and Wilkins, 1957.
27. Converse JM, Wood-Smith D. Horizontal osteotomy of the mandible. *Plast Reconstr Surg* 1964; 34:464.

28. Rosen HM. Aesthetic guidelines in genioplasty: The role of facial disproportion. *Plast Reconstr Surg* 1995; 95(3):463–469; discussion 470–472.

29. Rosen HM. Osseous genioplasty. In *Grabb and Smith's Plastic surgery*, 5th edn. Philadelphia: Lippincott-Raven, 1997; 705–710.

30. Frodel JL, Sykes JM. Chin augmentation/genioplasty: Chin deformities in the aging patient. *Facial Plast Surg* 1996; 12(3):279–283.

31. Seltzer HM, Feuerstein SS. Anatomic considerations in augmentation mentoplasty. In *Proceedings of the Fourth International Symposium on Plastic and Reconstructive Surgery of the Head and Neck.* St. Louis: Mosby-Yearbook Inc 1984; 442–447.

32. Zide BM, Pfeifer TM, Longaker MT. Chin surgery: I. Augmentation—the allures and the alerts. *Plast Reconstr Surg* 1999; 104(6):1843–1853; discussion 1861–1862.

33. Pearson DC, Sherris DA. Resorption beneath silastic mandibular implants. Effects of placement and pressure. *Arch Facial Plast Surg* 1999; 1(4):261–264; discussion 265.

34. Guyuron B, Kadi JS. Problems following genioplasty. Diagnosis and treatment. *Clin Plast Surg* 1997; 24(3):507–514.

CHAPTER 39

Otoplasty

Fred J Stucker, Neil M Vora, Timothy Lian

Modern otoplasty techniques fall into two broad surgical categories—cartilage sparing and cartilage cutting: There are of course many variations for each. The common goals of these procedures are to achieve a normal appearing ear with acceptable protrusion, symmetry, and form. The most commonly seen defect is a poorly developed or absent antihelical fold and an abnormally large concha. Patients with protruding ears will possess one or both of these characteristics.

Otoplasty techniques have evolved since it was first described in the literature in 1881.[1] Many of the original operations consisted of skin excision only which usually resulted in disappointment and poor long-term benefits. Luckett in 1910 introduced the revolutionary concept of managing the cartilage in order to achieve normal auricular form.[2] In 1963, Mustarde described the use of mattress sutures to create and maintain the antihelical fold.[3] Furnas in 1968, introduced a corrective method to address the deep conchal bowl by placing concha-mastoid sutures.[4] Stucker in 1977, developed a technique combining resection of cartilage with mattress suture placement.[5] These techniques and numerous variations have withstood the test of time and have become an integral part of the modern otoplasty.

ANATOMY

External Ear

The external ear is composed largely of elastic cartilage except for the lobule. The circumference of the pinna consists of the helix, tragus and lobule. The inner cartilaginous fold or convexities consist of the antihelix and two crura. The depression or concavity between the helix and antihelix is the scaphoid fossa. Between the two crura lies the fossa triangularis. The bowl of the ear is the concha (Fig. 39.1).

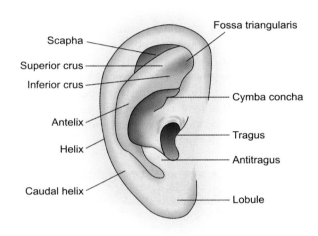

Fig. 39.1: Anatomy of auricle

Ligaments and Muscles

The pinna is attached to the skull by a series of three ligaments and muscles. The external muscles include the anterior, superior, and posterior auricularis. The intrinsic muscles include the helix, tragus, antitragus, transverse, and oblique muscles.

Nerves

The innervation of the ear is from four nerves which include the facial (VII), third division of trigeminal (V3), vagus (X) and greater auricular nerve (C2,3).

Vascular Supply

The blood supply to the ear is from the superficial temporal, posterior auricular, and occipital arteries. The venous drainage is via the posterior auricular, external jugular, superficial temporal and retromandibular veins.

EMBRYOLOGY

The embryological development of the auricle begins at approximately the sixth week of gestation. At this time the condensation of the mesoderm of the first and second brachial arches occurs, giving rise to the six Hillocks of His. The first arch contributes to the first three hillocks which give rise to the helix, helical crus, and tragus. The second arch contributes to the second three hillocks which give rise to the antihelix, antitragus, and lobule. The ear continues to develop even after birth. Adult size is reached between age 7 and 9 years.

PREOPERATIVE EVALUATION

An understanding of the anatomical features of the protruding ear and standard parameters of the normal ear (Table 39.1), allow the surgeon to effectively treat the patient's problem.[6,7] Deviation from the normal parameters and/or asymmetry will result in an abnormal appearing auricle. Recognizing the specific aberrant parameters will allow the surgeon to formulate a treatment plan. Photodocumentation should be obtained prior to surgical intervention.

Table 39.1: Normal parameters (Gluckman 1998; Nachlas 2002)	
• Auriculomastoid angle	20–35°
• Helical-mastoid distance	
Average	15–25 mm
Superior pole	10–12 mm
Middle (level of external auditory canal)	15–18 mm
Inferior (level of cauda helix)	20–22 mm
• Symmetry	

SURGICAL INDICATION

The most common deformity is the absence of the normal antihelical fold with a deep conchal bowl (Fig. 39.2). Generally, this finding is bilateral but can occasionally occur unilaterally. Most patients are children and are brought to the surgeon by their parents prior to entering school. The ideal age to correct ear deformities is when the cartilage has grown to its near-adult size typically between the ages of 4 and 6 years. If the patient is an older child or an adult, otoplasty with cartilage resection is frequently necessary (discussed in detail later). The following section describes a surgical technique combining cartilage resection with mattress suture placement.

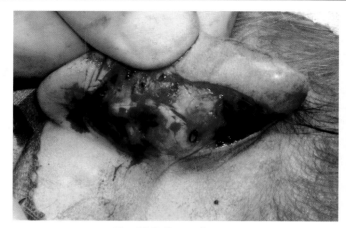

Fig. 39.2: Protruding ear

SURGICAL TECHNIQUE

Combined Technique

The patient is placed in a supine position. Subcutaneous injection of 1% lidocaine with epinephrine is used along the posterior portion of the pinna providing local anesthesia and hemostasis. As part of the draping process, a sterile orthopedic stockinet is placed over the head and endotracheal tube with openings for the ears (Fig. 39.3). This ensures sterility and allows for constant comparison of each side to insure symmetry of repair.

Next using a 15-blade scalpel, the postauricular skin is excised in a subdermal plane. Dissecting at this level, contrary to undue vascularity often mentioned, actually limits injury to the vessels in the subcutaneous tissues. This plane is easily dissected and reduces the possibility of postoperative hematomas. The amount of skin removed is determined by folding the pinna back and noting the superior and inferior fixation points needed

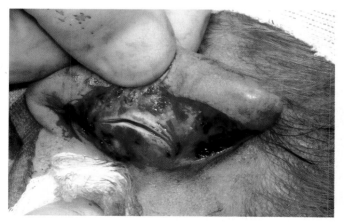

Fig. 39.3: Sterile stockinet placed over head with openings for ears

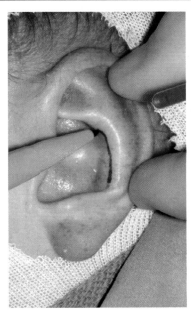

Fig. 39.4: Determining the location for the lateral conchal cartilage resection

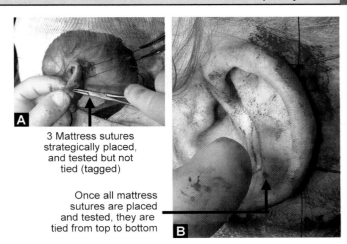

3 Mattress sutures strategically placed, and tested but not tied (tagged)

Once all mattress sutures are placed and tested, they are tied from top to bottom

Figs 39.6A and B: Folding the ear back

to hold the antihelical roll (Fig. 39.4). The skin excised is generally in the shape of an hourglass and is rarely removed from the mastoid surface. It is best to outline the skin to be excised before the local anesthetic is injected since the ballooning of the tissues may disrupt the design.

Next, the junction of the cauda helix and conchal cartilage are exposed and separated by sharp dissection (Fig. 39.5). Often a cleft is present and simple spreading action with an iris scissors results in separation. If fused, sharp dissection is used. This maneuver insures that the natural roll of the cauda is the dominant presentation of the operated auricle.

In patients with conchal excess, a lateral conchal cartilage resection is then performed.

Folding the ear back and noting the position of the antihelix help determine the location for the cartilage resection (Figs 39.6A and B). A crescent-shaped segment of cartilage, the width of which is determined by the

conchal excess, is removed from the lateral portion of the concha beneath the antihelix (Fig. 39.7). The incision extends longitudinally from the junction of the cauda helix with the conchal cartilage extending anteriorly below the inferior crus. Additional strips of cartilage can be removed until the ideal profile and antihelical height is obtained (Fig. 39.8). The cartilage resection eliminates the need for concha-mastoid sutures reducing the risk of meatal stenosis. The cauda helix is then sutured to the new leading edge of the concha. Occasionally, there is a need to trim excess cartilage of the cauda helix which if not addressed may result in a telephone ear deformity.

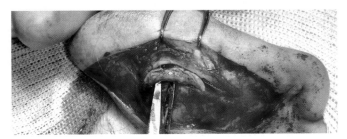

Fig. 39.5: Separation of cauda helix from lateral concha using sharp dissection

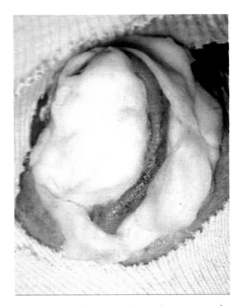

Fig. 39.7: Crescent-shaped segment of cartilage to be resected

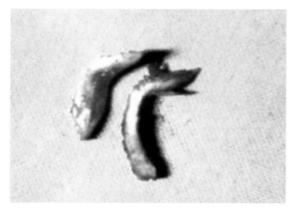

Fig. 39.8: Cartilage segment resected (*) using scalpel

Lastly, based on the techniques of Mustarde, three to four nylon mattress sutures are placed to recreate the antihelical fold. Braided sutures are to be avoided as they act as a gigli saw, cutting through the cartilage. Ensure that the suture is placed anterior enough to avoid a straight antihelix. For the novice, a Keath needle dipped in methylene blue may be used to mark the placement of the sutures. Following meticulous hemostasis, all the sutures are placed and permanently tied. No drains are employed. The postauricular skin incision is then closed with a running chromic suture. The same technique is used on the opposite ear.

Appropriately dressing the ear is a critical aspect of the procedure. The ear is liberally coated with ointment and a cotton ball placed in the concha. Cotton soaked in warm saline is placed into the folds and interstices of the ear and in the postauricular sulcus. Copious fluffs are placed and a bilateral mastoid dressing is applied. After one week, the dressing is removed and the patient instructed to wear a headband over the ears while sleeping to prevent inadvertent nocturnal trauma or displacement.

Results

As one reviews the literature, many techniques have been developed to manage the protruding ear. The best technique however is one that is reproducible, simple, and versatile. In the authors' practice, the lateral conchal cartilage resection with mattress sutures has been the preferred corrective method for the protruding ear for thirty-three years. As our experience has grown, the operation becomes more refined with improving results (Figs 39.9A to D).

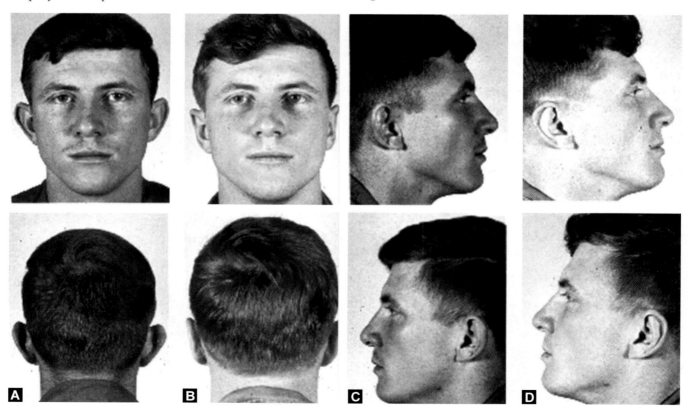

Figs 39.9A to D: (A, C)Preoperative photographs (B, D) Postoperative photographs

Advantages of the Combined Technique

There are numerous reasons for doing a combined cartilage-sparing and cartilage-resecting technique. First, removing strips of cartilage along the lateral portion of the concha provides a smooth transition from helix to antihelix. This combined with mattress sutures as described earlier recreate a natural appearing antihelical fold. Secondly, a reduction in the projection of the antihelix can be achieved with cartilage removal. By doing so, a telephone ear deformity is avoided. Lastly, with cartilage resection, there is no need for concha-mastoid sutures and the complication of meatal stenosis eliminated.

The reason cartilage resection is more common in the older child and adult stems from the inherent differences in the cartilage. As one ages the cartilage becomes less resilient, less pliable, and often calcified. Therefore in children, the cartilage will fold more easily while maintaining a natural appearance with smooth edges. Adults tend to have stiff, unyielding conchal cartilage, which require combined cartilage resection and suturing to achieve the desired result.

COMPLICATIONS

Early Complications

Early complications generally consist of hematomas and infections. Hematomas form due to blood accumulation between the skin and cartilage with no escape (Fig. 39.10). The causes include inadequate hemostasis or improper placement of the dressing. When such a complication occurs this can be managed with drainage in the office followed by bolster placement.

Infections rarely occur since most patients are treated with preoperative antibiotics. If a patient were to unfortunately develop an infection, he should be treated with antibiotics immediately. The most common organisms are *Staphylococcus aureus*, *Escherichia coli*, and *Pseudomonas aeruginosa*. When treatment is delayed, patients may develop chondritis resulting in cartilage necrosis and deformity.

Late Complications

Late complications occur several weeks to months following the operation. Suture failure, hypertrophic scars, and poor aesthetics are a few of the common delayed complications. Most suture failures occur within the first six months and are often preceded by a traumatic event. A secondary operation within the first year is required to re-establish proper auricle form and position.

Hypertrophic scar or keloid formation may occur along the postauricular incision (Fig. 39.11). African-Americans tend to develop keloids more frequently then Caucasians. Treatment may consist of steroid injections, scar revision, or skin grafting.

Numerous types of poor aesthetics result can occur following otoplasty. When using the lateral conchal cartilage resection technique, conchal skin bunching or redundancy may occur. If it persists, skin excision, as described by Smith et al will correct the problem.[8] Telephone ear deformity, conchal deformity, antihelical deformity, overcorrection, undercorrection and

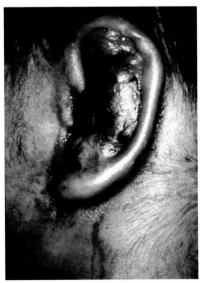

Fig. 39.10: Auricular hematoma

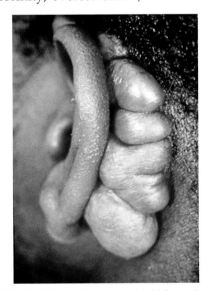

Fig. 39.11: Postauricular keloid formation

asymmetry can all occur and be aesthetically displeasing. Telephone ear deformity is caused by overcorrection of the midportion of the ear with inadequate flexion of the superior and inferior poles. Patients should undergo revision if the deformity is correctable and reassurance if not.

Summary

Patients with protruding ears are characterized by an absent antihelical fold, increased auriculomastoid angle and/or conchal excess. Many techniques for management of this problem have been described in the literature. It is important for the surgeon to familiarize himself/ herself with the various methods and develop one that can treat the majority of auricular deformities. The cartilage resection with mattress sutures is one such technique. This procedure is conservative, quickly learned, relatively free of complications and yields consistently good cosmetic results.

REFERENCES

1. Ely ET. An operation for prominence of the auricles. *Arch Opthalmol Otol* 1881; 10:97.
2. Luckett WH. A new operation for prominent ears based on the anatomy of the deformity. *Surg Gynecol and Obst* 1910; 10:635–637.
3. Mustarde JC. The correction of prominent ears using simple mattress sutures. *Br J Plast Surg* 1963; 16:170–176.
4. Furnas DW. Correction of prominent ears by concha-mastoid sutures. *Plast Reconst Surg* 1968; 42:189–192.
5. Stucker FJ, Christiansen TA. The lateral conchal resection otoplasty. *Laryngoscope* 1977; 87:58–62.
6. Gluckman JL, ed. *Renewal of Certification Study Guide in Otolaryngology—Head and Neck Surgery.* Iowa: Kendall/Hunt Publishing Company, 1998; 678–684.
7. Nachlas NE. Otoplasty. In Papel ID, ed. *Facial Plastic and Reconstructive Surgery.* New York: Thieme Medical Publishers, 2002; 309–321.
8. Smith R, Dickinson JT, Teachey WS. Medial conchal excision in otoplasty. *Laryngoscope* 1975; 85:738–750.

CHAPTER

40

Local Flaps in Facial, Head and Neck Surgery

Brad Woodworth, Terry A Day

Treatment and reconstruction of facial defects can be a complex and daunting task. The range of modalities employed is quite broad, ranging from secondary intention healing to free tissue transfers with micro-vascular anastomosis. There are a wide variety of local flaps available for each cutaneous defect although only a select few will accomplish the optimal aesthetic and functional outcome. This chapter will describe the variety of local flaps used to reconstruct defects of the head and neck as applied to the anatomic and functional units.

Ultimately, there is no one single local flap that is always applied to a particular defect of the facial region and head and neck. In some cases, healing by secondary intention may provide better results than attempting repair with a local flap that disrupts subunit boundaries. Some patients with recurrent cancer may benefit from a split thickness or full thickness skin graft rather than a complex local flap. Some complex defects with massive tissue loss are more appropriately repaired with a regional flap or free tissue transfer. With local flaps, skin with the same texture, quality, sebaceous character, and color can often fill a defect and give a patient their natural cosmetic appearance.

PHYSIOLOGY

Local flaps may be of skin, muscle, fascia, and fat. These flaps can be categorized based on vascular supply as random, axial, or free.[13] The random flaps are typically supplied via perforator vessels through fascia or muscle to the overlying skin of which the most distal perforators to the skin flap require division during elevation. The majority of local skin flaps in the facial region are classified as random pattern flaps and are not transferred with a named vessel. Axial flaps, however, receive blood supply through a direct cutaneous artery that is also elevated with the flap. Axial pattern flaps such as the

paramedian forehead flap or deltopectoral flap allow tissue to be transferred from more distant areas often without delay. The melolabial flap is one flap that can be transferred as a random skin flap or an axial flap (based on angular artery from the facial artery). Free tissue transfer is different from either axial or random flaps and represents the transfer of an axial pattern flap from a distant part of the body separating (dividing) the vascular supply and reanastomosing the arterial and venous supply to this tissue into respective vessels in the head and neck region.

Research[25] studies into the physiology of local flaps have led to increased survival with flap design and the use of flap delay.[1] Raising local flaps creates trauma to the tissues as well as stresses the neurovascular supply to the flap. The nutrient capillary network in the reticular dermis and AV shunts in papillary dermis provide the primary blood supply to the skin.[3] The blood supply to the skin is variable and is dependent on arteriolar pressure. Precapillary sphincters[66] increase flow to the skin by local hypoxemia and increased metabolic by-products while pre-shunt sphincters decrease flow to the skin by sympathetic contraction via norepinephrine.[22] Vessels travel via musculocutaneous arteries through the muscle or septocutaneous arteries through fascial septa. Septocutaneous arteries[65] usually run parallel to the skin thereby providing a larger surface area than the direct perforator musculocutaneous arteries.[58] Sensory nerves run in segmental fashion taking account for dermatome distribution, while sympathetic nerves are found near the cutaneous arterioles.[15]

The blood supply to a random cutaneous flap is derived from musculocutaneous arteries[2] near the base of the flap and the interconnecting subdermal plexus.[23] These flaps often have to be wider and shorter than axial pattern flaps. Axial pattern flaps have improved survival because of the incorporation of a septocutaneous artery along its axis. The surviving length is dependent on the length of this artery because of the relationship between the intravascular perfusion pressure and the critical closing pressure of the arterioles in the subdermal plexus. Partial interruption in the vascular supply reduces perfusion pressure to the skin.[54] This increases the risk of necrosis with increasing distance from the base of a flap. Beyond the first several days, neovascularization and wound healing lessen the flap's dependence on a pedicle.

PATIENT SELECTION/PREOPERATIVE EVALUATION

Most defects of the face are secondary to excision of skin cancer. Defects secondary to trauma, congenital malformations, or augmentation/cosmetic surgery are other possibilities but will not be the focus of this chapter. It is imperative that the facial plastic and reconstructive surgeon communicate with the other specialists such as head and neck oncologic or Mohs surgeon to determine the need for close monitoring of the primary site, risk of recurrence, potential for lymphatic metastases, and other issues which may alter the eventual outcome and survival.

Local flaps are not necessarily the best option for all skin defects of the face and head and neck region. Obviously, the cause of the defect predetermines the need for particular types of reconstruction. With malignancies, oncologic considerations are usually of primary importance. Flap reconstruction may also create new planes of scar that may serve as channels for cancer recurrence and spread. Malignancies associated with rapid local and regional spread may require additional treatment. Therefore, many skin cancers including melanoma may require close monitoring and mandate split thickness skin grafting for reconstruction of the defect. For other less aggressive cancers such as basal cell carcinoma, the surgeon may feel flap reconstruction is the best option because of the low likelihood of recurrence.

In the initial evaluation numerous issues that must be considered when evaluating a candidate for a local flap. Their occupation and avocations can often dictate the most appropriate reconstruction. Propensities for long hair, eyeglasses, or hats can be considerations for scar placement. Additionally, personal desires and expectations reflected in the chief complaint are often the most important aspect of the history. A patient with a defective ala may complain of nasal obstruction and doesn't care

as much for aesthetic outcome. In this case, functional considerations should be a higher priority than aesthetic ones.

A complete and thorough medical history and physical examination are necessary since a number of factors are known to increase complication risk, including smoking, hypertension, anticoagulation, peripheral vascular disease, diabetes mellitus, connective tissue disorders, chronic steroid use, and previous radiation therapy. Preoperative evaluation of comorbidities such as diabetes mellitus, chronic obstructive pulmonary disease, and heart disease is routine for general anesthesia, but often must be considered for local anesthesia as well. This can produce a significant amount of stress for the patient and should not be regarded as a risk-free procedure even in the outpatient setting. Diabetes, scleroderma, and smoking inhibit wound healing and should be weighed in reconstructive efforts. If reconstruction is planned for patients with these problems, they should be informed of the greater possibility of delayed wound healing and increased complications. A thorough physical examination must include an evaluation of the defect's location and size, depth and tissues involved, sensory/motor function, and the mobility, color, and texture of the surrounding skin. Analysis should be performed at rest and during voluntary and non-voluntary facial movements. Does the defect cross subunit boundaries?[21] Is there bone, muscle, or mucosa involved? Risks of the surgery must be discussed with the patients including flap necrosis, bleeding, infection, cancer recurrence, and the possibility of ending up with a larger defect secondary to complications. Consider all options when planning a reconstructive procedure of the facial region.

TREATMENT PLANNING

Once the full history and physical and work-up is complete, the procedure is scheduled. The patient is instructed to avoid all aspirin products, NSAIDS, Vitamin E, Gingko biloba and other antiocoagulants for at least two weeks prior to the procedure. It is often wise to document and complete your surgical plan at the time of evaluation in order to consider all possible options. A drawing depicting one's plan at the time of surgery facilitates incision placement once the patient is under anesthesia. For example, this may serve as a reminder of one of the planned incisions or flaps that provided a more functionally aesthetic result with smiling than could be delineated with the patient supine and sedated.

SURGICAL PREPARATION

The patient is and draped over the entire head and neck region, including areas that may be needed such as the thigh for a split thickness skin graft, ear for adjunctive cartilage graft, and possible regional or distant flap options. Eye protection is important and may require temporary tarsorrhaphy, corneal shield and corneal lubricant. Preoperative antibiotics are recommended but not always necessary. Allograft materials should be made available well in advance if considered for the reconstruction.[64] The wounds are marked with fine-point marking pens and measurements taken as needed with calipers. Local anesthesia is then injected along the lines of incision only after appropriate markings and measurements are performed.

INCISION PLACEMENT

Although incisions on the face heal very well due to an incredible vascular supply, the ideal incision is one that cannot be seen.[12] When possible the ideal incision is inside an orifice such as the mouth, eyelid, nose, or ear thus camouflaging the approach in certain circumstances. It may also be placed inside or along the hairline, but the potential for a receding hairline in males and transfer of hair-bearing skin should be considered.[48] The face is divided into distinct anatomic units with distinct aesthetic subunits even within these anatomic units. The cheek, forehead, eye, nose, lips, and ears are all separate units and placing incisions in the boundaries of these units is advantageous. If unable to place an incision in a boundary position, incisions should be placed along or parallel to the relaxed skin tension lines (RSTL) (Fig. 40.1).[46] These

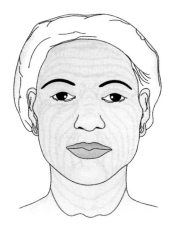

Fig. 40.1: Relaxed skin tension lines

are natural skin creases created by muscles of facial expression. Often, the eye perceives a long straight incision better than a broken line. This principle holds true on the face where it is often advantageous to break up an incision. These broken line incisions should still be made along RSTL if possible and should rarely if ever be perpendicular to a RSTL. Lines of maximum extensibility (LME) are usually perpendicular to the RSTL and represent the direction where closure is performed with the least tension. Local flaps should be designed with closure parallel to these lines.

CLASSIFICATION

Classification of flaps may be based on location of donor site, blood supply, direction of transfer, or shape. The location flaps are derived from include distant (free tissue transfer, regional (deltopectoral), or a local (melolabial) site. As described previously, the blood supply of flaps may be axial, random or free.[31] The direction or movement during transfer is classically used to describe the types of local skin flaps of the face and will be used here to detail the flap options in reconstruction of skin defects in the head and neck region. These are classified as advancement, rotation, and transposition flaps.

ADVANCEMENT FLAPS

Simple Advancement

The concept of advancement is best demonstrated with a simple elliptical excision.[38] Excising a lesion in an elliptical fashion results in a defect that can be closed via undermining of the opposing edges and approximation of those edges. This is the most basic concept of local advancement flaps. If the defect angles are greater than 30 degrees, this increases the chance of a standing cutaneous deformity also known as a 'dog ear'. When the elliptical closure does not fall into RSTL, a broken line closure or M-plasty can be used to break up the straight line closure and provide a more cosmetically appealing wound. An M-plasty can decrease tissue protrusion, save on the amount of skin excised and contribute to the aforementioned broken line technique.

Rectangular Advancement

Also known as a U-plasty, this technique involves advancing a rectangular portion of skin into a square-shaped defect. In reality, most defects are round so this flap can be rounded to fit the defect after advancement. An H-plasty is used when a single advancement will not fill the defect. This uses bilateral rectangular-shaped advancement flaps to close the defect between the two rectangles. Usually the ratio of the flap to the defect is 3 : 1. A 4 : 1 ratio and greater can be obtained if the flap is based on a named artery or delay is performed. This technique is most commonly performed in the forehead where RSTL allow favorable placement of these incisions. Disadvantages of these flaps are the relatively large number of incisions required relative to the defect size. Well planned Burow's triangles or Z-plasty can be installed anywhere along the incisions to relieve tension and standing cutaneous deformities, while also placing them strategically within RSTL or anatomic boundaries.

T-plasty

The O-T or A-T wound repairs change circular or triangular defects into T-shaped scars and essentially represent bilateral advancement flaps. A defect can then be closed by two flaps and this can allow incisions along favorable creases or lines of aesthetic units. The vertical portion of the scar may be more noticeable on certain parts of the face and it is used generally in specific areas including the forehead, lower eyelid, lip, and chin. This technique can be used in the central forehead where the vertical limb can be placed in the midline.

V-Y Advancement

This common technique uses a V-shaped flap that recoils away from the defect rather than pulls tissue towards a recipient site.[51] The incisions are closed with wound tension in an opposite direction forming a Y configuration. This is useful in lengthening the columella using local tissue alone with a favorable remaining scar.

Island Advancement

An island flap may function as an advancement, rotation or transposition flap allowing the skin flap to be circumferentially incised while the deep soft tissue remains connected to the underlying vascular supply.[33] Thus, the flap is actually disconnected from all surrounding skin thereby relying on a pedicle of subcutaneous tissue. This technique is useful for medium-sized defects of the upper lip or near the alar base, cheek, and nasal sidewall.

ROTATION FLAPS

This local flap involves rotation of an arc of tissue from an adjacent site into the recipient site. This is ideal for closing triangular defects, or when the RSTL are curvilinear, and also when the most skin laxity provides for rotation rather than advancement. These flaps are relatively large in size and usually requiring extensive undermining. Two rotation flaps can be used to close triangular, circular or square defects and often become a combination of rotation and advancement. This type of flap is often used for resurfacing large cheek defects with a cervicofacial rotation flap by carrying incision back down the ear and to the neck as needed. It is also useful for scalp defects using multiple rotation flaps.

O-Z Plasty

O-Z plasty is similar to the O-T or A-T advancement flap but incorporates double rotation flaps to close a circular defect.[35] This is useful in the eyelid where it allows minimal wound closure tension and redirects that tension along the long axis of the ellipse to direct tension parallel to the lid.

TRANSPOSITION FLAPS

A transposition flap involves lifting tissue from the donor site over a bridge of tissue to a separate recipient site. Many forms of transposition flaps exist while the versatility of these flaps permits the potential use in almost all situations. The most important element in design of transposition flaps is the pivot point rather than the geometry. The tissue must be pivoted in a way that prevents strangulation of the flaps blood supply and resultant tension related ischemia. Regional differences in mobility of tissue may also have a greater impact than the geometry. It is extremely important to spend time designing the transposition flap rather than modifying an improperly elevated flap poorly designed initially. Donor site issues often include pull on the eyebrow, hairline, lateral canthus, lower eyelid, nasal ala, upper lip, and lateral oral commissure. These flaps generally disperse wound tension over a large area, minimizing visible deformity and scar widening.

Z-plasty

This technique is widely used alone or in conjunction with other flaps to change the direction of tension on wound closure and lengthen a resulting scar.[26] This technique changes scar direction, interrupts scar linearity, and lengthens scar contracture. A 60° Z-plasty is the most common design, but angles between 30° and 90° are possible. Angles below 30° should not be used secondary to decreased tip vascularity. The goal is to provide maximum camouflage in RSTL. A general rule is that 30°, 60°, and 90° Z-plasty will respectively lengthen a scar 25%, 50%, and 75%. The Z-plasty also contributes to reorienting a scar into RSTL when using multiple Z-plasty for long scars. Oral competence can be restored secondary to orbicularis dysfunction or marginal mandibular nerve damage by transposing the oral commissure using Z-plasty technique.

Rhombic Transposition Flap

Originally called the Limberg flap,[57] this flap now has many variations (Figs 40.2A to C).[7] Although many use the term rhomboid flap interchangeably, an exact study of the geometry of this flap is essential to the understanding of flap dynamics and movement of tissue. In the Limberg flap, all the sides of the defect and the flap are the same length by definition. With a Limberg defect created, a line is drawn from one of the 120° angles to create a side of equal length that now becomes the new side to the flap.[8] This rhombic defect and flap are essentially four equilateral triangles. The Dufourmental flap[10] variation uses two isosceles triangles base to base, while the Webster 30° modification uses a 30° angle for the flap and an M-plasty at the base of the defect. This decreases tissue protrusion because the 60° angles of the defect have now been converted to two 30° angles as an M-plasty and shares the closure of the other angle with the flap. Rhombic flaps are one of the most common local flaps in the head and neck.[47]

Bilobed Flap

This flap can allow a 180° transfer of tissue (Fig. 40.3). This maximizes that the distance that skin can be moved. It transfers the tension of wound closure through a 90° arc instead of the normal 45-60° of the basic transposition flap.[17] Techniques that enhance the utility and application include placing Burow's triangles at the base, transposition of each flap over 45° instead of 90°, and wide peripheral undermining of the skin surrounding the defect, the flap and its donor site.[39] This flap is best suited for circular defects on the lateral aspect and lower third of the nose, but may be applied to large defects on the cheek in lieu of larger cervicofacial rotation flaps. Helical rim defects may be repaired with transfer of skin from the postauricular area. Disadvantages of this flap revolve around the incision sites that do not parallel RSTL or anatomic subunits.[63] The elevation of two flaps also contributes to a relatively lengthy scar. The commonly described 'pin-cushion' complication can be avoided when wide undermining is performed.

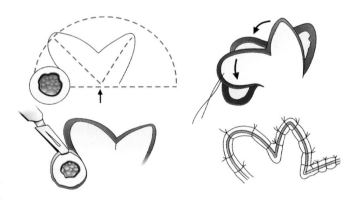

Fig. 40.3: The bilobed flap; it allows 180° transfer of tissue

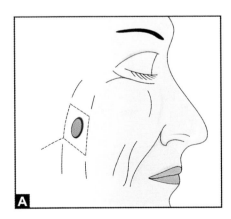
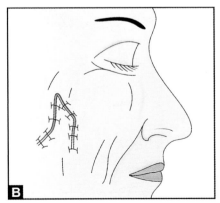
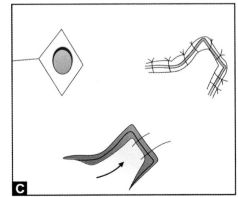

Fig. 40.2: The Limberg flap and its variations

Melolabial Flaps

Also called nasolabial flaps, this is one of the most widely used flaps for defects of the central face but can also be used intranasally and intraorally. They take advantage of extensibility of the medial cheek and a closure that remains within the borders of cosmetic units resulting in excellent cosmetic outcomes. These flaps allow enormous flexibility in design and movement and may be transposed or advanced and elevated with a random or axial blood supply. The flap can be based superiorly or inferiorly for various defects.

Superiorly based melolabial flaps may refill deep central and lateral nasal dorsal defects as well as defects of the nasal ala and tip (Figs 40.4A to C). However, this flap often results in blunting of the nasofacial sulcus, asymmetry of melolabial sulcus and distorted scar contracture thus requiring secondary revisions.

Inferiorly based melolabial flaps can repair deficits of the upper and lower lip, floor of the nose and columella. It is ideal for lateral upper lip defects that do not involve the vermilion of the lip. However, it can create scarring across alar-facial groove, trapdoor deformity, increase bulkiness of the upper lip, and obliterate the melolabial sulcus from the alar-facial sulcus to the lateral commissure.

Advancement melolabial flaps contribute to restoring the lateral aspect of nasal dorsum, lateral nasal ala defects not involving the alar rim, and defects which extend onto the cheek. To maintain the nasofacial sulcus, bolster sutures may be necessary while donor and recipient area closure lines usually fall in natural creases and shadows. The superior line prevails along the junction of the nasal dorsal and sidewall aesthetic subunits. Horizontal closure occurs near the nasal alar sulcus, while the donor site lies along the melolabial sulcus.

The melolabial interpolated flap is based on the angular artery and is used specifically for the recreation of the alar subunit in nasal reconstruction. Many sizes, shapes, and thicknesses can be created from this flap and advanced, rotated, or transposed into a variety of distal nasal defects.

Paramedian Forehead Flaps

The paramedian forehead flap and its variations have revolutionized reconstruction of the nose and are now widely used.[9] The paramedian forehead flap has a much narrower base than the median forehead flap and has greater freedom of rotation revealing a flap of greater effective length. This flap is pedicled on the supratrochlear artery which initial flows superficial to the corrugator and deep to the frontalis muscle but perforates the frontalis muscle near the eyebrow where it then begins its subcutaneous course. The distal aspect of this flap can be thinned based on the location of the pedicle distally to allow better contouring to the defect. The proximal dissection of skin near the pedicle may be as narrow as 1.2 cm which reduces donor site deformity in the glabellar area. This flap does not affect the mimetic musculature, has limited wound contraction, and usually does not require transfer of hair-bearing skin to the face. Donor site closure is achieved with flaps as wide as 4.5 cm, however, acceptable healing occurs by secondary intention in the distal forehead region. Tissue expansion has also been used to expand the size and lengthen this

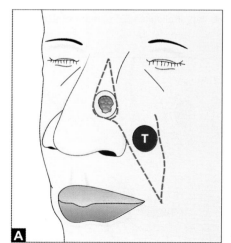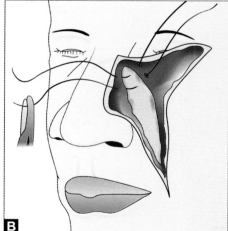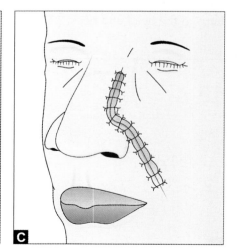

Figs 40.4A to C: Superiorly based melolabial flaps may refill deep central and lateral nasal dorsal defects as well as defects of the nasal ala and tip

flap.[59] A vertical scar in the central forehead does result and occasionally may have to be closed with a skin graft. However, 3 or 4 vertical fasciotomies on either side of the incision site may allow for another 1 cm of skin laxity. Major drawbacks include inadequate pedicle length in patients with a low forehead or widows peak and the requirement of a second operation three weeks later. Most commonly used for nasal defects larger than 2.5 cm in length, but may refill defects of the medial canthal region, upper/lower eyelid, cheek, melolabial region, or upper lip.[60] Total nasal reconstruction can be achieved with a combination of the paramedian forehead flap using adjunctive scalp, forehead and free flaps with bone and cartilage grafting. Menick has described a three stage forehead flap for more complex nasal defects that require additional subunit reconstruction.

Dorsal Nasal Flaps

Dorsal nasal skin can refill deficits of the lower nose that do not exceed 2 cm in diameter.[11] Originally described by Reiger, this flap pivots around a random pattern pedicle from the glabella/medial canthus down to the nasal/cheek junction and represents a modification of the V-Y flap. A vascular pedicle based on vessels near the inner canthus incorporating a vascular branch of the angular artery enables better narrowing of the pedicle and better rotation without restraint. If the rotation of this flap is to effectively reduce the tension of closure, then increasing the length of the sweep of the flap narrows the secondary defect and makes closure better. However, incisions then become quite extensive relative to the primary wound. This flap provides better skin match compared to forehead flaps or grafts that do not have the same skin quality, texture, sebaceous quality, color, or vascular patterns.[18] The incisions are well hidden in cosmetic junctions: alar crease, glabellar frown, nasofacial sulcus. It is important to realize the pull from the limited rotation on the nasal tip and alae which may be displaced secondary to inappropriate design. The axial based design and ensuring the flap reaches over the defect helps prevent this problem. This flap is ideally used for defects 2.5 cm or less medial or superior to the alar lobule.

DEFECT BASED APPROACH TO RECONSTRUCTION

Scalp Defects

Reconstruction of the scalp is required following excision of lesions, traumatic injuries, or for aesthetic correction of alopecia.[5] The goals of reconstruction involve coverage of exposed bone, restoration of symmetric contour, and appropriate distribution of hair bearing skin. Small defects less than 3 cm in diameter can be closed primarily or closed with advancement flaps and an additional galeotomy.[53] Intermediate-sized defects are best closed with local flaps, while regional/distant flaps and skin grafts are the best remedy for large defects. Tissue expansion is used more frequently in scalp reconstruction than other areas of the face and neck due to the limited mobility of the scalp. This technique involves serial expansion over time of a balloon inserted under the galea. This increases the surface area of skin to aid in reconstruction.[62] It does require an incision that may disrupt planning of local flaps in the future, thus, mandating that the surgeon plan the flap prior to insertion of the tissue expander.

The galea limits distensibility and produces stiffness within the tissue of the scalp.[6] Subsequently, closure of a scalp defect without leaving a secondary defect becomes difficult. The scalp is relatively tight over the vertex, while the tissue is more mobile encircling the cranium. The galea tends to dissipate into fascia in the areas overlying muscle resulting in more distensible tissue. Releasing incisions on the galea can increase the effective length of a local flap on the scalp.

Although the rotation flap has its limits for uses on the face, it is one of the most useful flaps in scalp reconstruction.[32] The length of an arcing incision should be greater than 4 times the length of a scalp defect in its greatest dimension. Increasing the arc of rotation increases the standing cutaneous deformity. Often the secondary defect has to be closed with a skin graft.

Transposition flaps should be designed so that the base lies in a loose scalp area, preferably over a known vascular supply.[67] Examples of these flaps include the temporoparietal and temporoparietal-occipital (Juri flap), and the parietal temporal postauricular vertical flap.

Advancement flaps are limited to the role of closing transposition flap donor sites and scalp reductions. The galea resists stretching with advancement but allows for greater wound closure tension since it protects from ischemia. Parallel releasing incisions can be made through the galea perpendicular to the direction of desired lengthening. U-plasty can close a small defect best if it is based in loose scalp tissue.

The use of multiple scalp flaps has been documented and successfully used for a variety of scalp and adjacent wounds.

FOREHEAD AND TEMPLE DEFECTS

The goals of reconstruction of the forehead encompass preservation of motor and sensory function, maintenance of normal boundaries of aesthetic units including natural frontal and temporal hairlines, maintenance of brow symmetry, and optimal scar camouflage.[24] The predominant muscle of the forehead is the frontalis muscle innervated by the temporalis branch of the facial nerve. It is most at risk over the zygomatic arch where it is very close to the skin surface. The nerve enters the frontalis muscle from the deep side in the forehead so it is much less likely to be transected here. The forehead aesthetic unit is defined as the juncture lines with the scalp superiorly, the temporal scalp and temple laterally, and the eyebrows and glabella inferiorly. Because flaps can be dissected out in the subcutaneous layer as well as under the frontalis, smaller flaps are better served within the subcutaneous layer while a larger defect is best repaired with a myocutaneous local flap. These can be broadly undermined in a relatively avascular plane.

Advancement flaps can maintain good contours, allow optimal scar placement, and usually allow adequate tissue for reconstruction. They do require extensive undermining and multiple incisions. Rotation flaps take advantage of the curvature of the skull, but have lengthy incision lines often diagonal to forehead creases. Transposition flaps play a lesser role, but may be used in the glabellar and lateral forehead area.

Midline Forehead

Primary repair of central forehead defects is best done in a vertical plane with an M-plasty inferiorly in the glabellar creases. This may cause some medial displacement of the brows. Large upper middle forehead defects can be closed with bilateral rotation flaps with incision in the hairline.

Paramedian Forehead

This section of the forehead is defined by the midline to the midbrow laterally. Reconstruction involves horizontal placement of incisions within the RSTL.[43] This area is restricted by the vertical height of the defect and hairline, degree of brow elevation, and lack of skin/scalp mobility. A second incision in the hairline with a galeotomy can increase mobilization and essentially create a bipedicled advancement flap. However, this can lower the hairline. When defects are too large for primary repair, a U or H-plasty is best. Placement of burow's triangles can be placed in glabellar creases.

Lateral Forehead

This subunit begins at mid brow and extends to lateral brow and upper temple. It is here where the frontal branch of temporal facial nerve is at greatest risk. Single or bilateral advancement flaps and A to T, O to T repairs are options here. Incisions can be well placed even with a vertical limb. A Burow's wedge advancement flap uses a triangular defect in the lateral brow by creating a curvilinear incision along the brow with rotation after a Burow's triangle is made in the crow's feet. O to Z rotation flaps are allowed secondary to the curvilinear RSTL in this region. Rhombic or 30° transposition flaps take advantage of the excess skin of the temple. Multiple angulations of these scars are well hidden in the concave surface of the temple.

Eyebrow

H-plasty in eyebrow defects allows for hidden scars in superior and inferior brow margins. Incisions have to be parallel to hair shafts otherwise there is a risk of alopecia. The V-Y advancement flap can be used in this region as well.

Temple

Adjacent tissue in the cheek and forehead is mobilized for reconstruction in this area. The RSTLs run obliquely from the lateral canthus and create increased tissue laxity in this area. Burow's wedge advancement flaps and rhombic flaps are especially useful here.

AURICULAR DEFECTS

Auricular defects occur as defects of cutaneous cover, with or without intact cartilaginous structure,[4] and full thickness defects.[52] Discussion is limited to the impact of local flaps in this area and will not be extended to repair of large defects and total auricular reconstruction.[40]

Conchal Bowl and Helix

The retroauricular island transposition flap or 'flip-flop' flap is well-suited for conchal reconstruction because of proximity and eliminates the necessity of a full thickness skin graft.[19] The retroauricular skin is transferred from posterior to anterior toward the concha followed by primary closure of donor site. Dissection is from posterior to anterior direction to maintain a thick subcutaneous pedicle. The vascular supply is based on the postauricular artery and vein. This flap can be bivalved when a need for lateral and medial skin coverage.[49]

Defects of root of helix can be reconstructed with a helical advancement flap. An incision made in the lateral helical rim is advanced in Y to V fashion to preserve contour of the ear. For larger defects a small Burow's triangle must be removed for adequate advancement.[55]

Upper Third

Superficial defects of the helical rim are best closed if the cartilage is excised to a full thickness defect and closed primarily if the defect is less than 0.15 cm in width and extends from the helical rim into the body of the auricle. Helical chondrocutaneous advancement flaps restore the helix when the defect is greater than 0.15 cm but less than 2 cm in width. Additional opposing advancement can be made by V-Y advancement of the root of the helix. For defects larger than 2 cm, better closure can be obtained with a retroauricular or preauricular tubed flap. First stage requires formation of skin tube leaving superior and inferior attachments. Second stage attaches tube to the auricle and the third stage involves flap inset. The aforementioned retroauricular island transposition flap is used for full thickness defects with an intact helical rim. Cartilage grafts with temporoparietal fascial flap and skin graft covering create better results for very large defects when portions of scapha, helix, and triangular fossa are missing.[68]

Middle Third

Defects of the middle third of the auricle less than 1.5 cm are repaired via wedge shaped excision and advancement. Helical chondrocutaneous advancement flaps are used for full thickness defects less than 2.5 cm. A tubed flap is used for defects greater than 2.5 cm but soft tissue defect only. Major defects involving helix and antihelix require cartilage grafting and two-stage retroauricular composite flap. The first stage involves retroauricular advancement flap that is advanced to lateral defect with a cartilage graft; usually conchal or septal cartilage is placed beneath the flap. Three weeks later, the flap is detached from the scalp and covers the medial aspect of the graft.

Lower Third

Laxity of skin in the lower third of auricle enables primary repair unless there is a total loss of lobule. With total loss of the lower one-third of the auricle, a composite flap containing conchal cartilage is embedded in the subcutaneous pocket below the auricle. Six weeks later the cartilage and overlying skin are elevated as a composite flap based on the remaining auricle.

EYELID DEFECTS

The restoration of the periorbital region involves several difficulties not addressed in other regions of the face.[14] The function of the eyelid is the major concern and techniques such as placing incisions in the RSTL often do not apply here. A basic elliptical excision in the RSTL will result in ectropion of the eyelid and create a hazardous situation for the patient.[61] Additionally, the unique anatomy of the eyelid creates special challenges for the surgeon.

Periorbital Skin

Advancement flaps are used mostly in the periorbital region and include standard rectangular flaps as well as V-Y advancement. The resulting parallel scars avoid deformities of the lid margins and use the available skin in the lid margins. Rhombic flaps can be used for periorbital defects, but they must be properly designed so that the wound tension vectors are horizontal instead of vertical to avoid displacement of the lid.

Partial Thickness Defects

Small partial thickness defects can be closed with local advancement flaps with horizontal wound tension. If the levator palpebra is torn then it should be advanced and reattached to the aponeurosis or tarsal plate, but if completely destroyed then frontalis can be advanced to suspend the aponeurosis or tarsus. For the lower eyelid, a laterally based transposition flap involves transposing a skin-muscle flap from the upper lid to the lower lid.

Full Thickness Defects

Primary closure for defects of 25% or less is most appropriate. Full vertical excision of the tarsus must occur to minimize tarsal buckling. The initial suture placed in the grey line approximates the lid margin. The tarsus and the orbicularis are closed next. In older individuals with significant lid laxity, up to a 40% defect can be closed. For slightly larger defects, a lateral cantholysis is needed. The superior crus is cut for upper lid defects and the lower crus for lower lid defects.

A Tenzel or semicircular flap can close larger lower lid defects up to 75%. A semicircle is drawn starting at the lateral canthus, with the apex of the semicircle in the opposite direction from the involved lid.

Wide undermining below the orbicularis is needed. After a canthotomy and cantholysis are performed, the curvilinear flap straightens out as it is advanced from lateral to medial.

Tarsoconjunctival flaps are useful for large defects of the upper and lower eyelid.[29] The Cutler-Beard technique is a two-stage full thickness tarsoconjunctival flap lid sharing procedure. A lower eyelid flap including skin, muscle, and conjunctiva is elevated under an intact margin to fill the deficiency in the upper eyelid. Autogenous cartilage or scleral graft can be placed between the muscle and conjunctiva of the flap. A lateral cantholysis aids with the reconstruction. The flap is divided after 6-10 weeks, and the unused portion is sutured to the donor site.

Tarsoconjunctival flaps can remedy large defects of the lower lid as well.[27] The Hughes tarsoconjunctival flap involves a transfer of the posterior lamella from the upper lid into the lower lid defect leaving 4 mm of tarsus intact in the upper lid margin.[28] Mullers muscle is not transferred with the flap. The flap is covered with a full thickness skin graft or advancement flap. The bridge is transected after 4-6 weeks 2-3 mm below estimated upper lid margin.

NASAL DEFECTS

Reconstruction should restore and preserve form and function. Aesthetic subunits consist of the nasal dorsum, nasal tip, columella, paired lateral nasal sidewalls, alar lobules, and the alar facets.[16] The preservation or recreation of these subunits is essential for providing optimal nasal appearance. The upper two-thirds of the nose are covered by thin, slightly mobile tissue, while the lower third is covered by thick, non-mobile sebaceous skin. If greater 50% of a subunit is missing in a defect, than it is better to replace the entire subunit. Each level of a defect must be addressed in reconstruction. For a full thickness defect of the ala for example, the inner lining must be replaced as well as the cartilage and skin. The cartilage supplies a supporting structure to prevent nasal valve collapse.

Local flaps such as a Banner flap[37] satisfactorily cover smaller defects of the dorsum and sidewalls. Ideally this flap is used for defects less than 2 cm because of the geometrical limitations of transposition of native tissue on the nose. Defects of the tip and ala have such thick poorly mobile skin that single lobe transposition flaps cause distortion of free margins secondary to excessive wound tension.[70,71] Rhombic flaps can close defects larger than the banner flap, but the angular nature of flap

incisions poses limitations for use on the nose. The bilobed flap of McGregor or Zitelli moves adjacent matching skin to the area of deficiency while filling the secondary defect with a second flap taken from the looser skin of the upper two-thirds of nose. These are best for small defects of the ala or nasal tip. The melolabial flap is one of the most versatile flaps used in nasal reconstruction.[20] The flap can be elevated with a superior- or inferior-based pedicle and can be based on the angular artery. Nasal defects 2.5 cm in diameter can be closed with this flap. A glabellar or dorsal nasal flap takes advantage of skin laxity in the glabellar region and acceptance of a vertical scar in this area. Island pedicle flaps must be of sufficient length and width to avoid undue tension, avoid flap ischemia, and allow a sufficient axis of rotation. These are mostly based in the nasolabial or glabellar areas.

Alar Subunit

If the deficit is less than 50%, a bilobed flap is adequate for reconstruction; if greater than 50%, the entire subunit is replaced with either a melolabial island flap or superiorly based melolabial flap.[36] Blood supply to the island flap is via perforaters from the facial artery near the alar base. To resurface with an island flap, a template of the opposite ala is recreated and then traced along the melolabial fold. Place the template low enough to ensure sufficient length of the pedicle to relieve tension on rotation. The flap is elevated while closing the donor site along the along the nasolabial crease. The flap is rotated inferiorly into nasal tip and trimmed only when adequate length is confirmed. The flap can be divided laterally and inset after 3-4 weeks. A superiorly based melolabial flap has the advantage of a larger size and the ability to extend to defects of both the ala and the tip. Effacement of the nasofacial sulcus and asymmetry at the nasolabial fold can be disadvantages. Nasal lining can be obtained from a bipedicled nasal mucosal flap. A cartilage graft for structural support helps prevent nasal valve collapse and also resists the upward contraction of the alar margin during the healing process.[50]

Columellar Subunit

Coverage of this defect, after appropriate cartilage grafting if needed, is accomplished with a pedicled island transposition flap based on the angular artery. This island flap is created in the nasal sidewall/nasofacial sulcus and advanced after undermining a tunnel, to the columellar strut. It is sutured to the tip skin superiorly, the base of the columella inferiorly and septal mucosa on both sides.

Tip Subunit

Cutaneous deficiencies less than 1.5-2 cm can be replaced with local flaps.[56] If greater than 2 cm and only the skin envelope is lost, a paramedian or median forehead flap is the best choice. In unusual circumstances, a scalping flap or even a free tissue transfer may be necessary.[69] Defects that involve cartilage and mucosal loss need replacement of those layers.[41,42]

Nasal Ala and Sidewall Subunits

These defects require the same strategy of replacing entire subunit and providing underlying cartilage grafts and inner nasal lining if there is a full thickness defect.[30] A paramedian forehead flap is the best choice for these defects.[45]

CHEEK DEFECTS

The cheek unit is defined laterally by the preauricular crease, superiorly by the infraorbital rim and superior border of the zygomatic arch, medially the nasofacial groove, melolabial crease, and labiomental sulcus, and inferiorly the boundary is the inferior mandibular border. It is further divided into medial, zygomatic, buccal, and lateral subunits.[44]

Medial Subunit

Tissue of the medial subunit is relatively thick and freely mobile. Small tissue defects along the nasofacial sulcus can be closed with advancement of lateral margin, but need a tacking suture to the periosteum to prevent blunting of the nasofacial sulcus. Larger defects require cheek rotation advancement flaps created by incising the infraorbital crease. These may also require periosteum tacking sutures to prevent blunting. Defects that cross the nasofacial sulcus should be repaired appropriately with two separate flaps to recreate separate aesthetic units. A bilobed flap can rotate tissue from the lateral cheek subunit with the second lobe harvested from postauricular region. Defects of the lower eyelid and upper medial subunit require special attention to prevent lid retraction. The superior rotation-advancement flap incision placed in the subciliary position allows for advancement of the remaining lower eyelid skin into the eyelid portion of the defect.

Buccal Subunit

Small to medium defects can be closed primarily or with transposition flaps. Transposition flaps can result in conspicuous scars because the posterior and superior subunit borders do not hide incisions well. Large defects can be served with cheek advancement or cervicofacial rotation flaps.

Zygomatic Subunit

Direct closure and transposition flaps can be used for small to medium defects. Lower eyelid distortion can result if tension vectors are in vertical position. Proper flap design and periosteal flap fixation sutures near the lateral canthus can alleviate this. The facial nerve must be protected in this region.

Lateral Subunit

Many defects in this area can be closed primarily with local advancement secondary to the relative laxity of anterior cheek tissue. Rhombic or bilobed flaps take advantage of cervical laxity along the inferior lateral border and can close small to medium defects. Large defects can be closed with advancement flaps or cervicofacial rotation advancement flaps.

LIP DEFECTS

The upper lip is divided into three aesthetic subunits – the philtrum and two lateral subunits, while the lower lip has one subunit only. The melolabial and labiomental creases separate the cheeks and chin from the lip subunits. The same principles hold true in lip reconstruction as other regions of the face. Plan incisions along subunits, creases, and RSTL and reconstruct entire subunits when possible. Goals include maintaining oral competence, providing sensation, allowing maximal oral aperture, and restoring acceptable anatomic proportions and aesthetic appearance.

Upper Lip

Small lesions of the vermilion can be excised with fusiform design based on RSTL and closed with simple advancement. These would be oriented vertically centrally and more obliquely laterally. Simple V-Y advancement flaps can release contracted areas of vermilion.

Upper lip cutaneous defects that are partial thickness can be reconstructed with a single stage perialar crescentic melolabial advancement flap best suited if the defect is near the alar base. Obliteration of the melolabial crease, pincushioning, and the advancement of non hair-bearing skin in males are disadvantages of this technique.

Defects in melolabial fold can be closed primarily. A to T repairs can be used when lesion is next to the vermilion. Partial thickness defects of philtrum are best closed by full thickness skin grafts or secondary intention. Larger lateral subunit defects can be repaired with an inferior based melolabial transposition flap.

With full thickness defects less than one-third of the lip, wedge excision with primary closure, carefully approximating mucosa, orbicularis, and skin is appropriate.[34] With defects one-third to two-thirds the size of the lip, attempts should be made to recreate an entire subunit. This can be done with the perialar crescentic flap for lateral subunit defects as in the partial thickness defect. An Abbe lip-switch flap is based on the labial artery and can be used to close lateral or philtral subunit defects. The Estlander modification of the Sabatini cross-lip flap is used when defects involve the commissure. This is a rotational flap that can be accomplished in one stage, with the potential drawback of rounding or blunting of the commisure that can be addressed with a later commisuroplasty. An Abbe flap can also be used for philtral defects and combined with a perialar crescentic advancement flap if the adjacent lateral subunit is involved. A Gillies fan flap based on labial vessels provides more tissue available for reconstruction than lip switch and advancement flaps. Bernard–von Burow design for total or subtotal upper lip reconstruction uses excision of triangles with advancement to recreate the upper lip.

Lower Lip

Vermilion and partial thickness defects can be closed primarily or with advancement flaps. Bilateral rectangular advancement flaps and melolabial flaps can be used. Wedge resection can be used in one half the length of the lower lip. Defects of up to one half the lower lip can be closed primarily after basic wedge excision with approximation of all three layers.

Centrally located lesions from one-half to two-thirds the length of lower lip may be reconstructed with the Karapandzic flap or bilateral advancement flaps. Attempts are made to preserve sensory and motor function by dissection and identification of the nerves lying inferior to the commissure. Flap height is equivalent to the height of the defect and is pedicled on labial vessels. Larger lateral lesions can be repaired with an Abbe flap with defects involving the commissure reconstructed with the Estlander flap.

Deficits greater than two-thirds of the lower lip may be reconstructed with the Gillies fan flap, Webster modification of the Bernard–von Burow flap, melolabial flaps and remote tissue flaps.

Total reconstruction of the lower lip requires the use of a free flap especially the radial forearm palmaris longus free flap with the use of a tongue flap to simulate the vermilion. This flap is given additional support by folding tissue over the suspended palmaris longus tendon which is sutured to the periosteum of the malar eminence and acts as a sling.

OTHER DEFECTS

In addition to the soft tissue defects which comprise the majority of procedures performed, defects of composite tissues and mucosa may be reconstructed with similar techniques. Reconstruction of these complex areas is beyond the scope of this chapter but should be understood in order for the reconstructive surgeon to use the ideal methods for each individual defect.

CONCLUSION

Techniques in soft tissue facial reconstruction continue to undergo aesthetic and functional improvements through modifications based on historical descriptions of flap design. The popularization of free tissue transfers and advanced techniques in local flaps have added a new dimension to the recreation of facial structures. Adherence to basic principles, however, is the cornerstone of proper and aesthetic reconstruction of facial structures. Restoration of aesthetic subunits, appropriate incision placement, preservation of function, and adherence to current techniques of reconstruction will facilitate appropriate management of patients with facial defects.

REFERENCES

1. Ahuja R. Geometric consideration in the design of rotational flaps in the scalp and forehead region. *Plast Reconstruct Surg* 1988; 81:900.
2. Al-Shunnar B, Manson PN. Cheek reconstruction with laterally based flaps. *Clin Plast Surg* 2001; 28(2):283–296.
3. Anden NA, Carlsson A, Haggendal J. Adrenergic mechanisms. *Ann Rev Pharmacol* 1969; 9:119.
4. Antia. N.H. and V.I. Buch. Chondroculaneous advancement flap for the marginal defect of the ear. *Plast Reconstruct Surg* 1967; 39:472.
5. Arnold PG, CS Randarathman CS. Multiple-flap scalp reconstruction orticochea revisited. *Plast Reconstruct Surg* 1981; 69(605).
6. Barron JN, Emmett AJJ. Subcutaneous pedicle flaps. *Br J Plast Surg* 1965; 18:51–78.
7. Becker FF. Rhomboid flap in facial reconstruction. New concept of tension lines. *Arch Otolaryngol* 1979; 105(10): 569–573.

8. Borges AF, The rhombic flap. *Plast Reconstruct Surg* 1981; 67:458.

9. Boyd CM, et al, The forehead flap for nasal reconstruction. *Arch Dermatol* 2000; 136(11):1365–1370.

10. Bray D. Clinical applications of the rhomboid flap. *Arch Otolaryngol* 1983; 109:37.

11. Burget GC, Menick FJ. The subunit principle in nasal reconstruction. *Plast Reconstruct Surg* 1985; 76(2):239–247.

12. Clark JM, Wang TD. Local flaps in scar revision. *Facial Plast Surg* 2001; 17(4):295–308.

13. Connor CD, Folko SW. Anatomy and physiology of local skin flaps. *Facial Plast Surg Clin North Am* 1996; 4:447–454.

14. Cutler NL, Beard C. A method for partial and total upper lid reconstruction. *Am J Ophthalmol* 1955; 39:1.

15. Cutting CA. Critical closing and perfusion pressures in flap survival. *Ann Plast Surg* 1982; 9:524.

16. Danahey, D.G. and P.A. Hilger, Reconstruction of large nasal defects. *Otolaryngol Clin North Am* 2001; 34:4.

17. Dinehart SM. The rhombic bilobed flap for nasal reconstruction. *Dermatol Surg* 2001; 27(5):501–504.

18. Elliott RJ. Rotation flaps of the nose. *Plast Reconstruct Surg* 1969; 44:147–149.

19. Eriksson E, Vogt PM. Ear reconstruction. *Clin Plast Surg* 1992; 19(637).

20. Fader DJ, Baker SR, Johnson TM. The staged cheek-to-nose interpolation flap for reconstruction of the nasal alar rim/lobule. *J Am Acad Dermatol* 1997; 37(4):614–619.

21. Flynn TC, Emmanouil P, Limmer B. Unilateral transient forehead paralysis following injury to the temporal branch of the facial nerve. *Int J Dermatol* 1999; 38:474–477.

22. Folkow B. Role of the nervous system in the control of vascular tone. *Circulation* 1960; 21:760.

23. Gottrup F, et al. A comparative study of skin blood flow in musculocutaneous and random pattern flaps. *J Surg Res* 1984; 37(6):443–447.

24. Grigg R. Forehead and temple reconstruction. *Otolaryngol Clin North Am* 2001; 34(3):583–600.

25. Hosal N, Turan E, Aras T. Lymphoscintigraphy inpectoralis major myocutaneous flaps. *Arch Otolaryngol Head Neck Surg* 1994; 120:659.

26. Hove CR, Williams EF 3rd, Rodgers BJ. Z-plasty: A concise review. *Facial Plast Surg* 2001; 17(4):289–294.

27. Hughes W. Total lower lid reconstruction: Technical details. *Trans Am Ophthalmol Soc* 1976; 74:321.

28. Jelks, GW and EB. Jelks, Prevention of ectropion in reconstruction of facial defects. *Otolaryngol Clin North Am* 2001; 34:4.

29. Jewett BS, Shockley WW. Reconstructive options for periocular defects. *Otolaryngol Clin North Am* 2001; 34:3.

30. Johnson TM, et al. The Rieger flap for nasal reconstruction. *Arch Otolaryngol Head Neck Surg* 1995; 121(6):634–637.

31. Johnson TM, Nelson BR. Aesthetic reconstruction of skin cancer defects using flaps and grafts. *Am J Cosmetic Surg* 1992; 9:253.

32. Juri J. Use of parieto-occipital flaps in the surgical treatment of baldness. *Plast Reconstruct Surg* 1975; 55:456.

33. Kobus K. Retroauricular secondary island flap. *Ann Plast Surg* 1985; 14(1):24–32.

34. Koshima I, et al. Free radial forearm osleocutaneous perforator flap for reconstruction of total nasal defects. *J Reconstr Microsurg* 2002; 18(7):585–588; discussion 589–590.

35. LeVasseur JG, Mellette JR. Applications of the double O to Z flap repair for facial reconstruction. *Dermatol Surg* 2001; 27(1):79–81.

36. Marchac D, Toth B. The axial frontonasal flap revisited. *Plast Reconstruct Surg* 1985; 76:686.

37. Masson JK, Mendelson BC. The banner flap. *Am J Surg* 1977; 134:419–423.

38. McGregor IA. Local skin flaps in facial reconstruction. *Otolaryngol Clin North Am* 1982; 15(1):77–98.

39. McGregor JC, Soutar DS. A critical assessment of the bilobed flap. *Br J Plast Surg* 1981; 34(2):197–205.

40. Mellette JR Jr. Ear reconstruction with local flaps. *J Dermatol Surg Oncol* 1991; 17(2):176–182.

41. Menick FJ. A 10-year experience in nasal reconstruction with the three-stage forehead flap. *Plast Reconstruct Surg* 2002; 109(6):1839–1855; discussion 1856–1861.

42. Menick FJ. A 10-year experience in nasal reconstruction with the three–stage forehead flap. *Plast Reconstr Surg* 2002; 109(6):1839–1855; discussion 1856–1861.

43. Menick FJ. Aesthetic refinements in use of forehead for nasal reconstruction: the paramedian forehead flap. *Clin Plast Surg* 1990; 17(4):607–622.

44. Menick FJ. Reconstruction of the cheek. *Plast Reconstruct Surg* 2001; 108(2):496–505.

45. Meyer R. Aesthetic refinements in nose reconstruction. *Aesthet Plast Surg* 2000; 24(4):241–252.

46. Miller PJ, Constantinides M. Simple and serial excisions. *Facial Plast Surg Clin North Am* 1998; 6:142.

47. Monheit GD. The rhomboid transposition flap re-evaluated. *J Dermatol Surg Oncol* 1980; 6(6):464–471.

48. Murakami CS, Nishioka GJ. Essential concepts in the design of local skin flaps. *Facial Plast Surg North Am* 1996; 4: 455–468.

49. Park SS, Hood RJ. Auricular reconstruction. *Otolaryngol Clin North Am* 2001; 34(4):713–738, v–vi.

50. Park SS, TA Cook. Reconstructive rhinoplasty. *Facial Plast Surg* 1997; 13:309.

51. Peled IJ, Wexler MR. The usefulness and versatility of V–Y advancement flaps. *J Dermatol Surg Oncol* 1983; 9(12): 1003–1006.

52. Ramirez OM, Heckler FR. Reconstruction ofnonmarginal defects of the ear with chondrocutaneous advancement flaps. *Plast Reconstruct Surg* 1989; 84:32.

53. Raposio E, Nordstrom RE. Tension and flap advancement in the human scalp. *Ann Plast Surg* 1997; 39(1):20–23.

54. Rees TD, Liverett DM, Guy CL. The effect of cigarette smoking on skin–flap survival in the face lift patient. *Plast Reconstruct Surg* 1984; 73(6):911–915.

55. Renard A. Postauricular flaps based on a dermal pedicle for ear reconstruction. *Plast Reconstruct Surg* 1981; 68:159.

56. Rieger R. A local flap for repair of the nasal tip. *Plast Reconstruct Surg* 1967; 52(361).

57. Rossi A, Jeffs JV. The rhomboid flap of Limberg—a simple aid to planning. *Ann Plast Surg* 1980; 5(6):494–496.

58. Sherman J. Normal arteriovenous anastomoses. *Medicine* 1963; 42:247.

59. Shumrick KA, Smith TL. The anatomic basis for the design of forehead flaps in nasal reconstruction. *Arch Otolaryngol Head Neck Surg* 1992; 118(4):373–379.

60. Siegle RJ. Forehead reconstruction. *J Dermatol Surg Oncol* 1991; 17:200.

61. Tenzel RR, Stewart WB. Eyelid reconstruction by the semi-circle flap technique. *Ophthalmology* 1978; 85:1164.

62. TerKonda RP, Sykes JM. Concepts in scalp and forehead reconstruction. *Otolaryngol Clin North Am* 1997; 30(4): 519–539.

63. Tramier H. Simple method of designing a bilobed flap. *Plast Reconstruct Surg* 2000; 105(7):2633–2634.

64. Tsur H, Daniller A, Strauch B. Neovascularization of skin flaps: Route and timing. *Plast Reconstruct Surg* 1980; 66:85.

65. Whetzel TP, Mathes SJ. Arterial anatomy of the face: An analysis of vascular territories and perforating cutaneous vessels. *Plast Reconstruct Surg* 1992; 89:591–603.

66. Wideman MR, Tuma R, Mayorvitz H. Defining the pre-capillary sphincter. *Microvasc Res* 1976; 12:71.

67. Yang CC et al. Reconstruction of children's scalp defects with the Orticochea flap. *Ann Plast Surg* 1992; 28(6):584–589.

68. Yang D, Morris SF. Vascular basis of the retroauricular flap. *Ann Plast Surg* 1998; 40(1):28–33.

69. Zitelli JA, Fazio MJ. Reconstruction of the nose with local flaps. *J Dermatol Surg Oncol* 1991; 17(2):184–189.

70. Zitelli JA. The bilobed flap for nasal reconstruction. *Arch Dermatol* 1989; 125(7):957–959.

71. Zitelli JA. The nasolabial flap as a single stage procedure. *Arch Dermatol* 1990; 126(1445).

The Nasal Tip

Stephen S Park, Brian F Perry

The nasal tip is conspicuously positioned in the center of the face and even subtle deformities can be immediately distracting, often overwhelming the other positive facial attributes that define beauty. Its aesthetic three-dimensional form is owed to a complex inter-relation between cartilage, bone, and soft tissue. The ideal nose is often considered the most normal nose, that is, one that blends in with the face and fails to call attention to it. In this sense, rhinoplasty is one of the most challenging surgical procedures because the most successful outcome is one that no one notices. From here, the nose can only fail in that it becomes distracting. Aberrancies in one or more of the supporting structures can produce an infinite array of tip deformities, including problems with projection, rotation, width, or symmetry. Preoperative evaluation not only involves recognition of the cutaneous deformity, that is, the features of the nose that the patient complains of, but must also include a careful analysis of the anatomic etiology that is underlying the external form. This critical step helps define the surgical options and creates a targeted surgical plan. The effects of each surgical maneuver, primary, secondary ones, and also the associated illusions created, must be anticipated. This chapter will review the analysis of nasal tip problems and present the surgical options frequently used.

AESTHETIC ANALYSIS

Nasal analysis includes not only the size and shape of the nose, but how it relates to the rest of the face, height, gender, and ethnicity. On frontal view, the tip lobule should reveal two, distinct tip-defining points that are detectable as reflections of light straddling a subtle bifidity to the tip. Their width should be proportional to the upper nose and facial shape, permitting the tip definition to gently blend into the aesthetic 'brow tip'

line. The supratip area should be contiguous with the sidewalls of the middle vault. Excessive fullness in this region is commonly referred to as the 'bulbous' tip and corresponds to the cephalic portion of the lateral crura, thus the ubiquity of the cephalic trim. On side view, one can appreciate a 'double break' as the profile transitions from the nasal tip to the infratip lobule segment and the columella. This double break is the natural curvature of the medial crura and contributes to the appropriate amount of columellar show (along with the length of the caudal septum and tip rotation).

Tip projection refers to the distance of the nasal tip from the coronal plane of the face, independent of the dorsum and length of the nose. It is an important landmark to assess, control, and preserve. Important determinants of tip projection are the size/shape of the lower lateral cartilages, the height of the caudal cartilaginous septum and its attachment to the medial crura. Different quantitative methods of assessing nasal tip projection have been described and are occasionally useful.[1,2] Under-projection of the nasal tip can lead to a flattened appearance to the midface, the illusion of a prominent dorsal hump, and flattening of the alar base and nostrils. On the other hand, over-projection of the tip can be evidenced by slit-like nostrils, nasal valve obstruction, and an overall narrow nose.

Tip rotation parallels the degree of inclination of the nasolabial angle. The normal angles are 90–100° for males and 100–105° for females. Shorter people can often tolerate more tip rotation than taller individuals. It is essential for surgeons to realize that tip rotation and projection are intimately related and manipulating one will inevitably impact the other.

Nasal symmetry will need to be carefully assessed when analyzing the nasal tip. Most patients will have some degree of asymmetry to the nasal tip. If the same technique is applied to both sides it may result in worsening of the asymmetry. If there is marked asymmetry, it may lend a twisted appearance to the entire nose.

STRUCTURAL ANALYSIS OF THE NASAL TIP

The structural analysis of the nose is done independently from the aesthetic evaluation, but the two must be brought together and the causal relationship between the two fully understood. Anatomic analysis of the nose begins with the overlying skin. The skin over the inferior third of the nose is characteristically thick and sebaceous, particularly in contrast to the soft tissues over the rhinion. Very thick skin, such as those found in African-Americans, may have a limited ability to contract and drape over a reoriented framework. As such, conventional rhinoplasty maneuvers will often be ineffective in refining the nasal tip and the amorphous or bulbous characteristic may persist. Under these circumstances, one often has to resort to augmentation techniques rather than resection or reorientation. Conversely, thin skin must alert the surgeon to the fact that even small cartilaginous irregularities become readily apparent. These imperfections can be distracting and gives the patient an 'operated' look. Grafts and cartilage borders will often require an additional cushion beneath the soft tissue envelop, such as acellular dermis.

The arterial supply to the tip skin is primarily through the paired columellar and lateral nasal arteries. There is a rich network of vascular channels in the subdermal layer and preserving its integrity is essential. Beneath the subcutaneous fat is the plane contiguous with the superficial musculo-aponeurotic system (SMAS) of the face. Surgical dissection beneath this layer ensures the preservation of the subdermal plexus.[3]

The paired lower lateral cartilages represent the major framework to the lower third of the nose and are most responsible for the size and shape of the tip (Figs 41.1A and B). Logically, surgical steps that manipulate these cartilages are the mainstay of nasal tip surgery. Each lower lateral cartilage consists of a medial and lateral crus, joined by a transitional segment known as the intermediate crus. Its complex, three-dimensional shape is suspended through specific ligaments and rests in an equilibrium of tension and vectors of force. Any destabilization or manipulation will disrupt this balance in a predictable manner and change the position and shape of the cutaneous tip. The 'tripod' concept is based on three supporting limbs that hold the tip in position.[4]

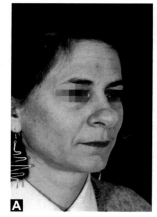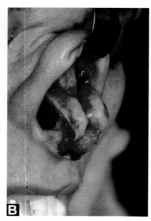

Figs 41.1A and B: (A) Oblique view of prominent nasal tip. (B) Intraoperative view showing patient's prominent lower lateral cartilages that form the nasal tip

The essence of tip rhinoplasty is the controlled alteration of these supporting vectors of the lower lateral cartilages and, thus its orientation in space.

The medial crura are intimately associated with the caudal septum through ligamentous attachments. The caudal strut is a stable foundation which supports the medial crura and provides tip projection and rotation. Disruption of these ligaments will immediately destabilize the tip and cause a loss of projection and rotation. The anterior nasal spine provides a platform for support and is a minor contributor to projection. The medial crura themselves have an intricate three-dimensional contour that gives shape to the columella.

The intermediate crura diverge from one another and are the structures responsible for the tip defining points. They are normally divergent from the medial crura and give rise to an appropriate width to the nasal tip. When the tip defining points are excessively divergent, it can create the unusually wide and bifid tip that appears trapezoidal on base view. This will disrupt the aesthetic 'brow-tip' line. Conversely, they can be too narrow, resulting in an unnatural and pointy tip. The ligamentous connection spanning the two intermediate crura rests on the anterior septal angle and helps support the tip in terms of projection.

The lateral crura are most responsible for the size and shape of the tip lobule and are the focus of most surgical maneuvers. They normally extend from the intermediate crura in a superior and lateral direction, lying in a plane close to the lateral nasal walls. They are not typically found in the alar lobule themselves. When the tip is bulbous, it may be due to the volume of the lateral crura or their orientation in space. Excessive volume will create

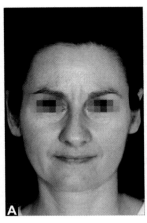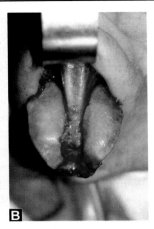

Figs 41.2A and B: (A) Anterior view of a patient with a broad and bulbous nasal tip. (B) Intraoperative view showing corresponding lower lateral cartilages. Note the coronal orientation to the lateral crura which cause the tip deformity

supratip fullness and can be refined through a resection of this area. On other occasions, the body of the lateral crus lies close to the coronal plane and this malorientation is the cause of a boxy and wide nasal tip (Figs 41.2A and B). Sutures may be used to reorient the lateral crura to refine the tip contour. Differentiating between these different causative factors is a pre-requisite to formulating a focused surgical plan.

Incisions and Approaches

A variety of incisions and approaches are used to perform rhinoplasty and their nomenclature should be used accurately. In order to prepare the nose, local anesthetic with epinephrine is injected throughout the nose with attention to the columella arteries, lateral nasal arteries, and external nasal nerves. When lateral osteotomies are anticipated, additional infiltration into that region will help. The total volume for complete anesthesia is rarely over 3 cc. The intercartilaginous incision is at the cephalic margin of the lower lateral cartilages, through the scroll and between the lateral crus and the upper lateral. This endonasal approach allows direct access to the upper two-thirds of the nose but requires a retrograde route to the nasal tip. Meticulous closure of this incision should be performed to minimize scarring that might lead to nasal valve narrowing.

Intracartilaginous incisions are made within the body of the lateral crus, parallel to its cephalic border. It can be carried through the cartilage itself for a direct excision of the cephalic border. This cartilage-splitting technique is associated with minimal soft tissue dissection over the nasal tip. An accurate identification of the caudal border of the lateral crus is a pre-requisite because the cartilage resection is made without direct vision of the remaining cartilage.

The marginal incision is along the caudal border of the lateral crus and gives access to the entire nasal tip. It is used with both the delivery approach and the external approach as well as with the endonasal insertion of small grafts. Closure of this incision should be performed with small bites in order to avoid distortion or notching along the alar margin.

The rim incision is along the caudal border of the alar lobule, inferior to the lateral crura. This incision is seldom used currently but may be needed during a functional rhinoplasty where an alar lobule batten graft is needed caudal to the lateral crus.

The transcolumellar incision is a part of the external approach and is usually made transversely across the narrowest portion of the mid-columella. The skin is characteristically thin in this area and care must be taken to avoid damage to the underlying medial crura. A broken or 'inverted V' design is often used to reduce notching along the lateral border as wound contracture occurs.

Surgical approaches to the nose are divided into endonasal or external. The endonasal route uses single intranasal incisions, either cartilage splitting or intercartilaginous, through which surgical maneuvers are performed. The advantage of this route is that it is the most direct and causes the least soft tissue distortion and swelling. Visualization is minimal and generally reserved for minimal tip manipulation. The *delivery approach* is a type of endonasal technique which uses the marginal and intercartilaginous incisions to gain access and visualization of the entire lateral crus. The cartilages are delivered extranasally as a bipedicled chondrocutaneous flap. This allows for complete visualization of the columellar skin without disruption. Disadvantages from this approach include two intranasal incisions and the fact that the cartilages are not being evaluated in a natural anatomic position. The latter can make it more challenging to reach an accurate diagnosis in terms of the anatomic etiology of cutaneous aberrancies.

The external approach uses a combination of the transcolumellar and marginal incision (Fig. 41.3). It provides an unprecedented exposure of the lower two-thirds of the nose, allowing visualization of the anatomy in its natural position and easy access for suture placement. There are disadvantages to this approach. Tip swelling and paresthesias can last for months. There is

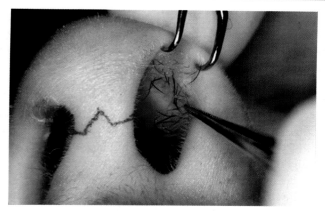

Fig. 41.3: Incisions for the external rhinoplasty approach. Inverted 'V' for the transcolumellar incision and marginal incision along the caudal border of the lateral crus (identified)

additional scarring from this approach that does not occur with the endonasal route. The transcolumellar scar generally heals remarkably well and is not an issue. The additional scarring that can be problematic occurs from the soft tissue dissection in areas that would otherwise not be violated. The significance of this scarring is that it may not be predictable and may not occur symmetrically. The progressive scarring and 'shrink wrap' effect of the subdermal dissection continues for years and can be the cause of twisting, asymmetry, bossae, or other irregularities. This must be considered prior to degloving the nose for relatively simple anatomic problems. Revision rhinoplasty is not necessarily an indication for the external approach because of the unpredictable scarring, especially when small camouflage grafts can be inserted endonasally.

SURGICAL TECHNIQUES

Tip Narrowing/Refinement

Refinement of the broad nasal tip is one of the more common goals in cosmetic rhinoplasty. Surgical options to achieve this can be categorized as:
• Volume reduction
• Cartilage reorientation
• Augmentation
• Soft tissue debulking

Choice of the appropriate technique depends on an accurate preoperative diagnosis in terms of the anatomic etiology.

Volume Reduction

Resection of the cephalic portion of the lateral crura is a common technique for narrowing the nasal tip. Often this

cephalic border is the culprit in tip bulbosity and its direct excision can have dramatic effects on the nasal tip. The primary effect is to narrow the supratip region and allow the tip lobule to blend in better with the upper nose. The secondary effects of such a maneuver is to create some cephalic tip rotation as well as de-projection. This technique was often referred to as the 'complete strip' procedure, because of the complete strip of cartilage left behind. Ancillary maneuvers were also performed that further narrowed the tip, such as excising triangles of cartilage from the remaining strip.

The secondary effects of this resection are the result of the 'dead space' that is created from this resection. Like any tissue void in the body, it is subject to natural wound contracture. This phenomenon continues for many years following surgery and is the cause of two long-term stigmata of a tip rhinoplasty, i.e. excessive columellar show due to alar retraction and nasal obstruction due to collapse of the nasal side wall and internal nasal valve. More contemporary techniques have emphasized cartilage preservation with an extremely conservative resection of the lateral crura. The technique is better characterized as a cephalic trim rather then a resection (Fig. 41.4).

A bilateral, vertical dome division and resection of the intermediate crura is a direct method of reducing volume and narrowing the tip lobule. This technique is warranted when the boxy nasal tip is due to an excessive amount of cartilage along the intermediate crus, especially oriented in an obtuse angle. Resection in this area with primary anastomosis is an effective and direct way of correcting this problem. Cartilaginous edges are reapproximated with simple stitches and often camouflaged with a tip graft (Figs 41.5A to E).

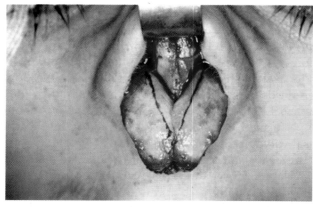

Fig. 41.4: Cephalic trim. Note the conservative resection and preservation of a majority of the lateral crus

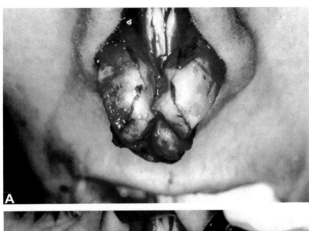

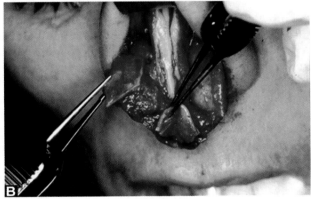

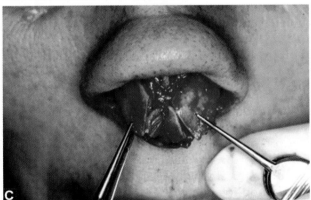

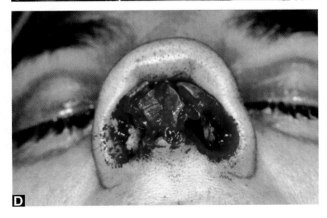

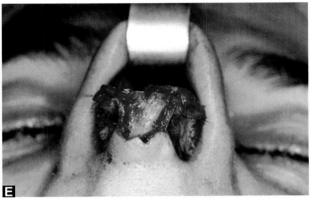

Figs 41.5A to E: Vertical dome division. (A) Vertical dome division and cephalic trim designed. (B) Wedge of cartilage from intermediate crura excised. (C) Reapproximation of cut edges reorients plane of lateral crura. (D) Tip deprojection occurs with VDD. (E) Tip graft

Reorientation

A more conservative and contemporary technique for refining the nasal tip is by cartilage reorientation rather then resection. Strategic placement of sutures can change the resting orientation of the lateral crura and consequently narrow and refine the tip lobule. A broad intermediate crus can be narrowed with a dome-binding' suture placed in a horizontal mattress fashion. The suture will pinch the medial and lateral crus together, narrowing the angle between the two, and creating a more discreet tip-defining point. The surgeon should be alert to the recurvature of the lateral crura because the dome binding suture can pull it inward and create valve obstruction. In these cases, a *lateral crural batten graft* placed between the cartilage and vestibular mucosa will straighten the curvature and allow refinement of the tip. This can also be used when the curvature of the lateral crura is the primary cause of the tip bulbosity.

Broadly splayed tip-defining points will create a wide nasal tip with a trapezoidal base. Interdomal sutures can be used to approximate the tip-defining points and create a narrower and less discreet tip lobule. Resorbable sutures can be used because the longevity from this maneuver comes from the scar contracture and 'shrink wrap' that occurs postoperatively (Representative Case 1).

Combination techniques of volume reduction and reorientation can be used for more significant deformities. The combination of a cephalic trim with dome binding sutures is a useful tandem. A vertical dome division with resection of the intermediate crura can be performed in such a way that the anastomosis will reorient the plane of the lateral crura. Excising the intermediate crus in a wedge-shaped with the base oriented superiorly, will allow the lateral crus to reorient its plane along the lateral nasal wall. The effect of this is decreased tip bulbosity (Representative Case 2).

Augmentation

Augmentation offers an effective way of improving tip definition. The amorphous tip may be best served with a strong tip graft that protrudes beyond the existing framework and creates a new scaffold for tip support. This graft can camouflage pre-existing asymmetries, form new tip-defining points, and effectively narrow the tip lobule. Tip grafts may be accurately sutured to the intermediate crura through the external approach or inserted into meticulous pockets through the endonasal route.

Soft Tissue Debulking

On rare occasions, it may be necessary to debulk some of the overlying soft tissue envelope in order to improve the amorphous nasal tip. This is often done in conjunction with strong augmentation grafts designed to push through the thick overlying skin. Thinning the soft tissue envelope may be necessary in patients with extremely thick skin, who paradoxically often have a poorly developed cartilaginous framework. This debulking must be done conservatively in order to avoid the subdermal vascular plexus and jeopardizing flap viability.

Tip Projection

Tip projection and de-projection are two effects that one must be able to control intraoperatively. Moreover, there should be sufficient support that will provide long-term projection and resist future collapse.

Increase in Tip Projection

Onlay grafts are as tip grafts or cap grafts, and are an effective way of directly improving tip projection. These autogenous cartilaginous grafts can be placed in discreet pockets or via the external approach with suture fixation.

Tip projection can also be enhanced by augmenting the medial crura of the lower lateral cartilages. This can be accomplished with a columella strut that reinforces that limb of the tripod. Similarly, that area can be reinforced with sutures placed between the medial crura and caudal cartilaginous septum. The sutures can be oriented in such a way that the medial crura climb-up the caudal septum.

Sutures can also be used in the interdomal region in an attempt to recruit a portion of the lateral crura towards the tip-defining point. This 'lateral crura steal' technique is effective for small degrees of augmentation. In a horizontal mattress fashion, sutures are passed between each lateral crus and re-approximated in the midline area. This technique will also create some degree of cephalic tip rotation.

Decrease in Tip Projection

One of the major tip support mechanisms is the ligamentous attachment between the medial crura and the caudal septum. A direct division of this supporting structure will allow the medial crura to slide posteriorly, thus decreasing tip projection. This effect can be taken further with a direct resection of a portion of the medial crura. A reduction of the lateral crura will also create a decreased in tip projection. This effect will be seen with a cephalic trim and, in a more dramatic fashion, with a direct resection of portion of the lateral crus (Representative Case 3).

Decreasing tip projection by reducing one of the limbs of the tripod will have some impact on tip rotation. If one desires a decrease in tip projection without rotation, one must either reduce all three limbs equally (that is, both lateral crura and medial crura) or perform a direct reduction of the intermediate crura. This type of vertical dome division along the tip-defining points will decrease tip projection in a linear dimension.

Tip Rotation

Rotation of the nasal tip is occasionally a secondary effect from a tip-narrowing maneuver. There are occasions where one needs to change the nasal labial angle and tip position via direct rotational maneuvers. The tripod concept is critical when considering the maneuvers that can affect tip rotation.

Increase in Tip Rotation

To increase tip rotation one can either shorten the two lateral limbs (lateral crura) or enhance the medial limb (medial crura). The techniques for shortening the lateral crura have been discussed under techniques of volume reduction. One may also slide the lateral crura in a posterior direction without direct resection. The medial crura can also be enhanced with suture techniques or columella struts. It is important to bear in mind the power of creating the illusion of tip rotation. Placing a 'plumping graft' of crushed cartilage within the nasal labial angle will make a more obtuse angle and the illusion of cephalic tip rotation. Similarly, a dorsal hump reduction will allow the nose to appear shorter and create the illusion of tip rotation (Representative Case 4).

Decrease in Tip Rotation

Once again, the tripod concept is applied when understanding surgical maneuvers for decreasing projection. Any maneuver that will lengthen the lateral limbs (lateral crura) or will shorten the medial limb (medial crura) will create a decrease in tip rotation. Dividing the ligamentous attachments between the medial crura and caudal septum is a simple and effective means of shortening the middle limb. One can also create the illusion of decreasing tip rotation by augmenting the nasal dorsum or supratip area. This will appear to lengthen the nose and create the illusion of decreased tip rotation. Direct onlay grafts to the infratip lobule will also impact the tip-defining point and the effective nasal labial angle. Dome-binding sutures and interdomal sutures can create some cephalic rotation of the tip by orienting them so that the superior sutures travel further than the inferior ones.

Complications

Complications from rhinoplasty can be acute or long term. The acute problems are similar to any nasal surgery and relate to epistaxis, swelling, ecchymosis, nasal obstruction, and rarely infection. Many problems specific to tip surgery can arise in the long-term. A great many of these are the consequence of continued scar contracture that occurs for many months, if not years, following surgery. Alar retraction with excessive columellar show is usually the result of an over-aggressive resection of the lateral crus and subsequent contracture of the dead space created. The correction often requires the placement of composite grafts into the vestibular lining.[5] This excessive tissue void is also the etiology of future valve problems and pinching in the middle nasal vault. The sheet of scar that envelopes the lower lateral cartilages will 'shrink wrap' around the tip and can buckle the remaining lower lateral cartilage, creating a bossae that protrudes through the nasal tip. Strong lower lateral cartilage, overly resected, with thin overlying skin, are risk factors for bossae formation.[6] Tip asymmetry can also occurs as a complication from scarring of the soft tissue envelope. One can view a rhinoplasty, particularly when done through the external approach, as a bilateral operation and the assumption is that the two sides heal

at a similar rate and with the same degree of scarring. When this does not occur evenly, twisting of the tip framework may ensue. The power of wound contracture cannot be overestimated.

Technical errors can lead to long-term complications such as a visible trans-columellar scar, twisting of tip grafts, or iatrogenic nasal obstruction from over aggressive dome-binding sutures. Prolonged tip edema can occur if soft tissue debulking was performed. If subcutaneous steroid injections are considered, they must be used extremely judiciously.

Summary

Surgery of the nasal tip remains one of the most challenging operations we perform. The successful outcome is predicated on an analysis that combines the cutaneous deformity with the structural and anatomic etiology. This exercise is a pre-requisite to formulating a targeted surgical plan. Many maneuvers are available to control the nasal tip and one should be able to position it precisely in the optimal orientation, rotation, and projection. Each technical step on the nasal tip will have a primary effect, secondary effect (particularly long-term effect), and tertiary illusions on the surrounding areas. The surgical plan should incorporate all these variables with the patient anticipation of long-term results.

Representative Cases

1. A young woman is unhappy with the appearance of her nose, particularly the width of the tip. Pre-operative views show the tip-defining points to be widely splayed and distracting from the facial beauty. Her dorsum is also slightly overprojected and there is a caudal septal deviation (Figs 41.6A to D). Intraoperative view demonstrating the widely distracted tip defining points (Fig. 41.7). Primary surgical maneuver to address the trapezoidal tip is an interdomal suture used to narrow the tip lobule. In addition, the following steps are performed: Open approach, dorsal reduction (bony and cartilaginous), cephalic trim, full transfixion incision. One year postoperatively, she is satisfied and without problems of nasal obstruction (Figs 41.8A to D).

2. A middle-aged schoolteacher is unhappy with the prominent nasal tip, especially with the attention it gets from the students. Her lower lateral cartilages are extremely strong and clearly visible, creating a prominent tip. She also has an overprojection to her dorsum, including her nasal tip. The tip projection is

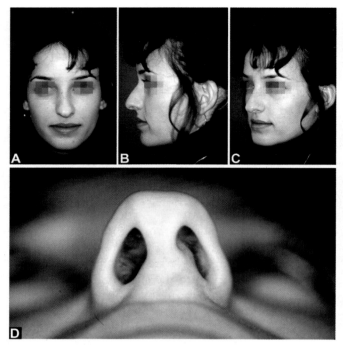

Figs 41.6A to D: Preoperative views of patient with wide tip: (A) Frontal view. (B) Lateral view. (C) Oblique view. (D) Base view

due to the over-development of her lower lateral cartilages and a volume reduction maneuver is warranted (Figs 41.9A to D). The corresponding intraoperative views show the cause of the nasal deformity as being an overgrowth of cartilage (Figs 41.10A and B). The primary surgical plan for tip deprojection and refinement is through a volume reduction along the intermediate crura, in the form of a vertical dome division. In addition, the wedge of cartilage excised is oriented with the base from the cephalic margin. This allows the lateral crural body

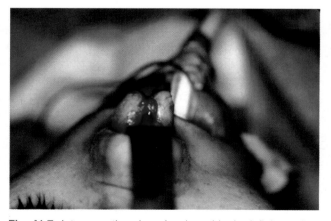

Fig. 41.7: Intraoperative view showing wide tip-defining points

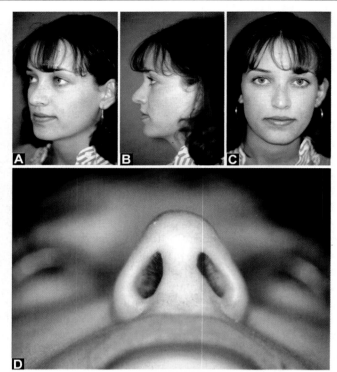

Figs 41.8A to D: One year postoperative views. Note how the beauty of her eyes becomes more apparent. (A) Frontal. (B) Lateral. (C) Oblique. (D) Base view

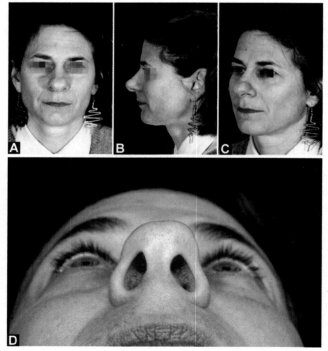

Figs 41.9A to D: Preoperative views of a middle-aged patient with a prominent and bulbous tip. (A) Frontal. (B) Lateral. (C) Oblique. (D) Base view

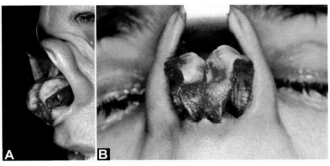

Figs 41.10A and B: Intraoperative views of overdeveloped lower lateral cartilages that cause the tip disfigurement

to be reoriented during the primary closure and dramatically decrease the tip bulbosity without over-resection of the crural strip. Additional maneuvers include dorsal reduction, tip grafting, full transfixion incision. One year postoperative surgery, she is doing well with a tip that is less conspicuous and without problems of alar retraction, excessive tip rotation, or valve collapse (Figs 41.11A to D).

3. A man unhappy with the overall size of his nose, particularly the overprojected dorsum and tip. Analysis reveals a prominent nasal tip with moderate bulbosity and overprojection. There is also a mild hump along the dorsum. He has no nasal obstruction (Figs 41.12A to D). The operative plan for decreasing his tip projection is through a combination of cephalic trim, full transfixion incision, and lowering of the

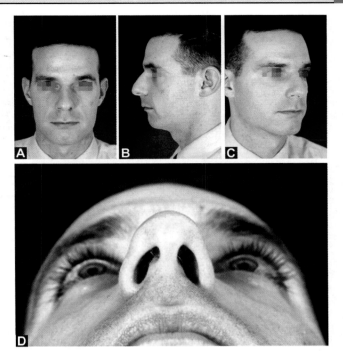

Figs 41.12A to D: Preoperative views of a gentleman with an over-projected tip and dorsum. (A) Frontal; (B) Lateral; (C) Oblique; (D) Base view

anterior septal angle. There was an interdomal suture placed to stabilize the tip. The dorsum was addressed with resection, lateral osteotomies, and finally bilateral spreader grafts (Fig. 41.13). Two years postoperative surgery he is doing well. Despite the spreader grafts, a small degree of narrowing along the middle third is visible (Figs 41.14A to D).

4. A young lady presents with complaints of the hump on her nose and small tip. Analysis shows a low radix,

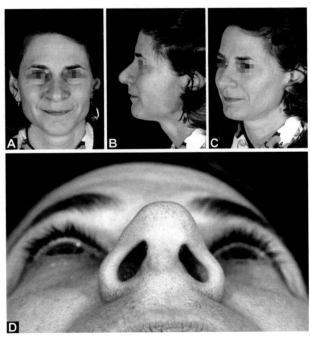

Figs 41.11A to D: One year postoperative views. (A) Frontal. (B) Lateral. (C) Oblique. (D) Base

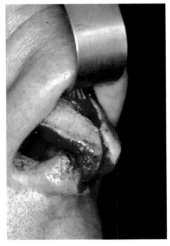

Fig. 41.13: Intraoperative view after cephalic trim, interdomal suture

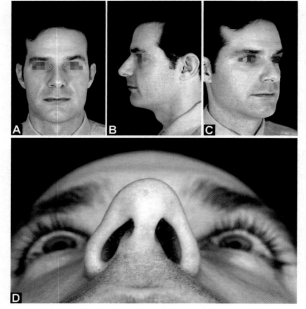

Figs 41.14A to D: Two years postoperative views. (A) Frontal view. (B) Lateral view. (C) Oblique view. (D) Base view

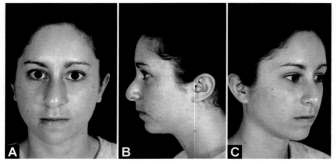

Figs 41.15A to C: Preoperative views of a ptotic nasal tip and low radix. (A) Frontal view. (B) Lateral view. (C) Oblique view

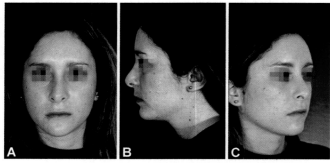

Figs 41.16A to C: Three years postoperative views. Tip rotation is improved and radix remains low. (A) Frontal view. (B) Lateral view. (C) Oblique view

slight overprojection of cartilaginous dorsum, and a ptotic tip (Figs 41.15A to C). Cephalic tip rotation was planned with a resection of the distal, dorsal septal cartilage along with conservative cephalic trimming and a columellar strut to enhance support to the medial crura. Three years later, she shows an improved profile although some deviation to the dorsum persists and the radix remains low (Figs 41.16A to C).

REFERENCES

1. Powell N, Humphreys B. *Proportions of the Aesthetic Face.* New York: Thieme-Stratton, 1984.
2. Crumley RL, Lancer R. Quantitative analysis of nasal tip projection. *Laryngoscope* 1988; 98:202–208.
3. Toriumi DM, Meuller RA, Grosch T et al. Vascular anatomy of the nose and the external rhinoplasty approach. *Arch Otolaryngol Head Neck Surg* 1996; 122:24–34.
4. Webster RC. Advances in surgery of the tip: Intact rim cartilage techniques and the tip-columella-lip esthetic complex. *Otolaryngol Clinic North Am* 1975; 8:615.
5. Tardy ME, Toriumi DM. Alar retraction: Composite graft correction. *Fac Plast Surg* 1989; 6(2):101–107.
6. Simons RL, Gall JF. Rhinoplasty complications. *Fac Plast Surg Clin North Am* 1994; 2(4):521–529.

Open (External) Septorhinoplasty Approach

Amita A Bagal, Etai Funk, Peter A Adamson

Initially a controversial operation, open rhinoplasty or external approach rhinoplasty has gained acceptance widely amongst accomplished rhinoplasty surgeons worldwide in recent years. While the earliest description of the external approach dates back circa 600 BC to Sushruta in India, Goodman and Charboneau of Toronto first popularized the approach in North America followed by Anderson, Wright, and others.[1-4] The greatest advantage of open or external approach rhinoplasty is superior exposure of the underlying nasal structures. The direct visualization of the cartilaginous and bony framework of the nose provided by the open rhinoplasty approach enables accurate diagnosis and precise correction of the underlying nasal deformity.

Open structure rhinoplasty is the other term used to describe an open or external approach rhinoplasty. The term 'structure' is added to describe a philosophy of rhinoplasty aimed at preserving existing support structures of the nose during an external approach rhinoplasty.[5] Suturing, reorientation of nasal cartilages, and grafting can help prevent weakening nasal structures and perhaps providing enhanced strength.

INDICATIONS

The indications for an open rhinoplasty approach are unique for each patient and surgeon depending on the surgeon's technique and experience. The open rhinoplasty approach is recommended for all rhinoplasties unless:
- An accurate preoperative diagnosis can be made
- The surgeon feels confident that the desired aesthetic and functional result can be obtained using a closed or endonasal approach.

CONTRAINDICATIONS

A relative contraindication may be previous rhinoplasty or nasal surgery in which the dermal tissues of the skin soft-tissue envelope (S-STE) have been thinned excessively, potentially having compromised the subdermal plexus blood supply. Unfortunately, this may be impossible to determine preoperatively.

Preservation of the lateral nasal artery is critical to maintain nasal tip vascular integrity. Additionally, cadaver studies have demonstrated that the lateral nasal artery is located 2–3 mm superior to the alar groove.[6] Therefore, bilateral alar base resection performed too cephalad may compromise nasal tip vascularity.

PREOPERATIVE ASSESSMENT

The initial consultation begins with a complete history, followed by a focused history of the nasal deformity. Functional and aesthetic concerns are documented. A history of mucosal problems including chronic rhinitis, allergic rhinitis, or sinusitis is obtained. The patient should be specifically questioned about previous nasal surgery. A complete head and neck examination is performed, followed by a detailed examination of the nose. The external contour of the nose is examined and palpated. A thorough examination of the internal nose is performed before and after decongestion with a topical vasoconstrictor. The nose is palpated internally to identify subtle septal deflections. With nasal endoscopy, occult posterior nasal pathology (not easily identified with anterior rhinoscopy alone) may be identified.

Digital photographs and/or computer-imaging are used to approximate the goals of the patient. The patient is educated regarding realistic expectations by viewing preoperative and postoperative rhinoplasty results. Patients are further educated with literature provided during the initial consultation. Nasal airflow studies and medical photographs are obtained prior to the second consultation. Preoperative photographic documentation is used to collect the standard preoperative rhinoplasty views: Frontal, right and left profile, basal, and right and left oblique.

A second planning session establishes and reiterates the aesthetic and functional goals of the rhinoplasty. The surgical protocols and risks are discussed. Patients are informed about postoperative edema and the need for patience up to a full year prior to complete resolution. Results of nasal airflows are reviewed. Drawing on patient photographs or employing a computer imager defines accurate aesthetic goals. After answering patient questions and concerns, written consent is obtained. The position of the columellar scar is drawn and reviewed with the patient on a graphic model in the surgical consent. The patient initials the drawing of the scar line. The intraoperative plan is outlined in detail on a preoperative rhinoplasty assessment worksheet.

INTRAOPERATIVE TECHNIQUE

Anesthesia

Most rhinoplasty patients are treated on an outpatient basis using a general anesthetic or intravenous sedation anesthesia. Patients are given an intravenous pre-operative antibiotic. Topical vasoconstriction using either cocaine 4% solution dose adjusted for the patient or oxymetazoline is applied to pledglets and placed in the nose for several minutes prior to infiltration of local anesthetic, only if deemed necessary. The local anesthetic with vasoconstriction facilitates hydrodissection and minimizes intraoperative blood loss. The nose is then infiltrated internally and externally with lidocaine (xylocaine), 1% with epinephrine (adrenalin), 1:100,000, mixed in equal parts with bupivacaine (marcaine), 0.5%, with epinephrine, 1:200,000. This provides long-acting anesthesia with a favorable vasoconstrictive effect.

Surgical technique

Incision and Exposure

An inverted-V transcolumellar, 'gull wing' incision is made initially with a No. 11 blade at the midcolumella and caudal to the medial crura. Precautions are taken to avoid damage to the underlying medial crura during incision placement by controlling the depth of the incision. The midcolumellar incision is joined to bilateral marginal incisions placed along the caudal margin of the lateral and intermediate crura. The marginal incisions extend in a paracolumellar fashion as a vertical marginal incision using a No. 15 blade. The vertical marginal incision should be made superficially to avoid damage to the medial and intermediate crura. The vertical marginal incision joins the lateral extent of the inverted-V transcolumellar incision at right angles. These angles are scored in order to reapproximate the incision appropriately upon closure. Next, using the converse scissors from the inferior extent of the vertical marginal incision and between the columellar flap and the caudal margin of the medial crura, the proper surgical plane is identified and the columellar flap is released.

The columellar flap is elevated initially with sharp scissors dissection. The use of skin hooks by surgeon and assistant greatly facilitate flap elevation. The columellar flap is elevated superolaterally to expose the domes, intermediate, and lateral crura bilaterally. The columellar flap is elevated directly over the lower lateral cartilages leaving a very thin layer of perichondrium in place. The dissection returns to the midline elevating the soft tissue over the anterior septal angle and middle third in a subareolar plane. The soft tissues over the osseous upper third of the nose are elevated. Blunt dissection in the subperichondrial and subperiosteal plane is used to elevate the thinner skin over the dorsum. Skin is elevated minimally, but enough to allow for favorable redraping. Dissection in the proper plane minimizes bleeding during this maneuver.

Occasionally, especially in thick-skinned patients with weak cartilages, identifying the caudal margin of the lateral crus may be challenging. In this situation, to avoid erroneous placement of the lateral extent of the marginal incision, performing only the vertical marginal and midcolumellar incisions and meticulously following the caudal margin of the intermediate and lateral crura during flap elevation facilitates desired exposure.

Occasionally, bleeding develops from the paired inferior columellar arteries arising from the superior labial artery branch of the facial artery. The brisk bleeding may obscure the field and is controlled by digital pressure or judicious bipolar cautery under direct visualization.

Septoplasty

The open approach is unique for its ability to provide access to the caudal and anterosuperior aspects of the septum. The upper lateral cartilages may be sharply dissected from the septum if extensive work in the middle third of the nose is anticipated.

Septoplasty is performed, if functional problems exist and to harvest septal cartilage if grafting is anticipated. Subtle septal deviations may become problematic postoperatively and are best-addressed during an initial procedure to prevent postoperative nasal airway obstruction. Sometimes, the septal work anticipated is minimal; however, tip correction necessitates an open approach for the rhinoplasty. In such cases, some surgeons prefer to do an endonasal approach for the septoplasty to preserve the support provided by the interdomal ligaments and soft tissue attachments between the medial crura and caudal septum. If an endonasal septoplasty is performed, the preoperative integrity of the columella is maintained, often obviating the need for a columellar strut, but limiting the ability to correct columellar and premaxillary deformities.

In the open approach, the anterior septal angle is approached from a superior direction. Soft tissue between the intermediate and medial crura is gently dissected down to the premaxilla using blunt dissection to identify the caudal-most portion of the quadrangular cartilage. Once the dissection is completed, the entire caudal septum is visualized. Furthermore, if the patient requires slight augmentation at the nasolabial angle, the soft tissue between the medial crura can be recruited as an inferiorly based flap and secured with a through-and-through premaxillary transfixion suture.[7] Bilateral complete submucoperichondrial and submucoperiosteal flaps are elevated providing wide exposure of the cartilaginous and bony septum.

Posterior septal deviations: Posterior deviations of the septum are examined to establish whether they are bony or cartilaginous. A high sub-radix cartilaginous deflection may create a residual dorsal deviation if not corrected, as it may prevent symmetrical infracturing of the nasal bones. Treatment of these deviations requires vertically shaving and scoring the cartilage on the concave side. If the deviation is of the bony septum, the bone may be excised or carefully mobilized to the midline, taking care not to fracture the perpendicular plate of the ethmoid superiorly.

Dorsal septal deviations: The open approach allows the most thorough examination of the dorsal septum. Dorsal septal deviations or curvatures may be treated by:

- Castellation or incision of the dorsal strut from above and below
- Upper lateral cartilage septal transfixion sutures strategically placed for correction of minor dorsal curvatures

- A unilateral spreader graft on the concave side of the septum
- Bilateral spreader grafts to structurally straighten the dorsum

Spreader grafts are rectangular cartilaginous grafts used to create width or improve function in the middle third of the nose. A unilateral spreader graft is placed by suture transfixion to the concave side of the curved dorsal septum. Occasionally, bilateral spreader grafts are applied to create width if the middle third of the nose is narrow, or to alleviate airway obstruction from internal valve collapse.[8,9]

Caudal septal deviations: The greatest advantage of the open approach is that it provides an undistorted view of the caudal septum. The additional exposure is clinically useful in diagnosing even subtle deviations. During standard septoplasty, cartilage excision may change the tension on the septal quadrangular cartilage, possibly resulting in curvatures or deflections not appreciated preoperatively. Furthermore, failure to diagnose a subtle caudal septal deviation after reducing a markedly bulbous tip may create a postoperative deformity and the appearance of a deviated nose. Releasing incisions of the inferior aspect of the caudal septum allow the deviated septum to swing to the midline and rest in the maxillary crest groove. Convexities of the caudal septum can also be scored until the cartilage straightens. The effect of these maneuvers is evident immediately without distortion from instrumentation.

Severe complete septal deformities: The severely deviated septum with multiple curvatures and fractures may require total septal reconstruction.[10] The entire cartilaginous septum is harvested en bloc leaving a dorsal strut. The harvested septal cartilage is used to design a graft restoring at least a 1.5 cm dorsal and caudal strut. The residual dorsal strut provides a buttress on which to replace, transfix, and secure the newly reconstructed septum.

Septal perforations: The open approach provides the required exposure to repair septal perforations. Symptomatic perforations up to 3 cm in diameter that bleed, whistle, or crust may benefit from repair by elevating superior and inferior septal advancement flaps. The repair of larger perforations is associated with a higher failure rate unless performed by experienced surgeons.

Closing the Septoplasty

After the septal deformity has been corrected, the submucoperichondrial flaps are apposed and transfixed with 4-0 plain gut sutures. If the caudal septum is released from the maxillary crest groove and realigned in the midline, additional transfixion is performed using a 4-0 polyglycolic acid suture (vicryl, ethicon, somerville, NJ).

Inferior Turbinate Outfracture

If preoperative nasal airway obstruction is present, fracturing the inferior turbinates laterally often improves the airway. Occasionally, more significant inferior turbinate hypertrophy with documented preoperative nasal airway obstruction necessitates submucosal dissection with removal of 1 cm of the anterior portion of the bone if the patient has not responded to medical therapy.[11]

Nasal Base

After septoplasty is completed, the nasal base is set. By addressing the nasal base first, the desired tip projection and rotation can be set, followed by appropriate dorsal reduction or augmentation. An exception to this operative sequence is the nose that has an excessively high dorsum creating a tension tip. The tip is drawn cephalad thereby increasing the nasolabial angle and distorting normal tip dynamics. Reducing the dorsum first in such cases alleviates the distorted tip dynamics. Applying the tripod concept of tip dynamics facilitates setting nasal length, projection, and rotation. The tripod concept considers the two medial crura as one leg of the tripod and each of the lateral crura as a separate leg thus creating a tripod structure.[12] Shortening or lengthening the tripod legs enables establishing appropriate nasal parameters. For a more sophisticated approach to the tip, the M-Arch Model is applied.[13]

Medial crura: Conservative soft tissue excision between the medial crura produces a slight degree of columellar narrowing. A wide columellar base, often resulting from inferior flare of the medial crural feet, may be improved by application of a buried, mattress suture to bunch the medial crural feet together. Intermediate curual horizontal mattress sutures can be placed if required to narrow a wide anterior columella or correct lobular bifidity. The open approach provides excellent exposure to excise premaxillary soft-tissue and narrow a prominent nasal spine. Complete removal of the nasal spine is not recommended.

The columellar strut is a type of graft used for aesthetic and functional purposes. The application of a cartilaginous columellar strut placed between the medial crura functions in many ways. Most importantly, a columellar strut restores the loss of tip support resulting from dissection between the medial and intermediate crura and disruption of the interdomal ligaments. Columellar strut application can also support weak-buckled medial crura, strengthen thin, flail medial crura, lengthen short medial crura, and enhance overall nasal tip support. Columellar struts are placed between the medial crura, above the premaxillary spine, under direct vision and secured with transfixion sutures of 4-0 polyglycolic acid through both medial crura, strut, and membranous caudal septum. The columellar strut should extend to, but not beyond the nasal spine. If the columellar strut extends below the nasal spine, the patient may experience a clicking sensation as the strut may flip from one side to the other. Angling the columellar strut in the inferior columella enables augmentation of the nasolabial angle or increasing columellar show. In noses with excess nasal length due to a long septum, caudal septal need to be shortened may be required prior to application of a columellar strut to prevent creating an iatrogenic hanging columella deformity.

Cartilaginous columellar batten grafts placed caudal to the medial crura are onlay grafts that may be suture fixated to increase columellar show or camouflage columellar asymmetries. Columellar batten grafts are shorter than infratip lobule or shield grafts.

Lateral crura: In most primary rhinoplasties, the cephalic margin of the superior aspect of the lower lateral cartilage is excised to refine or narrow the nasal lobule (Figs 42.1A to L). In comparison with endonasal approaches, the open approach provides superior exposure of the lower lateral cartilages allowing for a high degree of accuracy and symmetry when performing this maneuver. Frequently, upon intraoperative inspection, the lower lateral cartilages may have an intrinsic irregularity, asymmetry, or deformity that was not appreciated preoperatively due to relative tip symmetry on preoperative exam. Furthermore, symmetric and precise amounts of cartilage can be preserved using the external approach ensuring an intact strip of at least 7–9 mm for continued nasal support. The improved exposure minimizes potential violation of the scroll region (attachment of the cephalic margin of the lower lateral cartilage to the caudal margin of the upper lateral cartilage), a major tip support mechanism.

Lobule refinement: The open approach provides an unobstructed view of the nasal tip cartilages making it desirable for lobule refinement. The enhanced view

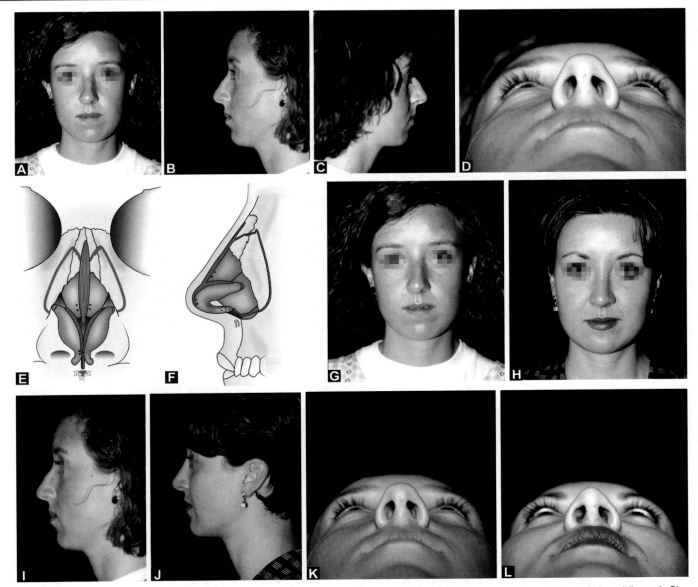

Figs 42.1A to L: This 19-year-old patient felt her nose was too large, too wide, and had an overprojected tip and dorsal 'hump'. She desired improvement of her retruded chin and flat cheeks. She had a conservative cephalic trim of lower lateral cartilage, lower lateral cartilage hinge cutback, deepening of the nasolabial angle, and columella strut. The dorsum was lowered several millimeters. She had a moderate size anatomic style silastic chin implant and large size anatomical style silastic cheek implants. Five year postoperative result, after open approach

enables the surgeon to perform aesthetic and functional maneuvers with a higher degree of accuracy. Maneuvers such as cephalic trim of the lateral crura, cartilage scoring, placement of double dome or single dome unit sutures, vertical crural division with crural reconstruction, and onlay grafting can be performed bimanually (Figs 42.2A to L). The maneuvers chosen depend on the patient's nasal deformity.

Specific Techniques for Lobule Reconstruction

Suture modification techniques: Placement of double dome unit sutures comprising 6-0 nylon may decrease an excessively wide domal angle to result in a more refined nasal tip appearance with a slight increase in tip projection. Variant anatomy may result in two aberrant lower lateral cartilages; individual single dome unit sutures can be used in this situation. When the domal

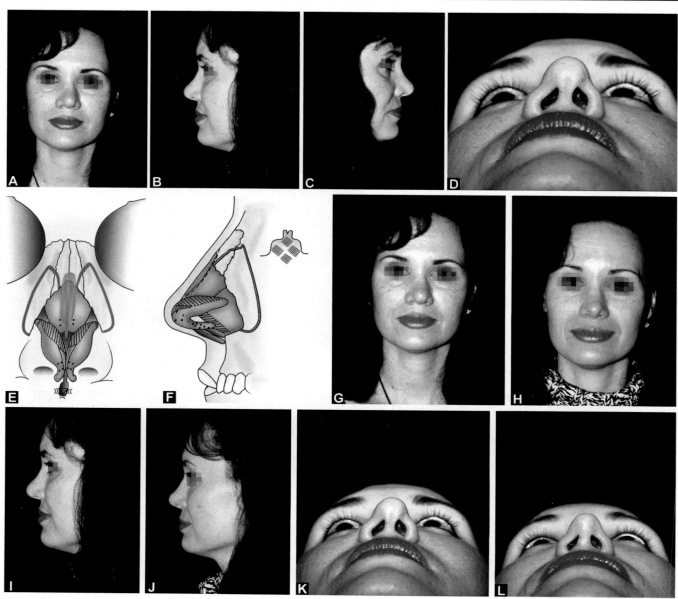

Figs 42.2A to L: This 38-year-old woman had two childhood nasal traumas and three previous septorhinoplasties. She felt her dorsal bridge was too wide, 'slooped', and crooked, the tip bulbous and the nostrils uneven. Scarring was marked at the intercartilaginous incision sites Airflow studies showed mild obstruction. Open approach revealed asymmetric resection of cephalic lower lateral cartilages and dorsal deficiency. The lobule was refined with minimal cartilage excision, single dome unit sutures, columellar strut, and nasolabial angle cartilage plumping graft. Conchal cartilage was transcutaneously fixed along the dorsum, soft tissue scar refined in the lobule and alar hooding corrected. One year postoperative result

angle is unusually obtuse, creating a broad domal arch, 'bunching' sutures may provide additional refinement. These 'bunching' sutures are double dome unit sutures placed more laterally on the lateral crura. Placing an intercrural suture between the intermediate crura can narrow a wide infratip lobule.

Vertical crural division: This is reserved for patients with noses that require deprojection and refinement of the nasal tip. The overprojection is typically due to an excessively long and broad lateral crural-medial crural arch complex that thrusts the nose forward creating deformity. Vertical crural division with overlap can be performed in the lobule (called vertical domal division), mid-lateral crus (called lateral crural overlay), or hinge region (called hinge cutback). Vertical crural division shortens the M-arch and usually causes deprojection of the tip. When performed cephalad to the tip defining point, rotation is achieved. Similarly, executing this maneuver caudad to the tip-defining point creates counter-rotation. It can also be useful to correct lobule asymmetries and broad lobular arches. The vestibular skin is meticulously dissected from the undersurface of the lower lateral cartilages prior to division. Reconstructing the crura using 6-0 nylon sutures in the lobule

or 4-0 polyglycolic acid transfixion sutures in the lateral crus after crural division restores structure and support.[14,15]

Grafting techniques: Cartilaginous grafts of septal or conchal cartilage can be sculpted and placed to increase tip projection, improve tip definition, lengthen the nose, camouflage asymmetries, and give a degree of apparent counter-rotation (Figs 42.3A to L).[16] The shield or infratip

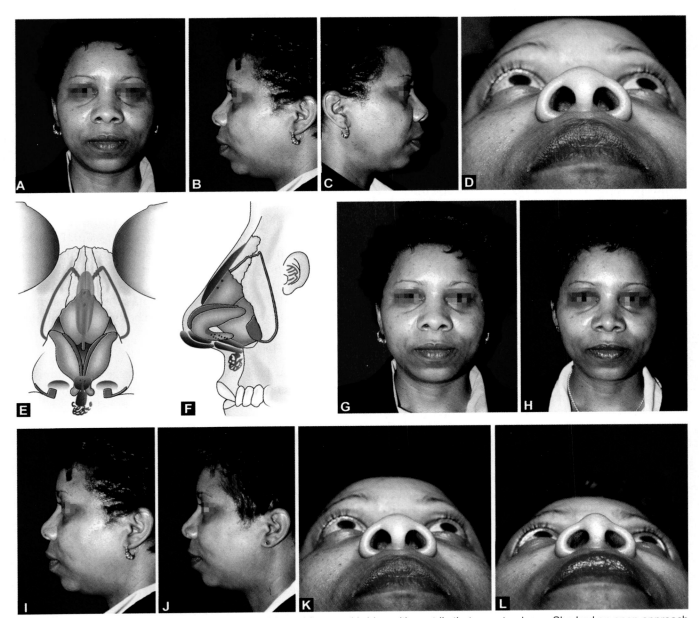

Figs 42.3A to L: This 48-year-old woman had a wide and flat nasal bridge with nostrils that were too large. She had an open approach septorhinoplasty to conservatively resect cephalic lower lateral cartilage and place a septal cartilage columellar strut, two -layered tip graft, and nasolabial angle plumping graft. Conchal cartilage was used to augment the dorsum. Bilateral alar base reduction was performed. One year postoperative result

lobule graft may be sculpted before or after suture fixation to the caudal aspect of the medial and intermediate crura using 6-0 nylon. The design (width, length, shape, and thickness) and position of the graft will determine the aesthetic effect created. The variable design of graft shape and position depend on the anatomical deformities to be corrected. Grafts can be used in primary rhinoplasty or secondary rhinoplasty. In secondary rhinoplasty especially, grafts help to restore structural support as well as improving aesthetics. Alar battens are overlay type grafts that are functional and/or aesthetic grafts used in lobule reconstruction to improve the appearance of supra-alar pinching and alleviate external valve collapse of primary or iatrogenic etiology.[17]

Nasal Dorsum

Profile alignment and modifications of the nasal dorsum are simplified by the open approach due to the improved exposure. A potential challenge for those unaccustomed to the open approach is the need to re-drape the S-STE to assess changes in the dorsum.[18] Precise amounts of dorsal cartilaginous septum can be reduced using the angled scissors. Moreover, localized dorsal prominences can be easily diagnosed as being cartilaginous or bony by direct inspection. Diamond rasps allow for a controlled, precise lowering of the bony dorsum. Fading, abbreviated medial osteotomies are performed under direct vision allowing precise placement and decreasing the potential for bony chips and a rocker deformity. When narrowing of the upper third of the nose, lateral osteotomies through an open approach can be performed similar to those using an endonasal approach. Low lateral osteotomies can be performed using a small pyriform margin incision.

Additional benefits of dorsal correction through an open approach include correction of dorsal irregularities through sculpting or suturing techniques, application of spreader grafts, and dorsal augmentation. Subtle irregularities of the dorsal septum and upper lateral cartilages can be precisely diagnosed and corrected under direct vision. Spreader grafts can be secured with 4-0 polyglycolic acid sutures directly to the septum for aesthetic and functional effects if indicated. While precise pocket grafting is slightly more challenging using the open approach, dorsal augmentation using autologous cartilage grafts can be performed with transcutaneous fixation of graft material for four days to ensure proper placement. Moreover, if dorsal augmentation is anticipated preoperatively, a limited elevation of the S-STE in the upper third of the nose can be performed.

Closure

Prior to closure the S-STE is re-draped and the nose is inspected critically to ensure optimal improvement in function and aesthetics. In certain cases of excessive subcutaneous tissue or dense scar formation, prudent, conservative excision of the supratip or tip region soft tissue (not the dermis) may improve S-STE re-draping and refinement. Graft position and stability are checked. The midcolumellar incision is closed first. If there is moderate tension, a subcutaneous suture may be required. Extending the vertical marginal incisions inferiorly and bilaterally may also reduce tension and facilitate closure. If the nose was markedly deprojected, the columellar flap may require judicious trimming of 1–1.5 mm to prevent a potential mild hanging columella postoperatively. The flap edges require precise realignment prior to closure. Most often, in the presence of minimal tension, the incision is closed with 6-0 nylon. Marginal incisions are closed with 4-0 chromic sutures. Placing the sutures laterally in the marginal incision avoids distorting the domes and tip. A meticulously closed incision yields a nearly imperceptible scar line.

At the conclusion of the operation, septal splints designed from exposed radiographic film are applied using 4-0 polyglycolic acid suture. The nose is taped externally using steri-strips. A water-resistant cast (Aquaplast™ Wyckoff, NJ) is applied. A single strip of vaseline gauze is lightly packed in both nasal vestibules.

Alar Base Reduction

A wide alar base, alar base flaring, large or asymmetric nostrils, hooded ala or thick ala can be reduced following closure to achieve ideal basal proportions.[19,20]

POSTOPERATIVE MANAGEMENT

Patients are followed closely in the initial postoperative period. Packing is removed on the first postoperative day. Early suture removal prevents unfavorable suture marks. Cast and splint are removed one week postoperatively. Nasal exercises are started following cast removal to ensure and maintain favorable positioning of nasal bones. The patient is followed-up closely for the first several weeks. Active exercise is avoided for 3 weeks and contact sports are avoided for 6 weeks. Follow-up should ensure resolution of tip edema and favorable healing of the scar line. Long-term follow-up of all rhinoplasty patients is strongly recommended. Postoperative photographic documentation should be performed at least at six months and one year. Patients are encouraged to return annually to photo-document long-term changes in nasal contour resulting from forces of wound contracture and to analyze critically the effectiveness of the surgical maneuvers employed.

RESULTS

Skin is a significant factor determining the ultimate aesthetic result irrespective of the rhinoplasty approach used, endonasal or open. Thick-skinned patients should be counseled preoperatively about the patience required for resolution of edema. Skin thickness may be appreciated by assessing preoperative sebaceous activity. Redraping and changes in cartilaginous contour can be appreciated more readily in thin-skinned individuals. Thin-skinned patients are more susceptible, however, to the appearance of subtle irregularities over time due to the forces of wound contracture.

A subjective dissatisfaction rate of 1% and objective unsatisfactory rate of 2% has been reported for the midcolumellar scar.[19] The greatest potential for unfavorable appearance of the scar is at the junction of the vertical marginal incisions and the transverse portion of the columellar incision. At this junction, forces of wound contraction tend to create a trapdoor effect giving the nostril a notched appearance and unfavorable scar. This effect can be alleviated by undermining the inferior columellar skin before closure and placing the angle suture full thickness in the inferior columellar flap and only partial thickness in the angle of the superior columellar flap, often thickened from edema.

Dissecting in the proper surgical plane minimizes the risk of prolonged postoperative edema, S-STE irregularities, and decreased flap viability.

The open approach only ensures improved exposure to correct nasal deformities; improved results occur only if appropriate rhinoplasty techniques are used as surgical experience accrues. The external approach must not be portrayed to the patient as being capable of obtaining unattainable results and creating unrealistic expectations. However, it appears that it may be associated with a lower revision rate than the endonasal approach.[14]

Advantages

Advantages of the open approach include superb exposure to the nasal cartilaginous and bony framework. The improved exposure allows for more precise diagnosis of deformities particularly of the caudal septum, dorsal septum, lower lateral cartilages, upper lateral cartilages, and the premaxillary spine. Surgical maneuvers can be performed bimanually. The open approach is also valuable for complex reconstructions including the cleft-lip rhinoplasty, saddle nose deformity, crooked nose deformity, and secondary rhinoplasty. Finally, the approach is educational for the novice and experienced surgeon. The open approach provides the opportunity for improved, accurate diagnosis.

Disadvantages

Disadvantages of the open approach include increased operating time. This slight increase is usually due to the time spent diagnosing and correcting deformities and performing a meticulous closure. Dissecting in the submuscular plane, avoiding tight dressings, gentle handling of the flap, and avoiding excess thinning of the flap with compromise of the subdermal plexus minimize concerns regarding flap viability. Finally, optimizing columellar scar camouflage requires proper incision planning and execution, meticulous closure technique, and gentle soft-tissue handling.

The open approach is a versatile approach and can be used for cosmetic and reconstructive rhinoplasty. Sound knowledge of nasal anatomy and function are prerequisites to safely performing an open approach rhinoplasty, just as they are for an endonasal rhinoplasty. The open approach, when used properly and carefully, is a powerful diagnostic tool and enables accurate correction of several different kinds of nasal deformities from subtle to complex. It has been shown that there has been an increasing acceptance and utilization of the open approach by facial plastic surgeons. Each surgeon, depending on his or her experience, should select the specific approach and technique required to achieve a satisfying result for the patients.

REFERENCES

1. Adamson PA, Smith O. Incision and scar analysis in open (external) rhinoplasty. *Arch Otolaryngol Head Neck Surg* 1990; 116(6):671
2. Adamson PA, McGraw B. Soft tissue premaxillary augmentation flap: how I do it. *Laryngoscope* 1991; 101(1).
3. Adamson PA. Open rhinoplasty. In *Facial Plastic and Reconstructive Surgery*, Papel ID and Nachlas, NE (eds) 1st ed St. Louis: Mosby Year Book. 1992; 295–304.
4. Adamson PA. Nasal tip surgery in open rhinoplasty. *Fac Plast Surg Clin North Am* 1993; 1:39–52.
5. Adamson PA, McGraw BL, Morrow TA. Vertical dome division in open rhinoplasty. Review of 116 cases. *Arch Otolaryngol* 1994; 120.
6. Adamson PA. The over-resected nasal dorsum. *Facial Plastic Surg Clin North Am* 1995; 3:407–419.

7. Anderson JR, Johnson CM, Adamson PA. Open rhinoplasty: an assessment. *Otolaryngol Head Neck Surg* 1982; 90:272–274.

8. Anderson JR. Surgery of the nasal base. *Arch Otolaryngol* 1984; 110:349.

9. Briant TDR, Middleton WG. The management of severe nasal septal deformities, *J Otolaryngol* 1978; 7(1):18.

10. Constantinides MS, Adamson PA. The long-term effects of open rhinoplasty on nasal airflow. *Arch Otolaryngol Head Neck Surg* 1996; 122.

11. Constantinides MS, Adamson PA. Vertical lobule division in open septorhinoplasty. *Face* 1997; 5(2):63–72.

12. Goodman WS, Charboneau PA. External approach to rhinoplasty. *Laryngoscope* 1974; 84:2195–2201.

13. Johnson CMJ, Toriumi DM. *Open structure rhinoplasty*. Philadelphia: WB Saunders 1990.

14. Rohrich RJ, Gunter JP, Friedman RM. Nasal tip blood supply: an anatomic study validating the safety of the trans-columellar incision in rhinoplasty. *Plast Reconstr Surg* 1995; 13:795–799.

15. Smith O, Adamson P, Tropper G, et al. The role of partial turbinectomy in aesthetic septorhinoplasty. Plastic and reconstructive surgery of the head and neck: proceedings of the fifth international symposium, Philadelphia, BC Decker, 1991.

16. Snell GED. History of external rhinoplasty. *J Otolaryngol* 1978; 7(1):6.

17. Toriumi DM. Mangement of the middle nasal vault. *Oper Tech Plast Reconstruct Surg* 1995; 2:16–30.

18. Toriumi DM, Mueller RA, Grosch T, Bhatacharyya TK, Larrabee WF: Vascular anatomy of the nose and the external rhinoplasty approach. *Arch Otolaryngol Head Neck Surg* 1996; 122:22–34.

19. Toriumi DM, Josen J, Weinberger M, Tardy ME. Use of alar batten grafts for correction of nasal valve collapse. *Arch Otolarygol Head Neck Surg* 1997; 123:802–808.

20. Wright WK, Kridel RWH. External septorhinoplasty: A tool for teaching and for improved results. *Laryngoscope* 1981; 91:945–951.

Soft Tissue Fillers of the Face and Liposuction of the Face and Neck

Daniel C Daube JR

Irritation from the sun, the aging process, gravity, wounding, tissue hypoxia from nicotine are some of the causes of collagen loss and tissue degeneration. There is a loss of tissue thickness, hydration, elasticity, and collagen is resorbed. In addition, to all of this supporting fat drifts, stretches and may even resorb. In addition, specific diseases can cause specific types of soft tissue loss of the face. For example, AIDS causes a specific pattern of facial lipoatrophy. There is malar and temporal wasting as seen with malnutrition, however, usually no loss of total body weight. This is why soft tissue replacement leads to a more youthful and healthy appearance.

THE PERFECT MATERIAL

Analysis and subsequent augmentation of facial soft tissue by physicians requires knowledge of patient requirements and characteristics of the material used to augment. This includes indications, expected results, and potential adverse effects of the material being used. Soft tissue fillers, biologic or synthetic, need to be costeffective, nontoxic, nonantigenic, nonmigrating, noninfectious, and noncarcinogenic. They need to be inert, just malleable enough at the time of surgery to be inserted and positioned, however closely they mimic the elasticity of the tissue. They would be easy to implant and should cause no donor site morbidity. They could be easily removed if desired. All current materials available cause (to some extent) an acute inflammatory response that creates a capsule around the implant. This is determined largely by the degree of antigenicity of each material and varies with each implant. The perfect material is yet to be identified.

Both synthetic and biologically derived materials exist. Although biologically derived materials have a better modulus of elasticity and, therefore, more closely

mimic human soft tissue, all of them inevitably resorb to some degree eventually. A characteristic of all non-absorbable implants at this time is the use of synthetically derived materials.

History

The history of materials used for soft-tissue augmentation of the face is accelerating as this is written. New technology and greater demand have spurred the creation of materials at an increased rate. Beginning in late 1800, there are reports of autologous tissue transfer in the face from the arm for soft-tissue augmentation. A decade later nonbiologic implants were attempted. In 1903, some of the materials tried included paraffin, vegetable oils, mineral oil, lanolin, and beeswax. However, when injected all of these materials created chronic inflammatory reactions and foreign body granulomas. Next, injectable silicone was used. However, aggressive injections and poor quality production created poor outcomes with silicone; and although there is a place for properly manufactured microdroplet silicone as an injectable in a limited amount, it is not used in the US.

International Scenario

Internationally, silicone is the most frequently injected material to date. However, there are a great number of materials being used internationally as injectables that are not FDA approved. A few of these include Artecoll (Artes Medical), Dermalive (Dermatech NZ), Bioplastique, Dermalive, and Profill. Artecoll is polymethyl methacrylate beads in collagen and is undergoing clinical trials in the US. Dermalive is acrylic beads suspended in hyaluronic acid and is also currently undergoing studies as a soft tissue filler. Dermadeep is a more robust form of Dermalive. Silskin (Alcon Labs) is medical grade silicone just as Silikon 1000 and is undergoing evaluation for facial soft tissue filling. Profill is also not yet available in this country. Bioplastique (vulcanized silicone rubber) causes unpredictable or exaggerated inflammatory responses and is not used in the US. In addition, hyaluronic skin fillers Restylane (Q-med) and Hylaform (Genzyme) are both used in Europe and may be used soon in the US as they appear to last longer with less reaction than bovine collagen.

NON-HUMAN BIOLOGIC MATERIALS

Injectable bovine collagen was first used in 1977. Approval by the FDA was granted in 1981 for Zyderm I (Collagen Corp). Collagen Corporation eventually developed Zyderm II and Zyplast in an attempt to create a longer lasting material *in vivo*. Prior to use, all of these require testing of a small amount of tissue in the forearm of the patient to receive the injection. Some physicians suggest a second test dose in the contralateral arm 2 to 3 weeks later as occasional false-negative tests do occur. After 6 weeks, the facial injections may then proceed assuming the test shows no hypersensitivity. Like all biologic injectables, collagen has a temporary effect; however, Zyplast, being the most stable, lasts the longest. The duration increases in less mobile areas of the face (up to 6 months in the glabella when injected with Botox) and is short-lived in the more mobile areas of the face (2 to 3 months in the lips). Complications include hypersensitivity, bruising, reactivation of herpes, bacterial infection, and soft tissue necrosis. Deep injections of the material seem to cause ischemic injuries in some patients (Table 43.1).

Autologous Tissue

Fat autografts were first attempted in 1893. With the advent of liposuction during the 1970s injected fat became more common. Its usefulness, however, is limited by its propensity to resorb quickly.

Cultured fibroblasts produce a material sold as Isolagen (Isolagen Co). The tissue taken from a biopsy or surgical specimen is sent to the company who then grows and processes the material. The longevity of the material is the same as bovine collagen. It is more painful to inject and requires 6 to 8 weeks to receive after the specimen has been sent. For these reasons, it is rarely used.

Autologen is similar to Isolagen except that a large amount of tissue is sent to the parent company (a facelift is generally enough tissue), and the material is extracted for injection. Again, the injections are quite painful if local anesthesia is not used, and the results, for the greater expense, are not longer lasting than bovine collagen. It should be noted that the process used to extract the injectable materials does not actually extract collagen from the tissue.

Gelatin matrix implants (Fibrel [Mentor]) have limited if any use because of the inconvenience of use. The kits contain a gelatin powder and epsilon amino-caproic acid, which must be mixed with the patient's own blood.

Table 43.1: Some biologically derived materials currently used for soft-tissue augmentation

Source	Product, injectable	Product, implantable	Manufacturer
Animal			
Collagen bovine	Zyderm, Zyplast, Zyplant		McGhan Medical
Human			
Allogenic (same species, different donor), homogenic			
skin	Dermalogen-injectable (no longer available)		Collagenesis
fascia	Fascian		Fascia Biosystems LLC
skin	Cymetra; micronized AlloDerm		
skin		Dermaplant, Implantable human matrix	Collagenesis
skin		AlloDerm (dermal sheeting)	Lifecell Corp
Autologous (same patient)			
	Isolagen		Isolagen Technologies
	Fat, dermis, fascia		self
	Autologen		Collagenesis

Perhaps if the results were permanent, this could be a more useful product; but like all biological implants, it resorbs.

Allografts

Fascia from cadavers is also sold as Fascian. This is an injectable product and comes in multiple particulate sizes. This may be advantageous because it requires no testing prior to injection. This is because the product is an allograft and no reactions have been reported. Some experts recommend the use of oral antibiotics at the time of injection and never inject into an infected area.

AlloDerm is an acellular dermal graft which may be transplanted without rejection for both reconstructive and cosmetic purposes and comes in multiple thicknesses and sizes. It has been used in nasal surgery for repair of septal as well as structural defects (saddle-nose deformities). It is used for minimization of the melolabial fold and marionette lines as well as lip augmentation, softening of the glabella, and filling of traumatic scarring of the face.

Dermalogen is currently on hold, human derived collagen.

NONBIOLOGIC MATERIALS

Occasionally soft-tissue defects are filled with advancing one's own skeletal framework as with the repositioning of the zygomatic complex for a malar deficiency. This approach will not be addressed except to say that it is a good approach where feasible (Table 43.2). The implant for this approach to stabilize the repositioning is usually of metal (three types used are vitallium, titanium, and stainless steel) or more recently polylactic acid (resorbable plating systems).

Polymers make up the remainder of the nonbiologic materials used at present. These are long repeating molecules and include the following:

Silicone

Silicone is not injected in the USA as some as the smaller polymers may induce systemic illness. Depending on the polymer length and cross linkage, silicone may be solid or liquid. Histologic studies show that the body reacts to it by encapsulation; therefore, underinjection is recommended as this encapsulation results in greater augmentation. However, because the degree of reaction by the host is unpredictable, the FDA has not approved this material for injection as it once did. Hardened silicone is often used in the cheek and chin as an implant. An injectable form of silicone is used outside of this country *bioplastique*, silicone (microbeads).

Polyethylene (HDPE)

Polyethylene (HDPE), known as MedPore, is stiff and is used in chin and cheek implantation. It is malleable with difficulty, provides good tissue ingrowth, and little shifting; for the same reasons, it is difficult to remove.

Other Materials

Some materials that are rarely if ever used for soft-tissue augmentation, are referred to below. Methyl methacrylate is a larger implant and is prone to fracture. A form used outside the US in an injectable form is Artecoll. HTR is similar to methyl methacrylate with a calcium hydroxide coating. Two mesh implants include supramid (Ethicon), a polyamide, and Mersaline (Ethicon), a polyester, have been used in the past; however, these two materials are not currently used. Materials such as Gore-Tex do not have the same degree of tissue ingrowth. Proplast is no longer available. Ceramics such as hydroxyapatite are used in ear surgery but have little role at the current time in soft-tissue augmentation.

The most commonly used nonbiologic soft-tissue filler currently is polytetrafluoroethylene. It comes in a nonexpanded form as Teflon paste; the expanded form Gore-Tex (e-PTFE), has been proven as safe and reliable. It has been used as a vascular graft for over twenty years. Limited ingrowth of tissue, soft, and low extrusion rates make it a useful material for soft-tissue augmentation. Various shapes are used to overcome some of its shortcomings. For example, tubes are extruded at a lesser rate than the nonhollowed rolls, cords, or solid shapes. This material is biocompatible, safe, and reliable.

Risks

Risk of cancer from any of the above materials in the head and neck area has never been reported except once: the case report was of squamous cell carcinoma at the site of a mandibular plate. In the head and neck region, none of the discussed materials have been shown in the literature

Table 43.2: Nonbiologically derived materials used for soft-tissue augmentation		
Material	*Name*	*Manufacturer*
Silicone	Silskin	
e-PTFE	SoftForm is replaced by UltraSoft	McGhan
	Advanta	Atrium Medical

to cause systemic illness either. There is a debate as to whether the effect of silicone charge on surrounding proteins, smaller silicone impurities, or effects of silicone on cholesterol metabolism may cause systemic disease; none of these has been proven or disproven. Hypersensitivity may occur, however, and has been confirmed with metal implants. Type IV reactions confirmed with patch testing has occurred with metal implants but not with polymers. Some side effects are difficult to distinguish from technical errors. These include infection, fistula, exposure, extrusion, displacement, implant fracture, seroma, persistent edema, pain, and inflam-matory reaction.

TECHNIQUE FOR INJECTABLE IMPLANTS

Many experts recommend oral antibiotics, antiviral agents, and Cox 2 inhibitors to minimize a post-inflammatory response. In addition, Botox may be injected with filler if dynamic lines are being treated. Under no circumstances should one inject into infected tissues. The depth of injection is determined by the result desired and the material being injected. When using biologic materials over-treatment is recommended and with synthetic materials undertreatment is best. The patient must be informed that they will feel irregularities. Application of ice immediately after injection will minimize the postprocedure swelling and, for that matter, prior to injection will minimize discomfort and also help with minimizing postprocedure swelling. Multiple sessions are required for all injectables. Some of these injectables require a field block or nerve block with lidocaine. Inject at body temperature. Check for allergies to antibiotics: some products are treated with antibiotics, for example, AlloDerm is packaged with gentamicin and other antibiotics as described in the packet insert.

Anatomic Considerations

It should be noted that the gray line between cosmetic and reconstructive surgery is occasionally blurred; thus these techniques discussed, although cosmetic in nature, are often used for reconstructive techniques when necessary.

Forehead, Glabellar and Forehead Lines

Botox and endoscopic browlift play a greater role in these areas than soft-tissue augmentation techniques; however, collagen injection may be used in the glabella with some caution. For tissue loss in the temple, Conform (a e-PTFE

manufactured in various sizes to fit and augment areas of the face as a surgical implant) may be used. AlloDerm is also an excellent alternative if no autologous tissue is available.

Nose

Again, this is an area where surgical manipulation of the native tissues is preferable to the introduction of soft tissue fillers; however, the situation does arise where these fillers are necessary. Some materials used include MedPore, silicone, collagen, and Gore-Tex. It is important to keep in mind that the stiffer the implant the greater the extrusion rate of the implant. Keeping this in mind, AlloDerm is an excellent choice for the dorsum as is all on the injectables. For camouflaging a bony dorsum both AlloDerm and e-PTFE work well: Both are available in various thicknesses.

Cheek

Cosmetic augmentation of the cheeks requires careful preoperative evaluation. In case of the cheek, the malar fat eminence descends with age and the buccal fat pad enlarges and shifts lateroinferiorly. The SMAS becomes increasingly elastic and lax resulting in increasing jowls. The lateral canthus of the eye turns downward secondary to this pull with decreasing elasticity and strength of the dermal tissues. There is resorption in the midface and decreasing vertical height accentuating the malar pouch.

Tissue repositioning is the best method to deal with these changes. However, occasionally ptosis procedures alone cannot address loss of subcutaneous bulk; implantation may then be used as an alternative. This is best accomplished with surgically implanted materials. Incisions to place implants are made either transconjunctival, subciliary, or transoral. The incisions used should be no longer than those required to place the implant. A carefully created pocket holds the implant in the proper position; and to help with this, the author suggests making marks on the freer elevator so that dissection can stop once these are reached. Too small a pocket, however, will result in bowing of the implant and is likewise a problem. Even with perfect technique, however, overtime the capsule may distort silicone implants and cause 'bowing' and the need for removal. The most common location where one can palpate an edge of these implants is along the infraorbital rim. For this reason, it is important that the surgeon pay particular attention to this area and secure it to the periosteum well. The most likely complication is asymmetry or malposition of the implants. Other than hard silicone implants, one may use Conform (see earlier in this chapter). For soft-tissue defects of the cheek, however, injectables and AlloDerm both work well.

Nasolabial Folds

The paranasal area is best treated with solid implants, as is most of the cheek area. The exception is depressions due to scarring. However, with issues such as acne scarring, it is often better to excise the depression or laser-abrade the surrounding tissue to camouflage rather than use tissue fillers especially since none are truly permanent.

Lips, Marionette Lines

Aesthetic surgery of the lips is evolving as a significant field in facial plastic surgery. Initial attempts at beautifying the lips probably started with Cleopatra, who would apply red color to her lips. Later, silicone was used to augment the soft tissue of the body and face, and the lips were no exception. Other materials were then developed which could be used to augment the lips. Some of these include collagen (bovine), Gore-Tex, and acellular human matrix (Table 43.3).

The lips are the most malleable and animate of all the facial features. They are the most pleasing feature of the lower third of the face. This presents the surgeon with a special set of circumstances. Specifically, many of the techniques we use on other areas of the face may not work on the lips because of their three-dimensional animate nature. With this in mind, there are many ways to augment the lips as well as change both their animate and/or repose shape. The surgeon must always be aware of how the static changes to the lip will change the animate aesthetics and function of the lip. Patients occasionally refer to this as 'kissability.' Generalizations about beautiful lips may be made; however, different cultural and generational perceptions exist: these too are not constant.

Table 43.3: Soft-tissue augmentation options for the lips

Temporary	
Autologous dermis	Resorption-rate is great
Tendons and fascia	Donor site morbidity
Fat	Unpredictable results
Collagen	Bovine, has long history of use
Autologen	Painful injections
Dermalogen	Inconsistent fluency of material
Permanent	
e-PTFE	UltraSoft is replacing SoftForm

As we age, the lips thin and the wet line moves caudally in reference to the dentition. In addition, the oral commissures begin to downturn and Cupid's bow flattens out. Thus, thin, flat, and poorly defined lips impart a sense of senility. There are specific procedures to address each of these labial signs of senility, and they may or may not include augmentation. However, when full, well-defined, and in proportion, they impart a sense of both beauty and youth.

All procedures of the lip may be done with local anesthetic as a field block, nerve block, or no anesthesia at all. The less the tissue is distorted (by local infiltration of anesthetic agent), the better. However, this should be balanced by the ability to use the epinephrine in the local to help with hemostasis. Because the lips are so sensitive, injections should be buffered with sodium bicarbonate and injected slowly. Once work begins, the lips will swell quickly because the histology of the epidermis in this area does not resist deformation well (thus the lips are soft). Placing ice on the lips after the procedure will help slow the swelling process over the next 24 hours.

During consultation with patients considering a surgical lip procedure, there must be defined goals in the surgeon's mind. First, is the patient a better candidate for temporary or permanent augmentation? For example, it is better to temporarily inject a patient who has had no prior cosmetic surgery and is unsure if they are going to do well with larger lips. These patients deserve a trial with bovine collagen or the newer cadaveric collagen. After this trial, if they are satisfied with the results, a more permanent method may be used. One might then move to AlloDerm, which is felt by most to be long-lasting, but perhaps not permanent.

Patients also need to be warned that the lips may look 'too large' after surgery. It will take 4 to 6 weeks for the swelling to resolve. If the lip is the appropriate size immediately after surgery, then it will be ultimately too small. The patient also needs to know this prior to surgery so that the surgeon is not asked to remove some or all of the implant prematurely.

Although not common, some persons do seek lip reduction or even subtle lip sculpting, such as augmenting only the lateral philthrum. This is the beauty of lip surgery as rhinoplasty; our imagination is the only true limit of our artistic ability.

Temporary Options

Temporary options are the safest initial treatment for most patients. Collagen, bovine and human, are both used for temporary augmentation. As a temporary measure, bovine collagen is an excellent option. It requires skin testing in the forearm prior to injection and, furthermore, is contraindicated in those with autoimmune diseases. The duration of the implant is a function of the specific type of collagen used, i.e. Zyderm I, Zyderm II, or Zyplast. Zyplast is the best choice if duration of results is the priority. The location of the injection is also important. The more mobile the area injected, the quicker the resorption time of the collagen implant. Finally, different individuals resorb the implant at different rates. It seems that those who have had multiple injections in the same spot have longer lasting results. If tattooing of the lip is to be done in the near future, however, it is not recommended that collagen be used. Instead inject after the tattooing has been done. In addition, the duration is a linear change and not a short-term phenomenon; this accounts for some of the variation in patient reports about the duration.

Human collagen has recently become available as an injectable augmentation option. To date there is limited experience; however, no testing will be required and the duration is projected to be much longer. One's own collagen can be used after harvesting and processing. This is a more expensive option and the processing can be unpredictable in the sense that occasionally no useful collagen is available. There is a limited time period the collagen must be used in as well. Finally, injection of the autologen is more painful than bovine collagen. Thus, the area must be injected with anesthetic prior to placement of the autologen.

Fat has been used for augmentation, however, as noted, due to relatively quick disappearance, requires multiple procedures.

AlloDerm sheets, which come from a single source at the present (LifeCell Corp) last much longer than the collagen and may give some permanent results as well. An advantage of this implant as opposed to Gore-Tex (discussed later) is that it is softer and is easier to augment in a more diffuse manner. The disadvantage is that at the present it appears to last 1 to 2 years on gross-inspection. It is relatively easy to implant although a touch-free method should be used. In addition, when healing, it may become lumpy; although this is almost always temporary. These products are impregnated with an antibiotic solution and allergies must be confirmed prior to implantation. It may be possible to obtain graft material free of antibiotic or with different antibiotic if the supplier is contacted with enough prior notice.

There are many reports of using the patient's own harvested fat, fascia, or dermis. Human collagen and autologous implants of dermis, fat, or fascia, however, are prone to reabsorption and often require an additional incision from the donor site.

Permanent Options

There are permanent solutions for augmentation as well. Gore-Tex (WL Gore Co) makes both solid implantable threads in different sizes as well as SoftForm, which is available in two sizes at present. Both are excellent for the vermilion border; however, the solid implants and the multi-string implants are not as natural in feel as the newer hollow-core implants. Two important cautions when placing these are precise placement and caution not to vary depth. Technically, all of these products are easy to place, but because SoftForm comes in its own delivery device, it is easier than the other forms. (There are other designs being created at this time as well). However, it cannot be emphasized enough that a touch-free technique must be used with all the implants. It is the author's preference to place these in the barrel of a 10 cc syringe filled with antibiotic solution and place the implant under negative pressure to saturate it with antibiotic. However, care must be taken to ensure that the patient has no allergy to the antibiotic used. If placed too superficially, it will extrude or create a white firm lump. The disadvantage of nonautologous implants is the risk of infection. The risks of migration, allergic reaction, and formation of a foreign body granuloma are always present. Although rarely reactive, this has been reported with Gore-Tex.

SoftForm is being replaced with UltraSoft (Tissue technologies) at the time of this publication because it is longer, softer, and available in larger sizes.

A liplift via the excision of subnasal skin to show greater maxillary incisors and roll the lip out to create a greater vertical red lip height relative to the upper sub-nasal lip is a relatively simple procedure (and satisfying to the patient) in a person with long upper lip. Thus, if the lowest horizontal third of the face is too long with showing of the mandibular dentition, this should be included as part of the treatment regimen. The incision is caudal to the nasal sill and minimally appreciated by the onlooker.

Lip advancement by excising the skin just above the upper lip vermilion border with advancement of the vermilion border itself yields poor definition of the white roll. For this reason, it is a poor choice unless the female patient is willing to outline her lips either daily or permanently. It is a poor choice for men in almost all cases.

Z-plasty of the upper and/or lower lip is an outstanding choice with or without an implant although the results are modest. The incisions must be relatively long for each arm of the plasty. Generally only 3 to 4 lengths can be created on each side of the central lip only. They should extend from the wet line to within 1 cm of the labial alveolar sulcus. If an implant is also being used, it may be placed later in a stage procedure or simultaneously if placed anterior to the Z-plasty, anterior to the wet line. If the latter approach is chosen, undermining of the lip will be limited at the time of surgery.

For the down-turned commissure, a corner lift may be used. This requires removing a small triangle of upper skin excised from the corner of the lips: In the author's experience, the results are subtle.

Other materials used for implantation include galea, the patient's own dermis, breast capsule, and de-epithelialized flaps. These have been used with variable success and have been described in the medical literature.

Some patients are not good candidates for lip augmentation by any of the methods discussed and camouflage may be a better option. A long-lasting option in this regard is the tattooing of the vermilion border of the lip with a darker color or even creating the pigment beyond the natural borders to give the appearance of larger and fuller lips. This can be an outstanding option for most of these patients and be used with other techniques, if desired.

There are many possible incisions that may be used to implant materials in the upper and lower lip. In addition, one must decide how much of the lip is to be augmented horizontally and vertically. It is often difficult to control lip projection, which will always occur with augmentation. In other words, should the vermilion border alone be augmented or should the wet line be enhanced as well? There are some general principles that should be followed regardless of the material being implanted. One single thread of material should never be used to stretch across the entire upper lip. This will result in an abnormal showing of the upper gingiva when the patient smiles. For this reason, it is usually necessary for the surgeon to place three incisions, one centrally and one at each commissure. The lower lip requires only two incisions; however, one may not want to go from commissure to commissure, but instead augment only the central region to create a 'pout.' Never place an implant under the incision.

In addition, the lips are extremely sensate. This will be altered by any invasive manipulation to some degree. This is most often temporary, but may be quite disconcerting for the patient. It may be severe enough to affect function, that is, speech or oral competence; however, this is rare.

If the implant becomes infected, treat with antibiotics first. Implanted materials that extrude must be trimmed under sterile conditions and the exit site-closed or extrusion may persist. The closure should allow for drainage and the patient informed as little movement of the lip is best. Bactroban ointment will also aid in healing. If the infection does not resolve, then the implant must be removed.

Risks

Results can still improve in many ways with increasing safety, predictability, consistency, and life of volume gain and change in shape. Ischemic injury and allergic reactions have both been reported.

Chin Augmentation

By far the most common method of chin augmentation is solid silicone implantation. There are other materials used including Gore-Tex and hydroxyapatite; however, silicone implants have the greatest data due to their popularity in the past.

Many of the problems lie not with the filler itself but the way it is used and the technique of implantation.

LIPOSUCTION OF THE HEAD AND NECK

Liposuction of the head and neck does not have the same popularity as liposuction of many other parts of the body but can assist the surgeon as an isolated procedure in facial rejuvenation or as an augmentation to concurrent procedures. The technique is not new dating back to 1976 when liposculpture was initiated by a gynecologist and not a plastic surgeon. Current techniques date back to 1986 when tumescent liposuction was initiated.

SURGICAL TECHNIQUES

Treatment of the neck with this technique gives a surgeon the best chances of success as the neck has the attributes of being the safest area to treat as well as the area that appears to accumulate fat at a faster rate than the other areas of the face and neck. Buccal fat extraction has been described; however, many surgeons do not recommend this as aging causes buccal depression and sagging and repositioning generally results in a better outcome.

Cervical Liposuction

After sedation is initiated, the areas to be liposuctioned are marked as well as the proposed cervicomental crease and the inferior border of the mandible. This procedure can be performed simultaneously with a facelift, endoscopic necklift, or in isolation. The area marked is then infiltrated with a diluted solution of lidocaine, sodium bicarbonate, and epinephrine. Next, a submental incision is made as well as bilateral postauricular incisions. The subdermal plane is then undermined from the inferior mandibular line down to the proposed cervicomental angle. Cannulas of various sizes and shapes are then used; however, their rotation is critical as is the use of the 'smart' hand. The 'smart' hand is the nondominant hand that pinches the skin as the hand using the liposuction cannula is maneuvered back and forth as a piston. The 'smart' hand can feel the depth and position of the cannula tip and may even be used to guide the tissues into position around the cannula as opposed to relying on only the direction of the cannula to find its path. One must be careful that each stroke is complete and that the distal or proximal line of the cannula is not treated out of proportion to the amount of fat present. After the procedure is completed, a pressure dressing is placed and removed at day one. I no longer recommend a prolonged pressure garment for the following week as I believe it may lead to unnatural positioning of the skin as it heals and may cause 'rippling;' however, many experts do use prolonged pressure dressing and are quite comfortable with this postoperative treatment. It goes without saying that preoperative and postoperative photography is important as the results, although consistently positive, often need to be reviewed with the patient months after surgery. This is especially true with heavy patients who may initially seek treatment to create a jawline but have an unspoken goal of a thinner lower face and neck. Even the best preoperative discussion may not communicate the expected results.

Liposuction in the lower neck for lipomas are not recommended as these are best treated with open procedures. If treated with liposuction, chylous leaks can easily be created.

Complications

Younger and healthier skin will contract sooner and more smoothly than older skin after submental liposuction; therefore, the best results are obtained in younger patients. Death due to pulmonary thromboembolism is the most severe complication; however, this has not been reported with cervical liposuction in isolation. It has only been reported when performed in combination with larger amounts of body liposuction. Other causes of death reported in the literature were anesthesia, sedation and medication, fat embolism, cardiopulmonary failure, massive infection, hemorrhage, electrolyte imbalance. These are related to the duration of procedure and amount of fat removed, which is usually small in facial procedures. Other articles list MI, CVA, and aspiration as well as pulmonary edema as possible complications. None of these involved facial liposuction. Morbidity of facial liposuction includes prolonged edema, ecchymosis, infection, skin irregularities, over- or under-treatment, hematomas, seromas, facial nerve injuries, cutaneous perforation of the cannula; all of which are rare when the technical aspects of the procedure are closely adhered to. Thus, facial liposuction seems to be a very safe and satisfying procedure.

Most of the significant risk factors, if not all, are due to a combination of general anesthesia with liposuction. Known risk factors include, aspirate volume, excessive IV fluids, hypothermia, and complications associated with general anesthesia. Therefore, tumescent technique under IV or little sedation when surgery is limited to the face and neck makes a great deal of sense. Tumescence reduces blood loss.

The use of lidocaine enables the surgeon to perform this procedure with sedation only; hydrostatic dissection of the tissue with a solution containing lidocaine is important in the case of mechanical disruption of the fat. Guidelines of an FDA application in 1946 suggested that lidocaine be used in a dose of 7 mg/kg of body weight: however, this not based on strong scientific evidence. The Guidelines for Liposuction Surgery issued by AACS in 2000 states that the maximum dose of lidocaine for liposuction is 55 mg/kg of body weight. With tumescent techniques, peak plasma levels of lidocaine are reached 12 to 14 hours after infiltration. It must be emphasized that this assumes coadministration with epinephrine which vasoconstricts the tissues and causes slower absorption. The lidocaine is metabolized via the p-450 cytochrome system. Therefore, any drugs that are likewise metabolized by this system (tetracycline, erythromycin) will delay the metabolism of the lidocaine. Suffice it to stay that the margin of safety for this drug when used for facial liposuction is very safe.

BIBLIOGRAPHY

1. Ahn M, Monhian N, Mass C. Soft tissue augmentation. *Fac Plast North Am* 1999; 7:35–41.
2. Aiache AE. Facial liposuction for rejuvenation. *Cosmetic Dermatol* 2002; 15:42–44.

3. Baker J, Singh S. Lip augmentation. *J Florida MA* 2000; 86: 14-16.

4. Burres SA. Lip augmentation with preserved fascia lata. *Dermatol Surg* 1997; 23(6):459–462.

5. Castor SA, To WC, Papay FA. Lip augmentation with AlloDerm acellular allogenic dermal graft and fat autograft: a comparison with autologous fat injection alone. *Aesthetic Plast Surg* 1999; 3:218–223.

6. Coleman SR. Facial recontouring with lipostructure. *Clin Plast Surg* 1997; 24:347–367.

7. Conrad K, MacDonald MR. Wide Polytef (Gore-Tex) implants in lip augmentation and nasolabial groove correction. *Arch Otolaryngol Head Neck Surg* 1996; 122:664–670.

8. De Benito J, Fernandez-Sanza I. Galea and subgalea graft for lip augmentation revision. *Aesthetic Plast Surg* 1996; 20(3): 243–248.

9. Gatti JE. Permanent lip augmentation with serial fat grafting. *Ann Plast Surg* 1999; 42:376–380.

10. Hernandez-Perez E, Valencia-Ibiett E. Analysis of liposuction-related complications and mortality in the United States and Latin America. *Cosmetic Dermatol* 15:23–27.

11. Hetter GT. *Lipoplasty, the theory and practice of blunt suction lipectomy.* Boston: Little Brown 1984.

12. Hoffmann C, Schuller-Petrovic S, Soyer HP, and Kerl H. Adverse reactions after cosmetic lip augmentation with permanent biologically inert implant materials. *J Am Acad Dermatol* 1999; 40:100–102.

13. Hubmer MG, Hoffmann C, Popper H, and Scharnagl E. Expanded polytetrafluoro-ethylene threads for lip augmentation induce foreign body granulomatous reaction. *Plast Reconst Surg* 1999; 103:1277–1279.

14. Isenberg JS. Permanent lip augmentation using autologous breast implant capsule. *Ann Plast Surg* 1996; 37(2):121–124.

15. Kostianovsky AS. Upper and lower lip augmentation by buried, de-epithelialized local flaps: an alternative to the use of foreign material implants when shortening the lips. *Aesthetic Plast Surg* 1996; 20:433–437.

16. Maloney BP. Cosmetic surgery of the lips. *Facial Plast Surg* 1996; 12(3):265–278.

17. Mass C, Denton A. Synthetic soft tissue substitutes. *Facial Plastic Surg Clin North Am* 2001; 9:219–227.

18. Mass C, Ericson T, McCalmont T. Evaluation of expanded polytetraflouroethylene as a soft-tissue filling substance: an analysis of design-related implant behavior using the porcine skin model. *Plast Reconst Surg* 101:1307–1314.

19. Ramirez A, Monhian N, Maas C. Current concepts in soft tissue augmentation *Facial Plast Clin North Am* 2000; 8: 235–251.

20. Rubin J, Yaremchuk M. Complications and toxicities of implantable biomaterials used in facial reconstructive and aesthetic surgery: A comprehensive review of the literature. *Plast Reconst Surg* 1997; 100:1336.

21. Teimourian B. Face and neck suction-assisted lipectomy associated with rhytidectomy. *Plast Reconst Surg* 1983; 72:627.

22. Tobin HA, Karas ND. Lip augmentation using an alloderm graft. *J Oral Maxillofac Surg* 1998; 56:722–727.

23. Wang J, Fan J, Nordstrom RE. Evaluation of lip augmentation with Gore-Tex facial implant. *Aesthetic Plast Surg* 1997; 21: 433–436.

Oromandibular Reconstruction

Gary Y Shaw

Successful mandibular reconstruction requires the head and neck and reconstructive surgeon to have a variety of skills and knowledge for. Perhaps no other head and neck reconstructive endeavor in the last fifty years has been so affected by the advent of new innovation and new technology. From the understanding of bony healing first elucidated in the 1940s and 1950s to the advent of biphase plating fixation to reconstructive plates, to the introduction of the myocutaneous flap, and more recently to the osteocutaneous microvascular free-flaps. This is to say nothing of the utility of antibiotics, hyperbaric oxygen and dental and osteal implants. With the advent of so many new emerging technologies, it is incumbent upon the mandibular reconstructive surgeon to accurately analyze mandibular defects and reconstruct using the most appropriate technique.

It is the goal of this chapter to review mandibular reconstruction techniques both old and new and emphasize appropriate applications.

PRINCIPLES OF MANDIBULAR RECONSTRUCTION

The recent decades have seen several shifts in perspective regarding mandibular reconstruction.[12] When one considers that early on, mandibular reconstruction was predominantly used for managing ballistic injuries and trauma. While these are still known to happen, the majority, more than 80%, are secondary to defects that are post-extirpative surgery. Mandibular reconstruction in the past was rarely performed at the time of primary extirpative surgery. Concern of intraoral contamination with subsequent infection, poor stability and an inability to accurately determine surgical margins in an expedient fashion, argued for staged delayed procedures. The advent of broad spectrum antibiotics, reconstructive plates, and vascularized bone tissue, frozen sections and other newer developments have created not only the ability, but the expectation to reconstruct at the time of primary mandibular excision.

The ideal mandibular reconstruction, like any reconstructive effort should, as closely as possible, restore premorbid form and function. In mandibular reconstruction, this entails the ability to:
- Restore mandibular continuity and facial contour
- Maintain mobility of the tongue
- Re-establish the buccal mandibular sulcus
- Rehabilitate and allow use of a functional denture
- Optimize mastication deglutition, and speech
- Restore sensation to resurfaced intraoral soft tissue in the lower lip.

While no single technique can be used for all mandibular defects, the size, shape and extent of the soft tissue will, to a large extent, determine the technique chosen.

Defect Classification

A thorough understanding of the oromandibular anatomy is essential. It is useful for the reconstructive surgeon to have a classification system to analyze and categorize defects. In general, these should be considered for analyzing both the bony defect as well as the soft tissue defect.

Bony Classification

The four main regions are the symphysis, body, ascending ramus, condylar process (Fig. 44.1).

The Symphysis

Promotes chin prominence and is chiefly responsible for the vertical height of the lower one-third of the face. In

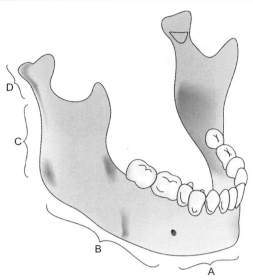

Fig. 44.1: Applied anatomy of the mandible demonstrating the four functional regions. (A) Symphysis; (B) Body; (C) Ascending ramus; (D) Condylar process

combination with the lower teeth, it also supports the lower lip. It serves as the attachment for the mylohyoid and the genial muscles necessary for tongue support. The mentalis muscle is also attached and serves as support for lower lip competence.

The Body

The body supports posterior dentition and through it runs the inferior alveolar nerve providing sensation to the teeth, gums; it exits as a mental nerve providing sensation to the lower lip and chin.

The Ramus

Key is the attachment of the suspensory muscles of mastication, namely the pterygoid, masseter sling, and temporalis muscle.

The Condyle

A uniquely complex surface allows the condyle to move in three planes, vertical, rotational and translational, relative to the base of skull articulation.

It is for these reasons that a fixation point for the remaining mandibular reconstruction be provided unless oncologically necessary. The coronoid, conversely, is often purposely removed in mandibular reconstruction to prevent uncontrolled upward and medial pull of the attached temporalis muscle, especially if prolonged inactivity and radiation producing fibrosis of this muscle is expected.

Soft Tissue Reconstruction

The overall success of oromandibular reconstructive surgery is often based on the quality of soft tissue reconstruction, as the bony defect form and function are paramount. Optimally, the soft tissue should be pliable and not bulky to facilitate tongue mobility and sulcus creation, yet vascularly hard enough to withstand intraoral bacterial contamination and support a lower dental prosthetic. The reconstructive construction planning should take into account not only the soft tissue loss but also previous surgical scars and previous or planned radiation therapy. Management of soft tissue defects, particularly in the secondary case may be proved by pre-surgical hyperbaric oxygen.[21] Historically, graft failures have been secondary to poor recipient tissue, underscoring the need for optimal soft tissue.[14] Previous irradiation is generally detrimental to bony reconstruction causing hypocellularity, hypovascularity and hypoxia. Hyperbaric oxygen has been shown to effectively reverse this. Marx et al recommends hyperbaric oxygen for all tissue beds which have received 5 kGy in the past. He noted the stimulation of the macrophage derived angiogensis factor (MDAF) which promotes early capillary ingrowth. Standard recommendations consist of placing the subject in a sealed chamber breathing 100% oxygen at 2.4 ATA for 90 minutes, six days a week for 20 sessions prior to grafting. Postoperatively, ten additional sessions are generally used to promote wound healing.

RECONSTRUCTIVE TECHNIQUE

A variety of reconstructive techniques are available to correct mandibular defects. For an isolated ramus defect in an edentulous patient, no reconstruction is necessary. Alternatively, a thorough soft tissue anterior defect requires extensive soft tissue and bony reconstruction which challenges the ability of all reconstructive surgeons. The various methods (and materials) used for modern mandibular reconstruction are described here.

Alloplast

Implants such as pins, trays, biphase fixation, and reconstructive plates have been used in mandibular reconstruction. The composition of alloplast (Figs 44.2A to C) is vitallium, stainless steel, reinforced dacron mesh, titanium, and more recently absorbable methylcellulose (Lactosorb®) plates. Early use consisted of Krischner wires or orthopedic Steinman pins inserted into the

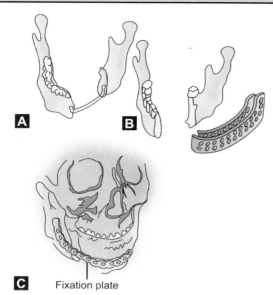

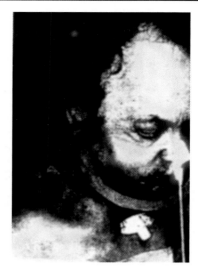

Fig. 44.4: Immediate postoperative period following immediate reconstruction of the mandible. Note Hall-Morris biphase stabilization and shoulder donor effect

Figs 44.2A to C: Alloplastic implants used in mandibular reconstruction. (A) Pins are used to maintain mandibular position; (B) Trays are used as spacers; (C) Plates and screws maintain mandible segments

intramedullary spaces of the proximal and distal segments to maintain a premorbid relationship of the bony segments. Nevertheless, because of the instability of these devices, they are currently rarely used. Trays or cribs of various materials, filled with particulate cancellous bone and marrow (PCBM), have been used since the 1950s[10] (discussed later in this chapter). The trays were fenestrated well to allow for cellular and vascular ingrowth from the recipient bed (Fig. 44.3).

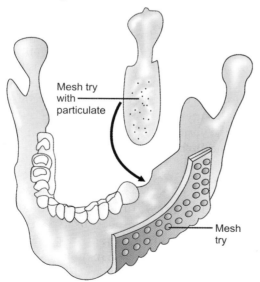

Fig. 44.3: Perforated titanium tray used in combination with corticocancellous chips in secondary mandibular reconstruction

External pin fixation[25] (Roger Anderson, Joe–Hall–Morris, biphase) (Fig. 44.4) introduced in 1949, is still used to fix comminuted mandibular fractures, principally from high-energy ballistic trauma.[15] It allows the surgeon to maintain correct position of residual segments, decreasing secondary infection and mandibular bony sequestration. After several weeks, allowing for soft tissue repair, the biphase is then removed and definitive mandibular reconstruction is undertaken.

Rigid plate fixation is used for bony defects as well as for securing bone grafts into position. The composition of the plate is determined by thickness and conformability. While more rigid plates offer more intrinsic strength, they are harder to configure. Three of the four bicortical screws in each segment will allow for the stabilization, generally one to five years.[6,9] Longer lasting plates (Thorp-titanium hollow screw reconstructive plates) introduced by Raveh[27] relies on expanse style fenestrated screws where plates do not rely on bony contact for fixation, but rather the plate screw expands into the hollow shell placed in the bone. This technique, in theory, avoids substantial subcortical resorbtion. Bony ingrowth into the screw itself ensures long-term stability.[20]

Bone Grafts

Autogenous Bone Grafts

The fundamental goal of bone grafting is to transfer osteocompetent cells to a tissue defect missing bone.[5,16] Basically three types of bone grafting exist:

- Non-vascularized block bone grafts
- Particulate cancellous bone and marrow (PCBM) which relies on either alloplastic trays or autogenic cribs[7]
- Vascularized bone grafts, either pedicled or free with microvascular anastomosis.

Free bone grafts are generally harvested from either rib, calvarium, or iliac crest.[8] They generally consist of cortical bone with an underlying cancellous portion.[24] The advantage of this type of graft is that it provides osteoblasts in the necessary strength to bridge defects. The main drawback is that it has very slow revas-cularization because of the inorganic minerals in the cortical bone plate, which in-term threatens the cancellous portion.

Particulate Cancellous Bone and Marrow Grafts

These were introduced by Boyer in the 1940s.[4] In this form of graft, transplanted cells, capable of forming new bone rather than mature osteocytes and hard bone matrix as does a block graft. Seminal work by Axhausen,[3] describes a dual phase of healing of bone grafts. In phase I, cells that survive the transplant, proliferate and lay down new osteoid. This process continues to approximately four weeks. This phase will determine the final size of the bone graft. Therefore, it is important to transplant an adequate amount of osteoblastic cells. Clinically, this is done by compacting the cancellous bone and marrow into as tight a paste as possible within the tray or crib. In phase II, remodeling and host cell replacement occurs.[4] This is actively mediated by bone morphogenic protein (BMP) which are in high concentration in cortical bone. Therefore cortical bone chips must be included in the PCBM slurry.[24] Phase II generally begins at two weeks, peaks at about six weeks and is generally over by six months. This two-phase process will produce viable bone at the recipient site if the site is adequately vascularized. Unlike block grafts where the active cancellous or osteoblastic cells are trapped within a cortical bone shield, PCBM chips are generally exposed to the nutrient tissue by being packed via a variety of carriers. Alloplastic cribs include titanium, vitallium, stainless steel and dacron mesh.[17] While there is uniform to allow fenestration for microvascular ingrowth. The existence of the crib however, makes vestibular sulcus and osteal implants difficult, but not impossible, to 'receive'. Hence, allogenic and autogenic cribs are generally preferred.[18] Allogenic cribs are manufactured from freeze-dried or gamma-radiated cadaver mandible.[19] The bone is hollowed and fenestrated and packed with PCBM, usually harvested

from the posterior iliac crest. Autogenic cribs are derived from taking either the resected mandible, exposing it to intraoperative radiation to render it sterile and then again, hollow, fenestrate and pack it with the bioactive PCBM. If a larger amount of mandible structure is needed, the patient's iliac crest can be harvested as a block graft. Marrow and particulate bone can be obtained from the graft as well, hollowing it out, fenestrating it and packing it with PCBM. The advantage of allogenic and autogenic cribs is the fact that the cortical structure will eventually degrade and this then simplifies subsequent sulcoplasties and placement of osteal implants. Generally about six months are required for adequate cortical degradation.

The above techniques use non-vascularized bone.[31] To this end, applications are generally used only in secondary reconstruction. Intraoral contamination would doom these grafts. Therefore, they are approached through an external incision and great care should be taken when exposing mandible stumps, to prevent oral contamination. Position the graft to promote mandibular continuity. This is aided by dentition fixation or biphase[36] fixation at the time of the extirpative surgery to maintain proper relationship. If the coronoid is still present, a corondectomy should be performed in order to prevent upward rotation and pull of the temporalis muscle. The block graft or alloplastic cribs are generally secured with reconstructive plate with three bicortical screws placed proximally distally.

Vascularized Bone Grafts

The advent of the regional pedicle myocutaneous flap with vascularized bone was a major breakthrough in mandibular reconstruction. For the first time, both soft and hard tissue defect could be replaced simultaneously. Moreover, since the blood supply is derived from distal vessels well out of the oral field, tissue could be reconstructed at the time of the original extirpative surgery. Five flaps have generally been used: pectoralis major with rib; trapezius with the spine of the scapula; latissimus dorsi with rib; sternocleidomastoid with clavicle; temporalis muscle with outer calvarium.

Pectoralis major: First described for mandibular reconstruction in 1979 by Ariyan,[1,2] it rapidly became the workhorse in the 1980s and much of the 1990s for head and neck reconstruction. It is still the flap of choice for surgeons who do not perform microvascular anastomosis or in patients where microvascular anastomosis is not feasible.[28] Its axial blood supply is derived from the lateral thoracic, superior thoracic, and anterior mammary perforators (Fig. 44.5A). Its skin muscle is harvested in the area between the nipple and the sternum. When bone was transferred it was generally the fifth or sixth rib or even a portion of the sternum.

Trapezius: This flap actually could be harvested as a superior flap based on perispinous perforators or a distal island flap based on descending branch of the transverse cervical artery which must be consciously spared during neck dissection.[30] The superior flap could include the spine and the scapula thus supplying bony tissue (Fig. 44.5B).

Latissimus dorsi: This flap is particularly useful for soft-tissue defects up to 14 cm² (Figs 44.5C and D). This flap is based on the descending branch of the thoracodorsal artery.[22] The skin panel is usually oblique paralleling the direction of the muscle fibers superior to lateral. The posterior and lateral portion of the sixth rib could be included as a bony attachment.

Sternocleidomastoid: This generally uses a muscle-only flap based on superior insertion in the occipital artery. A portion of the clavicle can be included, if the muscle branch from the superior thyroid artery is preserved. Its insertion point in the clavicle can be included for bony reconstruction (Fig. 44.5E).

Temporalis/calvarium: Based upon the superficial temporal artery and vein, the superficial investing fasci continues above the temporalis line as periostium providing blood supply to the outer table calvarium, generally in the parietal area (Fig. 44.5F). Frequently, full-thickness bone is harvested, split and the inner table secured back to the cranium to repair the bony defect. Frequently, the temporalis muscle is also included which when skin-grafted can supply soft tissue reconstruction.

While these vascularized pedicled composite flaps represented a quantum leap, they also had significant limitations. The bone was generally too small to support endosteal implants or dentures. The arc of rotation was significantly limited because of the pedicles and tension-free placement of soft tissue and bone was frequently difficult. The soft tissue itself was frequently not well-suited for the intraoral cavity, not being pliable and quite thick. Therefore, the contours of the oral cavity could not be easily reproduced. Finally, as a result of the profusion pressure in the distal portion of the flap, particularly those with a long axis of rotation, the pectoralis major, trapezius, and latissimus dorsi become tenuous the more superior the flap. The blood supply to the bone was purely periosteal and quite tenuous; none of the flaps provided endosteal blood supply.

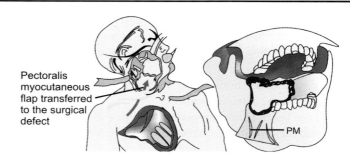

Fig. 44.5A: Pectoralis myocutaneous flap transferred to the surgical defect

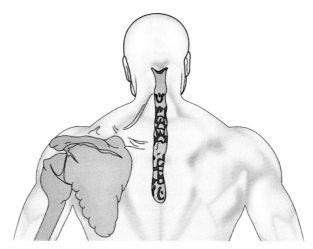

Fig. 44.5B: Tripartite blood supply to the trapezius muscle

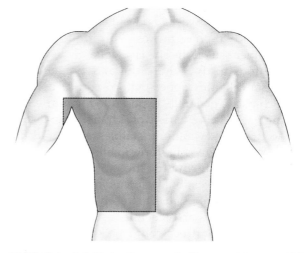

Fig. 44.5C: Potential skin territory supplied by vasculature supplying latissimus dorsi myocutaneous flap. This can measure 25 × 40 cm

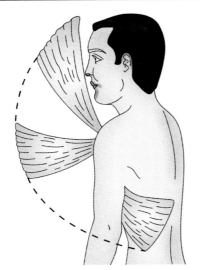

Fig. 44.5D: Arc of rotation of latissimus dorsi myocutaneous flap

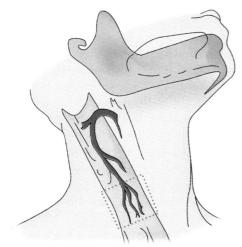

Fig. 44.5E: Sternocleidomastoid myocutaneous flap.
(A) Outline of flap and blood supply; (B) Flap within oropharynx

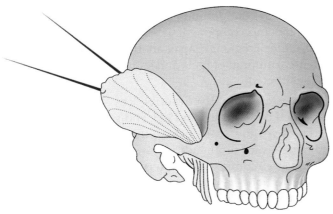

Fig. 44.5F: The temporalis muscle is elevated onto its deep vascular pedicle and reflected inferiorly

Microvascular Flaps

The advent of microvascular osteocutaneous flaps (Fig. 44.6) greatly increased the utility of vascularized flaps from oromandibular reconstruction.[38] These flaps have markedly improved vascularity of both soft tissue and bone. In many of these grafts the stock of bone is far superior to the regional flap bone, thus allowing for osseo-integrated implants and in general a more suitable cosmetic reconstruction. Many of the associated soft tissue to these flaps were thinner and more pliable, thus being able to reconstruct more faithfully the intraoral soft tissue. The blood supply to the bone is both periosteal and endosteal thus improving the survival of the vascularized bone graft. Finally, many of these flaps also allowed for sensation in the sensory nerve branches in the neuro-vascular pedicle, resensitized via anastomosis with either the lingual nerve or the inferior alveolar nerve, thus making deglutition more complete.

Free flaps have been used in mandibular recon-struction in the past;[37] however, these are rarely used today. These include the metatarsal graft, the dorsalis pedis, the humerus based upon the profunda brachii artery, rib based upon the intercostal artery and the ulna based upon the ulna artery. For various reasons, these grafts while potentially able to reconstruct defects have been found not well-suited for this type of reconstruction. The most popular free flaps used today are the radial forearm flap, scapular system free flaps, the fibula, and the ileum.

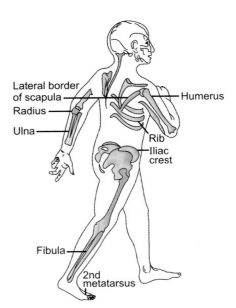

Fig. 44.6: Donor sites of vascularized bone flaps used in oromandibular reconstruction

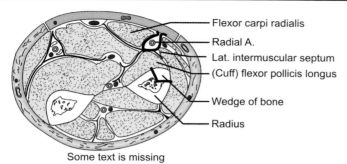

Some text is missing

Fig. 44.7A: Cross-section of forearm distal to insertion of pronator teres, showing anatomy of a composite osteofasciocutaneous flap

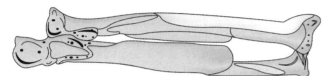

Fig. 44.7B: Longitudinal section showing extent of bone available for transfer

Radial forearm flap: Based upon the radial artery,[32] cephalic vein and antecubital nerve it provides a thin sensate large fasciocutaneous flap which can carry as much as 10 cm in length and 40% in circumference of the radial bone (Figs 44.7A and B). Reshaping of the bone is generally performed by ostectomy and osteotomy. Because it is short, however, it rarely matches remaining native mandible and therefore generally cannot support endosteal dental implants. Also a 40% fracture of the remaining radius bone has been described.

Scapular system: This area offers a wide variety of potential flaps. In this flap 10–12 cm of bone can be harvested from the lateral thoracic border. Scapular and parascapular cutaneous flaps can be included based on the circumflex scapular branches of the subscapular artery and vein[33] (Fig. 44.8). If the thoracodorsal branches are included, the

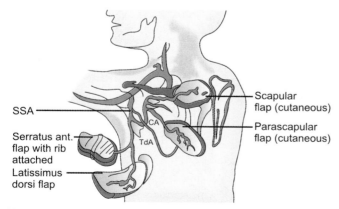

Fig. 44.8: The scapular flap system offers a wide array of skin, bone, and muscle components; CA, circumflex artery; SSA, subscapular artery; TdA, thoracodorsal artery

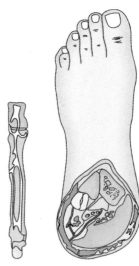

Fig. 44.9: The fibular osteocutaneous flap and its main blood supply. EDL, extensor digitorum longus; EHL, extensor hallucis longus; F, fibula; S, soleus; T, tibia; TA tibialis anterior; TB tibial posterior

latissimus dorsi and serratus anterior can also be included in this flap.[34] This allows for tremen-dous variation of placement of soft tissues. However, again the quality of the scapular bone is limited in both thickness and dimensions and because the patient must be positioned in a lateral decubitus position. This makes it difficult to perform two-team surgery using these flaps.

Fibula: The fibula osteocutaneous free flap is supplied by the peroneal artery and vein (Fig. 44.9). Its greatest advantage is that the bone is very thick and long (up to 25 cm). It is in fact the graft of choice for total mandibular reconstruction.[13] The blood supply is both endosteal and periosteal. The skin overlying the posterior crural septum is supplied by septocutaneous branches and thus is somewhat tenuous. The biggest drawback is the necessity for multiple ostectomies and osteotomies to create a mandibular configuration as well as the tenuousness of the cutaneous component. It is often used in conjunction with either a regional flap or another free flap when there is a great amount of bone and soft tissue that needs to be reconstructed.

Iliac crest: Originally described by Taylor in 1979,[35] modified by Ramastry in 1983, and widely promoted by Urken over the past decade, this flap provides many advantages for oromandibular reconstruction. Based on the deep circumflex iliac artery and vein, 14–16 cm of adequate bone can be harvested (Figs 44.10A to C). A complete heavy mandible can be fashioned.[39] The skin overlying the crest, however was quite thick and bulky and as originally described was not ideal for oral

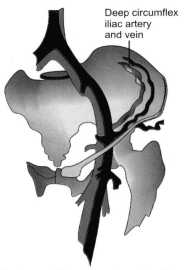

Fig. 44.10A: Anatomy of the deep circumflex iliac artery and vein

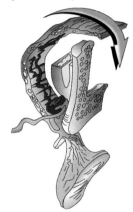

Fig. 44.10B: Design of internal oblique iliac crest osseomyocutaneous flap harvested from right hip for reconstruction of right hemimandible. This is a tripartite flap composed of bone, muscle and skin

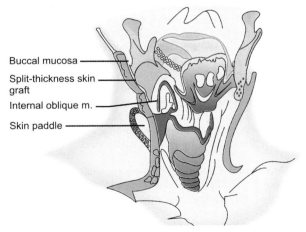

Fig. 44.10C: Cross-section of the internal oblique iliac crest bone flap in place. A split-thickness skin graft has been used to resurface the muscle and reconstruct the buccal and lingual sulci

reconstruction.[40,41] However, Ramastry in 1983 described the blood supply of the internal oblique muscle[26] which is generally thin and pliable, as being also supplied by branches of the deep circumflex artery and vein. Since this muscle can be skin-grafted and then used intraoral to create a sulcus at the time of original reconstruction. Donor site complications include gait disturbances and potential hernia.[29] Meticulous closure is necessary.

SENSORY RESTORATION

As mentioned earlier, restoration of sensory deficits (Fig. 44.11) will aid in deglutition postoperatively.[42] This includes two types of microneural reanastomosis. The first is cable grafting of the resected portion of the inferior alveolar nerve to the mental nerve to restore sensation to the lower lip. This is generally performed after extirpation and soft tissue reconstruction and prior to the bone inset by placing a cable graft harvested from either the greater auricular or, if longer the sural nerve in order to affect sensory deficits. Intraoral reneurotization can occur particularly with the radial forearm flap as well as the ulna and humerus flap. The antecubital nerve of the radial forearm flap is frequently reanastomosed with the lingual nerve, thus allowing for resensitization of the intraoral cavity. This is why many times this flap is often used as a fascocutaneous flap for intraoral reconstruction while a bony flap or even a bone graft is used for bony reconstruction.

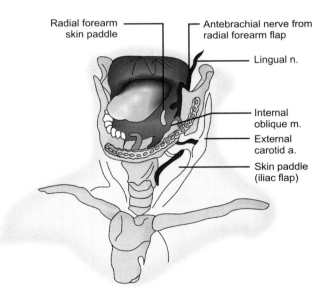

Fig. 44.11: Combination iliac crest/radial forearm flap used to provide sensory reinnervation of the oropharyngeal defects

New Frontiers

In the future, it is likely that the greatest advances in mandibular reconstruction would be made from basic research on bone induction, osteocyte culture techniques and genetic engineering (human genomes and other genetic tissue engineering) rather than development of newer and more sophisticated surgical techniques. The evolving field of distraction osteogenesis is also proving to be of considerable interest because clinical applications are currently being studied for mandibular reconstruction following tumor resection. Distraction osteogenesis[23] is a technique where new bone is created by physically stretching a developing callous between two bony ends and a favorable fracture. As the two fragments are gradually separated, the resulting gap is filled-in with an expanding callous that eventually develops into new bone (osteogenesis). These and other new developments will continue to push the frontier of mandibular reconstruction, potentially providing autogenous tissue, perfectly suited for the native mandible through less morbidity, perhaps even on an outpatient basis leading to a more rapid recovery and shorter hospital stay.

CONCLUSION

The reconstruction of oromandibular defects has seen tremendous advances in the past fifty years. Many techniques and technologies are available to the reconstructive surgeon. A sound analysis of the tissue defect, both hard and soft tissue is incumbent on determining which reconstructive technique to use. Often multiple techniques may be necessary to achieve optimal reconstruction. The ability to reconstruct all types of oromandibular defects and to optimize premorbid form and function, make it necessary for the reconstructive surgeon to either be fascicle and knowledgeable, or the ability to arrange for procurement through colleagues.

REFERENCES

1. Ariyan S. The pectoralis major myocutaneous flap. *Plast Reconstr Surg* 1979; 63:73.
2. Ariyan S. The sternocleidomastoid myocutaneous flap. *Laryngoscope* 1980; 90:976.
3. Axhausen W. The osteogenic phase of regeneration of bone—a historical and experimental study. *J Bone Jt Surg* 1956; 38-A:593.
4. Boyne PJ. Autogenous cancellous bone and marrow transplants. *Clin Orthop* 1970; 73:199.
5. Bradley PF. A two-stage procedure for re-implantation of autogenous freeze-treated mandibular bone. *J Oral Maxillofac Surg* 1982; 40:278–284.
6. Branemark PI, Lindstrom J, Hallen O et al. Osteointegrated implants in the treatment of the edentulous jaw. Experience from a ten-year period. *Sand J Plast Reconstr Surg* 1977; 1 (suppl 16).
7. Burwell RG. Studies in transplantation of bone VII. The fresh composite of homograft-autograft of cancellous bone. *J Bone Joint Surg* (B) 1964; 46:110.
8. Forrest C, Boyd B, Manktelow R et al. The free iliac crest tissue transfer: Donor site complications associated with eighty-two cases. *Br J Plast Surg* 1992; 45:89–93.
9. Frodel JL, Funk GF, Capper DT et al. Osseointegrated implants: A comparative study of bone thickness in four vascularized bone flaps. *Plast Reconstr Surg* 1993; 92:449–458.
10. Gaisford JC, Hanna DC, Gutman D. Management of the mandibular fragments following resection. *Plast Reconstr Surg* 1961; 28:192.
11. Gray JC, Elves MW. Early osteogenesis in compact bone isografts: A quantitative study of the contribution of the different graft cells. *Calcific Tissue Res Int* 1979; 29:225.
12. Gullane PJ, Holmes H. Mandibular reconstruction—new concepts. *Arch Otolaryngol Head Neck Surg* 1986; 112:714.
13. Hidalgo, D. Fibular free flap: A new method of mandible reconstruction. *Plast Reconstr Surg* 1989; 84:71.
14. Joseph DL, Shumrick DL. Risks of head and neck surgery in previously irradiated patients. *Arch Otolaryngol* 1973; 97:391–403.
15. Kellman RM, Gullane PJ. Use of the AO mandibular reconstruction plate for bridging of mandibular defects. *Otolaryngol Clin North Am* 1987; 20:519.
16. Kline SN, Rimer. Reconstruction of osseous defect with freeze dried allogenic and autogenous bone. Clinical and histological assessment. *Am J Surg* 1983; 146:471–482.
17. Komisar A, Worman S, Danziger E. A critical analysis of immediate and delayed mandibular reconstruction using AO plates. *Arch Otolaryngol Head Neck Surg* 1989; 115:830–835.
18. Kroll SS, Schusterman MA, Reece GP. Costs and complications in mandibular reconstruction. *Ann Plast Surg* 1992; 29:341–348.
19. Lawson W, Loscalzo L, Baek S, Biller HF, Krespi Y. Experience with immediate and delayed mandibular reconstruction. *Laryngoscope* 1982; 92–95.
20. Marx RE. A new concept in the treatment of osteoradionecrosis. *J Oral Maxillofac Surg* 1983; 41:351.
21. Marx RE, Ames R Jr. The use of hyperbaric oxygen therapy in bony reconstruction of the irradiated and tissue-deficient patient. *J Oral Surg* 1982; 40:412.
22. Maves MD, Panye WR, Shagets FW. Extended latissimus dorsi myocutaneous flap reconstruction of major head and neck cancer defects. *Otolaryngol Head Neck Surg* 1989; 92:551.
23. McCarthy JG, Schreiber J, Karp N et al. Lengthening of the mandibular bone by gradual distraction. *Plast Reconstr Surg* 1992; 8:1.
24. Molwem R. Cancellous chip bone grafts. *Lancet* 1944; 2:746.
25. Morris JH. Biphasic connector, external skeletal splint for reduction and fixation of mandibular fracture. *Oral Surg* 1949; 2:1382.
26. Ramasastry SS, Tucker JB, Swartz WM, Hurtwitz DJ. The internal oblique muscle flap: An anatomic and clinical study. *Plast Reconstr Surg* 1984; 73:721.

27. Raveh Y, Stich H, Sulter F. The use of titanium-coated hollow screw and reconstruction plate in bridging of lower jaw defects. *J Oral Surg* 1984; 42:281.

28. Russell RC, Feller AM, Elliott F et al. The extended pectoralis major myocutaneous flap: Uses and indications. *Plast Reconstr Surg* 1991; 88:814–823.

29. Selebian AH, Rappaport J, Allison G. Functional oromandibular reconstruction with the microvascular composite groin flap. *Plast Reconstr Surg* 1985; 76:819.

30. Shapiro MJ. Use of trapezius myocutaneous flaps in the reconstruction of head and neck defects. *Arch Otolaryngol* 1981; 107:333.

31. Simmons DJ, Lester PA, Ellasser JC. Survival of osteocompetent marrow cells *in vitro* and the effect of PHA stimulation on osteoinduction in composite bone grafts. *Proc Soc Exp Biol Medication* 1975; 148:986.

32. Soutar DS, McGregor IA. The radial forearm flap in intraoral reconstruction: The experience of 60 consecutive cases. *Plast Reconstr Surg* 1986; 78:1.

33. Swartz W, Banis J, Newton E, Ramasastry S, Jones N, Acland R. The osteocutaneous scapular flap for mandibular and maxillary reconstruction. *Plast Reconstr Surg* 1986; 77:530.

34. Swartz WM, Banis JC, Newton ED et al. The osteocutaneous scapular flap for mandibular and maxillary reconstruction. *Plast Reconstr Surg* 1986; 77:530.

35. Taylor GI, Townsend P, Corlett R. Superiority of the deep circumflex iliac vessels as the supply for free groin flaps: Clinical work. *Plast Reconstr Surg* 1979; 64:745.

36. Urist MR. The substratum for bone morphogenesis. *Develop Biol (Suppl)* 1970; 4:125.

37. Urken M. Composite free flaps in oromandibular reconstruction: Review of the literature. *Arch Otolaryngol Head Neck Surg* 1991; 117:724.

38. Urken ML, Buchbinder D, Sheiner A et al. Functional evaluation following microvascular oromandibular reconstruction of the oral cancer patient, a comparative study of reconstructed and non-reconstructed patients. *Laryngoscope* 1991; 101:935.

39. Urken ML, Buchbinder D, Vickery C, Weinberg H, Biller HF. The internal oblique iliac crest osteomyocutaneous microvascular free flap in head and neck reconstruction. *J Reconstr Microsurg* 1989; 5:203.

40. Urken ML, Buchbinder D, Weinberg H, Vickery C, Sheiner A, Biller HF. Primary placement of osseointegrated implants in microvascular mandibular reconstruction. *Otolaryngol Head Neck Surg* 1989; 101:56.

41. Urken ML, Vickery C, Weinberg H, Buchbinder D, Lawson W, Biller HF. The internal oblique iliac crest osteomyocutaneous free flap in oromandibular reconstruction—report of 20 cases. *Arch Otolaryngol Head Neck Surg* 1989; 115:339.

42. Wolford LM. Autogenous nerve graft repairs of the trigeminal nerve. In Lebanc JP, Gregg JM (eds) *Oral and maxillofacial surgery clinics of North America—trigeminal nerve injury diagnoses and management.* Philadelphia: WB Saunders 1992; 447–457.

Reconstruction of Facial Mohs Defects

45

William W Shockley

Currently non-melanoma skin cancers (NMSCs) account for 40% of all malignancies in the US, with more than one million new cases each year.[1] Basal cell carcinoma (BCC) makes up 75% of these tumors, while squamous cell carcinoma (SCC) comprises 20%.

The overwhelming majority of patients have a history of chronic sun exposure related to recreational or occupational activities.[2] The most important carcinogenic wavelengths for the induction of skin cancer come from ultraviolet B (UVB) light, although ultraviolet A (UVA) has also been implicated.[2,3] As the population ages and the ozone layer diminishes, the incidence for NMSC continues to increase. The average annual increase of BCC in the caucucian populations of the United States, Canada, and Australia ranges from 3 to 7%.[3] Sun exposure is the single most important causative factor for skin cancer, as demonstrated by the fact that 80% of NMSCs occur on the head, neck and back of the hands.[3]

Although the vast majority of skin cancers are small and may be readily treated in an office setting, certain high-risk lesions are referred for Mohs micrographic surgery. Once histologic clearance has been obtained by the Mohs surgeon, many of these patients are then referred for a reconstructive procedure. This chapter will highlight the issues related to these reconstructive efforts as they apply to the face, neck and scalp. It is beyond the scope of this chapter to serve as a compendium of reconstructive options. Instead, the author will emphasize the important principles that can be applied in this setting, using clinical examples to illustrate these tenets. There are several excellent texts devoted to nasal and facial reconstruction which can be of assistance in the decision-making process.[4–7] In reconstructing facial cutaneous defects, multiple options are available. It is up to the surgeon to select the one most appropriate for the clinical setting. These decisions should be based on thorough knowledge of the anatomy, the risk of recurrence, and the experience and expertise of the surgeon.

TREATMENT OF SKIN CANCER

Skin cancer can be treated by numerous modalities, all of which can be effective if proper selection is applied. Martinez and Otley categorize these treatment methods as superficial ablative techniques and full-thickness techniques. Superficial ablative techniques include electrodesiccation and curettage (ED&C) and cryotherapy. Full-thickness techniques include excisional surgery, Mohs micrographic surgery, and radiotherapy (Table 45.1).

In dermatology offices across the USA, the most common procedure for the treatment of low-risk skin cancers is electrodesiccation and curettage (ED&C). This procedure takes advantage of the fact that the neoplastic tissue (most often BCC) is more friable and curettes more easily than the adjacent dermis. Based on the 'feel' and texture of the tissue, curettage is undertaken until the tumor is removed and the firm resistance of the dermis is encountered. Electrodesiccation (monoterminal electrocautery) is undertaken following curettage. This adds superficial destruction, hemostasis, and inflammation (which contributes to tumor elimination).[1]

Table 45.1: Methods of treatment for non-melanoma skin cancer
Superficial ablative techniques
• Electrodesiccation and curettage
• Cryotherapy
Full-thickness techniques
• Surgical excision
• Radiotherapy
• Mohs micrographic surgery
Modified from Martinez and Otley, 2001[31]

Table 45.2: Five-year cure rate by treatment modality for primary and recurrent BCC and SCC

Treatment	Basal cell carcinoma (BCC)%		Squamous cell carcinoma (SCC)%	
	Primary	*Recurrent*	*Primary*	*Recurrent*
Electrodesiccation and curettage	92	60	96	NA
Cryotherapy	93	87	96	NA
Excision	90	83	92	77
Radiation	91	91	90	NA
All non-Mohs surgery methods	91	NA	92	NA
Mohs surgery	99	94	97	92

NA = not available

Courtesy: Nguyen and Ho, 2002[1]

The ED & C cycle is repeated 2–3 times for maximal cure rates. The results of the procedure are technique-dependent and cure rates are higher in more experienced hands.

Cryotherapy can also be used for low-risk lesions. This involves the application of liquid nitrogen. There are a number of variables affecting the level of tissue destruction, including the strength of the cryogen's delivery system, proximity of the spray to the tissue, freezing time, thawing time, and the number of freeze-thaw cycles.[1] Experience is required to balance tissue destruction, cure rate, and efficacy.

Surgical excision, Mohs surgery, and radiation therapy can all be applied to lesions with a higher level of risk. Recurrence rates are shown in Table 45.2. Excisional surgery may be performed in the office setting for well-circumscribed lesions. For a primary well-defined BCC or SCC which is less than 2 cm in diameter, the recommended margin of excision is 4 mm of normal appearing skin. Following these parameters, studies have shown that the expected cure rate is 95%.[8] Lesions larger than 2 cm, those with ill-defined borders and tumors with other high-risk factors should be excised with margins of 6 mm or greater.

Radiation therapy has comparable cure rates to excisional surgery and may be used as initial treatment for primary skin malignancies, less than 2 cm, which are well-defined. Adjunctive radiation is often recommended following surgery if there is deep tumor spread, perineural invasion, or regional lymph node metastasis.

MOHS SURGERY

For high-risk lesions, Mohs micrographic surgery remains the standard of care. Authors may differ as to the indications for Mohs, but this modality should be considered for lesions with ill-defined borders, tumors > 2 cm, recurrent tumors, high-risk histologic subtypes,

Table 45.3: Indications for Mohs surgery

- Recurrent tumors
- Large tumors (>2 cm in diameter)
- Incompletely excised tumors
- Tumors in high-risk locations
- Sites where tissue conservation is important
- Indistinct clinical margins
- Aggressive histological features
  - BCCs: Micronodular, infiltrative, morpheaform
  - SCCs: Poorly differentiated
  - Basosquamous carcinomas
- Perineural invasion
- Tumors arising in irradiated skin or chronic scars
- Adapted from Padgett and Hendrix, 2001.

and high-risk locations (temples, ears, periorbital, perioral, lips, and nose.[1] The commonly accepted indications for Mohs surgery are listed in Table 45.3.

Mohs surgery goes by several different names: Mohs chemosurgery, Mohs micrographic surgery, and microscopically oriented histologic surgery (MOHS). In this chapter we shall refer to the procedure as Mohs surgery. It is considered the gold standard for specially-selected NMSCs, as it is associated with the highest cure rates of all treatment modalities. In addition, it allows for the complete margin control, maximal tissue conservation, and provides a clinicohistologic correlation. The procedure itself requires not only prior training in the technical aspects, but also the ability to interpret the histologic findings on the tissue slices obtained. The basic tenet of Mohs surgery is the ability to review 100% of the peripheral and deep margins, thus maximizing tumor control. This is in contradistinction to standard frozen section margins, in which less than 1% of the margins are evaluated using the standard bread-slice or four-quadrant technique (Figs 45.1A and B).[9,10] The Mohs surgeon has specialized training not only in cutaneous oncology but also dermatopathology.

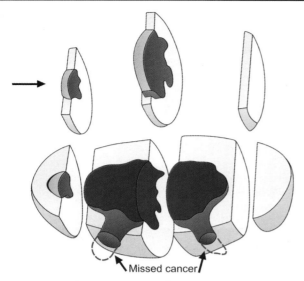

Fig. 45.1A: Bread-loaf tissue section method demonstrating subclinical extensions of missed cancer. Sections cut for microscopic examination (arrow) would show margins free of tumor (Johnson, 1996)[28]

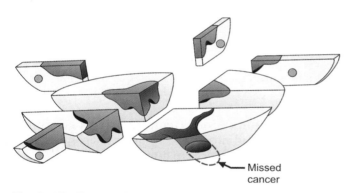

Fig. 45.1B: Four-quadrant tissue section method demonstrating subclinical extensions of missed cancer. Sections cut for microscopic examination (dots) would show peripheral and deep margins free of tumor (Johnson, 1996)[28]

Mohs Technique

The Mohs procedure is performed under local anesthesia in an outpatient setting. The first step is to curette the visible tumor. This is followed by excising a circular rim of tissue with 1–2 mm margins, including not only the cutaneous border but the tissue deep to the crater as well. Segments are then created for histologic review, being careful to mark, map, and orient each tissue slice.[10] The procedure is shown in Figures 45.2A and B.[9] Standard frozen section techniques are used, and the surgeon examines each histologic section. Because of the precise mapping and orientation, any tumor foci identified histologically can be accurately localized in the context of

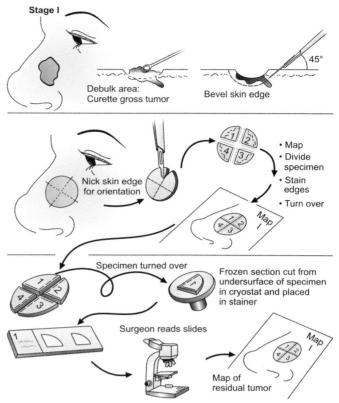

Fig. 45.2A: Schematic diagram of Mohs surgery technique for skin cancer excision. In this representation, frozen sections 2 and 3 are positive for tumor following stage I (Johnson, 1996)[28]

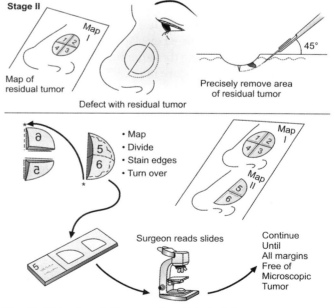

Fig. 45.2B: In stage II, the area of positivity is delineated and excised with another 2 mm margin. The process continues until all margins are free of microscopic tumor (Johnson, 1996)[28]

the newly created defect. In this way, the Mohs surgeon can 'chase the tumor' by following sequential histologic sections. Based on the tumor map, the surgeon excises another 1–2 mm of tissue in the area of the tumor positivity. The process continues in this fashion until all sections are free of tumor involvement.

Mohs surgery is an excellent technique which should be used whenever possible for high-risk lesions, providing an unparalleled cure rate, even for recurrent tumors. It provides maximal tissue sparing, and thus should be considered when lesions encroach upon specialized facial structures such as the nose, eyelid, ear, and lips. It should not be routinely used for low-risk lesions; however, as these may be expeditiously treated in an office setting using reliable and relatively inexpensive techniques, including ED&C, cryotherapy, and surgical excision.

Risk of Recurrence

As the reconstructive surgeon confronts each patient with a Mohs defect, the first issue to be addressed is whether construction should be undertaken. In the vast majority of cases, the Mohs procedure has proceeded smoothly and

the Mohs surgeon feels confident that the risk of recurrence is quite low. However, there must always be a dialogue between the Mohs surgeon and the recon-structive surgeon as to whether there are additional risk factors involved with the particular case. There are occasions which arise where both the Mohs surgeon and the reconstructive surgeon feel that there is a significant risk of recurrence, indicating that a temporizing measure may be more appropriate than definitive reconstruction. In these circumstances, it may be that the tumor was locally aggressive, that the pathology demonstrated worrisome features, or that the histology was difficult to evaluate and the margins are more suspect than in the usual situation. Perineural invasion is a finding that should be taken extremely seriously and postoperative irradiation should be anticipated.

As one tries to calculate the risk of recurrence, several factors need to be taken into consideration (Table 45.4).

It is well-known that certain sites of the head and neck are more prone to recurrence. The 'H zone' of the face has been identified as a region where recurrence rates are higher than adjacent areas (Fig. 45.3). This includes the nose, the perinasal and periorbital tissues as well as the preauricular and postauricular skin. Some authors

Table 45.4: Clinical and pathologic risk factors for recurrence of nonmelanoma skin cancer		
Low-risk	*High-risk*	*Clinical factors*
Tumor location, diameter	L < 20 mm	L ≥ 20 mm
	M < 10 mm	M ≥ 10 mm
	H < 6 mm	H ≥ 6 mm
Tumor borders	Well-defined	Poorly defined
Primary or recurrent tumor	Primary	Recurrent
Tumor at site of previous radiotherapy or chronic inflammatory process	No	Yes
Rapidly growing tumor (SCC)*	No	Yes
Immunosuppressant patient	No	Yes
Neurologic symptoms: pain, paresthesia, paralysis	No	Yes
Pathologic factors		
Tumor subtype (BCC)‡	Nodular, superficial	Metatypical, morpheaform
Degree of differentiation (SCC)*	Well-differentiated	Moderately or poorly-differentiated
Depth, Clark level or thickness (SCC)*	I, II, III or < 4 mm	IV, V or ≥ 4 mm
Perineural or vascular involvement	No	Yes

H = Areas at high-risk for recurrence, e.g. mask areas of face, chin, mandible, preauricular and postauricular skin and sulci, temples, ears, genitalia, hands, feet; L= Areas at low-risk for recurrence, e.g. trunk, extremities; M = Areas at middle risk for recurrence, e.g. cheeks, forehead, neck, scalp.

*Applicable only to squamous cell carcinoma
‡Applicable only to basal cell carcinoma

Modified from Miller and used by permission of the American Society for Dermatologic Surgery
Modified from: Martinez and Otley, 2001[31]

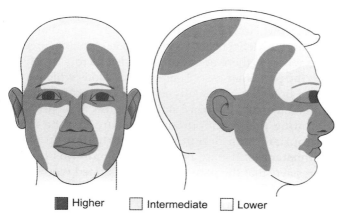

Higher ☐ Intermediate ☐ Lower

Fig. 45.3: Relative risk of recurrence and metastasis for non-melanoma skin cancer according to anatomic site (Martinez, 2001)[31]

have indicted sites of embryologic lines of fusion as being important in the prevalence of recurrence in these locations, while other authors have disputed this concept.

Recurrent tumors clearly have an added risk since these tumors have already demonstrated their ability to persist in spite of prior treatment. Thus the recurrence rate is even higher following the second attempt at eradication. For example, Mohs surgery for basal cell carcinoma in the untreated setting carries a recurrence rate of 1%, while recurrent lesions treated with Mohs have a recurrence rate of 6%.[1]

The clinical and histologic features of NMSCs play a significant role in the risk of recurrence as well. It is well-known that squamous cell cancers are generally more virulent than basal cell lesions. Squamous cell tumors are more prone to recurrence and are much more likely to metastasize; however, certain subtypes of basal cell carcinoma are notorious for subclinical extension and, thus, associated with higher rates of recurrence. These include micronodular, infiltrative and morpheaform BCCs.[2]

Host factors such as immunocompromised patients and those with genetic syndromes also place patients in a higher risk category.

Extensive actinic changes in the adjacent skin may not change the rate of recurrence but certainly enhances the development of multifocal disease.

As all of these prognostic factors are evaluated, the Mohs surgeon and reconstructive surgeon formulate a general assessment for the risk of recurrence. Although patients with lesions associated with increased risk of recurrence make up a small percentage of patients, these defects should be reconstructed in a fashion that allows for optimal surveillance or should be allowed to heal by secondary intention. Mohs defects following treatment of lesions associated with a low risk of recurrence can be considered for immediate and definitive reconstruction.

CONSIDERATIONS IN RECONSTRUCTION

Timing of Reconstruction

Timing of reconstruction is tied closely to the risk of recurrence. Patients considered at high-risk for recurrence are candidates for observation before definitive reconstruction takes place. This period of surveillance will minimize the risk of recurrence following reconstruction and provide a more secure setting for reconstruction. Even though Mohs surgery is associated with very low recurrence rates, there are specific identifiable risks that merit consideration of adjuvant treatment. The addition of postoperative radiation should be made on a case by case basis, but should generally be considered for perineural invasion, extensive soft tissue or bony invasion, or lymphatic spread.

The decision as to whether definitive reconstruction is indicated is also based on the reliability of the patient, as well as the complexity of the reconstruction, balanced with the patient's medical status. There are numerous clinical scenarios in which reconstruction will be inappropriate or unsatisfactory. In these cases, a prosthesis may be a more appropriate choice.

Once the decision to reconstruct has been made, the timing of reconstruction is based on whether reconstruction was a planned procedure to follow the Mohs surgery or whether this decision is being made following the creation of the Mohs defect. It is generally appropriate to reconstruct as soon as possible. However, it does not appear that waiting a few days to maximize patient and surgeon convenience has any deleterious effects. If a temporizing reconstruction is chosen, such as a split-thickness skin graft, it can be done immediately following the procedure. When a suitable period of observation has elapsed, definitive reconstruction can then be undertaken.

In some circumstances, reconstruction is mandatory regardless of the risk of recurrence. This includes massive orbitomaxillary defects, craniofacial defects, those which involve protection of the eye, and defects creating oral incompetence. Cutaneous tumors invading the maxilla require a maxillectomy, and often require free-flap reconstruction. Defects involving the lips must be reconstructed in order to re-establish oral competence. Periorbital and eyelid defects require reconstruction for satisfactory lubrication and protection of the eye.

Cutaneous Anatomy

In approaching the patient with a Mohs defect, it is important to keep in mind the variability of the cutaneous anatomy throughout the face, scalp and neck. There are significant differences in the thickness of the dermis, the sebaceous gland content, and the amount of subcutaneous tissue present. Eyelid skin is extremely thin and lies directly on the orbicularis muscle. Forehead skin consists of thick dermis with a thin layer of fat, whereas cheek skin has an extensive subcutaneous component. There are also topographical differences in the degree of skin elasticity. There is generally significant elasticity and redundancy in the cheek, lower face and neck; whereas, little elasticity exists in the forehead and even less in the scalp. The nose demonstrates different types of cutaneous tissue and these areas of varying skin thickness, texture, and elasticity have been divided into three zones.[11]

The adjacent cutaneous tissue may affect decision making as well. If the local tissues are traumatized or deficient, alternatives to flap reconstruction must be considered. Severe actinic damage, prior scarring from procedures such as cryotherapy, or radiation changes may play a role in these patients. Systemic problems can also affect tissue vascularity and flap survival. Diabetes, vascular disease, and smoking can all adversely affect the viability and healing of transferred tissues.

Patient Factors

Numerous patient factors come into play in the reconstructive decision-making process. Certainly the overall health status is important as one approaches surgical procedures. Some patients are best treated with a single simple procedure under local anesthesia or local with sedation. The desires and concerns of the patient must also be addressed. Some patients will simply desire avoidance of wound care with closure or grafting of the defect. Others may place a high aesthetic value on the reconstructive results and may be willing to undergo somewhat more complex or multistaged procedures in order to attain the most cosmetic result possible.

PRINCIPLES OF RECONSTRUCTION

Favorable Tension Lines

Principles of facial cosmetic surgery and reconstructive surgery have a great deal in common (Table 45.5). It is important to place incisions along relaxed skin tension lines (RSTLs) in order to camouflage scars. Recently the

Table 45.5: Facial cutaneous reconstruction: Ten basic principles

- Incisions in relaxed skin tension lines (RSTLs)
- Incisions at borders of aesthetic units
- Unit/subunit principles
- Thoughtful planning
- Contingency plan available
- Proper instrumentation
- Gentle tissue manipulation/undermining
- Careful flap elevation/inset
- Avoidance of tension on flap
- Postoperative wound care

term 'favorable tension lines' has been proposed to describe the facial lines which offer optimal locations for incision placement.

Unit/Subunit Principle

As reconstructive decisions are made, it is important to emphasize the concept of facial aesthetic units and subunits. The face can be divided into units based on facial structures, and each of these units is composed of subunits. For example, the upper lip can be considered as an aesthetic unit, but it can be divided into vermilion and cutaneous regions. The cutaneous component can be further divided into a central and two lateral subunits. Junctional sites at the boundaries of aesthetic units are optimal lines for incision placement. Likewise, the junction of facial subunits can be important in maximizing cosmesis and camouflaging incisions. Whenever possible, hiding incisions in the scalp or placing incisions at the periphery of the face, such as in the preauricular region and at the anterior hairline will also optimize results. In some instances, there should be a consideration of extending defects (by removing normal skin) in order to optimize this unit-subunit principle. The concept of normal tissue sacrifice is explained in the next section.

Some authors state that if a defect involves 50% or more of a subunit, the defect should be extended to encompass the entire subunit so that the reconstruction will look more natural. This axiom serves as a useful guideline, especially with respect to nasal defects. However, this concept must be individualized-based on the size and location of the defect, as well as the advisability with respect to the additional complexity of the reconstruction and the anticipated result. In observing the principle of aesthetic facial units, it may be necessary to use two or more flaps instead of one, in order to avoid crossing facial boundaries.

Planning

One of the most critical phases of facial cutaneous reconstruction is preoperative planning. Taking into account the size, depth, shape, and location of the deformity, the reconstructive surgeon considers the options and discusses the alternatives with the patient. If flap reconstruction is anticipated, the surgeon must determine which donor site provides suitable tissue for reconstruction and take into consideration the possible donor site deformities that could be encountered. In the case of skin cancer excision and reconstruction performed during the same setting, multiple options should be considered, since the size of the defect may be larger than anticipated based on tumor spread patterns. A thorough knowledge of flap physiology is important in order to optimize vascularity and minimize tension, contracture, and trapdoor deformity (pin-cushioning). Anticipation of tension vectors, tissue response to rotation and advancement, and potential traction on neighboring structures are all important factors in skin flap design. Whenever possible, the flaps should be inferiorly based in order to minimize the lymphedema that leads to the pincushion effect. This phenomenon leads to an increase in the thickness of the flap following healing and curvilinear contraction. Usually sharp angles are less noticeable than curved lines. This should be another consideration in flap design. The ability to visualize the optimal design and orientation of the flap and understand the expected changes that are associated with closure of the donor site, must become part of the expertise that is acquired by the reconstructive surgeon in training.

Symmetry

For defects in the midline and paramedian areas of the face, it is extremely important to observe symmetry and consideration should be given to enlarging the defect in order to make it symmetrical (Figs 45.4A to C). By creating a symmetrical defect and a symmetrically reconstructed facial structure, the observer is less likely to recognize scars and contour deformities and more likely to accept any changes in color, contour, or texture as variants of normal anatomy.

Technique

As with cosmetic surgery, sound surgical soft tissue principles are the keys to successful reconstruction. This includes: incision planning, gentle manipulation of the tissues, hemostasis, appropriate undermining and the use of proper instrumentation. It is also important to match the thickness of the flap to the depth of the defect. In fact, if 'pin-cushioning' is anticipated, the flap should be thinned such that its thickness is less than the depth of the defect. Flap thickness can be tailored just as the overall configuration of the flap is constructed to match the geometry of the defect.

Postoperative Care

The importance of postoperative care should not be underestimated. Although, there is little pharmacologic data available, there may someday be drugs which will improve flap survival. Early studies with steroids, oxygen radical scavengers, and rheostatic agents show promise.

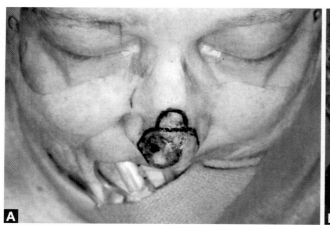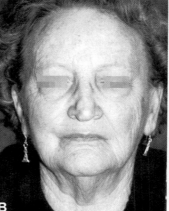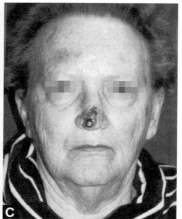

Figs 45.4A to C: (A) Mohs defect involving the nasal tip and supratip region. Note planned excision of additional skin in order to respect nasal subunits and enhance symmetry; (B) Nasal defect following Mohs surgery; (C) One year postoperative result following reconstruction with full-thickness skin graft from right melolabial region

Local wound care is important to provide optimal healing. Most surgeons have the patient clean the incision with half-strength hydrogen peroxide and then apply a thin layer of antibiotic ointment. This minimizes incisional inflammation and crusting. Occlusive dressings are an alternative to open wound care.

OPTIONS IN RECONSTRUCTION

Healing by Secondary Intention

As with primary closure, this option can always be considered. It is often used when the patient is in poor health and daily wound care can avoid a trip to the operating room. Secondary healing also allows for optimal observation for recurrence. If an area does not heal after a reasonable period of time, a biopsy should be considered. Clinical studies have documented that certain sites of the face provide more favorable cosmetic results following healing by secondary intention. Generally, such areas are concave and make-up the 'valleys' of the face such as the alar-facial junction, the medial canthal region, and the temporal region.

Becker and Adams reviewed their experience with 185 patients who had large Mohs defects of the head and neck region.[12] In this set of patients, all wounds were allowed to heal spontaneously. Postoperative reconstruction was performed as necessary following completion of healing. They concluded that large defects of the scalp, neck, or ear (except through-and-through defects) usually healed with acceptable cosmesis. However, large defects of the central cheek, lip, and chin-healed with poor cosmesis. They recommended that nasal defects be reconstructed immediately, but that other sites could be allowed to heal spontaneously, reserving reconstruction for those with poor results. In an earlier paper, Deutsch and Becker analyzed the results of secondary healing from Mohs defects involving the forehead, temple, and lower eyelid. Using a 0–3 rating system (0 = poor, 1 = fair, 2 = good, 3 = excellent), they concluded that many defects of the forehead and temple heal with acceptable results, while partial-thickness or small full-thickness wounds of the lower eyelid heal with excellent functional and cosmetic results.[13]

The disadvantage of secondary healing is that it involves at least daily wound care which can be quite problematic for many patients. Some older patients may have visual difficulties, arthritis and other infirmities that make dressing change difficult. For younger patients, this means wearing a bandage to their place of work for 4–6 weeks, interfering with their exercise regimen, making it socially impractical.

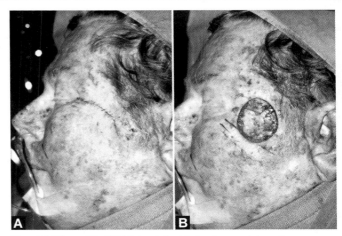

Figs 45.5A and B: (A) Mohs defect following excision of squamous cell carcinoma, left cheek and temple; (B) Immediate postoperative result following undermining of adjacent tissues and primary closure

Primary Closure

Although not as glamourous as a flap reconstruction, many defects can be closed with simple or extended undermining and primary closure. If at all possible, the closure should follow the RSTLs. This option is often overlooked, although proper case selection can yield a result superior to flap reconstruction (Figs 45.5A and B). Before embarking on a specific flap design, it is oftenwise to widely undermine the defect and see if primary closure is possible. For circular defects, a single suture can be placed at the midpoint of the skin on either side of the defect. This simple maneuver will demonstrate whether primary closure is feasible and will illustrate whether orientation of the suture line falls into a favorable skin tension line. Once the optimal line of closure is chosen, standing cutaneous deformities can be corrected. By creating a single linear or curvilinear scar, it is likely that a superior cosmetic result will be obtained.

Skin Grafts

Split-thickness Skin Grafts

In selected circumstances, a split-thickness skin graft may be the most appropriate choice for reconstruction. As alluded to previously, a split-thickness skin graft (STSG) is indicated for high-risk lesions where the defect needs to be observed for a suitable period of time. A split-thickness skin graft may be more suitable in a situation where a flap is either impractical (such as in the case of insufficient or unhealthy adjacent tissue) or when a flap procedure represents an overly complex reconstruction for the clinical setting. The advantage of a split-thickness skin graft is that compared to full-thickness grafts, it will more often survive on suboptimal tissues such as inburn patients or diabetics, or when only periosteum or peri-chondrium exits as a graft bed. Split-thickness skin graft survival rates generally surpass those for full-thickness grafts because of the lower metabolic needs of this thinner piece of tissue.

The major disadvantage of STSGs is the suboptimal cosmetic result. During the healing phase significant contraction occurs. The final result is a poor tissue match for the surrounding tissues and usually results as a 'sunken' or deficient area. STSGs tend to be pale, waxy, and somewhat stiff and flat.

Full-thickness Skin Grafts

Full-thickness grafts offer a better tissue match with respect to color, thickness and texture.[30,31] Since they include full-thickness dermis, they have a higher metabolic demand than split-thickness grafts and thus have a slightly diminished 'take' rate, especially if they are applied to a wound bed with a less than robust blood supply. However, these grafts generally have a more natural appearance with respect to the adjacent tissues. They also contract less since the full-thickness dermis provides more resistance to contractile forces. It should be noted however, that in many patients hyperpigmentation can occur and may be an unpreventable sequela. The most common sites for FTSG use include eyelid skin grafts for partial-thickness periocular defects and grafts used for small nasal defects involving the nasal tip.

Composite Grafts

Composite grafts may offer advantages over full-thickness grafts. Composite grafts are used routinely in hair restoration. The follicle-unit graft is a type of scalp micrograft that has become the preferred graft for many hair transplant surgeons.

Stucker has championed the use of perichondrial cutaneous grafts for reconstruction of nasal defects.[14,15] The advantage of the perichondrial cutaneous graft is that it offers a potentially superior color and texture match. It has been suggested that the perichondrium helps diminish contraction of the graft and may serve to enhance the color-matching capabilities of the graft.[14] Experimental data appears to corroborate these findings but prospective studies of a clinical nature are lacking. The most common donor site for perichondrial cutaneous grafts is the cymba concha. The donor site defect is reconstructed with a postauricular island flap.[15]

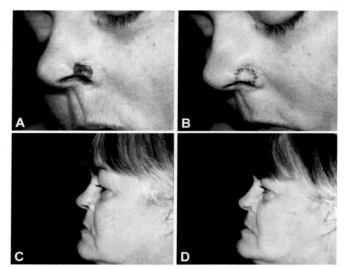

Figs 45.6A to D: (A) Turn-in flap has been rotated into position to serve as a base for the composite graft. (B) Chondrocutaneous composite graft from the left ear has been sutured into position. (C) Preoperative nasal defect six months following Mohs surgery. (D) Five-month result following reconstruction of nasal defect

For the most part, chondrocutaneous grafts have been abandoned because of their lack of reliability, significant contraction, and because modern nasal reconstruction emphasizes unit reconstruction. On occasion, however, a composite graft of skin and cartilage may be appropriate for small nasal alar defects (Figs 45.6A to D). The expected contraction that occurs with these grafts must be accounted for when planning a reconstruction.

LOCAL FLAPS

In most circumstances, local flaps provide a superior level of reconstruction. In the setting of cutaneous reconstruction for Mohs defects, local flaps serve as the gold standard for reconstruction, with a few notable exceptions (Table 45.6). Since adjacent tissue is being used, local flaps provide a superior color match, thickness and texture.

Table 45.6: Cutaneous flaps: Advantages and disadvantages
Advantages
• Superior tissue match (color, thickness, texture)
• Adjacent tissue as donor site
• Reliable blood supply
• Adjustable flap thickness vs defect
Disadvantages
• Facial donor site
• Potential for secondary deformity
• More likely to mask recurrence
• May be too thick for some sites

Flaps can be tailored with respect to size, shape and thickness, further optimizing cosmesis. If planned properly, these flaps tend to be extremely viable and highly reliable.

Disadvantages include the creation of another donor site and the potential downside of creating traction on neighboring facial structures, sometimes creating distortion. There is also a potential risk of masking a recurrence, thus causing a delay in diagnosis and potentially affecting the ultimate cure rate.

In specific cases, the optimal choice for reconstruction is a skin graft and not a flap. Examples include cutaneous defects involving the skin of the ear where only cartilage and perichondrium remain and eyelid defects in which only the skin is missing. In these circumstances, flaps tend to be overly bulky even with aggressive thinning.

Classification

Local flaps can be classified by their geometric pattern of transfer. Traditional nomenclature includes: Advancement, rotation, transposition, interpolation, and island flaps. However, an updated classification system is described below. Flaps can also be classified based on their blood supply as to whether they are axial (based on a specific named artery) or random (based on the subdermal plexus only). The reader is referred to several excellent texts and articles on the classification and dynamics of local flaps.[5,6,16]

Most local flaps are moved through a combination of pivoting and advancement, taking advantage of the geometry of rotation along with the intrinsic elasticity of the skin for the element of stretching (advancement). Thus many flaps are advancement-rotation flaps. In order to classify flaps by the method of transfer, the major mechanism of transfer is chosen as the primary descriptor. Although not universally accepted, many authors now recognize the classification system proposed in Table 45.7. Using this methodology, flaps are classified

Table 45.7: Flap classification

Pivotal flaps
- Rotation Flaps
- Transposition Flaps
- Interpolated Flaps

Advancement flaps
- Single Pedicle Advancement Flaps
- Bipedicle Advancement Flaps
- V-Y Advancement Flaps
- Y-V Advancement Flaps

Hinge flaps

primarily into three general categories: pivotal, advancement, or hinge.[17]

Pivotal Flaps

All pivotal flaps move toward the defect by rotating at the base of the flap around a pivotal point. Having a fixed base, pivotal flaps effectively shorten as they are rotated. It is estimated that the effective length of a pivotal flap moving through an arc of 180° is reduced by 40%. Pivotal flaps are divided into rotation, transposition, and interpolation flaps, based on their design and method of transfer.

Rotation flaps: Rotation flaps are designed in a curvilinear configuration, optimal for closure of triangular defects. The triangular defect also facilitates the avoidance of a dog-ear or standing cutaneous deformity. Since rotation flaps have a broad base, they tend to have a reliable blood supply. When possible, these flaps should be designed as inferiorly based in order to minimize flap edema and avoid a trapdoor deformity. Rotation flaps are useful for medial cheek defects, placing the incision at the junction of the cheek and periorbital aesthetic units. Large cheek defects can be reconstructed with cervicofacial rotation-advancement flaps. Scalp defects often lend themselves to reconstruction using scalp rotation flaps.

Transposition flaps: Transposition flaps represent the most common method of local flap reconstruction. In contradistinction to rotation flaps, transposition flaps have a straight linear axis. They can be designed so that one edge of the flap borders the defect, or such that only the base of the flap is contiguous with the defect. The latter circumstance is more common and allows construction of the flap at some distance from the defect, taking advantage of the ability to borrow skin from a site that offers greater tissue laxity and/or surface area. Transposition flaps can be designed in multiple sizes, shapes, and orientation. This includes single lobe flaps, bilobed flaps, note flaps, rhombic flaps, and Z-plasties.

Interpolation flaps: Interpolation flaps are pivotal flaps, also designed in a linear configuration, sharing some of the characteristics of transposition flaps. However, an interpolation flap has its base at some distance from the defect. For this reason, the flap must pass over (or under) intervening tissue. Therefore, in most circumstances, the pedicle must be divided at a later stage. The exception to this would be a flap which is partially de-epithelialized and this portion is tunneled or buried, avoiding a second stage. In the vast majority of cases, however, the interpolation flap is designed, elevated, and transposed into the defect, while maintaining its blood supply through a pedicle which is not contiguous with the defect. The paramedian forehead flap is the most well-known interpolation flap, ideal for resurfacing major nasal defects. The nasolabial flap, often used for reconstruction of alar defects, can be designed as a single lobe or as an island flap. In cases where staged procedures are planned, this represents another example of an interpolation flap.

Advancement Flaps

Advancement flaps are designed in a linear configuration and are moved into the defect by stretching the flap in a forward motion. In studying flap dynamics, it has been determined that primary and secondary movement of the tissues occur. Wound closure takes place as the flap stretches into the defect (primary movement), while the elasticity of the tissues adjacent to the defect also provides some movement in the opposite direction (secondary movement). Unlike rotation, transposition, or interpolation flaps, advancement flaps achieve tissue transfer along a single vector. Advancement flaps can be designed as: single pedicle, bipedicle, V-Y advancement flaps, or Y-V advancement flaps.

Single pedicle advancement flaps: A single pedicle advancement flap is created by parallel incisions, allowing a sliding motion of the flap along a single vector. In order to minimize standing cutaneous deformities, thorough undermining of the flap, flap base, and adjacent tissues is recommended. Dog-ears do occur, but can be dealt with by closure using the halving technique or by excising Burow's triangles anywhere along the length of the flap. The most common locations for the use of these flaps are in the forehead, the eyebrow region, the upper and lower lip, and the helix of the ear. Medial cheek defects are ideal for island advancement flaps. Based on a subcutaneous pedicle, the island flap is advanced into the defect, closing the secondary defect in a V-Y fashion.

Bipedicle advancement flaps: A bipedicle flap is a modification of the single pedicle advancement flap, where two flaps are created, designed, and advanced toward each other. This technique has limited indications but may be useful for selected forehead, lip, and scalp defects.

V-Y advancement flaps: The V-Y advancement flap is created in such a fashion that the flap is designed as a V, while closure of the apex of the defect 'pushes' the flap forward. Thus closure of the defect and adjacent tissue assumes a Y configuration. The V-Y flap is useful as a device to lengthen a structure (such as a shortened columella). It can also be used to release tissue which has been contracted. The latter circumstance might be exemplified by a contracted upper lip, where release through V-Y advancement re-establishes the contour of the vermilion border.

Y-V advancement flaps: This counterpart flap to the V-Y acts to move tissue in the opposite direction. In this case, the original incision is created as a Y, with the V-shaped portion of the flap being stretched forward and advanced into the Y-shaped defect. This may effectively shorten an overly long structure or may bring more tissue into an area which is deficient or contracted. Likewise, if redundancy exists at a specific site, the Y-V flap can efface or 'iron-out' this tissue excess as the tissue is advanced.

Hinge Flaps

The cutaneous hinge flap is designed to rotate around a base which faces the edge of the defect. Unlike the pivotal flaps, which rotate in the same plane as the defect, the hinge flap 'somersaults' into the defect on a hinged subcutaneous pedicle. These flaps go by various other names, including 'trapdoor', 'turn-in', 'turn-down', and 'turn-over' flaps. Reserved for full-thickness defects, these flaps turn into the defect and become lining tissue. Most commonly used for nasal defects, they can be designed to close defects involving the sinus, oral cavity, or pharynx. Since the hinge flap has a relatively limited blood supply, extra care must be taken in designing and elevating the flap. Under optimal circumstances, hinge flaps are based at the margin of a healed defect so that there is a mature subcutaneous pedicle at the hinge point. They can also be created at the edge of a fresh defect, but the subcutaneous pedicle will be more tenuous. As the flap is elevated, it is critical not to cut into the base of the flap. Instead, the base should remain thicker than the remainder of the flap, in order to minimize the risk of ischemic necrosis.

RECONSTRUCTION BY SITE

Scalp

The inelasticity of the forehead is exceeded only by the scalp. As everyone remembers from medical school, the scalp is made up of five layers which include: skin, subcutaneous tissue, galea aponeurosis, loose areolar tissue and periosteum. In analyzing scalp defects, the single most important finding is whether the periosteum is intact. A viable periosteal layer allows for a host of reconstructive options, including healing by secondary intention and skin grafting. However, whenever Mohs defects involve all layers of the scalp and leave bone exposed, it is important to obtain soft tissue coverage.

Optimal reconstruction of scalp defects is with a flap using the adjacent scalp tissue.

In rare circumstances, it may be appropriate to decorticate the outer table of the skull and apply a split-thickness skin graft; however, this does not represent a reliable method of reconstruction. Instead, if the scalp defect is down to bare bone and flap reconstruction is not possible, it is better to bur away the outer table and allow the wound to granulate. The wound can then heal by secondary intention or a STSG may be applied a few days later on the new bed of granulation tissue.

Under optimal circumstances, scalp flaps should be created in such a fashion that the donor site can also be closed. However, because of the inelasticity of the scalp, many local flaps that work perfectly well in the face and neck are not applicable to the scalp region. If donor site closure is not possible, a flap can still be designed to cover the defect with a split-thickness skin graft being placed over the donor site defect, taking advantage of the periosteal coverage in this location. Later the skin graft can be removed with either serial excision or scalp expansion techniques.

The author tends to prefer large rotation flaps whenever possible. The primary defect can usually be converted to a triangle and a large curvilinear rotation flap is designed. Because of the minimal stretching capabilities of the scalp tissue, the rotation flap should be at least four times that of the defect (Figs 45.7A to D). For defects in which the periosteum is intact, healing by secondary intention may also represent an option since this allows for significant wound contraction and recruitment of adjacent scalp tissues. This ultimately provides more hair-bearing tissue than if a STSG were used.

Forehead/Brows

Forehead defects can represent a reconstructive dilemma. Whenever possible, it is preferable to plan incisions along the natural horizontal lines of the forehead. However, it is also important not to use a flap which will itself cause distortion of the eyebrow. Generally, greater deformity results from brow asymmetry than from cutaneous forehead scars. For this reason, maintaining the natural brow position and contour takes precedence over the direction of forehead scars. Based on experience using the paramedian forehead flap, it has become apparent that a well-closed vertical scar is often cosmetically quite acceptable. For larger defects, especially those with bony exposure, reconstruction can be accomplished with a temporoparietal fascial flap with a split-thickness skin graft providing cutaneous coverage (Figs 45.8A to D). This works well in high-risk patients who are going to receive postoperative irradiation. Then, once the patient has undergone a suitable period of observation, definitive reconstruction can be entertained using tissue expansion techniques.

The eyebrow represents a unique anatomic structure. For small defects, the brow may simply be advanced and closed primarily. Women can camouflage minor deficits

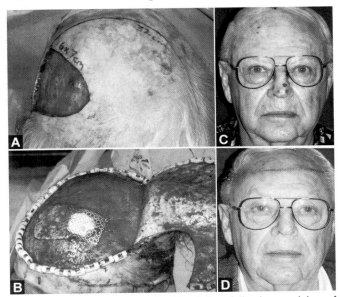

Figs 45.7A to D: (A) Large scalp defect following excision of recurrent squamous cell carcinoma. Circumference of planned scalp flap is 32 cm. (B) Scalp rotation flap has been elevated. Craniectomy was performed for bony invasion. (C) One-week postoperative result. (D) Five-month postoperative result

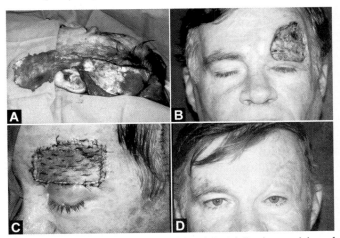

Figs 45.8A to D: (A) Extensive Mohs defect following excision of squamous cell carcinoma. There is exposed bone and postoperative radiation is anticipated. (B) Temporoparietal fascial flap has been elevated. (C) Immediate results following transposition of the flap and application of split-thickness skin graft to defect. (D) Six-month result following reconstruction and postoperative radiation

with make-up. Once again, it is most important to maintain brow position with respect to the opposite brow. For larger defects, hair transplant techniques may be applicable, although obtaining an optimal result can be quite difficult, as the density and orientation of the eyebrow hair is significantly different from the donor scalp. Multiple techniques have been described for brow reconstruction. This includes pedicled scalp flaps, microvascular tissue transfer, composite grafts (scalp strips), and hair transplant techniques. Juri reports that his preference is to use occipital scalp autografts in females, while in males a pedicled island flap from the parietal scalp is used.[18] Recent reports also confirm the utility of using follicular-unit micrografts for brow reconstruction.[19]

Eyelids/Periorbital Region

It is critical for the reconstructive surgeon to have a firm grasp of the anatomy of the eyelids, periorbital tissues, and lacrimal drainage system. If the surgeon has little experience in this area, it may be wise to enlist the assistance of an oculoplastic surgeon. In approaching these defects, it is important to remember that the eyelid is divided into two lamellae. The anterior lamella contains skin and muscle, while the posterior lamella contains conjunctiva, tarsal plates, and the lid retractors. These anatomic layers differ depending on the site of involvement. A cross-section of the eyelids reinforces this concept. The primary goal of reconstruction is protection of the cornea. Additional goals include an eyelid which is functional and is capable of providing eyelid lubrication as well as attaining an optimal cosmetic result. There are a multitude of options available and each will be applicable depending upon the involvement of the various lamellae as well as the size, shape, and depth of the defect.

In the region of the medial canthus, secondary healing should be a consideration; otherwise, a full-thickness skin graft or a thin local flap can be considered. It is beyond the scope of this chapter to discuss the gamut of reconstructive options available for eyelid defects, but this information is available from other sources.[5,20] Most commonly anterior lamellar defects can be reconstructed with a full-thickness skin graft, borrowing eyelid skin from the ipsilateral or contralateral upper eyelid. For through and through defects, a pentagonal excision and closure may be appropriate. For slightly larger defects, a lateral canthotomy and cantholysis is sufficient for closure of the defect. If this is insufficient, a Tenzel flap can be used to recruit enough tissue for reconstruction. Other

procedures include the use of composite grafts from the hard palate or the use of Alloderm, both of which will provide a conjunctiva-like surface along with the stiffness necessary to replace the tarsus.

For extensive subtotal eyelid defects, there are several procedures which involve transposition of upper or lower eyelid tissue. These flaps are performed in a two-stage fashion. The most familiar of these are the Hughes and Cutler–Beard procedures.[20] For total or near-total upper lid defects, the Cutler-Beard procedure offers a two-stage reconstruction in which a full-thickness flap of lower eyelid tissue is advanced into the defect and later divided at a second stage. The Hughes' flap is described for extensive lower eyelid defects. In this procedure, a tarsoconjunctival flap is created in the upper eyelid. Leaving a 4 mm strip of tarsus intact in the upper lid, the flap is transferred to the lower eyelid defect and sutured into position. Skin coverage of the defect is with a skin graft or local flap. At a second stage, the tarsoconjunctival flap is divided.

Cheek

The cheek offers anatomic features not found in the remaining portions of the face. The cheek has a surplus of subcutaneous tissue and as a result offers significant elasticity and laxity. The natural boundaries of the cheek include the periorbital region, the nose, the melolabial fold, the chin, neck, ear, and temporal region. Whenever possible, hair-bearing skin should be replaced with hairbearing skin. In males, a patch of non-hair-bearing skin placed within the beard area is readily identifiable.

The cheek offers many reconstructive advantages. Since it borders with the areas described above, there are multiple sites which allow optimal placement for incision lines at the junction of aesthetic units. Tissues of the cheek have a significant redundancy and flexibility, especially in older patients. For this reason, there tends to be enough adjacent tissue to readily reconstruct small to medium-sized defects.

For small defects, primary closure should always be considered but needs to be carefully-planned so that the ultimate scar lies along favorable skin tension lines. The direction of these lines changes with the location in the cheek, being more horizontal near the eyelid and more vertical near the melolabial fold.

For medium-sized defects, multiple flap options exist. These include: rotation, single lobe, bilobed, and rhombic flaps. For large medial cheek defects, island V-Y advancement flaps are quite useful. Sometimes, results can be further optimized by excising adjacent skin, bringing the line of closure to one of the aesthetic facial junctions. Cheek rotation, cervicofacial rotation flaps, and cervicofacial-pectoral flaps are reserved for larger defects.

Whenever possible, it is best to avoid distant flaps for isolated cutaneous defects. However, these flaps may be necessary for massive defects involving the maxilla, orbit and skull base. High-risk defects involving skin and subcutaneous tissue can be reconstructed with a split-thickness skin graft or allowed to heal by secondary intention, so long as ectropion is unlikely to result.

Temple

The temporal area should be approached with caution. Defects into the subcutaneous tissue often involve the temporal branch of the facial nerve. Patients are counseled prior to their Mohs procedure that the nerve is particularly vulnerable in this region and that forehead paralysis may result following eradication of the tumor. Thus, when the reconstructive surgeon evaluates the patient with a Mohs defect it is important to test facial nerve function and identify any resulting paresis or paralysis. The temporal region represents a danger zone with respect to the facial nerve because the temporal branch lies *within* the superficial musculoaponeurotic system (SMAS). If the nerve is intact following the Mohs procedure, extra caution must be taken in adjacent tissue undermining, flap creation and elevation.

As noted previously, the temple is one region that often heals with good to excellent cosmetic results following healing by secondary intention. In this author's experience, secondary healing typically provides a superior result to either a split-thickness skin graft or a full-thickness skin graft. Following this reasoning, primary closure, local flap reconstruction, or use of a cervicofacial flap tend to be the procedures utilized most often for defects involving this region.

Chin

The chin represents a midline facial structure in which a soft tissue mound overlies the symphysis of the mandible. It has a significant amount of subcutaneous tissue with a moderate amount of skin elasticity. Whenever possible, primary closure should be used but planning is necessary to optimize the direction of the scars. A vertical midline scar is quite acceptable. Scars at the periphery of the chin aesthetic unit are also optimal. It is important to observe or re-create the normal mentolabial crease. The author tends

to use rotation flaps based on the spherical nature of the chin as opposed to transposition flaps. On occasion, a large-bilobed flap or staged cervical visor flap may be useful for reconstruction of total or near total chin defects. For large defects of limited depth, a full-thickness skin graft may be satisfactory.[28]

Lip

In reconstructing the lip, it is important to carefully analyze the defect. Both the upper and lower lip have a cutaneous and a vermilion portion. Partial versus full-thickness defects of the lip may be managed differently. Options include: Primary closure, cutaneous advance-ment flaps, mucosal advancement flap, bilateral cuta-neous advancement flaps, lip interpolation techniques (Abbé and Estlander flaps),[29,30] as well as the Karapandzic flap. Recently reported has been the extended Abbé flap, which usesthe skin and soft tissues of the lower lip and chin.[16] Reconstruction of a central upper lip defect is shown in Figures 45.9A to D.

The Cervical Region

Except for massive defects, cutaneous defects of the neck are the most straightforward to reconstruct. Since there is usually significant laxity of the cervical soft tissues, primary closure is most often available and if not, extensive undermining allows for advancement and closure. Attention to the normal skin creases allows for the use of relaxed skin tension lines to optimize cosmetic results.

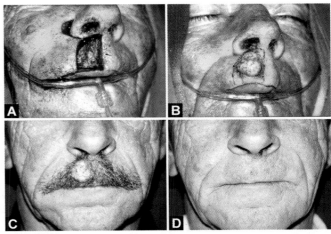

Figs 45.9A to D: (A) Keratoacanthoma of the upper lip. Note planned margins of excision. (B) Defect following excision. Advancement flap incisions along alar base and vermilion border. Crescentic peri-nasal excision to allow advancement of flap without nasal distortion. (C) Preoperative appearance. (D) Three-month postoperative result

On occasion, an extremely large defect can be resurfaced with a split-thickness skin graft.

Contracture often results with the ultimate defect being 50% of the original, thus allowing for delayed serial excisions of the graft. Extensive defects can also be addressed with a cervicopectoral or a deltopectoral flap.

Nose

Without question, the most significant advances in facial cutaneous reconstruction have come in the field of nasal reconstruction. Burget and Menick have advanced the modern principles of nasal reconstruction and have published several landmark papers in addition to a uniquely informative text.[4,11,21–24] Baker has further added to the literature with articles devoted to nasal reconstruction as well as the recent publication of his book devoted to nasal reconstruction.[7]

The nose is divided into subunits and it is important to respect these boundaries. It also may be important to extend the size of the defect in order to reach a subunit boundary. Reconstruction using the subunit principle avoids a 'patched' result. Likewise, it should be noted that there are different skin types throughout the regions of the nose with thick, sebaceous skin lying over the tip and ala while thin, mobile skin covers the dorsum and columella. As with other regions of the face, the size, depth and location of the nasal defect will determine which reconstructive options are most appropriate. Small defects, which are relatively superficial, may be amenable to a full-thickness skin graft or a perichondrial-cutaneous graft. Defects up to 1.5 cm involving the tip and ala may be reconstructed with a bilobed flap. Most surgeons use the

Zitelli's modification as shown in Figs 45.10A to D. Depending on size, significant alar defects should be reconstructed with a nasolabial island flap or paramedian forehead flap. Even alar defects with intact nasal lining require cartilaginous support to prevent alar collapse, contraction, and distortion (Figs 45.11A to D).

Complex nasal reconstruction is necessary for full-thickness defects. In these cases, the nasal lining must be replaced. This is combined with structural support by cartilage grafts and cutaneous coverage with a paramedian forehead flap. Nasal lining can be restored using bipedicled intranasal flaps, septal mucoperichondrial flaps, turbinate flaps, or a turn-in flaps. Staged procedures are required and revision surgery is often necessary for flap thinning and re-contouring. The paramedian forehead flap has become the workhorse for nasal reconstruction. Use of this flap is indicated for full-thickness defects, cutaneous defects > 1.5 cm, and for subtotal nasal defects. The island nasolabial flap is best reserved for isolated alar defects, while larger alar defects should be reconstructed using the paramedian forehead flap.[25]

Ear

Auricular defects can be problematic reconstructive cases. For those defects in which only the skin is missing and both the perichondrium and underlying cartilage are intact, a split-thickness or full-thickness skin graft may be in order.[32] Local flaps are generally too thick to allow visualization of the underlying contour of the auricular cartilage. If there is insufficient vascularity to sustain a split-thickness skin graft, small holes (2–4 mm in diameter)

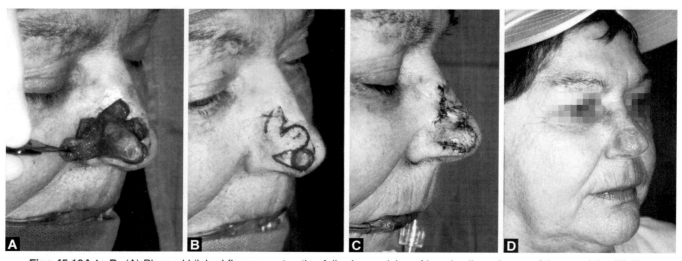

Figs 45.10A to D: (A) Planned bilobed flap reconstruction following excision of basal cell carcinoma of the nasal tip. (B) Flap elevated in the supra-perichondrial plane. (C) Immediate results following flap reconstruction. (D) Three-month postoperative result

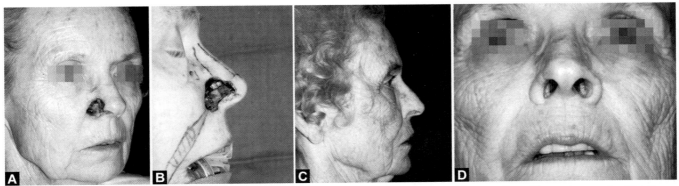

Figs 45.11A to D: (A) Nasal defect following Mohs surgery. (B) Cartilage graft sutured into position. Planned reconstruction is with nasolabial island flap. (C) Two-year postoperative result, lateral view. (D) Two-year postoperative result, base view

can be made in the cartilage itself to allow increased vascularity of the bed while not affecting the structural support of the cartilage. This author tends to use a full-thickness skin graft for defects in which the cartilage is missing and split-thickness skin grafts when only perichondrium exists as a graft bed.

Through and through defects offer a host of reconstructive options. For isolated, helical defects, a helical advancement flap is ideal. When the helix and antihelix are involved, a wedge resection and closure may work well. Otherwise, the star excision modification offers an alternative procedure that minimizes the 'buckling' that can occur with the standard wedge resection and closure. Another very useful option is the chondrocutaneous advancement flap as described by Antia and Buch.[26] The helical-antihelical defect in Figures 45.12A to C was reconstructed using this latter technique. For defects in the mid-portion of the ear involving the helix and antihelix, a postauricular flap can be designed, some-times in conjunction with a cartilage graft. A second stage is performed to create a postauricular surface and sulcus.

For conchal defects, the postauricular island flap offers an ideal reconstruction. The postauricular flap is designed around the postauricular sulcus, based on the postauricular artery. The flap is transposed from the back of the ear to the front and sutured into position. The donor site defect is closed in such a manner that the scar lies within the sulcus. Several reconstructive options are available for defects that involve the earlobe.

In those situations, where the entire ear is missing from trauma or oncologic surgery, it is very difficult to attain a satisfactory result using flaps, cartilage grafts, tissue expansion, or a temporoparietal flap with skin graft. Instead, osseointegrated implants may offer the best result in conjunction with a prosthetic ear.

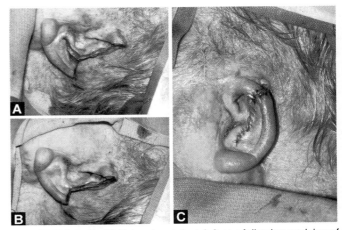

Figs 45.12A to C: (A) Extensive defect, left ear, following excision of basal cell carcinoma. (B) Inferiorly-based chondrocutaneous flap has been elevated. (C) Immediate postoperative result following reconstruction

REVISION PROCEDURES

Each patient should be counseled about the likelihood of revision procedures. Generally speaking, the more complex the reconstruction, the more likely that revision will be necessary. Likewise, areas that are most difficult to duplicate, such as the nose, eyelids, lips, and ear are more likely to need revision surgery. Initially, it is appropriate to simply wait and watch as the passage of time allows for maturation of the scars, softening of the involved tissues, and diminishing degrees of lymphe-dema.

Based on the deformity as well as the judgment and experience of the surgeon, a number of revision procedures may be applicable. One of the most common is a debulking or thinning procedure, often used in nasal reconstruction. Lesser degrees of persistent soft tissue fullness or excess may be ameliorated with the judicious use of steroid injections, using triamcinolone 10 mg per cc. In other situations, W-plasties and Z-plasties may be appropriate. For soft tissue deficits, autogenous grafts or allografts may be implanted.

CONCLUSIONS

In approaching the reconstruction of Mohs defects, it is important to make an initial assessment of the risk of recurrence.[27] Reconstruction can be undertaken if the risk is low. However, a period of observation should be entertained for the patient considered to be at high-risk for recurrence. Adjunctive therapy such as postoperative radiation should also be considered in selected circumstances.

As the initial assessment proceeds, it is important to take into account the patient's medical status, desires, capabilities and expectations. As is often the case, there is a balance between the ease of reconstruction and the results. For many patients, a simple, straightforward, and reliable procedure is preferable over a complex, multi-staged procedure, even though the latter may ultimately lead to a more refined cosmetic result.

The reconstructive surgeon and the patient must have an open dialogue prior to embarking on the course of reconstruction. Multiple options should be considered, including: healing by secondary intention, primary closure, skin grafts, local flaps, secondary delayed reconstruction, and a prosthesis. It is important to balance one's enthusiasm for reconstruction with the desires and expectations of the patient, especially in older patients. The necessity and nature of revision procedures should be anticipated and discussed as well. Ultimate success of facial cutaneous reconstruction lies in thoughtful planning, careful tissue handling, meticulous execution of the procedure, and attention to detail.

REFERENCES

1. Nguyen TH, Ho DQ. Nonmelanoma skin cancer. *Curr Treat Options Oncol* 2002; 3:193–203.
2. Padgett JK, Hendrix JD. Cutaneous malignancies and their management. *Otolaryngol Clin North Am* 2001; 34:523–553.
3. Gloster HM, Brodland DG. The epidemiology of skin cancer. *Dermatol Surg* 1996; 22:217–226.
4. Burget GC, Menick FJ, (Eds). *Aesthetic reconstruction of the nose.* St Louis: Mosby, 1994.
5. Larrabee WF, Sherris DA, (Eds). *Principles of facial reconstruction.* Philadelphia: Lippincott-Raven, 1995.
6. Baker SR, Swanson WA, (Eds). *Local flaps in facial recon-struction.* St Louis: Mosby, 1995.
7. Baker SR, Naficy S, (Eds). *Principles of nasal reconstruction.* St Louis: Mosby, 2002.
8. Wolf DJ, Zitelli JA. Surgical margins for basal cell carcinoma. *Arch Dermatol* 1987; 123:340–344.
9. Johnson TM, Nelson BR. Mohs surgery for cutaneous basal cell and squamous cell carcinoma. In *Basal and squamous cell skin cancers of the head and neck*, Weber RS, Miller MJ, and Goepfert H (Eds). Philadelphia: Williams and Wilkins, 1996; 147–155.
10. Snow SN, Madjar DD. Mohs surgery in the management of cutaneous malignancies. *Clin Dermatol* 2001; 19:339–347.
11. Burget GC. Aesthetic reconstruction of the tip of the nose. *Dermatol Surg* 1995; 21:419–429.
12. Becker GD, Adams AA. The management of large Mohs defects. *Ann Otol Rhinol Laryngol* 2000; 109:863–870.
13. Deutch BD, Becker FF. Secondary healing of Mohs defects of the forehead, temple and lower eyelid. *Arch Otolaryngol Head Neck Surg* 1997; 123:529–534.
14. Portuese W, Stucker F, Grafton W, Shockley W, Gage-White L. Perichondrial cutaneous graft. *Arch Otolaryngol Head Neck Surg* 1989; 115:705–709.
15. Stucker FJ, Shaw GY. The perichondrial cutaneous graft: A 12-year clinical experience. *Arch Otolaryngol Head Neck Surg* 1992; 118:287–292.
16. Murakami CS, Nishioka GJ. Essential concepts in the design of local skin flaps. *Facial Plast Surg Clin North Am* 1996; 4: 455–468.
17. Gluckman JL (Ed). *Renewal of Certification Study Guide in Otolaryngology—Head and Neck Surgery.* AAO-HNSF. Dubuque: Kendall/Hunt.1998.
18. Juri J. Eyebrow reconstruction. *Plast Reconstr Surg* 2001; 107:1225–1228.
19. Wang J, Fan J. Aesthetic eyebrow reconstruction by using follicular-unit hair grafting technique (Chinese). *Zhonghua Zheng Xing Wai Ke Ka Zhi* 2002; 18:101–103.
20. Jewett BS, Shockley WW. Reconstructive options for periocular defects. *Otolaryngol Clin North Am* 2001; 34:601–625.
21. Burget GC. Aesthetic restoration of the nose. *Clin Plast Surg* 1985; 12:463–480.
22. Burget GC, Menick FJ. The subunit principle in nasal reconstruction. *Plast Reconstr Surg* 1985; 76:239–247.
23. Burget GC, Menick FJ. Nasal reconstruction: seeking a fourth dimension. *Plast Reconstr Surg* 1986; 78:145–157.
24. Burget GC, Menick FJ. Nasal support and lining: The marriage of beauty and blood supply. *Plast Reconstr Surg* 1989; 84: 189–202.
25. Drisco BP, Baker SR. Reconstruction of nasal alar defects. *Arch Facial Plast Surg* 2001; 3:91–99.
26. Antia NH, Buch VI. Chondrocutaneous advancement flap for the marginal defect of the ear. *Plast Reconstr Surg* 1967;39: 472–477.
27. Hochman M, Lang P. Skin cancer of the head and neck. *Med Clin North Am* 1999; 83:261–282.
28. Johnson TM, Swanson N, Baker SR. Concepts of sliding and lifting tissue movement in flap reconstruction. *Dermatol Surg* 2000; 26:274–278.
29. Kriet JD, Cupp CL, Sherris DA, Murakami CS. The extended Abbé flap. *Laryngoscope* 1995; 105:988–992.
30. Larrabee WF, Makielski KH, (Eds). *Surgical Anatomy of the Face.* New York: Raven Press 1993.
31. Martinez JC, Otley CC. The management of melanoma and nonmelanoma skin cancer: A review for the primary care physician. *Mayo Clin Proc* 2001; 76:1253–1265.
32. Stucker FJ, Sanders KW. A method to repair auricular defects after perichondrial cutaneous grafting. *Laryngoscope* 2002; 112:1384–1386.